W9-CCK-554

■ CLINICAL TRIALS IN HEART DISEASE

■ ■ ■ A Companion to Braunwald's Heart Disease

Second edition

JoAnn E. Manson, MD, DrPH, FAHA, FACP
ELIZABETH F. BRIGHAM PROFESSOR OF WOMEN'S HEALTH AND PROFESSOR OF MEDICINE
HARVARD MEDICAL SCHOOL
Chief, Division of Preventive Medicine and
Co-Director of the Connors Center for Women's Health and Gender Biology
Brigham and Women's Hospital
Boston, MA

Julie E. Buring, ScD, FACE
PROFESSOR OF AMBULATORY CARE AND PREVENTION
HARVARD MEDICAL SCHOOL
Deputy Director, Division of Preventive Medicine
Brigham and Women's Hospital
Boston, MA

Paul M. Ridker, MD, MPH, FAHA, FACC
EUGENE BRAUNWALD PROFESSOR OF MEDICINE
HARVARD MEDICAL SCHOOL
Director, Center for Cardiovascular Disease Prevention
Brigham and Women's Hospital
Boston, MA

J. Michael Gaziano, MD, MPH, FACC
ASSOCIATE PROFESSOR OF MEDICINE
HARVARD MEDICAL SCHOOL
Chief, Division of Aging
Brigham and Women's Hospital
Director, Massachusetts Veterans Epidemiology Research and Information Center
Veterans' Administration Boston Healthcare System
Boston, MA

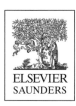

ELSEVIER
SAUNDERS

ELSEVIER
SAUNDERS

170 S Independence Mall W 300 E
Philadelphia, PA 19106-3399

Clinical Trials in Heart Disease: A Companion   ISBN 0-7216-0408-0
to Braunwald's Heart Disease

Notice

Medicine is an ever-changing field. Standard safety precautions must be followed, but as new research and clinical experience broaden our knowledge, changes in treatment and drug therapy may become necessary or appropriate. Readers are advised to check the most current product information provided by the manufacturer of each drug to be administered to verify the recommended dose, the method and duration of administration, and contraindications. It is the responsibility of the treating physician, relying on experience and knowledge of the patient, to determine dosages and the best treatment for each individual patient. Neither the publisher nor the editors assume any liability for any injury and/or damage to persons or property arising from this publication.

Previous edition copyrighted 1999
Library of Congress Cataloging-in-Publication Data

Clinical trials in heart disease: a companion to Braunwald's heart disease/[edited by]
JoAnn E. Manson . . . [et al.]. — 2nd ed.
   p.   ; cm.
  Companion to: Heart disease/edited by Eugene Braunwald. 2nd ed. 2004.
  ISBN 0-7216-0408-0
  1. Heart—Diseases—Research—Methodology.   2. Clinical trials.   I. Manson, JoAnn E.   II. Braunwald,
Eugene, 1929- Heart disease.
  [DNLM: 1. Heart Diseases—therapy.   2. Clinical trials. WG 210 C6417 2004]
  RC682.C585 2004
  616.1'2027—dc22

                               2003054492

Acquisitions Editor: *Anne Lenehan*
Editorial Assistant: *Vera Ginsburgs*
Publishing Services Manager: *Joan Sinclair*
Project Manager: *Mary Stermel*

Printed in The United States of America

Last digit is the print number: 9   8   7   6   5   4   3   2   1

This book is dedicated to family members Christopher, Jenn, Jeffrey M., Joshua, Jeffrey B., Susan, Andrew, Elena, Anne, Michaela, Dante, and Liam, for their unfailing support and forbearance.

JEM
JEB
PMR
JMG

Since the development of antibiotics in the middle of the last century, no area in clinical medicine has moved forward as rapidly as has cardiology. This has resulted from notable advances in cardiovascular biology and pathophysiology, as well as from the development of several classes of important new cardiovascular drugs and of a variety of effective new procedures and devices. The clinical impact of these new therapeutic modalities requires rigorous assessment in clinical trials, which have become *the* principal method of judging the efficacy and safety of interventions. Clinical trials serve as the critical interface between initial studies that have offered "proof of concept" of a therapeutic or preventive modality and its widespread clinical application. Clinical trials are also required for the registration of new drugs and devices. It is no exaggeration to say that the randomized clinical trial now provides the key to rational, evidence-based cardiac care and prevention of cardiovascular disease.

I am especially delighted that Drs. Manson, Buring, Ridker, and Gaziano, from the Preventive Medicine and Cardiovascular Divisions of Harvard Medical School's Department of Medicine and the Brigham and Women's Hospital have produced the second edition of this splendid volume—*Clinical Trials in Heart Disease*. The first section provides the understanding of the methods involved in the design, conduct, and interpretation of trials. The second section consists of a systematic review of the key cardiovascular treatment trials of coronary artery disease, especially acute coronary syndromes, arrhythmias, and heart failure. The third section details the growing number of trials designed to prevent or at least delay the development of cardiovascular disease.

This totally revised and expanded second edition provides an up-to-date review and analysis of this very important segment of cardiology. It should be of great interest not only to clinical trialists and trainees in this field, but to all physicians responsible for the care of patients with cardiovascular disease. I am proud that *Clinical Trials in Heart Disease* is a distinguished Companion to *Heart Disease: A Textbook of Cardiovascular Medicine*.

Eugene Braunwald, M.D.
Boston, MA

Cardiovascular disease (CVD) is the leading cause of death for adults worldwide.[1] In the United States, CVD is responsible for nearly 1 million annual fatalities, or two of every five deaths. CVD kills more Americans than the next seven causes combined—including cancer. Indeed, the average U.S. life expectancy would rise by nearly seven years if major forms of CVD could be eliminated. CVD also carries a tremendous economic burden, with direct health care costs and indirect costs from lost productivity estimated at $352 billion in the United States in 2003.[2]

Since the late 1960s, many developed countries have experienced a decline in CVD mortality, with reductions in the United States averaging about 2% each year. This favorable trend has been attributed to advances in both prevention[3] and treatment[4] of CVD. Despite more than three decades of sustained decline in mortality rates, however, CVD is expected to remain the number-one killer in the western world well into the 21st century.[5] Moreover, troubling recent evidence suggests that this long-standing secular decline in CVD mortality may be reaching a plateau or, in some groups such as African American women, even reversing. While age-adjusted death rates from coronary heart disease (CHD), which accounts for nearly half of CVD deaths in the United States, declined more than 3% per year between 1970 and 1990, the yearly rate of decline in CHD mortality slowed to 2.7% between 1990 and 1997. For stroke mortality, the deceleration of the annual rate of decline has been even more marked. After falling at a rate of 4.9% per year between 1970 and 1980, and 3.5% per year between 1980 and 1990, age-adjusted stroke mortality declined a mere 0.7% per year from 1990 to 1997.[6]

Another important cause of CVD death is congestive heart failure (CHF). It is the only category of CVD in which prevalence, incidence, and mortality have consistently *increased* over the past quarter-century in the United States.[6] Currently 4.6 million Americans suffer from CHF, and there are 550,000 new cases annually.[7] CHF is the leading hospital discharge diagnosis of men and women aged 65 years and older, and 30-day readmission rates for individuals with this condition are approaching 25%.[6]

Paralleling these trends is emerging evidence of an increasing prevalence of several CVD risk factors, which portends great difficulty in achieving further reductions in the incidence of CVD. Currently, two of every three U.S. adults are classified as overweight or obese, compared with fewer than one in four in the early 1960s.[8,9] The prevalence of diabetes is also on the rise; between 1990 and 2000, increases averaged 49% across all racial/ethnic groups.[10] The most recent estimates suggest that 7% of adults (1 in 15) have a diabetes diagnosis and that the prevalence of undiagnosed diabetes may be even higher.[11] And although the prevalence of smoking, elevated serum cholesterol, and untreated hypertension have each declined since the late 1970s, there has been little or no further reduction in the frequency of these cardiovascular risk factors within the last 10 years.[6,12] Similarly, the proportion of adults who report no leisure time physical activity has remained relatively stable at approximately 25% over the last decade, and about 75% have lower levels of activity than recommended.[13,14] Moreover, among U.S. adolescents, there are also trends toward increasing obesity,[15] smoking,[16] and physical inactivity.[14] In the aggregate, these secular changes, if not reversed, will have far-reaching consequences for future morbidity and mortality from CVD.

In developing countries, the proportion of worldwide deaths due to CVD is projected to climb from 28.9% to 36.3% between the years 1990 and 2020.[5] CVD is also predicted to jump from fourth to first in number of years of life lost, and from fifth to first as a cause of premature death and disability. These increases are related principally to a decline in competing causes of death, such as malnutrition and infectious diseases, which is allowing for population aging, as well as to a marked rise in cigarette smoking rates.[17]

Thus, the continuing enormous burden of CVD in developed countries, alarming trends in cardiovascular risk profiles of adolescents and adults, and the emerging increases in CVD in developing countries underscore the crucial need to redouble treatment and prevention efforts.[18]

Although equally important for both genders, such prevention and treatment efforts have lagged among women as compared with men. Until recently, CHD was widely perceived to be less of a public health problem for women than for men. While the incidence of CHD in women trails the incidence in men by 10 years for total CHD and by 20 years for more serious clinical events such as myocardial infarction (MI) and sudden death, CHD nevertheless becomes the leading killer of U.S. men by 45 years of age and of women by 65 years of age.[2] In fact, once women develop overt CHD, they have a markedly worse prognosis than men. Case-fatality rates are higher for women following both MI and myocardial revascularization procedures, with 38% of MIs in women but only 25% of MIs in men followed by death within one year.[2] Moreover, in 63% of women but in only 50% of men who died suddenly from CHD, there were no previous symptoms of this disease.[2] These gender differences are not entirely accounted for by differences in age. Additionally, secular declines in CVD and CHD mortality have been less pronounced among women than among men. Given the emerging epidemic of 'diabesity'[19] (i.e., obesity and diabetes) and the fact that diabetes appears to be a far more potent cardiovascular risk factor among women than among men,[20] boosting prevention and treatment efforts among women is necessary to forestall potentially widening gender disparities in cardiovascular outcomes.

Clinical trials are a powerful tool for evaluating the efficacy and safety of therapeutic and preventive interventions in both men and women. Such trials are, however, neither necessary nor desirable in all circumstances. For example, the benefits of pharmacologic treatment for malignant hypertension were so large and obvious in uncontrolled clinical observations that randomized trials would in fact have been unethical. Similarly, with respect to cigarette smoking and CVD, the totality of evidence derived from basic laboratory research, clinical investigation, and observational epidemiology was clearly sufficient for the U.S. surgeon general to declare smoking a cause of CHD—and smoking cessation an effective preventive measure—in the absence of clinical trial data. However, for many other therapeutic and preventive strategies, such as drug treatment of mild-to-moderate hypertension[21] or aspirin in the primary prevention of CVD,[22] the resulting effects are likely to be small to moderate (i.e., on the order of a 10% to 40% difference between treatment and control groups). While these differences may be very meaningful from a clinical or public health perspective, especially for such a common and serious disease as CVD, they are difficult to detect reliably in observational studies. Such effect sizes may easily be obscured by uncontrolled or uncontrollable confounding or biases inherent in cohort and case-control studies.[23] For this reason, clinical trials are the most reliable design strategy for evaluating definitively the many new promising hypotheses in the treatment and prevention of cardiovascular disease.

Indeed, with each new advance in cardiovascular medicine, randomized clinical trials generally, and those of large sample size in particular, have become even more crucial to achieving further gains. Therapeutic trials, which increasingly test new agents against already established treatments rather than inactive placebos, must be designed to detect ever decreasing benefit differences. Progress in treating acute MI, for example, has led to substantial decreases in short-term mortality following hospitalization for this condition, from approximately 20% in 1970 to 10% in 1995.[24-27] As a consequence, although a 20% mortality benefit in 1970 would have yielded an absolute reduction of four percentage points (from 20% to 16%), a new treatment today that confers a comparable 20% benefit would yield an absolute mortality reduction only half as great (a 2-percentage-point decrease, from 10% to 8%). Thus, the reliable detection of such a benefit today requires clinical trials of even larger sample sizes to rule out the statistical possibility that the play of chance accounts for any observed treatment effect. Clinical trials of large sample size are also crucial in evaluating promising primary prevention strategies, because participants in such trials are, by definition, at lower baseline risk of disease and will accrue outcomes at a much slower rate than those with a previous history of disease. Nevertheless, the discovery of effective primary prevention measures can have an even larger public health impact than successful treatments for already-ill patients, because preventive measures can be implemented broadly among a much larger proportion of the population.

No area of medicine has likely been the focus of more large-scale, randomized clinical trials than CVD. Efforts to compile listings of completed and ongoing trials in CVD have easily identified hundreds of investigations.[28-30] In the crowded alphabet soup of trial acronyms, more than a few selections have wound up serving multiple trial masters, with the popular choices ranging from the predictable (e.g., CARE, five separate trials listed) to the patently incongruous (e.g., BIGMAC, two separate trials listed).[30] Keeping up with the vast and seemingly exponentially expanding literature is a daunting task for increasingly busy academic researchers and clinical practitioners committed to applying scientifically sound, current knowledge to the care of their patients. Indeed, in the five years since the first edition of this book was published, progress has been occurring rapidly in many areas—for example, the efficacy and safety of postmenopausal hormone replacement therapy in the primary and secondary prevention of CHD have been called into question by the results of several large trials,[31-38] and trials of antioxidant vitamins have yielded conflicting results.[39]

This book, therefore, has been extensively revised and updated so that it may continue to serve as a comprehensive and state-of-the-art resource about clinical trials in CVD for those in research and in clinical practice. One third of the chapters are completely new, and the remainder have been substantially expanded since the first edition to reflect the recent explosion of trials in the field. Leading authorities in more than two dozen areas of cardiovascular treatment and prevention research provide clear distillations of current knowledge gleaned from clinical trials.

While large in number, clinical trials in cardiovascular disease vary in quality and in their ability to provide definitive evidence that can reliably guide clinical practice. Critically reviewing and synthesizing the results of such studies requires an understanding of their design and analysis. Section I provides an overview of these issues. The opening chapter places the contributions of clinical trials within a larger research context, emphasizing the importance of complementary evidence from basic laboratory research and observational epidemiology in arriving at sound clinical and public health policy decisions. The following chapters cover the basics of trial methodology, including the role of data monitoring boards, which are critical to the management of randomized trials.

Sections II and III provide substantive, critical assessments of clinical trials for the treatment and prevention of CVD. Section II reviews treatment trials for three common conditions: acute coronary ischemia, arrhythmias, and congestive heart failure. The latter two topics receive greatly expanded coverage here as compared with the first edition of the book. Prospects for the effective treatment of serious ventricular arrhythmias have recently brightened with the development of strategies that combine drug therapy with surgery and antiarrhythmic devices, such as implantable defibrillators. And, although the prognosis for heart failure patients remains poor, major therapeutic advances have been achieved in this area during recent years. Section III focuses on primary and secondary prevention trials. Primary prevention trials evaluate whether an agent or procedure can reduce the risk of developing CVD among those without prior CVD—either healthy individuals at usual risk or those already recognized to be at high risk of CVD. Secondary prevention trials, conducted among those with preexisting cardiovascular disease, determine the ability of an agent or procedure to ameliorate symptoms, prevent recurrence, or decrease CVD-related mortality. Secondary prevention trials can be distinguished from treatment trials in that, whereas treatment trials often take place in acute settings (e.g., thrombolytic therapy initiated immediately following myocardial infarction among hospitalized patients), secondary prevention trials evaluate chronic, long-term therapies, such as cholesterol reduction, antioxidant vitamin supplementation, physical activity, or weight loss. (Some agents, such as aspirin, are useful in both treatment and prevention settings, and are thus discussed in both Sections II and III.) Preventive strategies are assuming increasing importance in the face of constraints on health care resources in developed countries and the severely limited medical care available in developing countries now confronting the CVD pandemic.

ACKNOWLEDGMENTS

Collaboration and teamwork are critical elements in clinical trials of heart disease. So, too, were they vital in the preparation of this companion text to Braunwald's *Heart Disease*. The majority of chapter authors graciously accepted our initial invitation and provided outstanding comprehensive summaries of the current state of knowledge on clinical trials in their areas of expertise. Our medical editor, Shari Bassuk, ScD, performed yeoman's work. Her expert editing and superb organizational skills were crucial to the success of this project. At Elsevier, publisher Anne Lenehan and her assistant Vera Ginsburgs also provided invaluable assistance at all stages of production. Finally, we thank our families (in particular, Chris, Jenn, Jeffrey M., Joshua, Jeffrey B., Susan, Andrew, Elena, Anne, Michaela, Dante, and Liam) for their unfailing support and forbearance.

JoAnn E. Manson
Julie E. Buring
Paul M. Ridker
J. Michael Gaziano

REFERENCES

1. Murray CJL, Lopez AD: Mortality by cause for eight regions of the world: Global Burden of Disease Study. Lancet 1997; 349:1269-1276.
2. American Heart Association: Heart Disease and Stroke Statistics: 2003 Update. Dallas, Texas: American Heart Association, 2002.
3. Goldman L, Cook EF: The decline in ischemic heart disease mortality rates: An analysis of the comparative effects of medical interventions and changes in lifestyle. Annals of Internal Medicine 1984; 101:825-836.
4. Hunink MGM, Goldman L, Tosteson ANA, et al: The recent decline in mortality from coronary heart disease, 1980-1990. JAMA 1997; 277:535-542.
5. Murray CJL, Lopez AD: The global burden of disease: A comprehensive assessment of mortality and disability from diseases, injuries, and risk factors in 1990 and projected to 2020. Cambridge, MA: Harvard University Press, 1996.
6. Cooper R, Cutler J, Desvigne-Nickens P, et al: Trends and disparities in coronary heart disease, stroke, and other cardiovascular diseases in the United States: Findings of the National Conference on Cardiovascular Disease Prevention. Circulation 2000; 102:3137-3147.
7. National Heart Lung and Blood Institute: Morbidity & Mortality: 2000 Chart Book on Cardiovascular, Lung, and Blood Diseases. Bethesda, MD: National Heart, Lung, and Blood Institute, National Institutes of Health, 2000.
8. Flegal KM, Carroll MD, Ogden CL, Johnson CL: Prevalence and trends in obesity among US adults, 1999-2000. JAMA 2002; 288:1723-1727.
9. Flegal KM, Carroll RJ, Kuczmarski RJ, Johnson CL: Overweight and obesity in the United States: Prevalence and trends, 1960-1994. International Journal of Obesity 1998; 22:39-47.
10. Mokdad AH, Bowman BA, Ford ES, et al:. The continuing epidemics of obesity and diabetes in the United States. JAMA 2001; 286:1195-1200.
11. Harris MI, Flegal KM, Cowie CC, et al: Prevalence of diabetes, impaired fasting glucose, and impaired glucose tolerance in U.S. adults: The Third National Health and Nutrition Examination Survey, 1988-1994. Diabetes Care 1998; 21:518-524.
12. Arnett DK, McGovern PG, Jacobs DR, Jr., et al: Fifteen-year trends in cardiovascular risk factors (1980-1982 through 1995-1997): The Minnesota Heart Survey. American Journal of Epidemiology 2002; 156:929-35.
13. Barnes PM, Schoenborn CA: Physical Activity among Adults: United States, 2000. Advance Data No. 333. Hyattsville, MD: U.S. Department of Health and Human Services, Centers for Disease Control and Prevention, 2003.
14. U.S. Department of Health and Human Services: Physical Activity and Health: A Report of the Surgeon General. Atlanta, Georgia: U.S. Department of Health and Human Services, Centers for Disease Control and Prevention, National Center for Chronic Disease Prevention and Health Promotion, 1996.
15. Ogden CL, Flegal KM, Carroll MD, et al: Prevalence and trends in overweight among U.S. children and adolescents, 1999-2000. JAMA 2002; 288:1728-1732.
16. Johnson LD, Bachman JG, O'Malley PM: Cigarette smoking continues to rise among American teenagers in 1996. Ann Arbor, Michigan: University of Michigan News and Information Services, 1996.
17. Murray CJL, Lopez AD: The global burden of disease: Summary. Cambridge, MA: Harvard University Press, 1996.
18. Hennekens CH: Increasing burden of cardiovascular disease: Current knowledge and future directions for research on risk factors. Circulation 1998; 97:1095-1102.
19. Astrup A, Finer N: Redefining type 2 diabetes: 'Diabesity' or 'obesity dependent diabetes mellitus'? Obesity Reviews 2000; 1:57-59.
20. Manson JE, Spelsberg A: Risk modification in the diabetic patient. In: Manson JE, Ridker PM, Gaziano JM, et al, eds. Prevention of Myocardial Infarction. New York: Oxford University Press, 1996:241-273.
21. Hebert PR, Fiebach NH, Eberlein KA, et al: The community-based randomized trials of pharmacologic treatment of mild-to-moderate hypertension. American Journal of Epidemiology 1988; 127:581-590.
22. Hennekens CH, Buring JE, Sandercock P, et al: Aspirin and other antiplatelet agents in the secondary and primary prevention of cardiovascular disease. Circulation 1989; 80:749-756.
23. Hennekens CH, Buring JE: Observational evidence. Annals of the New York Academy of Science 1993; 703:18-24.
24. McGovern PG, Folsom AR, Sprafka JM, et al: Trends in survival of myocardial infarction patients between 1970 and 1985. The Minnesota Heart Survey. Circulation 1992; 85:172-179.
25. McGovern PG, Pankow JS, Shahar E, et al: Recent trends in acute coronary heart disease: Mortality, morbidity, medical care, and risk factors. New England Journal of Medicine 1996; 334:884-890.

26. Rosamond WD, Chambless LE, Folsom AR, et al: Trends in the incidence of myocardial infarction and in mortality due to coronary heart disease, 1987 to 1994. New England Journal of Medicine 1998; 339:861–867.

27. Goldberg RJ, Yarzebski J, Lessard D, et al: A two-decades (1975 to 1995) long experience in the incidence, in-hospital and long-term case-fatality rates of acute myocardial infarction: A community-wide perspective. Journal of the American College of Cardiology 1999; 33:1533–1539.

28. Astra AB: What's what: A guide to acronyms for cardiovascular trials. Goteborg, Sweden: Astra Hassle AB, 1996.

29. Parmley WW: TOTAL ABC CHAOS. Journal of the American College of Cardiology 1996; 27:1292.

30. Cheng TO: Acronyms of clinical trials in cardiology: 1998. American Heart Journal 1999; 137:726–765.

31. Hulley S, Grady D, Bush T, et al: Randomized trial of estrogen plus progestin for secondary prevention of coronary heart disease in postmenopausal women. Heart and Estrogen/progestin Replacement Study (HERS) Research Group. JAMA 1998; 280:605–613.

32. Grady D, Herrington D, Bittner V, et al: Cardiovascular disease outcomes during 6.8 years of hormone therapy: Heart and Estrogen/progestin Replacement Study follow-up (HERS II). JAMA 2002; 288:49–57.

33. Clarke SC, Kelleher J, Lloyd-Jones H, et al: A study of hormone replacement therapy in postmenopausal women with ischaemic heart disease: The Papworth HRT atherosclerosis study. British Journal of Obstetrics and Gynaecology 2002; 109:1056–1062.

34. Writing Group for the Women's Health Initiative Investigators: Risks and benefits of estrogen plus progestin in healthy postmenopausal women: Principal results From the Women's Health Initiative randomized controlled trial. JAMA 2002; 288:321–333.

35. Waters DD, Alderman EL, Hsia J, et al: Effects of hormone replacement therapy and antioxidant vitamin supplements on coronary atherosclerosis in postmenopausal women: A randomized controlled trial. JAMA 2002; 288:2432–2440.

36. ESPRIT Team: Oestrogen therapy for prevention of reinfarction in postmenopausal women: a randomised placebo controlled trial. Lancet 2002; 360:2001–2008.

37. Manson JE, Hsia J, Johnson KC, et al: Estrogen plus progestin and the risk of coronary heart disease. New England Journal of Medicine 2003; 349:523–534.

38. Michels KB, Manson JE: Postmenopausal hormone therapy: a reversal of fortune. Circulation 2003; 107:1830–1833.

39. Manson JE, Bassuk SS, Stampfer MJ: Does vitamin E supplementation prevent cardiovascular events? Journal of Women's Health 2003; 12:123–136.

CONTRIBUTORS

ROBERT ALLAN, PhD
Clinical Assistant Professor of Psychology in Psychiatry, Weill Medical College of Cornell University; Assistant Attending Psychologist in Psychiatry, New York Presbyterian Hospital, New York, New York.
Cardiac Psychology: Psychosocial Factors

ELLIOTT M. ANTMAN, MD
Associate Professor, Department of Medicine, Harvard Medical School; Director, Samuel A. Levine Cardiac Unit, Department of Medicine, Cardiovascular Division, Brigham and Women's Hospital, Boston, Massachusetts.
Direct Thrombin Inhibitors

SHARI S. BASSUK, ScD
Epidemiologist, Division of Preventive Medicine, Brigham and Women's Hospital, Boston, Massachusetts.
Antioxidant Vitamins

MALCOLM R. BELL, MBBS, FRACP
Professor of Medicine, Mayo Medical School; Consultant in Cardiovascular Diseases and Internal Medicine, Mayo Clinic and Mayo Foundation, Rochester, Minnesota.
Coronary Artery Bypass Surgery

JOHN A. BITTL, MD
Interventional Cardiologist, Ocala Heart Institute, Munroe Regional Medical Center, Ocala, Florida.
Direct Thrombin Inhibitors

JULIE E. BURING, ScD, FACE
Professor of Ambulatory Care and Prevention, Harvard Medical School; Deputy Director, Division of Preventive Medicine, Brigham and Women's Hospital, Boston, Massachusetts.
Contributions of Basic Research, Observational Studies, and Randomized Trials

CLAUDIA U. CHAE, MD, MPH
Instructor in Medicine, Harvard Medical School; Associate Physician, Division of Preventive Medicine, Brigham and Women's Hospital; Assistant in Medicine, Cardiology Division, Massachusetts General Hospital, Boston, Massachusetts.
Postmenopausal Hormone Replacement Therapy

DAVID E. CHIRIBOGA, MD, MPH
Fellow, Preventive Medicine, Department of Family Medicine and Community Health, University of Massachusetts Medical School, Worcester, Massachusetts.
Prevention Strategies: From the Office to the Community and Beyond

JEFFREY A. CUTLER, MD
Senior Scientific Advisor, Division of Epidemiology and Clinical Applications, National Heart, Lung, and Blood Institute, Bethesda, Maryland.
Comparative Features of Primordial, Primary, and Secondary Prevention Trials

DAVID L. DEMETS, PhD
Professor and Chair, Department of Biostatistics and Medical Informatics, University of Wisconsin, Madison, Wisconsin.
Principles of Data and Safety Monitoring Boards in Randomized Trials

JOHN P. DIMARCO, MD, PhD
Professor of Medicine, Internal Medicine, Cardiovascular Division, University of Virginia, Charlottesville, Virginia.
Drug Therapy for Ventricular Tachycardia and Ventricular Fibrillation

ERIC J. EICHHORN, MD
Adjoint Professor of Medicine, Department of Internal Medicine, University of Colorado Health Science Center, Denver, Colorado; Staff Physician; Director of Heart Failure Services, Medical City Dallas Hospital; Medical Director, Cardiopulmonary Research Science and Technology Institute, Dallas, Texas.
Beta Blockers

MARGARET C. FANG, MD
Clinical and Research Fellow in Medicine, Clinical Epidemiology Unit, Massachusetts General Hospital, Boston, Massachusetts.
Anticoagulant and Antiplatelet Drug Therapy in Atrial Fibrillation

GARY S. FRANCIS, MD
Director, Coronary Intensive Care Unit, Cardiology Department, Cleveland Clinic Foundation; Professor of Medicine, Ohio State University, Cleveland, Ohio.
Drugs Blocking the Renin-Angiotensin-Aldosterone System

LAURENCE S. FREEDMAN, PhD
Professor of Statistics, Department of Mathematics and Statistics, Bar Ilan University, Ramat Gan, Israel.
Methodology of Randomized Trials

LAWRENCE M. FRIEDMAN, MD
Assistant Director for Ethics and Clinical Research, National Heart, Lung, and Blood Institute, Bethesda, Maryland.
Comparative Features of Primordial, Primary, and Secondary Prevention Trials

J. MICHAEL GAZIANO, MD, MPH, FACC
Associate Professor of Medicine, Harvard Medical School; Chief, Division of Aging, Brigham and Women's Hospital; Director, Massachusetts Veterans Epidemiology Research and Information Center, Boston, Massachusetts.
Cholesterol Reduction; Aspirin, Other Antiplatelet Agents, and Anticoagulants; Antioxidant Vitamins

BERNARD J. GERSH, MB, ChB, DPhil
Professor of Medicine, Department of Internal Medicine, Mayo Medical School; Consultant, Department of Internal Medicine, Mayo Medical Center, Rochester, Minnesota.
Coronary Artery Bypass Surgery

C. MICHAEL GIBSON, MS, MD
Associate Professor of Medicine, Harvard University; Associate Chief of Cardiology, Beth Israel Deaconess Medical Center; Director, TIMI Angiographic Core Laboratory and Data Coordinating Center, Brigham and Women's Hospital, Boston, Massachusetts.
Angioplasty: Primary, Rescue, and Adjunctive Mechanical Interventions

HEATHER L. GORNIK, MD, MHS
Cardiology Fellow, Cardiovascular Division, Brigham and Women's Hospital, Boston, Massachusetts.
Adjunctive Medical Therapy

ERMINIA M. GUARNERI, MD, FACC
Medical Director, Integrative Medicine, Department of Cardiovascular Disease, Scripps Clinic, La Jolla, California.
Multiple Risk-Factor Intervention Trials

JACQUELINE A. HART, MD
Co-Medical Director, C.A.L.M. Program, Division of Cardiology, Newton-Wellesley Hospital, Newton, Massachusetts.
Multiple Risk-Factor Intervention Trials

JIANG HE, MD, PhD
Professor of Epidemiology and Medicine, Tulane University School of Public Health and Tropical Medicine, New Orleans, Louisiana.
Blood Pressure Reduction

ELAINE M. HYLEK, MD, MPH
Assistant Professor, Harvard Medical School; Associate Physician; Associate Chief, General Internal Medicine Division/Clinical Epidemiology Unit, Massachusetts General Hospital, Boston, Massachusetts.
Anticoagulant and Antiplatelet Drug Therapy in Atrial Fibrillation

JUHANA KARHA, MD
Clinical Fellow, Internal Medicine, Department of Medicine, Brigham and Women's Hospital, Boston, Massachusetts.
Angioplasty: Primary, Rescue, and Adjunctive Mechanical Interventions

CHARLES R. KERR, MD, FRCPC, FACC
Professor; Head, Division of Cardiology, Department of Medicine, University of British Columbia; Head, Division of Cardiology, Department of Medicine, St. Paul's Hospital, Vancouver, British Columbia, Canada.
Pacing

TOBIAS KURTH, MD, ScD
Instructor in Medicine, Department of Medicine, Harvard Medical School; Associate Epidemiologist, Divisions of Preventive Medicine and Aging, Department of Medicine, Brigham and Women's Hospital, Boston, Massachusetts.
Aspirin, Other Antiplatelet Agents, and Anticoagulants

J. MICHAEL MANGRUM, MD
Assistant Professor of Medicine, Department of Internal Medicine, Cardiovascular Division, University of Virginia, Charlottesville, Virginia.
Drug Therapy for Ventricular Tachycardia and Ventricular Fibrillation

JOANN E. MANSON, MD, DrPH, FAHA, FACP
Elizabeth F. Brigham Professor of Women's Health and Professor of Medicine, Harvard Medical School; Chief, Division of Preventive Medicine and Co-Director of the Connors Center for Women's Health and Gender Biology, Brigham and Women's Hospital, Boston, Massachusetts.
Postmenopausal Hormone Replacement Therapy; Antioxidant Vitamins

ELIZABETH MCNEILL, MD, MBChB, BSc (Hons), MRCP
Clinical Fellow in Electrophysiology, Department of Cardiology, University of British Columbia; Clinical Fellow in Electrophysiology, Department of Cardiology, St. Paul's Hospital, Vancouver, British Columbia, Canada; Specialist Registrar in Cardiology, Bristol Royal Infirmary (South West Deanery), Bristol, United Kingdom.
Pacing

SHAMIR R. MEHTA, MD, MSc (Epi), FRCPC, FACC
Assistant Professor, Department of Medicine, McMaster University; Staff Cardiologist (Interventional Cardiology), Hamilton Health Sciences, General Division, Hamilton, Ontario, Canada.
Aspirin and Thienopyridines

DAVID A. MORROW, MD, MPH
Instructor in Medicine, Harvard University; Associate Physician, Cardiovascular Division, Brigham and Women's Hospital, Boston, Massachusetts.
Heparin and Low–Molecular-Weight Heparin

CHARLES J. MULLANY, MB, MS
Professor of Surgery, Mayo Graduate School of Medicine, Mayo Clinic; Consultant, Division of Thoracic and Cardiovascular Surgery, Mayo Clinic-Saint Mary's Hospital, Mayo Clinic-Rochester Methodist Hospital, Rochester, Minnesota.
Coronary Artery Bypass Surgery

IRA S. OCKENE, MD
David and Barbara Milliken Professor of Preventive Cardiology; Director, Preventive Cardiology Program; Associate Director, Division of Cardiovascular Medicine, University of Massachusetts Medical School, Worcester, Massachusetts.
Prevention Strategies: From the Office to the Community and Beyond

PATRICK T. O'GARA, MD
Associate Professor, Department of Medicine, Harvard Medical School; Director, Clinical Cardiology, Brigham and Women's Hospital, Boston, Massachusetts.
Adjunctive Medical Therapy

E. MAGNUS OHMAN, MD, FRCPI, FACC
Ernest and Hazel Craige Professor of Cardiovascular Medicine, The University of North Carolina at Chapel Hill; Chief, Division of Cardiology; Director, University of North Carolina Heart Center, University of North Carolina Hospitals, Chapel Hill, North Carolina.
Glycoprotein IIb/IIIa Receptor Inhibitors

DEAN ORNISH, MD
Clinical Professor of Medicine, School of Medicine, University of California, San Francisco, California; Founder and President, Preventive Medicine Research Institute, Sausalito, California.
Multiple Risk-Factor Intervention Trials

RICHARD C. PASTERNAK, MD
Associate Professor of Medicine, Harvard Medical School; Director of Preventive Cardiology and Cardiac Rehabilitation, Department of Medicine-Cardiology Division, Massachusetts General Hospital, Boston, Massachusetts.
Prevention Trials of Smoking Cessation

SHARON C. REIMOLD, MD
Associate Professor, Department of Internal Medicine, University of Texas Southwestern, Dallas, Texas.
Drug Therapy for Supraventricular Tachycardia

PAUL M. RIDKER, MD, MPH, FAHA, FACC
Eugene Braunwald Professor of Medicine, Harvard Medical School; Director, Center for Cardiovascular Disease Prevention, Brigham and Women's Hospital, Boston, Massachusetts.
Aspirin, Other Antiplatelet Agents, and Anticoagulants

NANCY A. RIGOTTI, MD
Associate Professor, Department of Medicine, Harvard Medical School; Director, Tobacco Research and Treatment Center, Massachusetts General Hospital, Boston, Massachusetts.
Prevention Trials of Smoking Cessation

FRANK M. SACKS, MD
Professor of Cardiovascular Disease Prevention, Department of Nutrition, Harvard School of Public Health, Boston, Massachusetts.
Dietary Factors

STEPHEN SCHEIDT, MD
Professor of Clinical Medicine, Division of Cardiology, New York Weill-Cornell Medical Center, New York, New York.
Cardiac Psychology: Psychosocial Factors

BRET SCHER, MD
Clinical Fellow, Department of Cardiology, Scripps Clinic, La Jolla, California.
Multiple Risk-Factor Intervention Trials

RICHARD E. SCRANTON, MD, MPH
Instructor in Medicine, Harvard Medical School; Associate Physician, Division of Aging, Brigham and Women's Hospital; Clinician Investigator, Massachusetts VA Epidemiology Research and Information Center, New England VA Healthcare System, Boston, Massachusetts.
Cholesterol Reduction

DENISE G. SIMONS-MORTON, MD, PhD
Director, Clinical Applications and Prevention Program, Division of Epidemiology and Clinical Applications, National Heart, Lung, and Blood Institute, Bethesda, Maryland.
Comparative Features of Primordial, Primary, and Secondary Prevention Trials

DANIEL E. SINGER, MD
Professor of Medicine, Harvard Medical School; Chief, Clinical Epidemiology Unit, General Medicine Division, Massachusetts General Hospital, Boston, Massachusetts.
Anticoagulant and Antiplatelet Drug Therapy in Atrial Fibrillation

PETER R. SINNAEVE, MD, PhD
University of Leuven; Department of Cardiology, University Hospital Gasthuisberg, Leuven, Belgium.
Thrombolytic Therapy

KYOKO SOEJIMA, MD
Instructor, Cardiovascular Division, Department of Internal Medicine, Harvard Medical School; Associated Physician, Cardiovascular Division, Department of Internal Medicine, Brigham and Women's Hospital.
Arrhythmia Ablation

MARCIA L. STEFANICK, PhD
Professor of Medicine; Associate Professor of Gynecology
and Obstetrics, Stanford University, Stanford, California.
Physical Activity and Weight Loss

STEVEN R. STEINHUBL, MD
Associate Professor; Associate Director of Cardiac Catheterization Laboratory, Department of Medicine, University
of North Carolina, Chapel Hill, North Carolina.
Glycoprotein IIb/IIIa Receptor Inhibitors

LYNNE WARNER STEVENSON, MD
Associate Professor of Medicine, Department of Medi-
cine, Harvard Medical School; Co-Director, Cardiomyopa-
thy and Heart Failure Program, Department of Medicine,
Brigham and Women's Hospital, Boston, Massachusetts.
*Heart Transplantation and Mechanical Cardiac
Support*

WILLIAM G. STEVENSON, MD
Associate Professor, Cardiovascular Division, Department of Medicine, Harvard Medical School; Director,
Clinical Cardiac Electrophysiology Program, Cardiovascular Division, Department of Medicine; Director, Clinical Cardiac EP Fellowship Training Program, Brigham
and Women's Hospital, Boston, Massachusetts.
Arrhythmia Ablation

MICHAEL O. SWEENEY, MD
Assistant Professor of Medicine, Department of Cardi-
ology, Harvard Medical School; Cardiac Arrhythmia
Service, Brigham and Women's Hospital, Boston, Massa-
chusetts.
*Implantable Cardioverter-Defibrillators and Cardiac
Resynchronization Therapy*

W.H. WILSON TANG, MD
Fellow, Cardiovascular Medicine, Cleveland Clinic Foun-
dation, Cleveland, Ohio.
*Drugs Blocking the Renin-Angiotensin-Aldosterone
System*

K.K. STANLEY TUNG, MD, FRCP
Clinical Instructor, Department of Medicine, University
of British Columbia; Consultant, Clinical Cardiac Electro-
physiologist, Department of Cardiology, St. Paul's Hospi-
tal; Clinical Cardiac Electrophysiologist, Department of
Cardiology, Vancouver General Hospital, Vancouver,
British Columbia, Canada.
Pacing

FRANS VAN DE WERF, MD, PhD
Chairman, Department of Cardiology, K.U. Leuven; Chair-
man, Department of Cardiology, University Hospital
Gasthuisberg, Leuven, Belgium.
Thrombolytic Therapy

PAUL K. WHELTON, MD, MSc
Professor of Epidemiology and Medicine; Senior Vice
President for Health Sciences, Tulane University Health
Sciences Center, New Orleans, Louisiana.
Blood Pressure Reduction

HARVEY D. WHITE, DSc
Honorary Clinical Professor of Medicine, Department of
Medicine, University of Auckland; Director of Coronary
Care and Cardiovascular Research, Green Lane Hospital,
Auckland, New Zealand.
Direct Thrombin Inhibitors

JOHN A. YEUNG-LAI-WAH, MB, ChB, FRCPC, FACC
Clinical Associate Professor, Department of Medicine,
Division of Cardiology, University of British Columbia;
Director of Electrophysiology Laboratory, St. Paul's Hos-
pital, Vancouver, British Columbia, Canada.
Pacing

PAUL B. YU, MD, PhD
Clinical and Research Fellow, Cardiology Division, Massa-
chusetts General Hospital, Harvard Medical School,
Boston, Massachusetts.
Smoking Cessation

SALIM YUSUF, MBBS, FRCP, DPhil
Professor of Medicine, McMaster University; Director,
Population Health Research Institute; Department of
Cardiology, Hamilton Health Sciences, Hamilton, Ontario,
Canada.
Aspirin and Thienopyridines

CONTENTS

■ ■ ■ c h a p t e r **1**

Contributions of Basic Research, Observational Studies, and Randomized Trials*

Julie E. Buring

In cardiovascular disease, as in all areas of medicine, advances in our knowledge proceed on several fronts, optimally, simultaneously. Basic researchers provide biologic mechanisms to answer the crucial question of why an agent or intervention reduces the risk of premature death. Clinicians are providing enormous benefits to affected patients through advances in diagnosis and treatment, and they formulate hypotheses from their clinical experiences in case reports and case series. Clinical investigators address the relevance of basic research findings to affected patients and healthy people. Epidemiologists and statisticians, optimally collaborating with researchers in other disciplines, formulate hypotheses from descriptive studies and test these in analytic studies, both observational case-control and cohort studies, as well as, where necessary, randomized trials. The results of such studies answer the equally crucial and complementary question of whether an agent or intervention reduces premature morbidity or mortality. Thus, each discipline and, indeed, every strategy within a discipline provides importantly relevant and complementary information to a totality of evidence upon which rational clinical decisions for individuals and policy decisions for the health of the general public can be safely based.[1] It is crucial to consider the totality of evidence for any question because each research discipline has unique strengths and limitations.

BASIC RESEARCH

Basic laboratory and animal research has the unique strength of precision, in that it can achieve virtually complete control of exposures, environment, and even genetics. Because of this, basic research can provide the scientific underpinnings for all applied research in humans, with unique and crucial information concerning disease mechanisms. However, basic research also has the disadvantage of potential lack of relevance to free-living humans owing to such differences as species specificity, dose, and routes of administration of exposures. Thus, the results from basic research may differ so greatly from those that apply to free-living humans as to

render them of questionable direct relevance. The inability to predict the applicability of findings from a particular species of animals to humans was underscored by John Cairns, who wrote:

Who could have guessed that *Homo sapiens* would share with the humble guinea pig the unenviable distinction of being incapable of synthesizing ascorbic acid, or share with armadillos a susceptibility to the bacterium that causes leprosy, or that intestinal cancer usually occurs in the large intestine of humans and the small intestine of sheep?[2]

Because of such issues, the results from animal research may be limited in their ability to provide a reliable quantitative estimate of human disease risk. However, the precision possible in such research provides unique and crucial information, which is of great value in setting priorities for studies that test the relevance of animal research in free-living humans.[3]

Although basic research may add to our biologic understanding of why an exposure causes or prevents disease, only epidemiology allows the quantification of the magnitude of the exposure-disease relationship in humans and offers the possibility of altering risk through intervention. Indeed, epidemiologic research has often provided information that has formed the basis for public health decisions long before the basic mechanism of a particular disease was understood. In striving to identify factors that cause or prevent disease, laboratory testing and theoretic speculation about possible mechanisms are important, but no more so than direct, straightforward observation of what actually happens in human populations. If epidemiologic studies are well designed and conducted, and if the data are properly analyzed and interpreted, the studies can provide strong and reliable evidence on which to base clinical care of individual patients and, ultimately, policy decisions affecting the health of the general public.

EPIDEMIOLOGIC STUDIES

Epidemiology, because it is based directly on observations of free-living humans, has the unique advantage of relevance. However, for this same reason, epidemiologic studies have the potential disadvantage of imprecision. Indeed, in contrast with basic research, epidemiology is

---

*Based on Chapter 1 of the previous edition, Contributions of Basic Research, Observational Studies, and Randomized Trials, by Julie E. Buring and Charles H. Hennekens.

crude and inexact, because observations in free-living humans can never take place under the controlled conditions possible in the laboratory. Nonetheless, epidemiology contributes essential information to a totality of evidence, which then can support a judgment of a cause-effect relationship.

Making such a judgment involves several steps, the first being to establish whether there is a valid statistical association. To conclude that an association is valid, alternative explanations for the finding must be ruled out, including the potential roles of chance, bias, and confounding. If a valid statistical association is present, the question then becomes whether the relationship is one of cause and effect. To render this judgment, the totality of evidence from all sources must be considered, with particular attention to the strength of the association, the consistency of the evidence from different studies, and the existence of a plausible biologic mechanism to explain the findings.

The basic design strategies used in epidemiologic research can be broadly categorized according to whether such investigations focus on describing the distributions of disease or on elucidating its determinants. *Descriptive epidemiology* is concerned with the distributions of disease, including consideration of which populations or subgroups do or do not develop a disease, in what geographic locations a disease is most or least common, and how the frequency or occurrence of the disease varies over time. Information on each of these characteristics can provide clues leading to the formulation of an epidemiologic hypothesis that is consistent with existing knowledge of disease occurrence. *Analytic epidemiology* focuses on the determinants of a disease by testing the hypotheses formulated from descriptive studies, with the ultimate goal of judging whether a particular exposure causes or prevents disease.

There are a number of specific analytic study design options that can be employed. These can be divided into two broad design strategies: observational and interventional (i.e., randomized clinical trials). The major difference between the two approaches lies in the role played by the investigator. In *observational studies*, the investigator simply observes the natural course of events, noting who is exposed and nonexposed and who has and has not developed the outcome of interest. In randomized clinical trials, the investigators themselves allocate the intervention and then follow the subjects to determine the development of the outcome in each exposed group.

OBSERVATIONAL EPIDEMIOLOGIC STUDIES

There are two basic types of observational analytic investigations: case-control and cohort. In a *case-control study*, a case group, or series of patients who have a disease of interest, and a control group, or comparison series of people without the disease, are selected for investigation, and the proportions with the exposure of interest in each group are compared. In contrast, in a *cohort study*, subjects are classified on the basis of the presence or absence of exposure to a particular factor and then followed for a specified period to determine the development of disease in each exposure group.

Case-control and cohort studies are often criticized because of the potential for bias and confounding that is inherent in the fact that the design is observational. Because the use of a particular drug or treatment or the adoption of a certain lifestyle is self-selected, people who use that drug, for example, may be systematically different from those who do not in ways that will affect the outcome of interest. Moreover, because the outcome of interest has already occurred at the time exposure is assessed, case-control studies have the potential for bias in the selection of subjects into the study and in their recall of prior events. In a cohort study, the often-long latent period between exposure and disease can lead to bias owing to insufficient follow-up. However, despite these inherent limitations, many exposure-disease relationships have been well established from observational evidence.[4]

There are two chief strengths of observational evidence. The first relates to the evaluation of exposures that require long duration, and the second relates to detection of moderate- to large-sized effects, on the order of a 50% or greater difference in disease outcome. With respect to the evaluation of exposures that require long duration, one example of the strength of observational studies is the evaluation of the relationship between blood pressure and risk of myocardial infarction (MI). Basic research had suggested mechanisms for a benefit of blood pressure lowering on risks of stroke and MI, and observational studies had consistently demonstrated a statistically significant 40% to 45% increased risk of stroke and a 25% to 30% increase in risk of MI associated with a 6 mm Hg difference in diastolic blood pressure.[5] In contrast, although individual randomized trials of pharmacologic therapy of mild-to-moderate hypertension indicated that blood pressure lowering by 6 mm Hg resulted in a comparable 40% decrease in risk of stroke, there was a far smaller and less certain benefit on MI than that suggested by the observational evidence. The apparent inconsistency remained even after the availability of results from 14 individual randomized trials of drug therapy in 37,000 subjects. This led some researchers to conclude that treatment of hypertension did not reduce the risk of subsequent MI. However, a comprehensive overview, or meta-analysis, of the trials demonstrated that a decrease of 6 mm Hg in diastolic blood pressure significantly reduced stroke by 42% and MI by a smaller, but statistically significant, 14%.[6] A subsequent meta-analysis, which included three additional trials, demonstrated the reduction in risk of MI to be 16%.[7] The 14% to 16% reduction in risk of MI seen in the randomized trials over three to five years of treatment was about half the 28% reduction one would predict from the results of observational studies of blood pressure lowering over decades. This discrepancy may well have been due to chance but also could have been due to the fact that stroke risk immediately decreases following lowering of blood pressure levels, whereas MI risk may be affected by prolonged effects of hypertension on more chronic processes of atherogenesis and thus would require far longer than the usual three to five years of treatment in trials to observe the full impact. Thus basic research and observational studies with long durations of exposure have been crucial components of the totality of evidence concerning the relationship of blood pressure lowering with risk of MI.

The second strength of observational studies lies in evaluating associations where the relative risk is moderate to large—that is, where the increased (or decreased) risk is 50% or greater. In this regard, observational evidence has provided both necessary and sufficient information on which to judge a cause-effect relationship for a large number of questions of clinical importance and public health significance. Chief among these has been the health effects of cigarette smoking. Starting in 1950 with case-control studies by Doll and Hill in the United Kingdom[8] and Wynder and Graham in the United States,[9] observational epidemiologic studies established a clear association between smoking and lung cancer, with risks among long-term smokers about 20 times greater than those of nonsmokers. Based on their observational evidence, Doll and Hill judged smoking to be a cause of lung cancer years before there was any clear understanding of the actual mechanism of alterations in DNA by initiators or promoters of cancer. In 1964 the U.S. Surgeon General also judged smoking to be a definite cause of this disease, still years before the biologic mechanism was clearly understood.[10] Thus, although basic research is crucial to identify mechanisms to explain causal or preventive factors, direct answers to the questions of whether particular exposures are associated with risks of disease may derive from straightforward observation of what actually happens in free-living human populations.

With regard to smoking and coronary heart disease (CHD), the finding that current cigarette smokers have about an 80% increased risk of developing the disease has been consistently demonstrated during the last 30 years by different investigators in a large number of case-control and cohort studies involving millions of person-years of observation.[11] It is interesting that smoking was not judged to be a cause of CHD until much later than the judgment that it caused lung cancer. Part of this related to the lack of a clear biologic mechanism. However, another reason related directly to a limitation in interpreting the findings from any observational study, namely, that as the relative risk gets smaller, there is increasing concern that some factor other than the exposure being studied may explain all or at least part of the findings. For example, cigarette smokers may share other characteristics or lifestyle practices that independently affect their risk of CHD. Information can be collected on any potential confounding variables known to the investigator and then used in the data analysis to adjust for any impact of these factors. However, there can be no adjustment for the effects of unmeasured or unmeasurable confounding variables.

When a large effect is seen, such as with smoking and lung cancer, the amount of uncontrolled confounding may affect the magnitude of the relative risk estimate, making it, for example, as high as a 22-fold increased risk, or as low as an 18-fold increased risk, rather than the observed 20-fold increased risk. However, it is unlikely that complete control of confounding would materially change the conclusion that there is a strong positive association between smoking and lung cancer. Even in the case of current smoking and CHD, whereas uncontrolled confounding may mean that the true relative risk is as small as a 60% increased risk or as large as a twofold increased risk, instead of the 80% increased risk most consistently seen in observational studies, that range of uncertainty does not materially affect the conclusion that current cigarette smoking increases the risk of CHD. On the other hand, when the most plausible magnitude of benefit or harm is only 20% to 40%—as is the case with most promising interventions today—a small amount of uncontrolled confounding in an observational study could mean the difference between a relative risk of 0.8, indicating a 20% decreased risk; 1.0, indicating no effect; or 1.2, indicating a 20% increased risk. In such circumstances, randomized trials represent the most reliable research design strategy.

RANDOMIZED CLINICAL TRIALS

Randomized clinical trials, also referred to as *experimental studies* or *intervention studies*, may be viewed as a type of cohort study, because participants are identified on the basis of their exposure status and followed to determine whether they develop the disease. The distinguishing feature of the intervention design is that the exposure status of each participant is assigned by the investigator.

Intervention studies are often considered to provide the most reliable evidence from epidemiologic research because of the unique strength of randomization as the means of allocating exposure status in a trial. When participants are allocated to a particular exposure group at random, such a strategy achieves, on average, control of all other factors that may affect disease risk. Whereas such variables, if they are known to the investigators, could be controlled in the design, analysis, or both, of observational studies, the unique feature of randomization is that it also, on average, controls the effects of risk factors that are unrecognized or unmeasurable. It is this ability to control both known and unknown confounders that makes the randomized trial such a powerful epidemiologic strategy, especially for studying small-to-moderate effects. Of course, ethical concerns preclude the allocation of exposures that are known to be hazardous. Such exposures can properly be assessed in intervention studies only by attempts to eliminate them, as in the Multiple Risk Factor Intervention Trial,[12] which was designed to evaluate the effects of smoking cessation, blood pressure reduction, and cholesterol lowering on decreasing risk of CHD. There are also particular concerns of costs and feasibility for intervention studies. Nevertheless, when well designed and conducted, randomized clinical trials can indeed provide the most direct epidemiologic evidence on which to judge whether an exposure causes or prevents a disease.

If the treatments are allocated at random in a sample of sufficiently large size, intervention studies have the potential to provide a degree of assurance about the validity of a result that is simply not possible with any observational design option. It is rare that the introduction of a new treatment or procedure is accompanied by benefits as striking and as unequivocal as those that followed the introduction of the antibiotic penicillin, namely, an immediate reduction in death rates from pneumococcal pneumonia from about 95% to 15%. A randomized trial of the efficacy of penicillin seemed unnecessary because the mortality reduction was so large and immediate that it seemed clearly due to the drug itself. Most often, however, the effects of therapeutic or preventive measures are small to moderate, on the order of 20% to 40% differences in disease outcomes. Such effects can be extremely important from a clinical or public health standpoint, especially when the outcome of interest is mortality from common diseases. Although important, small-to-moderate differences are difficult to establish reliably from observational studies, because the magnitude of the observed effect of the treatment may be about the same as the amount of uncontrolled confounding. In these circumstances, the conduct of a randomized trial will yield the strongest and most direct epidemiologic evidence on which to base a judgment of whether an observed association is one of cause and effect.

A recent example that illustrates the contributions of the various types of research strategies to the totality of evidence relates to the evaluation of the role of postmenopausal hormones in the primary prevention of coronary heart disease (CHD). During the last 25 years, more than 40 observational epidemiologic analyses of estrogen therapy in postmenopausal women have been conducted. Taken together, these analyses suggest that women who take estrogen have a risk of CHD that is 20% to 50% lower than the risk among nonusers of estrogen therapy.[13-15] The potential for such a benefit is biologically plausible, in that randomized trials have shown that estrogen therapy reduces plasma levels of low-density lipoprotein (LDL) cholesterol, increases plasma levels of high-density lipoprotein (HDL) cholesterol, reduces levels of Lp(a) lipoprotein, inhibits oxidation of LDL, improves endothelial vascular function, and reverses postmenopausal increases in fibrinogen and in plasminogen activator inhibitor type I.[14,16,17] All of these changes are known or postulated to be associated with a reduced risk of CHD. At the same time, however, the basic research evidence has also suggested that estrogen therapy could have potentially adverse effects on cardiovascular biomarkers by increasing triglyceride levels; activating coagulation as a result of increases in factor VII, prothrombin fragments 1 and 2, and fibrinopeptide A; and increasing levels of the inflammatory marker C-reactive protein.[14,18]

As promising as the evidence from the observational studies appeared, the postulated benefit of estrogen therapy in the primary prevention of CHD was still unproven. As in any observational study, it may be, for example, that postmenopausal women who choose to take estrogen therapy have other medical or lifestyle characteristics that differ from those of nonusers of estrogen therapy. These characteristics may, in themselves, affect risk of CHD and thus account for some or all of the observed benefit of estrogen therapy. While adjustments can be made for known confounding variables for which data are collected, observational studies are unable to control for the potential effects of confounding variables not collected or known to the investigators, and when searching for the proposed modest-sized effects, the amount of uncontrolled confounding may be as large as the most likely effect.

For all these reasons, randomized trials of sufficient sample size and duration of treatment and follow-up were necessary to detect reliably any small-to-moderate sized effects of estrogen therapy. If the trials were large enough, the randomization process would, on average, evenly distribute known and unknown confounding variables among treatment groups. In addition, extremely large trials are necessary to avoid the possible uninformative null result of no benefit when in fact a modest-sized benefit truly exists.

The Women's Health Initiative, a randomized, double-blind, placebo-controlled primary prevention trial, was initiated to evaluate as one of its components the risks and benefits of hormone use in healthy postmenopausal women.[19] A total of 16,608 postmenopausal, 50- to 70-year-old women with an intact uterus were randomized to estrogen plus progestin versus a placebo. The primary outcome was CHD, with a primary adverse outcome of breast cancer, and a global index summarizing the balance of risks and benefits, including the two primary outcomes plus stroke, pulmonary embolism, endometrial cancer, colorectal cancer, hip fracture, and death due to other causes. After an average follow-up of 5.2 years, the Data and Safety Monitoring Board recommended stopping the trial of estrogen plus progestin, because the overall health risks clearly exceeded the health benefits[20] (a parallel component of estrogen alone versus a placebo in women who have had a hysterectomy is still ongoing, with a planned termination of March 2005). Specifically, estrogen plus progestin therapy increased breast cancer incidence by 26%, CHD incidence by 29%, stroke incidence by 41%, and doubled the incidence of pulmonary embolism, although the treatment decreased colorectal cancer by 37%, hip fracture by 34%, and endometrial cancer by 17%. Based on data from the Women's Health Initiative, in the context of data indicating similar lack of benefit from secondary prevention trials of hormone use,[16,21] the Women's Health Initiative investigators concluded that the risk-benefit profile found in the trial indicated that this regimen should not be initiated or continued for primary prevention of CHD.

SUMMARY

The evaluation of an epidemiologic hypothesis involves the consideration of the totality of evidence, including basic research, observational epidemiologic studies, and randomized clinical trials. Each of these strategies contributes unique and complementary information to the totality of evidence on which to base rational clinical decisions for individuals and policy decisions for the health of the general public.

For many if not most hypotheses, randomized trials are neither necessary nor desirable. For detecting small-to-moderate effects, however, they represent the most reliable research design strategy. Randomized trials certainly can be more difficult to design and conduct than observational epidemiologic studies, owing to their unique problems of ethics, feasibility, and costs. However, randomized trials that are sufficiently large, as well as carefully designed, conducted, and analyzed, can provide the strongest and most direct epidemiologic evidence on which to make a judgment about the existence of a cause-effect relationship.

REFERENCES

1. Hennekens CH, Buring JE: Epidemiology in Medicine. Boston, Little, Brown, 1987.
2. Cairns J: The treatment of diseases and the war against cancer. Sci Am 1985; 253:51-59.
3. Doll R, Peto R: The Causes of Cancer. New York, Oxford University Press, 1981.
4. Hennekens CH, Buring JE: Observational evidence. *In* Warren KS, Mosteller F (eds). Doing More Good than Harm: The Evaluation of Health Care Interventions. Ann NY Acad Sci 1993; 703:18-24.
5. MacMahon S, Peto R, Cutler J, et al: Blood pressure, stroke, and coronary heart disease: I. Prolonged differences in blood pressure: Prospective observational studies corrected for the regression dilution bias. Lancet 1990; 335:765-774.
6. Collins R, Peto R, MacMahon S, et al: Blood pressure, stroke, and coronary heart disease: II. Short-term reductions in blood pressure: Overview of randomized drug trials in their epidemiologic context. Lancet 1990; 335:827-838.
7. Hebert PR, Moser M, Mayer J, et al: Recent evidence on drug therapy of mild to moderate hypertension and decreased risk of coronary heart disease. Arch Intern Med 1993; 153:578-581.
8. Doll R, Hill AB: Smoking and carcinoma of the lung: Preliminary report. BMJ 1950; 2:739-748.
9. Wynder EL, Graham EA: Tobacco smoking as a possible etiologic factor in bronchiogenic carcinoma: A study of 684 proved cases. JAMA 1950; 143:329-336.
10. U.S. Department of Health, Education, and Welfare: Smoking and health: Report of the advisory committee to the Surgeon General of the Public Health Service. PHS Publication No. 1103. Bethesda, Md, U.S. Department of Health, Education, and Welfare; Public Health Service; Centers for Disease Control, 1964.
11. Hennekens CH, Buring J, Mayrent SL: Smoking and aging in coronary heart disease. *In* Bosse R, Rose C (eds). Smoking and Aging. Lexington, Mass, DC Heath, 1984, pp 95-115.
12. Multiple Risk Factor Intervention Trial Research Group: Multiple Risk Factor Intervention Trial: Risk factor changes and morbidity results. JAMA 1982; 248:1465-1477.
13. Barrett-Connor E, Grady D: Hormone replacement therapy, heart disease, and other considerations. Ann Rev Public Health 1998; 19:55-72.
14. Manson JE, Martin KA: Postmenopausal hormone-replacement therapy. N Engl J Med 2001; 345:34-40.
15. Nelson HD, Humphrey LL, Nygren P, et al: Postmenopausal hormone replacement therapy: Scientific review. JAMA 2002; 288:872-881.
16. Hulley S, Grady D, Bush T, et al: Randomized trial of estrogen plus progestin for secondary prevention of coronary heart disease in postmenopausal women. JAMA 1998; 280:605-613.
17. The Writing Group for the PEPI Trial: Effects of estrogen or estrogen/progestin regimens on heart disease risk factors in postmenopausal women: The Postmenopausal Estrogen/Progestin Intervention (PEPI) Trial. JAMA 1995; 273:199-208.
18. Ridker PM, Hennekens CH, Rifai N, et al: Hormone replacement therapy and increased plasma concentration of C-reactive protein. Circulation 1999; 100:713-716.
19. The Women's Health Initiative Study Group: Design of the Women's Health Inititative clinical trial and observational study. Control Clin Trials 1998; 19:61-109.
20. Writing Group for the Women's Health Initiative Investigators: Risks and benefits of estrogen plus progestin in healthy postmenopausal women: Principal results from the Women's Health Initiative randomized controlled trial. JAMA 2002; 288:321-333.
21. Mosca L, Collins P, Herrington DM, et al: Hormone replacement therapy and cardiovascular disease: A statement for healthcare professionals from the American Heart Association. Circulation 2001; 104:499-503.

Methodology of Randomized Trials

Laurence S. Freedman

Randomized clinical trials are the most reliable method available for comparing alternative preventive or therapeutic interventions. Since the conduct and publication of the earliest randomized trials in the 1940s, clinicians have increasingly accepted this method as the gold standard for evaluating new treatments. This trend has been more rapid in some specialties, such as cardiovascular disease and oncology, but the trend is evident in nearly all areas of medicine. In the last 15 years, a number of excellent textbooks have been published describing comprehensively the methodology of randomized trials.[1-3] This chapter discusses selected topics pertinent to cardiovascular disease trials.

Most of the issues surrounding the methodology of clinical trials revolve around three principles: *achieving unbiasedness, achieving adequate precision*, and, subject to these two principles, *increasing efficiency* (Table 2-1).

The main aim of any clinical trial should be to provide an estimate of the effect of a (usually new) treatment on clinical outcome compared with the effect achieved by another (usually standard) treatment. *Unbiasedness* means the ability of the trial—through proper design, conduct, and analysis—to obtain invariably the correct estimate of the treatment effect, given as large a number of participating subjects as desired. Many study designs, mostly nonrandomized, lead to bias and fail to satisfy the unbiasedness criterion. Furthermore, even when randomization is used, certain other design features or types of statistical analysis give biased results.

Unbiasedness is a theoretical, although nonetheless important, concept. In practice, the number of participating subjects is always limited. Limited sample sizes introduce *random error*, a type of error distinct from bias, into the estimation of the treatment effect. When the random error is large, the treatment effect cannot be accurately estimated, that is, estimated with good *precision*. The larger the sample size, however, the lower the random error and the better the precision of the estimate.

Important as they are, randomized clinical trials often require a large investment of money and time. Furthermore, many of these trials are financed by public money. It is therefore important for investigators to search continually for ways of reducing the costs of randomized clinical trials. There are many ways to design trials so they provide unbiased estimates of treatment effects with good precision. Two different designs that achieve unbiasedness and the same level of precision may have different costs. In particular, because the costs often depend heavily on the number of participating subjects, interest often focuses on how to achieve the same precision with fewer participants. The ratio of the reciprocals of the number of participants required by two designs to achieve the same precision is known as their *relative efficiency*. Clearly we should be interested in finding new designs with large efficiency relative to the standard design.

Table 2-1 shows how the eight topics discussed in this chapter relate to the three basic principles of unbiasedness, precision, and efficiency.

NEED FOR RANDOMIZATION

Until recently it was unusual to conduct formal medical experiments. However, lack of controlled experiments sometimes led to conflicting claims and even to adoption of treatments that later were demonstrated to be harmful, such as gastric freezing for duodenal ulcer.[4] A basic element of a controlled experiment is the use of a control group of patients who receive the standard therapy with which the new treatment is to be compared. The control group may be formed by a number of different methods, not necessarily involving randomization. Controls may be chosen from patients who refuse the new treatment or from patients who are not offered the new treatment. It is now quite widely accepted that patients who are offered and refuse a new treatment are likely to be characteristically different from those who accept, and are different in a manner that will affect their overall prognosis. Such prognostic differences naturally lead to bias in the comparison of the treatment with the control groups.

More controversial than using controls who refuse treatment is using *historical controls*, that is, patients who were treated with the standard therapy before the new treatment became available. Several problems arise when using this method. First, the eligibility criteria for the study of the new treatment may cause a different disease profile of patients from that in the historical control group. Friedman and associates[1] observe that an annual total mortality rate of 6% was anticipated in the control group of the Coronary Drug Project[5] based on rates from previous myocardial infarction (MI) patients. In fact, an annual mortality rate of approximately 4% was observed both in the control and in the treatment

■ ■ ■

TABLE 2-1   THREE PRINCIPLES IN CLINICAL TRIALS METHODOLOGY

Principles	Concept	Topics
Unbiasedness	Getting the correct estimate of treatment effect "with unlimited sample size"	Randomization Intention-to-treat analysis Handling missing outcome values
Precision	Getting an accurate estimate of the treatment effect	Sample size and statistical power Length of follow-up
Efficiency	Reducing costs subject to unbiasedness and good precision	Reducing noncompliance Factorial designs Surrogate endpoints

groups. If historical controls had been used, then the conclusion would have been that the new treatments were effective.

Gehan and Freireich[6] advocate the use of historical controls, particularly when the participants in the previous studies were chosen using similar criteria for eligibility and evaluation. However, even in these circumstances, time changes in the nature of the patients referred for treatment, in diagnostic criteria, or in supportive care can introduce hidden bias into the comparison. Byar and colleagues[7] report that, in the Veterans Administration Cooperative Urological Research Group trial of treatments for prostate cancer, patients admitted in the last half of the trial and randomized to estrogen had significantly better survival rates than the controls who entered in the first half of the trial. There was no survival difference, however, when the same patients allocated estrogen were compared with their concurrent control subjects.

Gehan and Freireich[6] advocate controlling for hidden biases by using a multivariate regression model to adjust for differences in known prognostic factors between the treatment and control groups. However, only if one has knowledge of all relevant prognostic factors can one be sure that this method will work. In reality, known prognostic factors for most chronic diseases account for only a small fraction (<15%) of the observed variation in clinical outcomes among patients.[8] Thus there is little hope of controlling for all hidden biases with this device. When the treatment difference is large, these biases may not be sufficient to mask the underlying difference, and a randomized design may not be necessary. However, for moderate and small treatment differences the biases found in historical controls are likely to distort the comparison and lead to erroneous results.

More recently, there has been much interest in using medical databases to evaluate the comparative effects of treatments.[9] This approach suffers from many of the problems of historical controls and more. Perhaps the most serious problem is that database information is rarely sufficient to describe *why* a patient receives a particular treatment. Very often, the choice of treatment is heavily confounded by the current health of the patient, including the extent of the disease, concurrent illnesses, and general fitness.[10] As a result, comparison often leads to apparent advantages for less invasive procedures, even after adjustment for known prognostic factors. Byar[11] describes the analysis of data from a thy-

roid cancer register that appeared to show that surgery followed by x-ray therapy was harmful compared with surgery alone. However, because it was unknown whether x-ray treatment was given selectively to those with an incomplete resection of the tumor, the result was not interpretable.

Allocating treatment to a patient by randomization avoids confounding of the treatment choice by the patient's state of health or by other characteristics that can affect prognosis. This property represents the principal advantage that randomization carries over other methods of forming a control group and is the reason the randomized, controlled trial is regarded as the gold standard of evaluation designs. However, the act of randomization does not by itself guarantee a trial to be free from hidden bias. For example, one sometimes prepares in advance a list of the treatments to be allocated in sequence as patients enter the trial. If the clinician in charge of entering patients into the trial has seen the list and remembers the next treatment to be allocated, then he or she has the possibility of encouraging or discouraging the next patient to enter, depending on the clinician's subjective opinion about the suitability of the treatment for that patient. Such selection can introduce bias and nullifies the advantage of randomization. It is therefore important that the randomized allocation remains unknown before the patient decides to enter the trial.

Another way in which bias can be introduced, even though randomized treatment allocation is used, is in the conduct of the outcome assessment. Often, to avoid biased assessment, a trial is designed to be double blind, that is, the control group receives an inert medication in place of the active medication received by the treatment group, and neither patients nor clinicians are informed whether they have been given the active or inert treatment (see Reference 2 for more details).

Another commonly encountered problem related to bias—the statistical analysis of the data—is discussed in the next section.

INTENTION-TO-TREAT ANALYSIS

The treatment protocol that is to be followed in a clinical trial comprises a number of details. For example, even in the simple case of use of aspirin for patients who have had an MI, the protocol would specify the dose and frequency of administration, the delay between the MI attack and starting the medication, and the duration of continuing the medication. Commonly, some patients do not receive the randomized treatment according to protocol. Treatment protocol deviations may involve minor changes in the dose or schedule, or they may involve gross departures, the most extreme being the failure to receive any of the medication. Similarly, patients allocated to the control group may not receive the standard treatment and may even receive the therapy offered to the treatment group.

A question arises at the time of statistical analysis regarding the handling of the data from patients who have deviated from the treatment protocol. On first consideration it seems natural to compare the outcomes of patients who have received the new treatment approximately according to protocol with those who have received the standard treatment approximately according to protocol. In this analysis, a patient allocated to the treatment group but receiving only standard therapy would be moved to the control group and vice versa. However, this analysis strategy, which is sometimes called *analysis by treatment received*, frequently introduces bias into the comparison.

The Coronary Drug Project Research Group[5] reported results of a comparison of clofibrate with a placebo given for up to five years to men with a previous MI. The investigators presented mortality rates according to whether or not subjects were more than 80% compliant with taking the allocated clofibrate capsules. The five-year mortality rate among the good compliers with clofibrate was 15.0%. Analysis by treatment received requires that this rate be compared with the total control group, because any noncompliance with a placebo should have no medical effect. The mortality rate in the total control group was 19.4%, and the difference between the two rates is statistically significant (P < 0.01). Thus from this analysis of compliers with the active drug one would conclude that clofibrate reduced the mortality rate in males following MI.

As pointed out in the same article, there was a strikingly lower mortality rate among good compliers with clofibrate (15.0%) than among poor compliers with clofibrate (24.6%). These data seem to support the conclusion that clofibrate reduces mortality. However, when the control group was considered, it was found that those who complied well with the placebo had a 15.1% mortality rate, nearly identical to that of the good compliers with clofibrate, whereas those who complied poorly with the placebo had a mortality rate of 28.2%, quite similar to the poor compliers with clofibrate. It is clear that the higher mortality rate in the placebo poor compliers compared with the placebo good compliers could not be caused by their failure to take placebo but must result from innate differences in the health and characteristics of poor versus good compliers. Consequently, it becomes clear that analysis by treatment received can cause serious biases in treatment comparisons.

An alternative strategy that avoids the bias introduced from using analysis by treatment received is to retain all patients in the group to which they are randomized, regardless of the treatment they received. This strategy has come to be known as *intention-to-treat analysis*, because when a patient is first randomized to a treatment group, the clinician intends to administer that treatment according to the protocol. Applying intention-to-treat analysis to the Coronary Drug Project example, the mortality in the total clofibrate group was 18.2% compared with 19.4% in the total control group, a difference that is not significant (P > 0.25). Thus in this example, when an unbiased analysis strategy is employed, the apparent treatment difference, seen when using analysis by treatment received, disappears.

When there is considerable noncompliance in a clinical trial, some argue that intention-to-treat analysis itself gives a biased (under)estimate of the real treatment difference. The truth of this statement depends on one's understanding of the term *real treatment difference*. If one means that the real difference is the difference that would occur under conditions of perfect compliance with the treatment protocol, then an intention-to-treat analysis would indeed underestimate this difference. However, the intention-to-treat analysis does provide an unbiased estimate of the treatment difference that would occur under the same compliance conditions as occurred in the trial. If the noncompliance that occurred in the trial were due to adverse side effects of the treatment or to the unpleasant nature of the treatment administration, then one might anticipate the same levels of noncompliance in general practice. In this instance the treatment effect under these same levels of noncompliance would be the most relevant effect to estimate.

Sometimes noncompliance is avoidable or at least can be reduced by modifications of the trial design. This topic is addressed later in this chapter.

HANDLING MISSING OUTCOME VALUES

As explained in the preceding section, intention-to-treat analysis involves a comparison of *all* of the patients entered into the trial, grouped according to the randomized treatment. In practice, intention-to-treat in this, its purest form, usually cannot be implemented, because the clinical outcomes of some of the patients are not ascertained. Patients without a value for their clinical outcome cannot be included in a standard analysis. Furthermore, their omission introduces the possibility of another form of selection bias: if the occurrence of missing data is in some way related to the value of the unobserved outcome, and the proportions of missing values in the two (randomized) treatment groups are unequal, then indeed omission of these patients from the analysis will create a biased comparison.

With a little reflection it becomes clear that occurrence of a missing clinical outcome could indeed be related to the true value of the outcome. For example, if the outcome in a secondary prevention trial is length of time between randomization and recurrent myocardial infarction or death, then loss to follow-up (with consequent missing information on outcome) can occur because a patient is feeling poorly and decides it is time to change doctors. In this case, occurrence of the missing outcome could be associated with a lower-than-average time before the patient experiences the primary disease event.

The best protection against bias arising from missing outcome data is to take all possible steps to minimize the occurrence of such missing data. Attention to methods of retaining patients on follow-up has been found to reap considerable benefits. These methods include systems for reminding patients about their scheduled visits, contacting the patients very soon after a no-show, and various incentives to attend clinic, such as providing transport where necessary. Trials in which the proportion of patients with missing outcome data is less than 10% are generally quite well protected from biases arising from missing data.

In addition, special methods of statistical analysis can help reduce the bias that may arise from missing outcomes. For example, suppose that missing outcomes are more common among elderly patients ($\geq$70 yr) and that recurrent MI or death is also more common in these patients. Then performance of the treatment comparison, *stratified according to age* (<70 yr and $\geq$70 yr), will reduce the level of bias compared with an unstratified comparison.

Another statistical strategy to reduce bias is to *impute* the missing values, that is, to estimate their values from other information, and then substitute these estimates into an intention-to-treat comparison of the treatments. This can be particularly effective in trials in which the outcome is measured repeatedly but in which the final measurement is the main interest. For example, in the Community Intervention Trial for Smoking Cessation,[12] a cohort of smokers was asked annually if they had quit smoking, the main outcome being quitting (yes or no) at the end of the fifth year. An individual's missing value at the final follow-up was imputed from his or her answers to the question in the previous years. When imputation is used, care must be taken to adjust the variance of the treatment difference upward, to account for the fact that imputed values are not exact, but, as estimates, are themselves subject to uncertainty.[13]

Many statistical methods for reducing the potential biases of missing outcome data in clinical trials are now available. For a recent review, see Reference 14.

SAMPLE SIZE AND STATISTICAL POWER

The precision with which we can estimate a treatment effect is directly related to the ability of the trial to detect reliably a real treatment difference as statistically significant. Trials with poor precision may be able to detect a large treatment effect but will have low probability of detecting moderate or small effects. The probability of detecting a given treatment difference is known as the *statistical power* of the trial.

Increasing the sample size improves the precision of the estimate of the treatment effect and increases statistical power. Suppose that we were designing a trial to prevent early deaths (events) following a first acute MI. Suppose we have evidence that with current standard therapy the five-week event rate will be approximately 12%. We expect that the new treatment will reduce this rate to 9%. Assuming that we will use a two-sided 5%

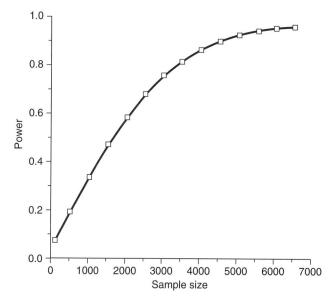

FIGURE 2-1. Effect of sample size on statistical power for detecting a reduction in event rate from 12% to 9% as statistically significant at the 5% level.

significance level, Figure 2-1 shows how sample size affects the statistical power. Clearly, small trials with fewer than 1000 patients have little chance of detecting the postulated reduction in event rate. To achieve a probability of at least 9 in 10 (power of 90%) of detecting the effect, we would need approximately 4500 patients or more in our trial.

The sample size requirements in a trial are extraordinarily sensitive to the magnitude of the treatment effect that one aims to detect. In the previous example, if we were unwilling to miss detecting a smaller reduction, say from 12% to 10%, and wished to have 90% power for that effect, then our sample size would need to be increased from 4500 to 10,300. Figure 2-2 shows in

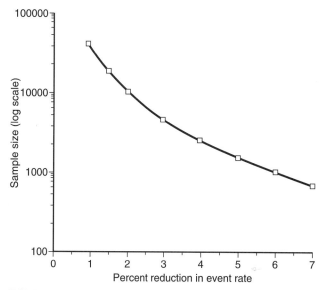

FIGURE 2-2. Sample size required for 90% power of detecting a given percent reduction in event rate as statistically significant (*e.g.*, 3% means that the event rate is reduced from 12% to 9%).

more detail the relationship between sample size requirements and the magnitude of treatment differences. The sample-size axis has been drawn on a logarithmic scale to accommodate the wide range of sizes. The rapid rise of sample size with decreasing treatment effect is readily appreciated.

Limited resources preclude us from designing all our trials with sample sizes that are large enough to be sure of detecting small effects. Nevertheless, for important questions involving common diseases carrying a risk of mortality, such an aim is only reasonable given the public health benefits that could result from even small improvements in therapy. The example par excellence of large trials conducted to detect small but worthwhile effects is the series of International Studies of Infarct Survival (ISIS) trials of treatment for MI. For example, the data from ISIS-2[15] showed 791 vascular deaths (9.2%) in the first five weeks among 8592 patients allocated streptokinase infusion compared with 1029 vascular deaths (12.0%) among 8595 patients allocated a placebo infusion. The difference of 2.8% is highly significant ($P > 0.00001$). Moreover, the 90% confidence interval for this difference is 2.0% to 3.6%, indicating a remarkably precise estimate of the vascular mortality reduction. Armed with such precise information, clinicians are far better equipped to form rational policies for managing the treatment of the many patients who suffer an MI.

For trials that do not have these large sizes, it is often possible to get a nonsignificant result even when a useful benefit really exists. To protect ourselves from premature discarding of such useful therapies, caution is required in our interpretation of nonsignificant results. Freiman and coworkers[16] have commented on this problem. They collected 71 published reports of randomized clinical trials that reported negative (*i.e.*, nonsignificant) results. Of these results 80% were not precise enough to exclude (using 90% confidence limits) the possibility of a 25% absolute reduction in the event rate. The authors concluded that "many of the therapies discarded as ineffective after 'negative' trials may still have a clinically meaningful benefit."

The antidote to the problem of prematurely discarding therapies, aside from increasing the size of trials, is to adopt caution in the interpretation of *nonsignificant* results. In the face of nonsignificant results it is best to focus on the confidence interval for the estimate of treatment effect. Treatment benefits that lie within this interval are quite consistent with the trial results. If the interval includes benefits that are clinically useful, then the nonsignificant result has not excluded a clinical benefit from the new treatment.

It is also prudent to reserve judgment concerning large, statistically significant treatment differences reported from small trials. In areas of medicine that have not seen dramatic improvements for many years, the emergence of a new treatment that is much superior to the standard is not a likely occurrence. For a small trial to demonstrate a statistically significant difference, the observed treatment difference must necessarily be large and is likely to overestimate the true difference. Thus, although it may be true that the new treatment does

have *some* added benefit, the small trial is likely to have seriously exaggerated the magnitude of this benefit.

Other factors in addition to sample size can strongly influence the statistical power of a trial. One of these factors—the duration of trial follow-up—is the topic of the next section.

LENGTH OF FOLLOW-UP

In the hypothetical example used in the previous section to illustrate the choice of sample size at the design stage of a trial, we postulated a control group five-week event rate of 12% compared with an anticipated treatment group rate of 9%, a 25% proportional reduction. For this trial at least 4500 patients are needed to attain good statistical power.

Suppose instead that we wished to design the trial based on a longer-term follow-up of patients, say two years. Previous data suggest that the control group event rate after two years will be about 20%. If the proportional reduction in events were maintained at 25%, then we would expect the two-year event rate of the experimental group to be about 15%. The number of patients needed to achieve a 90% power for detecting this effect is approximately 2500, compared with the 4500 calculated for the five-week follow-up design.

A useful rule of thumb related to this example is that the number of *events* rather than the number of patients is what really determines power. Thus the five-week design is expected to lead to 4500 × (12% + 9%)/2 or about 470 observed events, and the two-year design is expected to yield 2500 × (20% + 15%)/2 or about 440 events, demonstrating the approximately equal power of the two designs.

However, this rule of thumb is only valid under circumstances in which the same level of benefit from the treatment is expected to extend throughout the period of follow-up. In fact, several large trials of treatment following acute MI demonstrate that reductions in event rates are often limited to the early recovery period following MI. In ISIS-2,[15] the vascular mortality rate over the first 5 weeks was 12.0% in the control group and 9.5% in the aspirin group, a proportional reduction of 21%. In the course of the next 99 weeks (up to the end of the second year), the vascular mortality rate among the surviving patients was 9.1% in the control group and 9.7% in the aspirin group, indicating no further reduction in vascular mortality. Similarly, in the same trial, streptokinase reduced 5-week vascular mortality proportionally by 23%, but there was no observed reduction in vascular mortality among the survivors over the following two years.

Returning to the hypothetical example, if, anticipating a 25% proportional reduction in events throughout the period, we had planned the trial with 2500 patients followed for two years, but the reduction occurred only in the first five weeks with no effect thereafter, then the power of the trial would drop from the projected 90% to below 50%. Thus making optimistic assumptions about the duration of the treatment effect can lead to a seriously underpowered trial design. Generally speaking, prevention trials require longer analysis follow-up periods, whereas for treatment trials a shorter planned analysis period appears wise, as demonstrated by the examples just provided. A good understanding of the biology of the disease and the biologic mechanism of the intervention is the best guide to decisions regarding the appropriate follow-up period for the planned analysis of a trial.

REDUCING NONCOMPLIANCE

A section earlier in this chapter discussed patients' noncompliance with the therapy allocated by randomization, its impact on the statistical analysis of a trial, and the merits of intention-to-treat analysis versus analysis by treatment received. Noncompliance also affects the design of a trial. Its main effect is to reduce the treatment difference that is observed in the trial, and, as shown in Figure 2-2, this in turn necessitates an increase in the sample size to maintain good statistical power.

Returning again to the hypothetical trial in acute MI, suppose that the new treatment carried an acute side effect that made it intolerable to 20% of patients, and that these would have to terminate treatment almost immediately and cross over to receive the standard therapy. Assume also that those suffering the side effect carry the same prognosis as other patients. Using intention-to-treat analysis, the anticipated event rate in the treatment group will be increased from 9% under perfect compliance to $0.8 \times 9\% + 0.2 \times 12\% = 9.4\%$. This decreases the absolute reduction in event rate from 3% to 2.6% and necessitates an increase in sample size from 4500 to 6000 to maintain 90% power (see Fig. 2-2). Thus seemingly minor levels of noncompliance can necessitate substantial increases in the sample size and therefore the cost of the trial.

Noncompliance is a particularly important issue in prevention trials for several reasons. First, participants are healthy volunteers who are likely to be less motivated than patients to comply carefully with a prescribed treatment. Second, prevention interventions tend to involve longer-term medication than therapeutic interventions. Third, some prevention strategies require lifestyle changes, such as dietary modification and smoking cessation, that are difficult for people to achieve and maintain. Fourth, people in the control group may drift closer toward adopting the intervention of the treatment group as a result of population trends. All of these phenomena occurred in the Multiple Risk Factor Intervention Trial (MRFIT),[17] which involved dietary intervention, smoking cessation, and blood pressure reduction. This trial has since served as a lesson in the practical importance of noncompliance.

Considerable thought and effort are needed in first assessing the level of noncompliance that is likely, and then finding ways of reducing this level, if at all possible. If the noncompliance level is not assessed properly before the trial begins, then there is a danger that it will be underestimated, and the trial will consequently be seriously underpowered. If no effort is put into reducing

the noncompliance level, then the trial may be designed to be larger and more expensive than necessary.

An excellent example of coping with noncompliance was provided by the investigators of the Physicians' Health Study. This trial of aspirin and β-carotene for preventing cardiovascular disease and cancer, respectively, is being conducted in approximately 22,000 volunteer U.S. male physicians. The investigators arranged an 18-week run-in period during which potential participants were asked to take daily capsules similar to those used in the main trial.[18] Compliance at the end of the run-in period was assessed by questionnaires. Approximately 11,000 of the 33,000 volunteers decided not to participate in the main study, took less than two thirds of the capsules, or became ineligible during the run-in period and were not admitted to the trial. The investigators calculated that exclusion of these potentially noncompliant participants actually increased the power of the trial and reduced considerably the cost of the trial.

Another cost-efficient measure taken in the design of the Physicians' Health Study is discussed in the following section.

FACTORIAL DESIGNS

With the considerable amount of resources and money that are invested in large, long-term clinical trials, it is worth carefully considering whether the trial can be designed to answer more than one primary question about the therapy or prevention of disease. Factorial designs allow the effects of two or more interventions to be assessed in the same trial.

The simplest version of factorial designs is the 2×2 factorial design, which allows two separate treatments to be assessed. Suppose the new treatments are A and B and the control treatment is C. The design requires that at randomization one fourth of the patients are allocated treatment C, one fourth treatment A, one fourth treatment B, and one fourth a combination of treatments A and B (A + B). In this way one may estimate the effect of treatment A and of treatment B from the same trial. Moreover, if the effects of the treatments are *additive*, then the effects of treatment A and treatment B can both be estimated with the same precision as in a two-group trial of the same size. In other words, the 2×2 factorial design provides as much information about these treatments as would two separate equally sized trials, at approximately half the cost.

The reasoning underlying this surprising cost saving lies in the notion of additivity of effects. *Additivity* means that when considering the effect of treatment A, the difference between treatment A and treatment C is the same as the difference between treatment A + B and treatment B. Thus when estimating the effect of treatment A, we can employ information from all the patients participating in the trial. Treatment group A is compared with treatment group C to obtain one estimate of A's effect, while treatment group A + B is compared with treatment group B to obtain another independent estimate, and the two estimates are statistically combined. The effect of treatment B is estimated in an analogous manner, using comparisons of treatment groups B with C and treatment groups A + B with A.

This design has been used in a number of large trials recently. For example, ISIS-2 involved randomization to one month of daily aspirin (A), a one-hour intravenous infusion of streptokinase (B), both of these (A + B), or neither (C). Table 2-2 shows the five-week vascular mortality rates in the four groups, calculated from the information provided in the ISIS-2 Collaborative Group's report.[15] The treatment differences shown in the margins demonstrate that the additivity assumption is well supported in this trial, with the addition of streptokinase causing an estimated 2.8% to 2.9% absolute decrease in vascular mortality in the presence or absence of aspirin treatment, and the addition of aspirin causing an estimated 2.4% to 2.5% absolute reduction in vascular mortality whether or not streptokinase is given.

Another example of the use of a 2 × 2 factorial design is provided by the Physicians' Health Study, which was designed to study simultaneously the effects of aspirin on cardiovascular disease and β-carotene on cancer. In this case the factorial design takes on a new twist in that the two interventions targeted different diseases. The additivity assumption is again quite reasonable, because it would be unlikely (although not impossible) that a treatment targeting one disease would interact with another treatment's action on a different disease, and because the metabolic pathways and the hypothesized mechanisms of action of these agents are quite distinct.

The reason to be vigilant with respect to the additivity assumption is that the 2 × 2 design could be compromised if the effect of the combination of the treatments were *subadditive*.[19] Returning for the last time to the hypothetical example, suppose the effect of new treatment A in the absence of B is to reduce the event rate from 12% down to 9%, and that when B is given the event rate is 9% with or without treatment A. The combination effect is subadditive because A + B is no more effective than A alone or B alone. In our analysis of this 2 × 2 trial we would combine an estimated reduction of about 3% (A vs. C) with an estimated zero

reduction (A + B vs. B). The estimated overall reduction would then be approximately 1.5%, the average of the two estimates. In other words, introduction of the second treatment B into the design would reduce the magnitude of the treatment effect and consequently seriously reduce the power of the trial.

Conservative investigators have opposed the use of 2 × 2 factorial designs on the grounds that one cannot exclude the possibility of subadditivity. A more balanced view is that these designs should be avoided if the nature and postulated mechanisms of action of the treatments are similar or are likely to interact, but the designs should otherwise be encouraged. The experience with several such large trials in cardiovascular disease and in cancer prevention has so far been positive, with little or no evidence that negative interactions have compromised the results.

SURROGATE ENDPOINTS

Clinical trial investigators are continually searching for ways of reducing the duration and size of studies. One strategy that is commonly considered is changing the main outcome from a long-term clinical measure, such as survival time, to a measure or event that occurs sooner after treatment. The example that has captured the most attention in recent years has been the proposal to base clinical trials of treatments for HIV-infected patients not on time to progression to AIDS, but on short-term response (after six months or one year) of the patient's HIV RNA level.[20] Because such short-term outcomes are seen as *substituting* for the longer-term clinical outcome, they have been termed *surrogate endpoints*. It can be appreciated that the answers from such trials can be obtained much more quickly than from trials based on conventional clinical outcomes. In addition, because the surrogate endpoint is often measured on a continuous scale or is an event that occurs in greater proportions than the clinical endpoint, such trials can have greater statistical power and offer substantial savings in the number of patients required. In the case of HIV research, speeding the drug development process has been of paramount concern, both because of the seriousness of the AIDS epidemic and because of the large number of new treatments being developed. The attraction of surrogate endpoint trials in such a setting is evident.

The downside of surrogate endpoint trials is the doubt about whether the results of treatment comparisons based on the surrogate will indeed carry over to the clinical endpoint. Cardiologists will be particularly wary of this point following the widely publicized experience in the Cardiac Arrhythmia Suppression Trial (CAST).[21] The trial was designed to test the hypothesis that suppression of ventricular ectopy after a myocardial infarction reduces the incidence of sudden death. Patients in whom ventricular ectopy could be suppressed with encainide, flecainide, or moricizine were randomly assigned to receive either an active drug or a placebo. The patients assigned to receive encainide or its placebo numbered 857 (432 receiving active drug

■ ■ ■

TABLE 2-2 ESTIMATED 5-WEEK VASCULAR MORTALITY RATES IN THE 2 × 2 FACTORIALLY DESIGNED ISIS-2 TRIAL, SHOWING SUPPORT FOR THE ADDITIVITY ASSUMPTION

	Aspirin	No Aspirin	Difference
Streptokinase	8.1% (A + B)	10.5% (B)	−2.4% (A + B vs. B)
No streptokinase	10.9% (A)	13.4% (C)	−2.5% (A vs. C)
Difference	−2.8% (A + B vs. A)	−2.9% (B vs. C)	

Data from ISIS-2 Collaborative Group. Randomized trial of intravenous streptokinase, oral aspirin, both, or neither among 17,187 cases of suspected acute myocardial infarction: ISIS-2. Lancet 1988; 2:349–360.

and 425 receiving placebo), and 641 patients were assigned to receive flecainide or its placebo (323 to active drug and 318 to placebo). After a mean follow-up of 10 months, 89 patients had died: 59 of arrhythmia (43 receiving drug vs. 16 receiving placebo; P = 0.0004), 22 of nonarrhythmic cardiac causes (17 receiving drug vs. 5 receiving placebo; P = 0.01), and 8 of noncardiac causes (3 receiving drug vs. 5 receiving placebo). The use of encainide and flecainide was therefore discontinued because of excess mortality.

The CAST trial demonstrated that, although encainide and flecainide were successful in short-term suppression of ventricular ectopy, they were clinically harmful over the long term. This of course calls into question the central assumption underlying the use of surrogate endpoints. Fleming and DeMets[22] reinforce these doubts with further examples from trials in other clinical specialities. Biostatisticians have endeavored to create statistical criteria by which one may check empirically whether a particular surrogate endpoint can be relied upon to yield a trial result that translates to the conventional clinical endpoint.[23,24] However, to date, none of these methods have gained acceptance. Therefore, despite the fact that in a limited number of specialties (such as HIV research) certain surrogate endpoints are now accepted, it seems prudent to avoid their use as replacements for trials based on conventional clinical endpoints. They may be of greater use in Phase II-type studies that are designed to choose the most promising of several treatments for a conventional Phase III randomized trial.

CONCLUSION

The foundation principles of evaluation of clinical interventions rest on avoidance of biased comparisons, achieving adequate precision, and finding efficiencies in design. As new funding for health-care research becomes increasingly difficult to obtain, the pressure on large long-term studies will increase. Some of the most important questions regarding the prevention and treatment of common diseases, including cardiovascular disease, can be reliably answered only by such studies. Alternatives, such as historical control studies and database analyses, have been carefully considered. So far, for small-to-moderate treatment effects, these alternatives have been found to fall far short of the scientific standards that should be applied to evaluate one of our closest concerns, the maintenance of our own health.

REFERENCES

1. Friedman LM, Furberg CD, DeMets DL: Fundamentals of Clinical Trials, ed 2. Boston, John Wright, 1996.
2. Pocock SJ: Clinical Trials: A Practical Approach. Chichester, UK, John Wiley & Sons, 1983.
3. Meinert CL: Clinical Trials: Design, Conduct, and Analysis. Oxford, Oxford University Press, 1986.
4. Ruffin JM, Grizzle JE, Hightower NC, et al: A cooperative double-blind evaluation of gastric "freezing" in the treatment of duodenal ulcer. N Engl J Med 1969; 281:16-19.
5. Coronary Drug Research Group: Influence of adherence to treatment and response of cholesterol on mortality in the Coronary Drug Project. N Engl J Med, 1980; 303:1038-1041.
6. Gehan EA, Freireich EJ: Nonrandomized controls in cancer clinical trials. N Engl J Med 1974; 290:198-203.
7. Byar DP, Simon RM, Friedewald WT, et al: Randomized clinical trials: Perspectives on some recent ideas. N Engl J Med 1976; 295:74-80.
8. Korn EL, Simon RM: Measures of explained variation for survival data. Stat Med 1990; 9:487-503.
9. Hui SL, McDonald C, Katz B: Methods of using large databases in health care research: Problems and promises. Stat Med 1991; 10:505-674.
10. Miettinen OS: The need for randomization in the study of intended effects. Stat Med 1983; 2:267-271.
11. Byar DP: Why data bases should not replace randomized clinical trials. Biometrics 1980; 36:337-342.
12. The COMMIT Research Group: Community Intervention Trial for Smoking Cessation (COMMIT): I. Cohort results from a four-year community intervention. Am J Public Health 1995; 85:183-192.
13. Rubin DB: Multiple Imputation for Nonresponse in Surveys. Wiley, New York, 1987.
14. Patrician PA: Multiple imputation for missing data. Res Nurs Health. 2002; 25:76-84.
15. ISIS-2 Collaborative Group: Randomized trial of intravenous streptokinase, oral aspirin, both, or neither among 17,187 cases of suspected acute myocardial infarction: ISIS-2. Lancet 1988; 2:349-360.
16. Freiman JL, Chalmers TC, Smith H, et al: The importance of beta, the type II error, and sample size in the design and interpretation of the randomized control trial: Survey of 71 "negative" trials. N Engl J Med 1978; 299:690-694.
17. Neaton JD, Broste S, Cohen L, et al: The multiple risk factor intervention trial (MRFIT): VII. A comparison of risk factor changes between the study groups. Prev Med 1981; 10:519-543.
18. Lang JM, Buring JE, Rosner B, et al: Estimating the effect of the runin on the power of the Physicians' Health Study. Stat Med, 1991; 10:1585-1594.
19. Brittain E, Wittes J: Factorial designs in clinical trials: The effects of noncompliance and subadditivity. Stat Med 1989; 8:161-172.
20. Ghani AC, de Wolf F, Ferguson NM, et al: Surrogate markers for disease progression in treated HIV infection. J Acquir Immune Defic Syndr 2001; 28:226-231.
21. Echt DS, Liebson PR, Mitchell LB, et al: Mortality and morbidity in patients receiving encainide, flecainide, or placebo: The Cardiac Arrhythmia Suppression Trial. N Engl J Med 1991; 324:781-788.
22. Fleming TR, DeMets DL: Surrogate end points in clinical trials: are we being misled? Ann Intern Med 1996; 125:605-613.
23. Prentice RL: Surrogate endpoints in clinical trials: Definitions and operational criteria. Stat Med 1989; 8:431-440.
24. Daniels MJ, Hughes MD: Meta-analysis for the evaluation of potential surrogate markers. Stat Med 1997; 16:1965-1982.

Chapter 3

Comparative Features of Primordial, Primary, and Secondary Prevention Trials

Lawrence M. Friedman
Denise G. Simons-Morton
Jeffrey A. Cutler

The basic features of a good clinical trial apply whether the study population is healthy, at high risk of a disease or condition, or already stricken with the condition. These basic features include specification of the question being addressed, the intervention to be tested, and the primary outcome, as well as a properly justified sample size, randomization, unbiased measurement, and an intention-to-treat analysis. The differences in design and conduct of trials of primordial, primary, or secondary prevention are mostly matters of degree, rather than of kind.

Primary prevention is the prevention of the onset of disease. The primary prevention of risk factors is referred to as *primordial prevention*.[1] In the case of cardiovascular disease, primordial prevention would mean intervening to prevent the development of recognized risk factors, such as hypertension, elevated serum cholesterol level, or cigarette smoking. An example of a primordial prevention trial is the Child and Adolescent Trial for Cardiovascular Health (CATCH), a study of school-based interventions to lower fat in the diet, increase physical activity, and prevent smoking to reduce the likelihood of children developing risk factors in the future.[2]

Primary prevention also can be conducted in people at high risk for disease as a result of existing risk factors, with the aim of reducing the risk factors to decrease the probability of developing disease. Examples of primary prevention trials in high-risk populations are trials of blood pressure lowering in hypertensive people, such as the Hypertension Detection and Follow-up Program (HDFP)[3,4] and the Systolic Hypertension in the Elderly Program (SHEP)[5]; trials of lipid lowering in those with elevated blood cholesterol levels, such as the Lipid Research Clinics—Coronary Primary Prevention Trial (LRC-CPPT)[6,7] and the Air Force/Texas Coronary Atherosclerosis Prevention Study[8]; trials of smoking cessation in smokers[9,10]; and trials of reduction of several risk factors, such as the Multiple Risk Factor Intervention Trial (MRFIT).[11,12] Sometimes primordial prevention and primary prevention are combined in population-wide intervention strategies. Studies of community interventions to encourage lower-fat diets for reducing blood cholesterol, to foster smoking cessation and prevention, and to encourage physical activity are aimed at reducing the population distribution of risk factors associated with cardiovascular disease. The Minnesota Heart Health Program (MHHP),[13,14] the Stanford Five-Community Study,[15,16] and the Pawtucket Heart Health Program[17,18] are examples of studies of community interventions.

In *secondary prevention*, the disease or condition is already present. Secondary prevention trials include those that test strategies for early detection and treatment of subclinical disease, such as trials of screening mammography. Secondary prevention also includes interventions to forestall, delay, or reduce in intensity the sequelae of disease. Trials of interventions in patients with clinical coronary heart disease (CHD) or with acute myocardial infarction (MI) are secondary prevention studies. Examples include trials testing the effects on mortality of drug treatment of elevated cholesterol levels in men with previous MI, such as the Coronary Drug Project (CDP)[19,20] and the Scandinavian Simvastatin Survival Study (4S),[21,22] trials testing the effects of beta blockers in reducing mortality after acute MI,[23] trials of thrombolysis during acute MI,[24-26] and trials of angiotensin-converting enzyme inhibitors in people with heart failure[27] or coronary artery disease.[28]

STUDY DESIGN

The design of any clinical trial, as of any scientific study, starts with the primary objective, or main question to be answered. This main question drives whether the study will be one of primordial, primary, or secondary prevention. The conceptual framework for conducting prevention trials postulates that the natural history of disease goes from no or low risk, to elevated risk because of the presence of risk factors, to detectable disease, to disease sequelae (which may include mortality). Primordial, primary, and secondary prevention trials ask research questions at different places in this continuum. An example of how one topic can be addressed by any of the three types of studies is high blood cholesterol and heart disease. Trials to lower blood cholesterol level or prevent its increase in people who do not yet have hypercholesterolemia[2] are primordial prevention trials; trials testing approaches to lowering blood cholesterol level in people with hypercholesterolemia to prevent heart disease[7] are primary prevention trials in high-risk participants; and trials testing whether lowering cholesterol in patients with CHD will prevent a subsequent MI or mortality[21] are secondary prevention trials.

The study design traditionally used in clinical trials is that people are selected from the population at risk for developing the risk factor or disease in question and are randomly assigned (randomized) to either one or several intervention groups and a control group. Randomization of large numbers results in groups that tend to be comparable in factors that are known to be associated with the outcome of interest (e.g., age) as well as factors that are unknown and yet may be associated with the outcome of interest. Thus, the randomization process allows the inference that differences in outcomes are the result of the intervention being administered rather than of any other initial factors that may differ between the groups (i.e., potential confounders). The randomized, controlled trial is the preferred design for all types of intervention studies.

In all trials, an important consideration is the choice of control group. In addition to the research question, ethical, clinical, and logistic issues need to be considered to determine whether the control should be no treatment, placebo, usual or standard care, or best proven care. In primordial prevention trials, a "no treatment" control group may be more appropriate than in primary or secondary prevention trials. An example is the Pathways trial of obesity prevention in Native American schoolchildren,[29] in which children in the control schools were only measured, without any intervention provided (until after the study intervention period). In primary prevention trials, the severity of the condition and the duration of the study will influence whether or not the control group should incorporate an active treatment. The primary prevention trials PREMIER[30] and the Activity Counseling Trial[31] used "standard care" control groups—lifestyle recommendations for blood pressure control and physician advice for physical activity, respectively. Proven interventions are often used for the control group in secondary prevention trials, or in trials of high-risk primary prevention patients, if the research question is to determine the relative effectiveness of newer treatments compared with proven treatments; for example, diuretic treatment was used for the "active" control group in the Antihypertensive and Lipid-Lowering Treatment to Prevent Heart Attack Trial (ALLHAT).[32] In secondary prevention trials, even if a clinically popular treatment is unproved or only suspected of being useful, it may be difficult to justify not using it in the control group, as the participants are at higher risk of adverse consequences due to their condition. Although some may say that treatment guidelines should dictate the control group intervention, this conclusion is not necessarily the best one, and investigators should take into account whether the guidelines are evidence-based.

Generally, individual subjects are randomized into intervention and control groups. In some situations, however, entire groups, rather than individuals, may be randomized. These groups may be schools,[2] worksites,[33] medical practices,[34] or entire communities.[35,36] Group randomization (also called *cluster* or *unit randomization*) is often used in primordial or primary prevention trials, because such larger units are particularly relevant for interventions aimed at preventing or reducing risk factors. Trials in emergency treatment settings that have focused on early detection and treatment of disease have also been conducted using group randomization.[37,38] Advantages of randomizing groups include that (1) mass intervention techniques can be implemented, (2) the inherent social interaction within the group may reinforce adherence to the intervention, and (3) multilevel interventions can be tested (e.g., individual instruction for healthful eating plus cafeteria changes in food offerings). In group randomization, the primary sample size is considered the number of groups randomized, not the number of individuals in each group, although the latter does affect the study power.[39] The main disadvantage of group randomization is that if the group sizes are very large, as with communities, it may be difficult to find or afford to include enough communities to have adequate power and comparable intervention and control groups. Some studies have successfully recruited and randomized groups, such as schools, for a true randomized, controlled trial; for example, CATCH recruited and randomized 96 schools.[2] When fewer groups are being studied, matching of groups may be used, and randomization may be carried out within each matched pair.[40] Examples of studies randomizing within matched community pairs are the Community Intervention Trial (COMMIT) study of smoking cessation[35,36] and the Rapid Early Action for Coronary Treatment (REACT) trial.[37] Communities may be matched on the basis of size, location, or demographic characteristics of the population. If enough groups are included, this approach has the advantage of being a true randomized design and increases the likelihood that the intervention and control communities will be comparable on potential confounding factors.

Sometimes, rather than conducting a randomized, controlled trial, an investigator may undertake an intervention study with no control or comparison group. An effort is made to intervene in a participant or a community to see if changes occur, and the comparison is before and after intervention. An example is the Gothenborg study of community education to reduce delay in seeking care for acute MI symptoms (a secondary prevention question), which examined delay before and after the intervention.[41] It is unclear from a preintervention-to-postintervention design, however, whether changes are the result of the intervention or of other factors, such as secular trends. Other studies have been conducted in which a comparison group is chosen by some method other than randomization, often called a *quasi-experimental design*. An example is a school study for lowering fat in children's diets (a primordial prevention question) with two intervention and two comparison schools in which assignment was made by the investigator.[42] Although substantially better than not having any control, the quasi-experimental design suffers from some of the same problems as nonrandomized studies of individuals, in that various important characteristics may not be balanced between intervention and control groups. Whether they are used for primordial, primary, or secondary prevention studies, quasi-experimental designs do not eliminate biased allocation, or confounding from uncontrolled variables. Such studies, however, can be used to determine the feasibility of an intervention for primordial or primary prevention and to help estimate the treatment effect or to determine the side effects or dose of treatment for secondary prevention. A randomized, controlled trial could be conducted subsequently to provide a more definitive determination of the effect of intervention on outcome.

OUTCOMES

The primary outcome to be measured in any trial is directly linked to the research question being posed. Outcomes in trials of primordial or primary prevention often are the amount of change in a lifestyle behavior, a risk factor, or an intermediate or surrogate measure of disease. For example, the Activity Counseling Trial used physical activity level as an outcome,[31] and the Dietary Approaches to Stop Hypertension (DASH) and PREMIER studies used blood pressure level.[43,30] A surrogate measure may be a noninvasive assessment of subclinical disease; for example, assessment of atherosclerosis by carotid ultrasonography or some other measure of the disease process that would be a surrogate for a clinical outcome. Although changes in behaviors, risk factors, or disease measures are most commonly reported as average levels at the end of intervention (usually the least demanding choice for sample size), the rate of crossing a threshold value may better fit the idea of prevention and may also conform to clinical or pathophysiologic concepts (e.g., incidence of hypertension[44] or a critical arterial stenosis). The notion of slowing a disease process may be best satisfied by a measure of rate of change, although if change is not linear, such a rate may be difficult to define from multiple measurements during follow-up. Unless the trial is very large and long, the measurement of a clinical outcome (e.g., disease morbidity or mortality) in a primordial prevention trial usually is not feasible, because an insufficient number of clinical events will occur over the duration of the trial.

A trial of a primary prevention in a high-risk population or of secondary prevention may use surrogate disease endpoints but will more often have as its primary outcome major clinical events, such as acute MI or death. Regardless of the kind of study, the outcome selected should be one that is clinically relevant and likely to be reduced by the intervention to be tested. Sometimes, the separation between primordial, primary, and secondary prevention trials is blurred. In the area of blood pressure modification, the DASH[43] and DASH-Sodium[45] trials enrolled participants who had above optimal blood pressure but no hypertension, and participants who had hypertension but were otherwise healthy. DASH and DASH-Sodium showed that blood pressure could be lowered in both the hypertensive and nonhypertensive participants by means of reducing sodium intake and by a diet rich in fruits, vegetables, and whole grains and also low in fats, red meat, and sugar-containing products. Thus, the DASH trials combined primordial and primary prevention.

ALLHAT[32] was an example of combining primary and secondary prevention. ALLHAT enrolled more than 42,000 participants with hypertension, all of whom had additional risk factors and 25% of whom had been diagnosed with coronary heart disease (CHD). The primary goal of ALLHAT was to compare the effects of four antihypertensive agents on major CHD events (acute MI or CHD death).

All clinical trials have a primary outcome, which is directly related to the research question and is used to determine the power and sample size. Some trials have more than one primary outcome, in which case adjustments need to be made for multiple comparisons. For example, the Activity Counseling Trial (ACT)[31] had co-primary outcomes of self-reported physical activity level (a behavior) and measured cardiorespiratory fitness (a physiologic measure). Adjustments were made for two comparisons because there were two primary outcomes; additional adjustments were made for multiple comparisons because there were three randomized groups. In addition to the primary outcome, trials almost always have one or more secondary outcomes. These secondary outcomes will be similar in character to the primary outcomes for all types of trials but are usually not used to determine sample size or power. Quality of life as an outcome is useful in all kinds of trials, and cost-effectiveness is often an additional outcome, particularly for interventions tested in a clinical setting.

All trials also examine, to a greater or lesser extent, adverse effects of the interventions being tested. Adverse effects are perhaps less likely when the intervention is a change in lifestyle, but possible impairment of quality of life with such interventions may be considered an important outcome to detect.

For primordial prevention trials, one is less tolerant of adverse effects of an intervention than one would be for secondary prevention, or even primary prevention high-risk trials. Caution is needed to ensure that healthy people are not put at short-term risk to a degree that is unacceptable in an effort to prevent a possible future disease or condition. Possible harmful effects of lifestyle interventions include risk of musculoskeletal injury from an exercise program[31] or risk of delayed growth and development from a dietary intervention.[46] Drug treatment for any type of prevention carries potentially greater risks. Even drugs that are commonly used, such as aspirin, may not be worth testing for primordial prevention in those at low risk of developing heart disease in the short or medium term.

The Women's Health Initiative (WHI) trial of estrogen plus progestin tested whether this combination of hormone replacement therapy would reduce the occurrence of coronary heart disease in postmenopausal women with a uterus.[47] The trial was stopped earlier than planned because of small—though statistically significant—increases in incidence of breast cancer, heart disease, and stroke. The absolute increases in these outcomes were only seven or eight events per 10,000 person-years of exposure. Many of the millions of women who take hormone replacement therapy do so for the relief of menopausal symptoms, but others do so for the commonly supposed benefits of cardiovascular disease risk reduction. The WHI trial showed that the cardiovascular benefits do not, in fact, exist, so hormone replacement therapy should not be used for that purpose. Thus, women who wish to take the combination of estrogen and progestin need to decide if the symptomatic benefit is worth the small, but real, risk of serious adverse events, especially with long-term use.

STUDY SETTINGS AND POPULATIONS

The settings and participant enrollment strategies may be quite different for primordial, primary, or secondary prevention trials. Primordial prevention trials are generally conducted in community settings, such as schools or worksites. Primary prevention trials, such as smoking cessation in pregnant women, can be conducted in medical facilities[48,49] but also have been conducted in communities or in community settings. Medical settings, such as inpatient facilities (whether general medical, surgical, or special units, such as emergency departments, operating rooms, or coronary care units) would almost always be used for identifying participants and conducting secondary prevention trials. Primary or secondary prevention trials also could be implemented in outpatient facilities or physicians' offices. In the era of managed care with its controls on use of specialized services, such settings are becoming increasingly important.

In some trials, the intervention setting is the community, with the primary outcome occurring in a clinical setting. Examples include the Rapid Early Action for Coronary Treatment (REACT) trial,[37] which studied the effect of community-based intervention on delay time after symptoms of an acute myocardial infarction, and the Public Access Defibrillation (PAD) trial,[38] which is evaluating the effect of the use of automated external defibrillators on survival after out-of-hospital cardiac arrest in community units, such as apartment buildings and shopping malls. In both of these trials, the participants are those individuals who experience an event during the time period under study, the events being acute MI for REACT and cardiac arrest for PAD. Individual participants are not recruited in the traditional sense, but rather the communities and hospitals are recruited, and informed consent is obtained from persons experiencing events in order to obtain any additional data not already known.

Mass recruitment approaches, such as public service announcements and newspaper advertisements, should be helpful in both primordial and secondary prevention trials but may be less useful for primary prevention trials in high-risk populations. For primordial prevention trials, mass mailings and mass media may be used effectively to encourage large numbers of potentially eligible participants to contact the study investigator. For secondary prevention trials, most people will know if they have had an MI or been otherwise diagnosed with heart disease. However, for primary prevention trials in high-risk participants, most of the respondents to mass media or mailings may be incorrect or lacking in knowledge about their risk factor status, such as blood pressure or cholesterol levels, diabetes, or even family history. One exception is cigarette smoking as a risk factor. Nevertheless, even in primary prevention trials mass recruitment is effective at inducing large numbers of people to present themselves for in-person or telephone screening.

In clinical settings, potential participants are identified by record or chart review, by examining lists of patients who have undergone special procedures (surgical or diagnostic), or by referrals from physicians and other health care providers. Trials of high-risk participants could also identify people through community risk factor screening activities, such as at health fairs, worksites, apartment complexes, churches, or other areas where large numbers of people live, work, or congregate.

All three types of prevention trials require specific eligibility criteria for including participants in the study. Criteria are usually specified by defining both inclusion and exclusion criteria. In all cases, the eligibility criteria must create a study population that is relevant to the primary research question in terms of age, gender, and other characteristics. Eligibility criteria for primordial prevention trials are usually much broader than for primary and secondary prevention trials. For example, a primordial prevention trial may target all children in a school so that the only eligibility factors are age and attendance at a particular school. Examples of such primordial prevention trials are the CATCH and Pathways school-based trials.[2,29] In contrast, a primary prevention trial would require knowledge of an individual's risk factor status and therefore would require, for example, blood cholesterol or blood pressure levels that indicate a high-risk condition; the specific cutpoints for cholesterol and blood pressure and the method of measurement would also need to be specified. An example is the ALLHAT trial.[32] A primary prevention trial also would exclude someone with diagnosed disease, for example, CHD, because it is not possible to prevent a condition that already exists. A secondary prevention trial, by definition, requires that the clinical disease be present, so eligibility must contain the criteria by which one determines presence of disease. For example, self-reported prior MI may be sufficient, or confirmed acute cardiac ischemia by electrocardiographic tracing may be required.

The size of the study and the complexity of the eligibility criteria are not so much a function of whether the trial is primordial, primary, or secondary prevention, as they are a function of the primary question and the intervention being tested. For example, a primary prevention trial can be extremely large, with a simple intervention (e.g., aspirin) and broad eligibility criteria (e.g., no clinical evidence of heart disease, no indications for or contraindications to aspirin). On the other hand, it can be small, with a complicated intervention (e.g., a specially prepared diet given in a metabolic unit) and narrow eligibility criteria (e.g., a willingness to eat a specially prepared diet and no other food for some weeks). Similarly, a secondary prevention trial may be extremely large, with a simple intervention (e.g., aspirin), and broad eligibility criteria (e.g., physician's impression that the patient is suffering an acute MI). Alternately, a secondary prevention trial can be small, with an intervention requiring special training and experience (e.g., ablation of arrhythmia focus) and highly specific eligibility criteria (specified rhythm disturbance, resistance to pharmacologic therapy).

DURATION, EFFICACY, AND EFFECTIVENESS

The duration of a trial, and therefore the problem of maintaining participant involvement and adherence to the protocol, is not dependent on whether it is for primordial, primary, or secondary prevention. Depending on the nature of the question and intervention, primordial, primary, and secondary prevention trials may all be either short or long. If the outcome of interest is a clinical event, the primary prevention trial will need to be much larger and longer than the secondary prevention trial to accrue enough events for sufficient statistical power. In such a situation, the primary prevention trial may have more of a problem with competing risks. For example, in a primary prevention trial for cardiovascular disease, a greater proportion of the overall events may be noncardiovascular than in a secondary prevention trial in patients with acute MI. This competing risk may affect the ascertainment of the primary outcomes of interest. For primordial and primary prevention trials with risk factors (e.g., blood pressure) as the outcome, the duration is directly related to the research question in that some research questions specifically address the shorter- or longer-term effects of the intervention.

A distinction between studies of efficacy and effectiveness is sometimes made. An efficacy trial is one in which a well-controlled intervention is assessed under optimal circumstances with high compliance to ask how beneficial (or harmful) the regimen or procedure is itself. An effectiveness trial is conducted in circumstances more easily generalized and assumes that a certain proportion of the participants will not adhere to the regimen, either by failing to take the intervention as prescribed, or, if in the control group, by starting to take the intervention. Thus, an effectiveness trial more truly reflects a real-life situation. Only reasonably short studies or studies with irreversible mechanisms (e.g., surgery) that are also not widely available in general medical care can be done as efficacy trials because of the problem with long-term compliance to interventions in longer studies. Outcomes of an effectiveness trial are a function of both the efficacy of the intervention and the adherence.

Primordial, primary, or secondary prevention interventions can be tested either for efficacy or for effectiveness. For example, the Dietary Approaches to Stop Hypertension (DASH) study tested the efficacy of two dietary patterns compared with a reference diet in reducing elevated blood pressure.[43] All the food was provided to the participants, so the actual dietary intake had a high compliance for the patterns being tested. Similarly, DASH-Sodium,[45] which implemented the inter-

vention in a comparable way, is an efficacy trial. If the same dietary patterns were to be tested for effectiveness, dietary education would be delivered in a more typical situation, and the effect of the diet would be a function of both the diet itself and the compliance with the diet. An example of such a study is PREMIER,[30] a trial designed to see if the DASH diet can be successfully adopted in a "free-living" setting by participants who are also taught to adopt several other lifestyle changes important for blood pressure control. If the outcome is a clinical event, efficacy assessment is more feasible in a secondary prevention trial than a primary prevention trial. Because the high compliance necessary for an efficacy assessment may be reasonable only over the short term, participants with relatively high event rates are required (i.e., usually persons with an existing disease).

STUDY MANAGEMENT AND MONITORING

As with study design, study management and monitoring depend more on the nature of the intervention and outcome than on whether the study is one of primordial, primary, or secondary prevention. If the intervention is easy to perform and the outcome is simple to assess, then quality monitoring and assurance is not as extensive, regardless of the population being studied or the research question. When the intervention is more complex, however, quality assurance of intervention delivery is important, regardless of the size or type of study. For example, a small primordial prevention trial of exercise, with the outcome being long-term change in physical fitness, may require the same degree of quality assurance as a small secondary prevention trial of coronary artery stents for long-term vessel patency. Not only are the procedures of comparable complexity, but the data forms and assessment of adverse effects may also be comparable. Monitoring of adherence to the intervention and the protocol by the participants is also more similar than different, as long as the study sizes are similar and interventions are of similar complexity. A large, multicenter, primary prevention trial of aspirin with cardiovascular mortality as the outcome requires the same adherence assessment as a large, multicenter, secondary prevention trial of angiotensin-converting enzyme inhibitors with either total mortality or cardiovascular mortality as the outcome.

One possible difference in monitoring is that in primordial or primary prevention trials, the intervention may be more available to the control group, because the intervention consists of either a lifestyle change or use of a drug that is readily obtained, such as aspirin. Furthermore, compliance with lifestyle changes on the part of the intervention group may not be high. Therefore, primary prevention trials may be more likely to have crossovers, that is, intervention participants not receiving the full dose of intervention and control participants receiving some degree of intervention. In secondary prevention trials of physician-prescribed interventions, clinical decisions can also lead to large crossover rates, such as in medical treatment versus coronary artery bypass graft surgery.[50] Crossover rates do need to be carefully monitored, because if they are large, they can reduce the observed effect size and therefore the likelihood of detecting a significant effect. Anticipated crossover rates should be taken into account in determining the sample size for sufficient power to answer the primary question.

As noted earlier, data monitoring may be considerably different in primordial, primary, and secondary prevention trials. In primordial prevention trials, participants and investigators are less likely to accept serious or even bothersome adverse effects as the possible price of benefit. Not only does the likelihood of adverse events affect the choice of intervention, but it means also that if adverse trends emerge in the accumulating data, an investigator is more apt to stop the entire study before its planned end. An investigator might be willing to continue longer a study of high-risk patients, but not as long as a secondary prevention trial. Even in secondary prevention trials, there may be gradations, depending on the severity of the condition being studied. For example, a researcher would be willing to accept a fair amount of adverse events in the hope of improving duration or quality of life if testing an intervention in people with advanced heart failure, as opposed to a trial in patients with stable CHD. Another example would be the willingness to accept a fair amount of symptomatic hypoglycemia in diabetic patients if an intervention to normalize blood glucose levels might reduce cardiovascular events and death.

These monitoring concepts are often built into formal stopping guidelines of a trial. In primordial and primary prevention trials, the statistical boundaries for deciding if benefit or harm has been demonstrated may be asymmetric. That is, it would require more evidence to declare an intervention beneficial than harmful, with respect to the primary outcome. Even secondary prevention trials may employ asymmetric monitoring boundaries, but if the condition being studied is serious, an investigator may be willing to continue the trial even in the face of a strong adverse trend in the data because of the possibility that the trend may change with the accumulation of additional data.

ANALYSIS AND INTERPRETATION

For analysis and interpretation of results of the typical trial in which individuals are the unit of randomization, there are no important differences between primordial, primary, and secondary prevention studies. In all cases, the magnitude of effect one wishes to detect should be identified before the study begins based on the main research question of the study, and the magnitude of effect should be relevant either clinically or to public health. With primordial prevention trials, however, specifying effects important to public health may not be easy, because risk factors are not a measure of health, *per se*. For all three types of trials, existing evidence from prior studies should be used to determine event rates or, for continuous outcomes, variability in the measure, which are crucial components of power and sample size calculations.

As noted earlier, some trials generally, but not exclusively in primordial or primary prevention, employ group allocation. The power and sample size calculations and the analysis plans for such studies should take into consideration the design effects (i.e., the level of correlation between individuals within each unit randomized). The CATCH study, for example, used a two-stage analysis that took into account both the individual and school-level variance,[2] and the REACT study used a two-stage analysis that first determined rate of change over time within communities and then compared those rates between intervention and control communities.[37]

Trials sometimes use outcomes that yield more than one measure per randomized participant. An example is assessment of coronary artery lesion progression or regression. It may be important to assess more than one area of narrowing or a global evaluation of all coronary arteries. Because the lesions in an individual are not independent, it is, for example, inappropriate simply to count the total number of progressions or regressions. Statistical techniques allow one to take into account the degree of dependence among the lesions.[51] This is a similar analysis issue for group allocation, as mentioned earlier, in which correlations among individuals in each unit are likely to be present.

The standard analysis approach in all three types of trials is *intention-to-treat*, meaning that participants are all analyzed according to the group to which they are randomly assigned, regardless of adherence to the intervention. If group assignment is related to adherence, which it always can be, then analyzing only those who adhere creates biased assessments. With all three types of trials, researchers need to determine how to analyze those participants who are lost to follow-up. In trials with events as outcomes, follow-up time accumulated to the dropout date of those who are lost can be easily included. However, imputation of missing values is often a bigger issue in primordial and primary prevention trials that have continuous outcome measures (e.g., risk factors, such as blood pressure) than in primary or secondary prevention trials that have disease events as outcomes.

Interpretation of results in a randomized controlled trial is generally straightforward if the trial is conducted in a high-quality manner. That is, it is clear that the intervention caused the difference in outcomes between the randomized groups. However, there is often an issue of how much to generalize the results. For example, if an intervention is found to be effective for secondary prevention in participants with disease, can the effectiveness of that intervention be generalized to primary prevention in lower-risk participants? These are not easy questions to answer, and additional research is often needed to ensure that the results are, in fact, relevant to population groups not originally tested.

SUMMARY

Most of the design, management, and analysis features are common to all trials, whether they are primordial, primary, or secondary prevention types. Differences are more often a matter of degree than of kind. In all trials, the major issues are driven by the primary question posed. The study design best employed in all three types is the randomized, controlled trial. Even in primordial or primary prevention trials of whole communities, a randomized design is preferred. In all trials, eligibility criteria must be explicit. Primordial prevention trials often require recruitment methods that reach out to whole communities to recruit individuals or recruit entire communities for more broad-based interventions. Primary and secondary prevention trials, on the other hand, often recruit patients in clinical settings. All three types of trials could vary in duration and complexity of the intervention being tested. Primordial and primary prevention trials address questions of low-risk interventions and their effects on precursors or early manifestations of disease. Data monitoring for safety varies depending on the risk for adverse effects of the intervention being tested. Analysis methods are similar in that all randomized participants or groups should be analyzed according to the group (intervention or control) to which they are assigned.

REFERENCES

1. Expert Committee, Prevention in Childhood and Youth of Adult Cardiovascular Diseases: Time for Action: Report of a WHO Expert Committee, Technical Report Series No. 792. Geneva, World Health Organization, 1990.
2. Luepker RV, Perry CL, McKinlay SM, et al: Outcomes of a field trial to improve children's dietary patterns and physical activity: The Child and Adolescent Trial for Cardiovascular Health—CATCH Collaborative Group. JAMA 1996; 275:768-776.
3. Hypertension Detection and Follow-up Program Cooperative Group: Five-year findings of the hypertension detection and follow-up program: I. Reduction in mortality of persons with high blood pressure, including mild hypertension. JAMA 1979; 242:2562-2571.
4. Anonymous: Effect of stepped-care treatment on the incidence of myocardial infarction and angina pectoris: Five-year findings of the Hypertension Detection and Follow-Up Program. Hypertension 1984; 6(2 Pt 2):I198-I206.
5. (Systolic Hypertension in the Elderly Program) SHEP Cooperative Research Group: Prevention of stroke by antihypertensive drug treatment in older persons with isolated systolic hypertension: Final results of the Systolic Hypertension in the Elderly Program (SHEP). JAMA 1991; 265:3255-3264.
6. Lipid Research Clinics Coronary Primary Prevention Trial: The Lipid Research Clinics Coronary Primary Prevention Trial results: I. Reduction in incidence of coronary heart disease. JAMA 1984; 251:351-364.
7. Lipid Research Clinics Coronary Primary Prevention Trial: The Lipid Research Clinics Coronary Primary Prevention Trial results: II. The relationship of reduction in incidence of coronary heart disease to cholesterol lowering. JAMA 1984; 251:365-374.
8. Downs JR, Clearfield M, Weis S, et al: Primary prevention of acute coronary events with lovastatin in men and women with average cholesterol levels: Results of AFCAPS/TexCAPS. Air Force/Texas Coronary Atherosclerosis Prevention Study. JAMA 1998; 279:1615-1622.
9. Rose G, Hamilton PJ, Colwell L, et al: A randomised, controlled trial of antismoking advice: Ten-year results. J Epidemiol Community Health 1982; 36:102-108.
10. Rose G, Colwell L: Randomised, controlled trial of antismoking advice: Final (20-year) results. J Epidemiol Community Health 1992; 46:75-77.
11. Multiple Risk Factor Intervention Trial Research Group: Multiple risk factor intervention trial: Risk factor changes and mortality results. JAMA 1982; 248:1465-1477.
12. Multiple Risk Factor Intervention Trial Research Group: Mortality after 16 years for participants randomized to the Multiple Risk Factor Intervention Trial. Circulation 1996; 94:946-951.
13. Jacobs DR, Luepker RV, Mittelmark MB, et al: Community-wide prevention strategies: Evaluation design of the Minnesota Heart Health Program. J Chronic Dis 1986; 39:775-788.
14. Luepker RV, Murray DM, Jacobs DR, et al: Community education for cardiovascular disease prevention: Risk factor changes in the Minnesota Heart Health Program. Am J Public Health 1994; 84:1383-1393.
15. Farquhar JW, Fortmann SP, Maccoby N, et al: The Stanford Five-City Project: Design and methods. Am J Epidemiol 1985; 122:323-334.
16. Farquhar JW, Fortmann SP, Flora JA, et al: Effects of community-wide education on cardiovascular disease risk factors: The Stanford Five-City Project. JAMA 1990; 264:359-365.
17. Carleton RA, Lasater TM, Assaf A, et al: The Pawtucket Heart Health Program: I. An experiment in population-based disease prevention. RI Med J 1987; 70:533-538.
18. Carleton RA, Lasater TM, Assaf A, et al: The Pawtucket Heart Health Program: Community changes in cardiovascular risk factors and projected disease risk. Am J Public Health 1995; 85:777-785.
19. Canner PL, Klimt CR: The coronary drug project: Experimental design features. Control Clin Trials 1983; 4:313-332.
20. Canner PL, Berge KG, Wenger NK, et al: Fifteen-year mortality in coronary drug project patients: Long-term benefit with niacin. J Am Coll Cardiol 1986; 8:1245-1255.
21. The Scandinavian Simvastatin Survival Study Group: Design and baseline results of the Scandinavian simvastatin survival study of patients with stable angina and/or previous myocardial infarction. Am J Cardiol 1993; 71:393-400.
22. The Scandinavian Simvastatin Survival Study Group: Randomised trial of cholesterol lowering in 4444 patients with coronary heart disease: the Scandinavian simvastatin survival study (4S). Lancet 1994; 344:1383-1389.
23. Yusuf S, Peto R, Lewis J, et al: Beta blockade during and after myocardial infarction: An overview of the randomized trials. Prog Cardiovasc Dis 1985; 27:335-371.
24. Yusuf S, Collins R, Peto R, et al: Intravenous and intracoronary fibrinolytic therapy in acute myocardial infarction: Overview of results on mortality, reinfarction, and side effects from 33 randomized controlled trials. Eur Heart J 1985; 6:556-585.
25. Gruppo Italiano per lo Studio della Streptochinasi nell'Infarto Miocardico: Effectiveness of intravenous thrombolytic treatment in acute myocardial infarction: Gruppo Italiano per lo Studio della Streptochinasi nell'Infarto Miocardico (GISSI). Lancet 1986; 1:397-402.
26. ISIS-2 (Second International Study of Infarct Survival Collaborative Group): Randomized trial of intravenous streptokinase, oral aspirin, both, or neither among 17,187 cases of suspected acute myocardial infarction: ISIS-2. J Am Coll Cardiol 1988; 12(6 Suppl A):3A-13A.
27. Garg R, Yusuf S: Overview of randomized trials of angiotensin-converting enzyme inhibitors on mortality and morbidity in patients with heart failure: Collaborative group on ACE inhibitor trials. JAMA 1995; 273:1450-1456.
28. The Heart Outcomes Prevention Evaluation Study Investigators: Effects of an angiotensin-converting-enzyme inhibitor, ramipril, on cardiovascular events in high-risk patients. N Engl J Med 2000; 342:145-153.
29. Davis SE, Hunsberger S, Murray DM, et al: Design and statistical analysis for the Pathways study. Am J Clin Nutr 1999; 69(Suppl): 760S-763S.
30. The Writing Group of the PREMIER Collaborative Research Group: Effects of comprehensive lifestyle modification on blood pressure control: Main results of the PREMIER clinical trial. JAMA 2003; 89:2083-2093.
31. The Writing Group for the Activity Counseling Trial Research Group: Effects of physical activity counseling in primary care: The Activity Counseling Trial: A randomized controlled trial. JAMA 2001; 286:677-687.
32. Davis BR, Cutler JA, Gordon DJ, et al, for the ALLHAT Research Group: Rationale and design for the Antihypertensive and Lipid-Lowering Treatment to Prevent Heart Attack Trial (ALLHAT). Am J Hypertension 1996; 9:342-360.
33. Glasgow RE, Terborg JR, Hollis JF, et al: Take heart: Results from the initial phase of a work-site wellness program. Am J Public Health 1995; 85:209-216.
34. Ammerman A, Caggiula A, Elmer PJ, et al: Putting medical practice guidelines into practice: The cholesterol model. Am J Prev Med 1994; 10:209-216.
35. The COMMIT Research Group: Community Intervention Trial for smoking cessation (COMMIT): II. Changes in adult cigarette smoking prevalence. Am J Public Health 1995; 85:193-200.
36. The COMMIT Research Group: Community Intervention Trial for smoking cessation (COMMIT): I. Cohort results from a four-year community intervention. Am J Public Health 1995; 85:183-192.

37. Luepker RV, Raczynski JM, Osganian S, et al: Effect of a community intervention on patient delay and emergency medical service use in acute coronary heart disease: The Rapid Early Action for Coronary Treatment (REACT) trial. JAMA 2000; 284:60-67.

38. The PAD Trial Investigators: The Public Access Defibrillation (PAD) trial: Study design and rationale. Resuscitation 2003; 56:135-147.

39. Hsieh FY: Sample size formulae for intervention studies with the cluster as unit of randomization. Stat Med 1988; 7:1195-1201.

40. Martin DC, Diehr P, Perrin EB, et al: The effect of matching on the power of randomized community intervention studies. Stat Med 1993; 12:329-338.

41. Blohm M, Herlitz J, Hartford M, et al: Consequences of a media campaign focusing on delay in acute myocardial infarction. Am J Cardiol 1992; 69:411-413.

42. Simons-Morton BG, Parcel GS, Baranowski T, et al: Promoting physical activity and a healthful diet among children: Results of a school-based intervention study. Am J Public Health 1991; 81:986-991.

43. Appel LJ, Moore TJ, Obarzanek E, et al: A clinical trial of the effects of dietary patterns on blood pressure. N Engl J Med 1997; 336:1117-1124.

44. Hebert PR, Bolt RJ, Borhani NO, et al, for the Trials of Hypertension Prevention (TOHP) Collaborative Research Group: Design of a multicenter trial to evaluate long-term life-style intervention in adults with high-normal blood pressure levels: Trials of Hypertension Prevention (phase II). Ann Epidemiol 1995; 5:130-139.

45. Sacks FM, Svetkey LP, Vollmer WM, et al, for the DASH-Sodium collaborative research group: A clinical trial of the effect on blood pressure of reduced dietary sodium and the DASH dietary pattern (the DASH-Sodium trial). N Engl J Med 2001; 344:3-10.

46. The Writing Group for the DISC Collaborative Research Group: Efficacy and safety of lowering dietary intake of fat and cholesterol in children with elevated low-density lipoprotein cholesterol: The Dietary Intervention Study in Children (DISC). JAMA 1995; 273:1429-1435.

47. Writing Group for the Women's Health Initiative Investigators: Risks and benefits of estrogen plus progestin in healthy postmenopausal women: Principal results from the Women's Health Initiative randomized controlled trial. JAMA 2002; 288:321-333.

48. Ershoff DH, Mullen PD, Quinn VP: A randomized trial of a serialized self-help smoking cessation program for pregnant women in an HMO. Am J Public Health 1989; 79:182-187.

49. Mayer JP, Hawkins B, Todd R: A randomized evaluation of smoking cessation interventions for pregnant women at a WIC clinic. Am J Public Health 1990; 80:76-78.

50. Yusuf S, Zucker D, Peduzzi P, et al: Effect of coronary artery bypass graft surgery on survival: Overview of 10-year results from randomised trials by the Coronary Artery Bypass Graft Surgery Trialists Collaboration. Lancet 1994; 344:563-570.

51. Kelsey SF: Strategies for statistical analysis of angiographic data: Individual lesions versus individual patients. *In* Glagov S, Newman WP, Schaffer SA (eds). Pathobiology of the Human Atherosclerotic Plaque. New York, Springer-Verlag, 1990, pp 525-533.

Principles of Data and Safety Monitoring Boards in Randomized Trials

David L. DeMets

During the past three decades, clinical trials have evolved to become a major research methodology for clinical medicine. Many statistical principles have been applied to the design, conduct, and analysis of clinical trials, and these statistical methodologies continue to evolve as we apply clinical trials to an increasing array of research settings.[1-3] As the methodology for clinical trials began to develop, the National Institutes of Health (NIH) commissioned a task force to establish the administrative structure and process for conducting multicenter Phase III clinical trials, which are designed to establish the cost:benefit ratio of new therapies and interventions. This task force issued a report, known as the *Greenberg Report*,[4] in 1967. In addition to recommending a trial chair, the executive committee or steering committee headed by the trial chair, and a statistical or data coordinating center, the Greenberg Report also established the need for an independent Policy Advisory Board. This clinical trial model is illustrated in Figure 4-1. Although the functions of this board were not specified in detail, a subcommittee of this board focused on patient safety. Later this unit came to be known in most trials of the National Heart, Lung, and Blood Institute (NHLBI) at the NIH as the *Data and Safety Monitoring Board* (DSMB) or the *Data Monitoring Committee* (DMC).[5,6] In the current clinical trial structure, the DSMB is a critical component of the administrative structure in the comparative Phase III trial.[7-22] The DSMB is an independent group of experts who provide informed advice on the progress of a trial to the principal investigator or trial chair and to the sponsor of the trial. One possible outcome of a trial is early termination resulting from convincing evidence of benefit, harm, or equivalence of the treatments. This DSMB role has gained broader attention. As a result of a death of a young man in a gene therapy trial, the U.S. Secretary of Health and Human Services issued a directive that all human clinical trials sponsored by the NIH or regulated by the Food and Drug Administration (FDA) must have a monitoring plan.[23] For some trials, especially those with mortality or serious irreversible morbidity outcomes, an independent data and safety monitoring committee might be required. The NIH established guidelines or broadened the scope of existing guidelines,[24] and the FDA issued draft guidelines in November of 2001.[25] As a result, the activity in establishing DSMBs for both indus-

try and federally funded trials has increased. Although the DSMB has a 30-year history for multicenter trials,[5] the details of how a DSMB might function in a single-center trial have yet to be established; however, the principles should remain largely the same.

This chapter is a summary of the special role and responsibilities of the DSMB in monitoring a clinical trial. In particular, issues to be discussed include the rationale for data monitoring, the complexity of the decision process for early termination, the need for DSMB expertise, the constitution of a DSMB, and the format and content of DSMB meetings. There is no single or simple prescription for the role of a DSMB, but principles have emerged over the past three decades that seem useful. Examples from several cardiovascular trials are used to illustrate the issues that can arise in monitoring trials.

RATIONALE FOR DATA MONITORING

Clinical trials are designed to evaluate the usefulness of a newly emerging or an existing device, procedure, therapeutic treatment, or disease prevention strategy. The goal may be to establish the most effective dose or to identify side effects and toxicity. Patients who participate in these clinical trials trust that a trial will not continue if clear evidence of unacceptable adverse events or toxicity is observed. Furthermore, patients trust that a trial will not continue if convincing evidence of treatment benefit emerges and the risk:benefit ratio is favorable to treat. In addition, during their conduct, trials that evaluate the equivalence of two treatments may establish that one treatment is not worse than the other by a prespecified amount. In that case, patients would want to receive the treatment that is less invasive or costly or has fewer side effects. Thus, the trial might be terminated and the results presented. If a design flaw is identified early in the conduct, modifications should be made when possible to preserve the integrity of the trial and maximize its potential for success. Finally, trials that have little or no chance of achieving their stated goals, either primary or secondary, should be identified and considered for termination because further patient participation may be wasted effort. Thus, whether stated directly or implied in the informed consent, patients put their trust in the clinical trial process to consider these issues

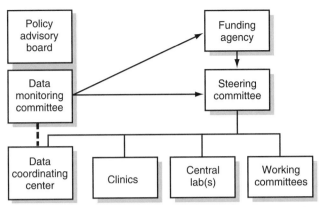

FIGURE 4-1. National Heart, Lung, and Blood Institute (NHLBI) clinical trial model[5] based on Greenberg's Heart Special Project Review.

while the trial is ongoing. Trials are both a patient and scientific investment. For these ethical and scientific reasons, data monitoring is an essential part of the clinical trial process.

Clinical trials often are classified into one of four categories. *Phase I trials* attempt to identify the maximum tolerated dose of a drug or biologic or the conditions for using a device. *Phase II trials* are designed to screen for possible biologic effectiveness and to identify side effects or toxicity rates. *Phase III trials* are the comparative trials, designed to test the effectiveness of a therapy and estimate the cost : benefit ratio. *Phase IV trials* typically are long-term follow-up studies to scrutinize approved or accepted therapies for potential harm not observed in the Phase III trial. By their design, Phase I and II trials have an inherent data-monitoring process because each step in their designs is based on the results of previous steps—that is, in Phase I trials, dose is not escalated until results of the current dose are known. In Phase II trials, if no positive results are observed in the first 12 to 24 patients, additional patients are not entered. Phase I and II trials typically do not have independent DSMBs perform the monitoring process; they rely on the investigators involved in the trial.

Phase III trials are larger, take longer to complete, and are more costly than Phase I or II trials because their goal is to provide a definitive answer to the treatment effectiveness question. Not all Phase III trials need to be monitored. However, if the primary or secondary outcomes involve mortality or irreversible morbidity or if safety issues could be a concern, then careful monitoring is critical and mandatory.[6,9,11,19,23] Balancing potential benefit with potential risks is exactly where the role of the DSMB is most important, and often that evaluation is complex and involves several factors.

MONITORING: A COMPLEX PROCESS

A clinical trial has several components, all of which must be functioning for success to be achieved. In the interim review of these components, if results suggest that a trial may need to be modified or terminated early, then several factors need to be taken into consideration before that decision is made.[22,26-29]

Early in the trial, administrative issues, such as the validity of design assumptions, recruitment success, and patient compliance, must be considered. Modifications to the design may be required, including changing entry criteria to improve recruitment, increasing sample size to compensate for lower-than-anticipated event rates or increased variability, or adjusting dosage to improve compliance. The purpose of these types of administrative analyses is to keep the design as close to the original goals as possible. If made early, such modifications have more of a chance to correct any identified problems.

Fleming[28] has noted that for a DSMB to carry out its responsibilities, the board must have relevant, high-quality data that are reasonably current. The Thrombolysis in Myocardial Infarction (TIMI) II trial[30] was designed to evaluate the use of a tissue plasminogen activator (t-PA), which is a thrombolytic agent, in percutaneous transluminal coronary angioplasty procedures. TIMI-I had established that t-PA was more effective in rapidly resolving blood clots. However, in the process of scaling up the manufacturing of the t-PA, a change in the methodology increased the potency of the agent. Thus, in the very early stages of TIMI-II, bleeding complications became a serious issue. Recruitment was suspended, and the matter was investigated. Ultimately a dose adjustment was made to account for the change in potency, and TIMI-II was completed successfully. However, it was critical that the data flow was rapid so timely decisions could be made before more bleeding complications had occurred. In the Diabetes Control and Complications Trial (DCCT),[31,32] a central laboratory with an excellent research record was unable to keep up with the volume of data generated by this very large trial and meet the turnaround required by the protocol on critical parameters for glucose control. Careful administrative monitoring quickly discovered this problem, and another laboratory was found with the necessary capability. Had this not been discovered early, patient safety could have been compromised.

Later in a trial, decisions often are related to early termination as a result of emerging evidence of benefit or harm. Previous experience suggests that this is a particularly complex decision process.[6,9,11,22,26] Comparability between the experimental and the control group needs to be examined carefully. Assessment of the primary, secondary, and side-effect measurements must be unbiased or the results will not be interpreted accurately. Lack of treatment effect may be the result of poor patient compliance to the protocol. Differential compliance rates may suggest bias. Another consideration is whether the results are internally consistent across other outcome measures and across risk groups or subgroups. Although magnitude of effect—either beneficial or harmful—may differ quantitatively, qualitative consistency is reassuring in terminating a trial early. External consistency with other trials or observational studies must be weighed as well. Finally, the risk : benefit ratio must be considered carefully. Benefit might be significant, but the toxicity (i.e., risk) is substantial, and these must be considered before a trial can be terminated and recommendations can be made. Early benefits that appear to wane with follow-up may not be considered important as the trial progresses.

Most trials measure numerous outcomes, and some outcomes may be measured repeatedly. Data monitoring requires repeated testing of these outcome measures, but this process also increases the chances of a false-positive result.[33,34] For example, if the nominal P (probability) value of 0.05 is used on each of five interim analyses, the true false-positive error is not 5% but almost 15%. Methods have been developed to guard against this, but they are limited mostly to one or two primary outcome measures. A common method, referred to as the *group sequential procedure*,[35-40] increases the level of evidence required at each interim analysis before statistical significance can be achieved. By being more conservative at each analysis, the overall trial false-positive error rate can be maintained at conventional levels (e.g., 0.05). There are several proposed group sequential methods, each producing different statistical criteria or interim boundaries for being conservative, although each can achieve the same overall false-positive error rate.[35-41] Another approach, referred to as *conditional power* or *stochastic curtailment*,[42,43] computes the probability (at an interim analysis) of reaching a statistically significant result—either for benefit or harm—if the trial continued to its scheduled end. If this probability is very low, the trial may be hopeless and not worth continuing. If this probability is extremely high, the results may be so overwhelming that continuation is not necessary. This method most often is used to compute the probability of recovering from an observed negative or harmful trend and of ever achieving a positive and statistically significant benefit. If this probability is very low considering a variety of reasonable, postulated treatment effects, then the trial is unlikely to demonstrate benefit and may in fact show harm.

Finally, the impact that any decision to terminate early will have on the practice of medicine and public health policy must be taken into account. Early termination that does not have an impact wastes the investment of patients, investigators, and sponsors. These factors are summarized in Table 4-1.

Given the number of factors that must be considered and weighed carefully, no single person would likely have all of the required expertise in clinical medicine,

epidemiology, biostatistics, clinical trials, and medical ethics. Furthermore, it is not likely that any single person would want responsibility for such a complex decision process. For that reason, major Phase III trials often are monitored through an independent committee, referred to here as the *DSMB*.[5,6,9,22,26,27]

To illustrate the complexity of the decision making, several cardiovascular trials with early termination are described briefly. Each presents different issues that a DSMB must be prepared for as a possibility. The Coronary Drug Project (CDP) compared several cholesterol-lowering drugs in men who recently had experienced a myocardial infarction (MI).[44] One of the drugs was clofibrate. As the interim data emerged and were reviewed by the DSMB, the standardized test statistic, or Z value, comparing mortality curves approached the nominal 0.05 boundaries on four occasions in favor of clofibrate, but these trends did not sustain themselves (Fig. 4-2). The horizontal boundaries correspond to using a 0.05 significance level or critical values of ± 2.0 for the test statistic at each analysis. The final comparisons produced nearly identical mortality curves.[26] This phenomenon is a consequence of repeatedly testing accumulating data, and the process leads to an increase in the false-positive error rate, as described earlier.[34] The CDP DSMB was well aware of this danger and did not respond prematurely in terminating this treatment arm and claiming a treatment benefit.

Another trial was terminated early because convincing evidence of treatment benefit emerged before the planned termination date. The Beta-Blocker Heart Attack Trial (BHAT) compared propranolol with placebo in a multicenter, randomized, double-blind trial.[45] A positive trend emerged early and continued to increase, eventually meeting statistical criteria used to control the false-positive error rate (Table 4-2). Whereas determining that a statistical boundary was crossed may not require much discussion, the monitoring process was still not

■ ■ ■

TABLE 4-1 EARLY TERMINATION CONSIDERATIONS

Baseline comparability
Unbiased evaluation
Compliance
Internal consistency
    Other outcomes
    Subgroups
External consistency
Benefit : risk
Length of follow-up
Public impact
Repeated testing
Multiple comparisons

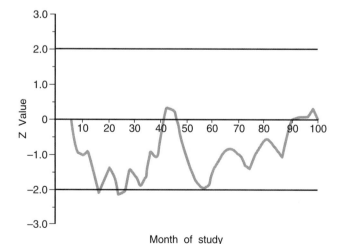

FIGURE 4-2. Interim analyses in the Coronary Drug Project if performed almost continuously. The horizontal lines at Z values of $+2.0$ and -2.0 represent the nominal 0.05 significance levels. The graph shows the interim standardized test statistic comparing event rates in the placebo group and the clofibrate group. A positive Z value indicates that placebo is better; a negative Z value indicates that clofibrate is better.

■ ▨ ■

TABLE 4-2   INTERIM ANALYSES FOR THE BHAT

Planned analysis	Calendar time (mo)	Total observed deaths (d)	Logrank Z	Critical boundary value*
1	11	56	1.68	5.88
2	16	77	2.24	5.04
3	21	126	2.37	3.79
4	28	177	2.30	3.19
5	34	247	2.34	2.64
6	40	318	2.82	2.30*
7	48	—	—	—

*If the logrank statistic (Z) exceeds the critical boundary value in absolute value, the mortality comparison is significant at the 0.05 level, adjusting for repeated testing.

simple for the BHAT DSMB.[46] Although propranolol appeared to be effective in the short follow-up period of 2 or 3 years, the question of how long a patient who is postinfarct should remain on propranolol had not been resolved. Issues listed in Table 4-1 had to be evaluated. In addition, other trials of beta blockers, such as the Norwegian Timolol Trial,[47] were becoming available and suggested that a placebo control may no longer be ethical when combined with the BHAT results. The BHAT DSMB had to consider what further information would be learned if the trial went to its planned termination date; it was determined that not enough information would be gathered to answer definitively the long-term question. Thus after considerable discussion, the BHAT DSMB recommended early termination for treatment benefit for the period observed.

In contrast to early termination for benefit, the Cardiac Arrhythmia Suppression Trial (CAST) was terminated very rapidly for unexpected but convincing evidence of treatment harm.[48] Cardiac arrhythmias are associated with sudden cardiac death, and drugs such as encainide and flecainide were known to be effective in suppressing arrhythmias. Drugs of this type were becoming widely used because of this effect. CAST was designed to evaluate the effect that suppressing arrhythmias with these drugs had on total mortality. The expectation was a reduction of mortality, but the magnitude of the effect was not anticipated. With only 10% to 15% of the expected deaths observed, the statistical comparison indicated a large effect but in the negative direction, contrary to expectation (Table 4-3). In addition, although the statistical criteria used to protect against false-positive errors were very conservative at this early stage of the trial, the test statistic for the mortality comparison already had been exceeded.[49,50] Given this dramatic result, which was contrary to conventional wisdom and expectation, the DSMB had to move quickly but carefully. A mistake in not terminating early would cause more deaths, but a mistake in jumping to a decision about treatment harm prematurely would cause confusion in a widely used treatment of a high-risk population. After weighing carefully all the evidence, including treatment group comparability, compliance, and outcome ascertainment, the DSMB concluded that CAST needed to be terminated and the results needed to be disseminated immediately.[50] However, these results caught the cardiology community by surprise, and patients receiving encainide and flecainide at the time had to be dealt with rapidly.

The most agonizing complex decision is the slowly emerging negative or harmful trend.[51] This occurred in two trials in congestive heart failure (CHF): the Prospective Randomized Milrinone Survival Evaluation (PROMISE) trial,[52] and the Prospective Randomized Flosequinan Longevity Evaluation (PROFILE)[53] trial. PROMISE was a randomized, double-blind, placebo-controlled trial testing the effect of a drug, milrinone, on total mortality for severe Class III and Class IV CHF. Milrinone had already been shown to be effective in exercise testing. The DSMB observed a negative trend early, but it was not as overwhelming as the CAST negative trend. As the PROMISE trend continued to become more negative, the ethical question arose whether this trial should prove harm or just that a positive benefit was not likely. In the trial setting, a neutral (or equivalent) result on mortality might mean that milrinone still could be used for its effect on exercise functioning. The DSMB determined that PROMISE should distinguish between a neutral result and a harmful effect. When the negative trend continued and passed the statistical criteria for significance, PROMISE was terminated early and the investigators concluded that milrinone had in fact a harmful effect on mortality. Later, another CHF trial, PROFILE, encountered similar challenges.[53]

■ ▨ ■

TABLE 4-3   CAST INTERIM RESULTS FOR ENCAINIDE AND FLECAINIDE

Time	Placebo†	Active†	Total†	Logrank	Lower critical boundary*
09/01/88	7 (576)	22 (571)	29 (1147)	−2.82	−3.18
03/30/89	9 (725)	33 (730)	42 (1455)	−3.22	−3.04*

*If the logrank statistic is below the lower critical boundary, the mortality comparison is significant at the 0.05 level.
†Number of deaths; sample size is shown in parentheses.

PROFILE was very similar in design to PROMISE, but it evaluated another drug, flosequinan, for a mortality effect. While the trial was just getting started, this drug was approved by the FDA because of its positive effect on exercise tolerance. However, as in PROMISE, the PROFILE DSMB began to observe a negative trend. In this instance, however, the drug had just been approved for use. Again, the DSMB had to weigh the impact of terminating a trial for not showing a beneficial effect or of waiting to distinguish between a neutral effect and a harmful effect. Because flosequinan had just been approved by the FDA, the DSMB concluded that PROFILE must distinguish between a neutral and a harmful result. Unfortunately, flosequinan, like milrinone, proved to have a statistically significant harmful effect on mortality.

In contrast with PROMISE and PROFILE, the Cooperative North Scandinavian Enalapril Survival Study (CONSENSUS) II trial terminated early with a negative trend that did not reach statistical significance.[54] CONSENSUS II was evaluating enalapril in the treatment of patients with MI. The primary outcome in this randomized, double-blind, placebo-controlled trial was 6-month total mortality. The sample size calculation assumed a one-sided, 0.05 significance level for treatment benefit. During the trial, conditional probabilities were to be calculated for accepting or rejecting the hypothesis of no treatment benefit. If this probability was very high (e.g., 90%), then the trial might be considered for early termination. In this case, a negative trend in 6-month mortality emerged, favoring placebo over enalapril (9.9% vs. 11.1%). This trend did not reach levels of statistical significance that proved treatment was harmful. However, the DSMB made a recommendation to terminate early on the basis that the trial was highly unlikely to show a positive benefit unless the current negative effect was reversed dramatically for the rest of the patient follow-up, and such a reversal would be extremely implausible.[55] This decision resulted in considerable discussion between investigators and the DSMB, but the recommendation was accepted by the investigators. In this instance, the issue for the CONSENSUS II investigators was whether termination was appropriate while not showing either benefit or harm. These types of negative trends require considerable judgment, expertise, and experience.

Another type of difficult and complex decision is whether to terminate a trial in which no apparent trends on the primary endpoint are emerging but other factors seem compelling for early stopping. The Physicians' Health Study (PHS) is an excellent example. The PHS was a trial of unique design in which more than 22,000 individual health physicians were randomized in a factorial design to receive β-carotene, aspirin, both, or neither.[56] The aspirin component was designed to test the effect on reducing total cardiovascular mortality, with total mortality and nonfatal MIs as secondary outcomes. After 5 years of the scheduled 7 years of follow-up, the aspirin component was terminated by the PHS DSMB[57] (results are shown in Table 4-4). Several factors played a role in the board's decision. The first issue was that the primary event rate of cardiovascular mortality in the placebo group was extremely low—less than 50% of that used in the design. As a result, the ability of the trial to detect the effect of aspirin on cardiovascular mortality was extremely low. The total mortality rate was also extremely low. From this perspective, the PHS had little or no chance of success with the primary goal unless the trial was extended for 10 or more years of follow-up. However, the effect of aspirin on the secondary outcome of fatal and nonfatal MIs—most of which were nonfatal—was overwhelmingly positive (44% reduction; P < 0.00001). This result had become increasingly positive as the trial progressed and ultimately exceeded the conservative statistical criteria used to control the false-positive error rate. However, additional events added to the complexity of the decision. A possible adverse risk of hemorrhagic stroke was observed in the aspirin group (23 vs. 12; P = 0.06). Although the number of hemorrhagic strokes was small, and the event rate was much lower than that of nonfatal infarctions, the consequences of a hemorrhagic stroke were nonetheless worrisome. As a further complication, aspirin was already approved as a secondary prevention for cardiovascular mortality in an MI population, and PHS physicians who had an MI during the trial began taking aspirin as a preventive measure. This further decreased the likelihood of detecting any aspirin effect on mortality. The DSMB decided the following:

The aspirin effect on nonfatal MI was important for public health.

The total mortality effect most likely would not be detected.

The stroke adverse-event rate was small and was already an expected risk for both primary and secondary use.

Not much more would be learned in the next 2 years of scheduled follow-up to resolve the stroke issue further.

Physician crossover from assigned treatment to aspirin was becoming increasingly nontrivial.

These were among the major factors that led to the early termination of the aspirin component.

CONSTITUTION OF A DSMB

As already indicated, the DSMB is an independent group of people that is not directly involved with the conduct of the trial and that has no special vested interest in the

■ ■ ■

TABLE 4-4   PHYSICIANS' HEALTH STUDY: 5-YEAR RESULTS

	Aspirin	Placebo	RR	P
Total mortality	217	227	0.96	0.64
Cardiovascular	81	83	0.96	0.87
Myocardial infarction	10	28	0.31	0.004
Nonfatal myocardial infarction	129	213	0.59	<0.00001
Total stroke	119	98	1.22	0.15
Ischemic	91	82	1.11	0.50
Hemorrhagic	23	12	2.14	0.06

RR, relative risk.

outcome.[4,5,6,9,22,27] The DSMB usually provides recommendations to the principal investigators of the trial, through its chair or executive committee, and to the sponsor (see Fig. 4-1). This reporting role should be stated clearly before the start of the trial. In some instances, the DSMB reports only to the study executive committee and not directly to the sponsor, whereas in other cases it may report to both. Either structure is feasible but must be understood at the initiation of the study. The DSMB usually is given the authority to make recommendations but not final decisions because it is primarily an advisory body to either sponsor, investigators, or both.

The authority to appoint the DSMB also must be identified in the protocol. Either the sponsor or the investigators may make the appointments. Because DSMB decisions ultimately impact on both sponsor and investigators, both parties ideally should agree to the appointments, regardless of who makes the invitation to individuals. Thus, it is recommended that this process be done jointly. As described by Armstrong and Furberg,[27] whatever reporting relationship is agreed to, the independence of the DSMB from both sponsor and investigator is in the best interest of the trial and the participants.

Given the complexity of most clinical trials and the decisions that must be made, the DSMB collectively must have expertise in the disciplines related to the disease, treatment, and populations being studied. This often requires both clinicians and laboratory scientists. In addition, the DSMB must have expertise in clinical trials, biostatistics, epidemiology, data management, and research ethics. NIH-sponsored trials traditionally appoint to the DSMB someone with medical ethics or sociology training to particularly reflect patients' point of view in the monitoring process. This is not as common in industry-sponsored trials. To cover this wide range of expertise, between three and seven people are likely to be needed. Often a DSMB of five members is adequate and is an ideal committee size for complex discussions. The chair of the DSMB should be someone either familiar with the specific scientific question being addressed or experienced in monitoring clinical trials and ideally should be an expert in both areas.

The DSMB should be kept independent of investigators entering or caring for patients in the trial.[12] Otherwise, the ethical dilemmas arise for the investigator as trends emerge or fail to emerge. Investigators should remain in equipoise about the benefits of the treatment until the trial is terminated.[58] Oncology trials as a routine used to share interim results with investigators. This practice, however, led to many trials not being completed presumably owing to investigators drawing inferences from nonsignificant trends.[59] Thus although the investigators have a great deal of relevant expertise, they should not be eligible for the DSMB.

Although the DSMB technically reports to either the investigators through their study chair or executive committee and to the sponsor, DSMB members must feel primarily responsible to the participants in the trial. During the conduct of the trial, they bear the major burden of monitoring patient safety, especially in double-blind trials. The next level of responsibility is to the investigators and to the integrity of the trial because investigators have turned over many of their concerns about the progress of the trial to the DSMB. Any DSMB will recognize the important role of the sponsor, whether it is federal or private, and will attempt to address those interests after those of the patient and investigator. Finally, the DSMB does not routinely interact with regulatory agencies, such as the FDA, but regulatory requirements must be recognized in DSMB deliberations and decisions.[25,60,61] However, although all of these four constituencies must be considered, their priority must be in the order described, starting with the participants in the trial.

Because the DSMB has the responsibility for monitoring the interim results of the trial and making recommendations about conduct, benefit, and safety to the investigators and sponsor, the DSMB members need to be independent of the trial[5,6,9,12,22,27]—that is, the DSMB members should not be entering patients into the trial or into any competing trials. Furthermore, they must be free of any real conflicts of interest, especially those that might appear to be financial. Conflict of interest in itself may not be bad unless it would influence decision making. Most scientists have some intellectual conflict just by being an expert in the field. However, undisclosed financial conflicts can be problematic. In addition to consulting and travel, another especially sensitive conflict is having financial investments in the company whose product is being tested by the trial. The members of the DSMB cannot have any financial investment in the sponsor. This policy has been described for one recent cardiovascular trial.[62] A good policy is for DSMB members to annually report their activities outside their own institution in terms of travel, speaking engagements, and honoraria for consulting, as well as any financial investments in the sponsor. These activities should be reviewed annually by the DSMB chair, the study chair, and the sponsor as appropriate. If the appearance of a conflict exists and cannot be resolved, the best action may be for that board member either to refrain from further activity on that issue or not continue on the DSMB.

In addition, representatives from the sponsor and the regulatory agency should not be members of the DSMB because they obviously are not independent.[5,6,9,12,22,27] Sponsor representatives have either a programmatic interest or a financial interest and thus cannot be totally independent. Furthermore, the DSMB is advisory either directly or indirectly to the sponsor, so it would be inconsistent for a DSMB member to also be independently advising his or her own institution. Similarly, representatives of regulatory agencies such as the FDA should also not be members of a DSMB. If the trial results are to be reviewed by the regulatory agency, it would be extremely awkward for the agency to fairly critique those results if they essentially participated in the trial decision making. This would be especially true if the trial was terminated early.

The roles of the regulatory agency and the DSMB are quite different. The DSMB primarily focuses on the conduct of a specific trial or set of trials. The regulatory agency must make judgments based on a much larger set of evidence, some of which may not even be fully known in scientific circles. Both sponsors and regulatory representatives may have a limited participation in DSMB meetings, according to guidelines on who should attend (described later). As Walters described it, the independence of the DSMB is not an end in itself but an essential means to achieving knowledge and maximum objectivity about new interventions, and the DSMB respects the patients making those contributions.[12] This is maximized by sponsors and regulators not being DSMB members.

In addition to being free of conflict of interest, DSMB members must be able to maintain absolute confidentiality. Interim data may reflect transient trends that, if shared, could be not only misleading but damaging to the trial, even precluding continuation. As already described, oncology trials demonstrated that routine presentation of interim data often precluded further recruitment as trends emerged.[59] Investigators may willingly turn over the monitoring responsibility to the DSMB, but it is only natural that they remain interested in how the trial is going and curious as to interim results. Thus, comments or inferences made by DSMB members in the presence of an investigator, sponsor, or regulator may be interpreted, correctly or incorrectly, and thus it is paramount that DSMB members are absolutely silent on DSMB matters outside their meetings. Even acknowledging that a DSMB member is going to a DSMB meeting sometimes can be informative to an interested party.

STATISTICAL ANALYSIS CENTER

To fulfill its monitoring responsibilities, the DSMB is heavily dependent on the statistical analysis and data management.[5,6] These activities may be accomplished in separate units, in a statistical analysis center and a data management center, or in a combined unit often referred to as a coordinating center. This center must have individuals with statistical, data management, and clinical trials expertise. The center is often responsible for the statistical aspects of the protocol design and for preparing the data collection instruments. At the conclusion of the trial, this center is involved in the preparation of final analyses and the trial publication. During the trial, it collects, enters, and edits the data in a timely manner and prepares interim reports for the DSMB. The DSMB also may request additional analyses from the statistical center as issues arise during its deliberations. Thus, the smooth working relationship between the DSMB and the statistical center is essential.[6,24]

DSMB MEETINGS

DSMB meetings should be held often enough so that patient safety can be protected but not so often that there is only a small increment in information from one meeting to the next. One guide is that the DSMB should meet at least once, and perhaps twice, per year. Another variation is a once-per-year meeting with an in-between

conference call meeting to at least review safety. From the statistical point of view, one guideline is to meet with every 20% increment in information (e.g., deaths or primary events). However, if events are slow in accruing, the once-to twice-per-year guideline should override because safety issues should not go on too long before review.

Expectation of attendance at DSMB meetings needs to be clearly understood at the beginning of the trial. Communication between the DSMB, investigators, and sponsor about some aspects of the trial progress and conduct is essential. Yet information on treatment comparisons for benefit or safety should not be shared among all parties. The NIH special report recommended that investigators not be aware of interim results because that knowledge may influence their decisions as to which patients to recruit or on the evaluation of treated patients, either influence biasing the trial and seriously damaging its scientific goal. In some special cases, such as Multiple Risk Factor Intervention Trial (MRFIT)[63] or BHAT,[45] the chair of the trial intentionally was selected to represent the investigators while not entering or taking care of patients in the trial. In those instances, the study chair has attended the DSMB meetings. For most NIH trials and some industry-sponsored trials (e.g., PROMISE and Prospective Randomized Amlodipine Survival Evaluation [PRAISE]), representatives of the sponsor have attended the entire DSMB meetings. However, the question of who should attend DSMB meetings has generated discussion for cardiovascular and noncardiovascular trials.[6,12] A general format has evolved that appears to meet the needs of all parties, using an open-session, closed-session, and executive-session process.[64]

During the open session, representatives from the investigators (usually the chair or co-chair), from the sponsor, and from the FDA may attend. During this session, information is shared on the conduct of the trial, including recruitment, compliance, data quality, and general operational issues. Exchange of this information may identify logistic problems or scientific issues that, if resolved early, may strengthen the trial and enhance the likelihood of a meaningful answer.

Following this interchange, the major portion of the DSMB meeting should be conducted in strict confidence in a closed session. Generally, only DSMB members plus representatives from the statistical center who present the interim analyses should be present. Traditionally, NIH-sponsored trials have an NIH representative at this closed session. Some industry-sponsored trials' representatives have been at the closed session (PROMISE, PRAISE), whereas others have not (GUSTO[65]). If sponsors do attend, they must not under any circumstances interfere with the business and responsibility of the DSMB. Furthermore, information learned at the closed session should not be shared with their colleagues within the sponsor. This requires a strong commitment and understanding by the sponsor with their designated trial representative. Walters[12] argues that neither sponsors nor regulators should attend the closed session, except when the sponsor is a federal agency such as the NIH. NIH project offices should be mostly representing the general public and the scientific community and not commercial interests. Even in this instance, however, NIH officials should have at most only a minor role in the DSMB deliberations. Otherwise, the DSMB soon loses the independence on which it is based.

An executive session at the end of each meeting, and during if necessary, is recommended where only DSMB members attend so that candid and frank comments can be made that may have been inhibited by the presence of any sponsor or statistical center representative at the closed session. Following the executive session, if held, the DSMB may return to open session to brief the study chair or Executive Committee as well as the sponsor as to their final recommendations.

DSMB REPORTS

Because the monitoring is a complex process and many factors must be considered, the data report presented to the DSMB must be both thorough and focused. Detailed analyses as to patient recruitment, baseline risk factors, treatment group comparability, compliance to therapy, primary and secondary outcomes, subgroup comparisons, and measures of safety and adverse events must be included. Graphic presentations whenever possible, with tables as backup, are recommended to make the most efficient use of the DSMB meeting. A standard format from meeting to meeting is also useful and should be developed early in the trial. As the trial progresses, new issues inevitably will arise so that a standard format will allow for new analyses to be included in a meaningful and efficient manner. Given the amount of data typically collected in a clinical trial, data reports can easily become voluminous and overwhelm a DSMB. DSMB reports with dozens or even hundreds of tables soon become uninformative. Graphs and executive type summaries with detailed tables in an appendix often serve the DSMB needs most effectively.

For an interim data report to be useful to the DSMB, the database itself must be relatively up to date.[28] A DSMB should be reluctant to make any decision, especially early termination decisions, based on data that are several months behind. Good standard practice should allow for a database to be delayed no more than 3 months. For mortality trials, information should be only a few days old if appropriate communication channels are developed. However, the need for current data for the interim analysis and the DSMB meeting may not be appreciated by investigators and sponsors, so this critical aspect must not be taken for granted. The Nocturnal Oxygen Therapy Trial (NOTT) evaluated continual versus nocturnal use of oxygen supplementation in patients with advanced chronic obstructive lung disease. NOTT reported[66,67] that a differential, perhaps biased, delay in reporting results from one or two centers almost led that DSMB to make a decision for early termination. However, an inquiry of all the clinical centers revealed a delay that modified the interim results. A premature early termination would have altered the inferences about the effectiveness of continual oxygen therapy. For trials such as CAST, reliable and updated interim results proved to be critical in the DSMB's ability to make rapid and correct decisions.

In presenting data to the DSMB, one issue is whether the DSMB should be blinded to treatment groups where possible.[11] Two approaches are being used successfully: One traditional approach is to label all tables by treatment identification or by codes (e.g., A vs. B) with codes known to the DSMB. Another is to label tables by these codes, which are consistent across all tables, except perhaps for those that may unblind the DSMB. This approach keeps the DSMB partially blind until a point is reached in the trial where a decision point may be approaching. The DSMB may want to discuss how knowledge of treatment assignment would affect their decision. Because decisions about early termination may not be symmetric, knowledge of whether an emerging, possibly convincing, trend is suggesting benefit or harm might make a difference in the decision. Thus, before any decision is made, the DSMB would unblind itself. The CAST DSMB used this latter approach. This latter approach allows any member of the DSMB to request that the code be broken at any time. Because the DSMB must keep strict confidence about the treatment comparisons, the tradeoff between these two approaches is mainly for the benefit of the DSMB, and the latter approach may require more reflection on how knowledge of the treatment code would change their decision. One approach that should not be considered is to have a data report that changes treatment code from table to table or between categories of tables for the purpose of ensuring that the DSMB is blind. For the DSMB to carry out its responsibility, it must assess the total risk : benefit profile, which can be done only with all tables presented consistently. Ultimately, however, the welfare of the patients is paramount, and the traditional approach where the DSMB knows the treatment code from the beginning is satisfactory and highly recommended.

Because each clinical trial has large databases that must be summarized and interpreted, most DSMB reports are somewhat lengthy, even where graphic presentations are used extensively. In addition, issues can be complex and may take several reviews of the report to grasp subtleties in the data. For that reason, statistical reports should be sent to the DSMB a few days prior to the meeting or conference call. Express mail is an efficient and secure method to distribute these confidential reports. DSMB reports should be accounted for carefully and collected by the statistical center following the meeting. This provides a little more assurance that these highly confidential data reports do not get left in a nonsecure place. This prior distribution of DSMB reports, however, places even more pressure on the data flow and data management process. Each delay forces the report to be more out of date and less useful to the DSMB.

EXTERNAL INFORMATION

During the conduct of a trial, additional information may become available that is relevant. This may be the discovery of new basic science or the results of other trials, perhaps in similar populations with a similar treatment. In some instances, it may even be the same population and the same treatment. The issue becomes how much the DSMB should take this into account in the monitoring of their trial. During the BHAT study, which tested a beta blocker drug in a postinfarct population, results of two other trials showing a treatment benefit became available, one using the drug timolol (Norwegian Timolol Trial[47]) and another trial using metoprolol.[68] Although the BHAT results had passed their own statistical criteria for termination for benefit, the discussion to terminate was not straightforward because it was not known how long the beta blocker therapy should be given. However, the results of the other two trials certainly gave the DSMB confidence about the 2-year results of BHAT. Given all the available information, both internal and external, the DSMB recommended that BHAT be terminated almost a year early.

Another cardiovascular trial that was testing arrhythmia-suppressing drugs, CAST, was terminated early because of an observed harmful effect. Conventional wisdom and practice in cardiology were to use this new class of drugs (encainide and flecainide), which was known to be highly effective in suppressing arrhythmias, and arrhythmias were known to be associated with sudden death and cardiovascular death. Quite early in the trial, the statistical evidence was strikingly showing a harmful effect of encainide and flecainide. In this instance, most of the external information favored these drugs' effectiveness, yet the DSMB had to rely heavily on the internal consistency of the CAST data to make their ultimate judgment.

Although external information should be used informally, such information should not be combined formally with the ongoing trial in a meta-analysis. An NIH-sponsored workshop discussed the concept of a formal sequential meta-analysis of all ongoing relevant trials. However, such an approach was not judged to be feasible[69] in most circumstances. Each trial should attempt to come to its own conclusions and use the external information as secondary support.

DOCUMENTATION OF THE DSMB

Because the DSMB plays such a central role in the conduct of Phase III trials with mortality or irreversible morbidity outcomes, the activities of the DSMB need to be documented carefully for scientific as well as regulatory reasons. Before the initiation of a trial, the DSMB should develop a brief guideline or charter on its operational procedures, including any statistical guidelines for early termination. The DSMB statistical reports for each meeting provide a summary of the analyses conducted. In addition, minutes of those DSMB meetings should be kept and filed along with the reports. Any correspondence between the DSMB and either the sponsor or the investigators also should be retained.

COMMUNICATION OF THE DSMB

In the event a decision is made to recommend a protocol modification or early termination, the DSMB must be prepared to communicate those recommendations quickly to the study chair and the sponsor as agreed. The rationale for the recommendation must be explained clearly along with the data analyses that led to the recommendation. This communication may require a special meeting between the full DSMB and the study executive committee in which the details of the DSMB report are discussed. However, there is usually not much time to prepare for such meetings, so communicating between the two chairs is the most efficient. If the sponsor was not present for the closed session of the DSMB meeting, then the sponsor must be fully briefed as soon as possible as well. In instances where an investigational new drug is being tested, communication between the DSMB and the FDA also may be requested. Because the final authority to modify a protocol or terminate the trial rests with the investigators and the sponsor, they must be given sufficient information to implement the recommendations as soon as possible.

CAST results were conveyed rapidly to both the FDA and investigators because of the harmful effects of the drugs being evaluated.[48-50] However, once the information was released, it became a challenge to get the detailed results through the peer review and into the scientific community rapidly. A special short presentation in a leading medical journal was arranged, and a more detailed manuscript followed as quickly as possible through regular peer review. Press coverage, however, caused the public and especially all the many patients on the drugs tested to get in touch with their physicians before many of those physicians were aware of the general CAST results, much less the detailed results. The PHS aspirin results appeared in the medical literature a few weeks following the DSMB recommendation for termination.[56] Generally, such rapid communication requires some anticipation by the DSMB that early termination might be possible and early drafts of manuscripts are prepared that can be modified at the time of the final decision. This was the case for both CAST and BHAT. In the PRAISE trial,[70] the chair of the DSMB and the director of the statistical center attended a briefing of the FDA by the sponsor to reflect their thoughts and deliberations.

Although the DSMB has typically no formal role in further dissemination of the trial results, many trial executive committees seek the advice and counsel of the DSMB in the preparation of the final manuscript. For example, the PRAISE chair met with the DSMB to get their advice on the conclusions of the trial, taking advantage of their extensive knowledge of the database and analyses. This interchange is especially prudent if the trial was terminated early based on the recommendations of the DSMB, and the essential features of their rationale need to be included. BHAT and CAST study chairs met with their DSMBs as well in preparation for dissemination of those results. In one NIH-sponsored trial,[71] some DSMB members were so displeased with the conclusions of the paper that they[72,73] took the unusual step of publishing their opinion that differed with that of the trial authors.

Hasty presentation of results shortly after termination can lead to mistaken conclusions or misunderstandings. Thus, as the DSMB senses that the trial may be terminated early, they should guide the statistical center and the chair of the trial in early preparation or at least rapid release of the information. In addition, the DSMB can provide the authors a first-pass peer review with their detailed knowledge of the trial and yet be somewhat independent. Through this interchange, the trial publication and communication of results likely will improve, which is to everyone's benefit.

SUMMARY

The concept of a DSMB has existed since the mid 1960s with the planning of the CDP. Since then, numerous DSMBs have existed for a wide variety of clinical trials across different diseases and sponsors. The success of the DSMB concept during this period has been outstanding. Confidentiality has been maintained. Trials have been terminated early for safety reasons or evidence of benefit or lack of feasibility. Although useful statistical guidelines exist for interpreting interim analyses, they are still limited, and the judgment and experience of the DSMB are essential to the clinical trial process.

REFERENCES

1. Friedman L, Furberg C, DeMets DL: Fundamentals of Clinical Trials, 3rd ed. St. Louis, Mosby, 1996.
2. Meinert CL: Clinical Trials: Design, Conduct, and Analysis, New York, Oxford University Press, 1986.
3. Pocock SJ: Clinical Trials: A Practical Approach. New York, John Wiley & Sons, 1983.
4. Heart Special Project Committee: Organization, Review, and Administration of Cooperative Studies (Greenberg Report): A Report from the Heart Special Project Committee to the National Advisory Council, May 1967. Control Clin Trials 1988; 9:137–148.
5. Friedman L: The NHLBI model: A 25-year history. Stat Med 1993; 12:425–432.
6. Ellenberg S, Fleming T, DeMets D: Data Monitoring Committees in Clinical Trials: A Practical Perspective. John Wiley & Sons, Ltd., West Sussex, England, 2002.
7. Ellenberg SS, Geller NL, Simon R, et al, (eds): Proceedings of Practical Issues in Data Monitoring of Clinical Trials. Bethesda, MD, January, 27–28, 1992. Stat Med 1993; 12:415–616.
8. Fleming TR: Evaluating therapeutic interventions: Some issues and experience. Stat Sci 1992; 7:428–456.
9. Fleming TR, DeMets DL: Monitoring of clinical trials: Issues and experiences. Control Clin Trials 1993; 14:183–297.
10. Hawkins BS: Data monitoring committees for multicenter clinical trials sponsored by the National Institutes of Health: I. Roles and membership of data monitoring committees for trials sponsored by the National Eye Institute. Control Clin Trials 1991; 12:424–437.
11. Task Force of the Working Group on Arrhythmias of the European Society of Cardiology: The early termination of clinical trials: Causes, consequences, and control. Circulation 1994; 89:2892–2907.
12. Walters L: Data monitoring committees: The moral case for maximum feasible independence. Stat Med 1993; 12:575–580.
13. O'Neill RT: Some FDA perspectives on data monitoring in clinical trials in drug development. Stat Med 1993; 12:601–608.
14. Peto R, Pike MC, Armitage P, et al: Design and analysis of randomized clinical trials requiring prolonged observations of each patient: I. Introduction and design. Br J Cancer 1976; 34:585–612.
15. Rockhold FW, Enas GG: Data monitoring and interim analyses in the pharmaceutical industry: Ethical and logistical considerations. Stat Med 1993; 12:471–480.
16. Williams GW, Davis RL, Getson AJ, et al: Monitoring of clinical trials and interim analyses from a drug sponsor's point of view. Stat Med 1993; 12:481–492.
17. Buyse M: Interim analyses, stopping roles, and data monitoring in clinical trials in Europe. Stat Med 1993; 12:509–520.
18. Wittes J: Behind closed doors: The data monitoring board in randomized clinical trials. Stat Med 1993; 12:419–424.
19. DeMets DL, Ellenberg SS, Fleming TR, et al: Data and safety monitoring board and acquired immune deficiency syndrome (AIDS) clinical trials. Control Clin Trials 1995; 16:408–421.
20. Liberati A: Conclusions: I. The relationship between clinical trials and clinical practice: The risks of underestimating its complexity. Stat Med 1994; 13:1485–1492.
21. O'Neill RT: Conclusions: II. The relationship between clinical trials and clinical practice: The risks of underestimating its complexity. Stat Med 1994; 13:1493–1500.
22. DeMets DL: Data monitoring and sequential analysis: An academic perspective. J AIDS 1990; 3(Suppl 2):S124–S133.
23. Shalala D: Protecting research subjects: What must be done. N Engl J Med 2000; 343(11).
24. National Institutes of Health: NIH policy for data and safety monitoring. NIH Guide, June 10. http://grants2.nih.gov/grants/guide/notice-files/not98-084.html, 1998. Accessed 08/07/03.
25. U.S. Food and Drug Administration (2001): Draft Guidance for Clinical Trial sponsors on the establishment and operation of Clinical Trial Data Monitoring Committees. Rockville, MD: FDA. http://www.fda.gov./cber/gdlns/clindatmon.htm. Accessed 08/07/03.
26. Coronary Drug Project Research Group: Practical aspects of decision making in clinical trials: The Coronary Drug Project as a case study. Control Clin Trials 1981; 2:363–376.
27. Armstrong PW, Furberg CD: Clinical trial data and safety monitoring boards: The search for a constitution. Circulation 1995; 91:901–904.
28. Fleming TR: Data monitoring committees and capturing relevant information of high quality. Stat Med 1993; 12:565–570.
29. Pocock SJ: Statistical and ethical issues in monitoring clinical trials. Stat Med 1993; 12:1459–1469.
30. The TIMI Study Group: Comparison of invasive and conservative strategies after treatment with intravenous tissue plasminogen activator in acute myocardial infarction. N Engl J Med 1989; 320:618–627.
31. Diabetes Control and Complications Trial Research Group: Diabetes Control and Complications Trial (DCCT): Design and methodologic considerations for the feasibility phase. Diabetes 1986; 35:530–545.
32. Diabetes Control and Complications Trial Research Group: The effect of intensive treatment of diabetes on the development and progression of long-term complications in insulin-dependent diabetes mellitus. N Engl J Med 1993; 329:977–986.
33. Armitage P: Interim analysis in clinical trials. Stat Med 1991; 10:925–937.
34. McPherson K: Statistics: The problem of examining accumulating data more than once. N Engl J Med 1974; 290:501–502.
35. Pocock SJ: Group sequential methods in the design and analysis of clinical trials. Biometrika 1977; 64:191–199.
36. Pocock SJ: Interim analyses for randomized clinical trials: The group sequential approach. Biometrics 1982; 38:153–162.
37. O'Brien PC, Fleming TR: A multiple testing procedure for clinical trials. Biometrics 1979; 35:549–556.
38. Lan KKG, DeMets DL: Discrete sequential boundaries for clinical trials. Biometrika 1983; 70:659–663.
39. DeMets DL, Lan KKG: Interim analyses: The alpha spending function approach. Stat Med 1994; 13:1341–1352.
40. DeMets DL, Lan KKG: The alpha spending function approach to interim data analyses. In Thall P (ed). Recent Advances in Clinical Trial Design and Analysis. Amsterdam, Kluwer Academic, 1995, pp 1–27.
41. DeMets DL, Ware JH: Asymmetric group sequential boundaries for monitoring clinical trials. Biometrika 1982; 69:661–663.
42. Lan KKG, Simon R, Halperin M: Stochastically curtailed tests in long-term clinical trials. Communicat Stat Sequent Analys 1982; 1:207–219.
43. Lan KKG, Wittes J: The B value: A tool for monitoring data. Biometrics 1988; 44:579–585.
44. Coronary Drug Project Research Group: The Coronary Drug Project: Design, methods, and baseline results. Circulation 1973; 47(Suppl 1):II–179.
45. Beta-Blocker Heart Attack Trial Research Group: A randomized trial of propranolol in patients with acute myocardial infarction: I. Mortality results. JAMA 1982; 247:1707–1714.

46. DeMets DL, Hardy R, Friedman LM, et al: Statistical aspects of early termination in the Beta-Blocker Heart Attack Trial. Control Clin Trials 1984; 5:362-372.

47. Norwegian Multicenter Study Group: Timolol-induced reduction in mortality and reinfarction in patients surviving acute myocardial infarction. N Engl J Med 1981; 304:801.

48. Cardiac Arrhythmia Suppression Trial (CAST) Investigators: Preliminary report: Effect of encainide and flecainide on mortality in a randomized trial of arrhythmia suppression after myocardial infarction. N Engl J Med 1989; 321:406-412.

49. Pawitan Y, Hallstrom A: Statistical interim monitoring of the Cardiac Arrhythmia Suppression Trial. Stat Med 1990; 9:1081-1090.

50. Friedman LM, Bristow JD, Hallstrom A, et al: Data monitoring in the Cardiac Arrhythmia Suppression Trial. Online J Curr Clin Trials 1993; Jul 31:Doc no 79.

51. DeMets DL, Pocock S, Julian DG: The agonising negative trend in monitoring clinical trials. Lancet 1999; 354: 1983-1988.

52. Packer M, Carver JR, Rodeheffer RJ, et al: Effect of oral milrinone on mortality in severe chronic heart failure. For the PROMISE Study Research Group. N Engl J Med 1991; 325:1468-1475.

53. Packer M, Rouleau J, Swedberg K, et al: Effect of flosequinan on survival in chronic heart failure: Preliminary results of the PROFILE study. Circulation 1993; 88(Suppl I):1-301.

54. Swedberg K, Held P, Kjekhus J, et al: Effects of early administration of enalapril on mortality in patients with acute myocardial infarction: Results of the Cooperative North Scandinavian Enalapril Survival Study II (Consensus II). N Engl J Med 1992; 327: 678-684.

55. Furberg C, Campbell R, Pitt B: Letter to the editor (on Consensus II). N Engl J Med 1993; 328:967-968.

56. Steering Committee for the Physicians' Health Study Research Group: Preliminary Report: Findings from the Aspirin Component of the Ongoing Physicians' Health Study. N Engl J Med 1988; 318:262-264.

57. Cairns J, Cohen L, Colton T, et al: Issues in the early termination of the aspirin component of the Physicians' Health Study: Data Monitoring Board of the Physicians' Health Study. Ann Epidemiol 1991; 1:395-405.

58. Freedman B: Equipoise and the ethics of clinical research. N Engl J Med 1987; 317:141-145.

59. Green S, Fleming T, O'Fallon J: Policies for monitoring and interim reporting of results. J Clin Oncol 1987; 5:1477-1484.

60. FDA Guideline: Guideline for the Format and Content of the Clinical and Statistical Sections of an Application. Bethesda, MD, Center for Drug Evaluation and Research, Food and Drug Administration, Department of Health and Human Services, July, 1988.

61. PMA Ad Hoc Committee on Interim Analysis: Interim analysis in the pharmaceutical industry. Control Clin Trials 1993; 14: 160-173.

62. Healy B, Campeau L, Gray R, et al: Conflict-of-interest guidelines for a multicenter clinical trial of treatment after coronary artery bypass graft surgery. N Engl J Med 1989; 320:949-951.

63. Multiple Risk Factor Intervention Trial Research Group: Multiple Risk Factor Intervention Trial: Risk factor changes and mortality results. JAMA 1982; 248:1465-1477.

64. DeMets DL, Fleming TR, Whitley RJ, et al: The Data and Safety Board and acquired immune deficiency syndrome (AIDS) clinical trials. Control Clin Trials 1995; 16:408-421.

65. GUSTO Investigators: An international randomized trial comparing four thrombolytic strategies for acute myocardial infarction. N Engl J Med 1993; 329:673-682.

66. Nocturnal Oxygen Therapy Group: Continuous or nocturnal oxygen therapy in hypoxemic chronic obstructive lung disease. Ann Intern Med 1980; 93:391-398.

67. DeMets DL, Williams GW, Brown BW Jr: A case report of data monitoring experience: The Nocturnal Oxygen Therapy Trial. Control Clin Trials 1982; 3:113-124.

68. Hjalmarson A, Elmfeldt D, Herlitz J, et al: Effect on mortality of metoprolol in acute myocardial infarction: A double-blind randomized trial. Lancet 1981; 2:823.

69. Pocock SJ: The role of external evidence in data monitoring of a clinical trial. Stat Med 1996; 15:1285-1293; discussion 1295-1297.

70. Packer M, O'Connor C, Ghali J: Effect of Amlodipine on Morbidity and Mortality in Severe Chronic Heart Failure. Presented at the American College of Cardiology Meeting, March 18, 1995, New Orleans.

71. Berson EL, Rosner B, Sandberg MA, et al: A randomized trial of vitamin A and vitamin E supplementation for retinitis pigmentosa. Arch Ophthalmol 1993; 111:761-772.

72. Marmor MF: A randomized trial of vitamin A and vitamin E supplementation for retinitis pigmentosa [comments]. Arch Ophthalmol 1993; 111:1460-1461.

73. Norton EWD: A randomized trial of vitamin A and vitamin E supplementation for retinitis pigmentosa [comments]. Arch Ophthalmol 1993; 111:1460.

■ ■ ■ chapter 5

Aspirin and Thienopyridines

Shamir R. Mehta
Salim Yusuf

RATIONALE FOR ANTIPLATELET THERAPY IN PATIENTS WITH ACUTE CORONARY SYNDROMES

Rationale for Acute Therapy

Platelets play a central role in the pathophysiology of arterial thrombosis. Following plaque disruption, erosion, or rupture, there are three essential steps involved in the formation of a platelet-rich thrombus: platelet adhesion, platelet activation, and platelet aggregation.

The first step, platelet adhesion, is mediated by adhesive proteins such as von Willebrand's factor. These adhesive proteins interact with platelet receptors (such as the glycoprotein [GP] 1b complex), which allow platelets in flowing blood to adhere to the site of injured endothelium.[1] The second step, platelet activation, is an important step involving several interrelated processes. Initially, platelet activation involves a change in the three-dimensional shape of the platelet, from a smooth discoid contour into a spiculated form.[2] This shape change greatly increases the membrane surface area of the platelet, on which thrombin generation occurs. Following this shape change, platelet activation involves degranulation or secretion of alpha and dense granules within the platelet, thereby releasing pro-thrombotic, inflammatory and chemo-attractant mediators, which propagate, amplify, and sustain the atherothrombotic process ("release reaction").[3] Platelet activation then leads to a conformational change in the GP IIb/IIIa receptor, converting the receptor into a form that can bind fibrinogen and link with other platelets (platelet aggregation).[4] The final step in the formation of the platelet-rich thrombus is platelet aggregation or the actual cross-linking of platelets by fibrinogen.

Rationale for Long-Term Therapy

In patients with acute coronary syndrome (ACS), an ongoing hypercoagulable state persists for several months. This is characterized by continued platelet activation and thrombin generation beyond the acute phase, which plays an important role in the pathogenesis of recurrent ischemic events. This is manifest clinically by a high rate of recurrent major ischemic events during long-term follow-up. For example, in a 6-month follow-up study of more than 8000 patients with unstable angina or (non-ST segment elevation myocardial infarction) NSTEMI, about 6% of patients developed a major cardiovascular event (CV death, myocardial infarction [MI], or stroke) between hospital discharge and 6 months.[6] Extended follow-up for up to 2 years indicated a continuing high event rate of approximately 6% to 8% per year.[7] This has focused attention on whether administration of long-term oral antiplatelet and antithrombotic strategies can reduce long-term events in patients with ACS.

Angioscopic, angiographic, and biochemical data help to characterize the ongoing stimulus for long-term cardiovascular events. First, angioscopic studies have shown that, despite the use of short-term antithrombotic therapies, coronary thrombi are still present at 30 days following an acute ischemic event, suggesting that longer term antithrombotic therapy may be required to reduce events, perhaps allowing passivation of the culprit lesion.[8] Second, there is good evidence to suggest that patients with ACS have, in addition to the culprit lesion, multiple complex coronary plaques that are associated with adverse clinical outcomes. In a careful angiographic study, patients who were found to have multiple complex coronary plaques had about an 11-fold increase in a recurrent ACS and about a 6-fold to 7-fold increase in adverse cardiac events compared to patients with only a single unstable plaque.[9] This suggests that plaque instability is caused by a widespread process that affects the entire coronary tree and is not a process confined to a single culprit lesion. Inflammation has been implicated as such a process.[10-12] In patients with ACS, intravascular ultrasound has confirmed the presence of multiple atherosclerotic plaque ruptures in the same patient, which are present simultaneously with the culprit lesion in other locations in the coronary tree.[12] These nonculprit ruptured plaques are often less severely stenosed and less calcified than the culprit, supporting the notion that ACS is associated with pan-coronary plaque destabilization. Third, biochemical studies have indicated persistent platelet hyperactivity and elevation of markers of the coagulation system, suggesting that the environment for thrombosis still is present many months after the initial event.[13-15] Fifth, as indicated earlier, long-term studies have demonstrated a significant increase in major cardiovascular events, despite modern-day treatments.[6,16] In addition, after stopping most short-term antithrombotic therapies there is no added benefit (and perhaps an increase in events with thrombin inhibitors), and further clinical events occur in both treatment and control groups, suggesting the need for longer term antithrombotic therapy.[17,18] These intriguing observations, when coupled with the emerging data on the importance of inflammation and coagulation in atherosclerosis and arterial thrombosis, support the concept that a generalized and persistent process is an important feature of future plaque disruption that causes further ischemic events.[19]

Thus, the elevated risk many months and years after the acute event may be related to the degree and multiplicity of atherosclerotic plaques, their location, and their cellular and biochemical characteristics. This chapter focuses primarily on the acute and long-term role of the oral antithrombotic therapies aspirin and thienopyridienes in ACS.

MECHANISM OF ACTION OF ASPIRIN AND THIENOPYRIDINES

Aspirin inhibits platelet cyclooxygenase by irreversible acetylation, thus preventing the formation of thromboxane A_2, which induces platelet aggregation. Because platelets are unable to generate new cyclooxygenase, enzyme inhibition lasts for the life of the platelet, or about 10 days. (Fig. 5-1) In vascular endothelial cells aspirin prevents the synthesis of prostacyclin, which inhibits platelet aggregation. However unlike platelets, endothelial cells can recover cyclooxygenase synthesis so that the inhibitory effects of aspirin may be of shorter duration than with platelets. In addition to antiplatelet effects, aspirin also has antiinflammatory effects, which may contribute to its clinical effectiveness in ACS.

The adenosine diphosphate (ADP) receptor antagonists, ticlopidine and clopidogrel, inhibit platelet activation, thereby preventing degranulation and the release of prothrombotic and inflammatory mediators from the platelet (Fig. 5-1). They also inhibit the activation of the

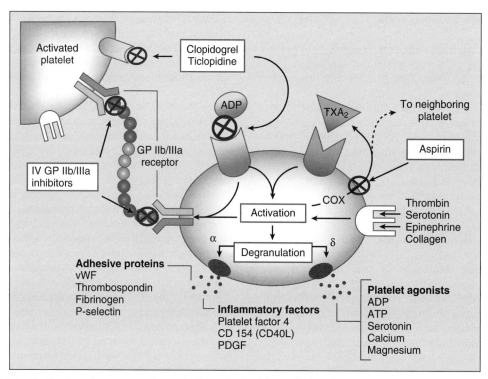

FIGURE 5-1. Platelet activation is an important early step in the pathophysiology of atherothrombosis. Platelet activation involves the following: (1) a shape change in which the platelet membrane surface area is increased greatly; (2) the secretion of proinflammatory, prothrombotic, adhesive, and chemotactic mediators ("release reaction"), which propagate, amplify, and sustain the atherothrombotic process; and (3) the activation of the glycoprotein IIb/IIIa receptor from its inactive form. Multiple agonists including thromboxane A_2 (TXA$_2$), adenosine diphosphate (ADP), thrombin, serotonin, epinephrine, and collagen can activate the platelet and thus contribute toward establishing the environmental conditions necessary for atherothrombosis to occur. Aspirin inhibits the production of TXA$_2$ by its effect on the enzyme cyclooxygenase 1 (COX1). The ADP receptor antagonists clopidogrel and ticlopidine prevent the binding of ADP to its receptor. The effect of combining aspirin and clopidogrel is synergistic in preventing platelet aggregation. Antithrombins such as unfractionated or low molecular weight heparin, hirudin, or bivalirudin are important in both interfering with thrombin-induced platelet activation and coagulation. The glycoprotein IIb/IIIa receptor antagonists act at a later step in the process by preventing fibrinogen-mediated cross-linking of platelets that already have become activated. Adapted from Mehta SR, Yusuf S: Short- and long-term oral antiplatelet therapy in acute coronary syndromes and percutaneous coronary intervention. J Am Coll Cardiol 2003; 41: 78S-87S.

GP IIb/IIIa receptor into the form that can bind fibrinogen and link platelets. These agents therefore act early in the sequence of events leading to the formation of the platelet thrombus, which results in effective inhibition of platelet aggregation. Specifically, they selectively and irreversibly inhibit the binding of ADP to the platelet ADP receptor $P2Y_{12}$.[20-22] The active metabolite of clopidogrel is a short-lived thiol derivative of the parent molecule.

ACUTE MYOCARDIAL INFARCTION

Aspirin

The International Study of Infarct Survival-2 (ISIS-2) was a 2×2 randomized double-blind trial of aspirin (ASA) versus placebo and streptokinase versus placebo in patients with acute myocardial infarction (AMI).[23] Aspirin was given in a dose of 162.5 mg immediately (with the first tablet crushed or chewed), followed by 162.5 mg daily for about 1 month. Overall 17,187 patients with suspected AMI presenting within 24 hours of symptom onset were randomized. There was a 23% reduction in vascular mortality at 1 month with aspirin versus placebo (804/8587, or 9.4% vs. 1016/8600, or 11.8%, relative risk [RR] 0.77, 2P < 0.00001) (Fig. 5-2). This reduction represents the avoidance of about 25 early deaths for every 1000 patients with AMI who are treated with aspirin for 1 month. The benefits at 1 month were maintained to at least 10 years of follow-up.[24] Further, there were additional reductions with aspirin in reinfarction (ARR 1.5%, 2P < 0.00001), cardiac arrest (ARR 1.2%, 2P < 0.001), and in stroke (ARR 0.4%, 2P < 0.01). These reductions translate into the avoidance of about

25 deaths and 10 to 15 nonfatal reinfarctions and strokes. The benefits of aspirin in ISIS-2 were similar irrespective of the delay from symptom onset to the start of treatment, indicating that aspirin should be given to all patients with AMI, even if they present late after the onset of symptoms. The benefits of aspirin were additive to the benefit of fibrinolysis with streptokinase, which itself reduced mortality by one-fourth (9.2% vs. 12.0%, RR 0.75, 2P < 0.00001). Thus in patients receiving both ASA and streptokinase versus neither agent, there was an impressive 42% reduction in vascular death (2P < 0.00001). In ISIS-2, major bleeding incidents (i.e., bleeds requiring transfusion) occurred with a similar frequency in the aspirin and placebo groups (0.4% vs. 0.4%), and there was no significant excess in cerebral hemorrhage with aspirin.

Thienopyridines

There have been no published trials comparing treatment with thienopyridines alone versus aspirin in the setting of ST elevation AMI. However, clopidogrel is recommended in patients who have absolute contraindications to aspirin. Although there have been no controlled studies, a loading dose of 300 mg of clopidogrel seems reasonable to achieve a rapid antiplatelet effect.

Combination of Aspirin and Clopidogrel

The effects of combination aspirin and clopidogrel are being tested in two randomized trials. In the Chinese Cardiac Society (CCS)-2 trial (also known as COMIT), approximately 30,000 to 40,000 patients with suspected AMI will be randomized to receive either clopidogrel 75 mg daily or placebo for 30 days in addition to aspirin and other standard therapies.[25] Treatment is for 1 month. The primary outcome of vascular mortality will be assessed at 1 month.

In the second trial, known as the Clopidogrel as Adjunctive Reperfusion Therapy—Thrombolysis In Myocardial Infarction 28 (or CLARITY-TIMI 28), 2200 patients with ST elevation AMI who are eligible for fibrinolytic therapy are being randomized to clopidogrel 300 mg loading dose within 10 minutes of fibrinolysis followed by 75 mg/day or matching placebo. Both groups will receive aspirin. The primary outcome is a combined angiographic/clinical composite of Thrombolysis in Myocardial Infarction (TIMI) glow grade 0 or 1 on the predischarge angiogram, death, or recurrent MI during the index hospitalization.

UNSTABLE ANGINA AND NON-ST SEGMENT ELEVATION MYOCARDIAL INFARCTION

Aspirin

There have been four key randomized trials testing the use of aspirin in unstable angina (Table 5-1).[26-29] These early studies were performed in the 1970s and 1980s, prior to the routine use of currently used therapies

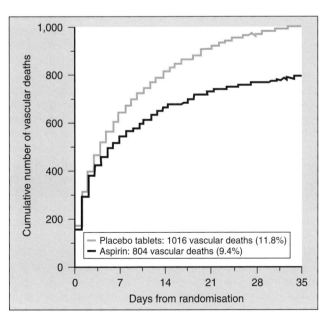

FIGURE 5-2. ISIS-2 Primary results of aspirin versus control comparison. Cumulative mortality from randomization to 35 days. (Modified from ISIS-2 [Second International Study of Infarct Survival] Collaborative Group. Randomised trial of intravenous streptokinase, oral aspirin, both, or neither among 17,187 cases of suspected acute myocardial infarction: ISIS-2. Lancet 1988; 2[8607]:349–360, with permission.)

■ ■ ■

TABLE 5-1   RANDOMIZED TRIALS OF ASPIRIN IN UNSTABLE ANGINA

Trial	Treatment	Follow-up	DEATH OR MYOCARDIAL INFARCTION		Relative risk reduction (%)	P
			Aspirin	Control		
Veterans Affairs Study, 1983[26]	ASA 324 mg daily vs. placebo	3 months	31/625 (5.0%)	65/641 (10.1%)	41	0.004
Canadian Study, 1985*[27]	ASA 325 mg 4 times daily or control	18 months (mean)	29/276 (10.5%)	41/279 (14.6%)	30*	0.072
Montreal Heart Study, 1988[28]	ASA 650 mg first dose then 325 mg twice daily for 6 days or placebo	6 days	6/243 (2.5%)	15/236 (6.4%)	63	0.04
RISC, 1990[29]	ASA 75 mg for 3 months or placebo	13 months	26/399 (6.5%)	68/397 (17%)	64	0.0001
Antithrombotic Trialists' Collaboration Meta-analysis†[30]	Various regimens vs. placebo/untreated control	Various durations	199/2497 (8.0%)	336/2534 (13.3%)	46	<0.0001

*Intention to treat analysis is presented. Mortality alone was reduced by 43%, P = 0.035.
†Endpoint reported is vascular death, myocardial infarction, or stroke. In addition to the trials in this table[26–29], this meta-analysis includes all trials of antiplatelet therapy in patients with unstable angina.
ASA, aspirin; RISC, Research Group on Instability in Coronary Artery Disease.

including heparin, clopidogrel, and GP IIb/IIIa antagonists. They were also performed prior to the widespread use of invasive procedures such as percutaneous coronary intervention (PCI) and coronary artery bypass graft (CABG) surgery, which are now commonly performed in patients with unstable angina and NSTEMI. Nevertheless, these trials individually demonstrated benefits of aspirin over placebo or untreated control in reducing ischemic events and have led to the universal recommendation of aspirin as standard therapy in ACS.

The first large study was the Veterans Affairs (VA) trial involving 1338 patients with unstable angina who were treated with 12 weeks of aspirin versus control.[26] It was performed between 1974 and 1981. This study demonstrated a 51% reduction in death or MI (10.1% in the placebo group vs. 5.0% with ASA, P = 0.004) in favor of 12 weeks of treatment with aspirin at a dose of 325 mg daily. Mortality was reduced in this trial from 3.3% to 1.6% (P = 0.054) with aspirin. In the Canadian Multicenter Trial aspirin therapy was given for much longer than in the VA trial, approximately 2 years after an episode of unstable angina.[27] This study of 555 patients was performed between 1979 and 1984. It demonstrated that aspirin (325 mg four times daily) was superior to control, with a 30% reduction in death or MI at 2 years (P = 0.072 in the intention-to-treat analysis) and a 43% reduction in death alone (P = 0.035). In the Montreal Heart study (N = 479), aspirin (325 mg twice daily) given for a very short period (only 6 days) reduced death or MI by 63% (6.3% vs. 2.6%, P = 0.04).[28] In the Research Group on Instability in Coronary Artery Disease (RISC) study, aspirin in a lower dose of 80 mg daily given for 1 year reduced death or MI by 49% in the 796 patients meeting the inclusion criteria (total of 945 patients randomized) up to 12 months (21.4% vs. 11%, P = 0.0001).[29]

In the Antithrombotic Trialists' Collaboration (ATC) overview,[30] among all patients who were at high risk for vascular events there was a 22% reduction in the composite of vascular death, MI, or stroke (13.2% vs. 10.7%, P < 0.0001). Vascular death alone was reduced by 15%

(P < 0.0001). Among the subset of patients with unstable angina, there was a 46% reduction in vascular events (13.3% vs. 8.0%, P < 0.0001) (Table 5-1).

Dose of Aspirin

In the acute situation of ACS, it seems reasonable to administer a loading dose of aspirin of about 150 to 325 mg to produce rapid and complete inhibition of thromboxane-mediated platelet aggregation.[31] With regard to aspirin dosing subsequent to the acute period, the ATC overview provides the most comprehensive data.[30] Among the three trials directly comparing doses of greater than 75 mg versus less than 75 mg of aspirin (total 3570 patients), there was no significant difference in vascular death, MI, or stroke between the two dose regimens (14.2% vs. 13.2%, P = NS). Among the trials that tested doses above 75 mg, there were seven trials totaling 3197 patients (with vascular disease) evaluating higher doses (500-1500 mg) versus lower doses (75-325 mg) of aspirin, with no significant differences in vascular death, MI, or stroke between the various doses (14.1% high dose vs. 14.5% low dose). Separating the trials of ASA versus control according to aspirin dose revealed that benefit was present in the 34 trials evaluating high aspirin doses (500-1500 mg) versus control (odds reduction 19%), the 19 trials evaluating moderate doses (160-325mg) versus control (odds reduction 26%), and the 12 trials evaluating lower doses (15-150 mg) versus control (odds reduction 32%). The three trials evaluating doses less than 75 mg versus control demonstrated a smaller effect (odds reduction 13%).

The benefit of aspirin in these early studies reinforced the concept that effective long-term antiplatelet therapy improves prognosis in patients after ACS and PCI. Despite the use of aspirin, however, recurrent events still remain high, prompting the search for newer agents, which can either replace aspirin or be added to aspirin in the long-term management of these patients.[6]

Safety

The main concern with aspirin is the increased risk of bleeding. The ATC meta-analysis demonstrated a 60% relative increase in major extracranial bleeding with antiplatelet therapy versus control (1.13% vs. 0.71%, OR 1.6, 95% CI 1.4–1.8). With regard to fatal or nonfatal intracranial hemorrhage, there was a significant increase with antiplatelet therapy compared to adjusted controls (217/48,571 [0.65%] vs. 162/48,681 [0.54%], relative increase 22%, 95% CI 3%–44%, P < 0.01).[30] However, this was balanced by a 30% reduction in fatal and nonfatal ischemic stroke (24%–35%, P < 0.0001). Overall, there was a significant 22% reduction in total fatal or nonfatal stroke [2501/66,860 (3.74%) vs. 3146/67,021 (4.75%), RR 0.78, SE 0.03].[30]

Thienopyridines

Both ticlopidine and clopidogrel have been studied in clinical trials in patients with atherosclerosis (including coronary artery disease, cerebrovascular disease, and peripheral arterial disease). The usefulness of ticlopidine, however, is limited by its potential to cause severe neutropenia in about 1% of patients, which necessitates close monitoring of blood counts, at least during the first few weeks or months of therapy.[32,33] Ticlopidine[34-36] and (to a much lesser extent) clopidogrel[37] very rarely have been associated with thrombotic thrombocytopenic purpura. In contrast to clopidogrel, the full antiplatelet action of ticlopidine is delayed for several days after commencement of therapy, limiting the usefulness of this agent in acutely ill patients and those undergoing nonelective PCI with stent implantation. By contrast, the effects of a 300-mg dose of clopidogrel are evident after only 2 hours, making it useful in both acute and chronic settings.[38]

In the setting of unstable angina, there has been one early randomized trial of ticlopidine for 6 months versus control in 662 patients. This study demonstrated a 46% reduction in the primary endpoint of cardiovascular death or MI with ticlopidine (P = 0.009).[39] This trial was conducted more than 10 years ago, prior to the routine use of aspirin in unstable angina, but demonstrated the clear potential for the ADP receptor antagonists to be effective in unstable angina.

In addition to this study, there have been several other studies of thienopyridines versus placebo or aspirin in a wide variety of patients with atherosclerotic disease (Table 5-2).[32,39-43] Specifically, there have been at least three moderate-sized trials of thienopyridines versus placebo or control in patients with atherosclerotic disease (one each in patients with unstable angina,[39] intermittent claudication,[40] and stroke[41]). Taken together, these three trials, totaling 2392 patients, demonstrate a 29% relative risk reduction (RRR) in vascular events (OR 0.71, 95% CI 0.0.58–0.86, P = 0.0006)[42] (see Table 5-2).

Data for a direct comparison of thienopyridine versus aspirin are dominated by the large CAPRIE study, which randomized 19,185 patients with previous MI, recent transient ischemic attack/stroke, or symptomatic peripheral vascular disease, to clopidogrel 75 mg/day or aspirin for a period of 1 to 3 years. At a mean of 1.9 years of follow-up, clopidogrel significantly reduced the primary outcome of vascular death, MI, or ischemic stroke compared with aspirin by 8.7% (95% CI 0.3%–16.5%).[43] A smaller study (TASS) randomized 3069 patients with cerebral ischemia to receive either aspirin or ticlopidine.[44] The results demonstrated a nonsignificant trend in favor of ticlopidine (RR 0.93, CI 0.79-1.09). Taken

■ ▪ ■

TABLE 5-2   CLINICAL TRIALS OF THIENOPYRIDINES VERSUS PLACEBO OR ASPIRIN IN PATIENTS WITH ATHEROSCLEROSIS

Trial, year	Setting	PRIMARY OUTCOME			Odds ratio	95% CI
		Definition	Thienopyridine (n/N)	Comparator (n/N)		
Thienopyridine versus placebo or control						
CATS 1989 (ticlopidine vs. placebo)[32]	Recent stroke	Death, MI, Stroke	106/525	134/528	0.74	0.56–0.99
Balsano 1990 (ticlopidine vs. control)[39]	Unstable angina	Death, MI	23/314	46/338	0.52	0.31–0.85
STIMS, 1990 (ticlopidine vs. placebo)[41]	Intermittent claudication	Death, MI, stroke	89/346	99/341	0.85	0.61–1.18
TOTAL*			**218/1185**	**279/1207**	**0.73**	**0.60–0.90***
Thienopyridine versus ASA						
TASS, 1989 (ticlopidine vs. ASA)[44]	Cerebral ischemia	Death, stroke	306/1529	349/1540	0.85	0.82–0.97
CAPRIE, 1996 (clopidogrel vs. ASA)[43]	Recent stroke, previous MI or PVD	Death, MI, stroke	939/9599	1021/9586	0.91	0.83–1.00
TOTAL*			**1245/11128**	**1370/11126**	**0.90**	**0.83–0.97†**

*P = 0.003.
†P = 0.009.
ASA, aspirin; CI, confidence interval; MI, myocardial infarction; CATS, Canadian American Ticlopidine Study; TASS, Ticlopidine Aspirin Stroke Study; STIMS, Swedish Ticlopidine Multi-center study; CAPRIE, Clopidogrel versus Aspirin in Patients at Risk of Ischemic Events.

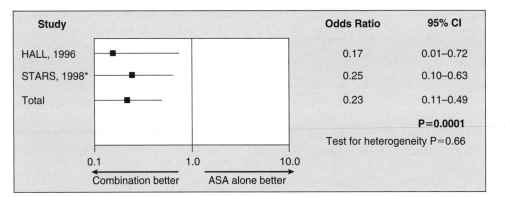

FIGURE 5-3. Death or myocardial infarction in trials of aspirin (ASA) + ticlopidine versus ASA alone after coronary artery stenting. (Modified from Mehta SR, Yusuf S, Clopidogrel in Unstable angina to prevent Recurrent Events [CURE] Study Investigators. The Clopidogrel in Unstable angina to prevent Recurrent Events [CURE] trial program: Rationale, design and baseline characteristics including a meta-analysis of the effects of thienopyridines in vascular disease. Eur Heart J 2000; 21:2033-2041, with permission.)

together, in these two head-to-head comparisons of thienopyridine versus ASA in patients with vascular disease (total N = 22,254 patients), thienopyridines were more effective than ASA in reducing the frequency of major ischemic events (OR 0.90, 95% CI 0.83-0.97, P = 0.009)[42] (see Tables 5-1 and 5-2).

Combination of Aspirin and Thienopyridines

Thienopyridines and aspirin act through complementary and independent mechanisms, and their combination can inhibit both ADP-induced platelet aggregation and thromboxane A_2 production.[45-47] The combination of these two antiplatelet strategies was initially studied in patients undergoing intracoronary stenting. In the two trials of ASA plus ticlopidine compared with aspirin alone there was a marked benefit of the combination in reducing death and nonfatal MI compared with ASA (OR 0.23, 95% CI 0.11-0.49, P = 0.0001). (Fig. 5-3)[48,49] ASA plus ticlopidine has been compared to an "active comparator" (i.e., ASA plus warfarin) in four randomized controlled trials in patients undergoing coronary artery stenting.[49-52] The combined results of these trials

demonstrate a 49% relative risk reduction in death or MI with use of ASA and ticlopidine (OR 0.51, 95% CI 0.33-0.78, P = 0.002) (Fig. 5-4). Several studies have compared the combination of clopidogrel and aspirin to ticlopidine and aspirin after coronary stenting, suggesting that the combination of aspirin and clopidogrel is better tolerated and at least as safe and effective as aspirin and ticlopidine.[53-57]

The Clopidogrel in Unstable Angina Recurrent Events (CURE) established the beneficial effects of clopidogrel in addition to aspirin in patients with non-ST segment elevation ACS.[58] CURE was a double-blind, placebo-controlled, international randomized trial of acute and long-term therapy with clopidogrel versus placebo in addition to aspirin and other standard therapies (including heparin, beta blockers, angiotensin converting enzyme [ACE] inhibitors, lipid-lowering therapies) in patients with non-ST segment ACS. Patients were eligible if they presented within 24 hours of chest pain onset and had evidence of ischemia (either elevated cardiac enzymes or troponin or electrocardiogram (ECG) changes such as ST-segment depression, T-wave inversion, or transient ST-segment elevation). Aspirin was administered to all patients in doses

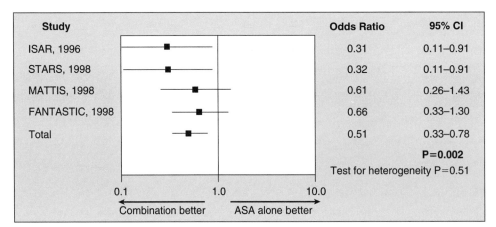

FIGURE 5-4. Death or myocardial infarction in trials of aspirin (ASA) + ticlopidine vs. ASA + oral anticoagulation after stenting. (Modified from Mehta SR, Yusuf S, Clopidogrel in Unstable angina to prevent Recurrent Events [CURE] Study Investigators. The Clopidogrel in Unstable angina to prevent Recurrent Events [CURE] trial program: rationale, design and baseline characteristics including a meta-analysis of the effects of thienopyridines in vascular disease. Eur Heart J 2000; 21:2033-2041, with permission.)

of 75 mg to 325 mg (median dose was 160 mg). Following randomization, there were no restrictions on the use of other procedures (such as percutaneous transluminal coronary angioplasty [PTCA] or CABG surgery) or medications, including the GP IIb/IIIa antagonists. Overall, 12,652 patients were recruited between December 1998 and September 2000 at 482 hospitals in 28 countries. Of patients, 5491 (44%) underwent angiography, 2072 (16.5%) underwent CABG, and 2658 (21.2%) underwent PCI.

The results demonstrated a highly significant 20% relative risk reduction in the first co-primary outcome of MI, stroke, or cardiovascular death in favor of clopidogrel over placebo (11.4% vs. 9.3%, RR 0.80, 95% CI 0.72-0.90; P = 0.00009) (Table 5-3, Fig. 5-5).[58] Consistent reductions were observed in all components of the primary composite endpoint, with a 7% reduction in cardiovascular death (5.5% vs. 5.1%, RR 0.93) and a 14% reduction in strokes (1.4% vs. 1.2%, RR 0.86), but the clearest effect was a 23% reduction in MI (6.7% vs. 5.2%, RR 0.77). Of these MIs, the most pronounced reduction was in large MIs (with ST elevation or Q waves), which were reduced by 40% (3.1% vs. 1.9%, RR 0.60, 95% CI 0.48-0.76). Consistent with this reduction in large MIs was a reduction in the use of thrombolytic therapy (2.0% vs. 1.1%, RR 0.57, P < 0.001) and in new-onset congestive heart failure after randomization (4.4% vs. 3.7%, RR 0.82, P = 0.026), emphasizing the clinical importance of this reduction in large MI (Table 5-3). During the initial hospitalization, there were reductions in a wide range of other ischemic events including refractory ischemia (defined as recurrent ischemia while on maximal medical therapy with ECG changes and requiring an intervention by midnight of the next day) (2.0% vs. 1.4%, RR 0.68, P = 0.007), additional severe ischemia (recurrent ischemia with ECG changes) (3.8% vs. 2.8%, RR 0.74, P = 0.003), or recurrent angina (any other chest pain in hospital) (22.9% vs. 20.9%, RR 0.91, P = 0.01).

The effects of clopidogrel became apparent very early after administration of the loading dose, with divergence in the Kaplan Meier Event curves occurring as early as 2 hours after randomization, indicating that the 300-mg loading dose produced a rapid and clinically apparent effect.[59] By 24 hours after randomization, there was already a highly significant 34% reduction in cardiovascular death, MI, stroke, or severe ischemia (RR 0.66, P = 0.003). At 30 days, clopidogrel reduced the first primary endpoint by 21% (P < 0.001).[37] Thus, the beneficial effects of clopidogrel become apparent very early, emphasizing the importance of giving the loading dose immediately after the diagnosis is made to obtain the greatest benefits in the largest number of patients.

In the CURE trial, patients were treated with study medication for a maximum of 1 year after randomization (mean follow-up 9 months). From day 31 up to 1 year, there was a highly significant incremental reduction of 18% in the primary outcome with clopidogrel (RR 0.82, P < 0.001).[59] This long-term benefit was in addition to the rapid early benefit observed (i.e., within the first 30 days).

The benefit of clopidogrel was observed in addition to standard therapies already used in unstable angina or NSTEMI, such as aspirin (used in 99.1%), beta blockers (used in 77.5%), ACE inhibitors (used in 48.9%), lipid-lowering therapy (used in 45.6%), and revascularization with either CABG or PTCA (performed in 38%).

When the CURE results are stratified according to the TIMI risk score, there are significant benefits across all levels of risk. Low-risk (4.1% vs. 5.7%, RR 0.71, ARR 1.6%, P < 0.03), intermediate-risk (9.8% vs. 11.4%, RR 0.71, ARR 1.6%, P < 0.02), and high-risk patients (15.9% vs. 20.7%, RR 0.73, ARR 4.8%, P < 0.003) all benefited, but the greatest absolute benefit was observed in the high-risk patients.[60]

In addition, patients who had a prior history of CABG had a large and highly significant benefit of clopidogrel (RR 0.55, 95% CI 0.43-0.72).[61] Those patients undergoing CABG surgery during the initial hospitalization in CURE had a consistent 19% reduction in the primary endpoint (95% CI 0.59-1.12). Thus, clopidogrel is effective over and above current therapies and across all patient risk levels, including those patients undergoing CABG surgery after randomization, emphasizing its value in a very wide spectrum of patients with ACS irrespective of other medical therapies or interventions used.

■ ■ ■

TABLE 5-3   MAIN RESULTS OF THE CLOPIDOGREL IN UNSTABLE ANGINA TO PREVENT RECURRENT EVENTS (CURE) TRIAL

	Placebo + ASA* (N = 6303) (%)	Clopidogrel + ASA* (N = 6259) (%)	Relative risk reduction (%)	P value
Cardiovascular death, MI, or stroke	9.3	11.4	20	0.00009
Cardiovascular death	5.1	5.5	7	
Stroke	1.2	1.4	14	
MI	6.7	5.2	23	<0.001
STEMI (Q-wave MI)	3.1	1.9	40	<0.001
Refractory ischemia†	2.0	1.4	32	0.007
Severe ischemia	3.8	2.8	26	0.003
Recurrent angina	22.9	20.9	9	0.01
Thrombolytic therapy	2.0	1.1	43	<0.001
Congestive heart failure with radiologic evidence	4.4	3.7	18	0.026

*In addition to other standard therapies.
†In hospital.
ASA, aspirin; MI, myocardial infarction; STEMI, ST-segment elevation myocardial infarction.

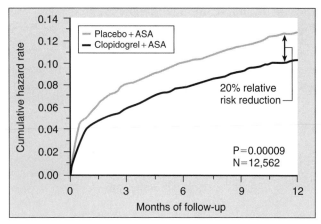

FIGURE 5-5. First co-primary outcome in CURE: cardiovascular death, myocardial infarction, or stroke from randomization up to 1 year of follow-up (mean 9 months). (Modified from The CURE Investigators. Effects of clopidogrel in addition to aspirin in patients with acute coronary syndromes without ST segment elevation. N Engl J Med 2001;345:494–502, with permission.)

In the CURE trial, there was no significant increase in life-threatening bleeding with clopidogrel compared with placebo (2.2% vs. 1.8%, RR 1.21, 95% CI 0.95–1.56, P = 0.13).[58] There were similar rates of fatal bleeding (0.2% vs. 0.2%), intracranial bleeding (0.1% vs. 0.1%), bleeding requiring surgical intervention (0.7% vs. 0.7%), and bleeding resulting in a large (>5 g/dL) decrease in hemoglobin (0.9% vs. 0.9%) between the clopidogrel and placebo groups.[58] There was a modest increase in major bleeding with clopidogrel as defined by the CURE criteria (3.7% vs. 2.7%, RR 1.38, 95% CI 1.13–1.67, P = 0.001) but no increase in TIMI major bleeding (1.08% vs. 1.15%, RR 0.94, 95% CI 0.68–1.30, P = 0.70).[58] Bleeding in CURE was significantly lower in both the aspirin-alone group and in the aspirin plus clopidogrel group when low-dose aspirin (<100 mg) was used, with no compromise in efficacy, compared with higher doses of aspirin.[62] Therefore, it is recommended that doses of aspirin of less than 100 mg are used together with clopidogrel therapy to achieve the largest benefit-risk ratio.[62]

PATIENTS WITH ACS UNDERGOING PCI

Aspirin

There are currently no randomized trials of aspirin in patients with ACS undergoing PCI. The current evidence for the use of aspirin in PCI comes from an early trial in patients with elective angioplasty. In this study of 376 patients undergoing mainly elective angioplasty, patients were randomized to receive either aspirin (990 mg) and dipyridamole (225 mg daily) or placebo starting 24 hours prior to angioplasty and continued for 4 to 7 months after.[63] Although there was no effect of antiplatelet therapy in reducing the frequency of restenosis, there was a large reduction in periprocedural Q-wave MI with antiplatelet therapy when started prior to the procedure (6.9% vs. 1.6%, P = 0.011). The benefits were likely the result of aspirin use, rather than dipyridamole,

which is known to precipitate myocardial ischemia in patients with coronary artery disease. In the only randomized trial of long-term aspirin therapy following angioplasty, aspirin (325 mg daily) given for 6 months was associated with a significant reduction in MI compared with placebo (5.7% vs. 1.2%, P = 0.03).[64]

Thienopyridines

There are no trials evaluating the Thienopyridines alone versus control specifically in patients with ACS undergoing PCI.

Combination Aspirin and Clopidogrel

The benefits of combination aspirin and clopidogrel in patients with ACS undergoing PCI were studied in the large PCI CURE study.[65] This prospectively planned substudy of the CURE trial examined whether patients randomized to clopidogrel derived benefit from pretreatment with dual antiplatelet therapy before angioplasty compared with aspirin and placebo and whether long-term therapy after PCI is superior to placebo. In total, 2658 patients were included.

Overall, from the time of randomization to the end of follow-up (up to 1 year), there was a highly significant 31% reduction in cardiovascular death or MI with clopidogrel pretreatment and long-term therapy after PCI (12.6% vs. 8.8%, RR 0.69, 95% CI 0.54–0.87, P = 0.002). (Fig. 5-6) There was a 30% reduction in the primary endpoint of cardiovascular death, MI, or urgent revascularization from the time of PCI to 30 days (6.4% vs. 4.5%, RR 0.70, P = 0.03). Because most patients in both groups receive open-label thienopyridine during this period, the benefit at 30 days after PCI reflects the impact of pretreatment with clopidogrel versus placebo in preventing major events after PCI. In the per protocol analysis, when only patients receiving an intracoronary

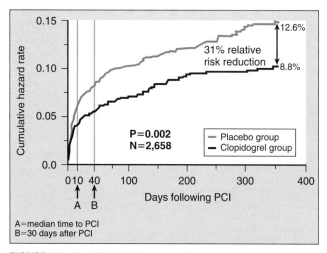

FIGURE 5-6. The PCI CURE Study overall results: cardiovascular death or myocardial infarction from time of randomization up to 1 year of follow-up. (Modified from Mehta SR, Yusuf S, Peters RJG, et al: Effects of pretreatment with clopidogrel and aspirin followed by long-term therapy in patients undergoing percutaneous coronary intervention: The PCI-CURE study. Lancet 2001;358:527–533, with permission.)

stent were examined (100% of whom received open-label thienopyridine after PCI), there was a 44% relative risk reduction in cardiovascular death, MI, or urgent target revascularization with clopidogrel pretreatment over placebo (P = 0.017) (Fig. 5-7).[66]

In the long term, there was a consistent benefit of clopidogrel over placebo from more than 30 days after PCI to end of follow-up, during which there was a significant reduction in cardiovascular death, MI, or rehospitalization (RR 0.86, P < 0.05). There was also a reduction in cardiovascular death or MI (RR 0.79, 95% CI 0.53-1.20) during this time period, which is consistent with the highly significant overall risk reduction in PCI CURE and the late (>30 days) benefit in the overall CURE trial (Fig. 5-4). Furthermore, in patients who had very early PCI (within 72 hours of admission, N = 544), there was a consistent 38% risk reduction in cardiovascular death or MI (95% CI 0.37-1.05, P = 0.076) compared in patients who had delayed intervention (risk reduction 29%, 95% CI 0.54-0.92, P = 0.01). The benefit of clopidogrel was identical regardless of whether patients underwent an intervention during the initial hospitalization (12.0% vs. 8.3%, RR 0.68, 95% CI 0.50-0.92, P = 0.01) or more electively, after discharge (13.8% vs. 9.8%, RR 0.70, 95% CI 0.48-1.02, P = 0.06). Thus, regardless of whether the intervention was performed early or delayed, there were consistent benefits of clopidogrel. Taken together therefore, the data from CURE and PCI CURE suggest that in patients with ACS, clopidogrel is beneficial when used long term, both in patients undergoing PCI and in those treated medically.

The Clopidogrel for Reduction of Events During Observation (CREDO) study randomized 2116 patients who were to undergo elective PCI to receive, in addition to aspirin, either clopidogrel given as a

300 mg loading dose prior to PCI then continued at 75 mg/day for 1 year or a placebo loading dose prior to the procedure, then clopidogrel 75 mg for 4 weeks if a stent was placed, followed by placebo for 1 year.[70] The aim of the study was to assess the effects of a loading dose of clopidogrel given prior to PCI (i.e., pretreatment) and to assess the value of long-term therapy with clopidogrel and aspirin for 1 year. Approximately two-thirds of patients had unstable angina or recent MI as the indication for PCI. About 24% of patients received prespecified IV GP IIb/IIIa antagonist and 22% received bail-out intravenous GP IIb/IIIa antagonist. Overall, the study did not demonstrate a benefit of clopidogrel pretreatment on the outcome of cardiovascular death, MI, or urgent revascularization at 30 days (RRR 18.5%, 95% CI 14.2%-41.8%, P = 0.23).[70] However, in a prespecified subgroup analysis, those pretreated greater than 6 hours prior to PCI did appear to derive benefit from pretreatment (RRR 38.6%, 95% CI -1.6%-62.9%, P = 0.051). These data are consistent with the benefits of pretreatment found in the PCI CURE study, in which the duration of pretreatment was much longer than 6 hours. At 1 year, there was a significant benefit of clopidogrel therapy compared with placebo in reducing the combined risk of death, MI, or stroke (RRR 26.9%, 95% CI 3.9%-44.4%, P = 0.02). There was consistency of benefit in a wide variety of subgroups, including those with and without ACS, diabetes, and use of intravenous GP IIb/IIIa antagonist. Overall, there was a nonsignificant trend toward an increase in major bleeding with clopidogrel (8.8% vs. 6.7%, P = 0.07), most of which was procedure related.[70]

PATIENTS WITH ACS UNDERGOING CABG

Aspirin

There are currently no randomized trials of aspirin in patients with ACS undergoing CABG surgery. However, a systematic review of 20 trials demonstrated that, in patients undergoing CABG surgery, there is a 46% reduction in graft occlusion (variably defined angiographically or clinically) with the use of antiplatelet therapy (mainly aspirin) compared with control administered for a mean of 7 months (P < 0.00001).[67]

Thienopyridine

There are no randomized trials of thienopyridines compared with placebo in patients with ACS undergoing CABG surgery. However, in an analysis of patients with prior CABG surgery, there was a significant benefit of clopidogrel over aspirin in reduction of vascular death, MI, stroke, or rehospitalization.[68]

Combination Aspirin and Thienopyridine

The largest and most comprehensive experience of patients with ACS undergoing CABG treated with the combination of aspirin and clopidogrel comes from the

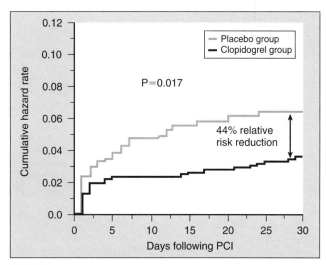

FIGURE 5-7. Effects of pretreatment with clopidogrel compared with placebo in stented patients (excludes those receiving open-label thienopyridine before percutaneous coronary intervention [PCI]). All patients received open-label clopidogrel or ticlopidine for a median of 30 days after PCI. Day 0 is the day of PCI. (Modified from Mehta SR, Zhao F, Yusuf S, Clopidogrel and percutaneous coronary intervention. Lancet 2002; 359:169, with permission.)

CURE trial. In this study, 2072 patients underwent CABG at a median of 25 days, with the effects of clopidogrel being consistent with the overall results of the CURE study on the primary outcome of cardiovascular death, MI, or stroke (14.5% clopidogrel vs. 16.2% placebo, RR 0.89, 95% CI 0.71–1.11).[61] Similar benefits were observed among the 1013 patients who underwent CABG during the initial hospitalization (RR 0.78, 95% CI 0.57–1.08). Overall, there was no significant increase in bleeding in patients undergoing CABG in the CURE study. However, most patients had stopped clopidogrel for various time periods prior to CABG. When clopidogrel was stopped more than 5 days prior to CABG, there was no excess in bleeding. When clopidogrel was continued to within 7 days of CABG, there was an increased bleeding risk (RR 1.55, P = 0.06).[61] There was no increase in TIMI major bleeding, regardless of whether clopidogrel was continued to within 5 days of surgery or not. Therefore, in the minority of patients who require CABG surgery after ACS, it is recommended to hold clopidogrel for about 5 days prior to surgery if possible.

CONCLUSION

Both aspirin and thienopyridines have been well studied in patients with ACS. In acute MI, there is good evidence that acute treatment with aspirin is effective in reducing major ischemic events. The combination of aspirin with the thienopyridine clopidogrel in acute MI is being investigated in large randomized trials. In patients with unstable angina or NSTEMI, aspirin is clearly superior to placebo in trials that were mostly conducted prior to the routine use of cardiac procedures such as PCI and CABG. These early studies have demonstrated that aspirin is beneficial in the treatment of unstable angina and NSTEMI, at a cost of a small increase in bleeding. The combination of aspirin and the thienopyridine clopidogrel has been studied in the largest trial in unstable angina and NSTEMI to date, the CURE study. This study demonstrated a clear benefit of aspirin and clopidogrel versus aspirin alone, with a highly significant 20% reduction in major ischemic events. There was a small excess in major bleeding, which was dependent on the dose of aspirin (with no significant excess in life-threatening or TIMI major bleeding) with combination therapy. A combined efficacy—safety endpoint (cardiovascular death, MI, stroke, and life-threatening bleeding) demonstrated clear benefit of clopidogrel over placebo. In those patients undergoing PCI, there was a 30% reduction in death or MI with aspirin and clopidogrel started prior to PCI followed by long-term therapy for a mean of 9 months, with no increase in major bleeding. The CREDO trial demonstrated a 27% relative risk reduction in death, MI, or stroke in patients treated with aspirin and clopidogrel for 1 year after PCI. In this study, two thirds of patients had unstable angina or recent MI. These trials suggest that the combination of aspirin and clopidogrel is beneficial in a broad range of patients with unstable angina and NSTEMI, regardless of management strategy.

REFERENCES

1. Sakariassen KS, Bolhuis PA, Sixma JJ: Human blood platelet adhesion to artery subendothelium is mediated by factor VIII-von Willebrand factor bound to the subendothelium. Nature 1979; 279:636–638.
2. Fox JE: The platelet cytoskeleton. Thromb Haemost 1993; 70:884–893.
3. Hoylaerts MF: Amplification loops: release reaction. In Gresele P, Page C, Fuster V, et al (eds). Platelets in thrombotic and non-thrombotic disorders. Cambridge University Press Cambridge, England, 2002.
4. Calvete JJ, Mann K, Schafer W, et al: Proteolytic of the RGD-binding and non RGD-binding conformers of platelet integrin GP IIb/IIIa: Clues for identification of regions involved in receptor's activation. Biochem J 1994; 298:1–7.
5. Mehta SR, Eikelboom JW, Yusuf S: Long term management of unstable angina. Eur Heart J 2000; 2(Suppl E):E6–E12.
6. Yusuf S, Flather M, Pogue J, et al: Variations between countries in invasive cardiac procedures and outcomes in patients with suspected unstable angina or myocardial infarction without initial ST elevation: OASIS (Organisation to Assess Strategies for Ischaemic Syndromes) Registry Investigators. Lancet 1998; 352:507–514.
7. Cronin L, Yusuf S, Flather M, et al: OASIS Registry 2-year follow-up: outcomes in patients with unstable angina or myocardial infarction without ST segment elevation admitted to hospitals with or without catheterization facilities. Eur Heart J 2000; 21:247.
8. Van Belle E, Lablanche JM, Bauters C, et al: Coronary angioscopic findings in the infarct-related vessel within 1 month of acute myocardial infarction: Natural history and the effect of thrombolysis. Circulation 1998; 90:26–30.
9. Goldstein JA, Demetrou D, Grines CL, et al: Multiple complex coronary plaques in patients with acute myocardial infarction. N Engl J Med 2000; 343:915–922.
10. Ross R: Atherosclerosis: An inflammatory disease. N Engl J Med 1999; 340:115–126.
11. Buffon A, Biasucci LM, Liuzzo G, et al: Widespread coronary inflammation in unstable angina. N Engl J Med 2002; 347:5–12.
12. Rioufol G, Finet G, Ginon I, et al: Multiple atherosclerotic plaque rupture in acute coronary syndrome: A three-vessel intravascular ultrasound study. Circulation 2002; 106:804–808.
13. Trip MD, Cats VM, van Capelle FJ, et al: Platelet hyperreactivity and prognosis in survivors of myocardial infarction. N Engl J Med 1990; 322:1549–1554.
14. Merlini PA, Bauer KA, Oltrona L, et al: Persistent activation of the coagulation mechanism in unstable angina and myocardial infarction. Circulation 1994; 90:61–68.
15. Flather MD, Weitz JI, Yusuf S, et al: Reactivation of coagulation after stopping infusions of recombinant hirudin and unfractionated heparin in unstable angina and myocardial infarction without ST elevation: Results of a randomized trial. OASIS Pilot Study Investigators. Eur Heart J 2000; 21:1473–1481.
16. Collinson J, Flather MD, Fox KA, et al: Clinical outcomes, risk stratification and practice patterns of unstable angina and myocardial infarction without ST elevation: Prospective Registry of Acute Ischaemic Syndromes in the UK (PRAIS-UK) Eur Heart J 2000; 21:1450–1457.
17. PURSUIT Trial Investigators: Inhibition of platelet glycoprotein IIb/IIIa with eptifibatide in patients with acute coronary syndromes. N Engl J Med 1998; 339:436–443.
18. OASIS-2 Investigators: Effects of recombinant hirudin (lepirudin) compared with heparin on death, myocardial infarction, refractory angina, and revascularisation procedures in patients with acute myocardial ischaemia without ST elevation: a randomised trial. Lancet 1999; 353:429–438.
19. Libby P: Current concepts of the pathogenesis of the acute coronary syndromes. Circulation 2001; 104:365–372.
20. Abbracchio MP, Burnstock G: Purinoceptors: Are there families of P2X and P2Y purinoceptors? Pharmacol Ther 1994; 64:445–475.
21. Hechler B, Leon C, Vial C, et al: The P2Y1 receptor is necessary for adenosine 5'-diphosphate-induced platelet aggregation. Blood 1998; 92:152–159.
22. Leon C, Hechler B, Vial C, et al: The P2Y1 receptor is an ADP receptor antagonized by ATP and expressed in platelets and megakaryoblastic cells. FEBS Lett 1997; 403:26–30.
23. ISIS-2 (Second International Study of Infarct Survival) Collaborative Group: Randomised trial of intravenous streptokinase, oral

aspirin, both, or neither among 17 187 cases of suspected acute myocardial infarction: ISIS-2. Lancet 1988; 2(8607):349-360.

24. Baigent C, Collins R, Appleby P, et al: ISIS-2: 10 year survival among patients with suspected acute myocardial infarction in randomized comparison of intravenous streptokinase, oral aspirin, both, or neither. BMJ 1998; 316:1337-1343.

25. Second Chinese Cardiac Study (CCS-2) Collaborative Group: Rationale, design and organization of the Second Chinese Cardiac Study (CCS-2): A randomized trial of clopidogrel plus aspirin, and of metoprolol, among patients with suspected acute myocardial infarction. J Cardiovasc Risk 2000; 7(6):435-441.

26. Lewis HD, Davis J, Archibald D, et al: Protective effects of aspirin against acute myocardial infarction and death in men with unstable angina. N Engl J Med 1983; 309:396-403.

27. Cairns J, Gent M, Singer J, et al: Aspirin, sulphinpyrazone, or both in unstable angina. N Engl J Med 1985; 313:1369-1375.

28. Theroux P, Ouimet H, McCans J, et al: Aspirin, heparin or both to treat unstable angina. N Engl J Med 1988; 319:1105-1111.

29. The RISC Group: Risk of myocardial infarction and death during treatment with low dose aspirin and intravenous heparin in men with unstable coronary artery disease. Lancet 1990; 336: 827-830.

30. Antithrombotic Trialists' Collaboration: Collaborative meta-analysis of randomised trials of antiplatelet therapy for prevention of death, myocardial infarction, and stroke in high risk patients. BMJ 2002; 324:71-86.

31. Reilly IAG, FitzGerald GA: Inhibition of thromboxane formation in vivo and ex vivo: Implications for therapy with platelet inhibitory drugs. Blood 1987; 69:180-186.

32. Gent M, Blakely JA, Easton JD, et al: The Canadian American Ticlopidine Study (CATS) in thromboembolic stroke. Lancet 1989; 1:1215-1220.

33. Gill S, Majumdar S, Brown NE, et al: Ticlopidine-associated pancytopenia: Implications of an acetylsalicylic acid alternative. Can J Cardiol 1997; 13:909-913.

34. Bennet C, Weinberg P, Rozenberg-Ben-Dror K, et al: Thrombotic thrombocytopenic purpura associated with ticlopidine: a review of 60 cases. Ann Int Med 1998; 128:541-544.

35. Kupfer Y, Tessler S: Ticlopidine and thrombotic thrombocytopenic purpura. N Engl J Med 1997; 337:1245 Letter.

36. Page Y, Tardy B, Zeni F, et al: Thrombotic thrombocytopenic purpura related to ticlopidine. Lancet 1991; 337:774-776.

37. Bennett CL, Connors JM, Carwile JM, et al: Thrombotic thrombocytopenic purpura associated with clopidogrel. N Engl J Med 2000; 342:1773-1777.

38. Herbert JM, Frechel D, Vallee E, et al: Clopidogrel, a novel antithrombotic agent. Cardiovasc Drug Rev 1993; 11:180-198.

39. Balsano F, Rizzon P, Violi F, et al: Antiplatelet treatment with ticlopidine in unstable angina: a controlled multicenter trial: the Studio della Ticlopidina nell'Angina Instabile Group. Circulation 1990; 82:17-26.

40. Balsano F, Coccheri S, Libretti A, et al: Ticlopidine in the treatment of intermittent claudication: A 21-month double-blind trial. J Lab Clin Med 1989; 114:84-91.

41. Janzon L, Bergqvist D, Boberg J, et al: Prevention of myocardial infarction and stroke in patients with intermittent claudication: Effects of ticlopidine: Results from STIMS, the Swedish Ticlopidine Multicentre Study. J Intern Med 1990; 227:301-308.

42. Mehta SR, Yusuf S, Clopidogrel in Unstable angina to prevent Recurrent Events (CURE) Study Investigators: The Clopidogrel in Unstable angina to prevent Recurrent Events (CURE) trial program: Rationale, design and baseline characteristics including a meta-analysis of the effects of thienopyridines in vascular disease. Eur Heart J 2000; 21:2033-2041.

43. The CAPRIE Steering Committee: A randomised, blinded, trial of clopidogrel versus aspirin in patients at risk of ischaemic events. Lancet 1996; 348:1329-1339

44. Hass WK, Easton JD, Adams HP, et al: A randomized trial comparing ticlopidine hydrochloride with aspirin for the prevention of stroke in high-risk patients: Ticlopidine Aspirin Stroke Study Group. N Engl J Med 1989; 321:501-507.

45. Bossavy JP, Thalamas C, Sagnard L, et al: A double-blind randomized comparison of combined aspirin and ticlopidine therapy versus aspirin or ticlopidine alone on experimental arterial thrombogenesis in humans. Blood 1998; 92:1518-1525.

46. Herbert J, Dol F, Bernat A, et al: The antiaggregating and antithrombotic activity of clopidogrel is potentiated by aspirin in several

experimental models in the rabbit. Thromb Haemost 1998; 80:512-518.

47. Cadroy Y, Bossavy JP, Thalamas C, et al: Early potent antithrombotic effect with combined aspirin and a loading dose of clopidogrel on experimental arterial thrombogenesis in humans. Circulation 2000; 101(24):2823-2828.

48. Hall P, Nakamura S, Maiello L, et al: A randomized comparison of combined ticlopidine and aspirin therapy versus aspirin therapy alone after successful intravascular ultrasound-guided stent implantation. Circulation 1996; 93:215-222.

49. Leon M, Baim D, Popma J, et al: A clinical trial comparing three antithrombotic drug regimens after coronary-artery stenting. N Engl J Med 1998; 339:1665-1671.

50. Schomig A, Neumann FJ, Kastrati A, et al: A randomized comparison of antiplatelet and anticoagulant therapy after the placement of coronary-artery stents. N Engl J Med 1996; 334:1084-1089.

51. Urban P, Macaya C, Rupprecht H, et al: Randomized evaluation of anticoagulation versus antiplatelet therapy after coronary stent implantation in high-risk patients: The Multicenter Aspirin and Ticlopidine Trial after Intracoronary Stenting (MATTIS). Circulation 1998; 98:2126-2132.

52. Bertrand M, Legrand V, Boland J, et al: Randomized multicenter comparison of conventional anticoagulation versus antiplatelet therapy in unplanned and elective coronary stenting: The Full Anticoagulation versus Aspirin and Ticlopidine (FANTASTIC) study. Circulation 1998; 98:1587-1603.

53. Moussa I, Oetgen M, Roubin G, et al: Effectiveness of clopidogrel and aspirin versus ticlopidine and aspirin in preventing stent thrombosis after coronary stent implantation. Circulation 1999; 99:2364-2366.

54. Muller C, Buttner HJ, Petersen J, et al: A randomized comparison of clopidogrel and aspirin versus ticlopidine and aspirin after placement of coronary-artery stents. Circulation 2000; 101:590-593.

55. Bertand ME, Rupprecht H-J, Urban P, et al: Double-blind study of the safety of clopidogrel with and without a loading dose in combination with aspirin compared with ticlopidine in combination with aspirin after coronary stenting: The clopidogrel aspirin international cooperative study (CLASSICS). Circulation 2000; 102:624-629.

56. Berger PB, Bell MR, Grill DE, et al: Frequency of adverse clinical events in the 12 months following successful intracoronary stent placement in patients treated with aspirin and ticlopidine (without warfarin). Am J Cardiol 1998; 81:713-718.

57. Mishkel GJ, Aguirre FV, Ligon RW, et al: Clopidogrel as adjunctive antiplatelet therapy during coronary artery stenting. J Am Coll Cardiol 1999; 34:1884-1890.

58. The CURE Investigators: Effects of clopidogrel in addition to aspirin in patients with acute coronary syndromes without ST segment elevation. N Engl J Med 2001; 345:494-502.

59. Yusuf S, Mehta SR, Zhao F, et al: Early and late effects of clopidogrel in patients with acute coronary syndromes. Circulation 2003: 107:966-972.

60. Budaj A, Yusuf S, Mehta SR, et al: Benefit of clopidogrel in patients with acute coronary syndromes without ST-segment elevation in various risk groups. Circulation 2002; 106:1622-1626.

61. Fox KAA, Mehta SR, Zhao F, et al: The risks versus benefits of clopidogrel treatment in acute coronary syndrome patients overall and those undergoing CABG: The CURE trial. Eur Heart J 2002; 23(Suppl) Abstract 2691:510.

62. Peters RJG, Mehta SR, Fox KAA, et al: The effects of aspirin dose when used alone or in combination with clopidogrel in patients with acute coronary syndromes: Observations from the Clopidogrel in Unstable angina to prevent Recurrent Events (CURE) study. Circulation 2003; 108:1682-1687.

63. Schwartz L, Bourassa MG, Lesperance J, et al: Aspirin and dipyridamole in the prevention of restenosis after percutaneous transluminal coronary angioplasty. N Engl J Med 1988; 318:1714-1719.

64. Savage MP, Goldberg S, Bove AA, et al: Effect of thromboxane A2 blockade on clinical outcome and restenosis after successful coronary angioplasty: Multi-Hospital Eastern Atlantic Restenosis Trial (M-HEART II). Circulation 1995; 93:3194-3200.

65. Mehta SR, Yusuf S, Peters RJG, et al:. Effects of pretreatment with clopidogrel and aspirin followed by long-term therapy in patients undergoing percutaneous coronary intervention: the PCI-CURE study. Lancet 2001; 358:527-533.

66. Mehta SR, Zhao F, Yusuf S: Clopidogrel and percutaneous coronary intervention. Lancet 2002; 359:169.

67. Collaborative overview of randomised trials of antiplatelet therapy—II: Maintenance of vascular graft or arterial patency by antiplatelet therapy. Antiplatelet Trialists' Collaboration. BMJ 1994; 308(6922):159-168.

68. Bhatt DL, Chew DP, Hirsch AT, et al: Superiority of clopidogrel versus aspirin in patients with prior cardiac surgery. Circulation 2001; 103(3):363-368.

69. Mehta SR, Yusuf S: Short- and long-term oral antiplatelet therapy in acute coronary syndromes and percutaneous coronary intervention. J Am Coll Cardiol 2003; 41:78S-87S.

70. Steinhubl SR, Berger PB, Mann JT, et al: Early and sustained dual oral antiplatelet therapy following percutaneous coronary intervention: A randomized controlled trial. JAMA 2002; 288: 2411-2420.

■■■c h a p t e r **6**

Heparin and Low–Molecular-Weight Heparin

David A. Morrow

The onset of unstable coronary disease usually occurs with erosion or rupture of an atherosclerotic plaque, exposing the highly procoagulant contents of the atheroma core to circulating platelets and coagulation proteins and culminating in formation of intracoronary thrombus.[1] In the majority of patients presenting with an acute coronary syndrome (ACS), the thrombus is partially obstructive, or only transiently occlusive, resulting in coronary ischemia without ST-segment elevation on the 12-lead electrocardiogram (unstable angina [UA] or non-ST elevation myocardial infarction [MI]). In the remaining approximately 15% of patients with ACS, the intracoronary thrombus completely occludes the culprit vessel causing an ST-segment elevation MI. Antithrombin and antiplatelet therapies aimed at halting the propagation of intracoronary thrombus and preventing recurrent thrombosis after initial therapy thus have become central to the early management of ACS.[2]

Coagulation Cascade as a Target for Therapy

Concomitant activation of platelets and the coagulation cascade contribute to the formation of flow-limiting coronary thrombus in ACS. When exposed to circulating blood, tissue factor produced by inflammatory monocytes within the atheroma binds to factor VII to initiate the extrinsic coagulation pathway and generate activated factor X (Xa) (Fig. 6-1).[3,4] Factor Xa converts prothrombin to thrombin (factor IIa), the key enzyme that generates fibrin from fibrinogen. Both factors Xa and IIa exert feedback interactions that enhance production of additional factor Xa as well as promote platelet activation and aggregation.[5] At each branch in this pathway, one molecule of activated enzyme is able to activate many molecules of its substrate protein, thereby amplifying each step in the coagulation cascade.

This cascade of proteins is restrained by several mechanisms, including the protein C system; tissue factor pathway inhibitor (TFPI); and the serine protease

inhibitor antithrombin (Fig. 6-1). Antithrombin exerts its inhibitory effect by binding to each of the serine proteases except VIIa (i.e., factors XIIa, XIa, IXa, Xa, and thrombin) to form highly stable, 1:1 complexes that are no longer capable of proteolysis. This interaction between antithrombin and key proteases in the coagulation cascade is enhanced substantially by endothelial cell proteoglycans. The catalytic action of endothelial proteoglycans is reproduced by the class of anticoagulant drugs called heparins.

Mechanisms of Action: Unfractionated and Low–Molecular-Weight Heparins

Unfractionated heparin (UFH) is a mixture of complex mucopolysaccharide chains of widely varying length and molecular weight (3,000–30,000 daltons) that typically is extracted for therapeutic use from porcine intestinal mucosa or bovine lung tissue. Low–molecular-weight heparin (LMWH) is manufactured by controlled chemical or enzymatic depolymerization of UFH to produce a more homogenous mixture of smaller chains (1000–10,000 daltons) with an average molecular weight (mean 4000–5000 daltons) that is approximately one-third that for UFH.[6] For heparins of either type, the interaction with antithrombin is mediated by binding of a unique pentasaccharide sequence on the heparin molecule and induces a conformational change in antithrombin that promotes a nearly 1000-fold increase in the affinity of antithrombin for factors Xa and IIa (Fig. 6-2).[7] Antithrombin that has been activated only by the specific pentasaccharide is capable of inhibiting factor Xa. However, for the heparin–antithrombin complex to bind to the heparin-binding domain of thrombin and exert its inhibitory action, an additional 13 saccharide residues are necessary (Fig. 6-2).[6]

In UFH, the majority of chains containing the pentasaccharide sequence are composed of at least 18 residues and thus are able to bind equally well to both thrombin and factor Xa, resulting in a ratio of anti-Xa:anti-IIa activity that is approximately 1.0, whereas in LMWH preparations only 25% to 50% of the chains are of

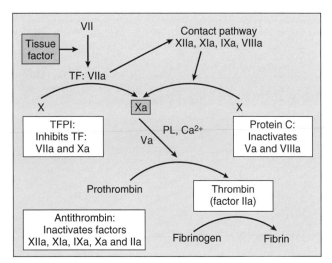

FIGURE 6-1. Summary of key participants in the coagulation cascade and its regulation. TF, tissue factor; TF: VIIa, tissue factor: VIIa complex; TFPI, tissue factor pathway inhibitor; PL, phospholipid; Ca^{2+}, calcium.

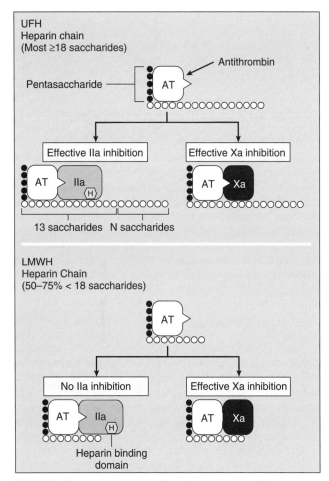

FIGURE 6-2. Activation of antithrombin (AT) and inhibition of factor Xa and thrombin (factor IIa) by unfractionated (UFH) and low-molecular-weight heparins (LMWH) (see text for details). Whereas the majority of chains in UFH are composed of at least 18 residues, in LMWH preparations, less than 50% of such chains are of adequate length to form a heparin–antithrombin–thrombin complex. Top and bottom panels depict representative heparin chains of >18 and <18 saccharides in length. H, heparin binding domain of thrombin.

sufficient length to stabilize the heparin-antithrombin-thrombin complex.[8] Because all chains with the requisite pentasaccharide are able to facilitate the binding of antithrombin to factor Xa, LMWHs carry a twofold to fourfold greater relative activity against factor Xa than against thrombin (i.e., a higher anti-Xa:anti-IIa activity ratio compared to UFH). Because there is amplification at each stage of the coagulation cascade with one molecule of factor Xa generating many molecules of activated thrombin, this enhanced relative activity against factor X may confer more effective inhibition of the coagulation cascade.

Other Differences Between Unfractionated Heparin and Low–Molecular-Weight Heparin

Although UFH has been a mainstay of anticoagulant therapy, it has a number of important limitations.[9] Most evident clinically is the relatively low and variable bioavailability that derives from extensive nonspecific binding to serum proteins, macrophages, and endothelial cells. The consequent fluctuation in anticoagulant activity necessitates frequent hematologic monitoring and poses a challenge to rapidly achieving and maintaining levels of anticoagulation within the target range. UFH also carries an appreciable risk of heparin-associated thrombocytopenia.[10,11] Heparin-related thrombocytopenia may occur in mild form in 10% to 20% of patients, with severe thrombocytopenia (platelet count <100,000) occurring in less than 2% of patients. Autoimmune heparin-induced thrombocytopenia with thrombosis occurs rarely (<0.2%) but carries very morbid complications.[12]

The LMWHs overcome a number of these deficiencies of UFH. LMWHs are subject to less nonspecific binding by blood constituents and plasma proteins and are less susceptible to neutralization by specific proteins such as platelet factor 4.[13-15] As a result, LMWHs exhibit more uniform bioavailability and more predictable levels of anticoagulation than UFH and thus may be administered subcutaneously without need for monitoring the activated partial-thromboplastin time (aPTT). Moreover, LMWHs also may have less propensity to stimulate, and even may act to suppress, platelet activation and aggregation.[16] LMWHs also appear to suppress coagulation through inhibition of the tissue factor-VIIa complex.[17,18] Specifically, whereas both UFH and LMWHs stimulate the release of TFPI, UFH appears to deplete blood levels of TFPI compared with LMWHs.[17-20]

There are now a number of available LMWH preparations that, based on differences in manufacturing, vary in the average length of their glycosaminoglycan chains and thus carry different relative anti-Xa:anti-IIa activities (Table 6-1). In addition, LMWH preparations vary with respect to their ionic form and release profile of TFPI.[6] The potential clinical impact of these differences should be considered in interpreting the individual and aggregate results of clinical trials of LMWH in ACS.[9]

TABLE 6-1 COMPARISON OF LOW–MOLECULAR-WEIGHT HEPARIN PREPARATIONS*

Generic name (trade name or synonym)	Mean molecular weight (daltons)	Anti-Xa: anti-IIa ratio	FDA indications
Enoxaparin (Lovenox, Clexane)	4200	3.8	**UA/NSTEMI**, DVT prevention/treatment
Nadroparin (Fraxiparine, Sleparina)	4500	3.6	**UA**, DVT prevention/treatment
Reviparin (Clivaparine)	4000	3.5	NA
Dalteparin (Fragmin)	6000	2.7	**UA/NSTEMI**, DVT prevention/treatment
Parnaparin (Fluxum, Minidalton)	4500–5000	2.4	NA
Ardeparin (Normiflo)	6000	1.9	DVT prevention
Tinzaparin (Innohep, Logiparin)	4500	1.9	DVT treatment with or without PE
Certoparin (Alphaparin, Sandoparin, Embolex)	4200–6200	†	NA

*In descending order of relative anti-Xa:anti-IIa activity.
†Published data not available.
FDA, Food and Drug Administration; UA, unstable angina; NSTEMI non-ST elevation myocardial infarction; DVT, deep venous thrombosis; NA, not applicable; PE pulmonary embolism.

TRIALS OF HEPARINS IN UNSTABLE ANGINA AND NON-ST ELEVATION MYOCARDIAL INFARCTION

Unfractionated Heparin

Although UFH has become entrenched in the clinical management of UA and non-ST elevation MI, the evidence from clinical studies directly testing its efficacy in this population is modest relative to that typically required for regulatory approval in the current era of large phase III cardiovascular trials. Nine randomized clinical trials have examined, with inconsistent results, the effect of UFH on the risk of death and/or recurrent ischemic events among patients with UA and non-ST elevation MI[21-29] (Table 6-2). These studies differed as to whether UFH was used alone or in combination with ASA (aspirin) and as to whether ASA was used as part of the control therapy. Four randomized trials included a comparison of UFH against placebo without ASA. In the first study to treat patients with UA early after presentation using a continuous infusion of UFH, treatment with heparin substantially reduced the risk of death or MI (0.8% vs. 13.6%, P = 0.0002) and refractory angina (8.5% vs. 22.9%, P = 0.002) compared with placebo.[23] Although two other small studies supported a similar reduction in ischemic events,[21,22] the largest of these four studies detected no advantage of UFH alone compared with placebo.[27] However, treatment with UFH in this trial was administered as intermittent bolus therapy beginning an average of 33 hours after presentation.[27] Although previous trials using intermittent bolus dosing indicated favorable effects,[21,22] at least one other clinical study has demonstrated less impact on recurrent ischemia and evidence of less inhibition of thrombin generation with intermittent boluses of UFH compared with a continuous infusion.[30]

Seven of the nine trials included study arms that compared treatment with UFH with or without ASA to ASA alone. Although one trial demonstrated a reduction in MI with UFH alone versus ASA,[24] none of the individual trials testing the addition of UFH to ASA have shown a significant effect on their respective primary efficacy endpoints (see Table 6-2). Nevertheless, two of these trials suggested an early benefit during the period of treatment with UFH.[26,27] Specifically, in the Antithrombotic Therapy in Acute Coronary Syndromes (ATACS) trial, patients treated with aspirin plus anticoagulation were at lower risk for death, MI, or recurrent angina at 14 days (10% vs. 27%, P = 0.004), but not at 3 months of follow-up (19% vs. 28%, P = 0.09).[26] Moreover, although pooled analyses of the data from this set of seven trials have provided slightly varied results owing to differences in the subset of trials included, together they suggest a 33% to 50% reduction in the risk of death or MI with combined antithrombin and antiplatelet therapy (Fig. 6-3).[26,31,32] For example, a pooled analysis of four trials considered by the American College of Cardiology and American Heart Association Guidelines Committee on Management of Unstable Angina demonstrated a 53% (95% CI, 12% to 77%) reduction in the risk of death or MI with the addition of UFH to treatment with ASA (Fig. 6-3).[32] This advantage comes with a detectable increase in minor but not major bleeding complications.[24,26,27]

On the basis of the overall directional consistency of these data and the strong pathobiologic rationale, the use of UFH (in combination with ASA) has been embraced in expert guidelines and in clinical practice for patients with non-ST elevation ACS.[32] Moreover, the results of subsequent placebo-controlled trials of LMWH have since provided additional support for the beneficial effects of antithrombin therapy in non-ST elevation ACS.

Dosing and Monitoring

The majority of benefit from UFH appears to be achieved during the period of intravenous (IV) administration and to be attenuated over the longer term[26,27] with a "rebound" increase in recurrent ischemic events on discontinuation suggested by several studies.[33,34] Because of the heterogeneity of anticoagulant effects of UFH, frequent monitoring of the aPTT is recommended[32]; however, few data exist to provide a definitive "therapeutic range." Small studies among patients with ACS have suggested that recurrent ischemic events occur more frequently in the setting of lower aPTT values and have supported a target range that is at least 1.5 times the mean control value.[35-37] The upper boundary of the target range is based on balancing effective anticoagulation versus the risk of bleeding.[38] In patients with STEMI treated with fibrinolytic the lowest rate of bleeding has been

TABLE 6-2 RANDOMIZED CLINICAL TRIALS EVALUATING THE EFFICACY OF UNFRACTIONATED HEPARIN (UFH) IN THE ACUTE MANAGEMENT OF PATIENTS WITH UNSTABLE ANGINA AND NON-ST ELEVATION MYOCARDIAL INFARCTION

Investigator/trial	Design	Size	UFH dosing	Comparator	Duration of treatment	Primary endpoint	Timepoint	Event rates (UFH vs. comparator)
DATA VS. PLACEBO								
Telford and Wilson, 1981[21]	Double-blind 2 × 2 (atenolol)	214	5000 U IVB + 5000 IV q6h	Placebo	7 days	New transmural MI	7 days	3.0% vs. 14.9%, P = 0.003
Williams et al, 1986[22]	Open-label	102	10,000 U IVB q6h	Placebo	2 days	Death, MI, RA	6 months	11.8% vs. 33.4%, P = 0.009
Theroux, 1988[23]	Double-blind 2 × 2 (ASA)	236*	5000 U IVB + 1000 U/h IV	Placebo	5–7 days	Death, MI, RA	5–7 days	9.3% vs. 26.3%, P < 0.001
RISC Group, 1990[27]	Double-blind 2 × 2 (ASA)	397*	5000 U IVB + 5000 IV q6h	Placebo	5 days	Death or MI	5 days	5.6% vs. 6.0%, P = 0.8
DATA VS. ASA								
Theroux et al, 1988[23]	Double-blind 2 × 2 (ASA)	243†	5000 U IVB + 1000 U/h IV + ASA	ASA 325 mg BID	5–7 days	Death, MI, RA	5–7 days	11.5% vs. 16.5%, P = 0.26
Theroux et al, 1993[24]	Double-blind extension of trial above	484	5000 U IVB + 1000 U/h IV (no ASA)	ASA 325 mg BID	5–7 days	MI	5–7 days	0.8% vs. 3.7%, P = 0.035
RISC Group, 1990[27]	Double-blind 2 × 2 (ASA)	399†	5000 U IVB + 5000 IV q6h + ASA	ASA 75 mg qd	5 days	Death or MI	5 days	1.4% vs. 3.7%, P = 0.14
Cohen et al, 1990 (ATACS Pilot)[25]	Open-label	69	100 U/kg IVB + infusion + ASA‡	ASA 325 mg qd	3–4 days	Death, MI or RA	12 weeks	43% vs. 25%, P = 0.11
Cohen et al, 1994 (ATACS)[26]	Open-label	214	100 U/kg IVB + infusion + ASA‡	ASA 162.5 mg qd	3–4 days	Death, MI, or RA	12 weeks	19% vs. 28%, P = 0.09
Holdright et al, 1994[28]	Single-blind	285	5000 U IVB + infusion + ASA	ASA 150 mg	2 days	Recurrent ischemia	2 days	18% vs. 24%, P = 0.18
Gurfinkel et al, 1995[29]	Single-blind	143	5000 U IVB + infusion + ASA	ASA 200 mg	5–7 days	Death, MI, RA, UR, major bleeding	5–7 days	63% vs. 59%, P = 0.6

*Because of the potential interaction between the effects of UFH and ASA, the data reported are restricted to UFH without ASA vs. placebo.
†Data are restricted to patients receiving UFH and ASA vs. ASA alone.
‡Patients were started on Coumadin after 2–3 days and continued for 12 weeks.
IVB, intravenous bolus; IV, intravenous; MI, myocardial infarction; RA, refractory angina; UR, urgent revascularization.

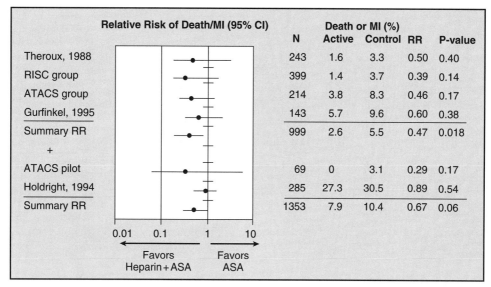

	N	Death or MI (%) Active	Control	RR	P-value
Theroux, 1988	243	1.6	3.3	0.50	0.40
RISC group	399	1.4	3.7	0.39	0.14
ATACS group	214	3.8	8.3	0.46	0.17
Gurfinkel, 1995	143	5.7	9.6	0.60	0.38
Summary RR	999	2.6	5.5	0.47	0.018
+					
ATACS pilot	69	0	3.1	0.29	0.17
Holdright, 1994	285	27.3	30.5	0.89	0.54
Summary RR	1353	7.9	10.4	0.67	0.06

FIGURE 6-3. Pooled analysis of trials comparing unfractionated heparin plus aspirin (ASA) to aspirin alone for the treatment of patients with non-ST elevation acute coronary syndromes. The first four trials are those considered by the American College of Cardiology/American Heart Association Guidelines Committee on Management of Unstable Angina.[2] The last two trials have been included in at least one other meta-analysis.[31] MI, myocardial infarction; RR, relative risk; CI, confidence interval.

observed in those achieving an aPTT between 50 and 70 seconds at 12 hours.[37] Higher levels of anticoagulation (aPTT > 2.0 times control) have not offered any detectable further reduction in recurrent ischemic events in patients presenting with UA/non-ST segment elevation myocardial infarction (NSTEMI).[39]

Weight-adjusted dosing of UFH has been suggested as a strategy to more rapidly achieve and reliably maintain target levels of anticoagulation.[40,41] Data from several randomized trials of weight-adjusted UFH in acute arterial and venous thrombotic disease have supported the superiority of a weight-based nomogram for rapidly achieving aPTT values above the target threshold.[40-43] The first weight-based nomograms to be evaluated did result in fewer patients with "sub-therapeutic" aPTT values at 6 to 8 hours.[40,41] However, the majority of patients (76%) had aPTT values above, rather than within, the target range.[41] These data prompted revision of several proposed weight-based nomograms to include less aggressive initial dosing.[41-43] A randomized study of one such nomogram (Fig. 6-4, Panel A) demonstrated that with a bolus of 60 U/kg IV and a 12 U/kg/hr infusion, compared with a standard nomogram, a higher proportion of patients achieved the target aPTT range of 45 to 70 seconds by 6 hours, with fewer patients exceeding the target range (Fig. 6-4, Panel B).[42] Notably, even with iterative refinement of such nomograms, only 75% of patients treated with UFH achieve aPTTs within an intended target range in the first 24 hours,[42] and even fewer (30%) maintain target levels of anticoagulation for 48 hours or longer.[43]

Guided by these data, current expert recommendations are for dosing of UFH based on the patient's weight with subsequent adjustments guided by a standardized nomogram to achieve a target range of 1.5 to 2.5 times the mean control aPTT (e.g. 45-75 sec for a laboratory with a mean control of 30 sec.[32] In clinical trials of UFH for UA/NSTEMI, UFH generally has been

continued for 2 to 5 days (Table 6-2). However, the optimal duration of treatment remains undefined.[32]

Low–Molecular-Weight Heparins

Based on the more predictable levels of anticoagulation, potential for improved efficacy, greater convenience, and logistic advantages for extended therapy that might sustain the early benefit achieved with antithrombin therapy, the LMWHs have been viewed as an attractive alternative to UFH for management of UA and NSTEMI.[9] Several LMWH preparations have been evaluated in randomized clinical trials, both in the acute phase of in-hospital management and for continued outpatient therapy.

Acute Medical Management

LMWH preparations have been compared both to ASA alone and combined therapy with UFH and ASA for the acute management of UA and NSTEMI (Table 6-3). In the first of such studies, nadroparin appeared to reduce the risk of recurrent cardiac ischemic events compared with UFH and ASA and was associated with fewer minor bleeding events (P = 0.01).[29] Subsequent trials with other LMWHs have expanded on these initial promising findings but have not provided uniform results when compared with UFH.

The safety and efficacy of dalteparin for patients with non-ST elevation ACS has been evaluated in two large randomized trials of similar general design but different control therapy (see Table 6-3).[44,45] In the acute phase of the Fragmin during Instability in Coronary Artery Disease (FRISC) trial,[44] administration of dalteparin, starting within 72 hours of symptoms and continuing for 6 days, reduced the risk of death or nonfatal MI at 6 days by 63% compared with placebo (Fig. 6-5). However, when the same regimen was tested in the Fragmin in Unstable Coronary Artery Disease (FRIC)[45] trial against active

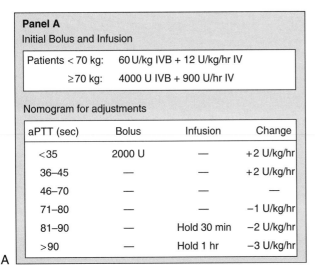

Panel A
Initial Bolus and Infusion

Patients < 70 kg:	60 U/kg IVB + 12 U/kg/hr IV
≥70 kg:	4000 U IVB + 900 U/hr IV

Nomogram for adjustments

aPTT (sec)	Bolus	Infusion	Change
<35	2000 U	—	+2 U/kg/hr
36–45	—	—	+2 U/kg/hr
46–70	—	—	—
71–80	—	—	–1 U/kg/hr
81–90	—	Hold 30 min	–2 U/kg/hr
>90	—	Hold 1 hr	–3 U/kg/hr

A

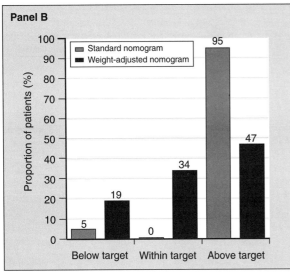

Panel B

B

FIGURE 6-4. Results of a randomized trial of a weight-based nomogram for dosing of unfractionated heparin (UFH). *A*: Weight-based nomogram. *B*: Proportion of patients achieving an aPTT within the target range by 6 hours. IVB, intravenous bolus; aPTT, activated partial thromboplastin time; hr, hour; min, minutes; sec, seconds. (Data from Hochman JS, Wali AU, Gavrila D, et al: A new regimen for heparin use in acute coronary syndromes. Am Heart J 1999;138:313–318, with permission.)

therapy with open-label UFH, dalteparin showed no reduction in death, MI, or recurrent angina (9.3% vs. 7.6% with UFH, P = NS). Results of a second large double-blind trial of nadroparin versus UFH and aspirin were similar to FRIC. Specifically, the Fraxiparine in Ischemic Syndrome (FRAXIS) trial showed comparable but not superior efficacy to UFH when nadroparin was administered for either 6 or 14 days after presentation with UA/NSTEMI.[46] Nevertheless, given low rates of bleeding and similar efficacy to UFH with dalteparin and nadroparin, both the FRIC and FRAXIS investigators concluded that these LMWHs are convenient and safe alternatives to UFH for the early management of UA/NSTEMI.

Two randomized, double-blind, parallel group trials have evaluated enoxaparin compared to UFH for the acute management of UA/NSTEMI. Both the Efficacy and Safety of Subcutaneous Enoxaparin in Non-Q-Wave Coronary Events (ESSENCE) and Thrombolysis In Myocardial Infarction (TIMI) 11B trials enrolled patients with rest symptoms in the prior 24 hours and randomly allocated them to treatment with enoxaparin 1 mg/kg subcutaneously twice daily or IV UFH.[47,48] In the ESSENCE trial, by 14 days patients treated with enoxaparin were at 20% lower risk of death, MI, or recurrent angina (Table 6-3). This benefit was sustained at 30 days and 1 year (13% relative risk reduction, P = 0.022) with directionally consistent effects with respect to each element of the composite endpoint and no evidence of a "rebound" increased in ischemic events after discontinuation of enoxaparin.[49] The TIMI 11B trial provided highly consistent evidence with a similar 24% reduction in the composite of death, nonfatal MI, or urgent revascularization, evident as early as 48 hours (Fig. 6-6).[48] A pooled analysis of the data from the 7081 patients enrolled in ESSENCE and TIMI 11B indicate an approximate 20% relative reduction in death or MI that is evident as early as 8 days and persists to 43 days of follow-up.[50,51]

The divergent results between trials of dalteparin and enoxaparin against active therapy have been challenging to interpret.[9] Differences in the enrollment criteria and design of these trials, as well as multiple differences in the biologic properties of the individual LMWHs, must be considered.[52] For example, it is plausible that with its greater relative anti-Xa:anti-IIa activity and potentially more potent inhibition of thrombin production, enoxaparin facilitates a greater early reduction in thrombus burden that translates into fewer subsequent ischemic events during long-term follow-up.[9] For these reasons, caution should be exercised in interpreting the results of analyses pooling these divergent trials.[53] Moreover, the possibility of clinically important differences in the effects of different LMWH preparations will remain unresolved in the absence of head-to-head comparison of the individual LMWH preparations. Preliminary results of one trial (Enoxaparin Versus Tinzaparin Trial [EVET]) comparing two LWMHs among patients with UA/NSTEMI demonstrated similar rates of bleeding, death, and rehospitalization for ACS but a lower rate of urgent revascularization through 30 days with enoxaparin compared with tinzaparin (16.3 vs. 26.1%, P = 0.019).[54] Enoxaparin also has been compared to a synthetic pentasaccharide (fondaparinux) that mimics the key region of heparins that bind to antithrombin. Although this agent has appeared more effective in preventing venous thrombosis,[55] no difference with respect to the risk of death or recurrent ischemic events was detected when compared to enoxaparin in a randomized trial among patients with UA (n = 1147) enrolled in the Pentasaccharide in Unstable Angina (PENTUA) trial.[56]

Taken together, the results of randomized trials of dalteparin, nadroparin, and enoxaparin have established these LMWHs as effective alternatives to UFH for the initial treatment of patients with non-ST elevation ACS. Moreover, existing data support a modest reduction (approximately 3% absolute) in death and recurrent ischemic events conferred by enoxaparin compared with UFH. As suggested by a cost-effectiveness analysis from the ESSENCE trial, it is possible that this reduction in recurrent ischemic events, along with reduced costs for

TABLE 6-3 RANDOMIZED CLINICAL TRIALS EVALUATING THE EFFICACY OF LOW–MOLECULAR-WEIGHT HEPARINS IN THE ACUTE AND CHRONIC PHASE MANAGEMENT OF PATIENTS WITH UNSTABLE ANGINA AND NON-ST ELEVATION MYOCARDIAL INFARCTION

TRIALS OF ACUTE-PHASE LMWH THERAPY

Investigator/trial	Design	Size	LMWH	Comparator	Acute-phase duration	Primary endpoint	Timepoint	Event rates
Gurfinkel et al, 1995[29]	Single-blind	219	Nadroparin 214 U/kg SC bid	UFH	5–7 days	MI, RA, UR, major bleed	7 days	22% vs. 63%, P = 0.0001
FRISC Study Group, 1996[44]	Double-blind	1506	Dalteparin 120 U/kg SC q12h*	Placebo	6 days	Death or MI	6 days	1.8% vs. 4.8%, P = 0.001
Klein et al, 1997 (FRIC)[45]	Open-label†	1482	Dalteparin 120 U/kg SC q12h	UFH	6 days	Death or MI	6 days	3.9% vs. 3.6%, P = NS
Cohen et al, 1997 (ESSENCE)[47]	Double-blind	3171	Enoxaparin 1 mg/kg SC q12h	UFH	2–8 days	Death, MI, or UR	14 days	16.6% vs. 19.8%, P = 0.019
Antman et al, 1999 (TIMI 11B)[48]	Double-blind	3910	Enoxaparin 30 mg IVB + 1 mg/kg SC q12h	UFH	3–8 days	Death, MI, or UR	8 days	12.4% vs. 14.5%, P = 0.048
FRAXIS Investigators, 1999[46]	Double-blind	3468	Nadroparin 86 U/kg IVB + 86 U/kg SC bid	UFH	6 days	Death, MI, RA, UA	6 days	14.8% vs. 14.9%, P = NS
Goodman, 2002 (INTERACT)[80]	Open-label	746	Enoxaparin 1 mg/kg SC q12h	UFH	4 days	Major bleeding‡	4 days	1.8% vs. 4.6%, P = 0.03

TRIALS OF EXTENDED LMWH THERAPY

Investigator	Design	Size	LMWH	Comparator	Chronic-phase duration	Primary endpoint	Timepoint	Event Rates
FRISC Study Group, 1996[44]	Double-blind	1506	Dalteparin 7500 U SC qd	Placebo	40 days	Death or MI	40 days	8.0% and 10.7%, P = 0.07
Klein et al, 1997 (FRIC)[45]	Double-blind	1482	Dalteparin 7500 U SC qd	Placebo	45 days	Death, MI, or RA	45 days	12.3% vs. 12.3%, P = NS
Antman et al, 1999 (TIMI 11B)[48]	Double-blind	3910	Enoxaparin 40 mg or 60 mg SC bid (based on weight)	Placebo	43 days	Death, MI, or UR	43 days	17.3% vs. 19.7%, P = 0.048
FRISC II, 1999[58]	Double-blind	2267	Dalteparin 5000 U or 7500 U SC bid (based on weight)	Placebo	90 days	Death or MI	30 days / 90 days	3.1% vs. 5.9%, P = 0.002 / 6.7% vs. 8.0%, P = 0.2
FRAXIS Investigators, 1999[46]	Double-blind	3468	Nadroparin 86 U/kg SC bid	UFH × 6 days	14 days	Death, MI, RA, UA	14 days	20.0% vs. 18.1%, P = NS

*Up to a maximum dose of 10,000 IU.
†FRIC was open-labeled during the acute phase and double-blinded during the chronic phase. ‡Death or MI was a secondary endpoint (5.0 vs. 9.0%, P = 0.03).
LMWH, low–molecular-weight heparin; UFH, unfractionated heparin; MI, myocardial infarction; RA, refractory angina; UR, urgent revascularization; NSTEMI, non-ST elevation myocardial infarction; UA, unstable angina.

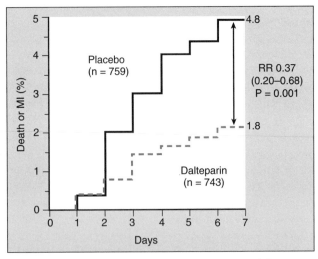

FIGURE 6-5. Kaplan-Meier plots of time to first event of the primary endpoint of death or myocardial infarction (MI) during treatment with dalteparin or placebo in the FRISC Trial. RR, relative reduction. (Modified from FRISC Study Group. Low-molecular-weight heparin during instability in coronary artery disease, Fragmin during Instability in Coronary Artery Disease (FRISC). Lancet 1996; 347:561–568, with permission.)

monitoring, may translate into an overall reduction in the costs of anticoagulant therapy with enoxaparin.[57] As such, the updated 2002 American College of Cardiology/American Heart Association (ACC/AHA) Guidelines for Management of UA/NSTEMI recommended *either* a LMWH administered subcutaneously or UFH given intravenously in conjunction with antiplatelet therapy (Class I, level of evidence A). The guidelines also included a Class IIa (level of evidence A) recommendation for enoxaparin as preferable to UFH for patients with UA/NSTEMI, unless a coronary artery bypass graft (CABG) is anticipated within 24 hours of initiation of treatment.[32]

Extended Anticoagulation with Low–Molecular-Weight Heparin

In light of consistent evidence from trials of UFH suggesting that the majority of benefit occurs during active therapy and that there may be an increased hazard on discontinuation of heparin, investigators have advanced the hypothesis that prolonged outpatient treatment with antithrombin might reduce the risk of recurrent ischemic events.[44,45,48] Given the ease and reliability of subcutaneous (SC) dosing of the LMWHs, they are particularly appealing for this purpose and have been assessed as extended therapy in five randomized double-blind trials (Table 6-3).

Dalteparin, enoxaparin, and nadroparin all have been tested for this purpose with similar negative results.[44-46,48,58] In FRISC and FRIC, dalteparin was continued from 6 to 45 days at a fixed dose, lower than that used in the acute phase, with progressive attenuation of any initial benefit and increased risk of minor bleeding (5.1% vs. 2.8% with UFH in FRIC). Similar findings emerged from the TIMI 11B trial in which there was no additional benefit beyond the acute phase of treatment but an increased rate of major bleeding compared with placebo (2.9% vs. 1.5%, P = 0.021) when enoxaparin was continued through 43 days.[48] Only the FRISC II trial, which used a more aggressive regimen of dalteparin dosed twice daily in two tiers based on body weight, has suggested any benefit from extended treatment.[58] In patients allocated to the conservative arm of this 2 × 2 trial of extended LMWH (3 months) versus placebo and early invasive versus conservative management strategies, dalteparin conferred an early 2.8% absolute reduction in the risk of death or MI that was evident at 30 days but was attenuated with time and no longer significant after 90 days (Fig. 6-7). These findings

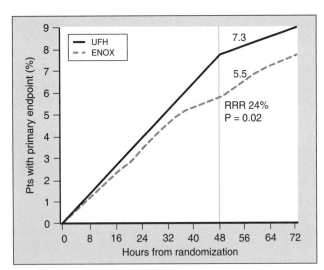

FIGURE 6-6. Kaplan-Meier plots of time to first event of the primary endpoint of death, myocardial infarction (MI), or urgent revascularization over the first few days of treatment with enoxaparin (Enox) and unfractionated heparin (UFH) in TIMI 11B. RRR, relative risk reduction; Pts, patients. (From Antman EM, McCabe CH, Gurfinkel EP, et al: Enoxaparin prevents death and cardiac ischemic events in unstable angina/non-Q-wave myocardial infarction: Results of the thrombolysis in myocardial infarction (TIMI) 11B trial. Circulation 1999; 100:1593–1601, with permission.)

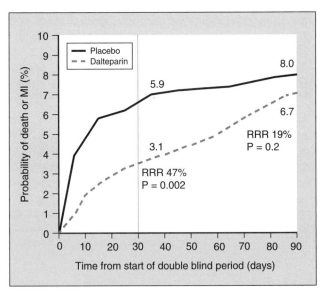

FIGURE 6-7. Probability of death or myocardial infarction (MI) over 3 months of therapy with dalteparin or placebo during the blinded treatment phase of the FRISC II trial. RRR, relative risk reduction. (From FRISC II Investigators: Long-term low-molecular-mass heparin in unstable coronary-artery disease: FRISC II prospective randomised multicentre study. Lancet 1999; 354:701–707, with permission.)

led the FRISC II investigators to conclude that with more frequent dosing, sustained therapy with dalteparin may be useful among patients managed with a conservative strategy or while awaiting delayed invasive evaluation.[58] However, for the majority of patients with UA and NSTEMI, extended use of LMWH beyond hospital discharge does not appear to be warranted.

Increased Efficacy of Low–Molecular-Weight Heparin in Specific Subgroups

Exploratory analyses from several trials have revealed subgroups that appear to derive particular benefit from the use of LMWHs, including some that may accrue benefit from prolonged outpatient therapy. Elevated levels of cardiac troponins have been shown in three trials to be useful for recognizing patients who are likely to benefit most from treatment with LMWHs.[58-60] Among patients with elevated levels of troponin I enrolled in TIMI 11B, in-hospital treatment with enoxaparin reduced the risk of death or recurrent ischemic events by approximately 50% compared with no detectable advantage among those with normal serial troponins.[60] Furthermore, observations from FRISC[59] and FRISC II[58] indicate that in the subgroup of patients with elevated levels of cardiac troponin T (66% of the population) prolonged treatment with dalteparin reduces the risk of recurrent cardiac events.

Lastly, other clinical indicators of high risk for death or recurrent ischemic events also identify patients who appear to derive the greatest *relative* as well as absolute benefit from treatment with enoxaparin. For example, when compiled in the TIMI Risk Score for UA/NSTEMI, seven clinical factors can be used to effectively stratify patients with respect to the risk of recurrent events as well as the benefit of treatment with enoxaparin (Fig. 6-8).[61]

Low–Molecular-Weight Heparins in Patients Undergoing Coronary Intervention

Despite the advantages of LMWH, some clinicians have been reluctant to switch from UFH to LMWHs because of uncertainty regarding the safety and efficacy of LMWHs in patients undergoing invasive evaluation or treatment with glycoprotein IIb/IIIa (GPIIb/IIIa) antagonists. This issue has taken on even greater importance in light of data supporting the superiority of early invasive versus conservative management of UA/NSTEMI and convincing evidence for the greater efficacy of timely primary angioplasty versus fibrinolysis for STEMI. Fortunately, the evidence base addressing the compatibility of LWMH with percutaneous coronary intervention (PCI) and GPIIb/IIIa inhibition is growing rapidly. To date the emerging evidence regarding use of LMWHs in these settings has been encouraging.[62]

Data from subgroup analyses in clinical trials of LMWHs for UA/NSTEMI have demonstrated similar rates of bleeding and recurrent ischemic events among patients undergoing initial medical treatment with LMWHs followed by transition to UFH for PCI.[63,64] For

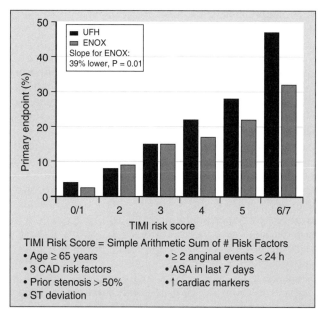

FIGURE 6-8. TIMI risk score for unstable angina/non-ST Elevation myocardial infarction (MI) reveals an increasing benefit of enoxaparin (ENOX) compared with unfractionated heparin (UFH) for the reduction of death, new MI, or urgent revascularization among patients enrolled in the TIMI 11B Trial. CAD, coronary artery disease. (Data from Antman EM, Cohen M, Bernink PJ, et al: The TIMI risk score for unstable angina/non-ST elevation MI: A method for prognostication and therapeutic decision making. JAMA 2000; 284:835–842, with permission.)

example, in a combined analysis from patients undergoing PCI in the TIMI 11B and ESSENCE trials, those who were randomized to enoxaparin and switched to UFH for PCI had similar rates of death or MI post-PCI (4.3% vs. 7.1%, P = 0.07) compared to those allocated to UFH.[63] In these studies (combined N = 1982), UFH generally was initiated 8 to 12 hours after the last dose of LMWH in anticipation of PCI.

LMWHs have been evaluated as the procedural anticoagulant in multiple nonrandomized open-label studies as well as in two randomized pilot trials. In one of the few randomized trials with active control therapy, reviparin given intravenously was associated with less frequent early thrombotic complications during complicated PCI (3.9% vs. 8.2%, P = 0.027) when compared to UFH for elective procedures in the Reduction of restenosis after percutaneous transluminal coronary angioplasty (REDUCE) trial.[65] In a randomized trial of enoxaparin versus UFH among 60 patients undergoing elective PCI, those receiving enoxaparin administered as a 1 mg/kg IV bolus had similar procedural outcomes to those treated with UFH.[66] Bleeding complications were infrequent in both groups (1/30 patients). The subsequent National Investigators Collaborating on Enoxaparin (NICE) 1 observational study of 828 patients undergoing elective or urgent PCI confirmed low rates of major bleeding with the same dosing regimen in a larger group of patients.[67] The 1.1% rate of major bleeding in NICE 1 may be contrasted with the 2.2% rate observed among patients randomized to UFH in the Evaluation of Platelet IIb/IIIa Inhibitor for Stenting (EPISTENT) trial.[68] When used in combination with abciximab for elective or urgent PCI in the NICE 4 study, enoxaparin at a dose of 0.75 mg/kg IV was associated with rates of major hemorrhage (0.6%), transfusion (1.8%), and thrombocytopenia (2.3%) that were similar to those reported in other contemporary interventional studies.[69] This same dosing strategy (0.75 mg/kg IV × 1) for enoxaparin has been studied in combination with eptifibatide in a randomized open-label trial using UFH as the control antithrombin for patients undergoing elective PCI.[70] In this pilot study (n = 261), patients treated with enoxaparin or UFH had similar rates of TIMI major bleeding (2.5% vs. 1.6%) and death, MI, or need for urgent revascularization through 30 days of follow-up (8.5% vs. 7.6%).[70] A recent study of enoxaparin administered as 0.5 mg/kg IV with and without glycoprotein IIb/IIIa inhibition indicates that this lower dose may be effective for procedural anticoagulation with lower rates of bleeding than observed in studies of 0.75 to 1.0 mg/kg.[71] Studies of dalteparin (60 IU/kg IV) in combination with abciximab also have suggested that dalteparin may be an acceptable alternative to UFH for procedural anticoagulation during PCI.[72]

Several studies have evaluated a strategy of transitioning patients from medical management of UA/NSTEMI to PCI while maintaining LMWH as the anticoagulant. Pharmacokinetic data indicate that therapeutic levels of anticoagulation are maintained within the first 8 hours after the prior dose of enoxaparin.[73,74] For example, among 293 patients receiving enoxaparin for UA/NSTEMI (1 mg/kg SC q12h) who underwent catheterization within 8 hours of the morning SC dose, 97.6% of patients were found to have anti-Xa activity above the lower boundary established for efficacy in trials of venous thromboembolism (0.5 IU/ml).[74] In this study, there were no abrupt closures or urgent revascularization attempts, and there was only one (0.8%) major bleeding event among the 132 patients who underwent PCI.[74] In patients undergoing PCI 8 to 12 hours after the preceding dose of enoxaparin, an additional bolus of 0.3 mg/kg IV achieved anti-Xa activity of 0.6 to 1.8 IU/ml in 96% of patients.[73] At 2 hours after the IV bolus, anti-Xa activity remained within the expected therapeutic range in 91% of patients.[73] Supported by these pharmacokinetic data, the NICE 3 study evaluated a strategy of continued anticoagulation with enoxaparin from presentation through completion of PCI.[75] No additional LMWH was administered for PCI performed within 8 hours of the last dose of SC enoxaparin, and 0.3 mg/kg was given intravenously if a procedure was to begin more than 8 hours after the most recent dose of LMWH.[75] Of the 700 patients enrolled in this observational study, the majority (645) received a GPIIb/IIIa inhibitor selected at the managing physician's discretion and 46% of patients underwent PCI. A preliminary report of the results of this uncontrolled study showed a rate of non-CABG bleeding (2.0%) that is similar to the cumulative experience from prior studies of GPIIb/IIIa inhibitors with UFH.[76]

Emerging technology has made available a method for point-of-care monitoring of anticoagulation with enoxaparin.[77] Additional studies will clarify the role of such measurements in routine clinical practice.

Use of Low–Molecular-Weight Heparin in Combination with GPIIb/IIIa Antagonists

An additional area of clinical interest is the safety and efficacy of combining LMWHs with GPIIb/IIIa antagonists for the medical management of ACS. Studied in the randomized, double-blind Antithrombotic Combination Using Tirofiban and Enoxaparin (ACUTE) I and II trials, treatment with the LMWH versus UFH in conjunction with tirofiban was associated with comparable, low rates of major bleeding (0.6% vs. 0.5%), as well as with more consistent inhibition of platelet aggregation in patients treated with enoxaparin.[78,79] At 30 days of follow-up, patients in the ACUTE II study (n = 525) randomized to enoxaparin had a significantly lower rate of recurrent angina or rehospitalization for UA (1.6% vs. 7.1%, P = 0.002). Such data indicate a possible advantage of LMWHs over UFH in combined antithrombin and antiplatelet therapy. These findings have been supported by a subsequent randomized, open-label trial of enoxaparin versus UFH in combination with eptifibatide for patients with UA/NSTEMI.[80] Results of the Integrilin and Enoxaparin Randomized Assessment of Acute Coronary Syndromes Treatment (INTERACT) trial indicate a lower rate of non-CABG major bleeding with enoxaparin (1.8% vs. 4.6%, P = 0.03).[80] Moreover, patients treated with enoxaparin had fewer episodes of recurrent ischemia detected by continuous ST monitoring and were at lower risk of death or nonfatal MI (5.0% vs. 9.0%, P = 0.03). In this study, 63% and 29% of patients underwent coronary angiography and PCI, respectively, by 30 days after enrollment (mean time to angiography, 4.1 days). Preliminary results of the Aggrastat to Zocor (A-to-Z) trial among 3987 patients with UA/NSTEMI treated with tirofiban and randomized to enoxaparin or UFH demonstrate that enoxaparin is non-inferior compared to UFH with respect to the risk of death, myocardial infarction, or refractory ischemia, and support similar safety of the two antithrombins.[81,82]

Data from at least one study including dalteparin provide observations regarding safety that are consistent with those for enoxaparin.[83] In the Global Use of Strategies to Open Occluded Coronary Arteries (GUSTO) IV ACS trial, 974 of 7800 patients enrolled were treated with dalteparin as an adjunct to therapy with abciximab or placebo for patients with non-ST elevation ACS. In a prespecified subgroup analysis, rates of non-CABG major bleeding were comparable among patients receiving LMWH and abciximab (1.3%) compared to those receiving either abciximab and UFH (0.8%) or LMWH and placebo (0.7%).[83]

On the basis of the available data, an international task force of experts has provided consensus guidelines for use of LMWH in non-ST elevation ACS and during PCI (Fig. 6-9).[62] Nevertheless, randomized data for patients undergoing early invasive management are few, and ongoing randomized studies of LMWH versus UFH in combination with GPIIb/IIIa inhibition are needed to provide additional information regarding the safety and clinical efficacy of LMWHs in the setting of contemporary therapy with potent antiplatelet agents and early invasive management. The Superior Yield of the New

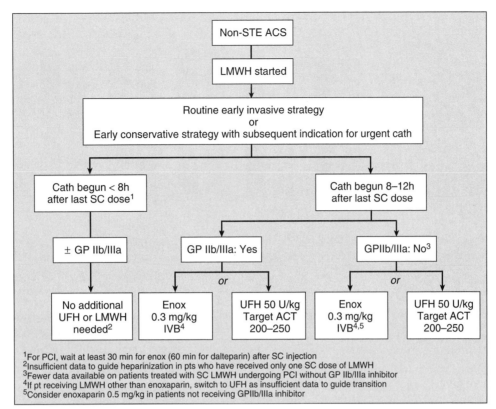

FIGURE 6-9. Algorithm for anticoagulation during percutaneous coronary intervention (PCI) among patients treated with low–molecular-weight heparin for non-ST elevation acute coronary syndromes. Non-STE ACS, non-ST elevation acute coronary syndrome; LMWH, low–molecular-weight heparin; Cath, cardiac catheterization; SC, subcutaneous; GP IIb/IIIa, glycoprotein IIb/IIIa receptor inhibitor; UFH, unfractionated heparin; Enox, enoxaparin; ACT, activated clotting time; IVB, intravenous bolus; pts, patients. (Modified from Kereiakes DJ, Montalescot G, Antman EM, et al: Low-molecular-weight heparin therapy for non-ST-elevation acute coronary syndromes and during percutaneous coronary intervention: an expert consensus. Am Heart J 2002; 144:615–624, with permission.)

Strategy of Enoxaparin, Revascularization, and Glycoprotein IIb/IIIa Inhibitors (SYNERGY) trial is enrolling approximately 8000 patients with UA/NSTEMI to be managed with an early invasive management strategy incorporating GPIIb/IIIa inhibition and randomly allocated to adjunctive treatment with UFH or enoxaparin administered in a strategy similar to that from NICE 3.[84] Such trials are needed to provide an important evidence base for clinicians managing patients with early-invasive and aggressive antiplatelet and antithrombin therapies.[62]

TRIALS OF HEPARINS IN ST-SEGMENT ELEVATION MYOCARDIAL INFARCTION

The potential benefits of acute therapy with antithrombins in ST-segment elevation MI (STEMI) are multiple, including preventing venous thromboembolic events and ventricular thrombus formation and facilitating more rapid and durable patency of the infarct-related artery. Nevertheless, the data from clinical trials have left sufficient questions to fuel continued debate. In particular, as reperfusion therapy has evolved, the relevance of data from previous clinical trials has become less certain. However, emerging placebo-controlled data with LMWHs used as an adjunct to contemporary reperfusion regiments are now providing additional support for acute administration of antithrombins in STEMI.

Unfractionated Heparin

Evidence for a reduction in venous thromboembolic events, stroke, and reinfarction with early administration of IV UFH originated from trials performed before the introduction of fibrinolytic therapy or the widespread and routine use of ASA, beta blockers, and angiotensin-converting enzyme inhibitors.[85] Together, data from 21 trials (n = 5459) of UFH versus placebo in patients with STEMI treated without aspirin and, for the majority, without fibrinolytic indicate 35 ± 11 fewer deaths, 15 ± 8 fewer reinfarctions, and 10 ± 4 fewer strokes per 1000 patients treated with UFH.[85,86] This 25% relative reduction in mortality came at the cost of 10 ± 4 additional episodes of major bleeding per 1000 treated.[85,86] These data support expert recommendations (Class IIa) for use of UFH in patients not treated with fibrinolytic therapy.[87]

Trials of Unfractionated Heparin as an Adjunct to Fibrinolysis

Owing to differences in the degree of systemic fibrinolysis between the nonspecific fibrinolytic agents (streptokinase, anistreplase, and urokinase) and the direct plasminogen activators (alteplase, reteplase, and tenecteplase), the degree of anticoagulation caused by production of fibrin degradation products and the

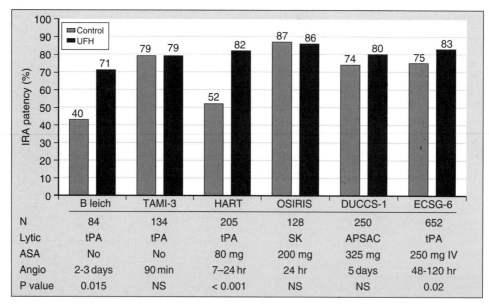

FIGURE 6-10. Rates of patency of the infarct-related artery (IRA) after fibrinolysis with and without adjunctive unfractionated heparin (UFH). Lytic, fibrinolytic; tPA, alteplase; SK, streptokinase APSAC, anistreplase; ASA, aspirin; IV, intravenous; Angio, indicates the timing of coronary angiography relative to the initiation of fibrinolytic; NS, not significant.

need for adjunctive antithrombin also may differ. As such, expert recommendations regarding the need for and route of administration of UFH generally have addressed these two groups of agents separately.[87] However, clinical trials evaluating UFH versus placebo as adjuncts to fibrinolysis were not all designed along these lines.

Angiographic Data

At least six clinical trials have provided angiographic assessment of the impact of UFH on patency of the infarct-related artery after initiation of fibrinolysis for STEMI (Fig. 6-10).[88–93] The varied results of these studies are challenging to interpret in light of important differences regarding the use of aspirin, the fibrinolytic and dose administered, and the timing of angiographic assessment. Overall, these data at least raise the possibility that adjunctive therapy with UFH may enhance late patency after the administration of alteplase. The available data to date do not support a very early (e.g., 60–90 minutes) advantage of treatment with UFH in establishing angiographic patency of the infarct-related artery in conjunction with fibrinolysis.[92] Furthermore, immediate IV administration of UFH showed no detectable advantage compared to delayed SC UFH with respect to patency at 90 minutes (60% vs. 54%, P = 0.15) or at 24 hours (80% vs. 77%, P = 0.6) in patients receiving streptokinase.[94]

Clinical Data

Data regarding the clinical efficacy of UFH as an adjunct to fibrinolysis are available both from several large randomized trials as well as the smaller angiographic studies (Table 6-4).[88–91,93,95–99] Although not relevant to contemporary management of STEMI because aspirin was not administered, the *Studio sulla Calciparina nell'Angina e nella Trombis ventricolare nell'Infarcto* (SCATI) trial included a subgroup of patients who were treated with

streptokinase and randomized to receive an IV bolus followed by SC UFH or placebo.[96] During in-hospital follow-up, UFH was associated with a trend toward lower mortality (4.6% vs. 8.8%, P = 0.08) and stroke (0% vs. 0.9%, P = 0.15).[96] The Gruppo Italiano per lo Studio della Sopravvivenza nell'Infarcto Miocardico (GISSI-2),[97] its international extension,[98] and the Third International Study of Infarct Survival (ISIS-3)[99] trials compared SC UFH to placebo as an adjunct to fibrinolysis with streptokinase, anistreplase, and alteplase in patients treated with ASA. In the larger of these two studies (ISIS-3), patients receiving SC UFH suffered four to five fewer deaths per thousand compared with placebo during the period of treatment; however, by 30 days this trend was no longer statistically significant.[99] Similarly, in GISSI-2, patients treated with UFH had no detectable reduction in mortality or reinfarction.[97,98] Combined data from these two large clinical trials demonstrate no detectable advantage of UFH compared with placebo with respect to mortality through 35 days (10.0% vs. 10.2%, P = 0.37) or reinfarction (3.0% vs. 3.3%, P = 0.06).[100] However, a statistically significant increase in the risk of noncerebral major hemorrhage (1.0% vs. 0.7%, P < 0.001) was apparent with UFH.[100] In a subsequent pooled analysis of approximately 68,000 patients with data on in-hospital mortality available from six randomized clinical trials, the addition of UFH (either SC or IV) to aspirin was associated with 5 ± 2 fewer deaths (P = 0.03) and 3 ± 1 fewer reinfarctions (P = 0.04) for every 1000 patients treated.[86] However, when the data are limited to those patients treated with fibrinolytic, no advantage of UFH is detected (Fig. 6-11).

Intravenous Unfractionated Heparin and Nonspecific Fibrinolytics

Intravenous administration of UFH was compared to SC administration among patients treated with streptokinase in the GUSTO I trial with no difference detected

TABLE 6-4 RANDOMIZED CLINICAL TRIALS EVALUATING THE EFFICACY OF UNFRACTIONATED HEPARIN IN THE ACUTE MANAGEMENT OF PATIENTS WITH ST-SEGMENT ELEVATION MYOCARDIAL INFARCTION TREATED WITH FIBRINOLYTIC

Investigator/trial	Design (fibrinolytic)	Size	UFH dosing	Comparator	Duration of treatment	Mortality (UFH vs. comparator)	Timepoint	Major bleeding (UFH vs. comparator)
DATA VS. PLACEBO								
ISIS-2 Pilot, 1987[95]	Open-label (SK)	204*	Delay 12 h 24,000 U/24 h IV	Placebo	2 days	6.7% vs. 11.0%, P = 0.3	Hosp	1.0% vs. 0%, P = NS
SCATI, 1989[96]	Open-label (SK)	443[†]	2000 U IVB + 12,500 U SC q12h	Placebo	Hospitalization	4.6% vs. 8.8%, P = 0.08	Hosp	1.8% vs. 0.9%, P = 0.4
Bleich et al, 1990[90]	Open-label (tPA)	95	5000 U IVB + 1000 U/h IV	Placebo	48–72 hr	13.0% vs. 10.2%, P = 0.7	Hosp	0.5% vs. 0.5%, P = 1.0
DATA VS. ASA								
ISIS-2 Pilot, 1987[95]	Open-label (SK)	209[‡]	Delay 12 h 24,000 U/24 h IV	ASA	2 days	7.5% vs. 5.8%, P = 0.6	Hosp	0% vs. 1.0%, P = NS
GISSI-2, 1990[97,98]	Open-label (SK/tPA)	20,891	Delay 12 h 12,500 U SC q12h	ASA	Hospitalization	8.5% vs. 9.0%, P = 0.29	Hosp	1.0% vs. 0.5%, P = 0.0002
OSIRIS-3, 1992[93]	Open-label (SK/tPA/AP)	41,299[§]	Delay 4 h 12,500 U SC q12h	ASA	7 days	9.1% vs. 9.5%, P = 0.17	Hosp	1.0% vs. 0.8%, P = 0.005
ECSG-6, 1992[89]	Double-blind (tPA)	652	5000 U IVB + 1000 U/h IV	ASA	2–5 days	2.8% vs. 3.4%, P = 0.6	Hosp	0.9% vs. 1.3%, P = 0.7
DUCCS, 1994[88]	Open-label (AP)	250	Delay 4 h 360 U/kg/24 h IV	ASA	4 days	9.4% vs. 4.9%, P = 0.17	14 days	10.9% vs. 5.7%, P = 0.14

*Data are restricted to study subjects who received a fibrinolytic without aspirin.

[†]Data are restricted to study subjects who received a fibrinolytic.

[‡]Data are restricted to study subjects who received both a fibrinolytic and aspirin.

[§]Data are restricted to study subjects who received a fibrinolytic and had mortality follow-up.

UFH, unfractionated heparin; SK, streptokinase; h, hour; IV, intravenous; Hosp, hospitalization; IVB, intravenous bolus; SC, subcutaneous; tPA, alteplase; ASA, aspirin; AP, anistreplase

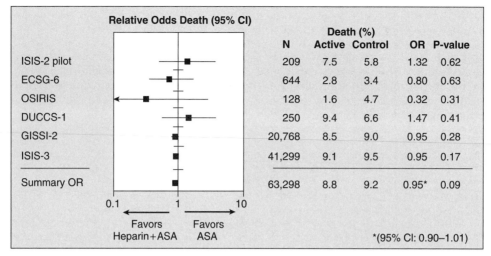

FIGURE 6-11. Pooled analysis of data from randomized trials of unfractionated heparin versus placebo as an adjunct to fibrinolysis for STEMI in trials that included routine administration of aspirin. Data are restricted to patients receiving fibrinolytic. OR, odds ratio; CI, confidence interval; ASA, aspirin. (Data from Collins R, MacMahon S, Flather M, et al: Clinical effects of anticoagulant therapy in suspected acute myocardial infarction: Systematic overview of randomised trials. BMJ 1996; 313:652–659, with permission; and individual trial references listed in Table 6-4.)

in mortality at 35 days (7.5% vs. 7.2%) and a statistically significant increase in severe bleeding (1.5% vs. 1.2%, P < 0.001).[101] Placebo-controlled data evaluating IV UFH as an adjunct to nonselective fibrinolytics are few. Among 250 patients receiving anistreplase in the Duke University Clinical Cardiology Studies (DUCCS)-1 trial, patients randomized to IV UFH had a higher rate of bleeding (32% vs. 17.2%, P = 0.006) with no difference in the primary endpoint of death, reinfarction, recurrent ischemia, or reocclusion of the infarct-related artery (P = 0.94).[88] Independently and considered together, the trials that have studied IV UFH against placebo with streptokinase and anistreplase have provided unpromising results.[86,100,102]

In light of the available data, routine administration of IV UFH within 6 hours of a nonselective fibrinolytic, such as streptokinase, is not recommended in the 1999 ACC/AHA Guidelines for Management of Acute MI.[87] However, *intravenous* administration of UFH may be considered on return of the aPTT to less than two times control (about 4–6 hours) for those at high risk for systemic embolic events (Class IIa) and *subcutaneous* administration considered for patients who are not deemed at high risk for systemic emboli (Class IIb).

Intravenous Unfractionated Heparin and Direct Plasminogen Activators

Adjunctive therapy with UFH for patients receiving agents with relatively higher fibrin-specificity (e.g., alteplase, reteplase, tenecteplase) has been supported by a stronger consensus of opinion; however, data from placebo-controlled clinical trials are sparse and exist only for alteplase. Angiographic data provide modest support for an increase in late patency with UFH in conjunction with alteplase (Fig. 6-10).[89-91] In addition, retrospective analyses from the LATE trial of patients treated with tPA (alteplase) 6 to 24 hours after onset of acute MI demonstrated lower 35-day mortality in patients treated with IV UFH at the physician's discretion compared to

those in which the physician elected to treat without UFH (7.6% vs. 10.4%).[103]

In the absence of randomized clinical trials designed to detect differences in clinical events, expert guidelines have concluded (Class IIa) that it "seems judicious to use heparin for ≥48 hours with alteplase."[87] No placebo-controlled data for adjunctive use of UFH exist with newer fibrin-specific fibrinolytics (reteplase and tenecteplase) because the phase III trials establishing their efficacy and safety each have used adjunctive IV UFH.[104,105]

Dosing and Monitoring

As in non-ST elevation ACS, the optimal dose of IV UFH to use in conjunction with fibrinolysis is not well defined. Exploratory analyses from large clinical trials have provided an evidence base on which to make reasonable clinical decisions.[87] Angiographic studies have shown a relationship between the aPTT and patency of the infarct-related artery 7 to 120 hours after fibrinolysis.[91,106] However, higher levels of anticoagulation are also associated with increased risk of major bleeding, including intracranial hemorrhage.[37,107] Patients at highest risk are those who are elderly, are female, have low body weight, have marked prolongation of the aPTT (>90–100 sec), or require invasive procedures.[108-112] Data from the GUSTO-1 trial suggest that the optimal clinical outcomes (death, reinfarction, stroke, and bleeding) were achieved among patients with an aPTT in the range of 1.5 to 2.0 times mean control.[37] Weight-adjusted initial dosing appears to be more reliable in achieving desired target levels of anticoagulation, and expert guidelines have moved toward lower caps for the initial bolus and infusion rates so as to avoid excessive levels of anticoagulation and the attendant bleeding risk.[42,87,107]

Similarly, the optimal duration of therapy with UFH is not defined and few randomized trials have addressed the issue. Based on the notion of allowing sufficient time for healing of ruptured intracoronary plaque, 3 to 5 days of anticoagulation had been an informal standard.

In a small trial of IV UFH continued for either 24 hours or through 7 to 10 days after fibrinolysis, no increase in ischemic events or coronary occlusion (19.8% vs. 18.9%) was apparent in the group receiving only 24 hours of anticoagulation.[113] However, given evidence for a "rebound" activation of thrombin after abrupt discontinuation of UFH, strategies for extended treatment with an antithrombin have been of substantial interest.

Low–Molecular-Weight Heparins

LMWHs have now been evaluated as an adjunct to fibrinolysis in at least eight clinical trials with at least three different fibrinolytics (Table 6-5). Together the results of these trials suggest an advantage of LMWHs in preserving late patency of the infarct-related artery and reducing the risk of reinfarction.

Angiographic Evidence

The initial randomized trials of LMWHs in STEMI were designed to evaluate angiographic endpoints, such as the success of epicardial and myocardial reperfusion both early and late after fibrinolysis. Data from three trials examining early angiographic endpoints have shown a modest trend toward higher rates of TIMI grade 3 flow but no definite advantage of LMWH with respect to early restoration of epicardial flow when compared with placebo or UFH (Fig. 6-12, Panel A).[114-116] Specifically, in the placebo-controlled Biochemical Markers in Acute Coronary Syndromes (BIOMACS)-II trial, patients (n = 101) treated with dalteparin and streptokinase showed a pattern of modestly higher rates of TIMI 3 flow at angiography in the first 20 to 28 hours (68% vs. 51%, P = 0.10).[114] Results were similar with enoxaparin versus active control (IV UFH) as an adjunct to alteplase (patency: 81.1% vs. 75.1% at 90 minutes) and tenecteplase (TIMI 3 flow: 51% vs. 50% at 60 minutes) in the Heparin and Aspirin Reperfusion Therapy (HART)-II and Enoxaparin and TNK-tPA with or without GPIIb/IIIa Inhibitor as Reperfusion Strategy in STEMI (ENTIRE)-TIMI 23 trials, respectively.[115,116] Nevertheless, the results of these studies indicate that early rates of patency are similar whether a LMWH or UFH is used as an adjunctive antithrombin to fibrinolysis.

Trials that have evaluated late patency suggest that the potential benefits of LMWH are more likely to reside with higher rates of durable reperfusion after fibrinolysis (Fig. 6-12, Panels B and C). When studied against placebo in conjunction with streptokinase in the Acute Myocardial Infarction-StreptoKinase (AMI-SK) trial, treatment with enoxaparin (30 mg IV bolus followed by 1 mg/kg SC every 12 hours for 3–8 days) was associated with increased patency (87.6 vs. 71.7%, P < 0.001) and TIMI 3 flow (70.3 vs. 57.8%, P = 0.01) at 8 days.[117] In the HART II trial, which included both early and late angiography after alteplase, the number of patients who experienced reocclusion of a patent infarct-related artery tended to be lower when treated with enoxaparin versus UFH (5.9% vs. 9.8%, P = 0.26, Fig. 6-12,

Panel C).[115] Angiography performed at 4 to 7 days after reperfusion with alteplase in the Assessment of the Safety and Efficacy of a New Thrombolytic Agent (ASSENT)-PLUS trial showed increased patency of the infarct-related artery (86.6% vs. 75.6%, P = 0.003) with a nonsignificant trend toward higher rates of TIMI 3 flow (69.3 vs. 62.5%, P = 0.16), and less visible thrombus (18.9 vs. 27.3%, P = 0.05) in patients treated with adjunctive dalteparin.[118]

Clinical Data

A potential clinical benefit of LMWHs as an adjunct to fibrinolysis has been supported by several trials, resulting primarily from reductions in recurrent ischemic events—an advantage that may be related to more durable patency of the infarct-related artery (IRA) (see Table 6-5). Three trials have examined LMWH versus placebo in patients with STEMI receiving streptokinase. Patients treated with dalteparin in the BIOMACS-II study had a lower incidence of recurrent ischemic episodes on continuous electrocardiogram monitoring (16% vs. 38%, P = 0.037).[114] Among the 496 patients studied in AMI-SK, those treated with enoxaparin were at lower risk of death, MI, or recurrent angina through 30 days (13.4 vs. 21.0%, P = 0.03).[117] Lastly, in the Fragmin in Acute Myocardial Infarction (FRAMI) trial, among 776 patients randomized to dalteparin or placebo, those treated with the LMWH had a reduced incidence of left ventricular thrombus or clinically apparent systemic embolism (14.2% vs. 21.9%, P = 0.03).[119]

Consistent, encouraging data have come from comparison of LMWH versus UFH as an adjunct to fibrinolysis (Table 6-5).[116,118,120,121] In the largest of these studies, the ASSENT-3 trial, 6095 patients were randomly allocated to a standard reperfusion regimen of full-dose tenecteplase with weight-adjusted UFH for at least 48 hours, full-dose tenecteplase with enoxaparin for 7 days, or reduced-dose tenecteplase with abciximab and UFH.[121] Patients allocated to the enoxaparin group were at significantly lower risk of death through 30 days or in-hospital reinfarction or ischemia compared with those treated with full-dose tenecteplase and UFH (relative risk 0.74; 95% CI 0.63–0.87).[121] This advantage was driven primarily by a reduction in reinfarction with enoxaparin (2.7% vs. 4.2%, P < 0.01) and was associated with an increased frequency of severe bleeding (3.0% vs. 2.2%, P < 0.01) but no detectable difference in intracranial hemorrhage (0.88% vs. 0.93%, P = 0.98). Major bleeding was particularly common in patients older than 75 years and was higher in those treated with either enoxaparin or abciximab. This observation of higher bleeding risk with enoxaparin in elderly patients receiving fibrinolysis was reinforced by findings from the ASSENT 3-Plus Trial (a prehospital extension of ASSENT 3).[122] Specifically, in patients older than 75 years, those receiving enoxaparin had a 6.7% rate of intracranial hemorrhage compared with 0.8% among patients treated with UFH (P = 0.01). No difference in the rate if intracranial hemorrhage was evident in

TABLE 6-5 RANDOMIZED CLINICAL TRIALS EVALUATING THE CLINICAL EFFICACY OF LOW–MOLECULAR-WEIGHT HEPARINS IN THE ACUTE MANAGEMENT OF PATIENTS WITH ST-SEGMENT ELEVATION MYOCARDIAL INFARCTION TREATED WITH FIBRINOLYTIC

Investigator/trial	Design (fibrinolytic)	Size	LMWH dosing	Comparator	Duration of LMWH	Clinical endpoint (primary or secondary)	Timepoint	Event rates (LMWH vs. comparator)
DATA VS. PLACEBO								
FRAMI, 1997[119]	Double-blind	517*	Dalteparin 150 U/kg SC q12h	Placebo	Hospitalization	Left-ventricular thrombus or systemic embolism	Hosp	14% vs. 22%, P = 0.03
BIOMACS-II, 1999[114]	Double blind (SK)	101	Dalteparin 100 U/kg SC + 120 U/kg 12 h	Placebo	24 hours	Episodes of ischemia on continuous ST monitoring	6–24 hr	16% vs. 38%, P = 0.04
AMI-SK, 2002[117]	Double-blind (SK)	496	Enoxaparin 30 mg IVB + 1 mg/kg q12h	Placebo	3–8 days	Death, re-MI, recurrent angina	30 days	13% vs. 21%, P = 0.03
DATA VS. UFH								
Baird et al, 1997[120]	Open-label (SK†)	300	Enoxaparin 30 mg IVB + 40 mg SC q8h	UFH × 4 days	4 days	Death, re-MI, readmission for ACS	90 days	25.5% vs. 36.4%, P = 0.04
ASSENT-PLUS, 2001[118]	Double-blind (tPA)	439	Dalteparin 120 U/kg SC q12h	UFH × 48 h	4–7 days	Reinfarction	30 days (7 days)	6.5% vs. 7.0%, P = ns (1.4% vs. 5.4%, P = 0.01)
ENTIRE-TIMI 23, 2002[116]	Open-label (TNK ± abciximab)	483	Enoxaparin ± 30 mg IVB + 0.3–1.0 mg/kg SC q12h‡	UFH × minimum of 36 h	8 days	Death or re-MI	30 days	4.4% vs. 15.9%, P = 0.005
ASSENT-3, 2001[121]	Open-label (TNK)	6095	Enoxaparin 30 mg IVB + 1 mg/kg SC q12h	UFH × 48 h	7 days	Death, in-hospital re-MI or refractory ischemia	30 days	11.4% vs. 15.4%, P = 0.0002

*Data are restricted to patients evaluable for the primary endpoint (776 patients were enrolled). †Predominantly SK and anistreplase (19 patients received alteplase)
‡Dose ranging for initial two doses followed by 1 mg/kg SC q12 h; clinical outcomes presented in this table are for LMWH vs. UFH pooled across all LMWH doses but restricted to patients receiving standard-dose TNK without abciximab.

LMWH, low–molecular-weight heparin; SC, subcutaneous; Hosp, hospitalization; h, hours; IVB, intravenous bolus; MI, myocardial infarction; UFH, unfractionated heparin; ACS, acute coronary syndrome; tPA, alteplase; TNK, tenecteplase.

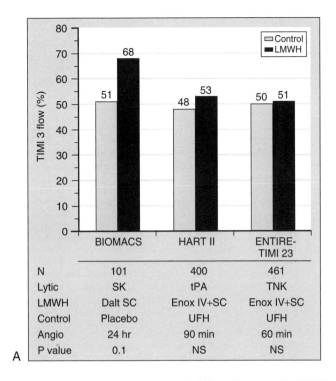

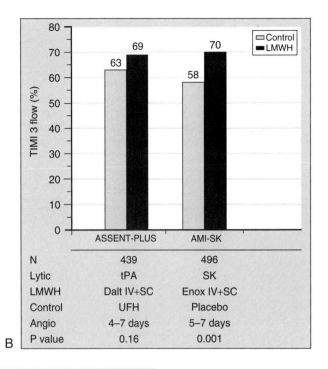

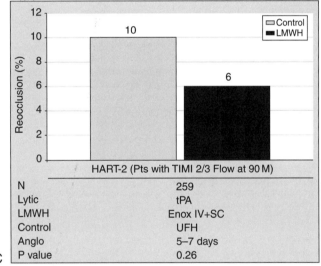

FIGURE 6-12. Angiographic trials evaluating low–molecular-weight heparins (LMWHs) as an adjunct to fibrinolysis. *A*: Assessment of early flow in the infarct-related artery. *B*: Assessment of late flow in the infarct-related artery. *C*: Assessment of reocclusion of the infarct-related artery. Lytic, fibrinolytic; SK, streptokinase; tPA, alteplase; TNK, tenecteplase; Dalt, dalteparin; SC, subcutaneous; Enox, enoxparin; IV, intravenous; UFH, unfractionated heparin; Angio, indicates the timing of angiography relative to initiation of fibrinolytic; NS, non-significant.

patients younger than 75 years. These preliminary findings have provided support for the benefits of antithrombin therapy in conjunction with fibrinolytics, including streptokinase, and have formed a basis for larger clinical trials that are ongoing.[123] At least one of these trails includes a reduction in the dose of enoxaparin among elderly patients.

When studied among patients ineligible for reperfusion therapy, combined therapy with enoxaparin and tirofiban was associated with a trend toward a lower rate of death, reinfarction, or recurrent ischemia compared to treatment with UFH along with or without tirofiban (OR 0.89, 95% CI 0.66 to 1.21).[124]

SUMMARY

The critical role of the coagulation cascade in acute ischemic heart disease continues to draw attention as a target for therapeutic intervention. Supported by a modest base of evidence from clinical trials and a strong pathobiologic rationale, UFH has been an inextricable component of care for patients with non-ST elevation and ST elevation ACS. Nevertheless, clinicians and researchers have sought alternative agents that might be free of the therapeutic and practical limitations of UFH. LMWHs are now supported by a robust and consistent body of clinical data for the acute management of UA/NSTEMI. Placebo-controlled trials of LMWHs have contributed additional, valuable support for the benefit of heparins in ACS, and randomized trials against UFH have shown similar (dalteparin, nadroparin) or superior (enoxaparin) efficacy with respect to ameliorating the risk of death and recurrent ischemic events. The database from trials of LMWHs in patients undergoing PCI, being treated with GPIIb/IIIa antagonists, or presenting with STEMI has been expanding with encouraging preliminary results. Additional randomized studies testing the safety and clinical efficacy of LMWHs in the setting of contemporary therapy with potent antiplatelet agents and routine invasive management are needed, and several are ongoing. These data will be important to clinicians as the use of LMWHs in the management of patients with ACS continues to increase.

REFERENCES

1. Lee RT, Libby P: The unstable atheroma. Arterioscler Thromb Vasc Biol 1997; 17:1859–1867.
2. Braunwald E, Antman EM, Beasley JW, et al: ACC/AHA guidelines for the management of patients with unstable angina and non-ST-segment elevation myocardial infarction: a report of the American College of Cardiology/American Heart Association Task Force on Practice Guidelines (Committee on the Management of Patients with Unstable Angina). J Am Coll Cardiol 2000; 36:970–1062.
3. Camerer E, Kolsto AB, Prydz H, et al: Cell biology of tissue factor, the principal initiator of blood coagulation. Thromb Res 1996; 81:1–41.
4. Moreno PR, Bernardi VH, Lopez-Cuellar J, et al: Macrophages, smooth muscle cells, and tissue factor in unstable angina. Implications for cell-mediated thrombogenicity in acute coronary syndromes. Circulation 1996; 94:3090–3097.
5. Dahlback B: Blood coagulation. Lancet 2000; 355:1627–1632.
6. Weitz JI: Low-molecular-weight heparins. N Engl J Med 1997; 337:688–698.
7. Danielsson A, Raub E, Lindahl U, et al: Role of ternary complexes, in which heparin binds both antithrombin and proteinase, in the acceleration of the reactions between antithrombin and thrombin or factor Xa. J Biol Chem 1986; 261:15467–15473.
8. Hirsh J, Warkentin TE, Raschke R, et al: Heparin and low-molecular-weight heparin: Mechanisms of action, pharmacokinetics, dosing considerations, monitoring, efficacy, and safety. Chest 1998; 114:489S–510S.
9. Antman EM: The search for replacements for unfractionated heparin. Circulation 2001; 103:2310–2314.
10. Warkentin TE, Chong BH, Greinacher A: Heparin-induced thrombocytopenia: Towards consensus. Thromb Haemost 1998; 79:1–7.
11. Deitcher SR, Carman TL: Heparin-induced thrombocytopenia: Natural history, diagnosis, and management. Vasc Med 2001; 6:113–119.
12. Warkentin TE, Levine MN, Hirsh J, et al: Heparin-induced thrombocytopenia in patients treated with low-molecular-weight heparin or unfractionated heparin. N Engl J Med 1995; 332:1330–1335.
13. Young E, Prins M, Levine MN, et al: Heparin binding to plasma proteins, an important mechanism for heparin resistance. Thromb Haemost 1992; 67:639–643.
14. Young E, Cosmi B, Weitz J, et al: Comparison of the non-specific binding of unfractionated heparin and low molecular weight heparin (Enoxaparin) to plasma proteins. Thromb Haemost 1993; 70:625–630.
15. Young E, Wells P, Holloway S, et al: Ex-vivo and in-vitro evidence that low molecular weight heparins exhibit less binding to plasma proteins than unfractionated heparin. Thromb Haemost 1994; 71:300–304.
16. Serra A, Esteve J, Reverter JC, et al: Differential effect of a low-molecular-weight heparin (dalteparin) and unfractionated heparin on platelet interaction with the subendothelium under flow conditions. Thromb Res 1997; 87:405–410.
17. Hansen JB, Sandset PM: Differential effects of low molecular weight heparin and unfractionated heparin on circulating levels of antithrombin and tissue factor pathway inhibitor (TFPI):
A possible mechanism for difference in therapeutic efficacy. Thromb Res 1998; 91:177–181.
18. Hansen JB, Naalsund T, Sandset PM, et al: Rebound activation of coagulation after treatment with unfractionated heparin and not with low molecular weight heparin is associated with partial depletion of tissue factor pathway inhibitor and antithrombin. Thromb Res 2000; 100:413–417.
19. Sandset PM, Bendz B, Hansen JB: Physiological function of tissue factor pathway inhibitor and interaction with heparins. Haemostasis 2000; 30:48–56.
20. Lupu C, Poulsen E, Roquefeuil S, et al: Cellular effects of heparin on the production and release of tissue factor pathway inhibitor in human endothelial cells in culture. Arterioscler Thromb Vasc Biol 1999; 19:2251–2262.
21. Telford AM, Wilson C: Trial of heparin versus atenolol in prevention of myocardial infarction in intermediate coronary syndrome. Lancet 1981; 1:1225–1228.
22. Williams DO, Kirby MG, McPherson K, Phear DN: Anticoagulant treatment of unstable angina. Br J Clin Pract 1986; 40:114–116.
23. Theroux P, Ouimet H, McCans J, et al: Aspirin, heparin, or both to treat acute unstable angina. N Engl J Med 1988; 319:1105–1111.
24. Theroux P, Waters D, Qiu S, et al: Aspirin versus heparin to prevent myocardial infarction during the acute phase of unstable angina. Circulation 1993; 88:2045–2048.
25. Cohen M, Adams PC, Hawkins L, et al: Usefulness of antithrombotic therapy in resting angina pectoris or non-Q-wave myocardial infarction in preventing death and myocardial infarction (a pilot study from the Antithrombotic Therapy in Acute Coronary Syndromes Study Group). Am J Cardiol 1990; 66:1287–1292.
26. Cohen M, Adams PC, Parry G, et al: Combination antithrombotic therapy in unstable rest angina and non-Q-wave infarction in nonprior aspirin users. Primary end points analysis from the ATACS trial. Antithrombotic Therapy in Acute Coronary Syndromes Research Group. Circulation 1994; 89:81–88.
27. The RISC Group: Risk of myocardial infarction and death during treatment with low dose aspirin and intravenous heparin in men with unstable coronary artery disease. Lancet 1990; 336:827–830.
28. Holdright D, Patel D, Cunningham D, et al: Comparison of the effect of heparin and aspirin versus aspirin alone on transient myocardial ischemia and in-hospital prognosis in patients with unstable angina. J Am Coll Cardiol 1994; 24:39–45.
29. Gurfinkel EP, Manos EJ, Mejail RI, et al: Low molecular weight heparin versus regular heparin or aspirin in the treatment of unstable angina and silent ischemia. J Am Coll Cardiol 1995; 26:313–318.
30. Neri Serneri GG, Gensini GF, Poggesi L, et al: Effect of heparin, aspirin, or alteplase in reduction of myocardial ischaemia in refractory unstable angina. Lancet 1990; 335:615–618.
31. Oler A, Whooley MA, Oler J, et al: Adding heparin to aspirin reduces the incidence of myocardial infarction and death in patients with unstable angina. JAMA 1996; 276:811–815.
32. Braunwald E, Antman EM, Beasley JW, et al: ACC/AHA 2002 guideline update for the management of patients with unstable angina and non-ST-segment elevation myocardial infarction: a report of the American College of Cardiology/American Heart Association Task Force on Practice Guidelines (Committee on the Management of Patients With Unstable Angina). Available at: http://www.acc.org/clinical/guidelines/unstable/unstable.pdf 2002. Accessed August 10, 2003.
33. Granger CB, Miller JM, Bovill EG, et al: Rebound increase in thrombin generation and activity after cessation of intravenous heparin in patients with acute coronary syndromes. Circulation 1995; 91:1929–1935.
34. Theroux P, Waters D, Lam J, et al: Reactivation of unstable angina after the discontinuation of heparin. N Engl J Med 1992; 327:141–145.
35. Melandri G, Branzi A, Traini AM, et al: On the value of the activated clotting time for monitoring heparin therapy in acute coronary syndromes. Am J Cardiol 1993; 71:469–471.
36. Tracy RP, Kleiman NS, Thompson B, et al: Relation of coagulation parameters to patency and recurrent ischemia in the Thrombolysis in Myocardial Infarction (TIMI) Phase II Trial. Am Heart J 1998; 135:29–37.
37. Granger CB, Hirsch J, Califf RM, et al: Activated partial thromboplastin time and outcome after thrombolytic therapy for acute myocardial infarction: Results from the GUSTO-I trial. Circulation 1996; 93:870–878.

38. Landefeld CS, Cook EF, Flatley M, et al: Identification and preliminary validation of predictors of major bleeding in hospitalized patients starting anticoagulant therapy. Am J Med 1987; 82:703–713.

39. Becker RC, Cannon CP, Tracy RP, et al: Relation between systemic anticoagulation as determined by activated partial thromboplastin time and heparin measurements and in-hospital clinical events in unstable angina and non-Q wave myocardial infarction. Thrombolysis in Myocardial Ischemia III B Investigators. Am Heart J 1996; 131:421–433.

40. Raschke RA, Reilly BM, Guidry JR, et al: The weight-based heparin dosing nomogram compared with a "standard care" nomogram. A randomized controlled trial. Ann Intern Med 1993; 119:874–881.

41. Hassan WM, Flaker GC, Feutz C, et al: Improved anticoagulation with a weight-adjusted heparin nomogram in patients with acute coronary syndromes: A randomized trial. J Thromb Thrombolysis 1995; 2:245–249.

42. Hochman JS, Wali AU, Gavrila D, et al: A new regimen for heparin use in acute coronary syndromes. Am Heart J 1999; 138:313–318.

43. Becker RC, Ball SP, Eisenberg P, et al: A randomized, multicenter trial of weight-adjusted intravenous heparin dose titration and point-of-care coagulation monitoring in hospitalized patients with active thromboembolic disease. Antithrombotic Therapy Consortium Investigators. Am Heart J 1999; 137:59–71.

44. FRISC Study Group: Low-molecular-weight heparin during instability in coronary artery disease, Fragmin during Instability in Coronary Artery Disease (FRISC). Lancet 1996; 347:561–568.

45. Klein W, Buchwald A, Hillis SE, et al: Comparison of low-molecular-weight heparin with unfractionated heparin acutely and with placebo for 6 weeks in the management of unstable coronary artery disease. Fragmin in unstable coronary artery disease study (FRIC). Circulation 1997; 96:61–68.

46. The FRAXIS Study Group: Comparison of two treatment durations of a low molecular weight heparin in the initial management of unstable angina of non-Q wave myocardial infarction: FRAXIS. Eur Heart J 1999; 20:1553–1562.

47. Cohen M, Demers C, Gurfinkel EP, et al: A comparison of low-molecular-weight heparin with unfractionated heparin for unstable coronary artery disease. Efficacy and Safety of Subcutaneous Enoxaparin in Non-Q-Wave Coronary Events Study Group. New Engl J Med 1997; 337:447–452.

48. Antman EM, McCabe CH, Gurfinkel EP, et al: Enoxaparin prevents death and cardiac ischemic events in unstable angina/non-Q-wave myocardial infarction. Results of the thrombolysis in myocardial infarction (TIMI) 11B trial. Circulation 1999; 100:1593–1601.

49. Goodman SG, Cohen M, Bigonzi F, et al: Randomized trial of low molecular weight heparin (enoxaparin) versus unfractionated heparin for unstable coronary artery disease: One-year results of the ESSENCE Study. Efficacy and Safety of Subcutaneous Enoxaparin in Non-Q Wave Coronary Events. J Am Coll Cardiol 2000; 36:693–698.

50. Antman EM, Cohen M, Radley D, et al: Assessment of the treatment effect of enoxaparin for unstable angina/non-Q-wave myocardial infarction. TIMI 11B-ESSENCE meta-analysis. Circulation 1999; 100:1602–1608.

51. Antman EM, Cohen M, McCabe C, et al: Enoxaparin is superior to unfractionated heparin for preventing clinical events at 1-year follow-up of TIMI 11B and ESSENCE. Eur Heart J 2002; 23:308–314.

52. Fareed J, Jeske W, Hoppensteadt D, et al: Low-molecular-weight heparins: Pharmacologic profile and product differentiation. Am J Cardiol 1998; 82:3L–10L.

53. Eikelboom JW, Anand SS, Malmberg K, et al: Unfractionated heparin and low-molecular-weight heparin in acute coronary syndrome without ST elevation: A meta-analysis. Lancet 2000; 355:1936–1942.

54. Michalis LK, Papamichail N, Katsouras C, et al: Enoxaparin versus tinzaparin in the management of unstable coronary artery disease (EVET Study) [abstract]. J Am Coll Cardiol 2001:365a.

55. Turpie AG, Gallus AS, Hoek JA: A synthetic pentasaccharide for the prevention of deep-vein thrombosis after total hip replacement. N Engl J Med 2001; 344:619–625.

56. Ferguson JJ: Meeting Highlights: American Heart Association Scientific Sessions 2001. Circulation 2002; 105:e37–41.

57. Mark DB, Cowper PA, Berkowitz SD, et al: Economic assessment of low-molecular-weight heparin (enoxaparin) versus unfractionated heparin in acute coronary syndrome patients: results from the ESSENCE randomized trial. Circulation 1998; 97: 1702–1707.

58. FRISC II Investigators: Long-term low-molecular-mass heparin in unstable coronary-artery disease: FRISC II prospective randomised multicentre study. Lancet 1999; 354:701–707.

59. Lindahl B, Venge P, Wallentin L: Troponin T identifies patients with unstable coronary artery disease who benefit from long-term antithrombotic protection. Fragmin in Unstable Coronary Artery Disease (FRISC) Study Group. J Am Coll Cardiol 1997; 29:43–48.

60. Morrow DA, Antman EM, Tanasijevic J, et al: Cardiac troponin I for stratification of early outcomes and the efficacy of enoxaparin in unstable angina: A TIMI 11B sub-study. J Am Coll Cardiol 2000; 36:1812–1817.

61. Antman EM, Cohen M, Bernink PJ, et al: The TIMI risk score for unstable angina/non-ST elevation MI: A method for prognostication and therapeutic decision making. JAMA 2000; 284:835–842.

62. Kereiakes DJ, Montalescot G, Antman EM, et al: Low-molecular-weight heparin therapy for non-ST-elevation acute coronary syndromes and during percutaneous coronary intervention: An expert consensus. Am Heart J 2002; 144:615–624.

63. Fox KAA, Antman EM, Cohen M: Are treatment effects of enoxaparin (low-molecular weight heparin) more marked in those undergoing percutaneous intervention: Results of the ESSENCE/TIMI 11B? [abstract]. Eur Heart J 2000; 21:3267A.

64. FRISC II Investigators: Invasive compared with non-invasive treatment in unstable coronary-artery disease: FRISC II prospective randomised multicentre study. Lancet 1999; 354:708–715.

65. Karsch KR, Preisack MB, Baildon R, et al: Low molecular weight heparin (reviparin) in percutaneous transluminal coronary angioplasty. Results of a randomized, double-blind, unfractionated heparin and placebo-controlled, multicenter trial (REDUCE trial). Reduction of Restenosis After PTCA, Early Administration of Reviparin in a Double-Blind Unfractionated Heparin and Placebo-Controlled Evaluation. J Am Coll Cardiol 1996; 28:1437–1443.

66. Rabah MM, Premmereur J, Graham M, et al: Usefulness of intravenous enoxaparin for percutaneous coronary intervention in stable angina pectoris. Am J Cardiol 1999; 84:1391–1395.

67. Young JJ, Kereiakes DJ, Grines CL: Low-molecular-weight heparin therapy in percutaneous coronary intervention: The NICE 1 and NICE 4 trials. National Investigators Collaborating on Enoxaparin Investigators. J Invasive Cardiol 2000; 12 Suppl E:E14–18.

68. The EPISTENT Investigators: Randomised placebo-controlled and balloon-angioplasty-controlled trial to assess safety of coronary stenting with use of platelet glycoprotein- IIb/IIIa blockade. Evaluation of Platelet IIb/IIIa Inhibitor for Stenting (EPISTENT). Lancet 1998; 352:87–92.

69. Kereiakes DJ, Grines C, Fry E, et al: Enoxaparin and abciximab adjunctive pharmacotherapy during percutaneous coronary intervention. J Invasive Cardiol 2001; 13:272–278.

70. Bhatt DL, Lee BI, Casterella PJ, et al: Safety of Concomitant Therapy with Eptifibatide and Enoxaparin in Patients Undergoing Percutaneous Coronary Intervention–Results of the Coronary Revascularization Using Integrilin and Single Bolus Enoxaparin Study. J Am Coll Cardiol 2003:41:20–25.

71. Choussat R, Montalescot G, Collet JP, et al: A unique, low dose of intravenous enoxaparin in elective percutaneous coronary intervention. J Am Coll Cardiol 2002; 40:1943–1950.

72. Kereiakes DJ, Kleiman NS, Fry E, et al: Dalteparin in combination with abciximab during percutaneous coronary intervention. Am Heart J 2001; 141:348–352.

73. Martin JL, Fry ETA, Serano A: Pharmacokinetic study of enoxaparin in patients undergoing coronary intervention after treatment with subcutaneous enoxaparin in acute coronary syndromes. The PEPCI Study. Eur Heart J 2001; 22 (Abstr Suppl):14.

74. Collet JP, Montalescot G, Lison L, et al: Percutaneous coronary intervention after subcutaneous enoxaparin pretreatment in patients with unstable angina pectoris. Circulation 2001; 103:658–663.

75. Ferguson JJ: Combining low-molecular-weight heparin and glycoprotein IIb/IIIa antagonists for the treatment of acute coronary syndromes: The NICE 3 story. National Investigators Collaborating on Enoxaparin. J Invasive Cardiol 2000; 12 (Suppl E):E10–13.

76. Ferguson JJ, 3rd: NICE-3 Preliminary Results. In: 22nd Congress of the European Society of Cardiology, 2000; Amsterdam, 2000.

77. Moliterno DJ, Hermiller JB, Kereiakes DJ, et al: A novel point-of-care enoxaparin monitor for use during percutaneous coronary intervention. Results of the Evaluating Enoxaparin Clotting Times (ELECT) Study. J Am Coll Cardiol 2003; 42:1132–1139.

78. Cohen M, Theroux P, Weber S, et al: Combination therapy with tirofiban and enoxaparin in acute coronary syndromes. Int J Cardiol 1999; 71:273-281.

79. Cohen M, Theroux P, Borzak S, et al; Randomized double-blind safety study of enoxaparin versus unfractionated heparin in patients with non-ST-segment elevation acute coronary syndromes treated with tirofiban and aspirin: The ACUTE II study. The Antithrombotic Combination Using Tirofiban and Enoxaparin. Am Heart J 2002; 144:470-477.

80. Goodman SG, Fitchett D, Armstrong PW, et al: Randomized evaluation of the safety and efficacy of enoxaparin versus unfractionated heparin in high-risk patients with non-ST-segment elevation acute coronary syndromes receiving the glycoprotein IIb/IIIa inhibitor eptifibatide. Circulation 2003; 107:238-244.

81. Blazing MA, De Lemos JA, Dyke CK, et al: The A-to-Z Trial: Methods and rationale for a single trial investigating combined use of low-molecular-weight heparin with the glycoprotein IIb/IIIa inhibitor tirofiban and defining the efficacy of early aggressive simvastatin therapy. Am Heart J 2001; 142:211-217.

82. SoRelle R: Late-breaking trials from the 52nd scientific sessions of the American College of Cardiology. Circulation 2003; 107:e9024.

83. Simoons ML: Effect of glycoprotein IIb/IIIa receptor blocker abciximab on outcome in patients with acute coronary syndromes without early coronary revascularisation: The GUSTO IV-ACS randomised trial. Lancet 2001; 357:1915-1924.

84. The SYNERGY trial: Study design and rationale. Am Heart J 2002; 143:952-960.

85. Collins R, MacMahon S, Flather M, et al: Clinical effects of anticoagulant therapy in suspected acute myocardial infarction: Systematic overview of randomised trials. BMJ 1996; 313:652-659.

86. Collins R, Peto R, Baigent C, et al: Aspirin, heparin, and fibrinolytic therapy in suspected acute myocardial infarction. N Engl J Med 1997; 336:847-860.

87. Ryan TJ, Antman EM, Brooks NH, et al: 1999 update: ACC/AHA Guidelines for the Management of Patients With Acute Myocardial Infarction: Executive Summary and Recommendations: A report of the American College of Cardiology/American Heart Association Task Force on Practice Guidelines (Committee on Management of Acute Myocardial Infarction). Circulation 1999; 100:1016-1030.

88. O'Connor CM, Meese R, Carney R, et al: A randomized trial of intravenous heparin in conjunction with anistreplase (anisoylated plasminogen streptokinase activator complex) in acute myocardial infarction: The Duke University Clinical Cardiology Study (DUCCS) 1. J Am Coll Cardiol 1994; 23:11-18.

89. de Bono DP, Simoons ML, Tijssen J, et al: Effect of early intravenous heparin on coronary patency, infarct size, and bleeding complications after alteplase thrombolysis: Results of a randomised double blind European Cooperative Study Group trial. Br Heart J 1992; 67:122-128.

90. Bleich SD, Nichols TC, Schumacher RR, et al: Effect of heparin on coronary arterial patency after thrombolysis with tissue plasminogen activator in acute myocardial infarction. Am J Cardiol 1990; 66:1412-1417.

91. Hsia J, Hamilton WP, Kleiman N, et al: A comparison between heparin and low-dose aspirin as adjunctive therapy with tissue plasminogen activator for acute myocardial infarction. Heparin-Aspirin Reperfusion Trial (HART) Investigators. N Engl J Med 1990; 323:1433-1437.

92. Topol EJ, George BS, Kereiakes DJ, et al: A randomized controlled trial of intravenous tissue plasminogen activator and early intravenous heparin in acute myocardial infarction. Circulation 1989; 79:281-286.

93. Col J: Infusion of heparin conjunct to streptokinase accelerates reperfusion of acute myocardial infarction: Results of a double-blind randomized study (OSIRIS). Circulation 1992; 86 (Suppl I):259.

94. The GUSTO Angiographic Investigators: The effects of tissue plasminogen activator, streptokinase, or both on coronary-artery patency, ventricular function, and survival after acute myocardial infarction. N Engl J Med 1993; 329:1615-1622.

95. ISIS (International Studies of Infarct Survival) pilot study investigators: Randomized factorial trial of high-dose intravenous streptokinase, of oral aspirin and of intravenous heparin in acute myocardial infarction. Eur Heart J 1987; 8:634-642.

96. The SCATI (Studio sulla Calciparina nell'Angina e nella Trombosi Ventricolare nell'Infarto) Group: Randomised controlled trial of subcutaneous calcium-heparin in acute myocardial infarction. Lancet 1989; 2:182-186.

97. Gruppo Italiano per lo Studio della Sopravvivenza nell'Infarto Miocardico: GISSI-2: A factorial randomised trial of alteplase versus streptokinase and heparin versus no heparin among 12,490 patients with acute myocardial infarction. Lancet 1990; 336:65-71.

98. The International Study Group: In-hospital mortality and clinical course of 20,891 patients with suspected acute myocardial infarction randomised between alteplase and streptokinase with or without heparin. Lancet 1990; 336:71-75.

99. ISIS-3 (Third International Study of Infarct Survival) Collaborative Group: ISIS-3: A randomised comparison of streptokinase vs tissue plasminogen activator vs anistreplase and of aspirin plus heparin vs aspirin alone among 41,299 cases of suspected acute myocardial infarction. Lancet 1992; 339:753-770.

100. Ridker PM, Hebert PR, Fuster V, et al: Are both aspirin and heparin justified as adjuncts to thrombolytic therapy for acute myocardial infarction? Lancet 1993; 341:1574-1577.

101. The GUSTO investigators: An international randomized trial comparing four thrombolytic strategies for acute myocardial infarction. N Engl J Med 1993; 329:673-682.

102. Mahaffey KW, Granger CB, Collins R, et al: Overview of randomized trials of intravenous heparin in patients with acute myocardial infarction treated with thrombolytic therapy. Am J Cardiol 1996; 77:551-556.

103. The LATE Study Group: Late Assessment of Thrombolytic Efficacy (LATE) study with alteplase 6-24 hours after onset of acute myocardial infarction. Lancet 1993; 342:759-766.

104. GUSTO III Investigators: A comparison of reteplase with alteplase for acute myocardial infarction. The Global Use of Strategies to Open Occluded Coronary Arteries (GUSTO III). N Engl J Med 1997; 337:1118-1123.

105. Assessment of the Safety and Efficacy of a New Thrombolytic (ASSENT) Investigators: Single-bolus tenecteplase compared with front-loaded alteplase in acute myocardial infarction: The ASSENT-2 double-blind randomised trial. Lancet 1999; 354:716-722.

106. Arnout J, Simoons M, de Bono D, et al: Correlation between level of heparinization and patency of the infarct-related coronary artery after treatment of acute myocardial infarction with alteplase (rt-PA). J Am Coll Cardiol 1992; 20:513-519.

107. Giugliano RP, McCabe CH, Antman EM, et al: Lower-dose heparin with fibrinolysis is associated with lower rates of intracranial hemorrhage. Am Heart J 2001; 141:742-750.

108. Antman EM: Hirudin in acute myocardial infarction. Safety report from the Thrombolysis and Thrombin Inhibition in Myocardial Infarction (TIMI) 9A Trial. Circulation 1994; 90:1624-1630.

109. The Global Use of Strategies to Open Occluded Coronary Arteries (GUSTO) IIa Investigators: Randomized trial of intravenous heparin versus recombinant hirudin for acute coronary syndromes. Circulation 1994; 90:1631-1637.

110. Sane DC, Califf RM, Topol EJ, et al: Bleeding during thrombolytic therapy for acute myocardial infarction: mechanisms and management. Ann Intern Med 1989; 111:1010-1022.

111. Berkowitz SD, Granger CB, Pieper KS, et al: Incidence and predictors of bleeding after contemporary thrombolytic therapy for myocardial infarction. The Global Utilization of Streptokinase and Tissue Plasminogen activator for Occluded coronary arteries (GUSTO) I Investigators. Circulation 1997; 95:2508-2516.

112. Krumholz HM, Hennen J, Ridker PM, et al: Use and effectiveness of intravenous heparin therapy for treatment of acute myocardial infarction in the elderly. J Am Coll Cardiol 1998; 31:973-979.

113. Thompson PL, Aylward PE, Federman J, et al: A randomized comparison of intravenous heparin with oral aspirin and dipyridamole 24 hours after recombinant tissue-type plasminogen activator for acute myocardial infarction. National Heart Foundation of Australia Coronary Thrombolysis Group. Circulation 1991; 83:1534-1542.

114. Frostfeldt G, Ahlberg G, Gustafsson G, et al: Low molecular weight heparin (dalteparin) as adjuvant treatment of thrombolysis in acute myocardial infarction—a pilot study: biochemical markers in acute coronary syndromes (BIOMACS II). J Am Coll Cardiol 1999; 33:627-633.

115. Ross AM, Molhoek P, Lundergan C, et al: Randomized comparison of enoxaparin, a low-molecular-weight heparin, with unfractionated heparin adjunctive to recombinant tissue plasminogen activator thrombolysis and aspirin: second trial of Heparin and Aspirin Reperfusion Therapy (HART II). Circulation 2001; 104:648-652.

116. Antman EM, Louwerenburg HW, Baars HF, et al: Enoxaparin as adjunctive antithrombin therapy for ST-elevation myocardial infarction: Results of the ENTIRE-Thrombolysis in Myocardial Infarction (TIMI) 23 Trial. Circulation 2002; 105:1642-1649.

117. Simoons M, Krzeminska-Pakula M, Alonso A, et al: Improved reperfusion and clinical outcome with enoxaparin as an adjunct to streptokinase thrombolysis in acute myocardial infarction. The AMI- SK study. Eur Heart J 2002; 23:1282.

118. Wallentin L, Bergstrand L, Dellborg M, et al: Low molecular weight heparin (dalteparin) compared to unfractionated heparin as an adjunct to rt-PA (alteplase) for improvement of coronary artery patency in acute myocardial infarction—the ASSENT Plus study. Eur Heart J 2003; 24:897-908.

119. Kontny F, Dale J, Abildgaard U, et al: Randomized trial of low molecular weight heparin (dalteparin) in prevention of left ventricular thrombus formation and arterial embolism after acute anterior myocardial infarction: the Fragmin in Acute Myocardial Infarction (FRAMI) Study. J Am Coll Cardiol 1997; 30:962-969.

120. Baird SH, Menown IB, McBride SJ, et al: Randomized comparison of enoxaparin with unfractionated heparin following fibrinolytic therapy for acute myocardial infarction. Eur Heart J 2002; 23:627-632.

121. Efficacy and safety of tenecteplase in combination with enoxaparin, abciximab, or unfractionated heparin: The ASSENT-3 randomised trial in acute myocardial infarction. Lancet 2001; 358:605-613.

122. Wallentin L, Goldstein P, Armstrong PW, et al: Efficacy and safety of tenecteplase in combination with the low-molecular-weight heparin enoxaparin or unfractionated heparin in the prehospital setting: The Assessment of the Safety and Efficacy of a New Thrombolytic Regimen (ASSENT)-3 PLUS randomized trial in acute myocardial infarction. Circulation 2003; 108:135-142.

123. White H: Further evidence that antithrombotic therapy is beneficial with streptokinase: Improved early ST resolution and late patency with enoxaparin. Eur Heart J 2002; 23:1233.

124. Cohen M, Gensini GF, Maritz F, et al: The safety and efficacy of subcutaneous enoxaparin versus intravenous unfractionated heparin and tirofiban versus placebo in the treatment of acute ST-segment elevation myocardial infarction patients ineligible for reperfusion (TETAMI): A randomized trial. J Am Coll Cardiol 2003; 42:1348-1356.

Thrombolytic Therapy

Peter Sinnaeve
Frans Van de Werf

The use of thrombolytic agents has dramatically changed the treatment of acute myocardial infarction (AMI) over the last two decades. As a result of the introduction of coronary care units in the 1960s and thrombolytic therapy in the 1980s,[1] short-term mortality in patients with ST-T-elevation AMI has decreased steadily over the last decades from more than 30% in the 1960s[2] to 5% to 6% in 2001 in patients randomized in thrombolytic trials[3,4] (Table 7-1). Nevertheless, data from contemporary registries suggests that mortality rates in daily practice outside clinical trials are significantly higher, ranging from 7%[5] to even 28%.[6] This difference between trials and routine practice probably reflects patient selection, underuse of reperfusion treatment, and high mortality rates in undiagnosed patients.[7]

Over the last few years, several attempts to improve on the shortcomings of current thrombolytic strategies have been tested in large clinical trials. These include the introduction of bolus administration of fibrinolytics and of novel, more potent antithrombotic cotherapies. For example, the combination of single-bolus administration of a thrombolytic agent and of a low–molecular-weight heparin not only is associated with low mortality rates, but its ease of administration makes it also very appealing for prehospital use. Ongoing clinical trials investigating prehospital thrombolysis or the combination of pharmacologic and mechanical interventions undoubtedly will further refine the therapeutic approach of AMI.

TRIALS OF THROMBOLYSIS IN ACUTE MYOCARDIAL INFARCTION

Pharmacologic reperfusion of occluded coronary arteries in patients was investigated as early as the 1950s.[8] In the 1960s and 1970s, several studies of intravenous thrombolytic therapy showed conflicting results, mainly because of small sample sizes, and different treatment protocols and endpoint analyses. A meta-analysis of these trials, however, showed a significant beneficial effect of thrombolytics on mortality.[9] Renewed interest in thrombolysis was aroused after DeWood unequivocally demonstrated that ST-elevation myocardial infarction (MI) is associated with coronary occlusion.[10] The initial trigger for acute coronary occlusion appeared to be thrombus formation following plaque rupture.[11] To dissolve these thrombi, plasminogen activators, which activate the blood fibrinolytic system, have to be infused. This strategy initiated the current era of the "open artery theory." Consequently, because there is a direct relation between early patency and decreased mortality,[12] immediate and complete reperfusion after onset of symptoms is the therapeutic goal. Indeed, 71% of patients with AMI who survived after thrombolysis demonstrated early reperfusion, whereas only 45% of patients who died after 24 hours had an open infarct-related artery.[13] However, Lincoff and Topol[14] indicated that the high patency rates reportedly associated with thrombolytic therapy are partly the result of endogenous fibrinolysis and initially are not occluded arteries at baseline. They conclude that optimal and long-term reperfusion occurs in only 25% of patients receiving front-loaded alteplase.

Initial thrombolytic regimens aimed at intracoronary administration of fibrinolytic drugs as a strategy to reduce systemic bleeding complications.[15-18] Nevertheless, logistic difficulties associated with routine intracoronary administration of thrombolytics to all patients presenting with an MI redirected interest toward the intravenous route of administration in the 1980s. However, because the majority of hospitals lacked a catheterization laboratory, renewed interest in systemic, intravenous thrombolytic therapy occurred. Subsequent trials have demonstrated a clear reduction in mortality after MI with intravenous fibrinolytic drugs. A meta-analysis of nine large randomized controlled trials, each with more than 1000 patients and totaling 58,511 patients, reported a significant 18% reduction in mortality with thrombolysis in the first 35 days after AMI.[19] This benefit was observed in nearly all patient subgroups, and the benefits of thrombolysis in improving survival of patients with AMI was sustained up to 10 years.[20,21] Consequently, current practice guidelines clearly advocate rapid restoration of normal epicardial blood flow and myocardial perfusion in the infarct zone.[22] Nevertheless, data from the Global Registry of Acute Coronary Events (GRACE) indicates that only 68% of all patients eligible for reperfusion therapy actually receive treatment, including 17% undergoing mechanical intervention, 43% receiving lytic therapy, and 8% receiving both treatments.[5]

■ ■ ■

TABLE 7-1 MORTALITY RATES OBSERVED IN LARGE TRIALS OF THROMBOLYSIS FOR ACUTE MYOCARDIAL INFARCTION

Trial	Year	No. of patients	Reference	Regimen	Mortality (%)
GISSI-1	1986	11,806	48	Streptokinase	10.7
ISIS-2	1988	17,186	50	Streptokinase	10.4
				Streptokinase+aspirin	8.0
GISSI-2	1990	20,891	42	Streptokinase	8.5
				Alteplase	8.9
ISIS-3	1992	41,299	43	Streptokinase	10.6
				Alteplase	10.3
				Anistreplase	10.5
GUSTO-I	1993	41,021	44	Streptokinase + SQ heparin	7.2
				Streptokinase + IV heparin	7.4
				Alteplase	6.3
				Alteplase + streptokinase	7.0
GUSTO-III	1997	15,059	60	Alteplase	7.2
				Reteplase	7.5
ASSENT-2	1999	16,949	73	Alteplase	6.2
				Tenecteplase	6.2
GUSTO-V	2001	16,588	4	Reteplase	5.9
				Reteplase + abciximab	5.6
ASSENT-3	2001	6,095	3	Tenecteplase + heparin	6.0
				Tenecteplase + enoxaparin	5.4
				Tenecteplase + abciximab	6.6

Indications and Contraindications for Thrombolysis

Administration of thrombolytic drugs generally is considered in patients younger than 76 years with typical chest pain of less than 12 hours duration presenting with electrocardiographic ST-segment elevations or new bundle branch block.[22] It is less clear whether patients presenting between 12 and 24 hours also benefit from thrombolytic therapy (discussed in detail later in this chapter).[23] In any case, patients presenting after 24 hours are generally not considered good candidates for thrombolytic therapy (class III). Likewise, patients older than 75 years of age often have been excluded from randomized trials, mainly because of an increased risk for bleeding complications. Nevertheless, elderly patients may benefit form thrombolytic therapy provided that they do not present with other contraindications (discussed in detail later in this chapter).[22,24]

The usual electrocardiographic criterion for administration of thrombolytic therapy is at least 0.1 mV of ST-segment elevation in two or more contiguous leads. Because mortality is significantly higher in patients with complete bundle branch block (23.6%), administration of a fibrinolytic agent is also recommended in this population. Indeed, thrombolysis in patients presenting with a new bundle branch block, obscuring ST-segment analysis, reduces mortality by 25%.[19] However, there is no evidence of benefit of thrombolytic therapy in patients presenting with normal electrocardiographic or ST-segment depression.[19]

Commonly established contraindications to thrombolytic therapy are in essence precautions to avoid excessive hemorrhage in patients with comorbidities that predispose for bleeding complications (Table 7-2). In these patients, including those with previous history of stroke, primary percutaneous coronary intervention (PCI) should be considered. Patients with AMI who underwent extensive cardiopulmonary resuscitation (CPR) have been excluded from many trials in throm-

■ ■ ■

TABLE 7-2 INDICATIONS AND CONTRAINDICATIONS FOR THROMBOLYTIC THERAPY

Indications	Contraindications
Ischemic-type chest pain	**Absolute**
—Within 12 hr of symptom onset (12-24 hr: Class IIb indication)	—Previous hemorrhagic stroke at any time
	—Nonhemorrhagic stroke >1 yr
—Age >75 yr (<75 yr: Class IIa indication)	—Intracranial neoplasm
	—Active internal bleeding
Electrocardiographic criteria	—Suspected aortic dissection
—ST-segment elevation ≥0.1 mV in at least two contiguous leads	**Relative**
	—Surgery or trauma (including head trauma) within past 2-4 wk
—(New) bundle branch block	—Uncontrolled hypertension on presentation (blood pressure >180/100 mm Hg)
	—Chronic severe hypertension
	—Prolonged cardiopulmonary resuscitation
	—Current use of anticoagulants with international normalized ratio of >2.3
	—Known bleeding diatheses
	—Recent internal bleeding (past 2-4 wk)
	—Noncompressible vascular punctures
	—Pregnancy
	—Active peptic ulcer
	—Previous use of streptokinase, APSAC (anisoylated plasminogen streptokinase activator complex), or staphylokinase

bolytic therapy because of a presumed increased risk of intrathoracic bleeding. However, trials have shown improved survival and more return of spontaneous circulation with administration of alteplase after initially failed CPR.[25,26] In another study, however, no such benefit could be demonstrated.[27]

Because a diastolic blood pressure higher than 110 mm Hg[28] and a systolic blood pressure higher than 175[19] at the time of presentation increases the risk for intracranial hemorrhage (ICH), patients with one of these criteria were usually not eligible for thrombolytic therapy. However, a history of systemic hypertension in itself does not predispose for ICH[29] and therefore should not represent a contraindication. Nevertheless, thrombolytic trials have adopted different approaches with regard to patients presenting with hypertension. In the third Assessment of the Safety and Efficacy of a New Thrombolytic Agent (ASSENT-3) trial, for example, patients were excluded only if they had a diastolic blood pressure higher than 110 mm Hg and/or systolic blood pressure higher than 180 mm Hg on *repeated* measurements.[3] Consequently, in this trial patients could still receive thrombolysis after successful treatment of their high initial blood pressure on admission. In contrast, patients were excluded after a single reading of diastolic blood pressure higher than 110 mm Hg and/or systolic blood pressure higher than 180 mm Hg in the fifth Use of Strategies to Open Occluded Coronary Arteries (GUSTO-V) study[4] and most TIMI (Thrombolysis In Myocardial Infarction) trials. Nevertheless, there is a substantial mortality benefit with thrombolysis in patients presenting with hypertension.[19] Thus, when primary PCI is not available, thrombolysis should still be considered in patients with high blood pressure on admission after initiation of antihypertensive treatment.

Evaluation of Reperfusion Therapy

Many clinical trials have used early (60- or 90-min) patency of the infarct-related vessel on angiography as the most important demonstration of successful thrombolysis. TIMI flow grade less than 3 in the infarct-related artery is associated with poor functional recovery of the left ventricle and increased mortality.[30,31] Nevertheless, angiography offers at best a snapshot view of the dynamic process of coronary occlusion and recanalization.[14] Furthermore, restored epicardial blood flow does not guarantee reperfusion at the tissue level. Indeed, myocardial tissue reperfusion correlates better with outcome than epicardial

coronary artery patency.[32,33] Failure to achieve early ST-segment recovery, a measure of adequate tissue perfusion, was associated with a worse 5-year outcome even in patients with TIMI grade 3 flow.[34] Angiographic assessment of myocardial perfusion ("myocardial blush") also correlates with mortality after thrombolysis. Thirty-day mortality was sevenfold higher in patients with patent epicardial infarct-related vessels but with decreased microvascular perfusion compared to those with normal microvascular flow.[35] Because new thrombolytic strategies aim at restoring stable flow at tissue level, future phase I and II trials in AMI will undoubtedly assess myocardial tissue flow in addition to epicardial coronary artery flow as a measure of successful reperfusion.

Thrombolytic Agents

Standard thrombolytic regimens (Table 7-3) suffer from several well-known limitations. The fibrinolytic agent needs 30 to 45 minutes on average to recanalize the infarct-related artery, and optimal TIMI grade 3 flow is only achieved in up to 60% of patients. Also, reocclusion as a result of prothrombotic effects is common,[36] occurring in 5% to 15% of successfully recanalized arteries.[37] Even when restored blood flow in the infarct-related artery is observed, microcirculatory reperfusion can still be absent ("no-reflow" phenomenon).[38,39] A further concern is bleeding complications, especially ICHs. Also, established thrombolytic regimens require continuous intravenous infusion, precluding efficient community or prehospital administration and potentially leading to dosing mistakes.[40] Finally, preexisting antibodies or immune response to some agents may reduce their fibrinolytic capacity or prohibit readministration.

Streptokinase

Streptokinase is a nonfibrinogen-specific fibrinolytic agent that indirectly activates plasminogen. Because of its lack of fibrin-specificity, streptokinase induces a systemic lytic state as circulating fibrinogen levels decrease below 20% of baseline.[41] As a consequence, heparin usually is not recommended in combination with streptokinase or other nonfibrin-specific fibrinolytics. In fact, no clear benefit of intravenous or subcutaneous heparin in combination with streptokinase was seen in large-scale trials.[42-44] Because streptokinase is produced by hemolytic streptococci, patients who receive streptokinase invariably

■ ■ ■

TABLE 7-3   CHARACTERISTICS AND DOSES OF FIBRINOLYTIC AGENTS

	Streptokinase	Staphylokinase	Alteplase	Reteplase	Lanoteplase	Tenecteplase	Saruplase
Fibrin-specificity	No	++++	++	+	+	+++	No
Half-life (min)	18-23	13 (PEGylated)	3-4	18	30	20	6-8
Administration (dose)	1-hr infusion (1.5 MU)	Single bolus (5 mg)	90-min infusion (15-mg bolus; 0.75 mg/kg IV [max 50] over 30 min, followed by 0.5 mg/kg over 60 min)	Double bolus (10 + 10 MU 30 min apart)	Single bolus (120 KU/kg)	Single bolus (<60 kg: 30 mg; 60-69.9 kg: 35 mg; 70-79.9 kg: 40 mg; 80-89.9 kg: 45 mg; >90 kg: 50 mg)	1-hr infusion (20 mg bolus, 60 mg IV over 1 hr)
Antigenicity	+++	+	No	No	No	No	No

develop antistreptococcal antibodies, precluding readministration.[45] Moreover, preexisting antistreptokinase antibodies impede reperfusion after treatment with streptokinase in patients with AMI.[46] However, hypotension, a frequent side effect of streptokinase, is more likely the result of bradykinin release than caused by an allergic reaction.[47]

The first large trial to show a significant reduction in mortality with a fibrinolytic agent was the landmark Gruppo Italiano per lo Studio della Streptochinasi nell' Infarto Miocardio (GISSI-1) trial.[48] In this study, 11,806 patients with an AMI presenting within 12 hours of symptom onset were randomized to either streptokinase or standard nonfibrinolytic therapy. In-hospital mortality was 10.7% in patients treated with intravenous streptokinase versus 13.1 in control patients, indicating 23 lives saved per 1000 patients treated. This benefit in mortality was preserved after 1-year and 10-year follow-up.[20,49] Another landmark trial, the Second International Study of Infarct Survival (ISIS-2), clearly showed a benefit of adding aspirin to streptokinase. Patients (n = 17,187) received 1.5 MU streptokinase, 160 mg aspirin daily for 1 month, both treatments, or neither.[50] Treatment with aspirin or streptokinase alone resulted in a significant reduction in mortality (23% and 24%, respectively), an effect that was additive, as witnessed by a 43% reduction in the combination group. Aspirin significantly reduced nonfatal reinfarction (1.0% vs. 2.0%) and was not associated with any significant increase in ICHs. Reinfarction rate was higher when streptokinase was used alone, an effect that was abolished when aspirin was added.

Tissue-Type Plasminogen Activator

Recombinant tissue-type plasminogen activator (alteplase, rt-PA) is a single-chain tissue-type plasminogen activator (t-PA) molecule, manufactured by recombinant DNA technology.[51] Alteplase requires a continuous infusion because of its short half-life. It also has considerable greater fibrin-specificity than streptokinase, but it nevertheless induces mild systemic fibrinogen depletion. Fibrin-specific agents such as alteplase increase the risk of reocclusion. In a pooled analysis of more than 1100 patients, the reocclusion rate was twice as high (13%) with alteplase than with nonfibrin-specific drugs.[52] As a consequence, concomitant treatment with heparin is needed in patients receiving alteplase.[22]

A 26% mortality reduction was seen after treatment with alteplase and heparin compared with placebo and heparin in the Anglo-Scandinavian Study of Early Thrombolysis (ASSET),[53] despite the absence of aspirin and the unusually long administration of alteplase in this study. Alteplase, given in a 3-hour dosing regimen, was subsequently shown to achieve significantly better patency scores than streptokinase.[52] Nevertheless, in the ISIS-3[43] and GISSI-2[42] trials, the 3-hour alteplase regimen was found to have an equal mortality rate as streptokinase. The question of which of the two fibrinolytic drugs is the most effective in terms of mortality reduction was answered in the first Global Use of Strategies to Open Occluded Coronary Arteries (GUSTO-1) trial.[44] In this trial that included more than 40,000 patients, a "front-loaded"

90-minute dosing regimen of alteplase was used, which had been shown to achieve higher patency rates than the 3-hour scheme.[54] Thirty-day mortality was 6.3% in patients receiving alteplase and intravenous heparin, compared to 7.4% in patients treated with streptokinase and intravenous heparin (P = 0.001).[44] This 1% lower 30-day mortality with front-loaded alteplase over streptokinase could be explained by a significantly higher TIMI flow grade 3 at 90 minutes: 54% versus 32% with streptokinase.[55]

Reteplase

Reteplase, a second-generation thrombolytic agent, was a first attempt to improve on the shortcomings of alteplase. It is a mutant of alteplase in which the finger, the kringle-1 domain, and epidermal growth factor domains were removed. This results in a decreased plasma clearance, allowing double-bolus administration. However, the removal of the finger domain diminishes fibrin specificity,[56] whereas inactivation by plasminogen activator inhibitor 1 (PAI-1) remains similar as with alteplase.

In two open-label randomized pilot trials, different doses of reteplase were evaluated in patients with AMI. In the Reteplase Angiographic Phase I International Dose-Finding (RAPID) I study,[57] patients treated with two boluses of 10 MU reteplase given 30 minutes apart had a significantly higher rate of TIMI-3 flow (63%) compared with patients treated with 100 mg alteplase over 3 hours (49%) (Fig. 7-1A). In RAPID II,[58] the same dose of reteplase was compared against 90-minute front-loaded alteplase in 324 patients. Again, reteplase achieved significantly higher TIMI-3 flow rates at 90 minutes than t-PA (60% vs. 45%). Total patency, defined as TIMI-2 or TIMI-3 flow rate, was also significantly higher in patients treated with reteplase (83% vs. 73% for alteplase).

Encouraged by these higher early patency rates, reteplase was compared with streptokinase (INJECT, or International Joint Efficacy Comparison of Thrombolytics) and alteplase (GUSTO-III) in two mortality trials. In the double-blind INJECT trial,[59] 6010 patients with AMI within 12 hours of symptom onset were randomized to either double-bolus reteplase (10 U), given 30 minutes apart, or 1.5 MU streptokinase over 60 minutes. Double-bolus reteplase was shown to be at least equivalent to streptokinase (35-day mortality 9.0% vs. 9.5%, respectively; 95% CI 1.98-0.96). In the GUSTO-III trial,[60] which was designed as a superiority trial, 15,059 patients were randomized to double-bolus reteplase (10 MU), given 30 minutes apart, or front-loaded alteplase (100 mg over 90 minutes) (Fig. 7-1B). Mortality at 30 days was again similar for both treatment arms (7.47% vs. 7.24%, respectively), as was the incidence of hemorrhagic stroke or other major bleeding complications. Similar mortality rates were maintained for both treatment groups at 1-year follow-up (11.2% vs. 11.1%, respectively).[61] Thus, higher TIMI-3 rates at 90 minutes with reteplase did not translate into lower short-term mortality rates. This might be explained in part by increased platelet activation and surface receptor expression with reteplase compared to alteplase.[62]

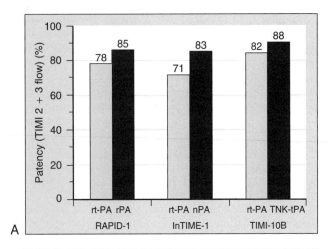

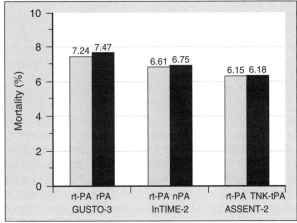

FIGURE 7-1. Patency and mortality rates in trials comparing alteplase with new thrombolytic agents. *Panel A:* Combined TIMI grade 2 and 3 flow rates at 90 minutes in trials comparing front-loaded alteplase with reteplase (RAPID-1),[57] lanoteplase (InTIME-1),[66] and tenecteplase (ASSENT-1).[72] *Panel B:* 30-day mortality rates in trials comparing front-loaded alteplase with reteplase (GUSTO-3),[60] lanoteplase (InTIME-2),[65] and tenecteplase (ASSENT-2).[73] rt-PA, alteplase; rPA, reteplase; nPA, lanoteplase; TNK-tPA, tenecteplase.

Lanoteplase

Lanoteplase (nPA) is a deletion mutant of alteplase by deleting its fibronectin fingerlike and epidermal growth factor domains and mutating Asn (117) to Gln (117),[63] leading to decreased plasma clearance and improved resistance to PAI-1.[64] However, these changes make lanoteplase less fibrin-specific compared to rt-PA.[65]

In the randomized double-blind intravenous nPA for the treatment of infarcting myocardium early (InTIME-1) trial,[66] 602 patients within 6 hours of symptom onset received weight-adjusted single-bolus lanoteplase (15–120 kU/kg) or front-loaded alteplase. Lanoteplase had a dose-dependent effect on coronary patency rates. The 60 kU/kg dose produced similar TIMI-3 flow rates compared with alteplase (44% vs. 37%) at 60 minutes. In the 120 kU/kg dose group, TIMI-3 flow rate was 47%. At 90 minutes, combined TIMI-2 and 3 flow was 72% and 83% for 60 and 120 kU/kg lanoteplase, respectively, compared with 71% for alteplase (Fig. 7-1A). In the InTIME-2 trial,[65] 15,078 patients were randomized in a

2:1 ratio to single-bolus lanoteplase (120 kU/kg) or accelerated alteplase. Thirty-day mortality was equivalent for both groups (6.75% vs. 6.61%; RR 1.02, upper limit of the one-sided 95% CI 1.137) (Fig. 7-1B). At 6 months and 1-year follow-up, mortality for both treatments remained similar (8.7% vs. 8.9% at 6 months, and 10.0% and 10.3% at 1 year).[65] Although the rate of combined hemorrhagic and ischemic strokes was not statistically different between the groups (1.87% for lanoteplase and 1.53% for alteplase), the rate of hemorrhagic strokes was significantly higher in patients treated with lanoteplase (1.12% vs. 0.64% for alteplase). Moreover, the incidence of mild bleedings was also significantly higher in the lanoteplase group (19.7% for lanoteplase vs. 14.8% for alteplase). The increased rate of ICH and minor bleeding complications with lanoteplase in the InTIME-2 trial possibly is related to the relatively high dose of lanoteplase and the lower fibrin-specificity. Lanoteplase is not investigated further, nor is it being developed for commercial use.

Tenecteplase

Tenecteplase (TNK-t-PA) is derived from alteplase after mutations at three places (**T**103, **N**117, **KHRR**296–299), which increases the plasma half-life, increases fibrin binding and specificity, and increases resistance to PAI-1. Its slower clearance allows convenient single-bolus administration. Higher fibrin specificity of tenecteplase can be explained by reduced efficiency of plasminogen activation in the presence of fibrinogen and fibrin degradation products, whereas efficiency in the presence of fibrin remains equivalent.[67] As a consequence, tenecteplase leads to faster recanalization compared to alteplase.[68] Tenecteplase also has higher thrombolytic potency on platelet-rich clots than its parent molecule.[69]

Efficacy of clot lysis was evaluated in the Thrombolysis In Myocardial Infarction (TIMI) 10A and 10B trials. In the TIMI 10A trial,[70] 113 patients with evolving MI within 12 hours of symptom onset received incremental doses of single-bolus tenecteplase (5–50 mg). The rate of TIMI-3 flow was 59% for the 30-mg group and 64% for the 50-mg group. Combined TIMI-2 and TIMI-3 flows were similar for all doses tested (85%). Levels of coagulation parameters were only affected to a small extent when compared with levels after treatment with alteplase. In the TIMI-10B trial,[71] 837 patients were randomized to single-bolus tenecteplase (30, 40, or 50 mg) or front-loaded alteplase (Fig. 7-1A). TIMI-3 flow rates were identical after single-bolus administration of 40 mg tenecteplase compared with alteplase (63%). The 50-mg dose of tenecteplase had to be discontinued early because of an excess of ICHs. The incidence of serious bleeding complications, however, decreased in both groups after adjustment of heparin dosing during the course of the study.

Concomitantly, the safety of single-bolus administration of tenecteplase was evaluated in the Assessment of the Safety and Efficacy of a New Thrombolytic Agent (ASSENT) 1 study.[72] In this study, 3325 patients received a single bolus of either 30 or 40 mg tenecteplase. The 50-mg dose was also discontinued and replaced by 40 mg because of the ICHs observed in the TIMI-10B study.[71] Death (6.4%) or severe bleeding complications (2.8%)

occurred in a low proportion of patients, without significant differences among the treatment groups. An ICH rate of 0.56% and 0.58% was observed in patients receiving 30 mg or 40 mg tenecteplase. This rate compares favorably with previous rates observed with alteplase.

In the double-blind ASSENT-2 trial,[73] 16,949 patients were randomized to single-bolus tenecteplase or weight-adjusted front-loaded alteplase (Fig. 7-1B). The dose of tenecteplase ranged from 30 to 50 kg according to body weight, based on the finding from the previous trials that 0.50 to 0.55 mg/kg tenecteplase yielded a similar efficacy and safety profile than front-loaded alteplase.[74] Specifically designed as an equivalency trial, this study showed that tenecteplase and alteplase were equivalent for 30-day mortality (6.18% vs. 6.15%, 90% CI 0.917–1.104). The two treatments did not differ significantly in any subgroup analysis, except for a lower 30-day mortality with tenecteplase in patients treated after 4 hours of symptom onset. Although the rates of ICH were similar for tenecteplase (0.93%) and rt-PA (0.94%), female patients, patients older than 75 years of age, and patients weighing less than 67 kg tended to have lower rates of ICH after treatment with tenecteplase.[75] Noncerebral bleeding complications occurred less frequently in the tenecteplase group, a difference that was even more apparent in high-risk females. Thus, increased fibrin specificity of TNK may induce both a better outcome in late-treated patients and fewer bleeding complications in high-risk patients.

Staphylokinase

Staphylokinase (STAR), a bacterial profibrinolytic agent readily available by recombinant DNA technology, is a 136 amino acid single-chain polypeptide with a unique structure and mechanism of action and of fibrin specificity.[76] Staphylokinase is highly selective for fibrinogen, in contrast with streptokinase.[77] Preclinical investigations showed attractive characteristics, including high thrombolytic potency. Staphylokinase is also very effective in dissolving platelet-rich thrombi and possesses a high fibrin specificity in human plasma. Although wild-type staphylokinase induces an antibody response, newer variants with reduced antigenicity have been shown to decrease the occurrence and magnitude of inactivating antibodies.[78]

In the STAR trial, a multicenter randomized trial, the effects of staphylokinase versus accelerated and weight-adjusted t-PA, were evaluated on early coronary artery patency in 100 patients with AMI.[79] Patients randomized to staphylokinase were given 10 mg or 20 mg over 30 minutes. TIMI-3 flow at 90 minutes was reached in 58% of patients treated with alteplase and in 62% of patients treated with staphylokinase. Staphylokinase proved to be highly fibrin-specific, preserving plasma fibrinogen, plasminogen and α_2-antiplasmin levels after infusions of 10 or 20 mg, whereas alteplase caused a very significant drop of fibrinogen (−30% at 90 minutes) and of plasminogen and α_2-antiplasmin (−60% at 90 minutes).

In the Collaborative Angiographic Patency Trial of Recombinant Staphylokinase (CAPTORS) trial,[80] patients with an AMI within 6 hours of symptom onset received one of three doses—15, 30, and 45 mg of staphylokinase (Sak42D variant) given as a bolus (20% of total dose)—followed by an intravenous infusion over a 30-minute period. Surprisingly, there was no difference in TIMI-3 patency rates between the three doses given (62%, 65%, and 63%, respectively). The lack of dose response possibly indicates that this study was operating on the flat part of the dose-response curve. No ICHs were observed. Staphylokinase did not significantly affect plasma fibrinogen and plasminogen levels irrespective of the dose, demonstrating its superior fibrin-specificity. α_2-Antiplasmin levels, however, showed a borderline significant reduction by dose (P = 0.053).

Because single-bolus administration has become the preferred regimen for treatment with thrombolytic agents, two staphylokinase variants with reduced immunogenicity and preserved lytic potency (Sak SY160 and SY161) have been derivatized with maleimide-polyethylene glycol (PEG) to reduce the plasma clearance by 2.5-fold.[81] PEGylated variants detected only one third of the antibodies generated by wild-type Sak in patients with AMI. Fourteen of the 18 patients who received an intravenous bolus of a reduced dose of 5 mg PEG-staphylokinase had TIMI grade 3 at 60 minutes (78%, 95% CI 55% to 91%).[82] Eleven additional patients received a 2.5-mg bolus of PEG-staphylokinase, resulting in TIMI grade 3 flow in seven patients at 60 minutes (63%, 95% CI 35% to 85%). Fibrinogen, plasminogen, and α_2-antiplasmin remained unchanged at 60 minutes in patients receiving both 2.5 and 5 mg PEG-staphylokinase, again indicating a high fibrin selectivity. An angiographic-controlled dose-finding trial (CAPTORS II) using single-bolus PEGylated staphylokinase (SY161) was completed in 2002.[83]

Saruplase

Saruplase is an unglucosylated single-chain recombinant urokinase-type plasminogen activator without immunogenicity. Although not fibrin-specific, it has a plasma half-life of 9 minutes.[84] In an initial trial, 20-mg bolus saruplase followed by a 60-mg infusion over 1 hour was demonstrated to yield TIMI-3 flow rates comparable to streptokinase.[85] In the Comparison Trial of Saruplase and Streptokinase (COMPASS) trial,[86] 3089 patients were randomized to saruplase or streptokinase. Thirty-day mortality tended to be lower in the saruplase group (5.7% vs. 6.7% for streptokinase). In contrast with the previous trial, however, ICHs were higher with saruplase (0.9% vs. 0.3% for streptokinase), although only a limited number of elderly patients were included in this trial. In the Bolus Administration of Saruplase in Europe (BASE) trial,[87] alternative administration regimens were tested: 192 patients with an AMI received a double bolus of 40 mg and 40 mg after 30 minutes, or a single bolus of 60 or 80 mg, or the standard regimen (a bolus of 20 mg and 60 mg IV infusion over 1 hour). At 90 minutes TIMI-3 flow was 73% with the 40-mg double bolus, 57% with the 80 mg bolus, only 36% with the 60-mg bolus, and 72% with the standard regimen, respectively. Although the double bolus of 40/40 mg resulted in the highest patency, it also had the highest complication rate. Saruplase was not approved for marketing in Europe.

Amediplase

Amediplase is a chimeric fusion protein consisting of the kringle 2 domain of t-PA and the catalytic domain of urokinase-PA. It is fibrin-specific, is nonimmunogenic, and can be given as a single bolus. In two angiographic studies (2k2 and 3k2),[88,89] TIMI flow grade 3 was obtained in more than 50% of the patients in a dose of ±1 mg/kg with a good safety profile. Currently, phase III trials are investigating the safety and efficacy of this fibrinolytic agent.

ANTITHROMBOTIC THERAPY

Unfractionated Heparin

Unfractionated heparin (UFH) has been standard adjunctive antithrombotic therapy with fibrin-specific fibrinolytics since GUSTO-1.[44] Although intravenous UHF does not improve early patency rates,[90] patency after alteplase is enhanced by UHF later because of an inhibition of early reocclusion.[91,92] However, the use of UFH has several drawbacks. The effectiveness of UFH is very variable in patients as a result of low bioavailability and variable clearance. This implies frequent assessment of the level of coagulation by monitoring activated partial-thromboplastin time (aPTT). UFH is also relatively ineffective in inhibiting clot-associated thrombin and factor X and does not reduce the generation of thrombin associated with fibrinolysis. This can result in rebound activation of the coagulation cascade after cessation of an infusion, increasing the risk of reocclusion.[93] Moreover, despite extensive experience with UFH in conjunction with thrombolytic therapy, the optimal dose of UFH remains uncertain. The current recommended regimens and aPTT targets are shown in Table 7-4.

The exact contribution of heparin to bleeding complications after reperfusion therapy still remains controversial. Gugliano and colleagues looked into different heparin dosing schemes and monitoring regimens in several studies.[94] In three of these trials (TIMI 9, GUSTO II, and TIMI 10B), heparin doses were reduced during the course of the trial, resulting in lower rates of ICHs. In the InTIME-2 study, ICH rates were lower after the introduction of an early aPTT time measurement at 3 hours during the course of the study, indicating that closer

monitoring of aPTT might be beneficial.[65] This stricter approach also has been adopted in the ASSENT-3 trial, which was also the first trial to incorporate the 1999 American College of Cardiology/American Heart Association (ACC/AHA) guidelines for heparin administration. Consequently, major bleeding complications but not ICH rates after treatment with tenecteplase and UFH were lower in ASSENT-3[3] when compared to ASSENT-2.[73]

Because third-generation thrombolytic agents have failed to decrease further mortality after MI, current trials have focused on the development and testing of strategies combining novel antithrombotic drugs with full-dose or reduced-dose thrombolytic agents. Because the formation and lysis of a coronary thrombus results from a complex interplay of different pathways involving platelets and the coagulation system, the use of agents that target each of these separate components could optimize clot lysis and prevention of reocclusion. Furthermore, a major drawback of fibrinolytic therapy is its plasmin-mediated procoagulant side effect. Therefore, better inhibition of new thrombin generation might improve efficacy of fibrinolysis. Because the glycoprotein IIb/IIIa receptor is the final common pathway of platelet aggregation, inhibition of this receptor also might enhance further clot lysis and prevent reocclusion.

Low–Molecular-Weight Heparin

LMWHs offer several advantages over UFH. They induce a more stable and predictable anticoagulant response that eliminates the need for aPTT monitoring, and the higher anti-Xa:IIa ratio is responsible for a better inhibition of new thrombin generation.[93] Studies have shown a reduction in reinfarction rates and enhanced late patency with the use of LMWH in acute coronary syndromes.[95] Furthermore, the subcutaneous administration and the longer half-life greatly facilitate the administration a LMWH when compared to UFH.

In the ASSENT PLUS trial, patients received the LMWH dalteparin or UFH, in combination with front-loaded alteplase. Reperfusion rates were assessed 4 to 7 days after study entry.[96] TIMI-3 flow rate tended to be higher in patients treated with dalteparin compared to UFH, with no excess in bleeding complications.

The Heparin Aspirin Reperfusion Trial (HART) II trial investigated the use of enoxaparin versus UFH in patients treated with front-loaded alteplase.[97] Enoxaparin was given as a 30-mg bolus followed by 1 mg/kg subcutaneously every 12 hours. As in ASSENT PLUS,[96] TIMI-3 flow rates at 5 to 7 days tended to be higher with LMWH. Among patients with TIMI grade 3 flow at 90 minutes, only 3.1% of patients receiving enoxaparin developed reocclusion at late angiography, compared with 9.1% in those treated with UFH.

In the ENTIRE-TIMI (Enoxaparin and Tenecteplase with or without glycoprotein IIb/IIIa Inhibitor as Reperfusion strategy in ST Elevation MI-Thrombolysis in Myocardial Infarction) 23 trial, 483 patients were randomized to the following: (1) full-dose tenecteplase and UFH; (2) full-dose TNK and enoxaparin (Table 7-4); (3) half-dose TNK, abciximab, and UFH; and (4) half-dose TNK, abciximab, and enoxaparin.[98] Enoxaparin

■ ■ ■

TABLE 7-4   HEPARIN DOSAGES

	Unfractionated heparin	Low–molecular-weight heparin (enoxaparin)
Bolus	60 U/kg (max 4000 U)	30 mg intravenously 1 mg/kg subcutaneously
Dosage	12 U/kg/hr (max 1000 U/hr)	1 mg/kg per 12 hr (max 100 mg for first 2 doses)
Target activated partial-thromboplastin time	50–70 s First measurement at 3 hr	NA
Duration	48 hr	Until hospital discharge or maximal 7 days

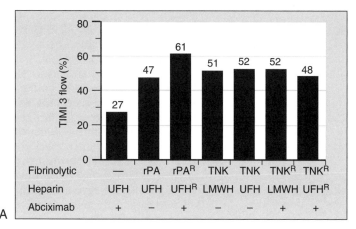
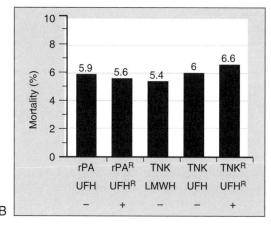

FIGURE 7-2. Patency (A) and mortality (B) in recent trials comparing full-dose fibrinolytics and reduced-dose fibrinolytics with abciximab or enoxaparin. TIMI flow rates were assessed at 60 to 90 minutes (median[62]) in the SPEED trial,[107] and at 60 minutes in the ENTIRE-TIMI 23 study.[98] Mortality rates indicate death at 30 days in GUSTO-5 and ASSENT-3. In the SPEED and GUSTO-5 trials, unfractionated heparin (UFH) was given as a 5000-U bolus followed by a 800 or 1000 U/hr infusion for patients weighing <80 or >80 kg, respectively, whereas a 60 U/kg UHF bolus followed by a 7 U/kg infusion was given in combination with abciximab. Full-dose reteplase (rPA) was given as a double-bolus of 10+10 U, whereas reduced-dose reteplase was given as a double bolus of 5+5 U. Enoxaparin dose represented in this graph is an intravenous bolus of 30 mg, followed by 1 mg/kg subcutaneous (max 100 mg). Reduced-dose and full-dose UFH in the ENTIRE and ASSENT-3 trials was 40 U (max 3000) or 60 U (max 4000) in bolus, followed by 7 U/kg (max 800 U) or 12 U/kg (max 1000 U) per hour for reduced dose or full dose, respectively. Full-dose and reduced-dose tenecteplase (TNK) was 0.53 mg/kg and 0.27 mg/kg, respectively.

achieved similar TIMI-3 flow rates compared to UFH at 60 minutes (Fig. 7-2A). Although this study was relatively small, a significant reduction in the composite endpoint of death and reinfarction at 30 days was seen with full-dose tenecteplase and enoxaparin (4.4%) compared to UFH (15.9%), largely because of a reduction in reinfarction rates (1.9% vs. 12.2%, respectively). Major hemorrhages were less frequent in the tenecteplase and enoxaparin group. The combination of half-dose tenecteplase, abciximab, and either enoxaparin or UFH tended to achieve more complete ST-segment resolution, but it did not further reduce the occurrence of postinfarct ischemic events when compared with full-dose tenecteplase and enoxaparin and was associated with more bleeding complications.

Enoxaparin also has been tested in combination with streptokinase in the Acute Myocardial Infarction-Streptokinase (AMI-SK) trial.[99] In this study, 496 patients with AMI were treated with streptokinase and enoxaparin (30-mg bolus and 1 mg/kg subcutaneous bid) or streptokinase and placebo for 3 to 8 days. In the enoxaparin group, ST-T segment resolution was faster and more complete at 180 minutes. Also, TIMI flow grade 3 rates at day 5 to 10 were higher in patients treated with enoxaparin (70% vs. 58% with placebo), confirming earlier reports that enoxaparin prevents reocclusion after treatment with streptokinase.[100]

Glycoprotein IIb/IIIa Antagonists

More potent antiplatelet therapy by inhibition of the glycoprotein IIb/IIIa receptor also offers opportunities for enhanced and sustained reperfusion.[101] Abciximab is a large chimeric mouse-human monoclonal antibody that binds and inactivates the glycoprotein IIb/IIIa receptor, whereas eptifibatide and tirofiban are smaller molecules that inhibit the glycoprotein IIb/IIIa receptor by mimicking certain amino acid sequences of fibrinogen.

Eptifibatide was tested with full-dose alteplase in the Integrilin to Minimize Platelet Aggregation and Coronary Thrombosis (IMPACT) II trial,[102] and with reduced-dose alteplase in the Integrilin and Low-dose Thrombolysis in Acute Myocardial Infarction (INTRO-AMI) trial.[103] In IMPACT-II, eptifibatide (bolus of 180 μg/kg followed by an infusion of 2.0 μg/kg/min for at least 12 hours) yielded better early TIMI-3 flow rates (66% vs. 39% with placebo). In the INTRO-AMI, the highest 60-minute reperfusion rates were seen in patients treated with double-bolus eptifibatide (10 minutes apart) followed by a 48-hour infusion and half-dose t-PA (60-minute TIMI-3 flow rate of 65% vs. 40% for full-dose alteplase alone). In the Integrilin and Tenecteplase in Acute Myocardial Infarction (INTEGRITI) trial,[104] patency was tested after half-dose tenecteplase plus various doses of double-bolus eptifibatide in 438 patients. The combination of eptifibatide (180 μg/kg bolus, 2 μg/kg/min infusion, and 180 μg/kg bolus 10 minutes later) tended to yield higher TIMI flow grade 3 rates and ST-segment resolution than tenecteplase alone but was associated with a higher rate of major bleeding complications and transfusions.

The combination of tirofiban with half-dose or full-dose tenecteplase was tested in 880 patients in the Fibrinolytics and Aggrastat ST-elevation Resolution (FASTER) trial.[105] Preliminary results in 324 patients showed significantly higher TIMI grade 2 and 3 flow rates and higher ST-resolution rates were observed the half-dose tenecteplase plus tirofiban (10 μg/kg bolus, 0.15 μg/kg infusion) when compared to full-dose tenecteplase alone, with similar bleeding rates in both groups.

In the TIMI-14 study, reperfusion rates were tested after half-dose alteplase with standard-dose abciximab versus standard-dose alteplase alone in 888 patients.[106] Abciximab with half-dose alteplase significantly enhanced reperfusion at 90 minutes in the TIMI-14 trial, with TIMI-3 flow in 72%, compared to 43% with alteplase alone. In the combination arms tested, better patency was observed when alteplase was given as a 15-mg bolus followed by a 1-hour infusion of 35 mg. TIMI-3 flow rates were significantly lower when alteplase was given as a single-bolus alone (38%) or as a bolus plus a 30-minute infusion (61%).

The effect of low-dose reteplase with abciximab on early reperfusion was tested in 528 patients in the Strategies for Patency Enhancement in the Emergency Department (SPEED) trial.[107] TIMI grade 3 flow rate was only 27% when abciximab was used in monotherapy and 47% with full-dose reteplase (10 + 10 U) alone. The highest TIMI-3 flow rate (61%) was observed in the group that received reduced double-bolus reteplase (5 + 5 U) in combination with abciximab and heparin (Fig. 7-2A). UFH was given as a 5000 U bolus followed by a 800 or 1000 U/hr infusion for patients weighing less than 80 or more than 80 kg, respectively, whereas a 40 or 60 U/kg UHF bolus followed by a 7 U/kg/hr infusion was given in combination with abciximab. Unfortunately, this benefit was at the expense of a substantial increase in major bleedings.[108]

Hirudin and Bivalirudin

In contrast with UFH, which inhibits only fluid-phase thrombin, hirudin and bivalirudin (or Hirulog) are direct thrombin-specific anticoagulants that inhibit both fibrin-bound and fluid-phase thrombin.[109] Because inadequately inactivated thrombin at the site of thrombus is in part responsible for the procoagulant side effect of thrombolysis, direct inhibition of thrombin thus might reduce the occurrence of ischemic complications after reperfusion. In patients with acute coronary syndromes, bivalirudin compared favorably against UFH with respect to mortality and MI rates.[110] In the GUSTO-IIb trial,[111] in 12,142 patients with acute coronary syndromes (ST elevation and non-ST elevation), recombinant hirudin provided a small but not significant advantage in the primary endpoint of 30-day mortality, nonfatal MI or reinfarction, as compared with UFH. In patients with AMI, hirudin yielded similar patency rates compared to UFH in the HIT-4 and TIMI-9b trials.[112,113] In the Hirulog and Early Reperfusion or Occlusion (HERO) 1 study, reperfusion rates were assessed in 412 patients receiving streptokinase with bivalirudin or UFH.[114] TIMI-3 flow rates were higher in the bivalirudin group (48%) than in the UFH group (35%), whereas there no increase in bleeding complications in patients receiving bivalirudin. Overall, a meta-analysis of 11 randomized trials showed a 15% reduction in mortality in acute coronary syndromes with direct thrombin inhibitors compared to UFH.[115]

Mortality and Safety Trials

HERO-2

In the HERO 2 trial, 17,073 patients were randomized to streptokinase and UFH or streptokinase and bivalirudin.[115,116] Bivalirudin was given as a bolus of 0.25 mg/kg followed by an intravenous infusion of 0.5 mg/kg/hr for the first 12 hours and 0.25 mg/kg/hr for the subsequent 36 hours. Reduction of the bivalirudin infusion was allowed only when the aPTT was higher than 150 seconds after 18 hours or higher than 120 seconds at 24 hours. UFH was given as a bolus of 5000 U followed by an infusion of 1000 U/hr (patients >80 kg) or 800 U/hr (patients <80 kg) for at least 48 hours, with an aPTT target of 50 to 70 seconds. Streptokinase was given as a 1.5 million unit infusion over 30 to 60 minutes, after the intravenous bolus of the antithrombotic therapy. All patients received aspirin (150–325 mg). Mortality at 30 days was not different for both regimens: 10.5% for bivalirudin and 10.9% for UFH. These mortality rates are higher than those observed in other contemporary thrombolytic trials, reflecting inclusion of more high-risk patients and longer time to treatment. However, when only patients randomized in Western countries were considered, overall mortality rate was only 6.7%. The reinfarction rate within 96 hours was significantly lower in the bivalirudin group (1.6% vs. 2.3% for UFH), suggesting that early and more efficient inhibition of thrombin can inhibit reocclusion. Mild to moderate bleeding complications were higher in the bivalirudin group, possibly because of higher aPTT values observed in the bivalirudin group, but ICH occurred infrequently in both groups (0.6% and 0.4% for bivalirudin and UFH, respectively). Thus, bivalirudin is efficient in reducing ischemic complications after thrombolysis with streptokinase for MI, without a significant increase in bleeding complications. Further studies investigating the role of this agent in combination with fibrin-specific fibrinolytics might be warranted.

GUSTO-V

In the GUSTO-V trial, an open-label noninferiority trial, 16,588 patients were randomized to either reteplase (administered in two boluses of 10 U 30 minutes apart) or half-dose reteplase (two boluses of 5 U 30 min apart) with weight-adjusted abciximab, a potent glycoprotein IIb/IIIa antagonist (0.25 mg/kg bolus followed by 0.125 μg/kg/min for 12 hours).[4] UFH was given as a 5000 U bolus followed by a 800 or 1000 U/hr infusion for patients weighing less than 80 kg or more than 80 kg, respectively, whereas a 60 U/kg UHF bolus followed by a 7 U/kg infusion was given in combination with abciximab. Target aPTT was between 50 and 70 seconds. All patients received aspirin (125–325 mg orally or 250–500 mg intravenously) at the time of randomization, followed by a daily dose of 75 to 325 mg. The primary endpoint was mortality at 30 days, whereas secondary endpoints were recurrent ischemia and reinfarction at 7 days. Thirty-day mortality rates were 5.9% for reteplase and 5.6% for the combined reteplase–abciximab group, thus fulfilling the criteria for noninferiority (Fig. 7-2B). One-year follow-up mortality rates were identical: 8.4%. Thus, the higher patency rates and the more complete ST-segment resolution with combination therapy reported in the SPEED trial[107] did not translate in lower mortality rates. The overall risk of bleeding, however, was significantly higher with reteplase and abciximab than with reteplase alone (24.6% vs. 13.7%), as were thrombocytopenia (2.9% vs. 0.7%) and the need for blood or platelets transfusion (5.7% vs. 4.0%). ICH rates were equal (0.6%) in the overall study population for both treatment arms, although in patients older than 75 years of age the rate of ICH was almost twice as high in the combination treatment arm (2.1% vs. 1.1% for standard-dose reteplase). Thus, combination therapy with reteplase and abciximab resulted in a significant reduction in ischemic complications after AMI, but this benefit was offset by an increased risk of bleeding complications, particularly in elderly patients.

ASSENT-3

In the ASSENT-3 study, the low–molecular-weight heparin (LMWH) enoxaparin, UFH, and abciximab were compared in combination with TNK-tPA.[3] Patients (n = 6095) with acute MI received either full-dose weight-adjusted single-bolus TNK-tPA with weight-adjusted enoxaparin (30-mg intravenous bolus followed by 1 mg/kg immediately and every 12 hours subcutaneous for 7 days) or UFH (40 mg/kg bolus [max 3000 U] followed by a 7 U/kg/hr infusion [max 800/hr]) or half-dose TNK-tPA with abciximab (0.25 mg/kg bolus followed by 0.125 µg/kg/min for 12 hours) and weight-adjusted low-dose UFH. Target aPTT was between 50 and 70 seconds. All patients received aspirin (150–325 mg). Primary endpoints were the composites of 30-day mortality, in-hospital reinfarction or refractory ischemia at 30 days (primary efficacy end point), and both of the previously mentioned items plus in-hospital ICH or major bleeding (primary efficacy plus safety endpoint). Both enoxaparin and full-dose tenecteplase and abciximab plus half-dose tenecteplase significantly reduced the risk for ischemic complications (reinfarction and refractory ischemia). Mortality at 30 days was 6.0% in the tenecteplase with UFH group, 5.4% in the tenecteplase with enoxaparin group, and 6.6% in the half-dose tenecteplase with abciximab group (Fig. 7-2B). A significant improvement in the primary efficacy and safety endpoint was seen with tenecteplase plus enoxaparin or with tenecteplase plus abciximab, when compared to standard tenecteplase and UFH. ICH rates were very similar in the three treatment arms, but major and minor bleeding complications, thrombocytopenia, and transfusions were more frequent with half-dose tenecteplase–abciximab. As in the GUSTO-V trial, patients older than 75 years experienced significantly more bleeding complications. In the tenecteplase plus enoxaparin group, no increase in thrombocytopenia but a modest increase in noncerebral bleeding complications was observed.

Which Thrombolytic Strategy Should Be Used?

Clearly, in both the GUSTO-V and ASSENT-3 trials, patients receiving reduced-dose fibrinolytic in combination with abciximab experienced fewer ischemic complications after AMI. However, this improvement was achieved at the cost of an increased incidence of bleeding complications, especially in the elderly. Moreover, the use of reduced-dose thrombolytics did not result in a lower ICH rate. Taking into account efficacy and safety in the total population including the elderly, the

ease of administration, and the lack of need of anticoagulation monitoring, combination of full-dose single-bolus tenecteplase plus enoxaparin emerges as an attractive reperfusion strategy for the emergency room and the prehospital setting. There seems to be no justification for the use of combination therapy in elderly patients at least at the doses used in GUSTO-V and ASSENT-3.

NEW TRENDS IN THROMBOLYTIC TRIALS

Noninferiority Trials

In the last two decades, the treatment of AMI has improved to the extent that new strategies or new agents at best can provide only a small additional advantage for mortality reduction. As a consequence, interests shifted toward showing noninferiority or "equivalence" for a new agent or treatment strategy versus standard or conventional treatment. Whereas equivalency trials intend to show that the difference between study and control treatments are small in either direction, noninferiority trials aim to demonstrate that a novel treatment is at least not worse than standard treatment.[117] After demonstrating noninferiority for a hard endpoint (e.g., mortality), a novel treatment might eventually be preferred over the existing treatment because of its more attractive pharmacodynamic profile, fewer side effects, or lower cost.[118]

Several thrombolytic trials adopted the noninferiority strategy to evaluate new treatments. They did not use the same definition of therapeutic noninferiority, mainly because of the lack of a widespread standard. The first large trial to incorporate noninferiority or equivalence was the INJECT trial, in which 6010 patients were randomized to either reteplase or streptokinase,[59] followed by the COBALT (Continuous Infusion versus Double-Bolus Administration of Alteplase),[119] COMPASS,[86] and ASSENT-2[73] trials.

Another shift in practice has been the use of composite endpoints instead of a single primary endpoint. For example, the ASSENT-3 study included only 6000 patients with a composite efficacy and a composite efficacy plus safety endpoint.[3,120] Such intermediate-size trials allow effective testing of new promising agents or combination of agents in appropriate doses before embarking on a definitive, larger scale mortality trials for registration.[120]

Globalization of Thrombolytic Trials

With the advent of mega-trials, thrombolytic trials also have become more worldwide.[121] Globalization has enabled us to include the large number of patients needed to demonstrate relatively small differences in critical endpoints. Randomization of patients from different countries has also given us more insight in outcomes for patients in different regions. Indeed, despite similar current guidelines for the treatment of MI,[22] outcomes greatly vary among different regions. In the GUSTO-1 trial, enrollment in the United States was a marginally significant predictor of better survival compared to other countries, which was explained by increased use of invasive procedures and other proven treatments.[122] Mortality rates at 30 days varied considerably more in the HERO-2 trial: 6.7% in Western countries, 9.6% in Eastern Europe, and 13.7% in Russia.[116] Mortality was also different in the In-TIME-II trial, with the lowest mortality in North America (5.7%) and the highest mortality in Latin America (10.1%), probably reflecting lower use of beta blockers, lipid-lowering drugs, and glycoprotein IIb/IIIa inhibitors as an adjunct to PCIs.[123] Moreover, non-Western contributing sites performed markedly less PCIs as a result of unavailability of on-site catheterization facilities.[124] Other differences that might explain different outcomes include variations in baseline characteristics. For instance, in GUSTO-1, GUSTO-3, and ASSENT-2 trials, non-U.S. patients were more likely to have higher Killip class and anterior localization of their MI.[121] Even so, international differences in mortality rates cannot be entirely accounted for by differences in concomitant therapies or baseline characteristics alone. This raises intriguing questions about genetic variability among different populations, including different susceptibility for thrombolytic or antithrombotic agents or potential underlying differences in disease processes. For instance, a substantially lower dose of alteplase is effective in Asian patients compared with that required in Western patients, even when correcting for body weight.[125] A dose-response study with tenecteplase is being conducted to explore efficacy and safety of fibrinolytic therapy for AMI in an Asian low-body-weight population.

FIBRINOLYTIC THERAPY AND THE RISK OF BLEEDING COMPLICATIONS

Intracranial Hemorrhages

Risk for bleeding complications, especially ICHs, remains a major concern with thrombolytic therapy. Risk factors or ICH include female sex, older age, lower body weight, high blood pressure on admission, African descent, and prior history of cerebrovascular disease and hypertension.[126] Over the past years, an increase in the incidence of ICH has been observed in thrombolytic trials, probably because of the inclusion of more patients at high risk such as the elderly and the more frequent use of revascularization procedures. Better and more frequent use of brain imaging may also have contributed to the increase in ICH rates observed in recent trials.[75]

Increased risk of ICH in women and in patients with low body weight may be caused by relative overdosing in these patients.[59,126] Many clinical trials have included a fixed dose of a thrombolytic agent. In the INJECT study, for example, fixed-dose double-bolus reteplase was compared with a fixed dose of streptokinase, and a higher rate of ICHs in patients with low body weight was observed.[59] In GUSTO-III, patients treated with (non–weight-adjusted) double-bolus reteplase had a higher risk of ICH and more major bleeding complications than those receiving weight-adjusted alteplase, although this difference may also be caused by the lower fibrin specificity of reteplase.[60] During the TIMI-

10A and 10B and ASSENT-1 trials, no weight-adjusted dosing was used, but analysis of TIMI 10B showed that there was a relationship between lower body weight and bleeding complications.[70-72] Recent studies have incorporated weight-adjusted dosing regimens.[74] Nevertheless, in the ASSENT-2 trial, even with a weight-adjusted dose for both tenecteplase and alteplase, more ICH was observed in patients with lower body weight.[75] ICH rates were almost twice as high in patients weighing less than 60 kg (2.24%) compared to patients weighing between 60 and 70 kg (1.15%). Rates of ICH did not differ between tenecteplase and alteplase throughout body-weight quartiles.[75,127]

Fibrin Specificity

Noncerebral bleeding complications also relate to fibrin specificity of the thrombolytic agent used. In the GUSTO-III study, double-bolus reteplase, which is less fibrin-specific than alteplase, carried a higher risk of major bleeds than weight-adjusted alteplase.[60] Likewise, in GUSTO-I more noncerebral bleeds were observed with streptokinase than with alteplase,[44] and in the InTIME-II trial, there was a higher rate of minor bleeding complications with the less fibrin-specific lanoteplase compared to alteplase.[65] Although ICH rates were similar in the ASSENT-2 trial (0.93% vs. 0.94%), significantly fewer bleeding complications and a lower need for blood transfusions were observed in the tenecteplase group, reflecting a better fibrin specificity of tenecteplase.[73]

Bolus Administration

Much controversy aroused when a meta-analysis showed increased risk of ICH with bolus administration of thrombolytic drugs.[128] This meta-analysis included all phase III trials comparing bolus administration versus continuous infusion of thrombolytic agents. Agents administered via bolus included anistreplase (ISIS-3),[43] reteplase (INJECT, GUSTO-III),[59,60] alteplase (COBALT),[119] tenecteplase (ASSENT-2),[73] saruplase (BASE),[87] and lanoteplase (InTIME-II).[65] The authors concluded that the overall odds ratio for ICH after bolus compared to infusion administration was 1.25 (95% CI 1.08–1.45, P = 0.003). However, the inclusion of different agents or different regimens has raised questions about the conclusions drawn from this meta-analysis. A similar meta-analysis comparing bolus versus infusion administration in phase II trials even showed a nonsignificant *lower* risk of ICH for bolus agents.[129] The different agents included in the analysis all have unique profiles as to fibrin specificity and pharmacodynamics. Also, different antithrombin strategies have been used in the trials included in this meta-analysis, whereas studies subsequent to those included in the analysis have incorporated a more conservative antithrombotic approach.[130] Furthermore, only two trials compared the very same agent in bolus versus continuous administration. When taking into account the data from the two agents that is currently available for bolus therapy (tenecteplase and reteplase) and there is no evidence of an increased risk ICH (odd ratio of 1.01 vs. alteplase).

Bleeding Complications in the Elderly

The use of thrombolytic therapy for AMI in the elderly remains controversial. Nevertheless, thrombolysis currently has a Class IIa indication for patients older than 75 years, according to the ACC/AHA guidelines.[22] In a recent registry study,[131] an excess mortality was observed in patients older than 75 years, possibly as a result of an excess of major bleeding complications. This excessive mortality might be explained in part by negative selection because fitter elderly patients might have been more amenable for primary angioplasty. Moreover, a substantial portion of elderly patients receiving thrombolytic therapy actually might have had one or more contraindications. An observational study showed that of the 719 elderly patients who were eligible for thrombolytic therapy, only 63% (455) actually received a thrombolytic drug, whereas of the 1940 patients who had contraindications, 280 (14.4) nevertheless received thrombolytic therapy.[132] This is apparently not without risk, as demonstrated by the higher mortality in patients older than 80 years of age receiving thrombolytic therapy versus those who did not. In addition, mortality increased significantly after thrombolysis in patients with contraindications, regardless of age.

Mortality rates in observational studies, however, are in contrast with findings from large randomized trials. Data from randomized trials undoubtedly favors thrombolysis versus conservative therapy. A reanalysis of the clinical outcomes by the Fibrinolytic Therapy Trialists (FTT) group in 3300 patients older than age 75 presenting within 12 hours of symptom onset with ST-segment elevation or bundle branch block revealed a significant 15% relative mortality reduction by fibrinolytic therapy.[24] This represents an absolute mortality reduction of 34 patients per 1000 randomized, in contrast with 16 per 1000 in those less than 55 years of age. Furthermore, data from the GISSI-1 study[48] suggests that the largest absolute benefit occurs in elderly patients because of their higher baseline risk.[133] It is interesting that lower ICH rates with tenecteplase in older patients in the ASSENT-2 study suggest that the timely use of more fibrin-specific agents might be preferable in older patients without contraindications for thrombolytic therapy.[75] Clearly, additional studies to reassess the safety and efficacy of thrombolytic therapy in the elderly are needed. This will become even more urgent in the near future because the percentage of elderly patients eligible for reperfusion therapies certainly will increase.

TIME-TO-TREATMENT AND THROMBOLYSIS

The greatest efficacy of thrombolysis is observed when therapy is initiated early after symptom onset[134] because infarct size clearly is related to the duration of coronary occlusion.[135] Current guidelines limit the use of thrombolytics to maximally 12 hours after symptom onset.[22] Although some controversy still exists about the efficacy of thrombolysis in patients presenting between 6 and 12 hours after the beginning of chest pain,[136] alteplase was shown to be still effective in patients presenting after 6 hours when compared to placebo.[23]

In the GUSTO-1 study, early thrombolysis was associated with lower mortality rates, but there was no benefit of alteplase over streptokinase in patients treated early.[137] However, streptokinase tends to be less efficient when started after 3 hours of symptom onset.[114,138,139] Indeed, the more fibrin-specific agents alteplase and reteplase did not show any difference in TIMI-3 flow rates in patients treated within or after 3 hours, whereas TIMI-3 rates dropped significantly after 3 hours after treatment with streptokinase and APSAC (anisoylated plasminogen streptokinase activator complex).[140] In the GUSTO-III trial, the mortality rate was higher in patients treated after 4 hours of symptom onset with reteplase, which is less fibrin-specific than alteplase.[60] Also, in the ASSENT-2 trial, mortality in patients treated after 4 hours of symptom onset was significantly lower after treatment with the more fibrin-specific tenecteplase compared to alteplase.[73] Thus, it seems reasonable to select thrombolytic agents with better fibrin-specific profile in patients presenting late, as stated in the 2002 guidelines of the European Society of Cardiology.[141]

Although the time required to identify and treat patients with AMI in the emergency department has decreased substantially, analysis from the GUSTO-I and GUSTO-III trials and from the second National Registry of Myocardial Infarction indicates that median time to treatment has not decreased over the years.[142,143] Faster reperfusion could be pursued through easier drug administration and prehospital treatment but also through implementation of critical pathways.[144,145] Expedited evaluation and management of admitted patients using these fast-track algorithms, based on data from randomized trials, have reduced door-to-drug times by half.[145,146] Easier and faster drug administration can be achieved with bolus administration of thrombolytics.[147] Bolus administration has indeed opened up new perspectives for prehospital treatment because earlier treatment may reduce death rates by salvaging more myocardium. A meta-analysis of six trials including more than 6400 patients observed a 1 hour time gain with prehospital treatment, resulting in a 17% mortality reduction.[148] Currently, the combination of single-bolus tenecteplase plus enoxaparin, which emerged as an easy and attractive therapy in the ASSENT-3 study, is being investigated in the prehospital setting in ±1600 patients in the ASSENT-3 Plus trial.

THROMBOLYSIS VERSUS PRIMARY PCI

In recent years, primary mechanical intervention has emerged as a valuable alternative for pharmacologic reperfusion therapy, especially in high-risk patients. Primary PCI offers several advantages over fibrinolytic therapy, including lower mortality rates and less ICH (Table 7-5).[149] Time to treatment remains as critical for mechanical revascularization as for thrombolysis.[150] Although higher door-to-balloon than door-to-needle times have been observed in clinical trials, primary PCI nevertheless results in lower 30-day mortality rates and

■ ■ ■

TABLE 7-5   COMPARISON OF THROMBOLYSIS VERSUS PRIMARY CORONARY INTERVENTION

	Thrombolysis	Primary PCI
Advantages	Widely available with broad access Little dependence on operator experience Can be given promptly and on site Simple to give in bolus format	Superior early patency Reduced residual stenosis, recurrent ischemia, and reinfarction Less intracranial hemorrhage Lower early mortality Superior in cardiogenic shock
Disadvantages	Systemic bleeding Intracranial hemorrhage	Critical dependence on operator experience Limited access Longer time to treatment

PCI, percutaneous coronary intervention.
Modified from Armstrong PW, Collen D. Fibrinolysis for acute myocardial infarction: Current status and new horizons for pharmacological reperfusion, part 2. Circulation 2001; 19;103:2987–2992, with permission.

ischemic complications. In the GUSTO-IIb trial, direct PCI demonstrated reduced mortality (5.7%) and reinfarction (4.4%) rates at 30 days when compared to front-loaded alteplase (7.0% and 6.5%, respectively), but this difference had dissipated by 6 months.[151] In a meta-analysis of 10 trials, 30-day mortality was 4.4% after primary PCI, compared to 6.5% after thrombolysis.[152] Initial success of primary PCI has been relatively hampered by reinfarction and late restenosis,[153] but recent trials have shown improved outcome with the use of stents in combination with glycoprotein IIb/IIIa antagonists.[154,155] Recent and preliminary data indicate that in patients admitted to community hospitals without a catheterization laboratory, immediate referral for primary PCI may yield a better outcome than on-site thrombolysis. The Danish Multicenter Randomized Study on Thrombolytic Therapy Versus Acute Coronary Angioplasty in Acute Myocardial Infarction-2 (DANAMI-2) showed a reduction of the composite endpoint of death, reinfarction, or disabling stroke in patients transferred for primary PCI compared to on-site thrombolysis.[156] Likewise, the Air-Primary Angioplasty in MI (Air-PAMI) trial showed that in 138 patients, major adverse cardiac events at 30 days were lower in high-risk patients who were transferred to a hospital with percutaneous transluminal coronary angioplasty (PTCA) compared to those treated with thrombolysis at a hospital without onsite PTCA.[157] Although there is clear evidence that primary PCI performed at the right time by the right (experienced) team is superior to thrombolysis, many issues remain to be solved regarding routine transfer of patients for primary PCI.

FUTURE PERSPECTIVES

Although several of the newer generation fibrinolytic agents offer theoretical advantages over alteplase, they appear not to be better than alteplase for reducing mortality. It is unlikely that there will be major advances in fibrinolytic drug development in the near future.[158] Of new thrombolytic agents currently in phase II testing, staphylokinase has the highest fibrin specificity; amediplase also has attractive properties, but their potential benefit over current third-generation fibrinolytic agents remains to be determined in larger trials.

Further improvement in pharmacologic reperfusion therapy will more likely come from improved antithrombotic cotherapies, novel drugs that target reperfusion injury or inflammation, timely administration by prehospital treatment, and the implementation of critical pathways.

Primary PCI can reduce mortality rates in qualified, high-volume centers, but much time often is wasted between diagnosis and intervention. Therefore, the future direction of reperfusion therapy might lie in combining pharmacologic and mechanical reperfusion strategies.[159] This combination, or "facilitated PCI," refers to a two-stage procedure of immediate administration of thrombolytic therapy, bridging the time necessary for transfer to a catheterization laboratory for urgent PCI. The rationale for this approach is that reperfusion can be obtained sooner than with PCI alone, whereas PCI can offer immediate recanalization in case of failed thrombolysis or improved TIMI flow grades when thrombolysis was not successful or was only partially successful. Indeed, early observations suggest that the combination of thrombolysis and glycoprotein IIb/IIIa antagonism facilitates percutaneous intervention.[108] Early experience from the Plasminogen-activator Angioplasty Compatibility Trial (PACT) trial suggests that this strategy leads to more frequent early recanalization, with greater left-ventricular function preservation.[160] Both full-dose tenecteplase plus enoxaparin and combination therapy with half-dose lytic plus a glycoprotein IIb/IIIa antagonist followed by immediate PCI are being tested in the setting of facilitated PCI.

CONCLUSION

Thrombolytic therapy significantly has improved outcome after AMI. Over the past years, new agents with several theoretic advantages over standard agents have been developed. Although they do not seem to decrease mortality, they are easier to administer and induce fewer side effects. Further improvement is expected from novel antithrombotic drugs, reduction of reperfusion injury, and reduced time to reperfusion through prehospital thrombolysis and facilitated percutaneous intervention. These strategies need to be tested in large clinical and mortality-driven trials.

REFERENCES

1. Braunwald E: Shattuck lecture—cardiovascular medicine at the turn of the millennium: Triumphs, concerns, and opportunities. N Engl J Med 1997; 337:1360-1369.
2. Sobel BE: Coronary thrombolysis and the new biology. J Am Coll Cardiol 1989; 14:850-860.
3. Efficacy and safety of tenecteplase in combination with enoxaparin, abciximab, or unfractionated heparin: The ASSENT-3 randomised trial in acute myocardial infarction. Lancet 2001; 358:605-613.
4. Topol EJ: Reperfusion therapy for acute myocardial infarction with fibrinolytic therapy or combination reduced fibrinolytic therapy and platelet glycoprotein IIb/IIIa inhibition: The GUSTO V randomised trial. Lancet 2001; 357:1905-1914.
5. Eagle KA, Goodman SG, Avezum A, et al: Practice variation and missed opportunities for reperfusion in ST-segment-elevation myocardial infarction: Findings from the Global Registry of Acute Coronary Events (GRACE). Lancet 2002; 359:373-377.
6. Kuch B, Bolte HD, Hoermann A, et al: What is the real hospital mortality from acute myocardial infarction? Epidemiological vs clinical view. Eur Heart J 2002; 23:714-720.
7. Wong CK, White HD: Has the mortality rate from acute myocardial infarction fallen substantially in recent years? Eur Heart J 2002; 23:689-692.
8. Fletcher A, Alkjaersig N, Smyrniotis F, et al: Treatment of patients suffering form early myocardial infarction with massive and prolonged streptokinase therapy. Trans Assoc Am Physicians 1958; 287-296.
9. Yusuf S, Collins R, Peto R, et al: Intravenous and intracoronary fibrinolytic therapy in acute myocardial infarction: Overview of results on mortality, reinfarction and side-effects from 33 randomized controlled trials. Eur Heart J 1985; 6:556-585.
10. DeWood MA, Spores J, Notske R, et al: Prevalence of total coronary occlusion during the early hours of transmural myocardial infarction. N Engl J Med 1980; 303:897-902.
11. Falk E, Shah PK, Fuster V: Coronary plaque disruption. Circulation 1995; 92:657-671.
12. Cannon CP, Braunwald E: GUSTO, TIMI and the case for rapid reperfusion. Acta Cardiol 1994; 49:1-8.
13. Ohman EM, Topol EJ, Califf RM, et al: An analysis of the cause of early mortality after administration of thrombolytic therapy. The Thrombolysis Angioplasty in Myocardial Infarction Study Group. Coron Artery Dis 1993; 4:957-964.
14. Lincoff AM, Topol EJ: Illusion of reperfusion. Does anyone achieve optimal reperfusion during acute myocardial infarction? Circulation 1993; 88:1361-1374.
15. Ganz W, Buchbinder N, Marcus H, et al: Intracoronary thrombolysis in evolving myocardial infarction. Am Heart J 1981; 101:4-13.
16. Kennedy JW, Ritchie JL, Davis KB, et al: Western Washington randomized trial of intracoronary streptokinase in acute myocardial infarction. N Engl J Med 1983; 309:1477-1482.
17. Rentrop KP, Blanke H, Karsch KR, et al: Initial experience with transluminal recanalization of the recently occluded infarct-related coronary artery in acute myocardial infarction—comparison with conventionally treated patients. Clin Cardiol 1979; 2:92-105.
18. Rentrop P, Blanke H, Karsch KR, et al: Selective intracoronary thrombolysis in acute myocardial infarction and unstable angina pectoris. Circulation 1981; 63:307-317.
19. Indications for fibrinolytic therapy in suspected acute myocardial infarction: Collaborative overview of early mortality and major morbidity results from all randomised trials of more than 1000 patients. Fibrinolytic Therapy Trialists' (FTT) Collaborative Group. Lancet 1994; 343:311-322.
20. Franzosi MG, Santoro E, De Vita C, et al: Ten-year follow-up of the first megatrial testing thrombolytic therapy in patients with acute myocardial infarction: Results of the Gruppo Italiano per lo Studio della Sopravvivenza nell'Infarto-1 study. The GISSI Investigators. Circulation 1998; 98:2659-2665.
21. Baigent C, Collins R, Appleby P, et al: ISIS-2: 10 year survival among patients with suspected acute myocardial infarction in randomised comparison of intravenous streptokinase, oral aspirin, both, or neither. The ISIS-2 (Second International Study of Infarct Survival) Collaborative Group. BMJ 1998; 316:1337-1343.
22. Ryan TJ, Antman EM, Brooks NH, et al: 1999 update: ACC/AHA Guidelines for the Management of Patients With Acute Myocardial Infarction: Executive Summary and Recommendations: A report of the American College of Cardiology/American Heart Association Task Force on Practice Guidelines (Committee on Management of Acute Myocardial Infarction). Circulation 1999; 100:1016-1030.
23. Late Assessment of Thrombolytic Efficacy (LATE) study with alteplase 6-24 hours after onset of acute myocardial infarction. Lancet 1993; 342:759-766.
24. White HD: Thrombolytic therapy in the elderly. Lancet 2000; 356:2028-2030.
25. Bottiger BW, Bode C, Kern S, et al: Efficacy and safety of thrombolytic therapy after initially unsuccessful cardiopulmonary resuscitation: A prospective clinical trial. Lancet 2001; 357:1583-1585.
26. Lederer W, Lichtenberger C, Pechlaner C, et al: Recombinant tissue plasminogen activator during cardiopulmonary resuscitation in 108 patients with out-of-hospital cardiac arrest. Resuscitation 2001; 50:71-76.
27. Abu-Laban RB, Christenson JM, Innes GD, et al: Tissue plasminogen activator in cardiac arrest with pulseless electrical activity. N Engl J Med 2002; 346:1522-1528.
28. Maggioni AP, Franzosi MG, Santoro E, et al: The risk of stroke in patients with acute myocardial infarction after thrombolytic and antithrombotic treatment. Gruppo Italiano per lo Studio della Sopravvivenza nell'Infarto Miocardico II (GISSI-2), and The International Study Group. N Engl J Med 1992; 327:1-6.
29. De Jaegere PP, Arnold AA, Balk AH, et al: Intracranial hemorrhage in association with thrombolytic therapy: Incidence and clinical predictive factors. J Am Coll Cardiol 1992; 19:289-294.
30. The effects of tissue plasminogen activator, streptokinase, or both on coronary-artery patency, ventricular function, and survival after acute myocardial infarction. The GUSTO Angiographic Investigators. N Engl J Med 1993; 329:1615-1622.
31. Van de Werf FJ, Arnold AE: Intravenous tissue plasminogen activator and size of infarct, left ventricular function, and survival in acute myocardial infarction. BMJ 1988; 297:1374-1379.
32. Ito H, Maruyama A, Iwakura K, et al: Clinical implications of the 'no reflow' phenomenon. A predictor of complications and left ventricular remodeling in reperfused anterior wall myocardial infarction. Circulation 1996; 93:223-228.
33. Santoro GM, Valenti R, Buonamici P, et al: Relation between ST-segment changes and myocardial perfusion evaluated by myocardial contrast echocardiography in patients with acute myocardial infarction treated with direct angioplasty. Am J Cardiol 1998; 82:932-937.
34. French JK, Andrews J, Manda SO, et al: Early ST-segment recovery, infarct artery blood flow, and long-term outcome after acute myocardial infarction. Am Heart J 2002; 143:265-271.
35. Gibson CM, Cannon CP, Murphy SA, et al: Relationship of TIMI myocardial perfusion grade to mortality after administration of thrombolytic drugs. Circulation 2000; 101:125-130.
36. Becker RC: Reocclusion following successful thrombolysis. Emerging concepts. Cardiology 1993; 82:265-273.
37. Topol EJ: Acute myocardial infarction: Thrombolysis. Heart 2000; 83:122-126.
38. Ito H, Tomooka T, Sakai N, et al: Lack of myocardial perfusion immediately after successful thrombolysis. A predictor of poor recovery of left ventricular function in anterior myocardial infarction. Circulation 1992; 85:1699-1705.
39. Maes A, Van de WF, Nuyts J, et al: Impaired myocardial tissue perfusion early after successful thrombolysis. Impact on myocardial flow, metabolism, and function at late follow-up. Circulation 1995; 92:2072-2078.
40. Cannon CP: Thrombolysis medication errors: Benefits of bolus thrombolytic agents. Am J Cardiol 2000; 85:17C-22C.
41. Collen D, Bounameaux H, De Cock F, et al: Analysis of coagulation and fibrinolysis during intravenous infusion of recombinant human tissue-type plasminogen activator in patients with acute myocardial infarction. Circulation 1986; 73:511-517.
42. GISSI-2: A factorial randomised trial of alteplase versus streptokinase and heparin versus no heparin among 12,490 patients with acute myocardial infarction. Gruppo Italiano per lo Studio della Sopravvivenza nell'Infarto Miocardico. Lancet 1990; 336:65-71.

43. ISIS-3: A randomised comparison of streptokinase vs tissue plasminogen activator vs anistreplase and of aspirin plus heparin vs aspirin alone among 41,299 cases of suspected acute myocardial infarction. ISIS-3 (Third International Study of Infarct Survival) Collaborative Group. Lancet 1992; 339:753–770.

44. An international randomized trial comparing four thrombolytic strategies for acute myocardial infarction. The GUSTO investigators. N Engl J Med 1993; 329:673–682.

45. Battershill PE, Benfield P, Goa KL: Streptokinase. A review of its pharmacology and therapeutic efficacy in acute myocardial infarction in older patients. Drugs Aging 1994; 4:63–86.

46. Juhlin P, Bostrom PA, Torp A, et al: Streptokinase antibodies inhibit reperfusion during thrombolytic therapy with streptokinase in acute myocardial infarction. J Intern Med 1999; 245:483–488.

47. Lew AS, Laramee P, Cercek B, et al: The hypotensive effect of intravenous streptokinase in patients with acute myocardial infarction. Circulation 1985; 72:1321–1326.

48. Effectiveness of intravenous thrombolytic treatment in acute myocardial infarction. Gruppo Italiano per lo Studio della Streptochinasi nell'Infarto Miocardico (GISSI). Lancet 1986; 1:397–402.

49. Long-term effects of intravenous thrombolysis in acute myocardial infarction: Final report of the GISSI study. Gruppo Italiano per lo Studio della Streptochinasi nell'Infarto Miocardico (GISSI). Lancet 1987; 2:871–874.

50. Mechanisms for the early mortality reduction produced by beta-blockade started early in acute myocardial infarction: ISIS-1. ISIS-1 (First International Study of Infarct Survival) Collaborative Group. Lancet 1988; 1:921–923.

51. Collen D: The plasminogen (fibrinolytic) system. Thromb Haemost 1999; 82:259–270.

52. Granger CB, Califf RM, Topol EJ: Thrombolytic therapy for acute myocardial infarction. A review. Drugs 1992; 44:293–325.

53. Wilcox RG, von der LG, Olsson CG, et al: Trial of tissue plasminogen activator for mortality reduction in acute myocardial infarction. Anglo-Scandinavian Study of Early Thrombolysis (ASSET). Lancet 1988; 2:525–530.

54. Neuhaus KL, Feuerer W, Jeep-Tebbe S, et al: Improved thrombolysis with a modified dose regimen of recombinant tissue-type plasminogen activator. J Am Coll Cardiol 1989; 14:1566–1569.

55. The effects of tissue plasminogen activator, streptokinase, or both on coronary-artery patency, ventricular function, and survival after acute myocardial infarction. The GUSTO Angiographic Investigators. N Engl J Med 1993; 329:1615–1622.

56. Hoffmeister HM, Kastner C, Szabo S, et al: Fibrin specificity and procoagulant effect related to the kallikrein-contact phase system and to plasmin generation with double-bolus reteplase and front-loaded alteplase thrombolysis in acute myocardial infarction. Am J Cardiol 2000; 86:263–268.

57. Smalling RW, Bode C, Kalbfleisch J, et al: More rapid, complete, and stable coronary thrombolysis with bolus administration of reteplase compared with alteplase infusion in acute myocardial infarction. RAPID Investigators. Circulation 1995; 91:2725–2732.

58. Bode C, Smalling RW, Berg G, et al: Randomized comparison of coronary thrombolysis achieved with double-bolus reteplase (recombinant plasminogen activator) and front-loaded, accelerated alteplase (recombinant tissue plasminogen activator) in patients with acute myocardial infarction. The RAPID II Investigators. Circulation 1996; 94:891–898.

59. Randomised, double-blind comparison of reteplase double-bolus administration with streptokinase in acute myocardial infarction (INJECT): Trial to investigate equivalence. International Joint Efficacy Comparison of Thrombolytics. Lancet 1995; 346:329–336.

60. A comparison of reteplase with alteplase for acute myocardial infarction. The Global Use of Strategies to Open Occluded Coronary Arteries (GUSTO III) Investigators. N Engl J Med 1997; 337:1118–1123.

61. Topol EJ, Ohman EM, Armstrong PW, et al: Survival outcomes 1 year after reperfusion therapy with either alteplase or reteplase for acute myocardial infarction: Results from the global utilization of streptokinase and t-PA for occluded coronary arteries (GUSTO) III trial. Circulation 2000; 102:1761–1765.

62. Gurbel PA, Serebruany VL, Shustov AR, et al: Effects of reteplase and alteplase on platelet aggregation and major receptor expression during the first 24 hours of acute myocardial infarction treatment. GUSTO-III Investigators. Global Use of Strategies to Open Occluded Coronary Arteries. J Am Coll Cardiol 1998; 31:1466–1473.

63. Nordt TK, Moser M, Kohler B, et al: Pharmacokinetics and pharmacodynamics of lanoteplase (n-PA). Thromb Haemost 1999; 82 (Suppl 1):121–123.

64. Ogata N, Ogawa H, Ogata Y, et al: Comparison of thrombolytic therapies with mutant tPA (lanoteplase/SUN9216) and recombinant tPA (alteplase) for acute myocardial infarction. Jpn Circ J 1998; 62:801–806.

65. Intravenous NPA for the treatment of infarcting myocardium early. InTIME-II, a double-blind comparison of single-bolus lanoteplase vs accelerated alteplase for the treatment of patients with acute myocardial infarction. Eur Heart J 2000; 21:2005–2013.

66. den Heijer P, Vermeer F, Ambrosioni E, et al: Evaluation of a weight-adjusted single-bolus plasminogen activator in patients with myocardial infarction: A double-blind, randomized angiographic trial of lanoteplase versus alteplase. Circulation 1998; 98:2117–2125.

67. Stewart RJ, Fredenburgh JC, Leslie BA, et al: Identification of the mechanism responsible for the increased fibrin specificity of TNK-tissue plasminogen activator relative to tissue plasminogen activator. J Biol Chem 2000; 275:10112–10120.

68. Binbrek A, Rao N, Absher PM, et al: The relative rapidity of recanalization induced by recombinant tissue-type plasminogen activator (r-tPA) and TNK-tPA, assessed with enzymatic methods. Coron Artery Dis 2000; 11:429–435.

69. Collen D, Stassen JM, Yasuda T, et al: Comparative thrombolytic properties of tissue-type plasminogen activator and of a plasminogen activator inhibitor-1-resistant glycosylation variant, in a combined arterial and venous thrombosis model in the dog. Thromb Haemost 1994; 72:98–104.

70. Cannon CP, McCabe CH, Gibson CM, et al: TNK-tissue plasminogen activator in acute myocardial infarction. Results of the Thrombolysis in Myocardial Infarction (TIMI) 10A dose-ranging trial. Circulation 1997; 95:351–356.

71. Cannon CP, Gibson CM, McCabe CH, et al: TNK-tissue plasminogen activator compared with front-loaded alteplase in acute myocardial infarction: Results of the TIMI 10B trial. Thrombolysis in Myocardial Infarction (TIMI) 10B Investigators. Circulation 1998; 98:2805–2814.

72. Van de Werf FJ, Cannon CP, Luyten A, et al: Safety assessment of single-bolus administration of TNK tissue-plasminogen activator in acute myocardial infarction: The ASSENT-1 trial. The ASSENT-1 Investigators. Am Heart J 1999; 137:786–791.

73. Single-bolus tenecteplase compared with front-loaded alteplase in acute myocardial infarction: The ASSENT-2 double-blind randomised trial. Assessment of the Safety and Efficacy of a New Thrombolytic Investigators. Lancet 1999; 354:716–722.

74. Wang-Clow F, Fox NL, Cannon CP, et al: Determination of a weight-adjusted dose of TNK-tissue plasminogen activator. Am Heart J 2001; 141:33–40.

75. Van de Werf FJ, Barron HV, Armstrong PW, et al: Incidence and predictors of bleeding events after fibrinolytic therapy with fibrin-specific agents. A comparison of TNK-tPA and rt-PA. Eur Heart J 2001; 22:2253–2261.

76. Collen D, Vanderschueren S, Van de Werf FJ: Fibrin-selective thrombolytic therapy with recombinant staphylokinase. Haemostasis 1996; 26 Suppl 4:294–300.

77. Collen D, Moreau H, Stockx L, et al: Recombinant staphylokinase variants with altered immunoreactivity. II: Thrombolytic properties and antibody induction. Circulation 1996; 94:207–216.

78. Laroche Y, Heymans S, Capaert S, et al: Recombinant staphylokinase variants with reduced antigenicity due to elimination of B-lymphocyte epitopes. Blood 2000; 96:1425–1432.

79. Vanderschueren S, Barrios L, Kerdsinchai P, et al: A randomized trial of recombinant staphylokinase versus alteplase for coronary artery patency in acute myocardial infarction. The STAR Trial Group. Circulation 1995; 92:2044–2049.

80. Armstrong PW, Burton JR, Palisaitis D, et al: Collaborative angiographic patency trial of recombinant staphylokinase (CAPTORS). Am Heart J 2000; 139:820–823.

81. Vanwetswinkel S, Plaisance S, Zhi-Yong Z, et al: Pharmacokinetic and thrombolytic properties of cysteine-linked polyethylene glycol derivatives of staphylokinase. Blood 2000; 95:936–942.

82. Collen D, Sinnaeve P, Demarsin E, et al: Polyethylene glycol-derivatized cysteine-substitution variants of recombinant staphylokinase for single-bolus treatment of acute myocardial infarction. Circulation 2000; 102:1766–1772.

83. Armstrong PW, Burton JR, Molhoek P: Patency trial of recombinant staphylokinase (CAPTORS II). J Am Coll Cardiol 2002; 281A.

84. Bar FW, Vermeer F, Michels R, et al: Saruplase in myocardial infarction. J Thromb Thrombolysis 1995; 2:195–204.

85. Randomised double-blind trial of recombinant pro-urokinase against streptokinase in acute myocardial infarction. PRIMI Trial Study Group. Lancet 1989; 1:863–868.

86. Tebbe U, Michels R, Adgey J, et al: Randomized, double-blind study comparing saruplase with streptokinase therapy in acute myocardial infarction: The COMPASS Equivalence Trial. Comparison Trial of Saruplase and Streptokinase (COMPASS) Investigators. J Am Coll Cardiol 1998; 31:487–493.

87. Bar FW, Meyer J, Boland J, et al: Bolus Administration of Saruplase in Europe (BASE), a Pilot Study in Patients with Acute Myocardial Infarction. J Thromb Thrombolysis 1998; 6:147–153.

88. Charbonnier B, Pluta W, De Ferrari G, et al: Evaluation of Two Weight-Adjusted Single Bolus Doses of Amediplase to Patients with Acute Myocardial Infarction: the 3k2 Trial (ABSTRACT). Circulation 2001; 107:II-538.

89. Vermeer F, Oldrovd K, Pohl J, et al: Safety and angiography data of Amediplase, a new fibrin specific thrombolytic agent, given as a single bolus to patients with acute myocardial infarction: the 2K2 Dose Finding Trial (ABSTRACT). Circulation 2001; 104:II-538.

90. Topol EJ, George BS, Kereiakes DJ, et al: A randomized controlled trial of intravenous tissue plasminogen activator and early intravenous heparin in acute myocardial infarction. Circulation 1989; 79:281–286.

91. Bleich SD, Nichols TC, Schumacher RR, et al: Effect of heparin on coronary arterial patency after thrombolysis with tissue plasminogen activator in acute myocardial infarction. Am J Cardiol 1990; 66:1412–1417.

92. Hsia J, Hamilton WP, Kleiman N, et al: A comparison between heparin and low-dose aspirin as adjunctive therapy with tissue plasminogen activator for acute myocardial infarction. Heparin-Aspirin Reperfusion Trial (HART) Investigators. N Engl J Med 1990; 323:1433–1437.

93. Antman EM: The search for replacements for unfractionated heparin. Circulation 2001; 103:2310–2314.

94. Giugliano RP, McCabe CH, Antman EM, et al: Lower-dose heparin with fibrinolysis is associated with lower rates of intracranial hemorrhage. Am Heart J 2001; 141:742–750.

95. Turpie AG, Antman EM: Low-molecular-weight heparins in the treatment of acute coronary syndromes. Arch Intern Med 2001; 161:1484–1490.

96. Wallentin L, Dellborg DM, Lindahl B, et al: The low-molecular-weight heparin dalteparin as adjuvant therapy in acute myocardial infarction: The ASSENT PLUS study. Clin Cardiol 2001; 24:I12–I14.

97. Ross AM, Molhoek P, Lundergan C, et al: Randomized comparison of enoxaparin, a low-molecular-weight heparin, with unfractionated heparin adjunctive to recombinant tissue plasminogen activator thrombolysis and aspirin: Second trial of Heparin and Aspirin Reperfusion Therapy (HART II). Circulation 2001; 104:648–652.

98. Antman EM, Louwerenburg HW, Baars HF, et al: Enoxaparin as adjunctive antithrombin therapy for ST-elevation myocardial infarction: Results of the ENTIRE-Thrombolysis in Myocardial Infarction (TIMI) 23 Trial. Circulation 2002; 105:1642–1649.

99. AMI-SK trial (unpublished). 2002.

100. Glick A, Kornowski R, Michowich Y, et al: Reduction of reinfarction and angina with use of low-molecular-weight heparin therapy after streptokinase (and heparin) in acute myocardial infarction. Am J Cardiol 1996; 77:1145–1148.

101. Gibson CM, de Lemos JA, Murphy SA, et al: Combination therapy with abciximab reduces angiographically evident thrombus in acute myocardial infarction: A TIMI 14 substudy. Circulation 2001; 103:2550–2554.

102. Ohman EM, Kleiman NS, Gacioch G, et al: Combined accelerated tissue-plasminogen activator and platelet glycoprotein IIb/IIIa integrin receptor blockade with Integrilin in acute myocardial infarction. Results of a randomized, placebo-controlled, dose-ranging trial. IMPACT-AMI Investigators. Circulation 1997; 95:846–854.

103. Brener SJ, Zeymer U, Adgey AA, et al: Eptifibatide and low-dose tissue plasminogen activator in acute myocardial infarction: The integrilin and low-dose thrombolysis in acute myocardial infarction (INTRO AMI) trial. J Am Coll Cardiol 2002; 39:377–386.

104. Giugliano RP, Roe M, Harrington R, et al: Combination reperfusion therapy with eptifibatide and reduced-dose tenecteplase for ST-elevation myocardial infarction: Results of the integrilin and tenecteplase in acute myocardial infarction (INTEGRITI) Phase II Angiographic Trial. J Am Coll Cardiol 2003; 41:1251–1260.

105. FASTER trial. (unpublished) 2002.

106. Antman EM, Giugliano RP, Gibson CM, et al: Abciximab facilitates the rate and extent of thrombolysis: results of the thrombolysis in myocardial infarction (TIMI) 14 trial. The TIMI 14 Investigators. Circulation 1999; 99:2720–2732.

107. Trial of abciximab with and without low-dose reteplase for acute myocardial infarction. Strategies for Patency Enhancement in the Emergency Department (SPEED) Group. Circulation 2000; 101:2788–2794.

108. Herrmann HC, Moliterno DJ, Ohman EM, et al: Facilitation of early percutaneous coronary intervention after reteplase with or without abciximab in acute myocardial infarction: Results from the SPEED (GUSTO-4 Pilot) Trial. J Am Coll Cardiol 2000; 36:1489–1496.

109. Weitz JI: Biological rationale for the therapeutic role of specific antithrombins. Coron Artery Dis 1996; 7:409–419.

110. Kong DF, Topol EJ, Bittl JA, et al: Clinical outcomes of bivalirudin for ischemic heart disease. Circulation 1999; 100:2049–2053.

111. A comparison of recombinant hirudin with heparin for the treatment of acute coronary syndromes. The Global Use of Strategies to Open Occluded Coronary Arteries (GUSTO) IIb investigators. N Engl J Med 1996; 335:775–782.

112. Antman EM: Hirudin in acute myocardial infarction. Thrombolysis and Thrombin Inhibition in Myocardial Infarction (TIMI) 9B trial. Circulation 1996; 94:911–921.

113. Neuhaus KL, Molhoek GP, Zeymer U, et al: Recombinant hirudin (lepirudin) for the improvement of thrombolysis with streptokinase in patients with acute myocardial infarction: Results of the HIT-4 trial. J Am Coll Cardiol 1999; 34:966–973.

114. White HD, Aylward PE, Frey MJ, et al: Randomized, double-blind comparison of hirulog versus heparin in patients receiving streptokinase and aspirin for acute myocardial infarction (HERO). Hirulog Early Reperfusion/Occlusion (HERO) Trial Investigators. Circulation 1997; 96:2155–2161.

115. Direct thrombin inhibitors in acute coronary syndromes: Principal results of a meta-analysis based on individual patients' data. Lancet 2002; 359:294–302.

116. White H: Thrombin-specific anticoagulation with bivalirudin versus heparin in patients receiving fibrinolytic therapy for acute myocardial infarction: the HERO-2 randomised trial. Lancet 2001; 358:1855–1863.

117. Siegel JP: Equivalence and noninferiority trials. Am Heart J 2000; 139:S166–S170.

118. Lesaffre E, Bluhmki E, Wang-Clow F, et al: The general concepts of an equivalence trial, applied to ASSENT-2, a large-scale mortality study comparing two fibrinolytic agents in acute myocardial infarction. Eur Heart J 2001; 22:898–902.

119. A comparison of continuous infusion of alteplase with double-bolus administration for acute myocardial infarction. The Continuous Infusion versus Double-Bolus Administration of Alteplase (COBALT) Investigators. N Engl J Med 1997; 337:1124–1130.

120. Van de Werf FJ: ASSENT-3: Implications for future trial design and clinical practice. Eur Heart J 2002; 23:911–912.

121. O'Shea JC, Califf RM: International differences in cardiovascular clinical trials. Am Heart J 2001; 141:866–874.

122. Van de Werf FJ, Topol EJ, Lee KL, et al: Variations in patient management and outcomes for acute myocardial infarction in the United States and other countries. Results from the GUSTO trial. Global Utilization of Streptokinase and Tissue Plasminogen Activator for Occluded Coronary Arteries. JAMA 1995; 273:1586–1591.

123. Giugliano RP, Llevadot J, Wilcox RG, et al: Geographic variation in patient and hospital characteristics, management, and clinical outcomes in ST-elevation myocardial infarction treated with fibrinolysis. Results from InTIME-II. Eur Heart J 2001; 22:1702–1715.

124. Llevadot J, Giugliano RP, Antman EM, et al: Availability of on-site catheterization and clinical outcomes in patients receiving fibrinolysis for ST-elevation myocardial infarction. Eur Heart J 2001; 22:2104–2115.

125. Ross AM, Gao R, Coyne KS, et al: A randomized trial confirming the efficacy of reduced dose recombinant tissue plasminogen activator in a Chinese myocardial infarction population and

demonstrating superiority to usual dose urokinase: The TUCC trial. Am Heart J 2001; 142:244-247.

126. Gurwitz JH, Gore JM, Goldberg RJ, et al: Risk for intracranial hemorrhage after tissue plasminogen activator treatment for acute myocardial infarction. Participants in the National Registry of Myocardial Infarction 2. Ann Intern Med 1998; 129:597-604.

127. Angeja BG, Alexander JH, Chin R, et al: Safety of the weight-adjusted dosing regimen of tenecteplase in the ASSENT-Trial. Am J Cardiol 2001; 88:1240-1245.

128. Mehta SR, Eikelboom JW, Yusuf S: Risk of intracranial haemorrhage with bolus versus infusion thrombolytic therapy: a meta-analysis. Lancet 2000; 356:449-454.

129. Eikelboom JW, Mehta SR, Pogue J, et al: Safety outcomes in meta-analyses of phase 2 vs phase 3 randomized trials: Intracranial hemorrhage in trials of bolus thrombolytic therapy. JAMA 2001; 285:444-450.

130. Armstrong PW, Granger C, Van de Werf FJ: Bolus fibrinolysis: risk, benefit, and opportunities. Circulation 2001; 103:1171-1173.

131. Thiemann DR, Coresh J, Schulman SP, et al: Lack of benefit for intravenous thrombolysis in patients with myocardial infarction who are older than 75 years. Circulation 2000; 101:2239-2246.

132. Soumerai SB, McLaughlin TJ, Ross-Degnan D, et al: Effectiveness of thrombolytic therapy for acute myocardial infarction in the elderly: Cause for concern in the old-old. Arch Intern Med 2002; 162:561-568.

133. Sherry S, Marder VJ: Mistaken guidelines for thrombolytic therapy of acute myocardial infarction in the elderly. J Am Coll Cardiol 1991; 17:1237-1238.

134. Cannon CP, Antman EM, Walls R, et al: Time as an Adjunctive Agent to Thrombolytic Therapy. J Thromb Thrombolysis 1994; 1:27-34.

135. Reimer KA, Lowe JE, Rasmussen MM, et al: The wavefront phenomenon of ischemic cell death. 1. Myocardial infarct size vs duration of coronary occlusion in dogs. Circulation 1977; 56:786-794.

136. White HD: Thrombolytic therapy for patients with myocardial infarction presenting after six hours. Lancet 1992; 340:221-222.

137. Newby LK, Rutsch WR, Califf RM, et al: Time from symptom onset to treatment and outcomes after thrombolytic therapy. GUSTO-1 Investigators. J Am Coll Cardiol 1996; 27:1646-1655.

138. Chesebro JH, Knatterud G, Roberts R, et al: Thrombolysis in Myocardial Infarction (TIMI) Trial, Phase I: A comparison between intravenous tissue plasminogen activator and intravenous streptokinase. Clinical findings through hospital discharge. Circulation 1987; 76:142-154.

139. Marder VJ, Sherry S: Thrombolytic therapy: current status (1). N Engl J Med 1988; 318:1512-1520.

140. Zeymer U, Tebbe U, Essen R, et al: Influence of time to treatment on early infarct-related artery patency after different thrombolytic regimens. ALKK-Study Group. Am Heart J 1999; 137:34-38.

141. Van de Werf F, Ardissino D, Betriu A, et al: Management of acute myocardial infarction in patients presenting with ST-segment elevation. The Task Force on the Management of Acute Myocardial Infarction of the European Society of Cardiology. Eur Heart J 2003; 24:28-66.

142. Gibler WB, Armstrong PW, Ohman EM, et al: Persistence of delays in presentation and treatment for patients with acute myocardial infarction: The GUSTO-I and GUSTO-III experience. Ann Emerg Med 2002; 39:123-130.

143. Goldberg RJ, Gurwitz JH, Gore JM: Duration of, and temporal trends (1994-1997) in, prehospital delay in patients with acute myocardial infarction: The second National Registry of Myocardial Infarction. Arch Intern Med 1999; 159:2141-2147.

144. Emergency department: Rapid identification and treatment of patients with acute myocardial infarction. National Heart Attack Alert Program Coordinating Committee, 60 Minutes to Treatment Working Group. Ann Emerg Med 1994; 23:311-329.

145. Cannon CP, Johnson EB, Cermignani M, et al: Emergency department thrombolysis critical pathway reduces door-to-drug times in acute myocardial infarction. Clin Cardiol 1999; 22:17-20.

146. Pell AC, Miller HC, Robertson CE, et al: Effect of "fast track" admission for acute myocardial infarction on delay to thrombolysis. BMJ 1992; 304:83-87.

147. Seyedroudbari A, Kessler ER, Mooss AN, et al: Time to treatment and cost of thrombolysis: A multicenter comparison of tPA and rPA. J Thromb Thrombolysis 2000; 9:303-308.

148. Morrison LJ, Verbeek PR, McDonald AC, et al: Mortality and pre-hospital thrombolysis for acute myocardial infarction: A meta-analysis. JAMA 2000; 283:2686-2692.

149. Armstrong PW, Collen D: Fibrinolysis for acute myocardial infarction: Current status and new horizons for pharmacological reperfusion, part 2. Circulation 2001; 19; 103:2987-2992.

150. Cannon CP, Gibson CM, Lambrew CT, et al: Relationship of symptom-onset-to-balloon time and door-to-balloon time with mortality in patients undergoing angioplasty for acute myocardial infarction. JAMA 2000; 283:2941-2947.

151. A clinical trial comparing primary coronary angioplasty with tissue plasminogen activator for acute myocardial infarction: The Global Use of Strategies to Open Occluded Coronary Arteries in Acute Coronary Syndromes (GUSTO IIb) Angioplasty Substudy Investigators. N Engl J Med 1997; 336:1621-1628.

152. Weaver WD, Simes RJ, Betriu A, et al: Comparison of primary coronary angioplasty and intravenous thrombolytic therapy for acute myocardial infarction: A quantitative review. JAMA 1997; 278:2093-2098.

153. Stone GW, Grines CL, Browne KF, et al: Implications of recurrent ischemia after reperfusion therapy in acute myocardial infarction: A comparison of thrombolytic therapy and primary angioplasty. J Am Coll Cardiol 1995; 26:66-72.

154. Montalescot G, Barragan P, Wittenberg O, et al: Platelet glycoprotein IIb/IIIa inhibition with coronary stenting for acute myocardial infarction. N Engl J Med 2001; 344:1895-1903.

155. Stone GW, Grines CL, Cox DA, et al: Comparison of angioplasty with stenting, with or without abciximab, in acute myocardial infarction. N Engl J Med 2002; 346:957-966.

156. DANAMI-2 trial. (unpublished). 2002.

157. Grines CL, Westerhausen DR, Jr., Grines LL, et al: A randomized trial of transfer for primary angioplasty versus on-site thrombolysis in patients with high-risk myocardial infarction: The Air Primary Angioplasty in Myocardial Infarction study. J Am Coll Cardiol 2002; 39:1713-1719.

158. Verheugt FW: GUSTO V: The bottom line of fibrinolytic reperfusion therapy. Lancet 2001; 357:1898-1899.

159. Cannon CP: Multimodality reperfusion therapy for acute myocardial infarction. Am Heart J 2000; 140:707-716.

160. Ross AM, Coyne KS, Reiner JS, et al: A randomized trial comparing primary angioplasty with a strategy of short-acting thrombolysis and immediate planned rescue angioplasty in acute myocardial infarction: The PACT trial. PACT investigators. Plasminogen-activator Angioplasty Compatibility Trial. J Am Coll Cardiol 1999; 34:1954-1962.

■■■c h a p t e r **8**

Direct Thrombin Inhibitors

John A. Bittl
Harvey D. White
Elliott M. Antman

The direct thrombin inhibitors comprise a successful case study in clinical trials research.[1-4] Proceeding systematically from a solid experimental foundation to large clinical trials, the development of these agents initially encountered several unexpected starts and stops.[5] Smaller efficacy effects than anticipated and unexpected safety differences among the various direct thrombin inhibitors punctuated their development. Compelling evidence from clinical trials has emerged since 1999, when the topic of direct thrombin inhibitors appeared in the first edition of *Clinical Trials in Cardiovascular Disease*.[1] Since then, the United States Food and Drug Administration (FDA) has approved three direct thrombin inhibitors—lepirudin, bivalirudin, and argatroban—as alternatives to heparin for a broad range of indications. Several other direct thrombin inhibitors—such as desirudin; melagatran; and the oral inhibitor, ximelagatran—have not been approved and marketed at the time of this writing but have entered the advanced stages of clinical development.

This chapter represents a major revision of the topic of direct thrombin inhibitors. The first section of this chapter outlines the pharmacologic actions of the three approved agents. The second section reviews the specific clinical settings in which direct thrombin inhibitors have been evaluated—ST elevation myocardial infarction (STEMI), unstable angina and non-ST elevation myocardial infarction (NSTEMI), percutaneous coronary interventions (PCI), heparin-induced thrombocytopenia (HIT), and deep venous thrombosis (DVT). This chapter emphasizes the indications for each agent for which the strongest clinical trial evidence exists and whenever possible describes clinical trials that are under way.

DIRECT THROMBIN INHIBITORS

Thrombus Formation

Acute coronary syndromes, such as MI or unstable angina, are associated with focal thrombosis in conjunction with atherosclerotic plaques and thus may be suitable indications for treatment with direct thrombin inhibitors.[4] The pathogenesis of the acute coronary syndromes is based on activation of tissue factor protein in disrupted atherosclerotic plaques, which combines with factors VIIa and Xa to form the prothrombinase complex.[6-9] This converts prothrombin to thrombin by splitting off the prothrombin fragment F1 + 2. The concentration of F1 + 2 thus reflects the extent of local thrombin generation.

Recruitment of platelets, fibrin, and red cells forms intravascular thrombus.[10] The relative proportion of each of these components in the arterial and venous systems depends on local hemodynamic factors. Arterial thrombi, which consist predominantly of platelets and thin fibrin strands, form under conditions of disturbed flow at sites of plaque rupture. Venous thrombi consist of red cells, large amounts of fibrin, and few platelets and form under conditions of stasis. The occlusive thrombi of STEMI,[11] as well as the instrumentation of coronary arteries during prolonged PCI procedures,[12] probably causes adjacent concretions of platelet-rich and fibrin-rich thrombus.

Thrombin participates in two central functions of thrombus formation—converting fibrinogen to fibrin and activating platelets.[13,14] The local activity of thrombin is reflected by the concentration of fibrinopeptide A, a fragment cleaved by thrombin from fibrinogen as it is converted to fibrin.

Although unfractionated heparin (UFH) has been used for several decades as the platform of anticoagulation, it has several limitations. UFH binds unpredictably to plasma proteins,[15] is only partially active against clot-bound thrombin,[16] is inhibited by platelet factor 4 released by activated platelets,[17] and also may cause the life-threatening syndrome known as heparin-induced thrombocytopenia and thrombosis (HITT).[18] The direct thrombin inhibitors have several theoretical and practical advantages over heparin.

Direct thrombin inhibitors do not require endogenous cofactors such as antithrombin for their anticoagulant effect. The direct thrombin inhibitors do not cause HITT, nor do they antigenically cross react with UFH. The direct thrombin inhibitors do not activate platelets,[19] are not inhibited by platelet factor 4,[17] and are equally potent against clot-bound thrombin as against soluble thrombin.[16]

The development of direct thrombin inhibitors has been based on the characterization of hirudin, the

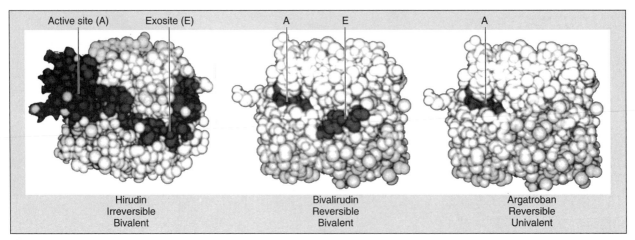

FIGURE 8-1. Space-filling molecular models of direct thrombin inhibitors *(dark gray)* are bound to the exosite-1 *(E)* and active site *(A)* of thrombin *(light gray)*. The prototypical direct thrombin inhibitor, hirudin, is a 65-amino-acid peptide that irreversibly binds to thrombin; bivalirudin is a specifically engineered 20-amino-acid peptide that binds reversibly to both sites; and argatroban is a small-molecule derivative that binds reversibly only to the active site of thrombin.

naturally occurring 65-amino-acid anticoagulant isolated from the salivary gland of the medicinal leech. The carboxy terminus of the bivalent inhibitors such as hirudin or bivalirudin binds to the substrate recognition site on thrombin, whereas the amino terminus blocks the active catalytic site of thrombin (Fig. 8-1). The univalent thrombin inhibitors, such as argatroban and efegatran, bind only to the active site of thrombin.

Experimental studies suggest that the bivalent inhibitors such as hirudin or bivalirudin are more effective anticoagulants than the univalent inhibitors. Inhibition of both the catalytic and the exosite domains of thrombin increases antithrombotic potency by several orders of magnitude over the inhibition of either domain alone.[20] This may translate into differences in clinical efficacy as well. A meta-analysis[21] of 35,970 patients in comparative trials with heparin in acute coronary syndromes or PCI showed a reduction in death or MI at 7 days (odds ratio 0.88 [95% confidence interval 0.80, 0.96]) and at 30 days (0.91 [0.84,0.99]) for the entire class of direct thrombin inhibitors (Fig. 8-2). Within the class of direct thrombin inhibitors, however, important differences were seen

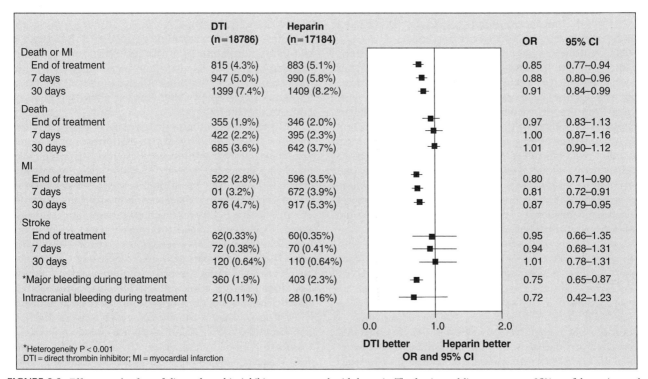

	DTI (n=18786)	Heparin (n=17184)		OR	95% CI
Death or MI					
End of treatment	815 (4.3%)	883 (5.1%)		0.85	0.77–0.94
7 days	947 (5.0%)	990 (5.8%)		0.88	0.80–0.96
30 days	1399 (7.4%)	1409 (8.2%)		0.91	0.84–0.99
Death					
End of treatment	355 (1.9%)	346 (2.0%)		0.97	0.83–1.13
7 days	422 (2.2%)	395 (2.3%)		1.00	0.87–1.16
30 days	685 (3.6%)	642 (3.7%)		1.01	0.90–1.12
MI					
End of treatment	522 (2.8%)	596 (3.5%)		0.80	0.71–0.90
7 days	01 (3.2%)	672 (3.9%)		0.81	0.72–0.91
30 days	876 (4.7%)	917 (5.3%)		0.87	0.79–0.95
Stroke					
End of treatment	62(0.33%)	60(0.35%)		0.95	0.66–1.35
7 days	72 (0.38%)	70 (0.41%)		0.94	0.68–1.31
30 days	120 (0.64%)	110 (0.64%)		1.01	0.78–1.31
*Major bleeding during treatment	360 (1.9%)	403 (2.3%)		0.75	0.65–0.87
Intracranial bleeding during treatment	21(0.11%)	28 (0.16%)		0.72	0.42–1.23

0.0   1.0   2.0
DTI better   Heparin better
OR and 95% CI

*Heterogeneity P < 0.001
DTI = direct thrombin inhibitor; MI = myocardial infarction

FIGURE 8-2. Efficacy and safety of direct thrombin inhibitors compared with heparin. The horizontal lines represent 95% confidence intervals. (From The Direct Thrombin Inhibitor Trialists' Collaborative Group: Direct thrombin inhibitors in acute coronary syndromes: Principal results of a meta-analysis based on individual patients' data. Lancet 2002;359:294–302, with permission).

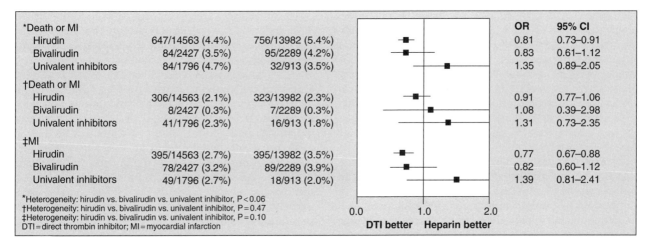

					OR	95% CI
*Death or MI						
Hirudin	647/14563 (4.4%)	756/13982 (5.4%)			0.81	0.73–0.91
Bivalirudin	84/2427 (3.5%)	95/2289 (4.2%)			0.83	0.61–1.12
Univalent inhibitors	84/1796 (4.7%)	32/913 (3.5%)			1.35	0.89–2.05
†Death or MI						
Hirudin	306/14563 (2.1%)	323/13982 (2.3%)			0.91	0.77–1.06
Bivalirudin	8/2427 (0.3%)	7/2289 (0.3%)			1.08	0.39–2.98
Univalent inhibitors	41/1796 (2.3%)	16/913 (1.8%)			1.31	0.73–2.35
‡MI						
Hirudin	395/14563 (2.7%)	395/13982 (3.5%)			0.77	0.67–0.88
Bivalirudin	78/2427 (3.2%)	89/2289 (3.9%)			0.82	0.60–1.12
Univalent inhibitors	49/1796 (2.7%)	18/913 (2.0%)			1.39	0.81–2.41

*Heterogeneity: hirudin vs. bivalirudin vs. univalent inhibitor, P < 0.06
†Heterogeneity: hirudin vs. bivalirudin vs. univalent inhibitor, P = 0.47
‡Heterogeneity: hirudin vs. bivalirudin vs. univalent inhibitor, P = 0.10
DTI = direct thrombin inhibitor; MI = myocardial infarction

0.0   1.0   2.0
DTI better   Heparin better

FIGURE 8-3. Efficacy of direct thrombin inhibitors compared with heparin, according to agent. The horizontal lines represent 95% confidence intervals. (From The Direct Thrombin Inhibitor Trialists' Collaborative Group: Direct thrombin inhibitors in acute coronary syndromes: Principal results of a meta-analysis based on individual patients' data. Lancet 2002; 359:294–302, with permission).

(Fig. 8-3). A reduction in death or MI was seen with hirudin (0.81 [0.73, 0.91]) and bivalirudin (0.83 [0.61, 1.12]) but not with univalent agents (1.35 [0.89, 2.05]). It was not certain whether the differences were caused by small numbers of subjects in some clinical trials, but statistical heterogeneity among the groups suggested that real differences do exist, favoring efficacy of bivalent over the univalent agents.[21] Other differences in the pharmacokinetics of the different thrombin inhibitors are highlighted in the next sections.

Hirudin

Lepirudin (Refludan, Berlex) is a recombinant derivative of native hirudin (Fig. 8-1). Lepirudin is similar to native hirudin except for substitution of leucine for isoleucine at the N-terminal of the molecule and the absence of a sulfate group on the tyrosine at position 63 ([Leu,[1] Thr[2]]-desulfatohirudin). Desirudin (Revasc, Aventis) is not marketed at this time but is similar to lepirudin, except that it contains valine substitutions for the first two N-terminal amino acids ([Val,[1] Val[2]]-63-desulfatohirudin).

The hirudins are irreversible inhibitors of thrombin, partially metabolized by hydrolysis, and excreted in urine with a terminal plasma elimination half-life ($t_{1/2}\beta$) of 1.3 hours in patients with normal renal function. The half-life of hirudin increases up to 150 hours in patients with renal failure.[22] The FDA-approved dosage of lepirudin is 0.4 mg/kg bolus, followed by 0.15 mg/kg/hr. If the serum creatinine level is greater than 1.5 mg/dL, the bolus should be reduced to 0.2 mg/kg. The infusion should be reduced by 50% in patients with creatinine levels of 1.6 to 2.0 mg/dL, by 70% in those with levels of 2.1 to 3.0 mg/dL, and by 85% in those with levels of 3.1 to 6.0 mg/dL. After thrombolytic therapy, the dose of lepirudin should be reduced to 0.2 mg/dL, followed by an infusion of 0.1 mg/dL/hr.

Hirudin is antigenic, eliciting an antibody response in approximately 45% of patients after 5 days of treatment.[23] The antibody response does not appear to reduce the anticoagulant effect of lepirudin. Instead, an enhanced anti-

coagulation effect has been observed and is caused by reduced renal clearance of hirudin–antihirudin antibodies,[24] requiring a reduction in the dose of hirudin to maintain a stable activated partial thromboplastin time (aPTT).

The hirudins prolong the aPTT and the activated clotting time (ACT) in a dose-dependent manner. In all reported clinical studies, the incidence of bleeding was greater in hirudin-treated patients that in control patients.[3] No neutralizing or reversing agent is available for lepirudin or desirudin.

Bivalirudin

Bivalirudin (Angiomax, The Medicines Company) was formally known as Hirulog. It is a 20-amino-acid peptide whose design is based on that of hirudin. Although its amino-acid sequence is much shorter than that of hirudin, its binding interactions with thrombin are similar and reversible.[25] Bivalirudin binds stoichiometrically to the catalytic site as well as to the substrate-binding exosite of thrombin (Fig. 8-1).

Bivalirudin does not bind to platelet factor 4, red blood cells, or plasma proteins (other than thrombin). It has a small volume of distribution (0.156 L/kg) and a half-life of 25 minutes. It is eliminated by a combination of renal excretion and inactivation by slow hydrolytic cleavage of the Arg_3-Pro_4 bond. Dosage adjustments are recommended in patients with glomerular filtration rates of less than 60 mL/min. Although no antidote exists, coagulation times return to baseline in about 1 hour after bivalirudin is stopped. The drug is partly hemodialyzable.

The dose of bivalirudin previously recommended during coronary angioplasty was 1.0 mg/kg, followed by an infusion of 2.5 mg/kg/hr. If concomitant treatment with a platelet-glycoprotein (GP) IIb/IIIa inhibitor is used, the recommended dose is 0.75 mg/kg, followed by an infusion of 1.75 mg/kg/hr (which is also the monotherapy dose commonly used in contemporary clinical trials reviewed in the following section, titled "Percutaneous Coronary Interventions: Bivalirudin"). The infusion of bivalirudin is reduced by 20% for patients with creatinine clearances of 30–60 mL/min, by 60% for creatinine clearances of 10–30 mL/min, and by 90% for patients on hemodialysis. Bivalirudin prolongs the aPTT and the ACT in a dose-dependent manner, allowing point-of-care assessment of the anticoagulant effect in the cardiac catheterization laboratory or at the bedside.

Argatroban

Argatroban (Novastan, GlaxoSmithKline) is a small-molecule direct thrombin inhibitor synthetically derived from L-arginine. Argatroban blocks the catalytic site of soluble and clot-bound thrombin (Fig. 8-1).

Argatroban is hepatically metabolized. No dosage adjustment is required for renal insufficiency. In the presence of normal hepatic function, the half-life of argatroban is 39 to 51 minutes. Its anticoagulant action is monitored by measuring the aPTT. The aPTT returns to normal within 2 hours of discontinuation of argatroban.

The starting dose of argatroban for medical conditions is 2 μg/kg/min. The recommended dose of argatroban for PCI is a loading dose of 10 mg followed by an infusion of 15 to 25 mg/hr. The aPTT and ACT should be monitored. If an infusion is used, it should be tapered to avoid rebound rather than being stopped abruptly.[26] No antidote or reversing agent exists for argatroban.

ST ELEVATION MYOCARDIAL INFARCTION

A coronary artery plaque that is moderately stenotic, relatively soft with a central core rich in lipids, and covered with a thin fibrous cap containing relatively small amounts of connective tissue and smooth muscle cells is referred to as a "vulnerable" plaque.[27] When it ruptures and exposes its contents to the bloodstream, platelets adhere to the subendothelial matrix, release adenosine diphosphate and thromboxane A_2, and amplify the generation of thrombin, resulting in the development of a platelet aggregate. In addition, the coagulation cascade is activated and fibrin strands are formed.[27] The culprit coronary artery becomes occluded by a thrombus containing both a fibrin mesh and platelet aggregates. When coronary blood flow is reduced sufficiently, patients experience ischemic discomfort. Complete occlusion of the culprit vessel produces ST segment elevation, and the majority of such individuals ultimately evolve a Q-wave MI.

Hirudins

Inadequate initial reperfusion of infarct-related arteries and reocclusion of successfully reperfused vessels continue to be important limitations of thrombolytic regimens for STEMI. In an effort to improve adjunctive regimens for use with thrombolysis, direct thrombin inhibitors have been evaluated in several clinical trials.

The Thrombolysis in Myocardial Infarction (TIMI) 5 study enrolled 246 patients with STEMI who were treated with front-loaded tissue plasminogen activator (tPA) and randomized to receive one of four ascending doses of recombinant desirudin (a bolus ranging from 0.15 mg/kg to 0.6 mg/kg followed by an infusion ranging from 0.05 mg/kg/hr up to 0.2 mg/kg/hr) versus heparin (a bolus of 5000 IU and an initial infusion of 1000 IU/hr titrated to an aPTT of 65–90 seconds).[28] At follow-up angiography carried out at 18 to 36 hours, infarct-artery patency was significantly more common in the desirudin-treated patients than in the heparin-treated patients. Reocclusion by 18 to 36 hours was seen in only 1.6% of patients taking desirudin compared with 6.7% of patients taking heparin (P = 0.07). No intracranial hemorrhages occurred in any of the desirudin dose groups; one patient of 86 (1.2%) in the heparin group had an intracranial hemorrhage. Major hemorrhage occurred predominantly at an instrumented site and ranged from 11.5% at the lowest dose of desirudin (0.05 mg/kg/hr infusion) to 29.4% at the highest dose of desirudin (0.2 mg/kg/hr infusion) as compared with 18.6% in heparin-treated patients. Analysis of the characteristics of the patients experiencing major bleeding suggested that an aPTT in excess of 100 seconds was associated with an increased risk of bleeding.

The TIMI 6 trial consisted of 193 patients treated with streptokinase for STEMI.[29] Patients were randomized to receive one of three doses of desirudin (boluses of 0.15, 0.3, and 0.6 mg/kg followed respectively by infusions of 0.05, 0.1, and 0.2/mg/kg/hr) versus heparin (bolus 5000 IU, initial infusion 1000 IU/hr). Major hemorrhage occurred during the initial hospitalization in 5.5%, 6.5%, and 5.6% of patients treated with the desirudin regimens described previously and in 5.6% of those treated with heparin. Death or nonfatal reinfarction occurred by hospital discharge in 8.8% of patients treated with heparin and 13.7%, 9.7%, and 5.7% of the three ascending desirudin dose groups. The trend toward a reduction in events with higher doses of desirudin persisted at 6 weeks after enrollment.

In the TIMI 9B trial,[30] 3002 patients with acute myocardial infarction (AMI) were treated with aspirin and either accelerated-dose tPA or streptokinase. They then were randomized within 12 hours of symptoms to receive either intravenous heparin (5000 IU bolus followed by infusion of 1000 IU/hr) or desirudin (0.1 mg/kg bolus followed by infusion of 0.1 mg/kg/hr). The infusions of both antithrombins were titrated to a target aPTT of 55 to 85 seconds and were administered for 96 hours. The primary endpoint (death, recurrent nonfatal MI, or development of severe congestive heart failure or cardiogenic shock by 30 days) occurred in 11.9% of the 1491 patients in the heparin group and in 12.9% of the 1511 patients in the desirudin group. The rates of major hemorrhage were similar in the heparin (5.3%) and desirudin (4.6%) groups. Intracranial hemorrhage occurred in 0.9% of the heparin group and 0.4% of the desirudin group. Patients in the desirudin group were significantly more likely to have an aPTT measurement within the target range over the first 96 hours of the trial.

In the Global Use of Strategies to Open Occluded Coronary Arteries (GUSTO) IIb trial,[31] 12,142 patients with acute coronary syndromes were randomized to receive either heparin or desirudin. Patients were stratified according to the presence of ST-segment elevation on the baseline electrocardiogram (4131 patients) or its absence (8011 patients), with the latter finding signifying unstable angina or non-Q-wave MI. At 24 hours, the combined incidence of death and MI was significantly lower in the group treated with desirudin than in the group treated with heparin (1.3% vs. 2.1%, P = 0.001). The primary composite endpoint of death, nonfatal MI, or reinfarction within 30 days was reached in 9.8% of the heparin group as compared with 8.9% of the desirudin group (P = 0.06). The predominant effect of desirudin was on MI or reinfarction and was not influenced by ST-segment status. There were no significant differences in the rates of serious or life-threatening bleeding complications, but desirudin therapy was associated with a higher incidence of moderate bleeding (8.8% vs. 7.7%, P = 0.03). When the results of the TIMI 9B and GUSTO IIb trials were combined, there was no reduction in mortality, but desirudin reduced the incidence of reinfarction by 14% (P = 0.024).[32]

The TIMI 9A,[33] GUSTO IIa,[34] and Hirudin for Improvement of Thrombolysis (HIT)-III[35] trials were the initial phase III trials testing the direct antithrombin desirudin versus heparin. The TIMI 9A and HIT-III trials focused on patients with STEMI, and GUSTO IIa enrolled patients with clinical presentations across the acute coronary syndrome spectrum. A feature common to all three trials was that they were stopped prematurely because of unacceptable rates of serious bleeding, particularly intracranial hemorrhage. This excessive rate of bleeding appeared to be the result of high levels of anticoagulation in both the heparin and desirudin groups in TIMI 9A and GUSTO IIa. Although a slightly lower dose of desirudin was used in HIT-III, it too was associated with an unacceptable rate of major hemorrhage. An important lesson learned from the hirudin trials was the necessity for monitoring the aPTT to adjust the infusion, much as is done with UFH. The risk of bleeding with hirudin is dose-related and is increased in patients with MI, congestive heart failure, renal insufficiency, liver injury, and recent surgery or recent stroke and after thrombolytic therapy.

Bivalirudin

Several trials have evaluated the adjunctive use of bivalirudin with streptokinase in patients with MI. Théroux and colleagues[36] compared low-dose bivalirudin (0.5 mg/kg/hr) and high-dose bivalirudin (1.0 mg/kg/hr) with heparin (bolus 5000 IU, infusion 1000 IU/hr). At 90 minutes, TIMI grade 3 flow was observed in 85% of the low-dose bivalirudin group, 61% of the high-dose bivalirudin group, and 31% of the heparin group (P = 0.008).

In the Hirulog and Early Reperfusion or Occlusion (HERO)-1 trial,[37] 298 patients with AMI were treated with bivalirudin or heparin as an adjunct to thrombolytic therapy. TIMI grade 3 flow was achieved by 90 minutes in 56% of 99 patients receiving high-dose bivalirudin (0.25 mg/kg bolus followed by 0.5 mg/kg/hr for 12 hours and then 0.25 mg/kg/hr), 49% of 99 patients receiving low-dose bivalirudin (0.125 mg/kg bolus followed by 0.25 mg/kg/hr for 12 hours and then 0.125 mg/kg/hr), and 35% of 100 patients receiving heparin (5000 IU bolus followed by 1000–2000 IU/hr). At 48 hours, reocclusion had occurred in 7% of the heparin group, 5% of the low-dose bivalirudin group, and 1% of the high-dose bivalirudin group (P = NS). By 35 days, death, cardiogenic shock, or reinfarction had occurred in 25 patients treated with heparin (17.9%), 19 patients treated with low-dose bivalirudin patients (14%), and 17 patients treated with high-dose bivalirudin (12.5%, P = NS). Two strokes occurred with heparin, none with low-dose bivalirudin, and two with high-dose bivalirudin. Major bleeding (40% from the groin site) occurred in 28% of the heparin group, 14% of the low-dose bivalirudin group, and 19% of the high-dose bivalirudin group (heparin versus low-dose bivalirudin, P < 0.01).

In the HERO-2 trial,[38] 17,073 patients with STEMI were randomized to receive either UFH or bivalirudin, given 3 minutes before streptokinase. The primary endpoint was 30-day mortality, and the major secondary endpoint was reinfarction (Fig. 8-4). The 30-day mortality

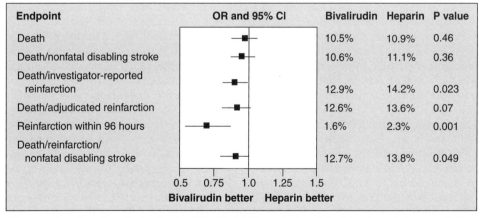

FIGURE 8-4. Key efficacy and net benefit endpoints in the HERO-2 trial. The endpoint of death is adjusted for sex and all factors in the GUSTO mortality risk model. The composite endpoints of death/investigator-reported reinfarction and death/reinfarction/nonfatal disabling stroke were not prespecified in the trial protocol. (From White, Hirulog, Early Reperfusion or Occlusion-2 Trial Investigators: Thrombin-specific anticoagulation with bivalirudin versus heparin in patients receiving fibrinolytic therapy for acute myocardial infarction: The HERO-2 randomised trial. Lancet 2001;358:1855–1863, with permission).

rates were 10.9% in the heparin group and 10.5% in the bivalirudin group (P = 0.88). The 30-day reinfarction rates were 3.6% in the heparin group and 2.8% in the bivalirudin group (P = 0.004). The overall rates of intracranial hemorrhage (0.5%) and transfusion were lower than in other recent trials,[39,40] although the HERO-2 population had greater risk factors for bleeding. Moderate bleeding and mild bleeding were more common with bivalirudin than with heparin (1.39% vs. 1.05%, P = 0.05; and 12.8% vs. 9.0%, P < 0.01, respectively). The aPTT in patients randomized to bivalirudin was about 40% longer than the optimal aPTT achieved in the heparin group (108 vs. 77 seconds at 12 hours, 80 vs. 77 seconds at 24 hours, P < 0.001). Statistical adjustment for the prolonged aPTTs explained 50% to 100% of the increase in bleeding observed with bivalirudin but did not affect the reduction in reinfarction. In addition, when an on-treatment analysis was performed, the increase in moderate bleeding observed with bivalirudin was not significant (1.4% vs. 1.1% with heparin, P = 0.062).[41]

Argatroban and Other Univalent Thrombin Inhibitors

In the Argatroban in Acute Myocardial Infarction (ARGAMI) trial,[42] argatroban was compared with heparin in patients receiving accelerated tPA for AMI. The study series consisted of an open-label dose-finding study (35 patients) followed by a placebo-controlled study with a double-dummy technique and 2:1 (argatroban: heparin) randomization. In the randomized study, 82 patients received argatroban (100-μg/kg bolus followed by 3 μg/kg/min for 72 hours) and 45 received heparin (5000 IU intravenous bolus followed by 1000 IU/hr infusion). Patency of the infarct-related artery with TIMI grade 2 or 3 flow was achieved by 90 minutes in 62 patients treated with argatroban (76%) versus 37 patients treated with heparin (82%, P = NS). The proportion of patients with TIMI grade 3 flow at 90 minutes was slightly higher in the heparin group (67%) than in the argatroban group (57%). Bleeding complications were observed in 16 patients treated with argatroban (19.5%) and in 9 patients treated with heparin (20.0%). One patient treated with heparin suffered a hemorrhagic stroke.

In the Promotion of Reperfusion in Myocardial Infarction Evolution (PRIME) trial,[43] the univalent thrombin inhibitor, efegatran, was compared with UFH as adjunctive therapy in MI. A total of 336 patients with AMI was randomized to receive one of five doses of efegatran or heparin for 72 to 96 hours, both with accelerated alteplase and aspirin. The primary endpoint (death, reinfarction, or TIMI grade 0–2 flow in the infarct artery from 90 minutes to discharge or 30 days) occurred in 53% of patients treated with heparin, in 54% of patients treated with efegatran overall (P = 0.90), and in 55% of patients given intermediate-dose efegatran (P = 0.74). Thus, the univalent inhibitor, efegatran, appeared to offer no clear advantage over heparin as an adjunct to thrombolysis for STEMI.

UNSTABLE ANGINA AND NON-ST ELEVATION MYOCARDIAL INFARCTION

Some patients with plaque rupture may sustain an NSTEMI[27] because no ST segment elevation occurs when the obstructing thrombus is subtotally occlusive, obstruction is transient, or a rich collateral network is present. The majority of such patients are diagnosed as having unstable angina, or if a serum cardiac marker indicative of myocardial necrosis is detected, they are considered to have a non-Q-wave MI.

The outcome of unstable angina and NSTEMI depends on the acuity at presentation and the severity of underlying coronary artery disease.[44,45] Patients with advanced age, elevated troponin levels, or greater electrocardiographic changes are more likely to have extensive underlying thrombus at the culprit lesion and a higher risk of complications with heparin therapy.

Lepirudin

In the Organisation to Assess Strategies for Ischemic Syndromes (OASIS) pilot study,[46] 909 patients with unstable angina or suspected AMI without ST elevation were randomized to receive either heparin (5000 IU bolus followed by 1000–1200 IU/hr), low-dose lepirudin (0.2 mg/kg followed by 0.10 mg/kg/hr), or medium-dose lepirudin (0.4 mg/kg followed by 0.15 mg/kg/hr) for 72 hours. The randomization to heparin versus lepirudin was performed in an open-label fashion, but the randomization to the two different doses of lepirudin was blinded. By 7 days, 6.5% of patients in the heparin group, 4.4% in the low-dose lepirudin group, and 3.0% in the medium-dose lepirudin group had suffered cardiovascular death, new MI, or refractory angina (P = 0.267 for heparin vs. low-dose lepirudin; P = 0.047 for heparin vs. medium-dose lepirudin).

In the OASIS-2 study,[47] 10,141 patients with unstable angina or suspected AMI without ST elevation were randomized to receive either heparin (5000 IU followed by 15 IU/kg/hr) or lepirudin (0.4 mg/kg and 0.15 mg/kg/hr) for 72 hours in a double-blind trial. The primary endpoint was cardiovascular death or new MI within 7 days (Table 8-1). By 7 days, 213 patients (4.2%) in the heparin group and 182 (3.6%) in the lepirudin group had suffered cardiovascular death or new MI (P = 0.077), whereas 340 (6.7%) versus 284 (5.6%), respectively, had suffered cardiovascular death, new MI, or refractory angina (P = 0.0125). These differences were observed primarily during the 72-hour treatment period. Although there was an excess of major bleeding requiring transfusion with lepirudin (1.2% vs. 0.7% with heparin, P = 0.01), there was no excess of life-threatening bleeding episodes (20 in each group) or strokes (14 in each group).

Pooled data from studies involving patients with acute coronary syndromes showed that the combined incidence of death and MI was lower with lepirudin than with UFH (Table 8-1).[3] The greater relative treatment effect during the lepirudin infusion, followed by a reduction in the magnitude of the drug effect, is consistent

■ ▓ ■

TABLE 8-1   LEPIRUDIN FOR ACUTE CORONARY SYNDROMES

	Heparin (n)	Lepirudin (n)	Relative risk (95% CI)	P
Cardiovascular death or MI at 7 days				
OASIS-1	18/371 (4.9%)	14/538 (2.6%)	0.54 (0.27–1.06)	0.07
OASIS-2	213/5058 (4.2%)	182/5083 (3.6%)	0.84 (0.69–1.02)	0.077
Total	231/5429 (4.3%)	196/5621 (3.5%)	0.81 (0.67–0.98)	0.039
Death or MI at 35 days				
OASIS-1	32/371 (8.6%)	33/538 (6.1%)	0.71 (0.44–1.14)	0.15
OASIS-2	388/5058 (7.7%)	345/5083 (6.8%)	0.87 (0.75–1.01)	0.06
Total	420/5429 (7.7%)	378/5621 (6.7%)	0.86 (0.74–0.99)	0.04

CI, confidence interval; MI, myocardial infarction; OASIS, Organisation to Assess Strategies for Ischemic Syndromes.
Modified from Greinacher A, Lubenow N: Recombinant hirudin in clinical practice: Focus on lepirudin. Circulation 2001; 103:1479–1484.

with rebound activation of the coagulation cascade after cessation of the infusion.

Bivalirudin

In the TIMI 7 trial,[48] 410 patients with unstable angina or NSTEMI were treated with one of four doses of bivalirudin for 72 hours (0.02, 0.25, 0.5, or 1.0 mg/kg/hr). Of the 160 patients treated with the lowest dose of bivalirudin, 10% suffered death or MI by hospital discharge compared with 3.2% of the 250 patients who received one of the higher doses of bivalirudin (P < 0.008). This difference in benefit between the low- and high-dose groups was sustained at 6 weeks, at which time death or MI had occurred in 12.5% of the low-dose group versus 5.2% of the high-dose group (P = 0.009). Of note, the patients receiving one of the three higher doses of bivalirudin exhibited a stable aPTT pattern, with 93% having values within a 30-second range throughout the study drug infusion. No intracranial hemorrhages occurred, but major spontaneous bleeding occurred in two patients (0.5%).

In the TIMI 8 trial,[49] 133 patients with unstable angina or non-Q-wave MI were randomized to receive either bivalirudin (0.1 mg/kg followed by 0.25 mg/kg/hr) or heparin (70 IU/kg followed by 15 IU/kg/hr) for 72 hours. The combined rates of death and MI were lower in the bivalirudin group at 14 days (2.9% vs. 9.2%) and at 30 days (4.4% vs. 12.3%). The rate of major hemorrhage was also lower in the bivalirudin group (0.0% versus 4.6%). The TIMI 8 trial was stopped prematurely by the sponsor based on a business decision after only 2.5% of the planned enrollment.[5,50]

Argatroban

In a pilot study involving 43 patients with unstable angina or non-Q-wave MI,[51] an intravenous infusion of argatroban (0.5–5.0 µg/kg/min for 4 hours) was monitored by sequential measurements of coagulation times and thrombin activity in vivo. Although significant dose-related increases in plasma drug concentrations and the aPTT occurred, no spontaneous bleeding was observed.

Myocardial ischemia did not occur during therapy, but nine of the 43 patients experienced an episode of unstable angina an average of 6 hours after the argatroban infusion was stopped. This early recurrent angina correlated significantly with a higher argatroban dose and with greater prolongation of the aPTT but not with other demographic, clinical, laboratory, and angiographic characteristics. This has been reported as an example of ischemic rebound in patients with unstable angina after abrupt cessation of argatroban therapy.[51] Tapering of argatroban infusions may prevent ischemic rebound.

PERCUTANEOUS CORONARY INTERVENTIONS

The use of platelet inhibitors during PCI has been a major therapeutic advance,[52-54] but an optimal anticoagulation regimen needs to be defined. Several case-control studies suggest that the odds of death, MI, or revascularization are reduced significantly with therapeutic as compared with subtherapeutic anticoagulation.[55-58] This observation has been extended by Chew and colleagues,[59] who evaluated the relation between ACTs and ischemic complications in 5216 patients in six randomized, controlled trials of new antithrombotic therapy during PCI. They observed that an ACT within the range of 350 to 375 seconds after heparin was associated with a 34% reduction in the combined incidence of death, MI, and target-vessel revascularization as compared with an ACT of 171 to 295 seconds by quartile analysis. These observations—along with those reported for subtherapeutic anticoagulation during a phase II study of bivalirudin during PCI (see later in this chapter)—support the requirement for therapeutic anticoagulation during PCI.

Hirudins

In the Hirudin European Trial Versus Heparin in the Prevention of Restenosis after PTCA (HELVETICA),[60] 1141 patients with unstable angina scheduled for angioplasty were given aspirin and randomized to one of

■ ▪ ■

TABLE 8-2   BIVALIRUDIN PHASE II STUDY: ACTUAL* AND IMPUTED ADVERSE CARDIAC EVENT RATES DURING PERCUTANEOUS TRANSLUMINAL CORONARY ANGIOPLASTY, BY DEGREE OF ANTICOAGULATION

	Imputed values	Groups 1–3	Groups 4–6
	No anticoagulation	Low-dose bivalirudin	Higher-dose bivalirudin
n	—	152	139
Dose of bivalirudin (mg/kg)	—	0.15–0.35	0.45–1.00
ACT >300 seconds (%)	0	27.9	79.1
Death, MI, revascularization, or AVC (%)	22.1	12.5	3.6

*Actual values from Topol EJ, Bonan R, Jewitt D, et al: Use of a direct antithrombin, hirulog, in place of heparin during coronary angioplasty. Circulation 1993; 87:1622–1629.
ACT, activated clotting time; AVC, abrupt vessel closure; MI, myocardial infarction.

three anticoagulation regimens: heparin (10,000 IU followed by 15 IU/kg/hr for 24 hours), desirudin (Revasc; 40 mg followed by 0.2 mg/kg/hr for 24 hours), or the identical desirudin regimen plus additional desirudin (40 mg administered subcutaneously twice daily for an additional 3 days). By 96 hours, 5.6% of the subcutaneous desirudin group versus 11.0% of the control group had died, suffered an MI, or undergone bypass surgery. By 6 months, 32.0% of the heparin group versus 33.7% of the combined desirudin groups had experienced major ischemic complications or undergone repeat revascularization.[60]

The HELVETICA Biochemical Substudy provided interesting insights into the comparison of the actions of heparin and desirudin.[60] Heparin therapy was associated with a reduction in the generation of thrombin, as determined by the levels of prothrombin fragment F1 + 2 (1.0 nM before balloon dilation vs. 0.9 nM after dilation), whereas hirudin administered intravenously and subcutaneously was associated with a slight increase in the levels of F1 + 2 (1.0 nM vs. 1.3 nM). Although hirudin was at least as effective as heparin in inhibiting activated thrombin, increased thrombin generation at the time of discontinuation of anticoagulant therapy theoretically increased the risk of "thrombin rebound," but this was not observed in the study.[60]

Limited experience has been reported with lepirudin during PCI. Manfredi and colleagues[61] described four patients with HITT who successfully underwent PCI with lepirudin used as the sole anticoagulant.

Bivalirudin

In an open-label dose-escalation Phase II study,[62] Topol and colleagues evaluated the safety and efficacy of bivalirudin as a substitute for heparin in 291 patients undergoing elective balloon angioplasty. Six ascending bolus doses (0.15, 0.25, 0.35, 0.45, 0.55, and 1.0 mg/kg of body weight) matched with six ascending infusion doses (0.6, 1.0, 1.4, 1.8, 2.2, and 2.5 mg/kg/hr) were evaluated in six groups of approximately 50 patients each. Bivalirudin produced a dose-dependent anticoagulant effect without increasing bleeding complications. The target ACT of greater than 300 seconds was achieved in 79% of patients in the three highest-dose groups versus 28% of patients in the three lowest-dose groups (Table 8-2). Major and minor angioplasty complications (including abrupt vessel closure, MI, or the need for emergency bypass surgery) were less common in the three highest-dose groups than in the three lowest-dose groups (3.6% vs. 12.5%). This study demonstrated that coronary angioplasty could be performed with a direct thrombin inhibitor in place of heparin and emphasized that adequate anticoagulation is required for the optimal performance of PCI.

In the Bivalirudin Angioplasty Study,[63,64] 4312 patients with unstable angina undergoing PCI were randomized to receive either bivalirudin or UFH. The randomization included a prestratified group of 741 patients with postinfarction angina.[65] Bivalirudin significantly reduced the incidence of clinical ischemic events (death, MI, or revascularization) in all patients (Table 8-3). The absolute

■ ▪ ■

TABLE 8-3   BIVALIRUDIN ANGIOPLASTY STUDY: CLINICAL ISCHEMIC ENDPOINTS IN HOSPITAL THROUGH SEVEN DAYS, BY TREATMENT GROUP

All patients	Bivalirudin (n = 2161)	Heparin (n = 2151)	Odds ratio (95% CI)	P
Death, MI, or revascularization	135 (6.2%)	169 (7.9%)	0.78 (0.62–0.99)	0.039
Post-infarction angina cohort	(n = 369)	(n = 372)		
Death, MI, or revascularization	18 (4.9%)	37 (9.9%)	0.47 (0.26–0.84)	0.009

CI, confidence interval; MI, myocardial infarction.
Modified from Bittl JA, Chaitman BR, Feit F, et al: Bivalirudin versus heparin during coronary angioplasty for unstable or post-infarction angina: The final report of the Bivalirudin Angioplasty Study. Am Heart J 2001; 142:952–959.

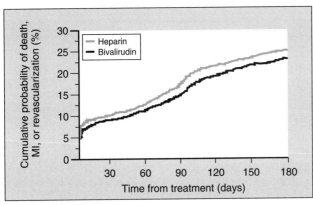

FIGURE 8-5. Probability of the combined endpoint of death, myocardial infarction, or revascularization within 180 days for all patients (Kaplan-Meier plot). (From Bittl JA, Chaitman BR, Feit F, et al: Bivalirudin versus heparin during coronary angioplasty for unstable or post-infarction angina: The final report of the Bivalirudin Angioplasty Study. Am Heart Journal 2001; 142:952–959, with permission.)

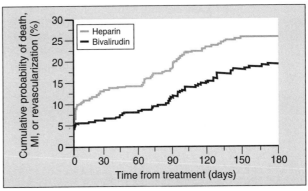

FIGURE 8-6. Probability of the combined endpoint of death, myocardial infarction, or revascularization within 180 days for patients undergoing coronary angioplasty within 2 weeks of myocardial infarction (Kaplan-Meier plot). (From Bittl JA, Chaitman BR, Feit F, et al: Bivalirudin versus heparin during coronary angioplasty for unstable or post-infarction angina: The final report of the Bivalirudin Angioplasty Study. Am Heart Journal 2001; 142:952–959, with permission.)

differences persisted between the two treatment groups at 90 days and 180 days (Fig. 8-5). Bivalirudin also significantly reduced the incidence of clinical ischemic events in patients with postinfarction unstable angina (Fig. 8-6) and significantly reduced the incidence of major bleeding events in all patients (Table 8-4).

The possibility of ischemic rebound was evaluated directly in the Bivalirudin Angioplasty Study.[63,64] After discontinuation of either heparin or bivalirudin at 18 to 24 hours, 25 of 2039 patients (1.2%) who had received heparin therapy experienced a major complication, whereas only seven of 2059 patients (0.3%) treated with bivalirudin experienced a complication.[66]

The safety of combining bivalirudin with routine abciximab and clopidogrel therapy was evaluated in phase A of the Comparison of Abciximab Complications with Hirulog Ischemia Events (CACHET) trial,[67] which showed that administration of full-dose bivalirudin (a 1 mg/kg bolus followed by 2.5 mg/kg/hr for up to 4 hours postprocedure) plus full-dose abciximab (n = 30) resulted in predictable anticoagulation, with ACTs of approximately 350 seconds and no excessive risk of hemorrhage or clinical ischemia.

These observations were extended in the CACHET B/C trial,[67] which evaluated heparin plus planned abciximab (n = 64) versus bivalirudin plus provisional abciximab (n = 144) in patients undergoing planned coronary stenting in a 2:1 randomization scheme. The use of bivalirudin (a 0.5–0.75 mg/kg bolus followed by 1.75 mg/kg/hr during the procedure) with provisional abciximab produced an immediate ACT of approximately 280 to 320 seconds and was associated with a lower combined incidence of death, MI, revascularization, or major hemorrhage than heparin plus planned abciximab (3.5% vs. 14.1%, P = 0.013). Among patients developing intraprocedural indications for provisional abciximab, comparable ischemic event rates were observed in both groups (5.9%).

The Randomized Evaluation in PCI Linking Angiomax to Reduced Clinical Events Part 1 (REPLACE-1) study[68] enrolled 1056 patients undergoing planned PCI. This was a randomized, open-label trial, designed to compare heparin with bivalirudin (a 0.75 mg/kg bolus followed by 1.75 mg/kg/hr during the procedure). Use of coronary stenting (84%) and GP IIb/IIIa inhibition (71%) remained at the discretion of the investigator.

■ ▦ ■

TABLE 8-4 BLEEDING ENDPOINTS IN HOSPITAL UP TO SEVEN DAYS, BY TREATMENT GROUP

All patients	Bivalirudin (n = 2161)	Heparin (n = 2151)	Odds ratio (95% CI)	P
Clinically significant bleeding	76 (3.5%)	199 (9.3%)	0.34 (0.26–0.45)	<0.001
Intracranial hemorrhage	1 (0.04%)	2 (0.09%)	0.50 (0.05–5.23)	0.624
Retroperitoneal bleeding	5 (0.2%)	15 (0.7%)	0.33 (0.13–0.87)	0.026
Red cell transfusion ≥2 units	43 (2.0%)	123 (5.7%)	0.34 (0.24–0.47)	<0.001
With >3 g/dL fall in Hb	41 (1.9%)	124 (5.8%)	0.33 (0.24–0.46)	<0.001
With >5 g/dL fall in Hb	14 (0.6%)	47 (2.2%)	0.29 (0.17–0.51)	<0.001

CI, confidence interval; Hb, hemoglobin.
Modified from Bittl JA, Chaitman BR, Feit F, et al: Bivalirudin versus heparin during coronary angioplasty for unstable or post-infarction angina: The final report of the Bivalirudin Angioplasty Study. Am Heart J 2001; 142:952–959.

Thienopyridines were administered before the procedure in 54% of patients. The combined endpoint of death, MI, or revascularization was reduced by 19% in the bivalirudin-treated patients at 48 hours. A 22% reduction in protocol-defined major bleeding and a 21% reduction in the composite quadruple endpoint of death, MI, revascularization, or major bleeding at 48 hours were observed. Among patients receiving GP IIb/IIIa inhibition, bivalirudin provided a further 16% reduction in death, MI, or revascularization at 48 hours.

The REPLACE-2 trial[69] enrolled 6010 patients undergoing PCI. This was a randomized, double-blind, double-dummy, active controlled trial comparing bivalirudin (0.75 mg/kg followed by 1.75 mg/kg/hr) and provisional GP IIb/IIIa inhibitors with heparin (65 U/kg bolus) and planned GP IIb/IIIa inhibitors in patients undergoing planned PCI. Provisional GP IIb/IIIa inhibitors were given to 7.2% of the bivalirudin patients. The primary endpoint was a "quadruple" composite endpoint consisting of the 30-day incidence of death, MI, urgent repeat revascularization, or in-hospital bleeding, and one secondary endpoint was the "triple" endpoint consisting of the 30-day incidence of death, MI, or urgent repeat revascularization.

In this equivalence trial,[69] all three prespecified statistical criteria for noninferiority were met. First, the quadruple endpoint occurred in 9.2% of patients treated with bivalirudin and provisional GP IIb/IIIa inhibitors versus 10.0% of those treated with heparin and planned GP IIb/IIIa therapy (OR 0.92 [0.77, 1.09]). Second, bivalirudin and provisional IIb/IIIa inhibition was superior to treatment with heparin alone (imputed). Third, the triple endpoint occurred in 7.6% of patients treated with bivalirudin and provisional GP IIb/IIIa inhibitors versus 7.1% of those treated with heparin and planned GP IIb/IIIa therapy (OR 1.09 [0.90, 1.32]. In-hospital major bleeding rates were reduced significantly with bivalirudin and provisional GP IIb/IIIa inhibitors as compared with heparin and planned GP IIb/IIIa inhibitors (2.4% vs. 4.1%).[69]

Argatroban

In a small series of patients undergoing angioplasty with either heparin (n = 15) or argatroban (n = 12), Suzuki and colleagues measured inflammatory and anticoagulation parameters.[70] Fibrinogen levels fell significantly with argatroban. The levels of prothrombin fragment 1 + 2 and thrombin antithrombin III complex increased markedly with both anticoagulants, but argatroban resulted in a more rapid return to the baseline levels than heparin treatment.

In the a series of 91 patients with HIT, Lewis and colleagues[71] described the use of argatroban as a substitute for heparin in during PCI. After PCI with argatroban Lewis and colleagues[71] observed death, MI, or urgent revascularization in 7.7% of patients at 24 hours. In this series of predominantly nonimmunulogic HIT, the mean platelet count was 193,000 and only 4 of 91 patients had noncoronary thrombosis. No additional follow-up beyond 24 hours was given in the report.[71] Argatroban

was evaluated in combination with abciximab for coronary stenting.

HEPARIN-INDUCED THROMBOCYTOPENIA AND HEPARIN-INDUCED THROMBOCYTOPENIA WITH THROMBOSIS

HIT occurs in two forms.[18,72] The first type is a mild, nonimmunologic form. It is defined by a 50% decrease in the platelet count to less than 150,000/mm^3. Profound thrombocytopenia is unusual. This form of HIT occurs in normal subjects, may recover spontaneously even during continuation of heparin, and is probably caused by platelet aggregation in vivo.

The severe form of HIT may be associated with arterial or venous thromboses (HITT). DVT, disseminated intravascular coagulation, pulmonary embolism, cerebral thrombosis, MI, or ischemic injury to the legs or arms can produce severe morbidity and mortality in approximately 50% of patients with HITT.[73]

The use of heparin is absolutely contraindicated in HITT. When HITT is diagnosed, early diagnosis and rapid management of patients are critical. Heparin should be stopped immediately, and another anticoagulant must be substituted to avoid thrombotic complications. Cross-reactivity between direct thrombin inhibitors and heparin has not been reported.

The low–molecular-weight heparins cannot be substituted for heparin in HITT because of cross-reactivity,[72] and administration of an oral anticoagulant such as warfarin (Coumadin) to patients with HITT may lead to venous limb gangrene.[74] Danaparoid (Orgaran, Organon, New Jersey) is a glycosaminoglycan antithrombotic consisting of a mixture of heparan sulfate (84%), dermatan sulfate (12%), and chondroitin sulfate (4%), which has an anti-Xa:anti-IIa ratio of 22:1. It is reasonable to use danaproid with caution in patients with HIT, but cross-reactivity between heparin and danaproid has been reported in 28% of patients with HIT.[75]

Lepirudin

Lepirudin has been designated as an orphan drug by the FDA for the indication of HIT. Approval of lepirudin for this condition was based on comparisons of historical controls with lepirudin-treated patients who had HITT antibodies and clinical symptoms, consisting of more than a 50% reduction in the platelet count or a new thromboembolic episode (Table 8-5).[3] No randomized comparison between control therapy and lepirudin for HITT has been performed—and probably could not be performed for ethical or logistical reasons.[3] The use of lepirudin has been associated with apparent 40% to 50% reductions in death, amputation, or new thromboembolic episodes, with only a slight increase in the risk of bleeding (Table 8-5).

The level of anticoagulation achieved by lepirudin in patients with HITT can be monitored by the aPTT. The aPTT should be measured before starting therapy, every

■ ■ ■

TABLE 8-5 DIRECT THROMBIN INHIBITORS FOR HEPARIN-INDUCED THROMBOCYTOPENIA

LEPIRUDIN STUDIES			
Study	Historical controls	HIT[83]	HITT[3]
N	120	82	112
Death, amputation, or new TE episode	52.1%	25.4%	31.9%
Bleeding	27.2%	39.1%	44.6%
Transfusion	9.1%	9.9%	12.9%

ARGATROBAN STUDIES[84]				
	HIT		HITT	
Study[84]	Historical controls	Argatroban	Historical controls	Argatroban
N	147	160	46	63
Death, MI, or new TE episode	38.8%	25.6%	56.5%	43.8%
Death	21.8%	16.9%	28.3%	18.1%
Amputation	2.0%	1.9%	8.7%	11.1%
New TE episode	15.0%	6.9%	19.6%	14.6%

HIT, heparin-induced thrombocytopenia; HITT, heparin-induced thrombocytopenia and thrombosis syndrome; TE, thromboembolic.

4 hours until a stable aPTT has been achieved, and at least once daily thereafter.

Bivalirudin

The experience with bivalirudin in patients with HITT is more limited than that with lepirudin. Chamberlin and colleagues[76] successfully administered bivalirudin to three patients with HITT without causing ischemic or bleeding complications. Bivalirudin also has been used for HITT and DVT.[77] Bivalirudin is currently available from the manufacturer in an FDA-monitored evaluation of HITT or HITT.

Argatroban

Argatroban has been tested in a series of 304 patients with HIT.[78] The patients received argatroban in an intravenous infusion of 2 μg/kg/min, adjusted to maintain the aPTT at 1.5 to 3.0 times the baseline value. Treatment was maintained for an average of 6 days. Clinical outcomes over 37 days were compared with outcomes in 193 historical control subjects with HIT (n = 147) or HITT (n = 46). The incidence of the primary efficacy endpoint (Table 8-5)—a composite of all-cause death, amputation, or new thrombosis—was reduced significantly in argatroban-treated patients with HIT (25.6% vs. 38.8% in control subjects, P = 0.014). In those with HITT, the primary efficacy endpoint occurred in 43.8% of argatroban-treated patients versus 56.5% of control subjects (P = 0.13). Argatroban-treated patients achieved therapeutic aPTTs generally within 4 to 5 hours of starting therapy and, compared with control subjects, had a significantly faster increase in platelet counts (P = 0.0001), which rose to greater than 100,000 or 1.5 times the baseline platelet count within 3 days of starting argatroban therapy.

In clinical trials of argatroban, severe hemorrhage occurred in approximately 2% of patients, a rate that compares favorably with historical controls treated with UFH. However, hematuria occurred in 12% of patients treated with argatroban, which is higher than the expected 1% rate with heparin. Allergic reactions including coughs or rashes occurred in 10% to 15% of patients treated with argatroban, mostly in those treated with thrombolytic or radiocontrast agents.

DEEP VENOUS THROMBOSIS

Hirudins

Experience with direct thrombin inhibitors to prevent or treat DVT is limited. In a randomized prevention trial performed at 31 centers in 10 European countries,[79] 2079 eligible patients were randomly assigned to receive desirudin or enoxaparin. The rate of proximal DVT was lower in the desirudin group than in the enoxaparin group (4.5 vs. 7.5%, P = 0.01, relative risk reduction 40.3%) and the overall rate of DVT was also lower (18.4 vs. 25.5%, P = 0.001, relative risk reduction 28.0%). The risk of bleeding was similar in the two treatment groups.

Bivalirudin

In a pilot study of primary prevention of DVT after orthopedic surgery,[80] 177 patients were treated with bivalirudin in an open-label, dose-escalation study. In patients receiving doses of 0.3 mg/kg twice daily to 1.0 mg/kg twice daily, the risk of proximal DVT was 20% (131 patients), whereas in those receiving doses of 1.0 mg/kg three times daily, the risk was 2% (46 patients). The risk of bleeding was low in this study and did not increase with escalating dose of bivalirudin.

Other Agents

Melagatran is a parenteral direct thrombin inhibitor and ximelagatran is an oral direct thrombin inhibitor unapproved at the time of this writing by the FDA but are in advanced phases of clinical development. Several clinical trials have evaluated these new direct thrombin inhibitors in patients at high risk for development of DVT. In a randomized, double-blind trial[81] involving patients undergoing total knee arthroplasty, ximelagatran 24 mg orally twice daily was compared with warfarin (target International Normalized Ratio [INR] 2.5) for prophylaxis against DVT. DVT occurred in 53 of 276 patients (19.2%) treated with ximelagatran versus 67 of 261 patients (25.7%) treated with warfarin (P = 0.07).[81] Major bleeding occurred in 1.7% of the ximelagatran-treated patients and in 0.9% of the warfarin-treated patients.

In another randomized trial[82] of 1495 patients undergoing total hip or knee replacement, four dose categories of sequential subcutaneous melagatran and oral ximelagatran were compared with subcutaneous dalteparin as prophylaxis against DVT. The frequency of DVT was lower in the highest dose of melagatran/ximelagatran (15.1%) than in the dalteparin group (28.2%).[82]

In the Stroke Prevention by Oral Thrombin Inhibitor in Atrial Fibrillation (SPORTIF II) trial,[85] ximelagatran was compared with warfarin for the primary prevention of systemic thromboembolism in nonvalvular atrial fibrillation. Three groups of patients received ximelagatran (n = 187) at 20, 40, or 60 mg twice daily, given in a double-blind fashion without routine coagulation monitoring. A fourth group received warfarin (n = 67), whose dosing was targeted to an INR of 2.0 to 3.0. One stroke and one episode of transient ischemic attack (TIA) occurred in patients treated with ximelagatran. Two episodes of TIA occurred in patients treated with warfarin. One major hemorrhage occurred in a patient treated with warfarin. A total of eight patients treated with ximelagatran (4.3%) had elevation of liver tests, which normalized on discontinuation of the study drug.[85]

CONCLUSIONS

Heparin is a nearly ubiquitous antithrombin whose clinical limitations are widely familiar to physicians.

As compared with heparin, the hirudin derivatives are associated with a reduction in the risk of MI during the period of drug infusion in patients presenting with unstable angina/NSTEMI. These agents also may reduce the risk of recurrent MI in patients presenting with STEMI requiring thrombolytic therapy. Monitoring of the aPTT and adjustment of the infusion are necessary to minimize the risk of bleeding, especially in patients with moderately reduced renal function.

If a substitute for heparin or platelet glycoprotein IIb/IIIa inhibitors is required for PCI, bivalirudin has a short half-life, a proven efficacy in a series of large clinical trials, and a low-risk profile that makes it the optimal choice for this indication.

For patients with renal failure and HIT who require PCI, bivalirudin with dose adjustment or argatroban is an alternative to heparin, but there are persistent concerns about the anticoagulant potency of the monovalent thrombin inhibitors relative to that of the bivalent inhibitors for acute coronary syndromes.

REFERENCES

1. Antman EM, Bittl JA: Direct thrombin inhibitors. In Hennekens CH, Buring JE, Manson JE, et al (eds): Clinical Trials in Cardiovascular Disease: A Companion to Braunwald's Heart Disease. Philadelphia, WB Saunders, 1999, pp 145-165.
2. Antman EM: The search for replacements for unfractionated heparin. Circulation 2001; 103:2310-2314.
3. Greinacher A, Lubenow N: Recombinant hirudin in clinical practice: Focus on lepirudin. Circulation 2001; 103:1479-1484.
4. Weitz JI, Buller HR: Direct thrombin inhibitors in acute coronary syndromes: Present and future. Circulation 2002; 105:1004-1011.
5. Califf RM: Publication policy, informed consent, and the randomized clinical trial. Am Heart J 2002; 143:187-188.
6. Wilcox JN, Smith KN, Schwartz SM, et al: Localization of tissue factor in the normal vessel wall and in the atherosclerotic plaque. Proc Natl Acad Sci 1989; 86:2839-2843.
7. Annex BH, Denning SM, Channon KM, et al: Differential expression of tissue factor protein in directional atherectomy specimens from patients with stable and unstable coronary syndromes. Circulation 1995; 91:619-622.
8. Banner DW, D'Arcy A, Chene C, et al: The crystal structure of the complex of blood coagulation factor VIIa with soluble tissue factor. Nature 1996; 380:41-46.
9. Toschi V, Gallo R, Lettino M, et al: Tissue factor modulates the thrombogenicity of human athersclerotic plaques. Circulation 1997; 95:594-599.
10. Hirsh J, Anand SS, Halperin JL, et al: Guide to anticoagulant therapy: Heparin. A statement for healthcare professionals from the American Heart Association. Circulation 2001; 103:2994-3018.
11. Mizuno K, Satomura K, Miyamoto A, et al: Angioscopic evaluation of coronary-artery thrombi in acute coronary syndromes. N Engl J Med 1992; 326:287-291.
12. Marmur JD, Merlinie PA, Sharma SK, et al: Thrombin generation in human coronary arteries after percutaneous transluminal balloon angioplasty. J Am Coll Cardiol 1994; 24:1484-1491.
13. Coughlin SR, Vu TK, Hung DT, et al: Characterization of a functional thrombin receptor. J Clin Invest 1992; 89:351-355.
14. Coughlin S: Thrombin signaling and protease-activated receptors. Nature 2000; 407:258-264.
15. Hirsh J, Foster V: Guide to anticoagulant therapy: Part I: Heparin. Circulation 1994; 89:1449-1468.
16. Weitz JI, Hudoba M, Massel D, et al: Clot-bound thrombin is protected from inhibition by heparin-antithrombin III but is susceptible to inactivation by antithrombin III-independent inhibitors. J Clin Invest 1990; 86:385-391.
17. Eitzmann DT, Chi L, Saggin L, et al: Heparin neutralization by platelet-rich thrombi: Role of platelet factor 4. Circulation 1994; 89:1523-1529.
18. Brieger DB, Mak KH, Kottke-Marchant K, Topol EJ: Heparin-induced thrombocytopenia. J Am Coll Cardiol 1998; 31:1449-1459.
19. Xiao Z, Théroux P: Platelet activation with unfractionated heparin at therapeutic concentrations and comparisons with a low-molecular-weight heparin and with a direct thrombin inhibitor. Circulation 1998; 97:251-256.
20. Kelly AB, Maraganore JM, Bourdon P, et al: Antithrombotic effects of synthetic peptides targeting various functional domains of thrombin. Proc Natl Acad Sci USA 1992; 89:6040-6044.
21. The Direct Thrombin Inhibitor Trialists' Collaborative Group: Direct thrombin inhibitors in acute coronary syndromes: Principal results of a meta-analysis based on individual patients' data. Lancet 2002; 359:294-302.
22. Vanholder R, Dhondt A: Recombinant hirudin: Clinical pharmacology and potential applications in nephrology. Biol Drugs 1999; 11:417-429.

23. Song X, Huhle G, Wang L, et al: Generation of anti-hirudin antibodies in heparin-induced thrombocytopenic patients treated with r-hirudin. Circulation 1999; 100:1528-1532.
24. Eichler P, Friesen HJ, Lubenow N, et al: Antihirudin antibodies in patients with heparin-induced thrombocytopenia treated with lepirudin: Incidence, effects on aPTT, and clinical relevance. Blood 2000; 96:2373-238.
25. Maraganore JM, Bourdon P, Jablonski J, et al: Design and characterization of hirulogs: A novel class of bivalent peptide inhibitors of thrombin. Biochemistry 1990; 29:7095-7101.
26. Gold HK, Johns JA, Leinbach RC, et al: A randomized, blinded, placebo-controlled trial of recombinant tissue-type plasminogen activator in patients with unstable angina pectoris. 1987; 75:1192-1199.
27. Libby P: Current concepts in the pathogenesis of the acute coronary syndromes. Circulation 2001; 104:365-372.
28. Cannon CP, McCabe CH, Henry TD, et al: A pilot trial of recombinant desulfatohirudin compared with heparin in conjunction with tissue-type plasminogen activator and aspirin for acute myocardial infarction: Results of the Thrombolysis in Myocardial Infarction (TIMI) 5 Trial. J Am Coll Cardiol 1994; 23:993-1003.
29. Lee LV: Initial experience with hirudin and streptokinase in acute myocardial infarction: Results of the Thrombolysis in Myocardial Infarction (TIMI) 6 Trial. TIMI 6 Investigators. Am J Cardiol 1995; 75:7-13.
30. Antman EM: Hirudin in acute myocardial infarction: Thrombolysis and Thrombin Inhibition in Myocardial Infarction (TIMI) 9B Trial. TIMI 9B Investigators. Circulation 1996; 94:911-921.
31. The Global Use of Strategies to Open Occluded Coronary Arteries (GUSTO) IIb Investigators: A comparison of recombinant hirudin with heparin for the treatment of acute coronary syndromes. N Engl J Med 1996; 335:775-782.
32. Simes RJ, Granger CB, Antman EM, et al: Impact of hirudin versus heparin on mortality and (re)infarction in patients with acute coronary syndromes: A prospective meta-analysis of the GUSTO-IIb and Timi 9b Trials (abstract). Circulation 1996; 94 Suppl I:I-430.
33. Antman E, for the TIMI 9A Investigators: Hirudin in acute myocardial infarction: Safety report from the Thrombolysis and Thrombin Inhibition in Myocardial Infarction (TIMI) 9A Trial. Circulation 1994; 90:1624-1630.
34. The Global Use of Strategies to Open Occluded Coronary Arteries (GUSTO) IIa Investigators: Randomized trial of intravenous heparin versus recombinant hirudin for acute coronary syndromes. Circulation 1994; 90:1631-1637.
35. Neuhaus KL, v Essen R, Tebbe U, et al: Safety observations from the pilot phase of the randomized r-hirudin for improvement of thrombolysis (HIT-III) study: A study of the Arbeitsgemeinschaft Leitender Kardiologischer Krankenhausärzte (ALK). Circulation 1994; 90:1638-1642.
36. Théroux P, Pérez-Villa F, Waters D, et al: Randomized double-blind comparison of two doses of Hirulog with heparin as adjunctive therapy to streptokinase to promote early patency of the infarct-related artery in acute myocardial infarction. Circulation 1995; 91:2132-2139.
37. White HD, Aylward PE, Frey MJ, et al: Randomized, double-blind comparison of hirulog versus heparin in patients receiving streptokinase and aspirin for acute myocardial infarction (HERO). Hirulog Early Reperfusion/Occlusion (HERO) Trial Investigators. Circulation 1997; 96:2155-2161.
38. White HD: Hirulog Early Reperfusion and Occlusion 2 Trial (HERO 2), European Society of Cardiology, Stockholm, September 3, 2001, 2001.
39. The Assessment of the Safety and Efficacy of a New Thrombolytic Regimen (ASSENT)-3 Investigators. Efficacy and safety of tenecteplase in combination with enoxaparin, abciximab, or unfractionated heparin: The ASSENT-3 randomised trial in acute myocardial infarction. Lancet 2001; 358:605-613.
40. Topol EJ: Reperfusion therapy for acute myocardial infarction with fibrinolytic therapy or combination reduced fibrinolytic therapy and platelet glycoprotein IIb/IIIa inhibition: The GUSTO V randomised trial. Lancet 2001; 357:1905-1914.
41. White HD, Chew DP: Bivalirudin: An anticoagulant for acute coronary syndromes and coronary interventions. Expert Opin Pharmacother 2002; 3:777-788.
42. Vermeer F, Vahanian A, Fels PW, et al: Argatroban and alteplase in patients with acute myocardial infarction: The ARGAMI Study. J Thromb Thrombolysis 2000; 10:233-240.
43. The Prime Investigators: Multicenter, dose-ranging study of efegatran sulfate versus heparin with thrombolysis for acute myocardial infarction: The Promotion of Reperfusion in Myocardial Infarction Evolution (PRIME) trial. Am Heart J 2002; 143:95-105.
44. Braunwald E: Unstable angina. A classification. Circulation 1989; 80:410-414.
45. Ahmed WH, Bittl JA, Braunwald E: Relation between clinical presentation and angiographic findings in unstable angina pectoris, and comparison with that in stable angina. Am J Cardiol 1993; 72:544-550.
46. Organisation to Assess Strategies for Ischemic Syndromes (OASIS) Investigators: Comparison of the effects of two doses of recombinant hirudin compared with heparin in patients with acute myocardial ischemia without ST elevation: A pilot study. Circulation 1997; 96:769-777.
47. Organisation to Assess Strategies for Ischemic Syndromes (OASIS-2) Investigators: Effects of recombinant hirudin (lepirudin) compared with heparin on death, myocardial infarction, refractory angina, and revascularisation procedures in patients with acute myocardial ischemia without ST elevation: A randomised trial. Lancet 1997; 353:429-438.
48. Fuchs J, Cannon CP, and the TIMI 7 Investigators: Hirulog in the treatment of unstable angina: Results of the Thrombin Inhibition in Myocardial Ischemia (TIMI) 7 Trial. Circulation 1995; 92:727-733.
49. Antman EM, McCabe CH, Braunwald E: Bivalirudin as a replacement for unfractionated heparin in unstable angina/non-ST-elevation myocardial infarction: Observations from the TIMI 8 Trial. Am Heart J 2002; 143:229-234.
50. White HD. Improved efficacy and less bleeding: Further evidence of a unique uncoupling of benefit and risk with bivalirudin. Am Heart J 2002; 143:189-192.
51. Gold HK, Torres FW, Garabedian HD, et al: Evidence for a rebound coagulation phenomenon after cessation of a 4-hour infusion of a specific thrombin inhibitor in patients with unstable angina pectoris. J Am Coll Cardiol 1993; 21:1039-1047.
52. Topol EJ, Mark DB, Lincoff AM, et al: Outcomes at 1 year and economic implications of platelet glycoprotein IIb/IIIa blockade in patients undergoing coronary stenting: Results from a multicentre randomised trial. Lancet 1999; 352:2019-2024.
53. The EPIC Investigators: Use of a monoclonal antibody directed against the platelet glycoprotein IIb/IIIa receptor in high-risk coronary angioplasty. New Engl J Med 1994; 330:956-961.
54. The EPILOG Investigators: Evaluation of PTCA to Improve Long-Term Outcome by c7E3 Glycoprotein IIb/IIIa Receptor Blockade (EPILOG). N Engl J Med 1997; 336:1689-1696.
55. Narins CR, Hillegass WB, Jr, Nelson CL, et al: Relation between activated clotting time during angioplasty and abrupt closure. Circulation 1996; 93:660-671.
56. McGarry TF, Gottlieb RS, Morganroth J, et al: The relationship of anticoagulation level and complications after successful percutaneous transluminal coronary angioplasty. Am Heart J 1992; 123:1445-1451.
57. Ferguson JJ, Dougherty KG, Gaos CM, et al: Relation between procedural activated coagulation time and outcome after percutaneous transluminal coronary angioplasty. J Am Coll Cardiol 1994; 23:1061-1065.
58. Bittl JA, Ahmed WH: Relation between the risk of abrupt vessel closure and the anticoagulant response to heparin or bivalirudin during coronary angioplasty. Am J Cardiol 1998; 82:50P-56P.
59. Chew DP, Bhatt DL, Lincoff AM, et al: Defining the optimal ACT during percutaneous coronary intervention: Aggregate results from six randomized controlled trials. Circulation 2001; 103:961-966.
60. Serruys PW, Herrman J-PR, Simon R, et al: A comparison of hirudin with heparin in the prevention of restenosis after coronary angioplasty. N Engl J Med 1995; 333:757-763.
61. Manfredi JA, Wall RP, Sane DC, et al: Lepirudin as a safe alternative for effective anticoagulation in patients with known heparin-induced thrombocytopenia undergoing percutaneous coronary interventions: Case reports. Cath Cardiovasc Intervent 2001; 52:468-472.
62. Topol EJ, Bonan R, Jewitt D, et al: Use of a direct antithrombin, hirulog, in place of heparin during coronary angioplasty. Circulation 1993; 87:1622-1629.
63. Bittl JA, Strony J, Brinker JA, et al: Treatment with bivalirudin (Hirulog) as compared with heparin during coronary angioplasty for unstable or postinfarction angina. N Engl J Med 1995; 333:764-769.

64. Bittl JA, Chaitman BR, Feit F, et al: Bivalirudin versus heparin during coronary angioplasty for unstable or post-infarction angina: The final report of the Bivalirudin Angioplasty Study. Am Heart J 2001; 142:952–959.

65. Bittl JA, Feit F: A randomized comparison of bivalirudin and heparin in patients undergoing angioplasty for postinfarction angina. Hirulog Angioplasty Study Investigators. Am J Cardiol 1998; 82:43P–49P.

66. Strony J, Ahmed WH, Meckel CR, et al: Clinical evidence for thrombin rebound after stopping heparin but not Hirulog (abstract). Circulation 1995; 92:I–609.

67. Lincoff AM, Kleiman NS, Kottke-Marchant K, et al: Bivalirudin with planned or provisional abciximab versus low-dose heparin and abciximab during percutaneous coronary revascularization: Results of the Comparison of Abciximab Complications with Hirulog for Ischemic Events Trial (CACHET). Am Heart J 2002; 143:847–853.

68. Lincoff AM, Bittl JA, Kleiman NS, et al: The REPLACE 1 Trial: A pilot study of bivalirudin versus heparin during percutaneous coronary intervention with stenting and GP IIb/IIIa blockade (abstract). J Am Coll Cardiol 2002; 39: in press.

69. Lincoff AM, Bittl JA, Harrington RA, et al: Bivalirudin and provisional glycoprotein IIb/IIIa blockade compared with heparin and planned glycoprotein blockade during percutaneous coronary intervention. JAMA 2003; 289:1638.

70. Suzuki S, Matsuo T, Kobayashi H, et al: Antithrombotic treatment (argatroban vs. heparin) in coronary angioplasty in angina pectoris: Effects on inflammatory, hemostatic, and endothelium-derived parameters. Thromb Res 2000; 98:269–279.

71. Lewis BE, Matthai WH, Cohen M, et al: Argatroban anticoagulation during percutaneous coronary intervention in patients with heparin-induced thrombocytopenia. Cath Cardiovasc Intervent 2002; 57:177–184.

72. Aster RH: Heparin-induced thrombocytopenia and thrombosis. N Engl J Med 1995; 332:1374–1376.

73. Warkentin TE, Levine MN, Hirsh J, et al: Heparin-induced thrombocytopenia in patients treated with low-molecular weight heparin or unfractionated heparin. N Engl J Med 1995; 332:1330–1335.

74. Warkentin TE, Elavathil LJ, Hayward CP, et al: The pathogenesis of venous limb gangrene associated with heparin-induced thrombocytopenia [see comments]. Ann Intern Med 1997; 127:804–812.

75. Koster A, Meyer O, Hausmann H, et al: In vitro cross-reactivity of danaparoid sodium in patients with heparin-induced thrombocytopenia type II undergoing cardiovascular surgery. J Clin Anesth 2000; 12:324–327.

76. Chamberlin JR, Lewis B, Leya F, et al: Successful treatment of heparin-associated thrombocytopenia and thrombosis using Hirulog. Can J Cardiol 1995; 11:511–514.

77. Reid T III: Hirulog therapy for heparin-associated thrombocytopenia and deep venous thrombosis (letter). Am J Hematol 1994; 45:352–353.

78. Lewis BE, Wallis DE, Berkowitz SD, et al: Argatroban anticoagulant therapy in patients with heparin-induced thrombocytopenia. Circulation 2001; 103:1838–1843.

79. Eriksson BI, Wille-Jorgensen P, Kalebo P, et al: A comparison of recombinant hirudin with a low-molecular-weight heparin to prevent thromboembolic complications after total hip replacement. N Engl J Med 1997; 337:1329–1335.

80. Ginsburg JS, Nurmohamed MT, Gent M, et al: Use of Hirulog in the prevention of venous thrombosis after major hip or knee surgery. Circulation 1994; 90:2385–2389.

81. Francis CW, Davidson BL, Berkowitz SD, et al: Ximelagatran versus warfarin for the prevention of venous thromboembolism after total knee arthroplasty. A randomized, double-blind trial. Ann Intern Med 2002; 137:648–655.

82. Eriksson BI, Bergqvist D, Kalebo P, et al: Ximelegatran and melagatran compared with dalteparin for prevention of deep venous thrombosis after total hip of knee replacement: The METHRO II randomised trial. Lancet 2002; 360:1441–1447.

83. Greinacher A, Janssens U, Berg G, et al: Lepirudin (recombinant hirudin) for parenteral anticoagulation in patients with heparin-induced thrombocytopenia. Heparin-Associated Thrombocytopenia Study (HAT) investigators. Circulation 1999; 100: 587–593.

84. Argatroban for treatment of heparin-induced thrombocytopenia. Med Let Drugs Ther 2001; 43:11–12.

85. Petersen P, Grind M, Adler J, et al: Ximelegatran versus warfarin for stroke prevention in patients with nonvalvular atrial fibrillation: SPORTIF II: A dose-guiding, tolerability, and safety study. J Am Coll Cardiol 2003; 41:1445–1451.

chapter 9

Glycoprotein IIb/IIIa Receptor Inhibitors

Steven R. Steinhubl
E. Magnus Ohman

Few therapeutic interventions of the last decade have had a greater impact on the treatment of patients with an acute coronary syndrome (ACS) than that of the glycoprotein (GP) IIb/IIIa antagonists. Although the central role of the platelet-rich thrombus in the pathophysiology of ACS has long been recognized, as has the efficacy of antiplatelet therapies such as aspirin and the thienopyridines in the treatment of patients with an ACS, these therapies are limited in their ability to acutely and completely prevent platelet aggregates from forming. Although nearly 100 agonists are known to stimulate platelet aggregation, only the thromboxane A_2 and adenosine phosphate (ADP) pathways specifically are inhibited by aspirin and the thienopyridines, respectively. Thus even with complete blockade of one or both of these pathways, platelet aggregates still may form, whereas complete inhibition of the GPIIb/IIIa receptor prevents platelet aggregation irrespective of the agonist.

The GP IIb/IIIa receptor (α_{IIb}/β_3) belongs to the integrin family of adhesion receptors found on many different cell types. Unlike other integrins, the GPIIb/IIIa receptor is found only on platelets and megakaryocytes.[1] Each platelet has approximately 80,000 GPIIb/IIIa receptors.[2] Studies in some animal models found that to achieve nearly complete inhibition of platelet aggregation and arterial thrombus formation, 80% or more of these receptors need to be blocked.[3] When activated, the receptor can bind adhesive proteins such as vitronectin, fibronectin, von Willebrand's factor and fibrinogen—the latter two being the principal proteins involved in platelet aggregation.[4,5] All of these adhesive proteins contain a common peptide segment that is involved in binding to the GPIIb/IIIa receptor, with the Arg-Gly-Asp (RGD) amino acid sequence present at least once in all of these proteins.[6] Elucidation of the function and structure of the GPIIb/IIIa receptor has led to the development of a number of antagonists, both parenteral and oral, which have been evaluated clinically in the treatment of patients with an ACS (Table 9-1).

PARENTERAL GPIIB/IIIA ANTAGONISTS

Abciximab

The first agent reported to inhibit the GPIIb/IIIa receptor was a murine monoclonal antibody developed by Coller and colleagues.[7] This original antibody has undergone considerable refinement to the present agent abciximab (ReoPro), a chimeric Fab fragment formed by combining the murine variable region with the constant regions of human immunoglobulin. Abciximab is unique from other GPIIb/IIIa receptor antagonists in that it is a noncompetitive inhibitor of the GPIIb/IIIa receptor, binding with pharmacodynamics that are consistent with nearly irreversible occupation of the GPIIb/IIIa receptor.[8] Because of this property, recovery of platelet function occurs slowly, with normalization of platelet aggregation requiring hours to days after completion of an infusion. Another unique property of abciximab is its integrin nonspecificity, interacting with other integrins including the vitronectin receptor ($\alpha_V\beta_3$) and the leukocyte integrin Mac-1 ($\alpha_M\beta_2$).[9,10]

The initial clinical evaluation of a monoclonal antibody directed against the GPIIb/IIIa receptor was a Phase I study of the murine antibody in patients with unstable angina,[11] which was followed by a double-blind randomized placebo-controlled pilot study of the chimeric antibody fragment in patients with unstable angina refractory to intensive medical therapy.[12] Following a baseline angiogram demonstrating a culprit lesion suitable for angioplasty, patients were randomized to placebo or a bolus of abciximab followed by an infusion for 18 to 24 hours until 1 hour after angioplasty. All patients also received heparin and aspirin. Patients treated with abciximab had fewer infarcts, fewer urgent interventions, and less mortality compared with patients receiving placebo without an excess of bleeding complications.

Eptifibatide

Eptifibatide (Integrilin) is a competitive inhibitor of the GPIIb/IIIa receptor with a rapid onset of action and a short half-life. It is a cyclic heptapeptide based on the RGD template but substitutes a lysine for an arginine creating a KGD sequence and increasing its specificity for GPIIb/IIIa.[13] Eptifibatide inhibits platelet aggregation in a dose-dependent fashion.[14,15]

Eptifibatide initially was evaluated in unstable angina in a Phase II randomized, double-blind safety and efficacy trial.[16] Two hundred and twenty-seven patients with unstable angina were randomized to one of three treatment groups: (1) low-dose eptifibatide (45-µg/kg bolus, 0.5-µg/kg/min infusion), (2) high-dose eptifibatide

■ ▥ ■

TABLE 9-1   CONTROLLED TRIALS EVALUATING GLYCOPROTEIN IIB/IIIA ANTAGONISTS IN PATIENTS WITH ACUTE CORONARY SYNDROMES

Agent	Trials
Monoclonal antibody	
Abciximab (ReoPro)	CAPTURE, GUSTO IV, GUSTO V, ASSENT 3
Cyclic peptide	
Eptifibatide (Integrilin)	PURSUIT
Nonpeptide mimetics	
Lamifiban	PARAGON A, PARAGON B
Tirofiban (Aggrastat)	PRISM, PRISM-PLUS
Orally active agents	
Orbofiban	OPUS-TIMI 16
Sibrafiban	SYMPHONY, 2nd SYMPHONY

(90-μg/kg bolus, 1.0-μg/kg/min infusion), or (3) placebo. All patients received a continuous heparin infusion, and patients receiving the study drug were given an aspirin placebo. The study drug was continued for 24 to 72 hours. The endpoint evaluated was the frequency and duration of ischemic episodes during the first 24 hours of drug infusion by continuous electrocardiogram (ECG) monitoring. There was a stepwise decrease in the number and duration of ischemic episodes in the low-dose and high-dose treatment groups compared with placebo, with the difference in the high-dose group reaching statistical significance. It is interesting that the doses used in this pilot study, as well as in early randomized trials of eptifibatide in percutaneous coronary intervention (PCI), subsequently were found to be insufficient to optimally inhibit platelet function because of an artifact of in vitro platelet aggregation testing.[17]

Lamifiban

Lamifiban is a low–molecular-weight, synthetic, nonpeptide, highly specific GPIIb/IIIa antagonist. Although not commercially available, it has undergone extensive evaluation in the ACS population. Lamifiban was initially studied in the Phase II dose-exploring Canadian Lamifiban Study.[18] In this study involving 365 patients, treatment groups included lamifiban bolus and infusions of 1, 2, 4, or 5 μg/min or placebo for 72 to 120 hours. During the infusion period, lamifiban (all doses combined) reduced the incidence of urgent revascularization compared with placebo (3.3% vs. 8.1%, P = 0.04). At 30 days, death or nonfatal infarction occurred in 8.1% of patients receiving placebo and in 2.5% of patients treated with the two highest doses of lamifiban (P = 0.03). Although inhibition of platelet aggregation was confirmed to be dose dependent, no clear dose-related clinical benefit was seen in this small study.

Tirofiban

Tirofiban (Aggrastat) is a small nonpeptide tyrosine derivative with a rapid onset of action and rapid reversal of effect after drug discontinuation. Like the other small

molecule agents, tirofiban is a specific inhibitor of the platelet fibrinogen receptor, with the level of platelet inhibition being dose-dependent.[19] Like eptifibatide, in vitro testing may have overestimated the level of platelet inhibition achieved in vivo by tirofiban as a result of calcium-dependent mechanisms.[20]

PHASE III TRIALS OF PARENTERAL GPIIB/IIIA ANTAGONISTS IN NON-ST ELEVATION ACUTE CORONARY SYNDROMES

Abciximab

Abciximab was the first agent to undergo large-scale evaluation in the ACS population, with a randomized placebo-controlled trial started in May of 1993 (Table 9-2).[21] The c7E3 Fab Antiplatelet Therapy in Unstable Refractory Angina (CAPTURE) study was scheduled to randomize 1400 patients with recurrent myocardial ischemia despite medical therapy with aspirin, heparin, and nitrates to abciximab or placebo. Recruitment was stopped after 1265 patients had been enrolled after predefined stopping rules had been met at a planned interim analysis. Eligible patients were required to have chest pain refractory to intensive medical therapy with associated ECG changes within 48 hours of enrollment. If a baseline angiogram identified a culprit lesion suitable for percutaneous intervention, the patient was randomized to an abciximab bolus (0.25 mg/kg) followed by an infusion (10 μg/min) or matching placebo. The infusion was continued for 18 to 24 hours until 1 hour after the angioplasty procedure. All patients continued to receive heparin and aspirin. During the infusion prior to angioplasty, progression to myocardial infarction (MI) occurred in 2.1% of patients receiving placebo and only 0.6% of abciximab-treated patients (P = 0.029). At 30 days following angioplasty the combined primary endpoint of death, MI, or urgent revascularization had occurred in 11.3% of abciximab patients and 15.9% of those receiving placebo (P = 0.012). By 6 months, however, there was some erosion in treatment benefit, with 242 events (death, repeat revascularization, or MI) occurring in the abciximab group and 274 events in those receiving placebo (P = 0.067). Also, there was an increased incidence of bleeding complications in the abciximab-treated patients, primarily involving the vascular access site, with 3.8% of abciximab-treated patients experiencing a major bleeding complication compared with 1.9% of patients receiving placebo (P = 0.043).

In the CAPTURE trial, serum samples from the time of randomization were available in 890 patients and analyzed for troponin T levels. A marked relationship between troponin elevation and treatment effect of abciximab was found (Fig. 9-1).[22] Normal baseline troponin levels were associated with an overall low event rate that did not differ based on randomization to placebo or abciximab. However, in troponin-positive patients, randomization to abciximab was associated with a relative risk of 0.32 for the ischemic endpoint (95% CI, 0.14–0.62, P = 0.002).

TABLE 9-2 PLACEBO-CONTROLLED TRIALS OF INTRAVENOUS GLYCOPROTEIN IIB/IIIA ANTAGONISTS IN PATIENTS WITH NON-ST ELEVATION ACUTE CORONARY SYNDROMES

Trial	Patients	Drug	Aspirin	Heparin	PTCA	Primary endpoint	% with endpoint		P value
							Control	IIb/IIIa Inhibitor	
CAPTURE[21]	1,265	Abciximab	Yes	Yes	Yes	Death, MI, or urgent revascularization at 30 days	15.9	11.3	0.012
GUSTO IV-ACS[23]	7,800	Abciximab	Yes	Yes—Unfractionated or low-molecular-weight heparin	Discouraged	Death or MI at 30 days	8.0	24-hour infusion—8.2% or 48-hour infusion—9.1%	NS for either
PURSUIT[29]	10,948	Eptibatide	Yes	Encouraged	Optional	Death or MI at 30 days	15.7	14.2	0.04
PARAGON[31]	2,282	Lamifiban	Yes	Randomized	Optional	Death or MI at 30 days	11.7	Low dose with heparin—10.3%	NS
PARAGON-B[32]	5,225	Lamifiban	Yes	Yes	Optional	Death, MI, or severe recurrent ischemia at 30 days	12.8	11.8	0.33
PRISM[34]	3,231	Tirofiban	Yes	Control arm only	Optional	Death, MI, or refractory ischemia at 48 hr	5.6	3.8	0.01
PRISM-PLUS[36]	1,560	Tirofiban	Yes	Yes	Optional	Death, MI, or refractory ischemia at 7 days	17.9	12.9	0.004

PTCA, percutaneous transluminal coronary angioplasty; MI, myocardial infarction.

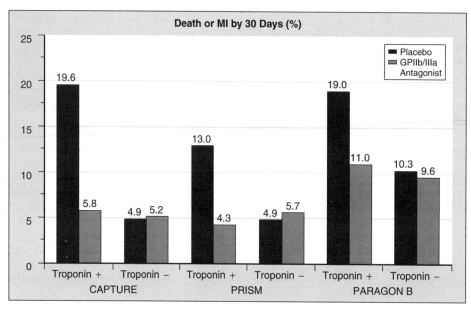

FIGURE 9-1. Thirty-day death and myocardial infarction rates in the CAPTURE, PRISM, and PARAGON-B trials based on baseline troponin status.

The early, pre-PCI benefit of an abciximab infusion compared with placebo in the CAPTURE trial, plus the clustering of adverse events around the intervention procedure, lead to the hypothesis that a prolonged infusion of abciximab without a revascularization procedure would be beneficial in an unstable angina population. This hypothesis was tested in the GUSTO (Global Use of Strategies To Open Occluded Coronary Arteries) IV-ACS trial in which 7800 patients presenting with chest pain associated with either ST-segment depression or positive markers of myocardial necrosis.[23] Patients were randomized to one of three arms: standard therapy with heparin (either unfractionated or low–molecular-weight), aspirin, nitroglycerin, and beta blockers; standard therapy plus a bolus (0.25 mg/kg) and 24-hour infusion (0.125 μg/kg/min) of abciximab, or standard therapy plus a bolus and 48-hour infusion of abciximab. Early revascularization was discouraged. Surprisingly, randomization to abciximab was not associated with any reduction in the occurrence of death or MI at 30 days; in fact, the trend was in the wrong direction, with the highest event rate in those patients randomized to a 48-hour infusion (Table 9-2). Outcomes at 1 year showed no change in this trend with a nonsignificant increase in mortality with a 48-hour (9.0%) or 24-hour abciximab infusion (8.2%) compared with placebo (7.8%).[24] Of note, randomization to a 48-hour abciximab infusion was associated with a statistically significant increase in 1-year mortality compared with placebo in patients who were troponin negative (8.5% vs. 5.8%, P = 0.02) and in those with elevated C-reactive protein at baseline (16.3% vs. 12.1%, P = 0.04). The clinical implications of these findings are not yet completely understood.

Whereas the results of GUSTO IV-ACS highlight the lack of benefit of abciximab in patients with ACS not treated with PCI, the results of CAPTURE as well as those of the three placebo-controlled PCI trials underscore the protective role of abciximab in patients with ACS undergoing a PCI. Although a significant benefit of abciximab compared to placebo was found for all patients enrolled in the EPIC (Evaluation of 7E3 in Preventing Ischemic Complications), EPILOG (Evaluation in PTCA to Improve Long Term Outcome with Abciximab GPIIb/IIIa Blockade), and EPISTENT (Evaluation of Platelet IIb/IIIa Inhibitor for Stenting) trials, when the ACS subgroup of patients from these trials were evaluated specifically, an even greater treatment effect was observed.[25] In the EPIC trial, a subgroup analysis of 489 patients with unstable angina demonstrated a significant reduction in the 30-day combined endpoint of death, MI, or urgent repeat revascularization by 62% in the abciximab bolus plus infusion group compared to placebo (4.8% vs. 12.8%, P = 0.012).[26] These findings are reinforced by results from the EPILOG trial, which enrolled 1328 patients with unstable angina as their indication for angioplasty. In patients treated with abciximab, there was a 60% reduction in the primary endpoint at 30 days compared with placebo (4.9% vs. 12.2%, P < 0.001).[27] In the EPISTENT trial, in patients with unstable angina within 48 hours prior to undergoing coronary stenting, randomization to abciximab was associated with a 58% relative decrease in the 30-day primary endpoint, from 12.7% to 5.4% (P = 0.004).[28]

The results of these trials strongly support the beneficial role of abciximab in patients undergoing coronary angioplasty for the treatment of unstable angina. The decrease in events with 24 hours of abciximab prior to PCI seen in the CAPTURE trial supports the early use of this agent but only in patients with refractory unstable angina in whom an early PCI is planned. Based on the results from GUSTO-IV ACS, prolonged treatment with abciximab in patients not undergoing a PCI is not of benefit, and potentially harmful, and should be avoided.

Eptifibatide

After clarification of the pharmacodynamics of eptifibatide, an enhanced dose designed to maintain platelet inhibition of more than 80% was evaluated in the PURSUIT (Platelet IIb/IIIa in Unstable Angina: Receptor Suppression Using Integrilin Therapy) trial.[29] This was a multicenter trial including nearly 11,000 patients with unstable angina or MI without ST segment elevation. Patients were randomized to an eptifibatide bolus (180 μg/kg) and infusion (2.0 μg/kg. min) or matching placebo for up to 72 hours. All patients received aspirin, and heparin use was encouraged, but the use of percutaneous revascularization was left to the discretion of the investigator. The primary combined endpoint of death or MI at 30 days was reduced from 15.7% in the placebo group to 14.2% in patients receiving eptifibatide (P = 0.04) (Table 9-2). The benefit of eptifibatide treatment was found to be greatest in the approximately 13% of patients who underwent an early (<72 hours) PCI.[30] As with the CAPTURE trial, an early benefit was seen in treated patients prior to their PCI, with a reduction from 5.5% in placebo-treated patients to 1.7% with eptifibatide treatment in the incidence of pre-PCI MI.

Lamifiban

Two doses of lamifiban, as well as the role of adjunctive heparin therapy, were studied in the Platelet IIb/IIIa Antagonism for the Reduction of Acute Coronary Syndrome Events in a Global Organization Network (PARAGON-A) trial.[31] Patients (n = 2282) were randomized to a 300-μg bolus and 1-μg/min infusion, 750-μg bolus and 5-μg/min infusion, or matched placebo for 72 hours and then subrandomized to either heparin or a heparin placebo. At 30-day follow-up there was not a significant difference between treatment groups in the combined endpoint of death or MI (Table 9-2). Surprisingly, those treated with the low-dose but not the high-dose lamifiban regimen displayed a trend toward benefit. Even more interesting was that at 6 months both high- and low-dose treatment arms had a decrease in the occurrence of death or MI compared with placebo but with only the low-dose arm reaching statistical significance (13.7% vs. 18.2%, P = 0.019). Analysis of the results of the heparin subrandomization also provided curious results: addition of heparin produced a trend toward benefit with low-dose lamifiban but not with high-dose lamifiban.

The PARAGON B study was designed to build on the results of PARAGON-A by carefully targeting drug levels by adjusting the infusion based on calculated creatinine clearance.[32] This study randomized 5225 high-risk patients with ischemic chest pain to receive either placebo or a lamifiban bolus (500 mg) followed by an infusion (1–2 mg/min based on calculated creatinine clearance) for 72 to 120 hours. All patients received aspirin and heparin, and 27% of patients underwent a PCI. At 30 days the combined endpoint of death, MI, or severe recurrent ischemia was only modestly reduced with lamifiban treatment (12.8% for placebo, 11.8% for lamifiban, P = 0.329) (Table 9-2). Unlike the PARAGON-A

trial, event rates in the placebo and treatment arms remained parallel out to 6 months, with a 1% absolute reduction in the composite of death or MI in the patients randomized to lamifiban (15.9% for placebo, 14.9% for lamifiban).

A prospectively defined substudy of PARAGON-B evaluated the treatment effect of lamifiban based on admission troponin status.[33] Troponin T was measured in 1160 patients enrolled in the study, with just more than 40% of patients having an abnormally elevated level at baseline. As in other trials, treatment with the GPIIb/IIIa antagonist significantly decreased death and MI in troponin-positive patients (19.4% for placebo, 11.0% for lamifiban, P = 0.01), with a minimal affect on troponin-negative patients (11.2% for placebo, 10.8% for lamifiban, P = 0.86) (Fig. 9-1). Despite the benefit seen in this subgroup, and although the overall absolute reduction in events was similar to that seen in other trials, there are no plans to market lamifiban at this time.

Tirofiban

Tirofiban has been evaluated in the treatment of patients with unstable angina in two multicenter, randomized trials. The Platelet Receptor Inhibition for Ischemic Syndrome Management (PRISM) trial compared heparin with tirofiban in 3231 patients with chest pain within the preceding 24 hours.[34] Patients were randomized to a 48-hour infusion of heparin (5000-U bolus and 1000-U/hr infusion adjusted to activated partial-thromboplastin time) or tirofiban (0.6 μg/kg/min for 30 minutes then 0.15 μg/kg/min for a mean of 47.5 hours) without heparin. All patients received aspirin unless contraindicated. Less than 2% of patients underwent a percutaneous revascularization during the 48-hour treatment period. The composite endpoint was the incidence of death, new MI, or refractory ischemia. At 48 hours, at just the completion of therapy, patients treated with tirofiban had a significant decrease in the composite endpoint compared with those receiving heparin, from 5.6% to 3.8% (P = 0.01) (Table 9-2). The greatest effect was seen in the reduction of refractory ischemia, defined as hemodynamic instability or angina with ECG changes. By 30 days, however, the treatment effect of tirofiban was largely lost, with the absolute difference in the composite endpoint (with the addition of readmission for unstable angina) being reduced from 17.1% in patients randomized to heparin to 15.9 in those receiving tirofiban (P = 0.34).

As in the CAPTURE and PARAGON-B trials, a substudy from the PRISM trial demonstrated a significant correlation between the therapeutic efficiency of tirofiban and baseline troponin status.[35] Overall, troponin-positive patients had a significantly higher 30-day event rate (13.0% death or MI in troponin-I-positive patients and 4.9% in troponin-I-negative patients, P < 0.001) (Fig. 9-1). Whereas no treatment effect of tirofiban was seen in troponin-negative patients, randomization to tirofiban in the troponin-positive cohort was associated with a significant decrease in the risk of death (adjusted hazard ratio 0.25, P = 0.004) and MI (adjusted hazard ratio 0.37, P = 0.01) at 30 days.

The Platelet Receptor Inhibition for Ischemic Syndrome Management in Patients Limited by Unstable Signs and Symptoms (PRISM-PLUS) trial was designed to evaluate tirofiban in "higher-risk" patients with unstable angina.[36] The trial enrolled 1915 patients and randomized them originally to three treatment arms: tirofiban (0.6 μg/kg/min for 30 minutes then 0.15 μg/kg/min) without heparin, heparin without tirofiban, or both tirofiban (0.4 μg/kg/min for 30 minutes then 0.10 μg/kg/min) and heparin. Study drug infusion was for a mean (±SD) of 71.3 ± 20 hours, with coronary angiography and revascularization performed when indicated after 48 hours. After 345 patients had been randomized to tirofiban only, this group was discontinued on the advice of the Data and Safety Monitoring Committee because of an excess in the mortality rate (4.6% vs. 1.1% for patients treated with heparin only). This increase in events is in contrast to the findings in the tirofiban-only arm of the PRISM trial and may be the result of a rebound phenomenon (because 70% of patients were already receiving heparin at the time of randomization) or the higher risk nature of the patients in PRISM-PLUS. For the remaining two treatment groups, the primary endpoint was the composite of death, MI, or refractory ischemia at 7 days. By 7 days, 90% of the patients had undergone angiographic evaluation and 54% had a revascularization procedure. The composite endpoint at 7 days was 12.9% for the 773 patients treated with tirofiban and heparin versus 17.9% among the 797 heparin-only cohort (P = 0.004) (Table 9-2). By 6 months there was some loss of treatment effect, but the difference for the composite endpoint remained significant (32.1% vs. 27.7%, P = 0.02).

The results of the PRISM and PRISM-PLUS trials reinforce the particularly important role of GPIIb/IIIa inhibition in the setting of a PCI in patients with an ACS. In the PRISM trial, in which only a small percentage of patients underwent angiography during study drug treatment, there was no significant sustained benefit of tirofiban therapy. In the PRISM-PLUS trial, as in the PURSUIT trial, patients treated with medical management experienced only a nonsignificant decrease in the 30-day composite endpoint with tirofiban treatment (14.8% vs. 16.8%, risk ratio 0.87, 95% confidence interval, 0.60 to 1.25), whereas randomization to tirofiban in patients undergoing angioplasty lead to a 45% reduction in the incidence of the combined endpoint at 30 days (8.8% vs. 15.3%, risk ratio 0.55, 95% confidence interval, 0.32 to 0.94).

The Role of Parenteral GPIIb/IIIa Antagonists in Non-ST Segment Elevation Acute Coronary Syndromes

The role of parenteral GPIIb/IIIa antagonists in the treatment of patients with ACS has been studied in placebo-controlled trials involving more than 31,000 patients. The results of a recent meta-analysis highlight some of the practical concerns remaining regarding how to best apply this proven therapy.[37] Although a statistically significant 9% relative reduction in the odds of death or MI was found in the analysis overall, this absolute 1% differ-

ence in thrombotic events (10.8% for IIb/IIIa antagonists vs. 11.8% for placebo, odds ratio 0.91, P = 0.015) was balanced by a 1% absolute increase in major bleeding complications (2.4% vs. 1.4%, P < 0.0001). Because the absolute treatment benefit is greatest in the highest-risk patients, and because the diagnosis of a suspected ACS encompasses a very heterogeneous population of patients, targeting those subgroups most likely to achieve the greatest benefit would optimize the effectiveness of GPIIb/IIIa antagonist therapy.

Objective evidence of myocardial ischemia, whether by ECG or cardiac markers, is indicative of risk in patients with ACS and is required for enrollment in all of the trials evaluating GPIIb/IIIa inhibitors in the treatment of these patients. These criteria preclude the extrapolation of the results of the trials discussed previously to all patients treated for an ACS because a substantial proportion of patients evaluated in emergency rooms for a suspected ACS do not have ECG changes, and an even greater percentage don't have elevated myocardial enzymes on presentation. In one series, nearly 40% of patients admitted with a suspected ACS did not have ECG changes, whereas the same was true for more than one-fourth of patients with a definite ACS.[38] Among patients with ACSs who have dynamic ECG changes, the type of ECG change is an important predictor of long-term outcome, with ST segment depression having a significantly worse long-term prognosis. In the GUSTO-IIb trial, patients with ST-segment depression had more than double the mortality rate of patients with T-wave inversion at 6 months (8.9% vs. 3.4%).[39] Therefore, the higher-risk group of patients, identified by their dynamic ST-segment depressions, would be most likely to derive the greatest benefit from starting GPIIb/IIIa antagonist therapy early in the treatment of their ACS.

Any abnormal elevation of cardiac markers, predominately troponins, at the time of presentation with an ACS appears to be the single most predictive objective criterion for an increased risk for death or (re)MI in the ensuing weeks, with several studies showing a direct association between the level of elevation and level of risk.[40,41] As noted in the individual trials listed previously, elevated myocardial markers also have been shown to identify a subgroup of patients with ACS who derive the greatest benefit from the addition of GPIIb/IIIa antagonist therapy (Fig. 9-1). However, patients fitting this criterion represent the minority of patients presenting with a possible ACS. In one study of patients presenting to an emergency room with chest pain, only 22% had an elevated troponin T.[42] In the PURSUIT trial, which included only patients with objective evidence of ischemia, more than 40% of patients had no elevation of CKMB (creatine kinase isoenzyme) at the time of enrollment.[41] Thus, patients with unstable angina who have elevated cardiac markers have an increased risk for recurrent events and represent a subgroup of patients more likely to benefit from the addition of a GPIIb/IIIa antagonist to their antithrombotic regimen.

Another subgroup of patients with ACS found to derive particular benefit from treatment with a GPIIb/IIIa antagonist are patients with diabetes mellitus. The presence of

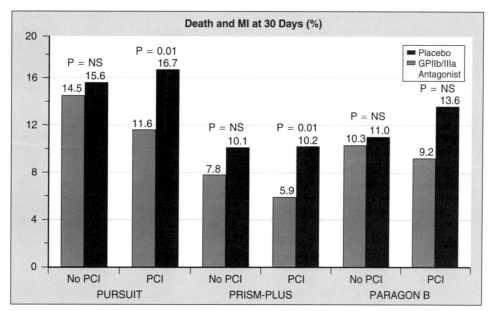

FIGURE 9-2. Death and myocardial infarction at 30 days based on randomization to placebo or a glycoprotein IIb/IIIa antagonist and whether a percutaneous coronary intervention (PCI) was performed in the PURSUIT, PRISM-PLUS, and PARAGON-B trials.

diabetes mellitus has been long recognized as a risk factor for adverse outcomes after an ACS, and this may at least in part be related to in vitro and ex vivo abnormalities of platelet function.[43] A meta-analysis of the 6458 patients with diabetes enrolled in the placebo-controlled ACS trials of GPIIb/IIIa antagonists found a striking benefit of treatment with a significant reduction in mortality at 30 days (4.6% vs. 6.2%, odds ratio 0.74, P = 0.007).[44] This mortality benefit of GPIIb/IIIa inhibitor treatment was even more pronounced among patients with diabetes undergoing a PCI (odds ratio 0.30, P = 0.002).

A consistent finding of all trials evaluating parenteral GPIIb/IIIa antagonists in patients with an ACS has been their markedly enhanced benefit in the subgroup of patients who underwent a PCI during treatment (Fig. 9-2). Based on the consistency of this finding among all trials, as well as the heightened benefit of treatment with a GPIIb/IIIa antagonist in patients with a diagnosis of unstable angina in the PCI trials with these agents, their use during a PCI in patients with unstable angina is supported solidly by the available data. However, the optimal time to start a GPIIb/IIIa antagonist in a patient who presents to the emergency room with a possible ACS remains less clear. A yet unresolved conflict regarding the optimal time to start a GPIIb/IIIa antagonist in a patient with ACS is the potential harm associated with a prolonged infusion of abciximab, as highlighted in the GUSTO IV-ACS results, and the proven superiority of abciximab over tirofiban in a PCI population, especially in the ACS subset of these patients, as shown in the TARGET trial.[45] Is there greater benefit derived from starting an infusion of eptifibatide or tirofiban in the emergency room, or from starting abciximab, or may be a higher PCI-dose of eptifibatide in the catheterization laboratory after the diagnostic angiogram is completed? Although analysis of the data from the CAPTURE, PRISM-PLUS, and PURSUIT trials found a benefit to

starting these agents early,[46] the magnitude of the benefit was small within the first 24 hours in all of these trials except the CAPTURE trial. This is likely because patients enrolled in this trial were more unstable because they were required to have recurrent ischemia despite antithrombotic therapy with heparin, aspirin, and intravenous nitroglycerin. Patients such as these, with refractory ischemia, represent a very high-risk subgroup of patients[47] in whom the early use of GPIIb/IIIa antagonists would be of greatest benefit. Likewise, high-risk patients who are likely to undergo a PCI but who will be medically stabilized for more than 24 hours may derive additional protection through starting a small-molecule GPIIb/IIIa receptor inhibitor early in their hospital course. It is this gap in the data that has led to the recommendations by the American College of Cardiology/American Heart Association Task Force on Practice Guidelines (Committee on the Management of Patients with Unstable Angina) that GPIIb/IIIa antagonists should be used in all high-risk patients eligible for such therapy, in particular those in whom revascularization is anticipated, but that such treatment can be initiated either early, or in the catheterization laboratory just prior to the PCI.[48]

PARENTERAL GPIIB/IIIA ANTAGONISTS IN ST-SEGMENT ELEVATION ACUTE MYOCARDIAL INFARCTIONS

With the success of the parenteral GPIIb/IIIa antagonists in the treatment of patients with a non-ST elevation ACS, in particular in those patients with troponin-positive thrombotic events, patients with an ST elevation acute MI would seem to represent an ideal cohort in whom improved antiplatelet protection with a GPIIb/IIIa antagonist would offer maximal benefit. However, trials in this population have not been uniformly positive, and the results to date seem to somewhat mimic those in the non-ST elevation ACS population in that the benefit is minimal in patients treated primarily medically, whereas the treatment effect is greatest in those undergoing a PCI, although even these results are mixed.

Primary angioplasty, with or without stenting, is associated with TIMI grade 3 epicardial flow in more than 90% of patients. However, recent studies have found that microvascular flow rather than epicardial flow following reperfusion is a more important determinant of long-term outcomes. Ito and coworkers[49] found that despite TIMI grade 3 epicardial flow in 126 patients following primary angioplasty, 37% had no microvascular flow as determined by myocardial contrast echocardiography. No reflow by myocardial contrast echocardiography was associated with a significant increase in left-ventricular end-diastolic volume as well as less functional recovery. In a second study, microvascular obstruction post-MI as demonstrated by magnetic resonance imaging was found in 17% of 30 patients with TIMI grade 3 flow and 60% of 10 patients with TIMI grade 0 to 2 flow.[50] These investigators found that microvascular obstruction was a more potent marker of postinfarction cardiovascular complications than epicardial flow. Two studies evaluating the filling and clearance of contrast in the myocardium during coronary angiography have confirmed that a large proportion of patients with TIMI grade 3 flow of the infarct-related epicardial artery do not achieve normal microvascular flow and that diminished microvascular flow is associated more strongly with mortality than epicardial flow.[51,52]

Glycoprotein IIb/IIIa Antagonists in Primary PCI

The microvasculature of the myocardium can be compromised in the setting of an acute MI through various mechanisms including distal embolization of platelet microaggregates and atherosclerotic debris and the release of potent vasoconstrictors from activated platelets and because of an inflammatory response to reperfusion injury. It is possible that the addition of a platelet glycoprotein IIb/IIIa receptor inhibitor could potentially decrease the platelet-associated aspects of microvascular injury. In confirmation of this, Neumann and colleagues compared coronary flow as measured by a Doppler wire in 200 patients undergoing stenting for an acute MI, half of whom were treated with abciximab and the other half with standard heparin.[53] Although residual stenoses did not differ between the two groups, abciximab treatment was associated with a significant improvement of peak coronary flow velocity as well as improved wall motion index and recovery of global left-ventricular function. This improved microvascular flow with abciximab translated into a significant decrease in the combined endpoint of death, re-MI, or urgent revascularization at 30 days and a strong trend toward decreased mortality at 6 months. These clinical benefits of abciximab in stenting for acute MI have been reinforced by the results of several randomized trials. In the ADMIRAL study, 300 patients with an acute MI were randomly assigned to either abciximab or placebo prior to PTCA and stenting.[54] At 24 hours TIMI grade 3 flow was improved significantly in abciximab-treated patients compared to those receiving placebo, from 82.5% to 92.0%. At 30 days the combined incidence of death, reinfarction, and target vessel revascularization also was reduced significantly, from 14.7% in controls to 7.3% in abciximab-treated patients. This benefit of GPIIb/IIIa inhibition was not confirmed, however, in the larger CADILLAC (Controlled Abciximab and Device Investigation to Lower Late Angioplasty Complications) trial.[55] In this trial 2081 patients were randomized to one of four treatment groups: (1) abciximab + stent, (2) placebo + stent, (3) abciximab + balloon, or (4) placebo + balloon. Abciximab therapy did not improve epicardial flow grade with either stents or balloon angioplasty, and at 6 months follow-up there was no difference in the combined endpoint.

Glycoprotein IIb/IIIa Antagonists with Fibrinolysis

Despite the recognized central role of the platelet in arterial thrombosis, fibrinolysis has been the cornerstone of pharmacologic reperfusion therapy for decades. Combined therapy with reduced-dose fibrinolytics plus a GPIIb/IIIa antagonist has been studied as a means of improving reperfusion and therefore long-term outcomes. Several dose-finding pilot studies with an angiographic endpoint have suggested improved reperfusion with combination therapy compared to standard fibrinolytics therapy. In the TIMI-14 trial abciximab was evaluated with alteplase or streptokinase.[56] In this study patients receiving half-dose alteplase plus abciximab achieved TIMI grade 3 epicardial flow in 76% of patients at 90 minutes compared to 57% of patients treated with alteplase alone. It is important that no increase in bleeding was noted with combination therapy. A similar, although nonsignificant, benefit of combination therapy was found in the Strategies for Patency Enhancement in the Emergency Department (SPEED) pilot trial that studied abciximab plus half-dose reteplase.[57] Here, 54% of the patients treated with half-dose reteplase plus abciximab achieved TIMI grade 3 epicardial flow compared with 47% of patients receiving reteplase alone. The Integrilin and Low-Dose Thrombolysis in Acute Myocardial Infarction (INTRO-AMI) study examined angiographic outcomes in patients treated with eptifibatide and reduced-dose alteplase.[58] Again, patients receiving combination therapy achieved significantly greater TIMI grade 3 epicardial flow, as well as improved microvasculature flow as determined by the TIMI frame count.

The clinical benefit of combination GPIIb/IIIa inhibition and half-dose fibrinolytics compared with fibrinolysis alone has been studied in the 16,588 patient GUSTO V trial.[59] Patients who were within 6 hours of an ST-segment elevation MI were randomized to standard dose reteplase or half-dose reteplase plus full-dose abciximab. Although the study was powered to demonstrate a mortality benefit at 30 days, no difference was found (5.9% for reteplase vs.

5.6% for reteplase plus abciximab, P = 0.43). However, there was a significant reduction in the key secondary endpoint of death plus nonfatal reinfarction with combination therapy (7.4% vs. 8.8%, P = 0.001). Somewhat surprisingly, however, this decrease in early reinfarction did not translate into an improvement in outcomes at 1 year.[60] Equally important, combination therapy was associated with an increased risk of nonintracranial bleeding complications, and there was a concerning trend toward an increased risk of intracranial hemorrhage in patients older than 75 years receiving combination therapy (2.1% vs. 1.1%, P = 0.07). The smaller Assessment of the Safety and Efficacy of a New Thrombolytic Regimen (ASSENT)-3 trial enrolled 6095 patients within 6 hours of onset of an ST elevation MI and randomized them to one of three treatment arms: full-dose tenecteplase and enoxaparin, half-dose tenecteplase plus abciximab and unfractionated heparin, or full-dose tenecteplase and unfractionated heparin.[61] The primary endpoint of this trial was the combined occurrence of death, in-hospital reinfarction, or in-hospital refractory ischemia. Compared to the control arm of tenecteplase and unfractionated heparin, both the enoxaparin and abciximab regimens were associated with a significant reduction in the combined endpoint at 30 days (11.4% for enoxaparin, 11.1% for abciximab, and 15.4% for control; P = 0.0002 for enoxaparin vs. control, and P < 0.0001 for abciximab vs. control), without an increase in bleeding complications.

The role for the routine use of GPIIb/IIIa antagonists in the treatment of patients suffering an acute ST elevation MI remains unclear. However, the results of several large-scale randomized trials such as Addressing the Value of Facilitated Angioplasty After Combination Therapy or Eptifibatide Monotherapy in Acute Myocardial Infarction (ADVANCE-MI) and Facilitated Intervention and Enhanced Reperfusion Speed to Stop Events (FINESSE) will aide in clarifying the optimal use of these agents in this setting.

THE IMPORTANCE OF THE LEVEL OF PLATELET INHIBITION ACHIEVED WITH GPIIB/IIIA ANTAGONISTS IN THE TREATMENT OF ACUTE CORONARY SYNDROMES

Based on the results in animal models, early dosing of GPIIb/IIIa antagonists was designed to achieve blockade of approximately 80% of platelet GPIIb/IIIa receptors and inhibit ADP-induced platelet aggregation to approximately 20% of baseline.[8,14,19] This dose was considered necessary to prevent ischemic complications in response to severe thrombotic provocations but also was recognized as being "highly speculative."[3] However, subsequent studies have suggested that a higher level of inhibition may be optimal, at least in the setting of a PCI.[62] There are limited data from ACS trials confirming the importance of achieving an adequate level of platelet inhibition. In the PARAGON-B trial, drug levels were carefully targeted in an ACS population.[63] Steady-state plasma concentrations of lamifiban were available in 1272 patients.[64] A trend

toward greater benefit with increasing plasma levels was found in the overall PARAGON-B population. However, the subgroup of troponin-positive patients with low plasma levels derived no benefit compared with patients randomized to placebo, whereas patients with target levels or greater of inhibition experienced a more than 50% relative decrease in ischemic events. Patients experiencing an acute thrombotic event may require greater doses of a GPIIb/IIIa antagonist to achieve adequate levels of platelet inhibition. In the TIMI-14 study of half-dose fibrinolytics plus full-dose abciximab 20 μM ADP-induced platelet aggregation was inhibited by more than 80% at 90 minutes in just more than half of the 51 patients studied.[65] These results suggest that the GPIIb/IIIa antagonists dosing may be more complex than previously believed, although further clinical testing is required.

ORAL GPIIB/IIIA ANTAGONISTS

The early benefit of parenteral therapy with GPIIb/IIIa antagonists, as well as the well-recognized long-term risk for thrombotic events in the ACS population despite chronic antiplatelet therapy with aspirin, led to the development and clinical evaluation of multiple orally active GPIIb/IIIa antagonists. Two of these agents, sibrafiban and orbofiban, have been evaluated in three large-scale, multicenter, randomized trials involving more than 25,000 patients with unstable angina or a non-Q-wave MI, with unexpectedly disappointing results (Table 9-3).

Sibrafiban was initially studied in the Phase II trial TIMI-12, which enrolled 329 patients post-ACS.[66] Patients were randomized to one of seven doses of sibrafiban ranging from 5 mg daily to 10 mg twice daily or aspirin for 28 days. This study found a dose-dependent inhibition of platelet aggregation with an associated risk of bleeding complications. Doses of 10 mg or more a day had a greater than 10% incidence of major or minor bleeding, leading to drug discontinuation in 10% to 18% of patients. Covariates that were identified to affect drug levels and therefore bleeding risk were renal function and body weight.

The Sibrafiban Versus Aspirin to Yield Maximum Protection from Ischemic Heart Events Post Acute Coronary Syndromes (SYMPHONY) trial compared a high- and low-dose regimen of sibrafiban with aspirin for 90 days in patients who have suffered an ACS (unstable angina, Q-wave or non-Q-wave MI) within the preceding 7 days.[67] To minimize bleeding complications, dosing was adjusted based on the patient's body weight and serum creatinine, as well as by protocol for minor bleeding events. The primary endpoint was the 90-day incidence of the composite of death, (re)infarction or severe recurrent ischemia. Despite an increase in major bleeding with high-dose sibrafiban (5.7% vs. 5.2% for low-dose sibrafiban and 3.9% for aspirin), no decrease in the composite event rate was seen. The Second SYMPHONY trial, which differed from the initial SYMPHONY trial by giving aspirin in combination with low-dose sibrafiban, was stopped prematurely at 6671 patients instead of the planned enrollment of 8400 following the disappointing results from SYMPHONY.[68] As in the SYMPHONY trial, Second SYMPHONY showed no significant difference in the composite endpoint among

■ ■ ■

TABLE 9-3   TRIALS OF ORAL GLYCOPROTEIN IIB/IIIA ANTAGONISTS IN ACUTE CORONARY SYNDROMES

Trial	Patients	Drug	Aspirin in treatment arm	Primary endpoint	% with endpoint		P value
					Control	IIb/IIIa inhibitor	
OPUS-TIMI-16[69]	10,288	Orbofiban, 50 mg BID, or 50 mg bid × 30 days, then 30 mg bID	Yes	Death, MI, severe recurrent ischemia or stroke at 10 mo	22.9	22.8 (50 bid) or 23.1 (50 bid, then 30 bid)	0.59 0.41
SYMPHONY[67]	9,169	Sibrafiban, 3 mg, 4.5 mg, or 6 mg bid based on weight and creatinine	No	Death, MI, severe recurrent ischemia at 90 days	9.8	10.1 (low-dose) or 10.1 (high-dose)	NS for either
Second SYMPHONY[68]	6,637	Sibrafiban, 3 mg, 4.5 mg, or 6 mg bid based on weight and creatinine	Low-dose arms only	Death, MI, severe recurrent ischemia at 90 days	9.3	9.2 (low-dose) or 10.5 (high-dose)	NS for either

MI, myocardial infarction.

treatment arms; however, there was a concerning, significant increase in the risk of death (odds ratio 1.83), MI (odds ratio 1.32), or the combination (odds ratio 1.43) in the high-dose arm.

The Orbofiban in Patients with Unstable Coronary Syndromes—Thrombolysis In Myocardial Infarction (OPUS-TIMI)[16] trial randomized 10,288 patients with unstable angina or non-Q-wave MI to receive 50 mg of orbofiban twice daily, 50 mg of orbofiban twice daily for 30 days then 30 mg twice daily, or placebo.[69] The trial was designed to evaluate 12,000 patients with treatment and follow-up for an average of 1 year but was stopped prematurely by the recommendation of the Data and Safety Monitoring Board because of an increase in 30-day mortality in the 50/30 orbofiban group compared with placebo. As in the SYMPHONY trials, treatment was associated with a significant increase in major bleeding (2.0% aspirin, 3.7% 50/30 orbofiban, P = 0.0004, and 4.5% for 50/50 orbofiban, P < 0.0001) but no difference in the primary endpoint.

The reason for the lack of benefit with prolonged GPIIb/IIIa inhibition is unknown. However, every trial of these agents, involving more than 40,000 patients, has found at least a trend toward increased mortality in those randomized to the oral GPIIb/IIIa antagonist, with a recent meta-analysis confirming a significant mortality risk.[70] There is some evidence that some of these agents actually may be prothrombotic, especially at lower concentrations achieved at trough levels.[71] There is even some suggestion of possible direct cardiotoxicity of these agents.[72] Currently, clinical trials with other agents of this class are no longer being pursued.

CONCLUSION

Despite tremendous advances in our understanding and treatment of ACS, the diagnosis still is associated with an unacceptably high risk of death or MI in the short term.

The central role of platelets in the pathophysiology of an ACS makes them an ideal target for therapeutic measures to prevent thrombotic adverse events in this population. The platelet GPIIb/IIIa receptor antagonists are currently the most effective agents available for preventing arterial thrombosis and its complications. The consistent relationship between troponin status and the benefit of treatment with GPIIb/IIIa antagonists give these agents the ability to be particularly affective when they are targeted to the appropriate population.

Despite the extraordinary clinical data surrounding these agents, several questions remain: in particular, the lack of benefit with the oral agents and long-term parenteral infusions without PCI. As new antiplatelet and anticoagulant regimens are developed and tested in the ACS population, the optimal role for the GPIIb/IIIa antagonists will continue to be refined but will likely remain an important component of the antithrombotic armamentarium.

REFERENCES

1. Plow EF, Ginsberg MH: Cellular adhesion: GPIIb/IIIa as a prototypic adhesion receptor. Prog Hemost Thromb 1989; 9:117-156.
2. Wagner CL, Mascelli MA, Neblock DS, et al: Analysis of GPIIb/IIIa receptor number by quantification of 7E3 binding to human platelets. Blood 1996; 88:907-914.
3. Coller BS, Scudder LE, Beer J, et al: Monoclonal antibodies to platelet GPIIb/IIIa as antithrombotic agents. Ann NY Acad Sci 1991; 614:193-213.
4. Plow EF, McEver RP, Coller BS, et al: Related binding mechanisms for fibrinogen, fibronectin, von Willebrand factor, and thrombospondin on thrombin-stimulated human platelets. Blood 1985; 66:724-727.
5. Andre P, Hainaud P, Bal dit Sollier C, et al: Relative involvement of GPIb/IX-vWF axis and GPIIb/IIIa in thrombus growth at high shear rates in the guinea pig. Arterioscler Thromb Vasc Biol 1997; 17:919-924.
6. Plow EF, D'Souza SE, Ginsberg MH: Ligand binding to GPIIb-IIIa: A status report. Semin Thromb Hemost 1992; 18:324-332.
7. Coller BS, Peerschke EI, Scudder LE, et al: A murine monoclonal antibody that completely blocks the binding of fibrinogen to platelets

produces a thrombasthenic-like state in normal platelets and binds to glycoprotein IIb and/or IIIa. J Clin Invest 1983; 72:325-338.

8. Tcheng JE, Ellis SG, George BS, et al: Pharmacodynamics of chimeric glycoprotein IIb/IIIa integrin antiplatelet antibody Fab 7E3 in high-risk coronary angioplasty. Circulation 1994; 90:1757-1764.

9. Simon DI, Xu H, Ortlepp S, et al: 7E3 monoclonal antibody directed against the platelet glycoprotein IIb/IIIa cross-reacts wth leukocyte integrin Mac-i and blocks adhesion to fibrinogen and ICAM-1. Arterioscler Thromb Vasc Biol 1997; 17:528-535.

10. Charo IF, Bekeart LS, Phillips DR: Platelet glycoprotein IIb-IIIa-like proteins mediate endothelial cell attachment to adhesive proteins and the extracellular matriz. J Biol Chem 1987; 262:9935-9938.

11. Gold HK, Gimple LW, Yasuda T, et al: Pharmacodynamic study of F(ab')2 fragments of murine monoclonal antibody 7E3 directed against human platelet glycoprotein IIb/IIIa in patients with unstable angina pectoris. J Clin Invest 1990; 86:651-659.

12. Simoons ML, de Boer MJ, van den Brand MJBM, et al: Randomized trial of a GPIIb/IIIa platelet receptor blocker in refractory unstable angina. Circulation 1994; 89:596-603.

13. Scarborough RM, Naughton MA, Teng W, et al: Design of potent and specific integrin antagonists. Peptide antagonists with high specificity for glycoprotein IIb-IIIa. J Biol Chem 1993; 368:1066-1073.

14. Harrington RA, Kleiman NS, Kottke-Marchant K, et al: Immediate and reversible platelet inhibition after intravenous administration of a peptide glycoprotein IIb/IIIa inhibitor during percutaneous coronary intervention. Am J Cardiol 1995; 76:1222-1227.

15. Harrington RA, Rios G, Kleiman NS, et al: Platelet function during integrilin administration in coronary angioplasty [abst]. Circulation 1993; 88:I-319.

16. Goldschmidt-Clermont PJ, Schulman SP, Bray PF, et al: Refining the treatment of women with unstable angina—a randomized, double-blind, comparative safety and efficacy evaluation of Integrelin versus aspirin in the management of unstable angina. Clin Cardiol 1996; 19:869-874.

17. Phillips DR, Teng W, Arfsten A, et al: Effect of Ca^{2+} on GP IIb-IIIa interactions with integrilin. Enhanced GP IIb-IIIa binding and inhibition of platelet aggregation by reductions in the concentration of ionized calcium in plasma anticoagulated with citrate. Circulation 1997; 96:1488-1494.

18. Theroux P, Kouz S, Roy L, et al: Platelet membrane receptor glycoprotein IIb/IIIa antagonism in unstable angina. The Canadian Lamifiban Study. Circulation 1996; 94:899-905.

19. Kereiakes DJ, Kleiman NS, Ambrose J, et al: Randomized, double-blind, placebo-controlled dose-ranging study of tirofiban (MK-383) platelet IIb/IIIa blockade in high risk patients undergoing coronary angioplasty. J Am Coll Cardiol 1996; 27:536-542.

20. Marciniak SJ Jr, Jordan RE, Mascelli MA: Effect of Ca^{2+} chelation on the platelet inhibitory ability of the GPIIb/IIIa antagonists abciximab, eptifibatide and tirofiban. Thrombosis & Haemostasis 2001; 85:539-543.

21. The CAPTURE Investigators: Randomised placebo-controlled trial of abciximab before and during coronary interventions in refractory unstable angina: The CAPTURE study. Lancet 1997; 349:1429-1435.

22. Hamm C, Heeschen C, Goldman B, et al: Benefit of abciximab in patients with refractory unstable angina in relation to serum troponin T levels. N Engl J Med 1999; 340:1623-1629.

23. The GUSTO IV-ACS Investigators: Effect of glycoprotein IIb/IIIa receptor blocker abciximab on outcome in patients with acute coronary syndromes without early coronary revascularization: the GUSTO IV-ACS randomised trial. Lancet 2001; 357:1915-1924.

24. Ottervanger JP, Armstrong PW, Barnathan ES, et al: Long term results after the glycoprotein IIb/IIIa inhibitor abciximab in unstable angina. One-year survival in the GUSTO IV-ACS (Global Use of Strategies To Open Occluded Arteries IV–Acute Coronary Syndrome) Trial. Circulation 2003; 107:437-442.

25. Kereiakes DJ, Lincoff AM, Tcheng J, et al: GPIIb/IIIa blockade during coronary intervention for unstable angina: Longer is not better. Am J Cardiol 1998; 82:95S.

26. Lincoff AM, Califf RM, Anderson KM, et al: Evidence for prevention of death and myocardial infarction with platelet membrane glycoprotein IIb/IIIa receptor blockade by abciximab (c7E3 Fab) among patients with unstable angina undergoing percutaneous coronary revascularization. J Am Coll Cardial 1997; 30:149-156.

27. The EPILOG Investigators: Platelet glycoprotein IIb/IIIa receptor blockade and low-dose heparin during percutaneous coronary revascularization. N Engl J Med 1997; 336:1689-1696.

28. The EPISTENT Investigators: Randomised placebo-controlled and balloon-angioplasty-controlled trial to assess safety of coronary stenting with use of platelet glycoprotein-IIb/IIIa blockade. Lancet 1998; 352:87-92.

29. The PURSUIT Trial Investigators: Inhibition of platelet glycoprotein IIb/IIIa with eptifibatide in patients with acute coronary syndromes. N Engl J Med 1998; 339:436-443.

30. Kleiman N, Lincoff A, Flaker G, et al: Early percutaneous coronary intervention, platelet inhibition with eptifibatide, and clinical outcomes in patients with acute coronary syndromes. Circulation 2000; 101:751-757.

31. The PARAGON Investigators. International, randomized, controlled trial of lamifiban (a platelet glycoprotein IIb/IIIa inhibitor), heparin, or both in unstable angina. Circulation 1998; 97:2386-2395.

32. The Platelet IIb/IIIa Antagonist for the Reduction of Acute coronary syndrome events in a Global Organization Network (PARAGON)-B Investigators: Randomized, placebo-controlled trial of titrated intravenous lamifiban for acute coronary syndromes. Circulation 2002; 105:316-321.

33. Newby LK, Ohman EM, Christenson RH, et al: Benefit of glycoprotein IIb/IIIa inhibition in patients with acute coronary syndromes and troponin T-positive status. The PARAGON-B Troponin T Substudy. Circulation 2001; 103:2891-2896.

34. The Platelet Receptor Inhibition in Ischemic Syndrome Management (PRISM) Study Investigators: A comparison of aspirin plus tirofiban with aspirin plus heparin for unstable angina. N Engl J Med 1998; 338:1498-1505.

35. Heeschen C, Hamm C, Goldman B, et al: Troponin concentrations for stratification of patients with acute coronary syndromes in relation to therapeutic efficacy of tirofiban. Lancet 1999; 354:1757-1762.

36. The Platelet Receptor Inhibition in Ischemic Syndrome Management in Patients Limited by Unstable Signs and Symptoms (PRISM-PLUS) Study Investigators: Inhibition with the platelet glycoprotein IIb/IIIa receptor with tirofiban in unstable angina and non-Q-wave myocardial infarction. N Engl J Med 1998; 338:1488-1497.

37. Boersma E, Harrington RA, Moliterno DJ, et al: Platelet glycoprotein IIb/IIIa inhibitors in acute coronary syndromes: A meta-analysis of all major randomised clinical trials. Lancet 2002; 359:189-198.

38. Klootwijk P, Hamm C: Acute coronary syndromes: Diagnosis. Lancet 1999; 353:10-15.

39. Savonitto S, Ardissino D, Granger C, et al: Prognostic value of the admission electrocardiogram in acute coronary syndromes. JAMA 1999; 281:707-713.

40. Hamm C, Ravkilde J, Gerhardt W, et al: The prognostic value of serum troponin T in unstable angina. New Engl J Med 1992; 327:146-150.

41. Alexander J, Sparapani R, Mahaffey K, et al: Association between minor elevations of creatine kinase-MB level and mortality in patients with acute coronary syndromes without ST-segment elevation. PURSUIT Steering Committee. Platelet Glycoprotein IIb/IIIa in Unstable Angina: Receptor Suppression Using Integrilin Therapy. JAMA 2000; 283:347-353.

42. Hamm C, Goldmann B, Heeschen C, et al: Emergency room triage of patients with acute chest pain by means of rapid testing for cardiac troponin T or troponin I. N Eng J Med 1997; 337:1648-1653.

43. Shukla SD, Paul A, Klachko DM: Hypersensitivity of diabetic human platelets to platelet activating factor. Thromb Res 1992; 66:239-246.

44. Roffi M, Chew DP, Mukherjee D, et al: Platelet glycoprotein IIb/IIIa inhibitors reduce mortality in diabetic patients with non-ST-segment-elevation acute coronary syndromes. Circulation 2001; 104:2767-2771.

45. Topol EJ, Moliterno DJ, Herrmann HC, et al: Comparison of two platelet glycoprotein IIb/IIIa inhibitors, tirofiban and abciximab, for the prevention of ischemic events with percutaneous coronary revascularization. N Eng J Med 2001; 344:1888-1894.

46. Boersma E, Akkerhuis M, Theroux P, et al: Platelet glycoprotein IIb/IIIa receptor inhibition in non-ST-elevation acute coronary syndromes. Early benefit during medical treatment only, with additional protection during percutaneous coronary intervention. Circulation 1999; 100:2045-2048.

47. Armstrong P, Fu Y, Chang W-C, et al: Acute coronary syndromes in the GUSTO-IIb trial. Prognostic insights and impact of recurrent ischemia. Circulation 1998; 98:1860-1868.

48. Braunwald E, Antman E, Beasley J, et al: ACC/AHA guideline update for the management of patients with unstable angina and non-ST-segment elevation myocardial infarction: a report of the American College of Cardiology/American Heart Association Task Force on

Practice Guidelines (Committee on the Management of Patients with Unstable Angina). Available at: http://www.acc.org/clinical/guidelines/unstable/unstable.pdf 2002.

49. Ito H, Maruyama A, Iwakura K, et al: Clinical implications of the 'no reflow' phenomenon. A predictor of complications and left ventricular remodeling in reperfused anterior wall myocardial infarction. Circulation 1996; 93:223-228.

50. Wu KC, Zerhouni EA, Judd RM, et al: Prognostic significance of microvascular obstruction by magnetic resonance imaging in patients with acute myocardial infarction. Circulation 1998; 97:765-772.

51. van't Hof AWJ, Liem A, Suryapranata H, et al: Angiographic assessment of myocardial reperfusion in patients treated with primary angioplasty for acute myocardial infarction. Myocardial blush grade. Circulation 1998; 97:2302-2306.

52. Gibson CM, Cannon CP, Murphy SA, et al: Relationship of TIMI myocardial perfusion grade to mortality after administration of thrombolytic drugs. Circulation 2000; 101:125-130.

53. Neumann FJ, Blasini R, Schmitt C, et al: Effect of glycoprotein IIb/IIIa receptor blockade on recovery of coronary blood flow and left ventricular function after the placement of coronary artery stents in acute myocardial infarction. Circulation 1998; 98:2695-2701.

54. Montalescot G, Barragan P, Wittenberg O, et al: Platelet glycoprotein IIb/IIIa inhibition with coronary stenting for acute myocardial infarction. N Eng J Med 2001; 344:1895-1903.

55. Stone GW, Grines CL, Cox DA, et al: Comparison of angioplasty with stenting, with or without abciximab, in acute myocardial infarction. N Eng J Med 2002; 346:957-966.

56. Antman EM, Giugliano RP, Gibson CM, et al: Abciximab facilitates the rate and extent of thrombolysis: Results of the Thrombolysis in Myocardial Infarction (TIMI) 14 trial. Circulation 1999; 99:2720-2732.

57. Strategies for Patency Enhancement in the Emergency Department (SPEED) Group: Trial of abciximab with and without low-dose reteplase for acute myocardial infarction. Circulation 2000; 101:2788-2794.

58. Brener SJ, Zeymer U, Adgey AAJ, et al: Eptifibatide and low-dose tissue plasminogen activator in acute myocardial infarction. J Am Coll Cardiol 2002; 39:377-386.

59. The GUSTO V Investigators: Reperfusion therapy for acute myocardial infarction with fibrinolytic therapy or combination reduced fibrinolytic therapy and platelet glycoprotein IIb/IIIa inhibition: The GUSTO V randomised trial. Lancet 2001; 357:1905-1914.

60. Lincoff AM, Califf RM, Van de Werf F, et al: Mortality at 1 year with combination platelet glycoprotein IIb/IIIa inhibition and reduced-dose fibrinolytic therapy vs. conventional fibrinolytic therapy for acute myocardial infarction: GUSTO V randomized trial. JAMA 2002; 288:2130-2135.

61. The Assessment of the Safety and Efficacy of a New Thrombolytic Regimen (ASSENT)-3 Investigators: Efficacy and safety of tenecteplase in combination with enoxaparin, abciximab, or unfractionated heparin: The ASSENT-3 randomised trial in acute myocardial infarction. Lancet 2001; 358:605-613.

62. Steinhubl S, Talley J, Braden G, et al: Point-of-care measured platelet inhibition correlates with a reduced risk of an adverse cardiac event following percutaneous coronary intervention. Results of the GOLD (AU-Assessing Ultegra) multicenter study. Circulation 2001; 103:1403-1409.

63. The PARAGON-B Investigators: Randomized, placebo-controlled trial of titrated lamifiban for acute coronary syndromes. Circulation 2002; 105:316-321.

64. Dyke C, Mahaffey KW, Berdan LG, et al: Optimal dosing of a glycoprotein IIb/IIIa antagonist with a simplified renal-based algorithm: Pharmacodynamic and clinical findings from PARAGON-B.[abst]. J Am Coll Cardiol 2001:343A.

65. Coulter SA, Cannon CP, Ault KA, et al: High levels of platelet inhibition with abciximab despite heightened platelet activation and aggregation during thrombolysis for acute myocardial infarction: Results from TIMI (Thrombolysis In Myocardial Infarction) 14. Circulation 2000; 101:2690-2695.

66. Cannon CP, McCabe CH, Borzak S, et al: Randomized trial of an oral platelet glycoprotein IIb/IIIa antagonist, sibrafiban, in patients after an acute coronary syndrome. Results of the TIMI 12 trial. Circulation 1998; 97:340-349.

67. The SYMPHONY Investigators: Comparison of sibrafiban with aspirin for the prevention of cardiovascular events after acute coronary syndromes: A randomised trial. Lancet 2000; 355:337-345.

68. Second SYMPHONY Investigators: Randomized trial of aspirin, sibrafiban, or both for secondary prevention after acute coronary syndromes. Circulation 2001; 103:1727-1733.

69. Cannon C, McCabe C, Wilcox R, et al: Oral glycoprotein IIb/IIIa inhibition with orbofiban in patients with unstable coronary syndromes (OPUS-TIMI 16) Trial. Circulation 2000; 102:149-156.

70. Chew D, Bhatt D, Sapp S, et al: Increased mortality with oral glycoprotein IIb/IIIa antagonists: A meta-analysis of the phase III multicenter randomized trials. Circulation 2000; 103:201-206.

71. Peter K, Schwarz M, Ylanne J, et al: Induction of fibrinogen binding and platelet aggregation as a potential intrinsic property of various glycoprotein IIb/IIIa ($\alpha_{IIb}\beta_3$) inhibitors. Blood 1998; 92:3240-3249.

72. Buckley CD, Pilling D, Henriquez N, et al: RGD peptides induce apoptosis by direct caspase-3 activation. Nature 1999; 397:534-539.

■■■c h a p t e r **10**

Adjunctive Medical Therapy

Heather L. Gornik
Patrick O'Gara

In the current era, the management of acute coronary syndromes (ACS) is dominated largely by the timely and appropriate use of invasive strategies and antithrombotic therapies. Nevertheless, anti-ischemic and other medical therapies have maintained a central role in both acute stabilization and secondary prevention. Much has been learned over the past four decades regarding the benefits and limitations of β-adrenoreceptor antagonists, angiotensin-converting enzyme (ACE) inhibitors, calcium channel blockers (CCBs), nitrates, magnesium, antiarrhythmic agents, and various metabolic factors in the treatment of acute myocardial infarction (AMI). This chapter summarizes the clinical trial evidence that supports the use of these adjunctive therapies in modern practice.

β-ADRENORECEPTOR ANTAGONISTS

The β-adrenergic receptor comprises two general classes of cell-surface protein complexes.[1] β-1 receptors reside on cardiac myocytes and the cells of the specialized conduction tissues, whereas β-2 receptors are found on vascular and bronchial smooth-muscle cells. These receptors mediate the interactions of endogenous and exogenous catecholamines with their target organs and act via G-coupled proteins to influence intracellular calcium handling. Blockade of cardiac β-1 receptors produces a variety of effects to decrease myocardial oxygen demand, including reductions in heart rate and contractility. Interference with both cardiac and hepatic β-receptors may blunt the adrenergic response to hypoglycemia and impair gluconeogenesis. β-2 receptor blockade may result in an increase in peripheral vascular resistance and bronchial smooth-muscle constriction. The latter may cause clinically significant bronchospasm. As with all pharmacologic agents, knowledge of potential contraindications and adverse effects is essential. The use of β receptor antagonists for their anti-ischemic, antiarrhythmic, and neurohormonal properties is substantiated by a significant body of evidence.[2-4]

Acute Phase of Myocardial Infarction

Since the first reported use of propranolol by P.J.D. Snow in 1965, several clinical trials have demonstrated the benefit of β-receptor antagonists in the treatment of AMI (Table 10-1).[5] It now has been more than two decades since the publication of the Goteborg Metoprolol Study of 1395 patients with suspected AMI randomized to intravenous followed by oral metoprolol or to placebo within a mean of 11.3 hours after symptom onset.[6] The study drug was continued for 90 days following randomization. The use of metoprolol was associated with a 36% reduction in total (all-cause) mortality at 90 days (P < 0.03). Subgroup analysis demonstrated similar reductions in total mortality in patients with definite MI, as confirmed by characteristic ECG changes or positive biomarkers.

The Metoprolol in Acute Myocardial Infarction (MIAMI) study investigators used a similar treatment strategy in a larger number of patients (n = 5778) treated for only 15 days.[7] There was no significant difference between groups in all-cause mortality, but there was a trend toward fewer recurrent myocardial infarctions (MIs) in patients allocated metoprolol (3.0% metoprolol vs. 3.9% placebo, RR 0.77, P = 0.08). In subgroup analysis, patients defined as high-risk (n = 2038) had a 29% reduction in total mortality with beta blocker therapy (6.0% metoprolol vs. 8.5% placebo, P = 0.033). This subgroup comprised patients characterized by advanced age, abnormal baseline electrocardiogram (ECG), prior cardiac history, diabetes mellitus, and treatment with diuretics or digitalis prior to study enrollment.

In the largest trial of β-receptor antagonists in the acute phase of MI, the First International Study of Infarct Survival (ISIS-1) investigators randomized 16,027 patients to intravenous followed by oral atenolol or open control within a mean of 5.0 hours after onset of symptoms.[8] Therapy was continued for a total of 7 days or until hospital discharge, and long-term follow-up data were available for a mean of 20 months after enrollment. The use of atenolol was associated with a 15% reduction in vascular mortality during the acute treatment period (P < 0.04). There was no significant difference in

■ ■ ■

TABLE 10-1   MAJOR TRIALS OF β-RECEPTOR ANTAGONISTS IN THE ACUTE PHASE OF MYOCARDIAL INFARCTION

Study (year of publication)	Drug and target dose	Study design	Number randomized	Timing of initial therapy	Duration of therapy	Total mortality
Goteborg Metoprolol Study (1981)[6]	Metoprolol 15 mg IV in divided doses followed by 100 mg PO bid	RCT	1,395	Mean 11.3 hr after onset of symptoms	90 days	8.9% placebo (62/697) 5.7% metoprolol (40/698) RR 0.64 (P < 0.03)
MIAMI (1985)[7]	Metoprolol 15 mg IV in divided doses followed by 100 mg PO bid	RCT	5,778	<7 hr after onset of symptoms	15 days	4.9% placebo (142/2901) 4.3% metoprolol (123/2877) RR 0.87 (P = NS)
ISIS-1 (1986)[8]	Atenolol 5–10 mg IV followed by 100 mg PO QD	RCT Open control	16,027	Mean 5.0 hr after onset of symptoms	7 days or until hospital discharge	*4.6% placebo (365/7990) 3.9% atenolol (313/8037) RR 0.85 (P < 0.04)
TIMI 2B (1991)[9]	Metoprolol Immediate therapy: 15 mg IV in divided doses followed by 100 mg PO bid Delayed therapy: 100 mg PO bid	RCT Factorial design	1,434	Either given immediately following t-PA (mean 3.3 hr after onset of symptoms) or given orally on hospital day 6	6 days intravenous therapy; oral metoprolol continued following discharge by both groups	†2.4% delayed metoprolol (17/714) 2.4% immediate metoprolol (17/720) RR 1.0 (P = NS)

*Endpoint of vascular mortality defined as death from myocardial infarction, stroke or other vascular cause, sudden death, and death from unknown cause.
†Mortality at 6 days. No significant difference in mortality at 6 days, 6 weeks, or 1 year.
IV, intravenously; PO, by mouth; BID, twice daily; RCT, randomized controlled trial; RR, relative risk; QD, daily; t-PA, tissue plasminogen activator.

mortality between the treatment and control groups following the discontinuation of atenolol. Of interest, there was also no significant difference between groups in the rates of reinfarction during hospitalization (2.5% atenolol vs. 2.8% placebo, P = NS).

The first major trial of the adjunctive use of β-receptor antagonists with reperfusion therapy in ST-segment elevation MI (STEMI) was the Thrombolysis in Myocardial Infarction (TIMI) 2B study.[9] In the TIMI 2 trial, patients received intravenous tissue-type plasminogen activator and were randomized to either a conservative or invasive strategy. The latter comprised either immediate or delayed (18–48 hour) angiography and balloon angioplasty as appropriate (TIMI 2A). In a factorial design, patients also were randomized to receive either immediate intravenous metoprolol followed by oral therapy or delayed therapy with oral metoprolol beginning on hospital day 6 (TIMI 2B). Metoprolol was continued indefinitely after hospital discharge. There were no significant differences in left-ventricular (LV) ejection fraction (EF) at discharge or in total mortality at 6 days, 6 weeks, or 1 year between patients randomized to immediate intravenous or delayed treatment with metoprolol. However, the use of immediate intravenous metoprolol was associated with significant reductions in the incidence of both recurrent chest pain and reinfarction (P ≤ 0.02). In a subgroup predefined as low risk, there were no deaths at 6 weeks among the immediate intravenous group, but there were seven deaths in the deferred metoprolol group (P = 0.007). It is important to note that the effect of immediate versus delayed therapy with metoprolol was the same regardless of randomization to an early-invasive or conservative strategy. TIMI 2B estab-

lished that in appropriately selected patients, beta blockers can be given safely with reperfusion therapy in the acute phase of MI and are associated with decreased myocardial ischemia and reinfarction in the first several weeks.

Secondary Prevention After Myocardial Infarction

Multiple clinical trials have demonstrated the efficacy of β-adrenergic receptor antagonists in the secondary prevention of death or recurrent infarction in MI survivors (Table 10-2). The Norwegian Multicenter Study Group randomized 1884 patients 7 to 28 days following confirmed MI to treatment with timolol or placebo.[10] Over a mean follow-up of 17.3 months, timolol treatment resulted in a 36% reduction in total mortality (P < 0.001), a 45% reduction in the cumulative incidence of sudden death (P = 0.0001), and a 38% reduction in the risk of reinfarction. The survival curves for the timolol and placebo groups continued to diverge over the first 2 years of follow-up.

The B-Blocker Heart Attack Trial (BHAT) demonstrated similar findings in 3837 patients randomized to propranolol or placebo 5 to 21 days following MI.[11,12] The total daily dose of study drug (60 or 80 mg PO tid) was based on serum propranolol levels. The trial was terminated early because of a 26% reduction in mortality (P < 0.005) and a 23% reduction in the combined endpoint of cardiac death plus nonfatal reinfarction (P < 0.01), at a mean follow-up of 25 months.

Throughout the 1970s and 1980s, a few trials investigated the use of beta blockers with intrinsic sympathomimetic activity (ISA) for secondary prevention.[2-4] As

TABLE 10-2   MAJOR TRIALS OF β-RECEPTOR ANTAGONISTS IN SECONDARY PREVENTION

Study (year of publication)	Drug and target dose	Study design	Number randomized	Timing of therapy after MI	Mean follow-up	Total mortality	Reinfarction
Norwegian Multicenter Study (1981)[10]	Timolol 10 mg PO BID	RCT	1884	7–28 days	17.3 mo	16.2% placebo (152/939) 10.4% timolol (98/945) RR 0.64 (P < 0.001)	15.0% placebo (141/939) 9.3% timolol (88/945) RR 0.62 (P < 0.001)
BHAT (1982)[11,12]	Propranolol 80 mg PO TID or 60 mg PO TID dose based on serum drug levels	RCT	3837	5–21 days	25 mo (early termination)	9.8% placebo (188/1921) 7.2% propranolol (138/1916) RR 0.74 (P < 0.005)	*13.0% placebo (249/1921) 10.0% propranolol (192/1916) RR 0.77 (P < 0.01)
APSI (1990)[13]	Acebutolol 200 mg PO BID	RCT	607	3–21 days	10.5 mo	11.0% placebo (34/309) 5.7% acebutolol (17/298) RR 0.52 (P = 0.019)	Data incomplete
CAPRICORN (2001)[14]	†Carvedilol Titrated to 25 mg PO bid	RCT	1959	3–21 days	15.6 mo	15.3% placebo (151/984) 11.9% carvedilol (116/975) RR 0.77 (P = 0.031)	5.8% placebo (57/984) 3.5% carvedilol (34/975) RR 0.59 (P = 0.014)

*"Coronary incidence" defined as recurrent nonfatal definite reinfarction plus cardiac death.
†Exerts Both alpha- and beta-blocking effects.
MI, myocardial infarction; PO, by mouth; BID, twice daily; RCT, randomized controlled trial; RR, relative risk; TID, three times daily.

a group, these trials failed to demonstrate the consistent reduction in overall mortality and reinfarction that had been demonstrated in the large trials of agents without ISA. There is the additional concern that these agents with ISA may be proarrhythmic. A possible exception was the Acebutolol et Prevention Secondaire de L'Infarctus (APSI) trial in which 607 patients were randomized 3 to 21 days after MI to acebutolol or placebo.[13] The trial was designed to enroll high-risk patients with an expected 1-year mortality rate of at least 20%. The trial was terminated early because of inadequate enrollment, especially of high-risk patients, but the investigators did report a 48% reduction in total mortality at a mean follow-up of 10.5 months. Despite these limited results, the use of β-adrenergic receptor antagonists with ISA in the early phases of AMI is not advocated.

The Carvedilol Post-Infarct Survival Control in LV Dysfunction (CAPRICORN) investigators studied an important group of patients excluded from previous secondary prevention trials, namely those with heart failure and LV systolic dysfunction.[14] Patients (n = 1959) with LVEF of 40% or less (mean 0.33) and compensated heart failure were randomized to either placebo or carvedilol 3 to 21 days after confirmed MI. There was a 23% reduction in total mortality and a 41% reduction in the rate of nonfatal reinfarction among carvedilol-treated patients. This trial more closely mimicked modern clinical practice because nearly half of patients enrolled were treated with either thrombolytic therapy or primary angioplasty,

86% of patients received aspirin, and 97% of patients received ACE inhibitors at the time of randomization. The results extended the proven benefits of beta blockade in chronic heart failure to patients with LV dysfunction in the recovery phase of AMI. Meta-analysis of earlier trials, in fact, had suggested that this relatively high-risk post-MI group derived the greatest relative benefit from β-receptor antagonists.[15,16]

Recommendations

In the absence of contraindications, all patients with AMI should receive treatment with an intravenous followed by an oral β-receptor antagonist. Therapy should be continued indefinitely unless intolerable side effects or specific contraindications intervene. Important contraindications include marked bradycardia, markedly prolonged PR interval (>0.24 seconds), advanced atrioventricular (AV) block, hypotension, decompensated heart failure, severe bronchospastic lung disease, brittle diabetes mellitus, and active Raynaud's disease. It is especially important to attempt initiation and maintenance of beta blocker therapy in patients with LV dysfunction or heart failure, as well as tachyarrhythmias, but only following stabilization and a period of proven compensation. The long-term benefit associated with beta blockers following MI reflects both their antiarrhythmic and anti-ischemic properties (Fig. 10-1).

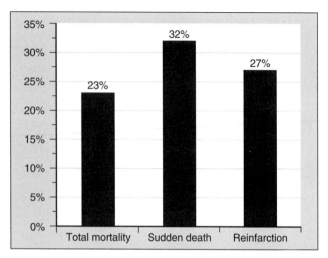

FIGURE 10-1. Reduction in recurrent events with long-term β-receptor antagonist therapy. (From Held PH, Yusuf S: Effects of beta-blockers and calcium channel blockers in acute myocardial infarction. Eur Heart J 1993; 14[Suppl F]:18–25, with permission.)

ANGIOTENSIN-CONVERTING ENZYME INHIBITORS

ACE inhibitors block the conversion of angiotensin I to angiotensin II (AT-2) and promote the formation of bradykinin.[1] In addition to their blood pressure–lowering effects, ACE inhibitors have the potential to counteract some of the myriad other effects of AT-2 on myocardial and vascular wall structure and function. It is important to recognize that there are non-ACE pathways by which AT-2 can be generated, which may attenuate the effectiveness of ACE inhibitors over time. Angiotensin receptor blockers (ARBs) often are substituted for ACE inhibitors when side effects intervene. To date, however, ARBs have not been studied extensively in the setting of AMI.

The early clinical trials of ACE inhibitors in MI can be segregated into two broad groups according to patient inclusion criteria. The nonselective trials (Table 10-3) enrolled all patients with suspected or proven MI, whereas the selective trials (Table 10-4) recruited patients with prespecified high-risk indicators, such as LV systolic dysfunction or anterior location of MI. These latter patients might be expected to derive relatively greater hemodynamic and neurohormonal benefit from the use of ACE inhibitors with less LV remodeling. There is substantial evidence for the use of ACE inhibitors in both the acute phase of MI and for the secondary prevention of recurrent events (Fig. 10-2). The long-term decrease in recurrent ischemic events reported in several clinical trials has sparked great interest in the vasculoprotective effects of these drugs.

Nonselective Trials

The Cooperative New Scandinavian Enalapril Survival Study II (CONSENSUS II) investigators examined the safety and efficacy of early enalapril administration among 6090 patients enrolled within 24 hours of MI onset.[17] Active therapy was given initially as intravenous enalaprilat followed by oral enalapril for 6 months. The trial was terminated prematurely as a result of an excess incidence of hypotension and death with intravenous enalaprilat. Only 48% of the patients enrolled in the trial were followed in blinded fashion for the intended 6-month duration of the study. As a result, neither a survival benefit nor a decrease in the rate of reinfarction was seen with enalapril therapy. There was no survival benefit for the prespecified high-risk subgroup of patients with anterior MI, and there was a disturbing trend toward increased

■ ■ ■

TABLE 10-3 MAJOR TRIALS OF ANGIOTENSIN-CONVERTING ENZYME INHIBITORS IN MYOCARDIAL INFARCTION WITH NONSELECTIVE ENROLLMENT

Study (year of publication)	Drug and target dose	Study design	Number randomized	Timing of therapy	Follow-up	Total mortality
CONSENSUS II (1992)[17]	Enalapril 1 mg IV enalalaprilat over 2 hr followed by 20 mg PO BID	RCT	6,090	Mean 15 hr after onset of symptoms Continued for 6 mo after enrollment	6 mo	9.4% placebo (286/3046) 10.2% enalapril (312/3044) RR 1.1 (P = NS)
GISSI-3 (1994)[18]	Lisinopril 10 mg PO QD	RCT 2 × 2 factorial design Open control	19,394	Within 24 hr of onset of symptoms Continued for 6 wk after enrollment	6 mo	7.1% control (673/9460) 6.3% lisinopril (597/9435) RR 0.88 (P = 0.03)
Chinese Cardiac Study (1995, 1997)[19,20]	Captopril 12.5 mg PO TID	RCT	14,962	Mean 16.6 hr after onset of symptoms Continued for 4 wk after enrollment	4 wk	9.7% placebo (730/7494) 9.1% captopril (681/7468) RR 0.94 (P = 0.20)
ISIS-4 (1995)[22]	Captopril 50 mg PO BID	RCT 2 × 2 × 2 factorial design	58,050	Median 8 hr after onset of symptoms Continued for 4 wk after enrollment	5 wk	7.7% placebo (2231/29022) 7.2% captopril (2088/29028) RR 0.93 (P = 0.02)

IV, intravenously; PO, by mouth; BID, twice daily; RCT, randomized controlled trial; RR, relative risk; QD, daily; TID, three times daily.

TABLE 10-4 MAJOR TRIALS OF ANGIOTENSIN-CONVERTING ENZYME INHIBITORS IN MYOCARDIAL INFARCTION WITH SELECTIVE ENROLLMENT

Study (year of publication)	Drug and target dose	Study design	Number randomized	Timing of therapy	Selection criteria	Follow-up	Total mortality	Reinfarction	Heart failure
SAVE (1992)[28]	Captopril 50 mg PO TID	RCT	2231	Mean 11 days post-MI Continued for 2 to 5 yr after enrollment	Recent MI with asymptomatic left ventricular systolic dysfunction (EF ≤ 0.40)	Mean 42 mo	24.6% placebo (275/1116) 20.4% captopril (228/1115) *RR 0.81 (P = 0.019)	15.2% placebo (170/1116) 11.9% captopril (133/1115) *RR 0.75 (P = 0.015)	Hospitalization for HF: 17.2% placebo (192/1116) 13.8% captopril (154/1115) *RR 0.88 (P = 0.019)
AIRE (1993)[29]	Ramipril 5 mg PO BID	RCT	2006	Mean 5.4 days post-MI Continued for at least 6 mo	Recent MI with clinical evidence of congestive heart failure	Mean 15 mo	22.6% placebo (222/982) 16.9% ramipril (170/1004) *RR 0.73 (P = 0.002)	9.0% placebo (88/982) 8.1% ramipril (81/1004) †RR 0.90	Severe or resistant HF: 18.1% placebo (178/982) 14.2% ramipril (143/1004) †RR 0.79
TRACE (1995)[30]	Trandolapril 4 mg PO QD	RCT	1749	Mean 4.5 days post-MI Continued for at least 2 yr	Recent MI with left ventricular systolic dysfunction (EF ≤ 0.35)	25–50 mo	42.3% placebo (369/873) 34.7% trandolapril (304/876) *RR 0.78 (P = 0.001)	12.9% placebo (113/873) 11.3% trandolapril (99/876) *RR 0.86 (P = 0.29)	HF requiring hospital admission, open-label ACE inhibitor, or resulting in death: 19.6% placebo (171/873) 14.3% trandolapril (125/876) *RR 0.71 (P = 0.003)
SMILE (1995)[32]	Zofenopril 30 mg PO BID	RCT	1556	Mean 15 hr after onset of symptoms Continued for 6 wk	Acute anterior MI ineligible for thrombolytic therapy	6 wk	6.5% placebo (51/784) 4.9% zofenopril (38/772) RR 0.75 (P = 0.19)	1.5% placebo (12/784) 1.4% zofenopril (11/772) RR 0.93 (P = NS)	Multiple signs of HF despite medical therapy requiring open-label ACE inhibitor: 4.1% placebo (32/784) 2.2% zofenopril (17/772) RR 0.54 (P = 0.018)

*Relative risk calculated by life-table analysis.
†P value not reported.
PO, by mouth; TID, three times daily; RCT, randomized controlled trial; MI, myocardial infarction; EF, ejection fraction; RR, relative risk; HF, heart failure; QD, daily; ACE, angiotensin-converting enzyme.

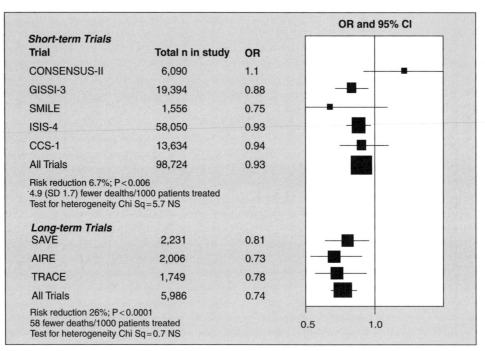

FIGURE 10-2. Effects of angiotensin-converting enzyme (ACE) inhibitors on mortality after myocardial infarction (MI). Results from short-term and long-term trials. (From Flather MD, Pfeffer MA: Angiotensin-converting enzyme inhibitors. In Hennekens CH, ed: Clinical Trials in Cardiovascular Disease: A Companion to Braunwald's Heart Disease. Philadelphia, WB Saunders, 1999, with permission).

mortality among patients age 70 years or older (17.3% enalapril vs. 14.7% placebo, P = 0.07). Because of inadequate follow-up and early termination, it is not known whether there would have been a longer-term benefit with enalapril in these patients.

The Gruppo Italiano per lo Studio della Sopravvivenza nell'Infarto Miocardico (GISSI-3) investigators randomized 19,394 patients within 24 hours of symptom onset in an open controlled trial with a 2 × 2 factorial design to test the efficacy and safety of lisinopril and nitroglycerin.[18] Patients received standard medical care (72% thrombolytics, 31% β-receptor antagonists, and 84% aspirin), standard medical care plus lisinopril, standard medical care plus nitroglycerin, or standard medical care plus lisinopril and nitroglycerin. MI was confirmed in 95% of patients. Study drugs were continued for 6 weeks after randomization, and 6-month follow-up data were available for more than 97% of patients. LV function are assessed by echocardiography at 6 months. Lisinopril therapy was associated with a 12% reduction in total mortality (P = 0.03) and a 10% reduction in the combined endpoint of death, heart failure, LV dysfunction (defined as EF ≤ 0.35), or severe echocardiographic regional wall motion abnormalities (P = 0.009). In contrast to the CONSENSUS II trial, there was a 12% reduction in the combined endpoint for elderly patients (P = 0.004). Reinfarction rates did not differ across groups. The combination of lisinopril and nitroglycerin was well tolerated and was associated with a 17% reduction in all-cause mortality (P = 0.021) and a 15% reduction in the combined endpoint (P = 0.003).

The Chinese Cardiac Study (CCS-1) investigators randomized 14,962 patients within 36 hours of MI presentation to captopril or placebo.[19,20] Only 26% of patients received thrombolytic therapy. Captopril was associated

with a nonsignificant 6% reduction in mortality at 4 weeks (P = 0.20). Patients with confirmed anterior MI derived the greatest benefit (RR 0.84, P = 0.02). The short-term use of captopril did not affect the rate of reinfarction, although there was a significant decrease in the risk of subsequent heart failure (RR 0.91, P = 0.01).[20] Two year follow-up demonstrated a more impressive benefit with a 14% reduction in all-cause mortality among patients treated with captopril for 4 weeks following AMI (P = 0.03).[21]

In the largest trial of ACE inhibitors in MI, the Fourth International Study of Infarct Survival (ISIS-4) Collaborative Group randomized 58,050 patients in a complex 2 × 2 × 2 factorial design to captopril, isosorbide mononitrate, intravenous magnesium infusion, or control during the first 24 hours of AMI.[22] The captopril and isosorbide mononitrate arms were placebo-controlled. MI was confirmed in 92% of patients. Seventy percent of patients were treated with thrombolytic therapy, 94% received aspirin, and 9% received intravenous beta blocker. Although the magnesium infusion was limited to the first 24 hours after enrollment, patients continued oral captopril, nitrates, or placebo for 4 weeks. There was a small (7%) but statistically significant reduction in total mortality at 5 weeks in patients treated with captopril (P = 0.02), resulting in an estimated five lives saved per 1000 patients treated for 1 month. The largest benefit was among patients with anterior MI. Of the total 143 fewer deaths in the captopril group, 44 occurred on day 0 or 1, suggesting that early therapy is important. This survival benefit persisted to 1 year. There was no significant interaction between captopril and treatment with either nitrates or magnesium. Hypotension requiring termination of study drug occurred in 10% of patients treated with captopril.

The ISIS-4 investigators also provided a meta-analysis of published trials of ACE inhibitors in the acute phase of MI. They reported a 6.5% reduction in short-term mortality risk among the more than 100,000 patients enrolled in 4 major and 11 small, underpowered trials (P = 0.006). This benefit translates to 4.6 fewer deaths per 1000 patients treated with ACE inhibitors. A more recent confirmatory meta-analysis estimated 4.8 fewer deaths per 1000 patients treated within the first 36 hours of MI at 30 days follow-up.[23] This benefit was greatest among patients with anterior MI, with a calculated 10.6 deaths avoided per 1000 patients treated.

More recently, the "nonselective" use of ACE inhibitors for primary and secondary prevention has been studied in high-risk vascular patients. The Heart Outcomes Prevention Evaluation (HOPE) investigators studied the effect of ramipril (goal 10 mg daily) and vitamin E on the development of MI, stroke, or cardiovascular death in high-risk patients in a 2 × 2 factorial design.[24] Patients (n = 9297) 55 years of age or older with either a history of coronary artery disease, stroke, peripheral arterial disease, or diabetes associated with at least one other cardiovascular risk factor were enrolled. Patients with heart failure or LVEF of less than 0.40, or MI or stroke within 4 weeks of enrollment, were excluded. At 5 years, the use of ramipril was associated with a 22% reduction in the primary composite endpoint of cardiovascular death, MI, or stroke (P < 0.001). There were similarly striking reductions in each of the individual components of this composite endpoint, as well as a 16% decrease in total mortality (P = 0.005). The recently reported findings of the European Trial on Reduction of Cardiac Events with Perindopril in Stable Coronary Artery Disease (EUROPA) support the use of ACE inhibitors for secondary prevention in low-risk patients.[25] Among 12,218 patients enrolled, there was a 20% reduction in the combined endpoint of death, MI, or cardiac arrest in patients randomized to perindopril (goal 8 mg/day) over 4.2 years of follow-up (P = 0.0003). In contrast to the HOPE trial, one third of patients enrolled were younger than 55 years of age and fewer patients had diabetes mellitus or hypertension. The Prevention of Events with Angiotensin-Converting Enzyme Inhibition (PEACE) trial, which is studying the use of trandolapril in similar low-risk populations, is ongoing.[26,27]

Selective Trials

Given the cumulative evidence of the important role of ACE inhibitors in the treatment of patients with LV dysfunction and heart failure, a number of trials were designed to identify subsets of patients with MI for whom the use of these drugs would result in relatively greater clinical benefit (Table 10-4). The Survival and Ventricular Enlargement (SAVE) investigators randomized 2231 patients with asymptomatic LV systolic dysfunction (EF ≤ 0.40%) 3 to 16 days after MI to captopril or placebo.[28] Thirty-three percent of patients received thrombolytic therapy and 17% were managed with percutaneous coronary intervention (PCI). Patients undergoing drug therapy were followed for at least 2 years. At a mean follow-up of 42 months, there was a 19% reduction in all-cause mortality (P = 0.019) and a 21% reduction in the risk of cardiac death (P = 0.014). The survival curves did not begin to diverge until approximately 1 year of treatment, suggesting the need for long-term therapy with ACE inhibitors for optimal clinical benefit. There was a 25% reduction in the risk of recurrent MI (P = 0.015) and a 22% reduction in the rate of hospitalization for heart failure (P = 0.019). There was no significant difference in the progression of LV dysfunction in patients treated with captopril. Captopril was well tolerated; 70% of surviving patients in the captopril group, compared to 73% in the placebo group, continued taking the study drug throughout the trial.

The Acute Infarction Ramipril Efficacy (AIRE) investigators studied the use of ramipril in patients with recent MI (2–9 days prior to randomization) and clinical evidence of heart failure (defined by the presence of pulmonary rales or a third heart sound on physical examination or pulmonary edema on chest radiograph).[29] LV function was not assessed. Patients were randomized to receive ramipril or placebo. Of the 2006 patients, 58% received thrombolytic therapy. At 15 months, there was a 27% reduction in total mortality among ramipril-treated patients (P = 0.002). In contrast to the SAVE trial, the survival curves began to diverge within the first few weeks after initiation of treatment. There was a 19% reduction in the composite of death and the first occurrence of severe heart failure, reinfarction, or stroke (P = 0.008). At 18 months, 40% of surviving patients had withdrawn from the study. The majority of patients who withdrew from the placebo group were receiving open-label ACE inhibitors.

The Trandolapril Cardiac Evaluation (TRACE) investigators randomized 1749 patients with recent MI and LV dysfunction (EF ≤ 0.35), approximately 60% of whom had evidence of heart failure, to either trandolapril or placebo.[30] Follow-up was extended to 2 years following enrollment of the last patient. There was a 22% reduction in all-cause mortality (P = 0.001) and a 24% reduction in sudden death (P = 0.03) among patients treated with trandolapril. There was a nonsignificant trend toward a lower rate of reinfarction in patients treated with trandolapril and a 29% reduction in severe heart failure (P = 0.003). As seen in the AIRE trial, the survival curves began to diverge at 1 month of treatment and continued to separate throughout the remainder of the follow-up period.

A recent meta-analysis of these three selective enrollment trials of long-term ACE inhibitor use following MI reported a 26% reduction in total mortality (P < 0.0001), a 20% reduction in the rate of reinfarction (P = 0.006), and a 27% reduction in the rate of readmission for heart failure (P < 0.0001).[31] The mortality reduction translates to 60 lives saved for every 1000 high-risk MI patients treated with ACE inhibitors.

The Survival of Myocardial Infarction Long-term Evaluation (SMILE) investigators enrolled 1556 high-risk patients with acute anterior MI who were ineligible for thrombolytic therapy.[32] Patients were randomized to zofenopril or placebo within 24 hours of symptom onset. Drug therapy was continued for 6 weeks, and surviving patients were followed for an additional year. There was a 34% reduction in the primary combined endpoint of death or severe heart failure at 6 weeks (10.6% placebo, 7.1% zofenopril, P = 0.018), although the difference in total mortality did not reach statistical significance (6.5% placebo, 4.9% zofenopril, P = 0.19). Despite discontinuation of zofenopril at 6 weeks, there was a 29% relative decrease in total mortality at 1 year (14.1% placebo, 10.0% zofenopril, P = 0.011).

Recent studies have begun to investigate the role of ARBs in the management of patients with MI. The Optimal Trial in Myocardial Infarction with the Angiotensin II Antagonist Losartan (OPTIMAAL) investigators enrolled patients within 10 days of MI with at least one of three additional features: clinical evidence of heart failure, LV systolic dysfunction, or presence of anterior Q waves on ECG.[33] Patients (n = 5477) were randomized to receive losartan (goal 50 mg daily) or captopril (goal 50 mg three times daily). At a mean 2.7 years of follow-up, there was a trend toward an increase in mortality in patients treated with losartan (RR 1.13, P = 0.07). There were no differences in the rates of reinfarction or hospital readmission. Fewer patients in the losartan group discontinued therapy (losartan 17% vs. captopril 23%, RR 0.70, P < 0.0001). The investigators concluded that traditional ACE inhibitors should remain the agent of first choice in patients surviving complicated AMI. Losartan could be considered an alternative for patients unable to tolerate ACE inhibitors.

Recommendations

The 1999 revised American College of Cardiology/American Heart Association (ACC/AHA) guidelines for the management of patients with AMI recommend initiation of oral ACE inhibitors within 24 hours of suspected or proven MI in all patients without contraindication.[34] Their use to the target doses reported in the major trials is especially appropriate for patients with anterior STEMI, clinical heart failure, or LV systolic dysfunction (EF < 0.40). Therapy should be continued indefinitely, particularly in patients with high-risk features. The HOPE trial has established the benefit of their long-term use in the chronic phase of MI, even among patients with preserved LV systolic function, and has extended their use to patients with atherosclerosis without documented coronary artery disease.[24] There is no role for the use of intravenous ACE inhibitors in the acute phase of MI. The precise timing of the initiation of an oral ACE inhibitor requires clinical judgment and an appreciation for the predicted tolerability of these agents in conjunction with other medical therapies.

CALCIUM CHANNEL BLOCKERS

The clinically available CCBs exert their pharmacologic effects predominantly via inhibition of L-type calcium channels, preventing the influx of calcium ions into various tissues.[1] Each agent has a given specificity for vascular smooth-muscle cells, myocardium, and the sinoatrial (SA) and AV nodes. CCBs have proved useful for the treatment of hypertension, chronic stable angina pectoris, supraventricular arrhythmias, and both coronary (Printzmetal's) and peripheral (Raynaud's) vasospasm.

The dihydropyridine CCBs, of which nifidipine is the prototype, act selectively on vascular smooth-muscle cells and have less effect on cardiac conduction and myocardial contractility.[1] These agents are potent vasodilators that reduce systemic vascular resistance and blood pressure. In the acute setting, when used as monotherapy, they may cause reflex tachycardia and a further increase in myocardial oxygen demand. This effect can be blunted by the concomitant administration of a β-receptor antagonist. Save for amlodipine, the use of dihydropyridines in patients with chronic LV systolic dysfunction generally is to be avoided.[35-38]

The nondihydropyridine CCBs, diltiazem and verapamil, have more potent effects on cardiac conduction and myocardial contractility.[1] In addition to their blood pressure–lowering effects, these agents cause SA and AV node slowing and depress myocardial contractility, especially in patients with established LV dysfunction.

The theoretic underpinnings for the use of CCBs in the treatment of myocardial ischemia are based on their unique properties.[1] In addition to decreasing myocardial oxygen demand by reducing heart rate (nondihydropyridine agents) and systemic blood pressure (all agents), they may prevent or relieve vasospasm and improve coronary blood flow. By reducing the influx of calcium, they also may attenuate myocardial reperfusion injury. Except in very isolated circumstances, CCBs do not as a rule augment diastolic relaxation.

Clinical Trials

Since the 1970s, numerous investigators have explored the potential role of CCBs in the treatment of myocardial ischemia (Table 10-5). Despite early enthusiasm, the evidence supporting the routine use of these agents in the treatment of ACS has been less than convincing. At present, they are used usually as second- or third-line therapy in patients with contraindications or inadequate responses to beta blockers, nitrates, or ACE inhibitors.

As summarized in Figure 10-3, CCBs have not been shown to reduce mortality after AMI. Similar findings also have been reported for patients with unstable angina.[39] In addition, there are data to suggest that these agents may be harmful in certain clinical situations, as is the case for the use of diltiazem in patients with pulmonary congestion.[40] Monotherapy with nifedipine in patients with ACS is to be avoided given the clear suggestion of excess mortality and/or reinfarction (Fig. 10-3). Meta-analyses of dihydropyridine trials have indicated a worrisome trend toward increased mortality when these agents are used in the setting of MI, particularly when administered in high doses.[3,41]

There is some evidence that the nondihydropyridine calcium antagonists, particularly diltiazem, may prevent refractory ischemia or reinfarction. In the Diltiazem Reinfarction Study, the use of diltiazem was associated with a 51% reduction in the incidence of reinfarction at 14 days (P = 0.03).[42] In the Diltiazem as Adjunctive

TABLE 10-5 TRIALS OF CALCIUM CHANNEL BLOCKERS IN ACUTE CORONARY SYNDROMES

Study (year of publication)	Drug	Indication	Number randomized	Timing of therapy	Total mortality	Recurrent ischemia or reinfarction
DAVIT I (1984)[89]	Verapamil	AMI	1436	Initiated immediately Continued for 6 mo	13.9% placebo (100/719) 12.8% verapamil (92/717) RR 0.93 (P = NS)	Reinfarction: 8.3% placebo (60/719) 7.0% verapamil (50/717) RR 0.84 (P = NS)
DAVIT II (1990)[45]	Verapamil	AMI	1775	9 days after admission Continued for up to 18 mo	*13.8% placebo 11.1% verapamil *RR 0.80 (P = 0.11)	First reinfarction: *13.2% placebo 11.0% verapamil *RR 0.77 (P = 0.04)
CRIS (1996)[90]	Verapamil	AMI	1073	13.8 days after admission Continued for up to 24 mo	5.4% placebo (29/542) 5.6% verapamil (30/531) *RR 1.06 (P > 0.1)	Reinfarction: 9.0% placebo (49/542) 7.3% verapamil (39/531) *RR 0.81 (P > 0.1)
Andre-Fouet, et al (1983)[91]	Diltiazem vs. propranolol	UAP	70	Initiated immediately Continued for up to 10 days	Too few events for analysis	Relief of angina: Benefit of diltiazem only in subset of patients with exclusive rest angina: 69% diltiazem (9/13) 0% propranolol (0/11) (P = 0.001)
Theroux, et al (1985)[92]	Diltiazem vs. Propranolol	UAP	100	Initiated immediately Continued for mean of 5.1 mo	No significant difference	No significant difference
Gobel, et al (1995, 1998)[93,94]	Diltiazem vs. IV TNG	UAP	121	Initiated immediately 48-hr continuous intravenous infusion	No deaths during 48-hr period	Composite endpoint of refractory angina or myocardial infarction: 41.0% nitroglycerin (25/61) 20.0% diltiazem (12/60) *RR 0.49 (P = 0.02)
Diltiazem Reinfarction Study (1986)[42]	Diltiazem	Non Q-wave MI	576	1–3 days after admission Continued up to 14 days or until discharge	3.1% placebo (9/289) 3.8% diltiazem (11/287) *RR 1.2 (P = NS)	Reinfarction: 9.3% placebo (27/289) 5.2% diltiazem (15/287) *RR 0.49 (P = 0.03)
Multicenter Diltiazem Postinfarction Trial Research Group (1988)[40]	Diltiazem	AMI	2466	3–15 days post-MI Continued for mean of 25 mo	10.0% placebo (124/1234) 10.3% verapamil (127/1232) *RR 1.02 (P = NS)	Combined endpoint cardiac death or reinfarction: 18.3% placebo (226/1234) 16.4% diltiazem (202/1232) *RR 0.90 (P = 0.26)
DATA (1998)[43]	Diltiazem	AMI treated with lytics	59	48-hr intravenous drug infusion initiated immediately Oral therapy continued for 4 wk	Too few events for analysis	Recurrent ischemia: 24.1% placebo (7/29) 3.3% diltiazem (1/30) *RR 11 (P = 0.02)
INTERCEPT (2000)[44]	Diltiazem	AMI treated with lytics	874	36–96 hr after onset of symptoms Continued for 6 mo	Cardiac death: 1.4% placebo (6/444) 1.6% diltiazem (7/430) *RR 1.26 (P = 0.67)	Combined endpoint nonfatal reinfarction or recurrent ischemia: 39.4% placebo (175/444) 30.7% diltiazem (132/430) *RR 0.80 (P = 0.05)
Gerstenblith, et al (1982)[95]	Nifedipine	UAP	138	Initiated immediately Continued for 4 mo	7.1% placebo (5/70) 10.3% nifedipine (7/68) †RR 1.45	Combined endpoint of sudden death, myocardial infarction, or angina requiring bypass surgery: 62% placebo (43/70) 44% nifedipine (30/68) RR 0.71 (P = 0.06)
Muller et al (1984)[96]	Nifedipine	UAP	126	Initiated immediately Continued for 14 days	0% placebo (0/63) 6.3% nifedipine (4/63) §(P = 0.13)	Myocardial infarction: 14.3% placebo (9/63) 14.3% nifedipine (9/63) RR 1.0 (P = NS)

TABLE 10-5   TRIALS OF CALCIUM CHANNEL BLOCKERS IN ACUTE CORONARY SYNDROMES—cont'd

Study (year of publication)	Drug	Indication	Number randomized	Timing of therapy	Total mortality	Recurrent ischemia or reinfarction
HINT (1986)[97]	Nifedipine	UAP	515	Initiated immediately Continued for 48 hr	Not reported	Recurrent ischemia or myocardial infarction: On maintenance beta blocker: RR 0.68 (P < 0.05) No maintenance beta blocker: RR 1.15 (P = NS)
Norwegian Nifedipine Multicenter Trial (1984)[98]	Nifedipine	Suspected AMI	227	Mean 5.5 hr after onset of symptoms Continued for 6 wk	8.7% placebo (10/115) 8.9% nifedipine (10/112) RR 1.03 (P = NS)	No difference in infarct size as measured by creatine kinase isoenzyme index
Muller et al (1984)[99]	Nifedipine	Suspected AMI	171	Mean 4.6 hr after onset of symptoms Continued for 14 days	0% placebo (0/82) 7.9% nifedipine (7/89) §(P = 0.018)	Confirmed infarction in patients with suspected myocardial infarction on admission: 75.0% placebo (36/48) 75.4% nifedipine (43/57) RR 1.0 (P = NS)
Trent Study (1986)[100]	Nifedipine	Suspected AMI	4491	Initiated immediately Continued for 4 wk	6.3% placebo (141/2251) 6.7% nifedipine (150/2240) RR 1.06 (P = NS)	Not studied
SPRINT (1988)[101]	Nifedipine	AMI	2276	Initiated 7–21 days after hospitalization Continued for up to 12 mo	5.7% placebo (65/1146) 5.8% nifedipine (65/1130) RR 1.02 (P = NS)	Reinfarction: 4.8% placebo (55/1146) 4.4% nifedipine (50/1130) RR 0.92 (P = NS)
SPRINT II (1993)[102]	Nifedipine	AMI	1006	Initiated up to 48 hr after admission Continued for up to 6 mo	15.6% placebo (79/508) 18.7% nifedipine (93/498) ‡RR 1.32 (P = NS)	Reinfarction: 4.2% placebo 5.1% nifedipine RR 1.21 (P = NS)

*Calculated by life-table analysis.
†Hypothesis testing not performed.
‡Adjusted relative risk via Cox proportional hazards model.
§Too few events to calculate relative risk.
AMI, acute myocardial infarction; UAP, unstable angina pectoris; IV TNG, intravenous nitroglycerin; t-PA, tissue-type plasminogen activator.

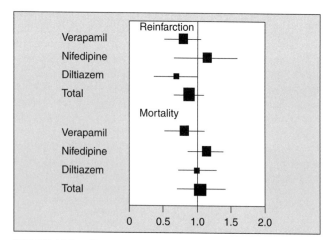

FIGURE 10-3. Effects of calcium channel blockers on reinfarction and mortality in acute myocardial infarction. (From Held PH, Yusuf S: Effects of beta-blockers and calcium channel blockers in acute myocardial infarction. Eur Heart J 1993; 14[Suppl F]:18–25, with permission.)

Therapy to Activase (DATA) and Incomplete Infarction Trial of European Collaborators Evaluating Prognosis post-Thrombolysis (INTERCEPT) studies, diltiazem was associated with significant decreases in the rates of recurrent ischemia and/or nonfatal reinfarction in patients receiving thrombolysis.[43,44] Verapamil use for up to 18 months following MI was associated with less reinfarction in the second Danish Verapamil Infarction Trial (DAVIT II) (RR 0.77, P = 0.04).[45]

Recommendations

Perhaps the only established role for CCBs in ACS is in the management of primary coronary vasospasm. Their routine use as adjunctive therapy in AMI or unstable angina is not recommended.[34,46] Pharmacologic agents of proven clinical benefit, namely β-receptor antagonists and ACE inhibitors, should be used preferentially. In patients with contraindications to β-receptor antagonists, a nondihydropyridine agent can be considered.

Nondihydropyridine CCBs should not be used in the setting of LV systolic dysfunction or heart failure. Dihydropyridine agents are contraindicated as monotherapy in the treatment of ACS.

NITROGLYCERIN

Nitrates and related compounds form a unique group of agents that have been used for decades in the treatment of angina pectoris and heart failure. Through complex biochemical pathways, nitrate compounds promote the generation of endogenous nitric oxide.[1] The major hemodynamic effects of nitrates include venodilation with an increase in venous capacitance, preload reduction, and a modest decrease in arterial blood pressure. Myocardial oxygen demand is reduced, consequent to the decrease in myocardial wall stress, and oxygen supply may be increased as a result of epicardial coronary and collateral vasodilation. Nitrates also may have a modest inhibitory effect on platelet aggregation. Continuous administration of nitrate compounds can result in drug tolerance with reduced hemodynamic effect. A nitrate-free interval often is required to ensure ongoing effectiveness.

Related nitrosovasodilators also exert their hemodynamic effects via the nitric-oxide cascade. Sodium nitroprusside is a direct nitric-oxide donor and a potent arterial vasodilator.[1] It is an effective afterload reducing agent and has been used in the treatment of hypertensive crisis and severe heart failure. It also has been studied as adjunctive therapy for MI, although its side effect profile, including the potential for coronary steal, the toxic accumulation of thiocyanate, and the capacity to cause severe hypotension, makes it a less attractive alternative.

Molsidomine is a unique nitric-oxide donor with hemodynamic properties similar to nitroglycerin.[1] It is not yet available for clinical use in the United States. Molsidomine is unlikely to result in therapeutic tolerance and may have more potent antiplatelet effects than nitroglycerin.[47]

Clinical Trials

A number of small clinical trials performed in the 1970s and 1980s investigated the efficacy of nitrates for the treatment of acute ischemia and MI. The majority of these trials were underpowered to detect differences in mortality, although there was a clear suggestion of survival benefit, especially for patients with anterior MI.[48] Two large meta-analyses of trials from the prethrombolytic era examined the efficacy of nitrate therapy in patients with AMI.

Yusuf and colleagues[49] reviewed 10 trials of intravenous vasodilators (seven trials of nitroglycerin and three trials of nitroprusside) in AMI and reported a significant 35% reduction in all-cause mortality. When the nitroglycerin trials were examined separately, the relative risk reduction reached 49% (Fig. 10-4). Although trials of oral nitrates were excluded from their final analysis, the authors determined that inclusion of the data from these trials would not have altered the findings substantially. In a cumulative and overlapping meta-analysis of 11 trials

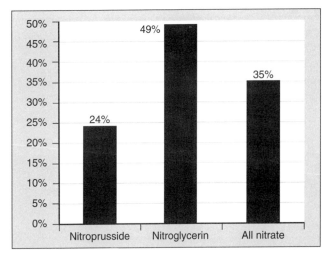

FIGURE 10-4. Reduction in mortality in pre-reperfusion era trials of nitrates in myocardial infarction. (From Yusuf S, Collins R, MacMahon S, et al: Effect of intravenous nitrates on mortality in acute myocardial infarction: An overview of the randomised trials. Lancet 1988; 1[8594]:1088–1092, with permission.)

of intravenous vasodilators, Lau and colleagues demonstrated a similar mortality reduction (43%).[50]

Several large randomized clinical trials of nitrates in AMI subsequently were designed and executed. The results were less impressive than anticipated, perhaps owing to the difficulty in showing a benefit with nitrates beyond what could be achieved with aspirin, reperfusion therapy, and beta blockade. The large, randomized clinical trials ("mega-trials") are summarized in Table 10-6.

The GISSI-3 investigators randomized 19,394 patients within 24 hours of MI onset to intravenous glyceryl trinitrate followed by a topical nitroglycerin patch or placebo for 6 weeks.[18] As discussed previously, the trial was a 2×2 factorial design with patients also randomized to receive lisinopril or open control. Although there was a slight but significant survival benefit with lisinopril, none was apparent with nitroglycerin. The use of nitroglycerin did not alter the rate of reinfarction or the incidence of the combined endpoint of death, heart failure, or LV systolic dysfunction. It is interesting to note that there was a small but significant reduction in the incidence of postinfarction angina (20% nitrates vs. 21.2% control, P = 0.033) and a 22% reduction in the development of cardiogenic shock (2.1% nitrates vs. 2.6% control, P = 0.009) among nitrate-treated patients. Combination therapy with nitrates and lisinopril was safe, with no excess of adverse events beyond those seen when the treatments were administered individually.

In the largest trial (n = 58,050) of nitrates in the treatment of MI, the ISIS-4 investigators randomized patients to oral isosorbide mononitrate or placebo within hours of the onset of chest pain.[22] As discussed previously, patients also were randomized in a complex factorial design to receive captopril, intravenous magnesium, or their corresponding placebos. There was no significant benefit observed with nitrate therapy on total mortality or the rate of reinfarction. In contrast to GISSI-3 study,

■ ■ ■

TABLE 10-6   MAJOR TRIALS OF NITRATES AND NITRIC-OXIDE DONORS IN MYOCARDIAL INFARCTION

Study (year of publication)	Drug	Study design	Number randomized	Timing of therapy	Follow-up	Mortality	Reinfarction
GISSI-3 (1994)[18]	Intravenous TNG followed by transdermal patch	RCT 2 × 2 factorial design Open control	19,394	Within 24 hr of onset of symptoms Continued for 6 wk after enrollment	6 mo	6.9% control (653/9442) 6.5% nitrates (617/9453) RR 0.94 (P = 0.28)	3.2% control (303/9442) 3.1% nitrates (292/9453) RR 0.96 (P = NS)
ISIS-4 (1995)[22]	Oral isosorbide mononitrate	RCT 2 × 2 × 2 factorial design	58,050	Median 8 hr after symptom onset Continued for 4 wk after enrollment	5 wk	7.5% placebo (2190/29032) 7.3% mononitrate (2129/29018) RR 0.97 (P = 0.30)	†3.9% placebo (1120/28522) 4.0% mononitrate (1143/28539) RR 1.02 (P = NS)
ESPRIM (1994)[51]	Intravenous linsidomine followed by oral molsidomine	RCT	4,017	Mean 7.9 hr after symptom onset Continued for 2 wk after enrollment	5 wk	8.8% placebo (176/2010) 8.4% molsidomine (168/2007) RR 0.96 (P = 0.66)	3.3% placebo (66/2010) 2.7% molsidomine (54/2007) RR 0.82 (P = 0.42)

TNG, glyceryl trinitrate; RCT, randomized controlled trial; RR, relative risk; NS, not significant.

there was no reduction in the incidence of postinfarction angina (15.0% mononitrate vs. 15.9% placebo, P = NS).

The European Study of Prevention of Infarct with Molsidomine (ESPRIM) investigators studied molsidomine in the acute phase of MI.[51] Patients (n = 4017) were randomized within hours of symptom onset to intravenous linsidomine, the active metabolite of molsidomine, for 48 hours or to placebo, followed by oral molsidomine or placebo for 12 days. Patients with Killip class III or IV heart failure were excluded. Fewer patients received thrombolytic therapy than in the GISSI-3 cohort (59%), whereas 88% of patients received aspirin and 92% of patients received heparin. At 35 days, the survival curves for molsidomine and placebo were superimposable. There was no effect of molsidomine on the rates of reinfarction or recurrent prolonged angina. Of note, there was an excess of hemorrhagic stroke associated with molsidomine treatment, occurring primarily in patients who also received heparin, aspirin, and thrombolytic therapy (10 patients in the molsidomine group vs. two patients in the placebo group, P = 0.021). The authors postulated that the antiplatelet properties of molsidomine may have contributed to the risk of stroke in patients receiving aggressive antithrombotic therapy and aspirin.

These randomized controlled trials largely have dispelled any prior notion of the life-saving role of nitrates in the treatment of AMI. A number of theories have been proposed to explain the discrepancy between the findings of the meta-analyses and those of the clinical trials, including the widespread nontrial use of nitrates among control patients. The use of proven therapies such as aspirin, thrombolytics, and beta blockers in these trials is an obvious point of departure from the earlier studies. Regardless of the cause(s) for this discrepancy, it is a powerful illustration of the value of randomized controlled trials to confirm or refute the findings generated by retrospective meta-analysis of nonrandomized data. The ISIS-4 investigators also performed a meta-analysis of all nitroglycerin trials, including 20 small trials of intravenous and oral therapy from the prethrombolytic era.[22]

When the data from the two mega-trials (GISSI-3, ISIS-4) were included, there was a modest 5.5% reduction in all-cause short-term mortality (P = 0.03), or approximately four lives saved per 1000 patients treated.

Recommendations

Sublingual nitroglycerin continues to have a central role in the treatment of angina and should be administered to all patients presenting with ACS unless contraindicated by hypotension or right ventricular infarction. Intravenous nitroglycerin should be provided to patients with MI who have ongoing chest discomfort and/or ischemia, particularly in the presence of hypertension or heart failure. It usually is continued for up to 48 hours, in concert with beta blockers and ACE inhibitors as appropriate.[34,46] Intravenous nitroglycerin should not be provided routinely in the absence of these indications. Oral nitrates are not recommended in the chronic phase of MI unless recurrent angina or heart failure intervene. As a result of case reports of profound hypotension and death, nitrates in any form are contraindicated within 24 hours of exposure to sildenafil (Viagra) or the related agent vardenafil (Levitra).

MAGNESIUM

The diverse physiologic and pharmacologic properties of magnesium make it an attractive potential treatment for myocardial ischemia. Magnesium is a potent coronary and peripheral arterial vasodilator with established antiarrhythmic efficacy, especially when used to treat polymorphic ventricular tachycardia. It may exert antiplatelet effects and attenuate reperfusion injury following coronary reflow.[1]

During the pre-reperfusion era, a number of small, underpowered clinical trials investigated the use of intravenous magnesium in the acute phase of MI. Although these trials were unable to show a consistent benefit of magnesium, meta-analysis suggested striking reductions in mortality and in the incidence of relevant arrhythmias.[50,52,53] These observations encouraged the design and execution of larger clinical trials to re-examine the efficacy of magnesium in MI.

Clinical Trials

Three large clinical trials have investigated the use of magnesium in MI (Table 10-7). The Leicester Intravenous Magnesium Intervention Trial (LIMIT-2) investigators randomized 2316 patients with suspected MI presenting within 24 hours of symptom onset to a 24-hour infusion of magnesium sulfate or placebo.[54] Of the patients, 74% were enrolled within 6 hours of symptom onset, 65% had confirmed MI, 65% received aspirin, and 35% were treated with thrombolytic therapy. Thrombolytic therapy, if administered, was initiated within 1 hour after the bolus of the study drug. Magnesium was associated with a 24% reduction in all-cause mortality at 28 days (P = 0.04) and a 25% reduction in the development of heart failure (14.9% placebo vs. 11.2% magnesium, P = 0.009). The magnesium infusion was well tolerated; flushing was the most commonly reported side effect. Although there was an increase in the incidence of sinus bradycardia with magnesium, there was no significant increase in the occurrence of advanced heart block or the need for temporary pacemaker insertion. The benefit of acute magnesium infusion reported by the LIMIT-2 investigators was sustained well beyond the initial period of treatment. There was a 16% reduction in all-cause mortality and a 21% reduction in cardiac death in magnesium-treated patients at 2.7 years.[55]

In a larger and more definitive trial of magnesium in AMI, the ISIS-4 investigators randomized 58,050 patients to receive a 24-hour intravenous infusion of magnesium sulfate or open control within 24 hours of presentation with AMI (median 8 hours).[22] Only 40% of patients were enrolled within 6 hours of symptom onset. As previously discussed, the magnesium arm of the study was a branch of a complex $2 \times 2 \times 2$ factorial design. In contrast to LIMIT-2, 70% of patients received thrombolytic therapy and 94% of patients received aspirin. There was no benefit with magnesium, but rather a trend toward a slight mortality excess at 35 days (RR 1.06, P = 0.07). There was no significant difference in mortality in the subgroup of more than 17,000 patients who did not receive thrombolytic therapy, nor was there a benefit in patients enrolled within 6 hours of symptom onset. Also in contrast to LIMIT-2, there was a 7% increase in the rate of development of congestive heart failure (P < 0.001) with magnesium. In a meta-analysis composed of nine early trials, LIMIT-2, and ISIS-4, no survival benefit with intravenous magnesium could be demonstrated.[22]

More recently, the Magnesium in Coronaries (MAGIC) trial enrolled 6213 high-risk MI patients, defined as age 65 years or older or unsuitable for acute reperfusion therapy.[56] Magnesium, or its corresponding placebo, was administered within 6 hours of symptom onset. Despite the careful study design and the very early administration of study drug, the results were disappointing. There was no effect of magnesium on 30-day mortality (RR 1.01, P = 0.96). No subgroup of patients was identified for whom treatment with intravenous magnesium was beneficial. No differences were found between magnesium and placebo in the incidence of treatable heart failure or clinically significant ventricular arrhythmias. The investigators concluded that there is no role for the routine administration of intravenous magnesium in high-risk patients with STEMI.

TABLE 10-7   MAJOR TRIALS OF INTRAVENOUS MAGNESIUM SULFATE IN MYOCARDIAL INFARCTION

Study (year of publication)	Infusion protocol	Study design	Number randomized	Timing of therapy	Follow-up	Mortality
LIMIT-2 (1992)[54]	8-mmol bolus over 5 min followed by 65 mmol over 24 hr	RCT	2,316	Within 24 hr of onset of symptoms	28 days	10.3% placebo (118/1150) 7.8% magnesium (90/1150) RR 0.76 (P = 0.04)
ISIS-4 (1995)[22]	8-mmol bolus over 15 min followed by 72 mmol over 24 hr	RCT $2 \times 2 \times 2$ factorial design Open control	58,050	Median 8 hr after onset of symptoms Study treatment started immediately after thrombolytic infusion	5 wk	7.2% control (2103/29039) 7.6% magnesium (2216/29011) RR 1.06 (P = 0.07)
MAGIC (2002)[56]	2-g bolus over 15 min followed by 17 g over 24 hr	RCT	6,213	Mean 3.8 hr after onset of symptoms Study drug started before percutaneous coronary intervention and before or during thrombolytic infusion	30 days	15.2% placebo (472/3100) 15.3% magnesium (475/3113) RR 1.01 (P = 0.96)

mmol, millimole; RCT, randomized controlled trial; RR, relative risk.

Recommendations

There is no role for the routine administration of intravenous magnesium in patients with AMI. Magnesium therapy should be provided for patients with significant hypomagnesemia from malnutrition, alcoholism, or prior diuretic therapy, particularly in the presence of ventricular ectopy. Intravenous magnesium therapy also should be provided for polymorphic ventricular tachycardia with a prolonged QT interval. Caution is advised in the setting of renal failure or high-grade AV block.

ANTIARRHYTHMIC THERAPY

Ventricular arrhythmias are a leading cause of death among patients with MI. Previously, there was great interest in the prophylactic use of antiarrhythmic agents in both the acute and chronic phases of MI. However, with the exception of amiodarone, trials of antiarrhythmic agents have been disappointing.

Lidocaine

Lidocaine, a Vaughan Williams class 1B antiarrhythmic agent, inhibits fast sodium channels and shortens the duration of the action potential in healthy cardiac tissue.[1] It is somewhat unique among antiarrhythmic agents because it acts selectively on ischemic myocardium to promote conduction block and to prevent reentrant circuits, which predispose to ventricular tachyarrhythmias. Lidocaine was shown in early studies to be highly effective in terminating ventricular tachycardia and suppressing ventricular ectopy in patients with MI.[57] Although the targeted use of lidocaine for high-grade ventricular ectopy in the setting of MI remains effective, its prophylactic administration to all patients with MI cannot be supported.

With rare exception, early trials investigating the efficacy of prophylactic lidocaine in MI were small, underpowered, and unable to document clinical benefit. During the late 1980s and early 1990s, a number of sophisticated meta-analyses were performed and demonstrated consistent findings.[50,58-60] Regardless of the route or timing of therapy, there was no demonstrable survival benefit associated with the prophylactic use of lidocaine. To the contrary, there was a disturbing trend toward increased mortality with its use in this fashion. Although meta-analysis has suggested a significant decrease in the incidence of ventricular fibrillation in patients with MI treated with lidocaine, this cumulative benefit was driven largely by the findings of one trial.[61] If this particular study were removed from the meta-analysis, no significant benefit of lidocaine in the prevention of ventricular fibrillation in MI was seen.[58] One meta-analysis, based on the findings of 18 randomized controlled trials, determined that 400 patients with MI would require prophylactic lidocaine to prevent one episode of ventricular fibrillation.[62]

In the most recent trial of the use of lidocaine in MI, Sadowski and colleagues[63] randomized 903 patients with STEMI in a 2 × 2 factorial design to lidocaine or open control and streptokinase with heparin or heparin alone. Patients were enrolled in the mid 1980s, although the trial was not published until 1999. Patients randomized to lidocaine received a series of intravenous boluses followed by a 48-hour continuous infusion. There was a 65% reduction in the incidence of ventricular fibrillation with lidocaine (2.0% lidocaine vs. 5.7% control, P = 0.004). This benefit was present regardless of whether patients were treated with thrombolytic therapy or heparin alone. Despite the reduction in the incidence of ventricular fibrillation, there was no associated survival benefit. In fact, there was a trend toward increased mortality in patients treated with lidocaine (9.7% lidocaine vs. 7.0% control, P = 0.145), corroborating the findings of earlier meta-analyses. In a related study, mexiletine, an oral class 1B agent, was associated with a trend toward increased mortality in patients with recent MI treated for a mean 9 months.[64]

The precise mechanism for the lack of survival benefit with lidocaine, especially in view of the observed reduction in ventricular ectopy, is not clear. Potential mechanisms include potentiation of ventricular arrhythmias (i.e., proarrhythmia), the precipitation of high-grade AV block, and other patient-specific toxicities. In addition, the incidence of death resulting from ventricular fibrillation after hospitalization for MI has declined considerably over the past 25 years as a result of the universal availability of external defibrillators in the coronary care unit as well as to the greater attention paid to the correction of electrolyte abnormalities.

Other Class I Agents

Class 1C antiarrhythmics inhibit fast sodium channels and slow conduction via the His-Purkinje system, resulting in a widened QRS complex.[1] They are effective in the treatment of supraventricular and ventricular arrhythmias and have been demonstrated to suppress premature ventricular contractions (PVCs) in patients following MI.[65] These agents have an increased potential for proarrhythmia, particularly at increased heart rates or states of increased sympathetic tone. They also are contraindicated in the setting of heart failure because of their potent negative ionotropic properties.

The Cardiac Arrhythmia Suppression Trial (CAST) investigated the potential benefit of the oral class 1C agents, encainide, flecainide, and moricizine, in the prevention of ventricular arrhythmias and death in high-risk patients following MI.[66,67] The CAST I trial was terminated early because of an excess risk of death in patients treated with encainide or flecainide. Additional patients were randomized to moricizine treatment as part of the Cast II trial.[68]

In CAST I, 1498 patients within 6 days to 2 years of MI with frequent premature ventricular contractions or nonsustained ventricular tachycardia received encainide or flecainide or placebo.[66,67] Patients were assigned to either encainide or flecainide based on the documented suppression of PVCs with these medications. Patients enrolled more than 90 days after MI were required to have LV systolic dysfunction (EF ≤ 0.40). At a mean follow-up of 10 months, there was more than a twofold increase in the risk of all-cause mortality or cardiac arrest in patients treated with either encainide or flecainide

(RR 2.38, P = 0.0001). There was a similar increase in the risk of death as a result of arrhythmia or cardiac arrest (RR 2.64, P = 0.0004). This finding persisted when data were analyzed for encainide and flecainide separately, as well as for the presence or absence of LV systolic dysfunction (EF > 0.30). The investigators concluded that use of prophylactic encainide or flecainide was of no benefit, and, in fact, was harmful in patients with MI at increased risk of ventricular arrhythmias.

The findings of CAST II were similarly disappointing. The trial enrolled patients 4 to 90 days after MI with LV systolic dysfunction (EF ≤ 0.40) and frequent PVCs or nonsustained ventricular tachycardia.[68] Patients received either low-dose oral moricizine or placebo during the first 2 weeks of enrollment and continued in the long-term phase of the study only if their PVCs had been suppressed with treatment. Patients from the CAST I trial with proven suppression of PVCs with moricizine also were included in the long-term phase of the CAST II trial. The CAST II trial was stopped early because of a marked increase in 14-day all-cause mortality among patients randomized to moricizine (2.5% moricizine vs. 0.45% placebo, RR 5.62, P < 0.02). In the 1155 patients who went on to the long-term phase of the study, there was no improvement in survival or in the incidence of cardiac arrest in patients treated with moricizine. Given the increase in short-term mortality associated with it use, as well as lack of any long-term benefit, moricizine cannot be recommended for the treatment of MI patients with ventricular ectopy.

Class III Agents

Class III agents exert their antiarrhythmic effects by blocking potassium channels and prolonging the repolarization phase of the action potential.[1] They are effective in the treatment of both supraventricular and ventricular arrhythmias. Of the agents in this class, amiodarone and sotalol have been investigated most thoroughly for the prevention of sudden death following MI. In addition to their class III properties, both of these agents are β-receptor antagonists.

d-Sotalol is a pure class III antiarrhythmic agent, without the beta blocker properties of its more commonly used isomer (d,l-sotalol).[1] The Survival with Oral d-Sotalol (SWORD) investigators studied the effect of d-sotalol on all-cause mortality in 3121 patients with recent or remote MI and LV dysfunction (EF ≤ 0.40) or symptomatic heart failure.[69] The study was terminated prematurely. At a mean 148 days follow-up, there was a 65% increase in the risk of death in patients randomized to active therapy (5.0% d-sotalol vs. 3.1% placebo, P = 0.006). The majority of excess deaths were attributed to pro-arrhythmia (3.6% d-sotalol vs. 2.0% placebo, RR 1.77, P = 0.008). Subgroup analysis demonstrated a consistent adverse effect of d-sotalol, regardless of concomitant beta blocker use or the number of days after MI. The risk of death associated with d-sotalol was more pronounced in the subgroup of patients with LVEF less than 0.30.

Although the limited experience with the isoforms of sotalol has been disappointing, the role of prophylactic amiodarone in patients following MI has been more promising. Amiodarone, in addition to having class III properties, is a β-receptor antagonist and CCB, and may exhibit class I antiarrhythmic properties.[1] Although highly effective in the treatment of arrhythmias, it has a worrisome side effect profile with a significant incidence of thyroid toxicity, peripheral neuropathy, and pulmonary and hepatic dysfunction with continued use.[70] A number of small, largely underpowered trials (n = 8) investigated the use of amiodarone following MI to prevent ventricular arrhythmias and sudden death.[60] Although only one trial demonstrated a clear benefit of amiodarone, meta-analysis demonstrated an overall 29% reduction in the risk of death among 1557 patients (P = 0.03).[60] Three subsequent clinical trials have provided additional insights.

The European Myocardial Infarct Amiodarone Trial (EMIAT) investigators randomized 1486 patients 5 days after confirmed MI to oral amiodarone (11.2-g oral load followed by 400 mg daily for 14 weeks and 200 mg daily for the duration of the study) or placebo.[71] All patients had documented LV dysfunction by nuclear imaging (EF ≤ 0.40) and 52% of patient had New York Heart Association Class II or III heart failure. Patients were followed for up to 2 years. At a median 21 months follow-up, there were no significant differences in the rates of total and cardiac mortality, although amiodarone was associated with a 35% reduction in the risk of arrhythmic death (P = 0.05). There were no episodes of torsades de pointes. Posthoc subgroup analyses have shown a trend toward improved survival among patients taking amiodarone who also received treatment with beta blockers.[72,73]

The Canadian Amiodarone Myocardial Infarction Arrhythmia Trial (CAMIAT) investigators enrolled 1202 patients within 6 to 45 days after confirmed MI.[74] Eligible patients had at least 10 PVCs per hour or at least one run of nonsustained ventricular tachycardia on monitoring. LV dysfunction was not a prerequisite. Patients were randomized to receive an oral loading dose of 10 mg/kg amiodarone over 2 weeks followed by 300 or 400 mg daily. The maintenance dose was reduced to as little as 200 mg daily if effective arrhythmia suppression was detected on ambulatory monitoring. Nearly 60% of patients received beta blockers. At a mean follow-up of 21.5 months, there was a 38.2% reduction in the risk of resuscitated ventricular fibrillation or arrhythmic death among patients treated with amiodarone (P = 0.029), although the associated reductions in total and cardiac mortality did not achieve statistical significance. As in the EMIAT trial, the benefit of amiodarone was greater in patients receiving beta blockers.

The Grupo de Estudios Multicentricos en Argentina (GEMICA) investigators randomized 1073 patients within the first 24 hours of MI to amiodarone (2.7 g intravenously over 48 hours and 600 mg orally twice daily for 4 days) or placebo followed by maintenance oral therapy (400 mg daily through day 90 followed by 200 mg daily).[75] The study protocol subsequently was modified after an interim data analysis indicated an increase in mortality in patients receiving the high-dose amiodarone load, possibly related to an excess incidence of hypotension. Patients enrolled after this adjustment received a modified amiodarone load (1.2 g intravenously over 48 hours and 800 mg orally once daily) followed by maintenance therapy (400 mg daily through day 90 followed by 200 mg daily) or placebo. More patients in the placebo group received β-receptor antagonists (59.7% amiodarone vs. 66.9% placebo, P = 0.008). For the entire cohort, no significant differences in total or cardiac mortality or in the incidence of sudden cardiac death were seen between the amiodarone and placebo groups at 6 months. There was a 46% reduction in the incidence of postinfarction angina in patients treated with amiodarone (P < 0.0001). Among the 516 patients randomized to high-dose amiodarone load or placebo, there was a significant increase in total mortality (16.3% amiodarone vs. 10.2% placebo, adjusted RR 1.72, P = 0.04). Among the 557 patients randomized to the modified amiodarone load or placebo, there were nonsignificant trends toward decreased total mortality (6.61% amiodarone vs. 9.47% placebo, adjusted RR 0.68, P = 0.20), cardiac mortality, and sudden cardiac death. The authors concluded that early administration of low-dose amiodarone may be considered if life-threatening arrhythmias warrant its use, although it should not be prescribed routinely for MI patients.

A recent meta-analysis comprising a total of 6553 patients from 13 trials, 89% of whom had a prior MI, reported a 13% reduction in total mortality (P = 0.030) and a 29% reduction in arrhythmic or sudden cardiac death (P = 0.0003) in patients treated with amiodarone.[70] The benefit was similar whether MI or heart failure was the dominant criterion for patient enrollment. At the end of 2 years, 41% of amiodarone-treated patients compared to 27% of control patients had discontinued drug therapy, largely because of an increased incidence of adverse drug events. The excess risk of pulmonary toxicity associated with amiodarone was 1% per year.

Recommendations

With the strong exception of β-receptor antagonists (class II antiarrhythmics), the routine prophylactic administration of antiarrhythmic agents following MI is not recommended. For patients with symptomatic or sustained ventricular arrhythmias in the acute phase of MI, treatment with lidocaine or amiodarone is indicated. Class 1C agents are contraindicated and should be discontinued in patients for whom these agents were prescribed prior to infarction. There is limited evidence that oral amiodarone may benefit a subset of post-MI patients at increased risk of sudden cardiac death, particularly those with heart failure or depressed LV function and high-grade ventricular ectopy. Any potential benefit of long-term amiodarone therapy must be weighed against the substantial risk of significant side effects. The dramatic benefits seen with implantable cardioverter-defibrillator (ICD) therapy in high-risk post MI patients have rendered previous discussions of antiarrhythmic agents largely moot.[76-78] ICD therapy clearly is preferred for appropriately selected patients with access to these devices.

METABOLIC FACTORS

There has been increasing interest in the development of other medical therapies to decrease morbidity and mortality following MI. Much of the work in this area has focused on the modulation of myocardial metabolism, with the ultimate goal of minimizing the extent of ischemic necrosis.

Insulin Therapy in Patients with Diabetes

It has long been recognized that patients with diabetes have a significantly worse prognosis after MI. Their hospital mortality rates are significantly higher than those for patients without diabetes. In addition, diabetes mellitus is associated with an increase in the incidence of heart failure, reinfarction, myocardial rupture, and conduction system disease.[79] Potential causes for this adverse prognosis include later presentation, a higher prevalence of multivessel coronary artery disease, and alterations in myocardial metabolism. Ischemic myocardium relies on the anaerobic metabolism of glucose rather than the aerobic metabolism of fatty acids to meet its energy needs. Cellular glucose transport is impaired in patients with diabetes, and fatty acids may be directly toxic to ischemic myocytes.[79] Correction of the relative insulin deficiency may improve glucose transport into ischemic myocytes, decrease circulating levels of free fatty acids, and lead to better outcomes.

In the largest trial of intensive insulin therapy in MI, the Diabetes Mellitus Insulin-Glucose Infusion in Acute Myocardial Infarction (DIGAMI) investigators randomized 620 patients with diabetes with suspected AMI within 24 hours of symptom onset to an intensive insulin regimen or control.[80] Patients randomized to intensive therapy received a continuous dextrose-containing intravenous insulin infusion for at least 24 hours using a prespecified protocol for rigorous glycemic control. Patients then received subcutaneous insulin injections four times daily for at least 3 months or their baseline therapy if randomized to the control group. All patients received standard therapy at the discretion of treating clinicians, including thrombolytics approximately 50%), beta blockers (70%), aspirin (80%), and ACE inhibitors (31%). Glycemic control was improved significantly in patients receiving intensive insulin therapy both during the initial 24 hours and at subsequent follow-up. Glycosylated hemoglobin values were significantly lower at 3 months follow-up (7.0% intensive therapy vs. 7.5% control, P < 0.01). Although there was no difference in mortality during hospitalization or at 3 months, there was a 29% reduction in all-cause mortality at 1 year in patients treated with intensive insulin therapy (18.6% intensive therapy vs. 26.1% control, P = 0.0273). There was a persistent 28% reduction in all-cause mortality at 3.4 years (P = 0.011) with one life saved for every nine patients treated with intensive therapy.[81] It is interesting that the benefit of intensive insulin therapy was highest among patients felt to be at low risk and in patients not previously treated with insulin.

Glucose-Insulin-Potassium Therapy in Nondiabetic Patients

Levels of circulating catecholamines are markedly elevated in patients with MI. Catecholamine excess is associated with increased levels of free fatty acids, which may potentiate myocardial necrosis.[79] During the 1960s and 1970s, multiple small clinical trials investigated the use of glucose-insulin-potassium (GIK) therapy in patients without diabetes as a means to suppress free fatty acid formation. Individually, these trials were not able to show a benefit with GIK therapy, but a subsequent meta-analysis of nine trials involving 1932 patients suggested a 28% reduction in in-hospital mortality in patients treated with GIK (P = 0.004).[82] Two recent randomized trials have reevaluated the efficacy of GIK therapy.

The Estudios Cardiologicos Latinoamerica Collaborative (ECLA) Group randomized 407 patients with suspected AMI within 24 hours of symptom onset to standard medical care or standard medical care plus one of two (high- or low-dose insulin) regimens of GIK for 24 hours.[83] Sixteen percent of patients had diabetes, and 62% were treated with reperfusion therapy, primarily thrombolytics. There was no significant difference in random blood glucose levels between the treatment and control groups. Although there was no significant reduction in in-hospital mortality with GIK, its use was associated with a 75% reduction in the incidence of electromechanical dissociation (P = 0.02) and a 41% reduction in the combined endpoint of death, severe heart failure, and nonfatal ventricular fibrillation (P = 0.03). Subset analysis identified a 66% reduction in in-hospital mortality among patients treated with GIK who had received reperfusion therapy (5.2% GIK vs. 15.2% control, P = 0.01), suggesting a possible role for GIK in preventing reperfusion injury. There was a sustained 33% reduction in mortality at 1 year among patients who received reperfusion therapy randomized to high-dose GIK (P = 0.046). GIK was well tolerated; phlebitis was the most commonly reported complication (16.8%) of patients.

The Multicenter Polish-GIK trial randomized 954 patients within the first 24 hours of suspected MI to either a 24-hour GIK infusion (insulin concentration intermediate to that of the high- and low-dose arms of the ECLA trial) or open control.[84] Six percent of patients had noninsulin requiring diabetes, and 59% of patients received thrombolytic therapy. The trial was stopped early following an interim analysis that demonstrated excess total mortality at 35 days among patients randomized to receive GIK (8.9% GIK vs. 4.8% control, RR 1.95, P = 0.01). There was a nonsignificant increase in cardiac mortality with GIK (6.5% GIK vs. 4.6% control, P = 0.20). The increase in total mortality associated with GIK infusion persisted at 6 months (11.1% GIK vs. 6.5% control, P = 0.01). The combined endpoint of death or any cardiac event at 35 days was similar in the two treatment groups. The investigators attributed the negative findings of this trial to either inadequate insulin dosing or to lower-than-expected mortality rate among control patients. The role of GIK infusion as adjunctive

therapy for patients without diabetes but with MI remains uncertain.

Hypothermia

Animal data have suggested that induction of mild hypothermia may reduce myocardial infarct size.[85] Hypothermia may promote cerebral salvage among comatose survivors of cardiac arrest.[86,87] A 2002 pilot study has investigated the safety and feasibility of endovascular cooling to induce mild hypothermia in patients with STEMI undergoing primary PCI.[88] Larger clinical trials are in development, including trials with thrombolytic therapy.

Recommendations

Whether novel therapies for myocardial protection in the setting of acute ischemia and reperfusion will have any additive role remains to be seen. Rigorous glycemic control in patients with diabetes may provide long-term benefit. GIK therapy and the selective use of hypothermia are not recommended.

CONCLUSION

Clinical trials have informed therapeutic decision making in the care of patients with AMI. Nitrates and β-receptor antagonists, in combination with antiplatelet and antithrombin strategies, remain the cornerstones of acute ischemia management. β-Receptor antagonists and ACE inhibitors provide powerful long-term benefit to the MI survivor, with reductions in recurrent MI and death and attenuation of LV remodeling. Calcium channel blockers, antiarrhythmic agents, and magnesium are not recommended for routine use. Further studies on the modification of metabolic factors are awaited.

REFERENCES

1. Opie LH, Gersh BJ, eds: Drugs for the Heart. ed 5. Philadelphia, W.B. Saunders Company, 2001.
2. Yusuf S, Peto R, Lewis J, Collins R, Sleight P: Beta blockade during and after myocardial infarction: An overview of the randomized trials. Prog Cardiovasc Dis 1985; 27(5):335-371.
3. Held PH, Yusuf S: Effects of beta-blockers and calcium channel blockers in acute myocardial infarction. Eur Heart J 1993; 14(Suppl F):18-25.
4. Freemantle N, Cleland J, Young P, et al: Beta Blockade after myocardial infarction: Systematic review and meta regression analysis. BMJ 1999; 318(7200):1730-1737.
5. Snow, PJ: Effect of propranolol in myocardial infarction. Lancet 1965; 2(7412):551-553.
6. Hjalmarson A, Elmfeldt D, Herlitz J, et al: Effect on mortality of metoprolol in acute myocardial infarction. A double-blind randomised trial. Lancet 1981; 2(8251):823-827.
7. The MIAMI Trial Research Group. Metoprolol in acute myocardial infarction (MIAMI). A randomised placebo-controlled international trial. Eur Heart J 1985; 6(3):199-226.
8. First International Study Group of Infarct Survival (ISIS-1) Collaborative Group. Randomised trial of intravenous atenolol among 16 027 cases of suspected acute myocardial infarction: ISIS-1. Lancet 1986; 2(8498):57-66.
9. Roberts R, Rogers WJ, Mueller HS, et al: Immediate versus deferred beta-blockade following thrombolytic therapy in patients with

acute myocardial infarction. Results of the Thrombolysis in Myocardial Infarction (TIMI) II-B Study. Circulation 1991; 83(2):422–437.

10. The Norwegian Multicenter Group. Timolol-induced reduction in mortality and reinfarction in patients surviving acute myocardial infarction. New Engl J Med 1981; 304(14):801–807.

11. Beta-Blocker Heart Attack Trial Research Group: A randomized trial of propranolol in patients with acute myocardial infarction. I. Mortality results. JAMA 1982; 247(12):1707–1714.

12. Beta-Blocker Heart Attack Trial Research Group. A randomized trial of propranolol in patients with acute myocardial infarction. II. Morbidity results. JAMA 1983; 250(20):2814–2819.

13. Boissel JP, Leizorovicz A, Picolet H, et al: Secondary prevention after high-risk acute myocardial infarction with low-dose acebutolol. Am J Cardiol 1990; 66(3):251–260.

14. Carvedilol Post-Infarct Survival Control in LV Dysfunction Investigators. Effect of carvedilol on outcome after myocardial infarction in patients with left-ventricular dysfunction: The CAPRICORN randomised trial. Lancet 2001; 357(9266):1385–1390.

15. Doughty RN, Rodgers A, Sharpe N, et al: Effects of beta-blocker therapy on mortality in patients with heart failure. A systematic overview of randomized controlled trials. Eur Heart J 1997; 18(4):560–565.

16. Heidenreich PA, Lee TT, Massie BM: Effect of beta-blockade on mortality in patients with heart failure: A meta-analysis of randomized clinical trials. J Am Coll Cardiol 1997; 30(1):27–34.

17. Swedberg K, Held P, Kjekshus J, et al: Effects of the early administration of enalapril on mortality in patients with acute myocardial infarction. Results of the Cooperative New Scandinavian Enalapril Survival Study II (CONSENSUS II). New Engl J Med 1992; 327(10):678–684.

18. Gruppo Italiano per lo Studio della Sopravvivenza nell'Infarto Miocardico. GISSI-3: Effects of lisinopril and transdermal glyceryl trinitrate singly and together on 6-week mortality and ventricular function after acute myocardial infarction. Gruppo Italiano per lo Studio della Sopravvivenza nell'infarto Miocardico. Lancet 1994; 343(8906):1115–1122.

19. Chinese Cardiac Study Collaborative Group: Oral captopril versus placebo among 13,634 patients with suspected acute myocardial infarction: Interim report from the Chinese Cardiac Study (CCS-1). Lancet 1995; 345(8951):686–687.

20. Chinese Cardiac Study Collaborative Group (CCS-1): Oral captopril versus placebo among 14,962 patients with suspected acute myocardial infarction: A multicenter, randomized, double-blind, placebo controlled clinical trial. Chinese Med J 1997; 110(11): 834–838.

21. Liu L: Long-term mortality in patients with myocardial infarction: Impact of early treatment with captopril for 4 weeks. Chinese Med J 2001; 114(2):115–118.

22. Fourth International Study of Infarct Survival (ISIS-4) Collaborative Group. ISIS-4: A randomised factorial trial assessing early oral captopril, oral mononitrate, and intravenous magnesium sulphate in 58,050 patients with suspected acute myocardial infarction. Lancet 1995; 345(8951):669–685.

23. ACE Inhibitor Myocardial Infarction Collaborative Group: Indications for ACE inhibitors in the early treatment of acute myocardial infarction: Systematic overview of individual data from 100,000 patients in randomized trials. ACE Inhibitor Myocardial Infarction Collaborative Group. Circulation 1998; 97(22):2202–2212.

24. Yusuf S, Sleight P, Pogue J, et al: Effects of an angiotensin-converting-enzyme inhibitor, ramipril, on cardiovascular events in high-risk patients. The Heart Outcomes Prevention Evaluation Study Investigators. New Engl J Med 2000; 342(3):145–153.

25. Fox KM and The European trial on reduction of cardiac events with perindopril in stable coronary artery disease investigators: Efficacy of perindopril in reduction of cardiovascular events among patients with stable coronary artery disease: Randomized, double-blind, placebo-controlled, multicentre trial (the EUROPA study). Lancet 2003; 362:782–88.

26. Pfeffer MA, Domanski M, Rosenberg Y, et al: PEACE Investigators: Prevention of events with angiotensin-converting enzyme inhibition (the PEACE study design). Am J Cardiol 1998; 82(3A): 25H–30H.

27. Pfeffer MA, Domanski M, Verter J, et al: PEACE Investigators: The continuation of the Prevention of Events with Angiotensin-Converting Enzyme Inhibition (PEACE) Trial. Am Heart J 2001; 142(3):375–377.

28. Pfeffer MA, Braunwald E, Moye LA, et al: Effect of captopril on mortality and morbidity in patients with left ventricular dysfunction after myocardial infarction. Results of the survival and ventricular enlargement trial. The SAVE Investigators. N Engl J Med 1992; 327(10):669–677.

29. The Acute Infarction Ramipril Efficacy (AIRE) Study Investigators: Effect of ramipril on mortality and morbidity of survivors of acute myocardial infarction with clinical evidence of heart failure. Lancet 1993; 342(8875):821–828.

30. Kober L, Torp-Pedersen C, Carlsen JE, et al: A clinical trial of the angiotensin-converting-enzyme inhibitor trandolapril in patients with left ventricular dysfunction after myocardial infarction. Trandolapril Cardiac Evaluation (TRACE) Study Group. New Engl J Med 1995; 333(25):1670–1676.

31. Flather MD, Yusuf S, Kober L, et al: Long-term ACE-inhibitor therapy in patients with heart failure or left-ventricular dysfunction: A systematic overview of data from individual patients. ACE-Inhibitor Myocardial Infarction Collaborative Group. Lancet 2000; 355(9215):1575–1581.

32. Ambrosioni E, Borghi C, Magnani B: The effect of the angiotensin-converting-enzyme inhibitor zofenopril on mortality and morbidity after anterior myocardial infarction. The Survival of Myocardial Infarction Long-Term Evaluation (SMILE) Study Investigators. New Engl J Med 1995; 332(2):80–85.

33. Dickstein K, Kjekshus J, Optimaal Steering Committee of the OPTIMAAL Study Group: Effects of losartan and captopril on mortality and morbidity in high-risk patients after acute myocardial infarction: The OPTIMAAL randomised trial. Optimal Trial in Myocardial Infarction with Angiotensin II Antagonist Losartan. Lancet 2002; 360(9335):752–760.

34. Ryan TJ, Antman EM, Brooks NH, et al: 1999 update: ACC/AHA guidelines for the management of patients with acute myocardial infarction. A report of the American College of Cardiology/American Heart Association Task Force on Practice Guidelines (Committee on Management of Acute Myocardial Infarction). J Am Coll Cardiol 1999; 34(3):890–911.

35. Packer M, Kessler PD, Lee WH: Calcium-channel blockade in the management of severe chronic congestive heart failure: A bridge too far. Circulation 1987; 75(6 Pt 2):V56–64.

36. Littler WA, Sheridan DJ: Placebo controlled trial of felodipine in patients with mild to moderate heart failure. UK Study Group. Br Heart J 1995; 73(5):428–433.

37. Packer M, O'Connor CM, Ghali JK, et al: Effect of amlodipine on morbidity and mortality in severe chronic heart failure. Prospective Randomized Amlodipine Survival Evaluation Study Group. [comment]. New Engl J Med 1996; 335(15):1107–1114.

38. Cohn JN, Ziesche S, Smith R, et al: Effect of the calcium antagonist felodipine as supplementary vasodilator therapy in patients with chronic heart failure treated with enalapril: V-HeFT III. Vasodilator-Heart Failure Trial (V-HeFT) Study Group. Circulation 1997; 96(3):856–863.

39. Held PH, Yusuf S, Furberg CD: Calcium channel blockers in acute myocardial infarction and unstable angina: An overview. BMJ 1989: 299(6709):1187–1192.

40. The Multicenter Diltiazem Postinfarction Trial Research Group: The effect of diltiazem on mortality and reinfarction after myocardial infarction. New Engl J Med 1988; 319(7):385–392.

41. Furberg CD, Psaty BM, Meyer JV: Nifedipine. Dose-related increase in mortality in patients with coronary heart disease. Circulation 1995; 92(5):1326–1331.

42. Gibson RS, Boden WE, Theroux P, et al: Diltiazem and reinfarction in patients with non-Q-wave myocardial infarction. Results of a double-blind, randomized, multicenter trial. New Engl J Med 1986; 315(7):423–429.

43. Theroux P, Gregoire J, Chin C, et al: Intravenous diltiazem in acute myocardial infarction. Diltiazem as adjunctive therapy to activase (DATA) trial. J Am Coll Cardiol 1998; 32(3):620–628.

44. Boden WE, van Gilst WH, Scheldewaert RG, et al: Diltiazem in acute myocardial infarction treated with thrombolytic agents: A randomised placebo-controlled trial. Incomplete Infarction Trial of European Research Collaborators Evaluating Prognosis post-Thrombolysis (INTERCEPT). Lancet 2000; 355(9217):1751–1756.

45. The Danish Study Group on Verapamil in Myocardial Infarction. Effect of verapamil on mortality and major events after acute myocardial infarction (the Danish Verapamil Infarction Trial II—DAVIT II). Am J Cardiol 1990; 66(10):779–785.

46. Braunwald E, Antman EM, Beasley JW, et al: ACC/AHA 2002 guideline update for the management of patients with unstable angina and non-ST-segment elevation myocardial infarction—summary article: A report of the American College of Cardiology/American Heart Association task force on practice guidelines (Committee on the Management of Patients with Unstable Angina). J Am Coll Cardiol 2002; 40(7):1366-1374.

47. Drummer C, Valta-Seufzer U, Karrenbrock B, et al: Comparison of anti-platelet properties of molsidomine, isosorbide-5-mononitrate and placebo in healthy volunteers. Eur Heart J 1991; 12(4):541-549.

48. Jugdutt BI, Warnica JW: Intravenous nitroglycerin therapy to limit myocardial infarct size, expansion, and complications. Effect of timing, dosage, and infarct location. Circulation 1988; 78(4):906-919.

49. Yusuf S, Collins R, MacMahon S, et al: Effect of intravenous nitrates on mortality in acute myocardial infarction: An overview of the randomised trials. Lancet 1988; 1(8594):1088-1092.

50. Lau J, Antman EM, Jimenez-Silva J, et al: Cumulative meta-analysis of therapeutic trials for myocardial infarction. New Engl J Med 1992; 327(4):248-254.

51. European Study of Prevention of Infarct with Molsidomine (ESPRIM) Group: The ESPRIM trial: Short-term treatment of acute myocardial infarction with molsidomine. Lancet 1994; 344(8915):91-97.

52. Teo KK, Yusuf S, Collins R, et al: Effects of intravenous magnesium in suspected acute myocardial infarction: Overview of randomised trials. BMJ 1991; 303(6816):1499-1503.

53. Horner SM: Efficacy of intravenous magnesium in acute myocardial infarction in reducing arrhythmias and mortality. Meta-analysis of magnesium in acute myocardial infarction. Circulation 1992; 86(3):774-779.

54. Woods KL, Fletcher S, Roffe C, et al: Intravenous magnesium sulphate in suspected acute myocardial infarction: Results of the second Leicester Intravenous Magnesium Intervention Trial (LIMIT-2). Lancet 1992; 339(8809):1553-1558.

55. Woods KL, Fletcher S: Long-term outcome after intravenous magnesium sulphate in suspected acute myocardial infarction: The second Leicester Intravenous Magnesium Intervention Trial (LIMIT-2). Lancet 1994; 343(8901):816-819.

56. Magnesium in Coronaries Trial (MAGIC) Investigators: Early administration of intravenous magnesium to high-risk patients with acute myocardial infarction in the Magnesium in Coronaries (MAGIC) Trial: A randomised controlled trial. Lancet 2002; 360(9341):1189-1196.

57. Gianelly R, von der Groeben JO, Spivack AP, et al: Effect of lidocaine on ventricular arrhythmias in patients with coronary heart disease. New Engl J Med 1967; 277(23):1215-1219.

58. MacMahon S, Collins R, Peto R, et al: Effects of prophylactic lidocaine in suspected acute myocardial infarction. An overview of results from the randomized, controlled trials. JAMA 1988; 260(13):1910-1916.

59. Hine LK, Laird N, Hewitt P, et al: Meta-analytic evidence against prophylactic use of lidocaine in acute myocardial infarction. Arch Intern Med 1989; 149(12):2694-2698.

60. Teo KK, Yusuf S, Furberg CD: Effects of prophylactic antiarrhythmic drug therapy in acute myocardial infarction. An overview of results from randomized controlled trials. JAMA 1993; 270(13):1589-1595.

61. Lie KI, Wellens HJ, van Capelle FJ, et al: Lidocaine in the prevention of primary ventricular fibrillation. A double-blind, randomized study of 212 consecutive patients. New Engl J Med 1974; 291(25):1324-1326.

62. Antman EM, Berlin JA: Declining incidence of ventricular fibrillation in myocardial infarction. Implications for the prophylactic use of lidocaine. Circulation 1992; 86(3):764-773.

63. Sadowski ZP, Alexander JH, Skrabucha B, et al: Multicenter randomized trial and a systematic overview of lidocaine in acute myocardial infarction. Am Heart J 1999; 137(5):792-798.

64. International Mexiletine and Placebo Antiarrhythmic Coronary Trial (IMPACT) Research Group. International mexiletine and placebo antiarrhythmic coronary trial: I. Report on arrhythmia and other findings. J Am Coll Cardiol 1984; 4(6):1148-1163.

65. Cardiac Arrhythmia Pilot Study (CAPS) Investigators. Effects of encainide, flecainide, imipramine and moricizine on ventricular arrhythmias during the year after acute myocardial infarction. Am J Cardiol 1988; 61(8):501-509.

66. Cardiac Arrhythmia Suppression Trial (CAST) Investigators. Preliminary report: Effect of encainide and flecainide on mortality in a randomized trial of arrhythmia suppression after myocardial infarction. New Engl J Med 1989; 321(6):406-412.

67. Echt DS, Liebson PR, Mitchell LB, et al: Mortality and morbidity in patients receiving encainide, flecainide, or placebo. The Cardiac Arrhythmia Suppression Trial. New Engl J Med 1991; 324(12):781-788.

68. Cardiac Arrhythmia Suppression Trial II (CAST) Investigators. Effect of the antiarrhythmic agent moricizine on survival after myocardial infarction. New Engl J Med 1992; 327(4):227-233.

69. Waldo AL, Camm AJ, deRuyter H, et al: Effect of d-sotalol on mortality in patients with left ventricular dysfunction after recent and remote myocardial infarction. The SWORD Investigators. Lancet 1996; 348(9019):7-12.

70. Amiodarone Trials Meta-Analysis Investigators. Effect of prophylactic amiodarone on mortality after acute myocardial infarction and in congestive heart failure: Meta-analysis of individual data from 6500 patients in randomised trials. Lancet 1997; 350(9089):1417-1424.

71. Julian DG, Camm AJ, Frangin G, et al: Randomised trial of effect of amiodarone on mortality in patients with left-ventricular dysfunction after recent myocardial infarction: EMIAT. European Myocardial Infarct Amiodarone Trial Investigators. Lancet 1997; 349(9053):667-674.

72. Boutitie F, Boissel JP, Connolly SJ, et al: Amiodarone interaction with beta-blockers: Analysis of the merged EMIAT (European Myocardial Infarct Amiodarone Trial) and CAMIAT (Canadian Amiodarone Myocardial Infarction Trial) databases. The EMIAT and CAMIAT Investigators. Circulation 1999; 99(17):2268-2275.

73. Janse MJ, Malik M, Camm AJ, et al: Identification of post acute myocardial infarction patients with potential benefit from prophylactic treatment with amiodarone. A substudy of EMIAT (the European Myocardial Infarct Amiodarone Trial). Eur Heart J 1998; 19(1):85-95.

74. Cairns JA, Connolly SJ, Roberts R, et al: Randomised trial of outcome after myocardial infarction in patients with frequent or repetitive ventricular premature depolarisations: CAMIAT. Canadian Amiodarone Myocardial Infarction Arrhythmia Trial Investigators. Lancet 1997; 349(9053):675-682.

75. Elizari MV, Martinez JM, Belziti C, et al: Morbidity and mortality following early administration of amiodarone in acute myocardial infarction. GEMICA study investigators. Eur Heart J 2000; 21(3):198-205.

76. Buxton AE, Lee KL, Fisher JD, et al: A randomized study of the prevention of sudden death in patients with coronary artery disease. Multicenter Unsustained Tachycardia Trial Investigators. New Engl J Med 1999; 341(25):1882-1890.

77. Moss AJ, Hall WJ, Cannom DS, et al: Improved survival with an implanted defibrillator in patients with coronary disease at high risk for ventricular arrhythmia. Multicenter Automatic Defibrillator Implantation Trial Investigators. New Engl J Med 1996; 335(26):1933-1940.

78. Moss AJ, Zareba W, Hall WJ, et al: Prophylactic implantation of a defibrillator in patients with myocardial infarction and reduced ejection fraction. The Multicenter Automatic Defibrillator Implantation Trial 2 Investigators. New Engl J Med 2002; 346(12):877-883.

79. Jacoby RM, Nesto RW: Acute myocardial infarction in the diabetic patient: Pathophysiology, clinical course and prognosis. J Am Coll Cardiol 1992; 20(3):736-744.

80. Malmberg K, Ryden L, Efendic S, et al: Randomized trial of insulin-glucose infusion followed by subcutaneous insulin treatment in diabetic patients with acute myocardial infarction (DIGAMI study): Effects on mortality at 1 year. J Am Coll Cardiol 1995; 26(1):57-65.

81. Malmberg K: Prospective randomised study of intensive insulin treatment on long term survival after acute myocardial infarction in patients with diabetes mellitus. DIGAMI (Diabetes Mellitus, Insulin Glucose Infusion in Acute Myocardial Infarction) Study Group. BMJ 1997; 314(7093):1512-1515.

82. Fath-Ordoubadi F, Beatt KJ: Glucose-insulin-potassium therapy for treatment of acute myocardial infarction: An overview of randomized placebo-controlled trials. Circulation 1997; 96(4):1152-1156.

83. Diaz R, Paolasso EA, Piegas LS, et al: Metabolic modulation of acute myocardial infarction. The ECLA (Estudios Cardiologicos

Latinoamerica) Collaborative Group. Circulation 1998; 98(21): 2227-2234.

84. Ceremuzynski L, Budaj A, Czepiel A, et al: Low-dose glucose-insulin-potassium is ineffective in acute myocardial infarction: Results of a randomized multicenter Pol-GIK trial. Cardiovasc Drugs Ther 1999;13(3):191-200.

85. Dae MW, Gao DW, Sessler DI, et al: Effect of endovascular cooling on myocardial temperature, infarct size, and cardiac output in human-sized pigs. Am J Physiol Heart Circ Physiol 2002; 282(5): H1584-591.

86. The Hypothermia after Cardiac Arrest Study Group: Mild therapeutic hypothermia to improve the neurologic outcome after cardiac arrest. New Engl J Med 2002; 346(8):549-556.

87. Bernard SA, Gray TW, Buist MD, et al: Treatment of comatose survivors of out-of-hospital cardiac arrest with induced hypothermia. New Engl J Med 2002; 346(8):557-563.

88. Dixon SR, Whitbourn RJ, Dae MW, et al: Induction of mild systemic hypothermia with endovascular cooling during primary percutaneous coronary intervention for acute myocardial infarction. J Am Coll Cardiol 2002; 40(11):1928-1934.

89. The Danish Study Group on Verapamil in Myocardial Infarction: Verapamil in acute myocardial infarction. The Danish Study Group on Verapamil in Myocardial Infarction. Eur Heart J 1984; 5(7):516-528.

90. Rengo F, Carbonin P, Pahor M, et al: A controlled trial of verapamil in patients after acute myocardial infarction: Results of the calcium antagonist reinfarction Italian study (CRIS). Am J Cardiol 1996; 77(5):365-369.

91. Andre-Fouet X, Usdin JP, Gayet C, et al: Comparison of short-term efficacy of diltiazem and propranolol in unstable angina at rest—a randomized trial in 70 patients. Eur Heart J 1983; 4(10):691-698.

92. Theroux P, Taeymans Y, Morissette D, et al: A randomized study comparing propranolol and diltiazem in the treatment of unstable angina. J Am Coll Cardiol 1985; 5(3):717-722.

93. Gobel EJ, Hautvast RW, van Gilst WH, et al: Randomised, double-blind trial of intravenous diltiazem versus glyceryl trinitrate for unstable angina pectoris. Lancet 1995; 346(8991-8992): 1653-1657.

94. Gobel EJ, van Gilst WH, de Kam PJ, et al: Long-term follow-up after early intervention with intravenous diltiazem or intravenous nitroglycerin for unstable angina pectoris. Eur Heart J 1998; 19(8):1208-1213.

95. Gerstenblith G, Ouyang P, Achuff SC, et al: Nifedipine in unstable angina: A double-blind, randomized trial. New Engl J Med 1982; 306(15):885-889.

96. Muller JE, Turi ZG, Pearle DL, et al: Nifedipine and conventional therapy for unstable angina pectoris: A randomized, double-blind comparison. Circulation 1984; 69(4):728-739.

97. Holland Interuniversity Nifedipine/Metoprolol Trial (HINT) Research Group: Early treatment of unstable angina in the coronary care unit: A randomised, double blind, placebo controlled comparison of recurrent ischaemia in patients treated with nifedipine or metoprolol or both. Br Heart J 1986; 56(5):400-413.

98. Sirnes PA, Overskeid K, Pedersen TR, et al: Evolution of infarct size during the early use of nifedipine in patients with acute myocardial infarction: The Norwegian Nifedipine Multicenter Trial. Circulation 1984; 70(4):638-644.

99. Muller JE, Morrison J, Stone PH, et al: Nifedipine therapy for patients with threatened and acute myocardial infarction: A randomized, double-blind, placebo-controlled comparison. Circulation 1984; 69(4):740-747.

100. Wilcox RG, Hampton JR, Banks DC, et al: Trial of early nifedipine in acute myocardial infarction: The Trent study. BMJ (Clin Res Ed) 1986; 293(6556):1204-1208.

101. The Israeli SPRINT Study Group: Secondary prevention reinfarction Israeli nifedipine trial (SPRINT). A randomized intervention trial of nifedipine in patients with acute myocardial infarction. Eur Heart J 1988; 9(4):354-364.

102. Goldbourt U, Behar S, Reicher-Reiss H, et al: Early administration of nifedipine in suspected acute myocardial infarction. The Secondary Prevention Reinfarction Israel Nifedipine Trial 2 Study. Arch Intern Med 1993; 153(3):345-353.

Chapter 11

Angioplasty: Primary, Rescue, and Adjunctive Mechanical Interventions

Juhana Karha
C. Michael Gibson

HISTORICAL PERSPECTIVE

Management of acute myocardial infarction (AMI) has been predicated on the time-dependent open-artery hypothesis—the notion that early, full, and sustained reperfusion results in improved clinical outcomes. This hypothesis has been confirmed by large-scale megatrials with angiographic substudies that have linked improved 90-minute patency profiles to improved left-ventricular function and in turn to improved mortality.[1,2] Initial efforts to restore antegrade flow to occluded vessels began with the administration of intracoronary thrombolytic agents in the late 1970s and the early 1980s.[3-5] These recanalization trials and the intracoronary route of thrombolytic administration were demanding logistically, and they soon were replaced by trials involving the simpler and more rapid intravenous route of thrombolytic administration in 90-minute patency trials such as the Thrombolysis In Myocardial Infarction (TIMI) phase 1 and the European Cooperative Study Group (ECSG) trials in the mid 1980s.[6,7] Up to the mid 1980s, the cardiac catheterization laboratory had served predominantly as a diagnostic tool in the setting of AMI. In more recent years, however, its role as a therapeutic modality has been expanding rapidly. Initially, the potential therapeutic role of the cardiac catheterization laboratory was perceived as only supplementary to the pharmacologic approach. It seemed reasonable that balloon angioplasty performed after thrombolytic administration would improve flow and reduce the risk of reocclusion and reinfarction. However, in several randomized prospective trials undertaken in the late 1980s, the combination of intravenous thrombolysis coupled with immediate angioplasty did not confer any clinical benefit over thrombolysis alone with deferred angioplasty.[8-10] Prompted by nonrandomized observational data on primary angioplasty, several randomized prospective trials set out to compare thrombolytic administration and primary angioplasty as separate reperfusion strategies and showed that primary angioplasty was associated with a reduction in the composite endpoint of death, recurrent myocardial infarction (MI), and intracranial hemorrhage (ICH).

Unfortunately, the data from these trials soon became obsolete given the rapid expansion in the scope of both mechanical and pharmacologic methods to achieve acute coronary reperfusion. Recent work has produced advances in the field of stenting, more potent and more fibrin-specific thrombolytic agents, and newer antiplatelet and antithrombin agents. In addition to progress within the two strategies, there has been a rebirth in considering a combined approach, termed "facilitated" percutaneous coronary intervention (PCI). The goal of facilitated PCI is to take advantage of the speed with which pharmacologic strategies open the artery and the more definitive and sustained patency achieved by a mechanical intervention. Research in this area is being undertaken, and if effective in general principle, the numerous specific permutations of facilitated PCI will require ongoing reevaluation.

This chapter reviews trial data pertaining to the following: (1) primary balloon angioplasty versus thrombolysis, (2) the use of new thrombolytic regimens, (3) advances in primary angioplasty including stenting, and (4) combined approach with rescue and facilitated angioplasty. Whenever appropriate, the limitations of existing data and the critical need for future research in these rapidly evolving fields are discussed.

PRIMARY BALLOON ANGIOPLASTY VERSUS THROMBOLYSIS WITH STREPTOKINASE AND t-PA

The initial strategy to open acutely occluded arteries in MI used the thrombolytic agent streptokinase, administered either directly to the culprit coronary artery or systemically via the intravenous route. Multiple large randomized trials had established that thrombolytic therapy was associated with improved survival in AMI compared with conservative management.[11-13] At first the cardiac catheterization laboratory served only a diagnostic function in the management of AMI. However, as reocclusion and recurrent infarction remained serious limitations of

■ ■ ■

TABLE 11-1   POOLED DATA FROM RANDOMIZED PROSPECTIVE TRIALS EVALUATING THE EFFECTIVENESS OF THROMBOLYSIS FOLLOWED IMMEDIATELY BY ROUTINE ADJUNCTIVE PTCA VERSUS THROMBOLYSIS ALONE WITH DEFERRED PTCA

	PREDISCHARGE LVEF		30-DAY MORTALITY	
	Immediate PTCA	Deferred PTCA	Immediate PTCA	Deferred PTCA
TAMI 1	53%	56%	4/99 (4%)	1/98 (1%)
ECSG	51%	51%	12/183 (7%)	5/184 (3%)
TIMI 2A	50%	49%	15/195 (8%)	10/194 (5%)
Total experience	50%*	51%*	31/382 (8%)†	16/476 (3%)

*These values represent weighted averages for the respective columns of trial data.
†P = 0.04 for mortality of immediate PTCA vs. deferred PTCA.
PTCA, percutaneous transluminal coronary angioplasty; LVEF, left-ventricular ejection fraction; TAMI 1, Thrombolysis and Angioplasty in Myocardial Infarction, phase 1 trial; ECSG, European Cooperative Study Group; TIMI 2A, Thrombolysis in Myocardial Infarction, phase 2A.

the thrombolytic strategy, interest developed in the potential therapeutic benefit that adjunctive mechanical revascularization could offer. Initially, the question was answered in several large randomized prospective trials, which demonstrated that the combination of routine adjunctive angioplasty immediately following thrombolysis did not improve clinical outcomes when compared with a strategy of thrombolysis alone coupled with deferred angioplasty[8-10] (Table 11-1). It thus became the consensus in the cardiology community that there did not appear to be a role for routine adjunctive conventional angioplasty in all patients following thrombolysis for AMI.

Catheter-based therapies offered a mechanical approach to recanalization, and many nonrandomized observational studies showed that primary angioplasty was associated with improved infarct-related artery (IRA) patency and favorable mortality rates.[14-37] These encouraging results with primary angioplasty prompted an interest in the direct comparison with thrombolysis. Weaver and others[38] subsequently performed a meta-analysis on 10 prospective randomized trials comparing primary angioplasty with thrombolysis in the setting of acute ST elevation myocardial infarction (STEMI). The meta-analysis comprised 2606 patients, and about two thirds of them were made up of the study populations from the Global Use of Strategies to Open Occluded Coronary Arteries 2B (GUSTO 2B) trial,[39] the Primary Angioplasty in Myocardial Infarction (PAMI) trial,[40] and the Zwolle trial[41] (Table 11-2). Primary angioplasty was associated with improved clinical outcomes compared with thrombolytic therapy using streptokinase or tissue plasminogen activator (t-PA). In three of the trials t-PA was infused according to a 90-minute "accelerated" dosing regimen. Mortality at 30 days or at hospital discharge in the angioplasty group (1290 patients) was 4.4%, compared with 6.5% in the thrombolysis group (1316 patients), corresponding to a 34% relative risk reduction [RRR] (P = 0.02). The combined endpoint of death or nonfatal reinfarction also was reduced in the primary angioplasty group compared with thrombolysis: 7.2% versus 11.9% (RRR 42%; P < 0.001). Stroke risk was reduced in the angioplasty arm by 65% (0.7% vs. 2.0%; P = 0.007). The mean time to treatment was 26 minutes

longer for patients treated with primary angioplasty than for those treated with thrombolysis. This may be less than the time delay associated with primary angioplasty in the community setting. The operators in these trials were experienced, and it is unclear how much of the incremental benefit associated with angioplasty was related to this. An important limitation of this meta-analysis is the relatively short length of follow-up of up to 30 days. In the GUSTO 2B trial the benefit seen at 30 days in the composite outcome (death, nonfatal reinfarction, and nonfatal disabling stroke) with angioplasty was attenuated and no longer statistically significant at 6 months.[39] The Zwolle study group has analyzed outcomes through 5 years of follow-up, and in the 395 patients there was a significantly lower mortality (13% vs. 24%; RR 0.54; P = 0.01) and reinfarction rate (6% vs. 22%; RR 0.27; P < 0.001) in the primary angioplasty group.[42] Two-year follow up of the PAMI trial also has shown persistent benefits with angioplasty over thrombolysis. The combined endpoint of death or nonfatal reinfarction was 14.9% in the angioplasty group, compared with 23.0% in the thrombolysis group (P = 0.034).[43]

ADVANCES IN THROMBOLYSIS

There have been several advances in the field of thrombolysis after this first wave of clinical trials compared the efficacy and safety of thrombolysis and primary angioplasty in AMI. It was evident from the initial studies that primary angioplasty when compared with thrombolytic administration resulted in greater IRA patency as measured by the number of arteries with normal TIMI grade 3 flow and lower incidence of reocclusion and reinfarction. Thrombolysis also is complicated by a risk of hemorrhagic stroke. To overcome these deficiencies, newer agents and dosing regimens were developed, and adjunctive antiplatelet and antithrombotic therapies were evaluated.

The TIMI phase 1 trial[6] and the ECSG trial[7] showed that t-PA (alteplase) resulted in improved coronary flow when compared with streptokinase. The GUSTO 1 trial established that a 90-minute (so-called front-loaded) t-PA dosing regimen was associated with improved early and

TABLE 11-2 POOLED DATA FROM RANDOMIZED PROSPECTIVE TRIALS EVALUATING THE EFFECTIVENESS OF PRIMARY PTCA VERSUS THROMBOLYSIS IN ACUTE MYOCARDIAL INFARCTION

Trialist	Number of patients	30-day mortality	Reinfarction	CABG
O'Neill, 1986				
Angioplasty	29	2 (6.8%)	2 (7%)	—
Thrombolysis (IC SK)	27	1 (3.7%)	4 (15%)	—
Ribeiro, 1993				
Angioplasty	50	3 (6.0%)	4 (8.0%)	1 (2.0%)
Thrombolysis (IV SK)	50	1 (2.0%)	5 (10.0%)	6 (15.0%)
Gibbons, 1993				
Angioplasty	47	2 (4.3%)	0 (0.0%)	6 (13.0%)
Thrombolysis (Duteplase)	56	2 (3.6%)	2 (3.6%)	7 (13.0%)
Grines, 1993				
Angioplasty	195	5 (2.6%)	5 (2.6%)	16 (8.0%)
Thrombolysis (3-hr t-PA)	200	13 (6.5%)	13 (6.5%)	24 (12.0%)
De Boer, 1994*				
Angioplasty	152	3 (1.9%)	2 (1.3%)	—
Thrombolysis (IV SK)	149	11 (7.4%)	15 (10.1%)	—
GUSTO II, 1996				
Angioplasty	565	32 (5.7%)	25 (4.5%)	47 (7.5%)
Thrombolysis (90-min t-PA)	573	40 (7.0%)	37 (6.5%)	47 (8.2%)
STOP-AMI, 2000				
Angioplasty	71	3 (4.2%)	5 (7.0%)	1 (1.4%)
Thrombolysis (90-min t-PA)	69	5 (7.2%)	9 (13.0%)	1 (1.4%)
DANAMI 2, 2002				
Angioplasty	790	52 (6.6%)	13 (1.6%)	—
Thrombolysis (90-min t-PA)	782	59 (7.6%)	49 (6.3%)	—
Total experience				
Angioplasty	1899	102 (5.4%)[†]	56 (2.9%)[‡]	71 (7.7%)[§]
Thrombolysis	1906	132 (6.9%)	134 (7.0%)	85 (9.0%)

*Includes 142 patients previously reported by Zijlstra F, de Boer MJ, Hoorntje JCA, et al. A comparison of immediate coronary angioplasty with intravenous streptokinase in acute myocardial infarction. N Eng J Med 1993; 328:680–684.
†P = 0.023 for angioplasty vs. thrombolysis.
‡P < 0.0001 for angioplasty vs. thrombolysis.
§P = 0.15 for angioplasty vs. thrombolysis.
PTCA, percutaneous transluminal coronary angioplasty; CABG, coronary artery bypass graft; IV SK, intravenous streptokinase; t-PA, tissue plasminogen activator.

sustained IRA patency and a survival benefit when compared with streptokinase.[1] Both streptokinase and t-PA are administered as intravenous infusions. Reteplase (r-PA) and tenecteplase (TNK-t-PA) are newer thrombolytics that are given as intravenous boluses. The rationale for use of bolus thrombolytics is simpler and more rapid administration. TNK-t-PA (tenecteplase) is a genetically engineered variant of t-PA with greater fibrin specificity. It also has slower plasma clearance and greater resistance to plasminogen activator inhibitor-1 than alteplase. The TIMI 10B[44] and Assessment of the Safety and Efficacy of a New Thrombolytic Agent (ASSENT) 2[45] trials showed that weight-based single-bolus TNK-t-PA is as efficacious as accelerated alteplase but is simpler to administer and safer with less bleeding.

Whereas r-PA and TNK-t-PA represent newer thrombolytic monotherapies, there has been recent effort to combine low-dose thrombolytic therapy with glycoprotein IIb/IIIa inhibitor agents. Theoretically, combination therapy with glycoprotein IIb/IIIa inhibitors may improve outcomes by countering the possible prothrombotic state that thrombolytic agents may induce. They also may allow for reduced doses of thrombolytics, thus potentially lowering the intracranial hemorrhage risk. Multiple randomized trials have shown that combination

therapy with glycoprotein IIb/IIIa inhibitors and reduced-dose thrombolytics (as well as reduced-dose unfractionated heparin [UFH]) is associated with improved TIMI 3 flow rates compared with standard-dose thrombolytics (TAMI 8 [Thrombolysis and Angioplasty in Myocardial Infarction], TIMI 14, SPEED [Strategies for Patency Enhancement in the Emergency Department, GUSTO 4 pilot], INTRO-AMI [Integrilin and Low-dose Thrombolysis in Acute Myocardial Infarction]).[46-50] A pooled analysis of data from the dose-confirmation phase of these trials (TIMI 14, SPEED, and INTRO-AMI) shows that in 650 patients the 60- to 90-minute TIMI 3 flow was 56% with thrombolysis alone versus 64% with the combination (thrombolytic plus glycoprotein IIb/IIIa inhibitor) (Fig. 11-1). The TIMI 3 flow difference of 8% in the pooled analysis could be expected to translate to a 30-day mortality benefit of 0.4% based on the GUSTO 1 results (in which a 22% difference in TIMI 3 flow was associated with a 1.1% 30-day mortality difference).[1,2] Indeed, the potential mortality benefit of combination therapy of half-dose r-PA with full-dose abciximab was assessed in the GUSTO 5 trial of 16,588 patients with AMI.[51] As predicted by the previously mentioned patency data, 30-day mortality (the primary endpoint in the trial) differed by 0.3% (5.6% vs. 5.9%; P = 0.43). Combination therapy

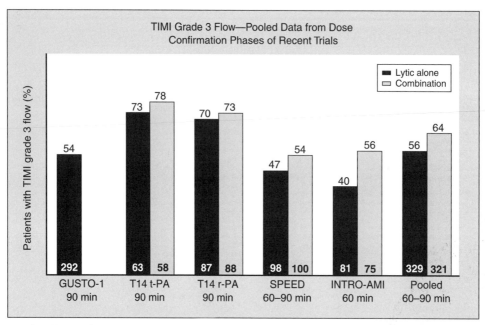

FIGURE 11-1. TIMI grade 3 flow in the setting of thrombolysis for acute myocardial infarction (MI) by use of combined therapy with glycoprotein IIb/IIIa inhibitors. Shown here are pooled data from dose confirmation phases of recent trials. Combined therapy resulted in 8% improvement in TIMI grade 3 flow (64% vs. 56%). The numbers within each bar denote the total number of patients treated. Also shown is the GUSTO-I trial in which 54% patients had TIMI grade 3 flow.

was associated with a lower rate of reinfarction at 7 days, but this endpoint was driven primarily by a reduction in the incidence of unblinded on-site investigator determination of recurrent ST segment deviation, which was not adjudicated. Combination therapy was associated with a higher incidence of bleeding complications and need for transfusion. There was also a significant interaction between age older than 75 years and increased risk of ICH (2.1% vs. 1.1%; P < 0.05).

Another combination therapy trial, the ASSENT 3 trial, studied half-dose TNK-t-PA with full-dose abciximab in acute STEMI.[52] Patients (n = 6095) were randomized to TNK plus enoxaparin, TNK plus abciximab (with reduced dose of UFH), or TNK plus UFH. The primary endpoint was the 30-day composite endpoint of death, reinfarction, and refractory ischemia. Combined therapy with abciximab was associated with a reduced risk of the composite endpoint by 28% (11.1% vs. 15.4%; P < 0.0001), and this was the result of fewer recurrent infarctions (2.2% vs. 4.2%; P < 0.001) and lower rates of refractory ischemia (3.2% vs. 6.5%; P < 0.0001) with no mortality difference (6.6% vs. 6.0%). The incidence of major bleeding doubled with the use of abciximab (4.3% vs. 2.2%; P = 0.0005). Similar to what was observed in the GUSTO 5 trial with respect to ICH, there were more adverse events among patients older than age 75 and among patients with diabetes who received abciximab. In contrast to abciximab, enoxaparin was well tolerated and was not associated with an increased incidence of adverse events or bleeding complications. Similar to abciximab, enoxaparin was superior to UFH with 26% RRR in the primary composite endpoint (11.4% vs. 15.4%; P = 0.0002).

Whereas the aforementioned trials studied the combination of reduced dose thrombolytic with either abcix-

imab or enoxaparin, the ENTIRE-TIMI 23 trial assessed the potential benefit of combining all three drugs: reduced dose TNK, abciximab, and enoxaparin. The trial randomized patients with acute STEMI in a 2 × 2 design to full-dose TNK-t-PA versus reduced-dose TNK-t-PA plus abciximab, with a subrandomization to either enoxaparin versus UFH.[53] The three-way combination of reduced-dose TNK, abciximab, and enoxaparin was not associated with a reduction in the 30-day incidence of death or reinfarction compared with the other regimens. Similar to what was observed in ASSENT 3, adjunctive enoxaparin was superior to UFH both in the setting of successful thrombolysis and with rescue PCI. Enoxaparin was associated with a lower 30-day combined endpoint of death or reinfarction (4.9% vs. 11.3%; P = 0.01) compared with UFH. This difference was predominantly the result of a lower reinfarction rate (1.8% vs. 8.2%; P = 0.002). Similar to what was observed in the prior studies, the combined strategy of half-dose TNK-t-PA plus abciximab was associated with more major bleeding.

To date, the combination of reduced-dose lytic and abciximab has offered limited clinical benefits but is associated with the disadvantage of increased bleeding and ICH in those patients older than age 75 years. It must be kept in mind that abciximab largely used as medical therapy in these STEMI trials. It also must be kept in mind that as medical therapy in unstable angina/non-STEMI, abciximab actually was associated with a higher rate of mortality at 48 hours in the GUSTO 4 trial (0.8% in the abciximab arms vs. 0.3% in the placebo arm, P < 0.05).[54] It is unclear if similar results would be observed with other glycoprotein IIb/IIIa inhibitors, which have been associated with clinical benefits as medical therapy. At the time of this writing, trials are planned to assess the efficacy of eptifibatide in combination with low-dose thrombolysis. With respect to antithrombotic agents, adjunctive enoxaparin appears to be more efficacious than UFH, while maintaining a similar safety profile. While enoxaparin does not currently have U.S. Food and Drug Administration (FDA)–approved labeling for the indication of AMI, trials are under way to prospectively assess enoxaparin as an adjunct to any of the FDA-approved thrombolytic agents (e.g., the EXTRACT [Enoxaparin and Thrombolysis Reperfusion for Acute Myocardial Infarction Treatment] trial).

ADVANCES IN PERCUTANEOUS CORONARY INTERVENTION

Interventional cardiology has seen many advances in the last decade, most notably the advent of drugs that inhibit the platelet glycoprotein IIb/IIIa receptor and new device technology with intracoronary stenting. The use of adjunctive abciximab in the setting of AMI has been assessed in several trials. The RAPPORT (ReoPro and Primary PTCA Organization and Randomized Trial) study randomized 483 patients undergoing primary angioplasty for acute STEMI to either adjunctive abciximab or placebo. There was no significant benefit in the prespecified primary endpoint of the study, the 6-month incidence of death, or recurrent MI.[55] The earlier 30-day combined endpoint of death, reinfarction, or urgent target vessel revascularization, however, was lower in the abciximab group (58% vs. 11.2%; P = 0.03; [at 6 months, 11.6% vs. 17.8%; P = 0.05]). Major bleeding also was increased in the abciximab arm.

The Abciximab before Direct angioplasty and stenting in Myocardial Infarction Regarding Acute and Long-term Follow-up (ADMIRAL) trial randomized 300 patients with acute STEMI to early adjunctive abciximab versus placebo.[56] All patients then went on to primary angioplasty with stenting. Abciximab achieved higher rates of TIMI grade 3 flow immediately before, immediately after, and 6 months after the primary PCI (TIMI 3 flow 16.8% vs. 5.4% [P = 0.01], 95.1% vs. 86.7% [P = 0.04], and 94.3% vs. 82.8% [P = 0.04], respectively). This improvement in TIMI grade 3 flow was associated with improved clinical outcomes, and the primary composite endpoint of death, reinfarction, and urgent culprit vessel revascularization was lower in the abciximab group both at 30 days (6.0% vs. 14.6%; P = 0.01) and at 6 months (7.4% vs. 15.9%; P = 0.02). The left-ventricular ejection fraction (LVEF) at 24 hours after primary angioplasty was improved among patients who received abciximab (LVEF 57.0% vs. 53.9%; P < 0.05) and the difference persisted at 6 months (61.1% vs. 57.0%; P = 0.05). In contrast to the RAPPORT trial, there was no excess bleeding with abciximab (0.7% vs. 0%).

Intracoronary stenting during routine angioplasty has been associated with a reduced incidence of restenosis.[57,58] The scaffolding provided by the stent tacks up dissection planes and tears, restores laminar flow, relieves intraluminal obstruction, and better accommodates the intimal hyperplasia that follows PCI. Observational studies documented the feasibility of stenting as an adjunct to primary angioplasty.[59-61] PAMI Stent assessed the efficacy of stenting compared with conventional balloon angioplasty in a randomized trial of 900 patients. Placement of a heparin-coated Palmaz-Schatz stent was compared with conventional balloon angioplasty in acute STEMI.[62] Post-PCI angiography revealed that stenting was associated with greater luminal diameter than balloon angioplasty (2.56 mm vs. 2.12 mm; P < 0.001), but somewhat paradoxically with lower rates of TIMI grade 3 flow (89.4% vs. 92.7%; P = 0.10). Restenosis at 6 months was less common in the stent group (20.3% vs. 33.5%; P < 0.001). The primary clinical composite endpoint of death, reinfarction, disabling stroke, and ischemia-driven target vessel revascularization at 6 months was reduced in the stent group (12.6% vs. 20.1%; P < 0.01), but the entire difference was to the result of a reduced need for revascularization. In fact, stenting was associated with a significantly higher rate of mortality at 6 months among those patients who at baseline had an occluded artery (6.0% vs. 2.1%, P < 0.05).[63] The underlying mechanism responsible for the higher mortality rate was not clear. Other smaller studies also have compared stents to conventional balloon angioplasty,[64-69] but no clear pattern in mortality has emerged.

The more recent Stent versus Thrombolysis for Occluded Coronary Arteries in Patients with Acute Myocardial Infarction (STOP AMI) trial showed that percutaneous revascularization strategy with stenting and glycoprotein IIb/IIIa inhibition in AMI was associated with reduced infarct size and improved clinical endpoint at 6 months when compared with front-loaded t-PA.[70] Patients (n = 140) were randomized, and infarct size was determined by nuclear imaging. The median infarct size in the stent plus abciximab group was 14.3%, which was significantly smaller than in the thrombolytic therapy group (median size of 19.4%; P = 0.02). The reperfusion therapies also were compared in their ability to salvage myocardium at risk on the initial nuclear scan. The salvage index was significantly greater with the stenting plus abciximab group (0.57 vs. 0.26; P < 0.001). The secondary endpoint was a clinical composite of death, reinfarction, and stroke at 6 months, and the percutaneous strategy was associated with a better outcome (8.5% vs. 23.2%; P = 0.02). Other trials also have shown that primary angioplasty with stenting improves coronary perfusion and reduces clinical events when compared with thrombolysis.[71-73]

The Controlled Abciximab and Device Investigation to Lower Late Angioplasty Complications (CADILLAC) trial built on the smaller trials of abciximab in primary PCI (RAPPORT and ADMIRAL) and also assessed the efficacy of intracoronary stent placement[74] (Table 11-3). It is important to note that a patient could be enrolled in the CADILLAC trial if a tight stenosis was present and ST-segment elevation was not required for entry.

Patients with AMI (n = 2082) were randomized in a 2 × 2 design to stenting versus balloon angioplasty and abciximab versus placebo. It should be noted that unlike ADMIRAL, in which abciximab could be administered before the intervention, abciximab was administered at the time of intervention in the CADILLAC trial.

■ ■ ■

TABLE 11-3   POOLED DATA FROM RANDOMIZED PROSPECTIVE TRIALS
EVALUATING THE EFFECTIVENESS OF STENTING IN PRIMARY ANGIOPLASTY

Trialist	Number of patients	6-month mortality	Reinfarction	Revascularization
PAMI Stent, 1999				
Angioplasty	448	12 (2.7%)	10 (2.2%)	76 (17.0%)
Abciximab	—	—	—	—
Stenting	452	19 (4.2%)	11 (2.4%)	35 (7.7%)
Stenting plus abciximab	—	—	—	—
CADILLAC, 2002				
Angioplasty	518	23 (4.5%)	9 (1.8%)	81 (15.7%)
Abciximab	528	13 (2.5%)	14 (2.7%)	73 (13.8%)
Stenting	512	15 (3.0%)	8 (1.6%)	43 (8.3%)
Stenting plus abciximab	524	22 (4.2%)	12 (2.2%)	27 (5.2%)
Total experience				
Angioplasty	966	35 (3.6%)	19 (2.0%)	157 (16.3%)
Abciximab	528	13 (2.5%)*	14 (2.7%)	73 (13.8%)†
Stenting	964	34 (3.5%)	19 (2.0%)	78 (8.1%)
Stenting plus abciximab	524	22 (4.2%)	12 (2.2%)	27 (5.2%)

Abciximab group underwent balloon angioplasty.
* P < 0.0001 for abciximab vs. stenting plus abciximab.
† P < 0.0001 for abciximab vs. stenting plus abciximab.

Exclusion criteria included cardiogenic shock, vein graft occlusion, greater than 12 hours of symptom duration, and vessel diameter less than 2.5 mm. Given these myriad exclusion criteria, it is notable that nearly a quarter of the patients were excluded from the study. The technical success rate was high (94% to 97%) and did not vary according to reperfusion strategy. Crossover to stenting in the study was permitted only in the event of suboptimal percutaneous transluminal coronary angioplasty (PTCA) results (16% of PTCA cases).

The primary endpoint was the combined outcome of death, reinfarction, disabling stroke, or ischemia-driven revascularization of the culprit artery at 6 months. Stenting was associated with a significantly reduced risk of the primary endpoint (20.0%, 16.5%, 11.5%, and 10.2% for PTCA, PTCA plus abciximab, stenting, and stenting plus abciximab, respectively; P = 0.03 for the comparison of stenting vs. PTCA plus abciximab), but this was entirely the result of the reduction in ischemia-driven revascularization of the culprit artery. Stenting was associated with a reduced incidence of angiographic restenosis (40.8% vs. 22.2% with balloon angioplasty; P < 0.001). The risk of target vessel reocclusion was reduced significantly with the use of abciximab compared with placebo (0.4% at 30 days compared with 1.4%; P < 0.001). Abciximab also was associated with a greater need for blood transfusions and more thrombocytopenia.

Thienopyridine administration prior to the PCI and delayed administration of abciximab until the time of PCI both may have contributed to the diminished efficacy of abciximab. An overriding concern is the fact that the mortality rate in this trial is much lower than that in other STEMI trials, again raising important questions as to the risk of the patients and the number of patients with a bona fide STEMI. It is notable that patients were enrolled in the trial if there was a tight culprit stenosis and an associated wall motion abnormality. In the absence of ST-segment elevation, these patients may have had unstable angina/non-STEMI or even stable angina with a tight epicardial stenosis. Many earlier trials of abciximab in the unstable angina arena were driven by a reduction in recurrent MI with careful surveillance of post-PCI creatine kinase (CK) release. In the setting of acute STEMI, recurrent infarction can be notoriously difficult to ascertain. Similarly, if patients without ST elevation were enrolled and if surveillance CK data were not collected, then recurrent MIs may likewise not have been detected as frequently as in other unstable angina trials. Because patients who did not have ST-segment elevation were enrolled in the trial, the results of the CADILLAC trial should not be incorporated into meta-analyses or pooled analyses of STEMI. The mortality results are also important in light of the PAMI Stent trial finding of unexpected increased 6-month mortality associated with stenting as compared with balloon angioplasty.[62] It is noteworthy that the 30-day mortality in the CADILLAC trial was lowest in the conventional primary balloon angioplasty plus abciximab group (1.1%). The corresponding mortality in the stent arms was between 2.2% and 2.7% (P = 0.31). Similar findings now have been observed at 1 year. These results fell far short of the hope that the use of lower profile stents in this study would have allowed the stent group to have mortality no higher than in the angioplasty group. It also had been hypothesized that the inhibition of platelet glycoprotein IIb/IIIa receptor would ameliorate the presumed process of thromboembolism, but the findings of this trial that abciximab had no effect on mortality or reinfarction makes that less likely.

It should be noted that the higher mortality in the PAMI Stent trial was observed during the era when higher balloon inflation pressure was used, when the more rigid Palmaz-Schatz stent was used, and when there was an emphasis on oversizing the stent, following the principle that "bigger is better." One possible mechanism for the increased mortality associated with stenting in the PAMI Stent trial is neurologically mediated spasm of the culprit coronary artery. Placement of an oversized intracoronary stent deployed at high pressures to provide good strut apposition may precipitate an increase in the α-adrenergic tone of the distal coronary bed. Gregorini and others[75] have demonstrated that the corrected TIMI frame counts 15 minutes after stent placement are worse than prior to stent placement, and likewise, there is an abrupt decline in regional wall motion. Importantly, α-adrenergic blockade improved the recovery of flow and wall motion in the setting of primary PCI with stenting.

ANGIOPLASTY VERSUS THROMBOLYSIS

A pharmacologic approach to the management of acute STEMI has several benefits. Thrombolytic agents are widely and rapidly available. There is no "learning curve" associated with their use, and they are suitable among patients in whom the coronary anatomy would preclude a percutaneous intervention. A major limitation of thrombolytic administration is the increased incidence of hemorrhagic stroke, although this risk may not be present with other pharmacologic approaches.

An advantage of primary angioplasty is the fact that this approach is associated with improved rates of TIMI grade 3 flow and lower rates of reocclusion. Reocclusion is associated with higher mortality rates and is the Achilles' heel of thrombolytic therapy.[76] It is notable that over the first day in GUSTO 2B, the thrombolytic strategy actually tended to have a lower mortality, and it was not until later, when reocclusion had begun to occur, that the primary angioplasty strategy pulled ahead. The lower rates of reocclusion and intracranial hemorrhage associated with primary angioplasty are the two main pathophysiologic mechanisms that drive the current superiority of this strategy (if achieved quickly).[77] Another often unrecognized advantage of primary angioplasty is the fact that it may offer early triage for patients who might benefit from surgical bypass grafting.

Despite these potential advantages, a critical challenge associated with primary angioplasty remains its timely implementation, measured by the door-to-balloon time, the time from patient arrival until the artery is opened by the balloon. Analysis of data from the Second National Registry of Myocardial Infarction (NRMI 2) demonstrated a clear association between door-to-balloon time and in-hospital mortality.[78] A door-to-balloon time of less than 60 minutes served as the reference cohort among 27,080 patients with ST-segment elevation MI evaluated between 1994 and 1998. For door-to-balloon times less than 2 hours, there was no increased mortality risk compared with a door-to-balloon time of less than 60 minutes. However, the adjusted odds of in-hospital mortality were increased significantly by 41% to 62% for patients with door-to-balloon times longer than 2 hours (OR 1.41 for 121–150 minutes; P = 0.01; OR 1.62 for 151–180 minutes; P < 0.001). Consistent with these registry findings, the randomized GUSTO 2B trial also demonstrated that prolonged enrollment-to-balloon times were associated with 30-day mortality.[77]

The NRMI 2 registry experience also demonstrated that higher institution volume is associated with improved clinical outcomes in the setting of primary PCI. Among the 661 centers that performed primary PCI, the adjusted in-hospital mortality was lower among hospitals with higher annual institutional volumes of primary PCI cases. Among hospitals in which one to three primary angioplasty cases were performed monthly, the relative odds of in-hospital mortality after multivariate adjustment were 0.86, compared with hospitals in which less than one case was performed monthly (8.0% vs. 6.2%, P = 0.03). Among busier hospitals that performed more than three primary PCIs per month, the relative odds were even lower at 0.67 (8.0% vs 4.7%, P < 0.001). This relationship is similar to that identified between institutional volume and the clinical outcomes associated with elective PCI.[79,80]

In another NRMI 2 study, 450 interventional hospitals and 257,602 patients were analyzed over the same time period (1994–1998).[81] The hospitals instead were divided into quartiles of volume (with the top quartile composed of institutions that performed >33 cases per year). Lower institutional volumes again were associated with higher in-hospital mortality in this analysis based on quartiles: 7.7%, 7.5%, 7.0%, and 5.7%. The RRR after multivariate adjustment was 28% when the top and bottom quartiles were compared (P < 0.001), representing 2.0 fewer deaths per 100 patients treated. It is notable that the door-to-balloon time was shorter in high-volume centers in both NRMI 2 studies. In contrast, there was no relationship between hospital volume and mortality among patients treated with thrombolysis (7.0% vs. 6.9%).

In a third study involving the NRMI 2 and 3 registries, primary angioplasty and thrombolytic strategies were compared stratified by institutional angioplasty volume in 62,299 patients at 446 hospitals.[82] In both high- and intermediate-volume centers, primary angioplasty was associated with lower in-hospital mortality (3.4% vs. 5.4%; P < 0.001; and 4.5% vs. 5.9%; P < 0.001, respectively) compared with thrombolysis. However, in low-volume centers (<17 primary angioplasty cases per year) there was no survival difference between the two reperfusion strategies (in-hospital mortality of 6.2% vs. 5.9% for PTCA and thrombolysis, respectively; P = 0.58). These data provide support for instituting minimum volume standards for the performance of primary angioplasty.

Up until the present time, the availability of on-site coronary artery bypass surgery has been required for a site to be credentialed in primary angioplasty. However, as interventional techniques have improved (especially with the advent of intracoronary stenting), the incidence of complications requiring emergency coronary artery bypass grafting (CABG) has decreased. As a result, questions have arisen as to whether the availability of on-site emergency cardiac surgery should be mandatory. To test whether primary angioplasty can be extended to the community hospital setting in the absence of on-site CABG, the C-PORT trial randomized 451 patients with acute STEMI presenting to 11 community hospitals between 1996 and 1999 without cardiac surgery backup to either thrombolytic therapy with front-loaded t-PA or primary

PCI.[83] The primary endpoint, the composite endpoint of death, reinfarction, and stroke was reduced at 6 months among patients randomized to the interventional strategy (12.4% vs. 19.9%; P = 0.03). Although there were trends favoring primary PCI in each of the three individual endpoints, only reinfarction reached statistical significance (5.3% vs. 10.6%; P = 0.04). Blood transfusion was more common in the primary PCI group. This study demonstrates the feasibility of performing primary PCI in a community hospital setting without cardiac surgery backup. Limitations of the study include the fact that it was stopped prematurely, and it is unclear how many interim looks were taken at the data.

The DANish Multicenter Randomized Study on Thrombolytic Therapy Versus Acute Coronary Angioplasty in AMI (DANAMI) 2 trial evaluated the efficacy of transferring patients between hospitals in a dedicated system of operators with varying degrees of experience in Denmark. The study enrolled patients with more than 4 mm of ST elevation from both dedicated PCI centers as well as from referring hospitals (transfer distance up to 95 miles with mean distance of 35 miles; transfer time up to 3 hours). Patients (n = 1562) were randomized to one of three strategies: primary PCI (with no transfer), transfer to another hospital for primary PCI, or 100 mg of front-loaded t-PA. The primary endpoint was a 30-day composite of death, reinfarction, and stroke. The study was stopped early because of the large reduction in reinfarction associated with the interventional strategy (1.6% vs. 6.3%; P < 0.0001) compared with thrombolysis. This resulted in a 45% RRR in the primary combined endpoint (8% vs. 14%; P = 0.0003), but there was no difference in the incidence of death or stroke. The results were similar in the transfer and nontransfer groups.

As has been observed in most recent trials comparing primary PCI with thrombolytic therapy, the results of the composite endpoint are driven by a reduction in the risk of recurrent MI. One vexing problem common to primary angioplasty trials is that they are not blinded, and so biases can be introduced easily. The rate of rescue/adjunctive PCI was much lower in DANAMI 2 (2.5%) when compared with other contemporary thrombolytic therapy trials, namely, GUSTO 5, ASSENT 3, and ENTIRE-TIMI 23 (rates of about 7% to 11%).[51-53] Likewise, the rates of reinfarction were also lower in these contemporary thrombolytic trials (range 1.8% to 4.2%) compared with the relatively high rate (6.3%) observed in the DANAMI 2 trial.

Although door-to-balloon times of up to 3 hours were permitted in the DANAMI 2 study, the actual time delays were much less, with an average door-to-balloon time of 114 minutes among patients transferred for primary PCI. This delay of 114 minutes obviously falls within the 120-minute window that was identified as the transition point for a significant increase in mortality in the NRMI 2 registry. Unfortunately, interhospital transfer in the United States is much slower than that reported in DANAMI 2. In the first 12 months of the NRMI 4 study (October 2000–September 2001) the median door-to-balloon time for transferred patients was 198 minutes (25th percentile 137 minutes, 75th percentile 281 minutes), and only 4.8% of patients had door-to-balloon time less than 90 minutes (NRMI 4 Transfer-In Annual Report 2002). This limits the practical application of the DANAMI 2 results in the United States.

RESCUE ANGIOPLASTY

If thrombolytic therapy is not effective (i.e., if TIMI grade 0 or 1 flow is present), a "rescue" or "salvage" angioplasty may be performed to restore flow. The angiographic substudy of the GUSTO trial linked full reperfusion to improved clinical outcomes,[2] and consequently an aggressive approach to mechanically restore flow to a persistently occluded vessel appears quite reasonable. The RESCUE trial was a randomized prospective trial that examined the benefits of conventional angioplasty following failed thrombolysis.[84] This trial enrolled 151 patients from 20 centers with TIMI grade 0 or 1 flow a mean of 4.5 hours after MI. Generalization of results from this trial are unfortunately somewhat limited because enrollment was restricted to patients with their first anterior wall MI. There was no difference in outcome for the prespecified primary endpoint of the trial, the resting LVEF at 30 days following the MI (40% in the rescue angioplasty group vs. 39% in the conservative group, P = NS). The mortality rate in patients treated with rescue angioplasty was 5.1%, which did not differ significantly from the 9.6% for those not treated with rescue angioplasty. As a secondary endpoint, death and congestive heart failure were analyzed together, and there was a trend for reduced incidence in the rescue angioplasty group (6.4%) compared with the group not treated with rescue angioplasty (16.6%, P = 0.055).

The combined TIMI 10B (tenecteplase vs. alteplase trial) and TIMI 14 (comparison of adjunctive abciximab vs. placebo in the setting of thrombolysis) experience has been analyzed to assess this issue in the more modern era of glycoprotein IIb/IIIa inhibition and stenting.[85] This retrospective observational study of 1938 patients with acute STEMI classified the interventions as rescue angioplasty (295 patients) or adjunctive angioplasty (424 patients), depending on the 90-minute angiogram TIMI flow grade (0 or 1 for a rescue procedure, 2 or 3 for an adjunctive one). The intervention was considered delayed (481 patients, 22 with TIMI 0 or 1 flow) if it was performed more than 150 minutes after symptom onset. Patients (n = 738; 55 of them with TIMI 0 or 1 flow) did not undergo a PCI at all. Among the patients with a closed culprit artery (TIMI 0/1), performance of a rescue PCI was associated with a trend toward lower 30-day mortality when compared with conservative post-thrombolysis management (6% vs. 17%; P = 0.01; after adjustment, P = 0.28). The adjunctive and delayed PCI groups had similar outcomes. Among the patients with normal (TIMI 3) flow on a 90-minute angiogram, PCI was associated with reduced incidence of death or reinfarction when compared with conservative therapy (adjusted multivariate model odds ratio 0.46; P = 0.02). Both death and reinfarction as outcomes alone had trends favoring the PCI group that did not reach statistical significance (P = 0.09 and P = 0.06, respectively). These results show that with newer techniques and procedures, early intervention after thrombolysis (with or without adjunctive abciximab therapy) may be associated with excellent outcomes. This finding should be confirmed in a large-scale randomized trial.

Whereas the previous study focused on the 30-day outcomes, in 2002 the association of rescue and adjunctive PCI with 2-year clinical outcomes were examined.[86] Previously we had demonstrated that improved flow both at an epicardial and tissue level was associated with better in-hospital and 30-day survival,[2,87,88] and this study evaluated the relationship of these flow indices on 2-year outcomes. Two-year follow-up data were available in 583 patients in 49 centers. Improved epicardial flow (represented by TIMI flow grade [TFG] and corrected TIMI frame count [CTFC]) and improved tissue-level perfusion (represented by TIMI myocardial perfusion grade [TMPG]) on the 90-minute angiogram that preceded the PCI all were associated with improved 2-year survival. For TFG 2/3, the Cox hazard ratio was 0.41 (P = 0.001); CTFC, Cox hazard ratio 0.92 per 10-frame decrease (P = 0.02); TMPG 2/3, Cox hazard ratio 0.51 (P = 0.038). These associations remained significant after multivariate analysis correcting for previously identified correlates of death. These findings suggest complementary mechanisms for the improved outcomes—both epicardial and tissue-level restoration of perfusion before PCI independently predict long-term survival. This finding supports the notion that not all TIMI 3 flow is equal. The 90-minute angiogram readily allows prognostication based on the previously mentioned flow indices (TFG, CTFC, TMPG). Moreover, the benefit from early restoration of flow is independent of a subsequent mechanical intervention.

After the 90-minute angiogram, PCI was performed at the discretion of operators and was not randomized. Performing a rescue PCI in the case of closed (TFG 0 or 1) arteries resulted in improved 2-year survival as compared with conservative management (P = 0.03) (Fig. 11-2). There was also a trend toward survival benefit with adjunctive PCI of patent (TFG 2 or 3) arteries (P = 0.11, multivariate P = 0.07) (Fig. 11-3). These data indicate that

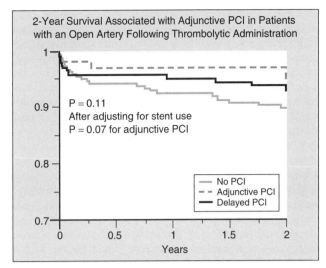

FIGURE 11-3. Kaplan-Meier survival curves for 2-year mortality by use of adjunctive and delayed percutaneous coronary intervention (PCI). Mortality trended lower in patients who underwent adjunctive and delayed PCI after 90-minute angiography (log-rank P = 0.2).

in the era of stenting, glycoprotein IIb/IIIa inhibition, and newer antiplatelet agents, rescue PCI for a closed vessel (TFG 0/1) is associated with improved 2-year survival. These data provide impetus for trials of facilitated PCI, in which a pharmacologic approach would be used to reestablish patency early, and a mechanical approach would follow to preserve and improve on this early patency.

"FACILITATED PCI"

Early trials that combined angioplasty and thrombolysis yielded disappointing results.[8-10,89] The failure of routine adjunctive angioplasty to improve outcomes in the setting of thrombolytic therapy for acute STEMI was thought to be the result of intramural hemorrhage in the arterial wall, which may have increased the incidence of abrupt closure. These trials preceded the introduction of stents, novel antiplatelet agents, and ACT (activated clotting time) monitoring. As a result of these advances, there has been renewed interest in evaluating a strategy termed "facilitated PCI." The goal of this strategy is to take advantage of the speed of patency offered by pharmacologic agents and the improved and preserved patency offered by a mechanical approach.

The early PAMI experience demonstrated that the achievement of TIMI 3 flow before primary PCI is associated with improved clinical outcomes independent of TIMI 3 flow following PCI.[90] The PACT trial[91] (n = 606) was designed to assess prospectively the potential benefit of improving patency prior to primary PCI with half-dose (50 mg) t-PA. Half-dose t-PA prior to the PCI was associated with improved coronary patency (TIMI grade 2 or 3 flow 61% vs. 34%; P = 0.001) and flow (TIMI grade 3 flow 33% vs. 15%) compared with placebo. There was no difference in the incidence of TIMI grade 3 flow following the PCI. There was no increase in the risk of safety endpoints such as the risk of stroke or major hemorrhage,

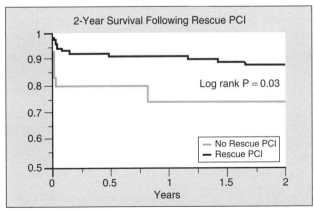

FIGURE 11-2. Kaplan-Meier survival curves for 2-year mortality by use of rescue percutaneous coronary intervention (PCI) in patients with TIMI flow grade (TFG) 0/1 at 90 minutes. Mortality was lower in patients who underwent rescue PCI after 90-minute angiography (log-rank P = 0.03).

although the trial was not powered to detect a difference in the risk of intracranial hemorrhage. Those patients with TIMI grade 3 flow before the PCI had improved left-ventricular function at discharge compared with those patients who had to wait to get the artery open with the balloon (62% vs. 57%, P < 0.05). Although clinical outcomes were not statistically significantly improved with half-dose t-PA in the PACT trial, this may have been in part because primary PCI was performed so quickly, in less than an hour in most cases. As discussed later, future trials of facilitated PCI will focus on those patients where time delays are involved.

In a retrospective substudy analysis, the SPEED investigators examined the efficacy of "facilitated PCI" in a small dose ranging trial of combination therapy (90). An interesting paradox arose in this analysis. Those patients who underwent rescue or adjunctive PCI in the trial had improved outcomes. However, it is notable that PCI was performed more often among patients who had received thrombolytic monotherapy (r-PA alone) rather than combination therapy with a glycoprotein IIb/IIIa inhibitor. Thus, a regimen that achieves inferior patency rates may trigger the more frequent performance of rescue or adjunctive PCI, which in turn may be associated with better outcomes.

FUTURE DIRECTIONS

As advances are made in both the pharmacologic and the interventional management of MI, different permutations of the two strategies will require ongoing evaluation in randomized clinical trials. If a technique shows promise in trials at high volumes with experienced operators, the generalizability of the results then will need to be confirmed in the community setting.

As noted earlier, the combined approach of pharmacologic and percutaneous interventions holds promise. A number of clinical trials are investigating facilitated PCI in the setting of AMI: Addressing the Value of Facilitated Angioplasty After Combination Therapy or Eptifibatide Monotherapy in Acute Myocardial Infarction (ADVANCE-MI), TITAN (TIMI 34), ASSENT 4, and Facilitated Intervention and Enhanced Reperfusion Speed to Stop Events (FINESSE).

REFERENCES

1. An international randomized trial comparing four thrombolytic strategies for acute myocardial infarction. The GUSTO investigators [see comments]. N Engl J Med 1993; 329:673-682.
2. The effects of tissue plasminogen activator, streptokinase, or both on coronary-artery patency, ventricular function, and survival after acute myocardial infarction. The GUSTO Angiographic Investigators [see comments] [published erratum appears in N Engl J Med 1994 Feb 17;330(7):516]. N Engl J Med 1993; 329:1615-1622.
3. Rentrop KP, Blanke H, Karsch KR, Kreuzer H: Initial experience with transluminal recanalization of the occluded infarct related artery in acute myocardial infarction: Comparison with conventionally treated patients. Clin Cardiol 1979; 2:92-102.
4. Khaja F, Walton JA, Brymer JF, et al: Intracoronary fibrinolytic therapy in acute myocardial infarction: Report of a prospective randomized trial. N Engl J Med 1983; 308:1305-1311.
5. Kennedy JW, Ritchie JL, Davis KB, Fritz JK: Western Washington randomized trial of intracoronary streptokinase in acute myocardial infarction. N Engl J Med 1983; 309:1477-1482.
6. The thrombolysis in myocardial infarction (TIMI) trial: TIMI Study Group. N Engl J Med 1985; 310:932-936.
7. Verstraete M, Bernard R, Bory M, et al: Randomized trial of intravenous streptokinase in acute myocardial infarction: Report from the European Cooperative Study Group for recombinant tissue type plasminogen activator. Lancet 1985; 1:842-847.
8. Topol EJ, Califf RM, George BS, et al: A randomized trial of immediate versus delayed elective angioplasty after intravenous tissue plasminogen activator in acute myocardial infarction. N Engl J Med 1987; 317:581-588.
9. Simoons ML, Col J, Betriu A, et al: Thrombolysis with tissue plasminogen activator in acute myocardial infarction: No additional benefit from immediate percutaneous coronary angioplasty. Lancet 1988; 1:197-203.
10. Immediate vs delayed catheterization and angioplasty following thrombolytic therapy for acute myocardial infarction. TIMI II A results. The TIMI Research Group. JAMA 1988; 260:2849-2858.
11. Effectiveness of intravenous thrombolytic treatment in acute myocardial infarction: Gruppo Italiano per lo Studio della Streptochinasi nell'Infarto Miocardico (GISSI). Lancet 1986; 1:397-402.
12. Randomized trial of intravenous streptokinase, oral aspirin, both, or neither among 17,187 cases of suspected acute myocardial infarction: ISIS-2. ISIS-2 (Second International Study of Infarct Survival) Collaborative Group. J Am Coll Cardiol 1988; 12:3A-13A.
13. Indications for fibrinolytic therapy in suspected acute myocardial infarction: Collaborative overview of early mortality and major morbidity results from all randomised trials of more than 1000 patients. Fibrinolytic Therapy Trialists' (FTT) Collaborative Group [published erratum appears in Lancet 1994 Mar 19;343(8899):742] [see comments]. Lancet 1994; 343:311-322.
14. Rothbaum DA, Linnemeier TJ, Landin RJ, et al: Emergency percutaneous transluminal coronary angioplasty in acute myocardial infarction: A 3 year experience. J Am Coll Cardiol 1987; 10:264-272.
15. Marco J, Caster L, Szatmary IJ, Fajadet J: Emergency percutaneous transluminal coronary angioplasty without thrombolysis as initial therapy in acute myocardial infarction. Int J Cardiol 1987; 15:55-63.
16. Flaker GC, Webel RR, Meinhardt S, et al: Emergency angioplasty in acute myocardial infarction. Am Heart J 1989; 118:1154-1160.
17. Ellis SG, O'Neill WW, Bates ER, et al: Coronary angioplasty as primary therapy for acute myocardial infarction 6 to 48 hours after symptom onset: Report of an initial experience. J Am Coll Cardiol 1989; 13:1122-1126.
18. Bittl JA: Indications, timing, and optimal technique for diagnostic angiography and angioplasty in acute myocardial infarction. Chest 1991; 99:150S-156S.
19. Williams DO, Holubkov AL, Detre KM, et al: Impact of pretreatment by thrombolytic therapy upon outcome of emergency direct angioplasty for patients with acute myocardial infarction (abstract). J Am Coll Cardiol 1991; 17:337A.
20. Grines CL, Meany TB, Weintraub R, et al: Streptokinase angioplasty myocardial infarction trial: Early and late results (abstract). J Am Coll Cardiol 1991; 17:336A.
21. Jaski BE, Cohen JD, Trausch J, et al: Outcome of urgent percutaneous transluminal coronary angioplasty in acute myocardial infarction: Comparison of single vessel versus multivessel coronary artery disease. Am Heart J 1992; 124:1427-1433.
22. Rogers WJ, Dean LS, Moore PB: Outcome of patients managed with primary PTCA versus lytic therapy in a multicenter registry (abstract). J Am Coll Cardiol 1993; 21:330A.
23. Himbert D, Juliard JM, Steg PG, et al: Primary coronary angioplasty for acute myocardial infarction with contraindication to thrombolysis. Am J Cardiol 1993; 71:377-381.
24. O'Keefe JHJ, Bailey WL, Rutherford BD, Hartzler GO: Primary angioplasty for acute myocardial infarction in 1,000 consecutive patients: Results in an unselected population and high risk subgroups. Am J Cardiol 1993; 72:107G-115G.
25. Nakagawa Y, Iwasaki Y, Nosaka H, et al: Serial angiographic follow-up after successful direct angioplasty for acute myocardial infarction: Single center experience (abstract). Circulation 1993; 88:I-106.
26. Dussaillant G, Martinez A, Marchant E, et al: Primary coronary angioplasty as early reperfusion treatment of acute myocardial infarction. Rev Med Chil 1994; 122:401-407.

27. Sarkis A, Badaoui G, Kassab R, et al: Primary angioplasty at the stage of acute myocardial infarction. J Med Liban 1994; 42:100-104.
28. Helmreich G, Kratzer H, Baumgartner H, Kuhn P: Primary angioplasty in acute myocardial infarction. Wien Klin Wochenschr 1994; 106:507-512.
29. Chamorro H, Ducci H, Methei R, et al: Primary coronary angioplasty as treatment choice in the 1st 6 hours following acute myocardial infarction. Rev Med Chil 1995; 123:727-734.
30. Every N, Douglas W, Parsons L, Martin JS: Direct PTCA vs. thrombolysis: Immediate and one year outcome and procedure utilization for the two treatment strategies. MITI Project Investigators. Circulation 1995; 92:I-138.
31. Brodie B, Stuckey T, Weintraub R: Timing and mechanism of death after direct angioplasty for acute myocardial infarction (abstract). J Am Coll Cardiol 1995; 27:295A.
32. Wharton TP, Schmitz JM, Fedele FA, et al: Primary angioplasty in acute myocardial infarction at community hospitals without cardiac surgery: Experience in 195 cases (abstract). Circulation 1995; 92:I-138.
33. Jhangiani AH, Jorgensen MB, Mansukhani PW, et al: Community practice of primary angioplasty for myocardial infarction (abstract). J Am Coll Cardiol 1996; 27:61A.
34. Patel S, Reese C, O'Connor RE, Doorey AJ: Adverse outcomes accompanying primary angioplasty (PTCA) for acute myocardial infarction (AMI)—dangers of delay (abstract). J Am Coll Cardiol 1996; 27:62A.
35. Caputo RP, Lopez JJ, Stoler RC, et al: The effect of institutional experience on the outcome of primary angioplasty for acute MI (abstract). J Am Coll Cardiol 1996; 27:62A.
36. Neuhaus KL, Vogel A, Harmjanz D, et al: Primary PTCA in acute myocardial infarction: Results from a German multicenter registry (abstract). J Am Coll Cardiol 1996; 27:62A.
37. Cannon CP, Costas TL, Tiefenbrunn AJ, et al: Influence of door to balloon time on mortality in 3.648 patients in the second national registry of myocardial infarction (NRMI 2) (abstract). J Am Coll Cardiol 1996; 27:61A.
38. Weaver WD, Simes RJ, Betriu A, et al: Comparison of primary coronary angioplasty and intravenous thrombolytic therapy for acute myocardial infarction: A quantitative review. JAMA 1997; 278:2093-2098.
39. A clinical trial comparing primary coronary angioplasty with tissue plasminogen activator for acute myocardial infarction. GUSTO IIb Investigators. N Engl J Med 1997; 336:1621-1628.
40. Grines CL, Browne KF, Marco J, et al: A comparison of immediate angioplasty with thrombolytic therapy for acute myocardial infarction. The Primary Angioplasty in Myocardial Infarction Study Group. N Engl J Med 1993; 328:673-679.
41. de Boer MJ, Hoorntje JC, Ottervanger JP, et al: Immediate coronary angioplasty versus intravenous streptokinase in acute myocardial infarction: Left ventricular ejection fraction, hospital mortality and reinfarction. J Am Coll Cardiol 1994; 23:1004-1008.
42. Zijlstra F, Hoorntje JC, de Boer MJ, et al: Long-term benefit of primary angioplasty as compared with thrombolytic therapy for acute myocardial infarction. N Engl J Med 1999; 341:1413-1419.
43. Nunn CM, O'Neill WW, Rothbaum D, et al: Long-term outcome after primary angioplasty: Report from the primary angioplasty in myocardial infarction (PAMI-I) trial. J Am Coll Cardiol 1999; 33:640-646.
44. Cannon CP, Gibson CM, McCabe CH, et al: TNK-tissue plasminogen activator compared with front-loaded alteplase in acute myocardial infarction: Results of the TIMI 10B trial. Thrombolysis in Myocardial Infarction (TIMI) 10B Investigators. Circulation 1998; 98:2805-2814.
45. Single-bolus tenecteplase compared with front-loaded alteplase in acute myocardial infarction: The ASSENT-2 double-blind randomised trial. Assessment of the Safety and Efficacy of a New Thrombolytic Investigators. Lancet 1999; 354:716-722.
46. Kleiman NS, Ohman EM, Califf RM, et al: Profound inhibition of platelet aggregation with monoclonal antibody 7E3 Fab after thrombolytic therapy. Results of the Thrombolysis and Angioplasty in Myocardial Infarction (TAMI) 8 Pilot Study. J Am Coll Cardiol 1993; 22:381-389.
47. Antman EM, Giugliano RP, Gibson CM, et al: Abciximab facilitates the rate and extent of thrombolysis: Results of the thrombolysis in myocardial infarction (TIMI) 14 trial. The TIMI 14 Investigators. Circulation 1999; 99:2720-2732.
48. Antman EM, Gibson CM, de Lemos JA, et al: Combination reperfusion therapy with abciximab and reduced dose reteplase: Results from TIMI 14. The Thrombolysis in Myocardial Infarction (TIMI) 14 Investigators. Eur Heart J 2000; 21:1944-1953.
49. Trial of abciximab with and without low-dose reteplase for acute myocardial infarction. Strategies for Patency Enhancement in the Emergency Department (SPEED) Group. Circulation 2000; 101:2788-2794.
50. Brener SJ, Zeymer U, Adgey AA, et al: Eptifibatide and low-dose tissue plasminogen activator in acute myocardial infarction. J Am Coll Cardiol 2002; 39:377-386.
51. Reperfusion Therapy for Acute Myocardial Infarction with Fibrinolytic Therapy or Combination Reduced Fibrinolytic Therapy and Platelet glycoprotein IIb/IIIa Inhibition: The GUSTO V Randomised Trial. Lancet 2001; 357:1905-1914.
52. Efficacy and safety of tenecteplase in combination with enoxaparin, abciximab, or unfractionated heparin: The ASSENT-3 randomised trial in acute myocardial infarction. Lancet 2001; 358:605-613.
53. Antman EM, Louwerenburg HW, Baars HF, et al: Enoxaparin as adjunctive antithrombin therapy for ST-elevation myocardial infarction: Results of the ENTIRE-Thrombolysis in Myocardial Infarction (TIMI) 23 Trial. Circulation 2002; 105:1642-1649.
54. Effect of glycoprotein IIb/IIIa receptor blocker abciximab on outcome in patients with acute coronary syndromes without early coronary revascularisation: The GUSTO IV-ACS randomised trial. The GUSTO IV-ACS Investigators. Lancet 2001; 357:1915-1924.
55. Brener SJ, Barr LA, Burchenal JE, et al: Randomized, placebo-controlled trial of platelet glycoprotein IIb/IIIa blockade with primary angioplasty for acute myocardial infarction. ReoPro and Primary PTCA Organization and Randomized Trial (RAPPORT) Investigators. Circulation 1998; 98:734-741.
56. Montalescot G, Barragan P, Wittenberg O, et al: Platelet glycoprotein IIb/IIIa inhibition with coronary stenting for acute myocardial infarction. N Engl J Med 2001; 344:1895-1903.
57. Serruys PW, de Jaegere P, Kiemeneij F, et al: A comparison of balloon-expandable-stent implantation with balloon angioplasty in patients with coronary artery disease. N Engl J Med 1994; 331:489-495.
58. Fischman DL, Leon MB, Baim DS, et al: A randomized comparison of coronary-stent placement and balloon angioplasty in the treatment of coronary artery disease. N Engl J Med 1994; 331:496-501.
59. Garcia-Cantu E, Spaulding C, Corcos T, et al: Stent implantation in acute myocardial infarction. Am J Cardiol 1996; 77:451-454.
60. Saito S, Hosokawa G, Kunikane K, et al: Primary stent implantation without Coumadin in acute myocardial infarction. J Am Coll Cardiol 1996; 28:74-81.
61. Monassier J-P, Hamon M, Elias J, et al: Early versus late coronary stenting following acute myocardial infarction: Results of the STENTIM I study. Cathet Cardiovasc Diagn 1997; 42:243-248.
62. Grines CL, Cox DA, Stone GW, et al: Coronary angioplasty with or without stent implantation for acute myocardial infarction. Stent Primary Angioplasty in Myocardial Infarction Study Group. N Engl J Med 1999; 341:1949-1956.
63. Lansky AJ, Stone GW, Mehran R, et al: Impact of baseline TIMI flow on outcomes after primary stenting versus primary PTCA in acute myocardial infarction. Results from PAMI Stent. J Am Coll Cardiol 1999; 33:368A.
64. Saito S, Hosokawa G, Tanaka S, Nakamura S: Primary stent implantation is superior to balloon angioplasty in acute myocardial infarction. Catheter Cardiovasc Interv 1999; 48:262-268.
65. Suryapranata H, Ottervanger JP, Nibbering E, et al: Long term outcome and cost-effectiveness of stenting versus balloon angioplasty for acute myocardial infarction. Heart 2001; 85:667-671.
66. Rodriguez A, Bernardi V, Fernandez M, et al: In-hospital and late results of coronary stents versus conventional balloon angioplasty in acute myocardial infarction (GRAMI trial). Am J Cardiol 1998; 81:1286-1291.
67. Antoniucci D, Santoro GM, Bolognese L, et al: A clinical trial comparing primary stenting of the infarct-related artery with optimal primary angioplasty for acute myocardial infarction. J Am Coll Cardiol 1998; 31:1234-1239.
68. Suryapranata H, van't Hof AW, Hoorntje JC, et al: Randomized comparison of coronary stenting with balloon angioplasty in selected patients with acute myocardial infarction. Circulation 1998; 97:2502-2505.
69. Maillard L, Hamon M, Khalife K, et al: A comparison of systematic stenting and conventional balloon angioplasty during primary percutaneous transluminal coronary angioplasty for acute myocardial infarction. J Am Coll Cardiol 2000; 35:1729-1736.
70. Schomig A, Kastrati A, Dirschinger J, et al: Coronary stenting plus platelet glycoprotein IIb/IIIa blockade compared with tissue

plasminogen activator in acute myocardial infarction. N Engl J Med 2000; 343:385-391.

71. Le May MR, Labinaz M, Davies RF, et al: Stenting versus thrombolysis in acute myocardial infarction trial (STAT). J Am Coll Cardiol 2001; 37:985-991.

72. Vrachatis AD, Alpert MA, Georgulas VP, et al: Comparative efficacy of primary angioplasty with stent implantation and thrombolysis in restoring basal coronary artery flow in acute ST segment elevation myocardial infarction: Quantitative assessment using the corrected TIMI frame count. Angiology 2001; 52:161-166.

73. Ribichini F, Steffenino G, Dellavalle A, et al: Comparison of thrombolytic therapy and primary coronary angioplasty with liberal stenting for inferior myocardial infarction with precordial ST-segment depression. J Am Coll Cardiol 1998; 32:1687-1694.

74. Stone GW, Grines CL, Cox DA, et al: Comparison of angioplasty with stenting, with or without abciximab, in acute myocardial infarction. N Engl J Med 2002; 346:957-966.

75. Gregorini L, Marco J, Kozakova M, et al: Alpha-adrenergic blockade improves recovery of myocardial perfusion and function after coronary stenting in patients with acute myocardial infarction. Circulation 1999; 99:482-490.

76. Ohman EM, Califf RM, Topol EJ, et al: Consequences of reocclusion after successful reperfusion therapy in acute myocardial infarction. TAMI Study Group. Circulation 1990; 82:781-791.

77. Berger PB, Ellis SG, Holmes DR, Jr., et al: Relationship between delay in performing direct coronary angioplasty and early clinical outcome in patients with acute myocardial infarction. Circulation 1999; 100:14-20.

78. Cannon CP, Gibson CM, Lambrew CT, et al: Relationship of symptom-onset-to-balloon time and door-to-balloon time with mortality in patients undergoing angioplasty for acute myocardial infarction. JAMA 2000; 283:2941-2947.

79. Jollis JG, Peterson ED, DeLong ER, et al: The relation between the volume of coronary angioplasty procedures at hospitals treating Medicare beneficiaries and short-term mortality. N Engl J Med 1994; 331:1625-1629.

80. Hannan EL, Racz M, Ryan TJ, et al: Coronary angioplasty volume-outcome relationships for hospitals and cardiologists. JAMA 1997; 277:892-898.

81. Canto JG, Every NR, Magid DJ, et al: The volume of primary angioplasty procedures and survival after acute myocardial infarction. N Engl J Med 2000; 342:1573-1580.

82. Magid DJ, Calonge BN, Rumsfeld JS, et al: Relation between hospital primary angioplasty volume and mortality for patients with acute MI treated with primary angioplasty vs thrombolytic therapy. JAMA 2000; 284:3131-3138.

83. Aversano T, Aversano LT, Passamani E, et al: Thrombolytic therapy vs primary percutaneous coronary intervention for myocardial infarction in patients presenting to hospitals without on-site cardiac surgery. JAMA 2002; 287:1943-1951.

84. Ellis SG, Ribeiro da Silva E, Heyndrickx GR, et al: Randomized comparison of rescue angioplasty with conservative management of patients with early failure of thrombolysis for acute anterior myocardial infarction. Circulation 1994; 90:2280-2284.

85. Schweiger MJ, Cannon CP, Murphy SA, et al: Early coronary intervention following pharmacologic therapy for acute myocardial infarction (the combined TIMI 10B-TIMI 14 experience). Am J Cardiol 2001; 88:831-836.

86. Gibson CM, Cannon CP, Murphy SA, et al: Relationship of the TIMI myocardial perfusion grades, flow grades, frame count, and percutaneous coronary intervention to long-term outcomes after thrombolytic administration in acute myocardial infarction. Circulation 2002; 105:1909-1913.

87. Gibson CM, Murphy SA, Rizzo MJ, et al: Relationship between TIMI frame count and clinical outcomes after thrombolytic administration. Thrombolysis In Myocardial Infarction (TIMI) Study Group. Circulation 1999; 99:1945-1950.

88. Gibson CM, Cannon CP, Murphy SA, et al: Relationship of TIMI myocardial perfusion grade to mortality after administration of thrombolytic drugs. Circulation 2000; 101:125-130.

89. O'Neill WW, Weintraub R, Grines CL, et al: A prospective, placebo-controlled, randomized trial of intravenous streptokinase and angioplasty versus lone angioplasty therapy of acute myocardial infarction. Circulation 1992; 86:1710-1717.

90. Stone GW, Cox D, Garcia E, et al: Normal flow (TIMI-3) before mechanical reperfusion therapy is an independent determinant of survival in acute myocardial infarction: Analysis from the primary angioplasty in myocardial infarction trials. Circulation 2001; 104:636-641.

91. Ross AM, Coyne KS, Reiner JS, et al: A randomized trial comparing primary angioplasty with a strategy of short-acting thrombolysis and immediate planned rescue angioplasty in acute myocardial infarction: The PACT trial. J Am Coll Cardiol 1999; 34:1954-1962.

■ ■ ■ c h a p t e r **12**

Coronary Artery Bypass Surgery

Malcolm R. Bell
Charles J. Mullany
Bernard J. Gersh

Acute coronary syndromes (ACS) account for almost 1.5 million hospital admissions per year in the United States and approximately 2.5 million worldwide. ACS include unstable angina and non-ST segment elevation myocardial infarction (NSTEMI).[1] The initial management of patients includes hospitalizing the patient and prescribing aspirin, heparin (unfractionated or low–molecular-weight), nitrates, and beta blockers. More recently, the use of intravenous platelet glycoprotein IIb/IIIa inhibitors also has been advocated,[1] as has the use of the oral antiplatelet drug clopidogrel.[2] Although the relative benefits and safety of an early-invasive approach (i.e., early coronary angiography followed by early revascularization when appropriate) have been controversial, the results of recent trials have proved that this approach is superior to the conservative (medical) management in patients with ACS.[3-5]

Revascularization for ACS is performed with either percutaneous coronary intervention (PCI) or with coronary artery bypass surgery. Initial angiography will uncover a wide spectrum of findings. Coronary artery disease severity varies from single-vessel disease to multivessel or left-main stenosis. In a minority of patients, no significant obstructive coronary disease is found. The majority of patients found to have single-vessel disease have PCI performed as the preferred method of revascularization, and PCI is also performed frequently in patients with two- and even three-vessel disease after identifying an assumed "culprit vessel."

However, in general, the indications for PCI and surgery in ACS are similar to those for stable angina.[1] Although emphasis is placed on the short-term outcome of patients in the setting of ACS, the long-term outcome of patients is just as important. Guidelines for revascularization strategies for patients with significant obstructive coronary artery disease have been developed from randomized trials of both medicine versus surgery[6] and surgery versus PCI.[7,8] It should be noted that although many of the patients in these trials had stable effort angina, many other patients had presented with unstable angina and were included in these trials. For example, 64% of patients enrolled in the randomized Bypass Angioplasty Revascularization Investigation (BARI) trial

had unstable angina at entry.[8] However, no formal post hoc analysis of such subsets of patients has been published. Therefore, physicians generally follow these guidelines when they are required to choose the optimal revascularization strategy for patients with ACS. High-risk patients with left-ventricular systolic dysfunction, patients with diabetes mellitus, and those with two-vessel disease with severe proximal left anterior descending involvement (particularly if not easily approachable with PCI) or severe three-vessel or left-main disease should be considered for coronary artery bypass surgery. Selected patients with diabetes with single-vessel disease or without diffuse disease and with good left-ventricular function also can be considered for PCI.[9] Most other patients can be revascularized by PCI if technically feasible lesions are identified.

This discussion focuses on the outcomes of patients with ACS (unstable angina or NSTEMI) who have surgical revascularization. The use of multiple and potent antiplatelet agents and anticoagulation with heparin also needs to be considered in terms of safety and risks of intraoperative and postoperative bleeding. The frequency with which emergency coronary bypass surgery is required after failed PCI in modern times has fallen significantly with the introduction of coronary stents. Although the outcome of patients undergoing such emergency surgery has improved a little over the years, morbidity and mortality remain high.[10] Because this event is now so infrequent and contemporary outcome data are so scant, it will not be discussed further.

CORONARY ANGIOGRAPHY AND SURGICAL REVASCULARIZATION

The spectrum of coronary artery disease severity identified at coronary angiography performed in patients with ACS is summarized in Table 12-1. Three-vessel disease is found in approximately 30% of patients with a range of 15% to 48%, depending on the patient population studied. Significant left-main disease is identified in approximately 10% of patients. Such patients usually are

■ ▪ ■

TABLE 12-1   CORONARY ANGIOGRAPHIC FINDINGS IN PATIENTS IN SELECTED RECENT TRIALS OF ACUTE CORONARY SYNDROMES IN WHICH EARLY CORONARY ANGIOGRAPHY WAS MANDATED IN AT LEAST ONE RANDOMIZED GROUP

Trial (no. of patients)	SEVERITY OF CORONARY ARTERY DISEASE				
	1-VD	2-VD	3-VD	LMCA	LVEF
TIMI IIIB[48]					
Early-invasive arm (726)	38%	29%	15%	4%	0.59
VANQWISH[15]					
Invasive arm (431)	21%	26%	40%	8%	0.53 ± 0.15
Conservative arm (106)	19%	19%	48%	13%	0.52 ± 0.16
FRISC II[11]					
Invasive arm (1201)	30%	26%	23%	8%	14% <0.45
Noninvasive arm (585)	26%	28%	30%	8%	12% <0.45
TACTICS[3]					
Invasive arm (1085)	NR	NR	34%	9%	NR
RITA 3[4]					
Invasive arm (865)	33%	24%	22%	NR	NR

VD, vessel disease; LMCA, left-main coronary artery; LVEF, left-ventricular ejection fraction; NR, not reported.

considered for coronary artery bypass surgery based on prior randomized trials that compared medicine to surgery.[6]

Although PCI is often performed in patients with three-vessel disease, coronary artery bypass surgery might be preferred in patients with depressed left-ventricular function or if the patient has diabetes mellitus.[8] Thus it can be expected that in both selected and nonselected patients undergoing coronary angiography during their index hospitalization, many will be found to have coronary anatomy more suited for coronary artery bypass surgery than for either PCI or for medical therapy. Furthermore, some patients with one- or two-vessel disease may not have anatomy well suited for PCI, and these patients also occasionally may be referred for surgery rather than PCI.

Table 12-2 shows the proportion of patients from a number of recent large prospective trials of ACS who had coronary angiography performed followed by either PCI or coronary artery bypass surgery. Coronary angiography in these trials was either mandated in the invasive arm or performed for clinical indications in the comparison arm. Angiography was performed in about 98% overall in the invasive arms and from 16% to 64% in the conservative arms. Both percutaneous and surgical revascularization procedures were used more frequently in the patients who were randomized to the early invasive groups than in the more conservatively managed groups. PCI was performed more commonly than coronary artery bypass surgery, and its overall use was approximately 30% to 40%. In comparison, coronary

■ ■ ■

TABLE 12-2   PROPORTIONS OF PATIENTS WITH ACUTE CORONARY SYNDROMES WHO UNDERWENT INITIAL REVASCULARIZATION WITH EITHER CORONARY ARTERY BYPASS SURGERY OR PERCUTANEOUS CORONARY INTERVENTION

Trial	Number of patients	Coronary angiogram (%)	PCI performed (%)	CABG performed (%)
TIMI IIIB[48]				
Early invasive	740	98	38	25
Early conservative	733	64	26	24
GUSTO IIB[49]	8011	57	18	14
VANQWISH[15]				
Invasive strategy	462	96	21	21
Conservative strategy	458	48	12	19
FRISC II[11]				
Invasive strategy	1201	98	43	36
Noninvasive strategy	1235	47	18	19
TACTICS-TIMI 18[3]				
Invasive strategy	1114	97	41	20
Noninvasive strategy	1106	51	24	13
RITA 3[4]				
Intervention strategy	895	97	35	21
Conservative strategy	915	16	7	4

PCI, percutaneous coronary intervention; CABG, coronary artery bypass graft.

artery bypass surgery was performed in approximately 25% of patients.

Whereas PCI often can be performed at the time of coronary angiography, or shortly afterward, coronary artery surgery typically is delayed in comparison. Such delays can be anticipated because of simple logistics as well as availability of resources (e.g., number of surgeons, operating rooms). The timing of surgery is typically more delayed in European centers compared with centers in the United States, primarily as a result of fewer available resources and problems with long waiting lists. In the recently reported TACTICS-TIMI 18 (Treat angina with Aggrastat and determine Cost of Therapy with an Invasive or Conservative Strategy-Thrombolysis in Myocardial Infarction) trial,[3] which predominantly enrolled patients at hospitals in the United States, the median delay to surgery from randomization was about 3.5 days. In contrast, in the recently reported British RITA-3 (Revascularization Intervention to Treat Angina) trial, surgery was performed at a median of 22 days, with only about half of the patients who had been selected for surgery undergoing their procedure during the index hospitalization.[4] In the Scandinavian FRISC II (Fragmin and Fast Revascularization during Instability in Coronary artery disease) trial the median delay to surgery was 7 days.[11]

Therefore, it can be reasonably expected that a significant proportion of patients who present with ACS will be found to have coronary disease severe enough to warrant the consideration of surgical revascularization during, or soon after, their index hospitalization. More extensive disease, and thus disease more likely to be treated surgically, often can be predicted by simple clinical parameters prior to angiography. These include a history of prior MI, diabetes mellitus, history of heart failure and peripheral vascular disease.[12]

MORTALITY ASSOCIATED WITH SURGICAL REVASCULARIZATION

There is surprisingly a paucity of recent data concerning the outcome of patients who undergo surgical revascularization for unstable angina or NSTEMI. Two very early randomized trials comparing coronary artery bypass surgery to medical therapy were conducted in the United States 25 to 30 years ago. The first was the National Cooperative Study Group that randomized almost 300 patients but excluded those with recent infarction or those older than 70 years of age.[13] Mortality for the group undergoing surgery was 5%; for those receiving medical therapy, it was 3%. The second trial was the Veterans Administration Cooperative Study that randomized almost 500 patients to either surgery or medical therapy.[14] This trial had similar entry criteria but enrolled only men. Mortality was 4.1% among the surgical patients in this study. Overall 2-year survival appeared to be similar among the patients randomized to surgery or medical therapy, but among patients with lower left-ventricular ejection fractions (LVEFs), survival was significantly better in those who had undergone surgical revascularization.

Those earlier studies were performed at a time when surgical techniques were less advanced than they are at present. Improvements in surgical technique, including use of predominantly arterial grafts, improved myocardial protective measures, and better adjunctive and convalescent medical care and therapy, can be expected to have had favorable influences on the outcome of patients undergoing surgical revascularization in the current era.

It is helpful to review the outcome of patients who were selected for surgical revascularization in some of the large trials listed in Tables 12-1 and 12-2. The surgical mortality of patients who underwent surgery in the FRISC II trial was 2.1% among the invasive group and 1.7% among patients who were initially conservatively treated.[11] Thirty-day mortality was 3.0% among all patients who underwent surgery in the RITA-3 trial.[4] These results need to put in perspective when comparing them to the earlier outcomes discussed previously. These more recent trials enrolled older patients, many more women, and many patients who had presented with NSTEMI.

The only anomalous trial result was that from the VANQWISH (Veterans Affairs Non-Q Wave Infarction Strategies in Hospital) trial, which reported a 30-day surgical mortality of 11.6% among the 95 patients who were referred for surgery in the invasive-strategy group.[15] The mortality was only 3.5% in the 87 patients who eventually were referred for surgery from the conservative-strategy group. Nevertheless, the high mortality seen in this trial resulted in much debate and controversy. The operative mortality of 11.6% was clearly higher than the average of 3.2% calculated in a large meta-analysis of coronary artery bypass surgery trials conducted approximately 20 or more years ago.[7] Although the latter analysis included data from perhaps a more stable population, many patients in these early trials had presented with unstable angina; moreover, patients with recurrent or persistent ischemia, or those with evidence of significant heart failure, were excluded from the VANQWISH trial. The VANQWISH surgical mortality was also significantly higher than in either the National Cooperative Group or Veterans Administration trials discussed earlier.[13,14] No satisfactory explanation has been forthcoming, and perhaps the most important lesson to be learned is that patients must be carefully selected, optimal adjunctive medical therapy must be used, and experienced surgical teams must be used when patients with recent infarction are being considered for early surgical revascularization.

Two other relatively recent surgical series also deserve some scrutiny. The studies were retrospective analyses of patients treated in the setting of unstable angina at two European centers. The first was reported from Belgium and included 474 patients who underwent coronary surgical revascularization during a 7-year period from 1986 to 1993.[16] The average age of these patients was 65 years, with the oldest being 85 years of age. There was a high prevalence of use of arterial conduits (83%) including single, bilateral, and sequential internal thoracic arterial grafts and inferior epigastric arterial grafts. Use of intraaortic balloon counter pulsation support was almost 20%. This patient series included 68 patients who were operated on as emergencies (14%). In-hospital mortality was relatively high (6.8%), although mortality was somewhat lower in the later period of observation. Longer aortic cross-clamp time was the single most important predictor of worse outcome followed by need for urgent transfer from intensive care, presence of left-ventricular aneurysm, female sex, greater number of diseased vessels, and reoperation.

The second of the two European studies was a retrospective analysis of 853 patients who had coronary artery bypass surgery for unstable angina at the Karolinska Hospital in Stockholm, Sweden.[17] The importance of this study was the demonstration of declining surgical mortality over time. Of patients, 28% had postinfarction angina, whereas the remainder had Braunwald class B angina.[18] Age range of patients extended to 84 years with a mean of 64 years. All surgeries were performed urgently; 4% were considered emergencies. Approximately 10% of patients had heart failure and reduced left-ventricular function. Three-vessel disease and left-main coronary disease were present in 61% and 18% of patients, respectively. The internal thoracic artery was used in 92% of patients, and a mean of 3.6 distal anastomoses was performed. Overall 30-day mortality was 5.9%, declining from a high of 9.7% in 1990 to 2.6% in 1995. Significant predictors of a fatal outcome included a history of prior coronary artery bypass surgery, congestive heart failure, emergency procedure after failed coronary angioplasty, and extended aortic cross-clamp times (especially if longer than 60 minutes). The outcome of patients with respect to survival and survival free of infarction was significantly better if the internal thoracic artery had been used. The decline in mortality was not explained by any differences in patient characteristics over time and was concluded to be the result of improved operator technique and better periprocedural care.

In summary, excellent results can be anticipated in selected patients referred for coronary artery bypass surgery who have presented with an ACS. However, a subset of high-risk patients can be identified who will require more intensive care (Table 12-3). These include patients who are treated in the setting of emergency procedures, have had prior coronary artery surgery, and who undergo longer and more difficult procedures resulting in longer aortic cross-clamp times. Use of arterial conduits, particularly in situ thoracic arteries, should be used whenever possible because, in addition to improved long-term outcomes, short-term outcomes also appear to be improved with their use.

A recently published analysis of surgical outcomes of patients with unstable angina provided a comparison

■ ■ ■

TABLE 12-3   RISK FACTORS FOR EARLY MORTALITY AFTER CORONARY SURGICAL REVASCULARIZATION IN PATIENTS WITH ACUTE CORONARY SYNDROMES

Prior coronary artery bypass graft surgery
Prolonged aortic cross-clamp duration
Number of diseased vessels requiring revascularization
Left-ventricular aneurysm
Congestive heart failure
Emergency surgery for failed percutaneous coronary intervention
Female sex

with patients who had undergone PCI. The trial was randomized by design, and this analysis was a post hoc one of the subset of 450 patients with unstable angina comparing 226 patients assigned to surgery and 224 to PCI.[19] Almost one-third of patients had three-vessel disease, and left-ventricular function was relatively preserved. Stents were used in almost all of the PCIs, with an average of almost 2.5 lesions treated per patient. Arterial conduits were used in almost all surgical patients to bypass the left anterior descending coronary artery (94% of cases). Hospital mortality was similar for both groups, as was 1-year event-free survival in terms of death, myocardial infarction (MI), and stroke. One-year mortality was 2.2% among surgical patients and 2.7% among patients in the stent group. The only significant difference was in the greater frequency of repeat revascularization procedures in the stent group compared with the surgical group (16.8% vs. 3.6%, respectively).

Finally, some further appreciation of the outcome of patients who undergo surgical revascularization after presenting with unstable angina can be obtained from the recent Veterans Affairs' AWSOME (Angina With Extremely Serious Operative Mortality Evaluation) study.[20,21] This trial enrolled patients who had angina refractory to medical therapy who were then randomized to either PCI or coronary artery surgery. This trial, however, cannot be considered to be one of ACS because the entry criteria included only patients with medically refractory angina who also were considered to be at high risk for coronary artery bypass surgery. However, it is likely that many patients in the trial did have unstable angina at entry. Furthermore, approximately one-third of patients had suffered an MI within 7 days of randomization.

Patients (n = 232) were randomized to coronary artery bypass surgery and included 23% with LVEF of less than 0.35, 33% with two-vessel disease, and 50% with three-vessel disease. Left internal thoracic arterial grafts were used in 70% of patients (approximately one third of patients had previously had coronary artery bypass surgery), whereas 3.2% had a right internal thoracic arterial graft and 2.9% had a radial arterial graft. The 30-day mortality was 5%, compared with 3% for those undergoing angioplasty (stent use of 54%). The 3-year survival was similar between the two randomized groups (79% for those who underwent surgery and 80% for those who had angioplasty performed). Freedom from unstable angina was similar for the two groups, although the need for repeat revascularization was significantly lower among surgically treated patients. Registry data from the same trial (physician-directed or patient-choice treatments) revealed similar outcomes.[22] Furthermore, no significant differences were found in short- or long-term survival among patients with diabetes with respect to their revascularization assignment.[23] Thus, both surgical and percutaneous revascularization approaches are associated with similar outcomes; the registry data would suggest that good clinical judgment with respect to assessment of patients' suitability and risk for each approach is likely to be reliable in patients with certain clinical or angiographic characteristics.

A summary of guidelines for choosing surgical or percutaneous revascularization procedures for patients with

TABLE 12-4 SUMMARY OF GUIDELINES FOR MODE OF CORONARY REVASCULARIZATION IN PATIENTS WITH ACUTE CORONARY SYNDROMES

Coronary disease severity	Optimal revascularization choice
Left-main disease	
Surgical candidate	CABG
Not surgical candidate	PCI
Three-vessel disease	
LVEF <0.50 and diabetes	CABG
LVEF <0.50 and proximal LAD	CABG
LVEF <0.50 and no diabetes or proximal LAD	CABG or PCI
LVEF >0.50 and with or without diabetes or proximal LAD	CABG or PCI
One- or two-vessel disease	
Proximal LAD and LVEF <0.50	CABG (or PCI if one-vessel disease)
Proximal LAD and LVEF >0.50	CABG or PCI
No proximal LAD and significant ischemia on noninvasive testing	PCI (if feasible)
No proximal LAD and minimal ischemia on noninvasive testing or inadequate medical therapy	None
Prior CABG with saphenous graft stenoses	
Multiple stenoses, especially with involvement of the graft to the LAD	CABG
Focal stenoses (single)	PCI
Focal stenoses (multiple) but poor surgical candidate	PCI

CABG, coronary artery bypass graft; PCI, percutaneous coronary intervention; LEVF, left-ventricular ejection fraction; LAD, left anterior descending.
Modified from Braunwald E, Antman EM, Beasley JW. ACC/AHA 2002 Guideline Update for the Management of Patients With Unstable Angina and Non-ST-Segment Elevation Myocardial Infarction Bethesda, MD, American College of Cardiology, 2002.

ACS is presented in Table 12-4 and is modified from the American College of Cardiology/American Heart Association (ACC/AHA) practice guidelines (www.acc.org).

BLEEDING RISKS

The initial medical treatment of patients treated for ACS includes the use of potent antiplatelet and antithrombotic agents. Antiplatelet therapy with aspirin combined with heparin, either unfractionated or low–molecular-weight, is the mainstay of the initial medical management for these patients. Use of aspirin is ubiquitous among patients with coronary artery disease, and most cardiac surgeons are currently comfortable with its use prior to coronary artery bypass surgery. Indeed, better surgical outcomes have been demonstrated when aspirin is used. Heparin is used intraoperatively, and its use prior to surgery is generally not associated with any significant risk of serious bleeding. More potent antiplatelet therapy with platelet glycoprotein IIb/IIIa inhibitors is also recommended as additional therapy for most patients.[1] More recently, the early administration of clopidogrel has been recommended as an additional antiplatelet agent.[1,2] Although these therapies have proven benefits in terms of early outcome, they have the potential to complicate the outcome of patients who undergo early coronary artery bypass surgery because of the associated risks of bleeding.

Platelet Glycoprotein IIb/IIIa Inhibitors

There is a significant reduction in mortality and MI among patients with ACS who are treated with IIb/IIIa inhibitors in addition to aspirin and heparin.[24,25] The use of tirofiban and eptifibatide in patients with ACS now is recommended in the published ACC/AHA guide-lines for the management of ACS.[1] A third IIb/IIIa inhibitor, abciximab, is approved only for use during PCI; therefore, it will be an issue only with respect to coronary artery bypass surgery in the rare case of failed PCI requiring emergency surgery. It currently is not recommended for the treatment of patients with ACS except when PCI is performed.[1] The requirement of red-cell and platelet transfusions is significantly higher when abciximab has been used immediately before coronary artery bypass surgery.[26]

In the PURSUIT (Platelet IIb/IIIa in Unstable angina: Receptor Suppression Using Integrelin Therapy) trial, more than 10,000 patients with ACS were randomized to receive either an infusion of eptifibatide or placebo.[25] Surgical outcomes were subsequently reported from 78 patients who required immediate or emergency coronary bypass surgery within 2 hours of discontinuing the study medication; 46 of these patients had been receiving placebo, whereas the remaining 32 had received eptifibatide.[27] Major bleeding, defined as an absolute decrease of 15% in the hematocrit or 5 g/dL reduction in hemoglobin, was reported in 64% and 63% of patients, respectively. There was no difference in the need for blood transfusions, which were required in more than half of the patients, and no difference in platelet transfusions, which were given in about one third of patients. Mortality was 6.3% and 6.5%, respectively.

A greater number of patients in the PURSUIT trial underwent less emergent surgery.[28] The primary endpoint of the trial was death and MI at 6 months and, among the patients who had coronary artery bypass surgery performed during the index hospitalization, was significantly lower in the group who had received eptifibatide (27.6%) than in the placebo group (32.7%). The eptifibatide infusions were discontinued an average of 66.5 hours prior to surgery with a range of 18 to 184 hours. As with the experience of the emergency cases, there was no significant difference in major bleeding. The reduction in the primary endpoints was much greater among patients who underwent surgery who had their study drug stopped only within 72 hours of surgery compared with those who had it stopped for a longer period. Thus, from these data, it appears that the use of eptifibatide prior to coronary artery bypass surgery poses no additive risk of bleeding.

Coronary artery bypass surgery was performed on an urgent basis in approximately 3% of patients in the PRISM-PLUS (Platelet Receptor Inhibition in Ischemic Syndrome Management in Patients Limited by Unstable Signs and Symptoms) trial. No excess of moderate to severe bleeding requiring transfusion was seen in the tirofiban–heparin group (4 of 11 patients) compared with the heparin-alone group (7 of 17 patients) (Stolz R. of Merck & Co., Inc., personal communication). The half-lives of tirofiban and eptifibatide are approximately 2 hours, and the antiplatelet activity is even more rapidly reversible. Therefore, cessation of these drugs within a few hours of surgery should suffice to minimize risks of periprocedural bleeding. Discontinuing them too early in an unstable patient may result in overall worse outcome because of the higher risk of acute MI and death. There is no widespread use of "point-of-care" or other laboratory tests that measure the degree of antiplatelet activity of the glycoprotein IIb/IIIa inhibitors during or after their administration. Such tools would likely be very helpful in guiding therapy in these unstable patients prior to surgery.

Low–Molecular-Weight Heparin

Low–molecular-weight heparin (LMWH) is gradually replacing unfractionated heparin (UFH) in hospital use because of its ease of use, its more predictable anticoagulant effect with greater bioavailability, and its slightly lower risk of heparin-associated thrombocytopenia. Furthermore, results of two trials comparing enoxaparin to UFH in patients with ACS have shown that the former was more efficacious in terms of reduction in coronary events.[29,30] LMWH is usually administered as a bolus injection, subcutaneously, once or twice a day and has a longer half-life than UFH. Minor bleeding appears to be more frequent with LMWH than UFH, and reversal with protamine cannot be fully relied on. These issues could have important implications for patients treated with LMWH who subsequently require urgent or emergency coronary artery bypass surgery.

The largest retrospective surgical study of patients with ACS comparing pretreatment with UFH to pretreatment with enoxaparin was reported from the Hospital for Latter Day Saints (Salt Lake City, Utah).[31] The outcomes of 1008 patients who received UFH, stopped just prior to entering the operating room, were compared with 151 patients who had been receiving enoxaparin with the last dose administered a mean of about 15 hours prior to open heart surgery. UFH was used during surgery in all patients. Concomitant use of clopidogrel or ticlopidine, or glycoprotein IIb/IIIa inhibitors, was infrequent. Transfusion requirements of red cells or platelets were similar for each group. However, reoperation for bleeding complications was required significantly more frequently in the enoxaparin group compared with the UFH group (7.9% vs. 3.7%, respectively); this difference remained significant even after adjustment for various pertinent baseline differences. However, the study's conclusions are limited to some extent by its retrospective nature, lack of randomization, and relatively small size.

A British surgical study has also raised concerns of increased bleeding risks with concurrent use of LMWH.[32] Patients with unstable angina who underwent coronary artery bypass surgery less than 12 hours after their last Fragmin injections, had significantly more bleeding, but not more reoperations, than either those who had their surgery delayed beyond 12 hours or those who had received only UFH.

The use of UFH is currently recommended over LMWH if coronary artery surgery is planned within the following 24 hours,[1] but further studies are clearly required to fully evaluate the safety of proceeding with open-heart surgery in patients being treated with LMWH. One of the fundamentally important issues is the general unavailability of specific monitoring tools to assess the extent of anticoagulation in these patients. Routine coagulation tests such as prothrombin time, activated partial prothrombin time, and activated clotting time do not provide useful information to guide therapy. Although monitoring tests that measure anti-Xa activity and anti-IIa activity are being introduced slowly, they are not widely available and furthermore there is no consensus on their use to guide therapeutic decisions (e.g., the timing of surgery, need for additional anticoagulation, or effectiveness of reversal). Reversal of the anticoagulant effect of LMWH with protamine is also not as predictable as it is for UFH. With the increasing use of LMWH in patients with ACS, there is clearly an urgent need for more formal studies and guidelines for the management of patients who will require surgery.

Clopidogrel

The antiplatelet thienopyridine derivatives, ticlopidine and now more frequently clopidogrel, are used routinely as an adjunct to aspirin to prevent stent thrombosis after intracoronary stent placement. Clopidogrel has been advocated for the initial treatment of ACS based on the results of the CURE (Clopidogrel in Unstable angina to prevent Recurrent Events) trial.[2] In this large trial, patients were randomized to receive 300 mg of clopidogrel followed by 75 mg of clopidogrel per day or a matching placebo, in addition to aspirin, for 3 to 12 months. Bleeding, major and minor, was significantly more frequent with use of clopidogrel than placebo. In the initial trial publication, no significant excess in major bleeding after coronary artery bypass surgery with use of clopidogrel was reported. However, most patients in the CURE trial had had their clopidogrel discontinued prior to surgery. No excess in major bleeding was observed among those who had surgery more than 5 days later. Although no detailed analysis was provided for the patients who had surgery within 5 days of discontinuing clopidogrel, an overall excess of bleeding was evident (9.6% vs. 6.3%).

Since the introduction and now widespread use of clopidogrel, many cardiac surgeons have voiced concern about the potential increased risk of serious bleeding in patients taking clopidogrel and who then undergo open heart surgery. The only published experience of such patients since the CURE publication is from Hongo and colleagues.[33] Theirs was a prospective analysis of a non-randomized consecutive cohort of 224 patients undergoing elective coronary artery bypass surgery. Bleeding complications were compared between 59 patients who had received clopidogrel within at least 7 days of surgery and 165 patients who had not received clopidogrel. Bleeding was measured by chest tube drainage volumes and blood-product transfusions. Reoperation for bleeding was performed more than 10 times more frequently in the group of patients who had received clopidogrel (6.8% vs. 0.6%). These findings raise significant concern about performing coronary artery bypass surgery on patients who have taken clopidogrel within the prior few days, particularly if the surgery is not urgent.

At hospitals where an early-invasive approach is generally followed for patients with ACS, the question of whether to start clopidogrel prior to coronary angiography is an important one. It is important to recognize that in the CURE trial, clopidogrel was not started until a mean of 14 hours after admission, IIb/IIIa inhibitors were not used, and more than one fourth of the patients were not receiving heparin at the time of drug initiation. Furthermore, coronary angiography was performed a mean of 8 days after admission, with interventions performed even later (PCI and coronary artery bypass surgery). Overall, the management of patients in the CURE trial should be considered very conservative compared with the usual management of patients with ACS in the United States and many other countries. If patients are to undergo early angiography (i.e., less than 24 or 48 hours after admission), it would probably be wise to not begin clopidogrel until coronary angiography has documented the coronary anatomy; this approach has also been recommended by the ACC/AHA guidelines committee.[1] Almost all patients can be stabilized on heparin, with LMWH being superior to UFH, and many also can receive an adjunctive IIb/IIIa inhibitor. Many patients may be found to have coronary disease best suited for surgical revascularization. If these patients already have been administered clopidogrel, their surgical morbidity will be increased significantly unless their surgery is delayed by at least 5 to 7 days, at which time the antiplatelet effect of clopidogrel should be minimal. If medical treatment does not include the use of a IIb/IIIa inhibitor and coronary angiography is likely to be delayed by a few days, particularly if coronary artery bypass surgery is unlikely to be performed or delayed by a week or so, then clopidogrel is likely to be useful.

RECENT ADVANCES IN REVASUCULARIZATION TECHNIQUES

Off-Pump Coronary Artery Bypass

Although the majority of coronary artery bypass surgery is still performed with cardiopulmonary bypass, an increasing number of patients is undergoing revascular-ization with the off-pump technique (OPCAB).[34] The possible advantages of this technique include shorter intensive care and hospital stays,[35,36] decreased blood product requirements,[37,38] better preservation of renal function,[39] less cost when compared with conventional bypass techniques,[40] and perhaps a reduction in neurologic complications. However, the data regarding neurologic events after off-pump surgery are conflicting. In a small randomized study of 281 patients, the 30-day incidence of stroke was not statistically different in the conventional coronary artery bypass surgery group compared with the off-pump surgical group (1.4% vs. 0.7%).[38] However, a review of the Society of Thoracic Surgeons' database of more than 100,000 coronary artery bypass surgical procedures from 1998 to 1999, showed that neurologic complications occurred statistically less frequently in the off-pump surgical group compared with the conventional group (1.25% vs. 1.99%, P < 0.001).[39]

Although initial experience with off-pump coronary bypass procedures was restricted to low-risk patients with single- or double-vessel disease,[41,42] experience has shown that the patients most likely to benefit from this technique are higher risk, older patients who are more susceptible to the risks of cardiopulmonary bypass.[35] However, concern still exists regarding the long-term outcome of the procedure, particularly with regard to long-term patency of grafts, recurrence of angina, and need for further interventions. One retrospective analysis has reported that patients treated with off-pump techniques have a higher risk of recurrent angina at 1 year when compared with patients having on-pump procedures.[36] Moreover, revascularization is not always complete in patients in whom off-pump techniques have been used.[43] At this time coronary artery bypass surgery, using conventional cardiopulmonary bypass techniques, still remains the gold standard for surgical myocardial revascularization.

Patients with unstable coronary symptoms most likely to benefit from off-pump surgical revascularization surgery are elderly patients with well-preserved left-ventricular function and stable hemodynamics. Patients with poor left-ventricular function, unstable hemodynamics, and calcified coronary arteries or intramyocardial vessels are better served by coronary artery bypass surgery using conventional cardiopulmonary bypass techniques. If, during an off-pump surgical revascularization, the surgeon feels that the patient might be harmed by inadequate or suboptimal revascularization, or if there is deterioration in the hemodynamics, then the operation should be converted to a standard cardiopulmonary bypass procedure.

Drug-Eluting Stents

This discussion has focused on the indications and use of surgical revascularization for ACS with emphasis placed on following the currently accepted recommendations for surgical revascularization rather than PCI in certain clinical and angiographic subgroups of patients (Table 12-4). One of the major limitations of PCI, with balloon angioplasty or stent placement, is the risk of restenosis, and in-stent restenosis is particularly difficult to treat.

Recently, stents have been developed with drug-eluting properties, with antiproliferative drugs, such as sirolimus and paclitaxel, incorporated onto polymerized stents. These stents then slowly "elute" the specific drug over a few weeks; the antiproliferative properties of these drugs then retard or prevent the proliferation of neointimal tissue that is the hallmark of in-stent restenosis. Clinical trials have confirmed the enormous potential for such stents to significantly lower in-restenosis rates in carefully selected patients.[44-47] However, large-scale trials will be required to prove that these new stents will be equivalent or superior to coronary artery bypass surgery in patients with severe multivessel disease, left-main disease, or diabetes. Depending on the results of these trials, these drug-eluting stents could have a major influence in the future on the choice of revascularization strategy in many patients with ACS.

REFERENCES

1. Braunwald E, Antman EM, Beasley JW, et al: ACC/AHA 2002 guideline update for the management of patients with unstable angina and non-ST-segment elevation myocardial infarction: Summary article. J Am Coll Cardiol 2002; 40:1366-1374.
2. The CURE investigators: Effects of clopidogrel in addition to aspirin in patients with acute coronary syndromes without ST-segment elevation. N Engl J Med 2001; 345:494-502.
3. Cannon CP, Weintraub WS, Demopoulos LA, et al: Comparison of early invasive and conservative strategies in patients with unstable coronary syndromes treated with the glycoprotein IIb/IIIa Inhibitor Tirofiban. N Engl J Med 2001; 344:1879-1887.
4. Fox KAA, Poole-Wilson PA, Henderson RA, et al: Interventional versus conservative treatment for patients with unstable angina or non-ST-elevation myocardial infarction: The British Heart Foundation RITA 3 randomized trial. Lancet 2002; 2002:743-751.
5. Wallentin L, Lagerqvist B, Husted S, et al: Outcome at 1 year after an invasive compared with a non-invasive strategy in unstable coronary-artery disease: The FRISC II invasive randomized trial. Lancet 2000; 356:9-16.
6. Yusuf S, Zucker D, Peduzzi P, et al: Effect of coronary artery bypass graft surgery on survival: Overview of 10-year results from randomized trials by the Coronary Artery Bypass Graft Surgery Trialists Collaboration. Lancet 1994; 344:563-570.
7. Pocock SJ, Henderson RA, Rickards AF, et al: Meta-analysis of randomised trials comparing coronary angioplasty with bypass surgery. Lancet 1995; 346:1184-1189.
8. The BARI investigators: Comparison of coronary bypass surgery with angioplasty in patients with multivessel disease. N Engl J Med 1996; 335:217-225.
9. Detre KM, Guo P, Holubkov R, et al: Coronary revascularization in diabetic patients: A comparison of the randomized and observational components of the bypass angioplasty revascularization Investigation (BARI). Circulation 1999; 99:633-640.
10. Seshadri N, Whitlow PL, Acharya N, et al: Emergency Coronary Artery Bypass Surgery in the Contemporary Percutaneous Coronary Intervention Era. Circulation 2002; 106:2346-2350.
11. The FRISC II investigatoirs: Invasive compared with non-invasive treatment in unstable coronary-artery disease: FRISC II prospective randomized multicentre study. Lancet 1999; 354:708-715.
12. Gibbons R, Chatterjee K, Daley J, et al: ACC/AHA/ACP-ASIM Guidelines for the management of patients with chronic stable angina: A report of the American College of Cardiology/American Heart Association Task Force on Practice Guidelines (Committee on the Management of Patients with Chronic Stable Angina). J Am Coll Cardiol 1999; 33:2092-2197.
13. Unstable angina pectoris: National Cooperative Study Group to Compare Surgical and Medical Therapy. Am J Cardiol 1978; 42:839-848.
14. Luchi R, Scott S, Deupree R: Comparison of medical and surgical treatment for unstable angina pectoris. Results of a Veterans Administration Cooperative Study. N Engl J Med 1987; 316:977-984.
15. Boden WE, O'Rourke RA, Crawford MH, et al: Outcomes in patients with acute non-Q-wave myocardial infarction randomly assigned to an invasive as compared with a conservative management strategy. N Engl J Med 1998; 338:1785-1792.
16. Louagie YAG, Jamart J, Buche M, et al: Operation for unstable angina pectoris: Factors influencing adverse in-hospital outcome. Ann Thorac Surg 1995; 59:1141-1149.
17. Bjessmo S, Hammar N, Sandberg E, et al: Reduced risk of coronary artery bypass surgery for unstable angina during a 6-year period. Eur J Cardiothorac Surg 2000; 18:388-392.
18. Braunwald E. Unstable angina. A classification. Circulation 1989; 80:410-414.
19. de Feyter PJ, Serruys PW, Unger F, et al: Bypass surgery versus stenting for the treatment of multivessel disease in patients with unstable angina compared with stable angina. Circulation 2002; 105:2367-2372.
20. Morrison DA, Sethi G, Sacks J, et al: A multicenter, randomized trial of percutaneous coronary intervention versus bypass surgery in high-risk unstable angina patients. The AWESOME (Veterans Affairs Cooperative Study #385, angina with extremely serious operative mortality evaluation) investigators from the Cooperative Studies Program of the Department of Veterans Affairs. Control Clin Trials 1999; 20:601-619.
21. Morrison DA, Sethi G, Sacks J, et al: Percutaneous coronary intervention versus coronary bypass graft surgery for patients with medically refractory myocardial ischemia and risk factors for adverse outcomes with bypass: A multicenter randomized trial. J Am Coll Cardiol 2001; 38:143-149.
22. Morrison DA, Sethi G, Sacks J, et al: Percutaneous coronary intervention versus coronary bypass graft surgery for patients with medically refractory myocardial ischemia and risk factors for adverse outcomes with bypass. The VA AWESOME multicenter registry: Comparison with the randomized clinical trial. J Am Coll Cardiol 2002; 39:266-273.
23. Sedlis SP, Morrison DA, Lorin JD, et al: Percutaneous coronary intervention versus coronary bypass graft surgery for diabetic patients with unstable angina and risk factors for adverse outcomes with bypass: Outcomes of diabetic patients in the AWESOME randomized trial and registry. J Am Coll Cardiol 2002; 40:1555-1566.
24. The PRISM-PLUS study investigators: Inhibition of the platelet glycoprotein IIb/IIIa receptor with tirofiban in unstable angina and non-Q-wave myocardial infarction. N Engl J Med 1998; 338:1488-1497.
25. The PURSUIT trial investigators: Inhibition of platelet glycoprotein IIb/IIIa with eptifibatide in patients with acute coronary syndromes. N Engl J Med 1998; 339:436-443.
26. Singh M, Nuttall G, Ballman K, et al: Effect of abciximab on the outcome of emergency coronary artery bypass grafting after failed percutaneous coronary intervention. Mayo Clin Proc 2001; 76:784-788.
27. Dyke C, Bhatia D, Lorenz T, et al: Immediate coronary artery bypass surgery after platelet inhibition with eptifibatide: Results from PURSUIT. Platelet Glycoprotein IIb/IIIa in Unstable Angina: Receptor Suppression Using Integrelin Therapy. Ann Thorac Surg 2000; 70:866-871; discussion 871-872.
28. Marso SP, Bhatt DL, Roe MT, et al: Enhanced efficacy of eptifibatide administration in patients with acute coronary syndrome requiring in-hospital coronary artery bypass grafting. Circulation 2000; 102:2952-2958.
29. Cohen M, Demers C, Gurfinkel EP, et al: A comparison of low-molecular-weight heparin with unfractionated heparin for unstable coronary artery disease. N Engl J Med 1997; 337:447-452.
30. Antman EM, McCabe CH, Gurfinkel EP, et al: Enoxaparin prevents death and cardiac ischemic events in unstable angina/non-Q-wave myocardial infarction: Results of the Thrombolysis In Myocardial Infarction (TIMI) 11B Trial. Circulation 1999; 100:1593-1601.
31. Jones HU, Muhlestein JB, Jones KW, et al: Preoperative use of enoxaparin compared with unfractionated heparin increases the incidence of re-exploration for postoperative bleeding after open-heart surgery in patients who present with an acute coronary syndrome: Clinical investigation and reports. Circulation 2002; 106:19I-22.
32. Clark S, Vitale N, Zacharias J, et al: Effect of low molecular weight heparin (fragmin) on bleeding after cardiac surgery. Ann Thorac Surg 2000; 69:762-765.
33. Hongo RH, Ley J, Dick SE, et al: The effect of clopidogrel in combination with aspirin when given before coronary artery bypass grafting. J Am Coll Cardiol 2002; 40:231-237.

34. Mack M, Duhaylongsod F: Through the open door! Where has the ride taken us? J Thorac Cardiovasc Surg 2002; 124:655–659.

35. Al-Ruzzeh S, Nakamura K, Athanasiou T, et al: Does off-pump coronary artery bypass (OPCAB) surgery improve the outcome in high-risk patients? A comparative study of 1398 high-risk patients. Eur J Cardiothorac Surg 2003; 23:50–55.

36. Arom K, Flavin T, Emery R, et al: Safety and efficacy of off pump coronary bypass grafting. Ann Thorac Surg 2000; 69:704–710.

37. Ascione R, Williams S, Lloyd C, et al: Reduced postoperative blood loss and transfusion requirement after beating-heart coronary operations: A prospective randomized study. J Thorac Cardiovasc Surg 2001; 121:689–696.

38. van Dijk D, Nierich A, Jansen E, et al: Early outcome after off-pump versus on-pump coronary bypass surgery. Circulation 2001; 104:1761–1766.

39. Cleveland J, Shroyer L, Chen A, et al: Off-pump coronary artery bypass grafting decreases risk-adjusted mortality and morbidity. Ann Thorac Surg 2001; 72:1282–1289.

40. Nathoe H, van Dijk D, Jansen E, et al: A comparison of on-pump and off-pump coronary bypass surgery in low-risk patients. N Engl J Med 2003; 348:394–402.

41. Benetti F, Naselli G, Wood M, et al: Direct myocardial revascularization without extracorporeal circulation. Chest 1991; 100:312–316.

42. Haase M, Sharma A, Fielitz A, et al: On-pump coronary artery surgery versus off-pump exclusive arterial coronary grafting: A matched cohort comparison. Ann Thorac Surg 2003; 75:62–67.

43. Sabik J, Gillinov A, Blackstone E, et al: Does off-pump coronary surgery reduce morbidity and mortality? J Thorac Cardiovasc Surg 2002; 124:698–707.

44. Morice M-C, Serruys PW, Sousa JE, et al: A randomized comparison of a sirolimus-eluting stent with a standard stent for coronary revascularization. N Engl J Med 2002; 346:1773–1780.

45. Grube E, Silber S, Hauptmann KE, et al: TAXUS I: Six- and twelve-month results from a randomized, double-blind trial on a slow-release paclitaxel-eluting stent for de novo coronary lesions. Circulation 2003; 107:38–42.

46. Sousa JE, Costa MA, Abizaid AC, et al: Sustained suppression of neointimal proliferation by sirolimus-eluting stents: One-year angiographic and intravascular ultrasound follow-up. Circulation 2001; 104:2007–2011.

47. Sousa JE, Costa MA, Sousa AGMR, et al: Two-year angiographic and intravascular ultrasound follow-up after implantation of sirolimus-eluting stents in human coronary arteries. Circulation 2003; 107:381–383.

48. The TIMI IIIB investigators: Effects of tissue plasminogen activator and a comparison of early invasive and conservative strategies in unstable angina and non-Q-wave myocardial infarction. Results of the TIMI IIIB Trial. Thrombolysis in myocardial ischemia. Circulation 1994; 89:1545–1556.

49. The GUSTO IIb investigators: A comparison of recombinant hirudin with heparin for the treatment of acute coronary syndromes. N Engl J Med 1996; 335:775–782.

■ ■ ■ chapter 13

Drug Therapy for Ventricular Tachycardia and Ventricular Fibrillation

J. Michael Mangrum
John P. DiMarco

For many years it was believed that controlled clinical trials for patients with sustained ventricular arrhythmias should not be performed because of ethical considerations. When invasive techniques for studying cardiac arrhythmias were introduced, however, it became clear that previous treatment strategies for patients with ventricular arrhythmias based solely on anecdotal experience were not optimal and that randomized trials evaluating therapy should be conducted. This chapter provides a review of clinical trials dealing with the acute management and the primary and secondary prevention of sustained ventricular tachycardia (VT) and ventricular fibrillation (VF).

SUSTAINED MONOMORPHIC VENTRICULAR TACHYCARDIA: ACUTE THERAPY

Sustained monomorphic VT may have a variety of clinical presentations and may be caused by several electrophysiologic mechanisms. In patients with structurally normal hearts, sustained episodes of VT that are sensitive to intravenous adenosine and/or verapamil have been described. These arrhythmias are rarely encountered in clinical practice, and no randomized trials dealing with these arrhythmias have been conducted. When sustained VT produces hemodynamic collapse or degenerates rapidly into VF, acute management consists of antiarrhythmic therapy as an adjunct to electrical cardioversion and defibrillation, as described later in this chapter, for victims of cardiac arrest. When sustained VT is well tolerated, randomized trials comparing antiarrhythmic drugs are possible, but only a few such studies have been reported.

Griffith and colleagues[1] studied 24 patients with inducible sustained VT induced during serial electrophysiologic studies. Of these 24 patients, 20 had coronary artery disease with prior myocardial infarction (MI); 3 had no structural heart disease, and 1 had a nonischemic cardiomyopathy. Of the 24, 12 were receiving chronic amiodarone therapy. VT was induced with pro-grammed stimulation. The tachycardia had a stable cycle length and electrocardiographic morphology and was hemodynamically well tolerated. The effects of intravenous adenosine (50–250 µg/kg), lidocaine (1.5 mg/kg), disopyramide (2 mg/kg, ≤150 mg), flecainide (2 mg/kg, ≤150 mg), and sotalol (1 mg/kg) were assessed after appropriate washout intervals during serial studies of the same induced tachycardia in each patient. Termination of the induced VT was seen with the following frequencies: adenosine, 0%; lidocaine, 30%; disopyramide, 50%; flecainide, 55%; and sotalol, 36%. Although flecainide was the most effective, it produced serious adverse reactions in 25% of the patients who received it. Sotalol (4 of 4), flecainide (4 of 4), disopyramide (4 of 4), and lidocaine (3 of 4) were most effective in patients without coronary disease.

Gorgels and colleagues[2] compared the efficacy of lidocaine and procainamide for termination of hemodynamically tolerated spontaneous, monomorphic VT in a small randomized, parallel study. The study included 29 patients; 25 had ischemic heart disease. Procainamide (10 mg/kg at 100 mg/min) and lidocaine (1.5 mg/kg, over 2 minutes) were administered during stable VT. Patients whose arrhythmia did not terminate after the first drug or those who later developed a recurrent episode received the alternate drug. Procainamide at this dose was effective in 12/15 patients. Lidocaine was effective in only 3/15 (P < 0.01) (Fig. 13-1). When all initial and crossover episodes were considered, lidocaine terminated 6 of 31, whereas procainamide terminated 38 of 48 (P ≤ 0.001). Minor side effects were noted after two procainamide and two lidocaine infusions.

No controlled trials on the use of intravenous amiodarone in stable, hemodynamically tolerated VT are available. However, based on the experience with intravenous amiodarone in patients with unstable VT and cardiac arrest cited later in this chapter, current Advanced Cardiac Life Support guidelines list amiodarone as the drug of choice for patients with stable VT and poor left-ventricular ejection fractions and list procainamide as the drug of choice for patients with preserved ejection fractions.

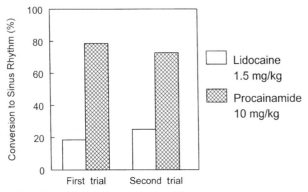

FIGURE 13-1. Lidocaine and procainamide in sustained monomorphic ventricular tachycardia (VT). Lidocaine was infused over 2 minutes, and procainamide was infused at 100 mg/min. Drugs were randomly assigned for the first trial. Patients whose arrhythmias failed to terminate or who developed recurrent episodes received the alternate drugs in the second trial. (Data from Gorgels APM, van den Dool A, Hofs A, et al: Comparison of procainamide and lidocaine in terminating sustained monomorphic ventricular tachycardia. Am J Cardiol 1996; 78:43–46.)

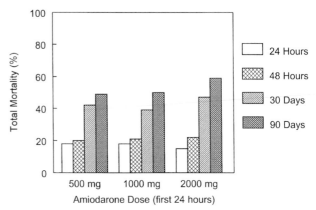

FIGURE 13-2. Mortality in patients receiving intravenous amiodarone. Mortality was high in all dose groups with no clear dose response observed. (Data from Levine JH, Massumi A, Scheinman MM, et al: for the Intravenous Amiodarone Multicenter Trial Group. Intravenous amiodarone for recurrent sustained hypotensive ventricular tachyarrhythmias. J Am Coll Cardiol 1996; 27:67–75.)

AMIODARONE IN UNSTABLE VENTRICULAR TACHYCARDIA

Amiodarone has emerged as the first-choice drug for pharmacologic management of many life-threatening arrhythmias. Early anecdotal studies suggested that intravenous amiodarone could be effective in patients with recurrent incessant VT that had failed to respond to conventional antiarrhythmic therapy.

Three large controlled trials of the relative safety and efficacy of intravenous amiodarone have been conducted.[3] All three trials enrolled patients who had experienced at least two episodes of hemodynamically unstable VT and VF within 24 hours of entry. Patients had failed trials with at least lidocaine and procainamide, and their arrhythmias were not caused by correctable drug or electrolyte abnormalities. The patients enrolled in these trials were critically ill. The mean left-ventricular fraction was 30%, and approximately 25% were either mechanically ventilated or using an intraaortic balloon pump. Most patients had coronary artery disease, and 11% were in the acute phase of a MI. In this critically ill population, a placebo-controlled study design was not feasible so the trials either used a range of amiodarone doses or compared intravenous amiodarone to bretylium, an agent previously recommended as second-line therapy in these patients.

The first reported randomized trial on intravenous amiodarone reported by Levine and colleagues[4] was a dose-ranging trial using doses of 500, 1000, and 2000 mg in the first 24 hours. The drug was administered as an initial bolus followed by a continuous infusion. Supplemental boluses were permitted in this and in the other two studies. The primary endpoint was freedom from recurrent VT or VF. Secondary endpoints included time to first recurrence of tachyarrhythmia and mortality. The authors observed no statistically significant dose-response relationship. With the three doses used in this study 41%, 45%, and 53% of the patients were free of recurrent VT during the first 24 hours. Mortality was

high in the trial and not statistically different between the groups at either 24 hours, 48 hours, 30 days, or 90 days (Fig. 13-2).

Because no significant difference was observed over a 24-hour dose range of 500 to 2000 mg, a second trial[5] was conducted using a lower range of doses: 125, 500, and 1000 mg/day. The 125-mg dose group had more VT events per hour, had a shorter time to first events, and received more supplemental bolus doses than did the 500- and 1000-mg dose groups. There were no differences in 24- or 48-hour mortality between the groups.

The third major study of the efficacy of intravenous amiodarone reported by Kowey and colleagues[6] was a double-blind comparison of two doses of amiodarone (125 and 1000 mg/first 24 hours) and bretylium (2500 mg/first 24 hours). High-dose amiodarone and bretylium were superior to low-dose amiodarone in an intention-to-treat analysis. It should be noted that a substantial portion of the bretylium patients crossed over to amiodarone as a result of drug-induced hypotension. Again, there was no differences in 48-hour survival between the three groups.

These three trials confirmed the role of intravenous amiodarone in patients with hemodynamically unstable VT and VF. Mortality in these trials was high at short-term follow-up, and mortality was not related to the acute efficacy of the drug. A later report by Fogel and colleagues[7] demonstrated that even patients who survived to hospital discharge remained at high (long-term) risk with a mortality of about 20% in the first year after discharge.

AMIODARONE IN CARDIAC ARREST

The role of antiarrhythmic drugs in the setting of cardiac arrest remains controversial. Early defibrillation is the key to survival, and antiarrhythmic drugs are thought to play a secondary role.[8] In this setting, however, antiarrhythmic drugs may be used either to facilitate defibrillation or to prevent immediate or early recurrence of VF or VT after initial cardioversion or defibrillation.

In view of the beneficial effects of amiodarone in patients with unstable ventricular arrhythmias in-hospital, it was logical that the drug be studied in the setting of out-of-hospital cardiac arrest. The Amiodarone in Out-of-Hospital Resuscitation of Refractory Sustained Ventricular Tachyarrhythmias Trial (ARREST)[9] was conducted in Seattle and suburban King County Washington. Cardiac arrest victims with VF or pulseless VT who had not been resuscitated after three or more transthoracic shocks were randomized to receive 300 mg of intravenous amiodarone or placebo. The primary endpoint for the trial was survival to hospital admission. Five hundred and four patients were entered into the trial. The mean time to drug administration after the start of the resuscitation attempt was relatively long (42 minutes). Patients in the amiodarone group were more likely to survive to hospital admission than patients in the control group (44% vs. 34%, P = 0.03), but there was no difference in survival to hospital discharge (13.4% vs. 13.2%, P = NS) (Table 13-1).

The Amiodarone Versus Lidocaine in Prehospital Ventricular Fibrillation Evaluation Trial (ALIVE)[10] compared amiodarone and lidocaine in out-of-hospital cardiac arrest victims with shock-resistant VF. Amiodarone (5 mg/kg estimated body weight) or lidocaine (1.5 mg/kg) was infused as a rapid bolus. The study enrolled 347 subjects who had persistent or recurrent VF after initial defibrillation. From the time of rescue squad dispatch, the mean time to drug administration was 25.8 minutes. The primary endpoint was survival to hospital admission. Survival to hospital discharge was a secondary endpoint. Second drug doses were permitted as clinically indicated. Amiodarone resulted in better survival to hospital admission (22.8% vs. 12.0%, P = 0.009). However, only 9 of 180 (5%) of the amiodarone-treated patients versus 5 of 167 (3%) lidocaine-treated patients (P = 0.34) were discharged from the hospital alive (see Table 13-1).

SELECTION OF ANTIARRHYTHMIC THERAPY

The introduction of invasive electrophysiologic studies during the 1970s had a strong influence on the way cardiologists selected antiarrhythmic therapy. Numerous uncontrolled observational studies suggested that sup-pression of the ability to induce VT during serial electrophysiologic testing correlated with long-term outcome.[11] Serial electrophysiologic testing was believed to be more reliable than approaches based on ambulatory monitoring. A small, randomized trial from the University of Calgary reported by Mitchell and colleagues[12] supported this hypothesis. The results of this trial were inconclusive, however, because of its small size and because many patients in this study eventually received amiodarone therapy that was not electrophysiologically guided.

The Cardiac Arrest in Seattle: Conventional Versus Amiodarone Drug Evaluation (CASCADE)[13] study randomly assigned 228 out-of-hospital cardiac arrest survivors to either conventional (i.e., Vaughn-Williams Class I) antiarrhythmic drug therapy selected by electrophysiologic study or empiric amiodarone therapy. Although the initial trial design had proposed using cardiac mortality as the primary endpoint, a high mortality in both arms early in the trial caused the investigators to permit implantable cardioverter defibrillator (ICD) therapy at the investigator's direction. Using a final composite endpoint of cardiac mortality, syncope, ICD shock, or resuscitated cardiac arrest, empiric amiodarone appeared superior to conventional drug therapy selected by serial electrophysiologic testing. In the latter group, suppression of VT induction did not predict outcome.

The Electrophysiologic Study Versus Electrocardiographic Monitoring Trial (ESVEM)[14,15] was a large, multicenter randomized trial designed to compare the relative accuracies of strategies based on serial electrophysiologic studies and serial ambulatory monitoring in patients with sustained ventricular arrhythmias. All 486 patients entered into the study had both an inducible sustained ventricular arrhythmia at electrophysiologic study and at least 10 premature ventricular contractions per hour during a 48-hour ambulatory monitor at baseline. Serial testing was performed during drug administration. Drugs were administered in random sequence and included imipramine, mexiletine, procainamide, quinidine, sotalol, pirmenol, and propafenone. Effective drug therapy was predicted in 77% of patients in the ambulatory monitoring arm versus only 45% of patients in the invasive arm. However, there was no significant difference between the two approaches using an endpoint of death or arrhythmia recurrence. The overall event rate was quite high: 58% at 2 years. When the response rates to the various drugs were compared, sotalol was associated with the best clinical outcomes.

ESVEM had many limitations. The electrophysiologic study protocol used was not representative of that used by many laboratories during that period. Several of the drugs used (imipramine, pirmenol, mexiletine) were never standard drugs for monotherapy in patients with sustained ventricular arrhythmias. Amiodarone, now the most commonly used antiarrhythmic drug for this indication, was not included in the trial. Much of the follow-up during the trial was in patients not receiving the therapy selected initially. This made interpretation of the intention-to-treat analysis used in the study difficult. There also appeared to be extensive pre-enrollment bias against trial participation at many of the centers. Despite these limitations, the ESVEM data accelerated the shift

■ ■ ■

TABLE 13-1 AMIODARONE IN OUT-OF-HOSPITAL CARDIAC ARREST

	Number of patients	Survival to hospital admission	Survival to hospital discharge
ARREST[9]			
Amiodarone	246	108 (43.9%)*	33 (13.4%)†
Placebo	258	89 (34.5%)*	34 (13.2%)†
ALIVE[10]			
Amiodarone	180	41 (22.8%)‡	9 (5.0%)†
Lidocaine	167	20 (12.0%)‡	5 (3.0%)†

*P = 0.03.
†P = NS.
‡P = 0.009.

toward use of empiric amiodarone and ICD therapy as the primary treatment modalities in patients with prior VT or VF.

ANTIARRHYTHMIC DRUGS VERSUS ICD THERAPY FOR SECONDARY PREVENTION

The introduction and evolution of the ICD during the 1980s marked a dramatic turning point in the management of life-threatening ventricular arrhythmias. Early observational studies established that the ICD could successfully terminate spontaneous episodes of VT and VF.[16] The introduction of transvenous lead systems, which eliminated the need for thoracotomy, made clinical trials comparing drug therapy and ICD therapy feasible.

The Antiarrhythmics Versus Implantable Defibrillator Trial (AVID)[17] compared drug therapy using either empiric amiodarone or electrophysiologically guided sotalol and ICD therapy in 1016 patients who had survived an episode of VF or VT with cardiac arrest, hypotension, or syncope. Almost all of the patients in the drug treatment arm received amiodarone. The primary endpoint was total mortality. In the ICD group, survival was 89.3%, 81.6%, and 75.4% after 1, 2, and 3 years, respectively. This was superior to survival in the drug therapy group, which was 82.3%, 74.7%, and 64.1% (P < 0.02), respectively, at the same time points. Separation of the survival curves was noted in the first 9 months after randomization, and this benefit was for the most part maintained throughout subsequent follow-up.

The Canadian Implantable Defibrillator Study (CIDS)[18] also compared amiodarone to ICD therapy. Entry criteria were similar to those in AVID with the exception that patients with syncope of unknown cause and inducible VT could be enrolled. The prespecified primary endpoint was mortality resulting from arrhythmia. Total mortality was a secondary endpoint. The study enrolled 659 patients. Arrhythmic mortality and total mortality were lower in the ICD group (8.3%/year and 3.0%/year) compared to the amiodarone group (10.2% and 4.5%), but these differences did not achieve statistical significance.

The final secondary prevention trial comparing drug therapy to ICD therapy was the Cardiac Arrest Study Hamburg (CASH).[19] Only patients with resuscitated cardiac arrest were enrolled in the trial. The original design was a four-way comparison of therapy with one of three drugs—amiodarone, metoprolol, or propafenone—or an ICD. The primary endpoint was all-cause mortality. Increased mortality with propafenone noted early in the trial led to discontinuation of that arm of the trial. A total of 288 patients were included in the three remaining arms of the trial. Compared to the study populations in AVID and CIDS, the patients enrolled in CASH were younger, had a higher mean ejection fraction, and were more likely to have no structural heart disease. Total and arrhythmic mortality rates were lower in the ICD group (7.7%/year and 1.5%/year) compared to the amiodarone group (9.4%/year and 5.1%/year), but these differences were not significant because of the small size of the trial. There were no differences in survival between the amiodarone and metoprolol groups.

■ ■ ■

TABLE 13-2 ICD VERSUS AMIODARONE: SECONDARY PREVENTION TRIAL META-ANALYSIS[20]

	AVID[17]	CASH[19]	CIDS[18]
Number of patients			
Amiodarone	509	92	331
ICD	507	99	328
All deaths (annual rate)			
Amiodarone	122 (16.5%)	35 (9.4%)	98 (10.2%)
ICD	80 (10 %)	37 (7.7%)	83 (8.3%)
Arrhythmic deaths (annual rate)			
Amiodarone	55 (7.4%)	19 (5.4%)	43 (4.5%)
ICD	24 (3.0%)	7 (1.5%)	30 (3.0%)

ICD, implantable cardioverter defibrillator.

The data from AVID, CIDS, and CASH have been combined in a meta-analysis that compared ICD therapy with amiodarone therapy.[20] This analysis showed that the estimates of ICD benefit in the three studies were consistent with each other (Table 13-2). The summary hazard ratio (ICD vs. amiodarone) for death from any cause was 0.72 (95% CI 0.60-0.87, P = 0.0006). For arrhythmic death, the hazard ratio was 0.50 (95% CI 0.37-0.67, P < 0.0001). ICD therapy prolonged survival by a mean of 4.4 months over 6 years of follow-up. Almost all benefit from ICD therapy was seen in those patients with left-ventricular ejection fractions at or below 35%. For patients with higher ejection fractions, there was no survival advantage associated with ICD therapy.

ANTIARRHYTHMIC DRUG COMPARISONS

A number of randomized trials have been published comparing the long-term efficacy of selected antiarrhythmic drugs in patients with prior sustained VT or VF. The original trial design for these studies used mortality and/or recurrence of sustained arrhythmia as the primary endpoint. As ICD therapy became more widely used, appropriate ICD therapy was adopted as an primary or secondary endpoint. In populations with an ICD in situ, comparison of an antiarrhythmic drug to placebo became possible. Events in antiarrhythmic drugs studies in ICD patients may be complex to interpret because there is not a 1:1 relationship between even "appropriate" ICD therapies and clinical events in control groups without an ICD.

The Amiodarone vs. Sotalol Study Group[21] reported an open-label, randomized comparison of chronic sotalol and amiodarone therapy in patients who had failed therapy with class I antiarrhythmic drugs. The amiodarone dose was 1200 mg/day initially with a final dose of 396 ± 69 mg/day. After an initial titration, the chronic sotalol dose was 491 ± 163 mg/day. Events during the first 3 weeks of amiodarone loading were not counted. Neither electrophysiologic studies nor ambulatory monitoring was used to guide therapy. Sixteen of 30 patients randomized to amiodarone successfully completed 1 year of therapy, compared to 16 of 29 patients randomized to sotalol.

There was no difference in mortality rate or the incidence of serious adverse drug reactions between the groups.

Steinbeck and colleagues[22] compared empiric metoprolol and electrophysiologically guided therapy with propafenone, flecainide, sotalol, or amiodarone in 170 patients with sustained VT, VF, or syncope with VT. Fifty-five patients who manifested no inducible arrhythmia at a baseline electrophysiologic study received empiric metoprolol. The 115 patients with inducible VT were randomized to empiric metoprolol or guided therapy. The primary endpoint was death or recurrence of sustained arrhythmia. Suppression of arrhythmia induction during serial testing was achieved in 29 of 61 patients; 18 of these 29 patients were taking sotalol. It should be noted that amiodarone was always the last drug tested. Among those with inducible VT, there was no difference in outcome between the metoprolol-treated group and the guided-therapy group. Suppression of VT during guided therapy was a predictor of outcome, but a "healthy responder" phenomenon cannot be excluded. The group of patients who had no inducible VT at baseline had better outcomes.

The ESVEM trial,[15] as mentioned earlier, examined the acute and long-term efficacy of six antiarrhythmic drugs selected during serial trials using either ambulatory monitoring or electrophysiologic testing. A drug efficacy prediction was achieved in 77% using the ambulatory monitoring approach and in 45% using the electrophysiologic approach. Mexiletine was the most frequently effective drug using ambulatory monitoring, and sotalol was the most frequently effective drug during electrophysiologic testing (Table 13-3). Long-term outcomes were better with sotalol selected with either technique.

Pacifico and colleagues[23] compared sotalol and placebo in 352 patients with sustained VT or VT who had either a new ICD implant or a recent implantable defibrillator shock. The primary endpoint was either death from any cause or delivery of a first ICD shock. There were four deaths in the sotalol group versus seven in the placebo group, but none of these resulted from arrhythmia. According to Kaplan-Meier estimates, 60% of patients in the sotalol group versus 46% in the placebo group had not reached the primary endpoint at 12 months (P < 0.001 by log-rank test) for a reduction of risk of 48% with sotalol.

Seidl and colleagues[24] compared sotalol and metoprolol in 70 patients after implantation of an ICD. The primary endpoint was appropriate ICD intervention during a follow-up of 26 ± 16 months. There were three (8.6%) deaths in the metoprolol group compared with six (17.1%) deaths in the sotalol group (P = 0.287). Actuarial survival free of VT recurrence was significantly higher in the metoprolol group compared to the sotalol group at 1 and 2 years (83% and 80% vs. 57% and 51%, respectively, P = 0.016).

Sotalol was compared to dofetilide in 135 patients with inducible sustained VT by Boriani and colleagues.[25] Patients received both drugs in randomized sequence, and drug efficacy was assessed acutely with programmed ventricular stimulation. Testing on both drugs was completed in 128 patients. Forty-six (35%) patients responded to dofetilide, compared with 43 (33.6%) who responded to sotalol. There was only a poor positive concordance (23 patients) between test results on the two drugs. A total of 67 patients, 41 taking dofetilide and 26 taking sotalol, entered the long-term phase of the study. Three patients in each group developed recurrent VT. Withdrawal of therapy for lack of efficacy or side effects was more common with sotalol than with dofetilide (37.0% vs. 23.8%).

PRIMARY PREVENTION OF SUDDEN CARDIAC DEATH

The goal of primary prevention of sudden cardiac death is to apply effective therapy to "at risk" patients prior to any sustained ventricular arrhythmias. Although most sudden cardiac deaths occur in patients without known cardiac disease, the greatest incidence occurs in groups with known risk factors.[26] The high-risk group most commonly enrolled in primary prevention trials is composed of patients with significant left-ventricular dysfunction, prior MI, and a history of significant ventricular ectopy.

The earliest primary prevention trials sought to determine if beta blockers would improve overall survival after a MI.[27-29] In addition to overall mortality reduction with beta blockers, most of these trials demonstrated a reduction in sudden cardiac death. This chapter will not discuss these trials in detail but will review some of the most important primary prevention trials using antiarrhythmic drugs or ICD therapy (Table 13-4).

Antiarrhythmic Drugs Versus Placebo

The Cardiac Arrhythmia Suppression Trial (CAST)[30] was a pioneering randomized, placebo-controlled trial on the ability of antiarrhythmic therapy to reduce sudden cardiac death. All patients in this study had a history of MI, some reduction in left-ventricular function, and six or more ventricular premature beats (VPBs) per hour. The underlying hypothesis of this trial was that suppression of VPBs by an antiarrhythmic medication would reduce the risk of sudden cardiac death. Therefore, after an initial titration phase to determine VPB and nonsustained VT suppressibility by study drug, 1498 patients were randomly assigned to drug (flecainide or encainide) or placebo. After an average follow-up of 9.7 months, total mortality was 7.7% in the flecainide/encainide groups vs. 3.0% in the placebo group;

■ □ ■

TABLE 13-3   IN-HOSPITAL EFFICACY OF ANTIARRHYTHMIC DRUGS IN ESVEM[15]

Agent	Ambulatory monitoring	Electrophysiologic testing
Imipramine (n = 129)	45%	10%
Mexiletine (n = 226)	67%	12%
Pirmenol (n = 109)	55%	19%
Procainamide (n = 158)	50%	26%
Propafenone (n = 220)	48%	14%
Quinidine (n = 157)	59%	16%
Sotalol (n = 234)	56%	35%

■ ■ ■

TABLE 13-4 PRIMARY PREVENTION TRIALS IN POST–MYOCARDIAL INFARCTION PATIENTS

Trial	Design	RESULTS		
		Harm	Neutral	Benefit
"Beta blockers"[27-29]	"Beta blockers" vs. placebo			X
CAST I[30]	Flecainide/encainide vs. placebo	X		
CAST II[31]	Moricizine vs. placebo	X		
BASIS[32]	"Class I" vs. amiodarone vs. placebo	X		X (Amio)
SWORD[37]	d-Sotalol vs. placebo	X		
Julian et al[36]	d, l-Sotalol vs. placebo		X	
EMIAT[34]	Amiodarone vs. placebo		X	
CAMIAT[35]	Amiodarone vs. placebo		X	
DIAMOND-MI[38]	Dofetilide vs. placebo		X	
ALIVE[39]	Azimilide vs. placebo		X	
MADIT I[40]	ICD vs, no Rx			X
MUSTT[41]	ICD/antiarrhythmic drugs vs. no Rx			X
CABG-Patch[42]	ICD vs. no Rx		X	
MADIT II[44]	ICD vs. no Rx			X

death from arrhythmias was 4.5% in the encainide/flecainide groups and 1.2% in placebo. Hence, despite VPB suppression, there was an increase in total mortality and sudden cardiac death in the drug treatment group.

In the Cardiac Arrhythmia Suppression Trial II (CAST-II),[31] moricizine also was shown to suppress VPBs, but drug therapy resulted in increased mortality in the short term and no beneficial effect long term. Based on these two studies, use of flecainide, encainide, and moricizine should be avoided in post-MI patients. CAST brought to our attention the fact that subtle proarrhythmia may occur late during antiarrhythmic therapy even in patients thought to be responders during the initial phase of treatment.

The VPB suppression theory was tested with other antiarrhythmic agents in the Basel Antiarrhythmic Study of Infarct Survival (BASIS)[32] study. In this study 312 patients with a recent history of a MI were randomized to receive either antiarrhythmic drug–guided therapy by continuous electrocardiographic (ECG) monitoring, amiodarone, or placebo for 12 months. Quinidine or mexiletine was used as first-line drugs with flecainide, propafenone, disopyramide, ajmaline, or D,L-sotalol being used as second-line agents. After 1 year of follow-up, there was no mortality benefit over placebo derived from antiarrhythmic drug therapy guided by ECG monitoring. However, a 61% reduction in mortality was seen in the amiodarone group as compared to placebo (5.1% vs. 13.2%; P = 0.048). Even after long-term follow-up of 84 months, the early benefit of amiodarone resulted in a reduction in probability of death from 45% for placebo to 30% for amiodarone.[33]

Unfortunately two other larger studies evaluating amiodarone in the post-MI population have not confirmed this overall mortality benefit. The European Myocardial Infarct Amiodarone Trial (EMIAT)[34] and the Canadian Amiodarone Myocardial Infarction Trial (CAMIAT)[35] trials were randomized, placebo-controlled trials evaluating amiodarone in the post-MI patient with a reduction in left-ventricular ejection fraction of more than 40% or with 10 or more premature ventricular contractions/hour by continuous ECG monitoring, respec-

tively. In EMIAT 743 patients were randomized to receive either amiodarone or placebo. After a median follow-up of 21 months, all-cause mortality was similar (103 patients in the amiodarone group vs. 103 in the placebo group), but there was a reduction in arrhythmic deaths with amiodarone (33 vs. 50 patients; P = 0.05). In CAMIAT 606 patients were assigned to the amiodarone group and 596 to the placebo group. After a mean follow-up of 1.8 years, overall mortality was not significantly different (37 vs. 50 deaths for the amiodarone group and placebo group, respectively; P = 0.13). However, the authors noted a relative risk reduction of 38.2% of arrhythmic death or resuscitated VF.

Other Vaughn-Williams Class III antiarrhythmic agents—sotalol, dofetilide, and azimilide—also have been evaluated in primary prevention trials. Julian and colleagues[36] randomized 1456 patients who survived an acute MI to treatment with D,L-sotalol versus placebo. After a mean follow-up of 12 months, the mortality rate was 7.3% in the sotalol group and 8.9% in the placebo group. Although the use of sotalol resulted in an 18% reduction in mortality, this reduction was not statistically significant.

In the Survival With Oral d-Sotalol Trial (SWORD)[37], d-sotalol, which has effects on repolarization without producing β-adrenergic blockade, was compared to placebo in a randomized, double-blind study of patients with a MI, ejection fraction of 40%, or less and New York Heart Association (NYHA) class II–III heart failure. A total of 3121 patients were randomized. The study was terminated prematurely because of excess mortality in the d-sotalol group compared to the placebo group (5.0% vs. 3.1%, respectively). The event rate in SWORD was lower than anticipated, and this trial's outcome highlights the problems inherent in using a drug with some proarrhythmic potential in a low- or moderate-risk group.

In the Danish Investigation of Arrhythmia and Mortality on Dofetilide trial (DIAMOND-MI),[38] the effects of dofetilide on mortality and morbidity was evaluated in patients with left-ventricular dysfunction and recent MI. A total of 1510 patients were randomized and followed-up after 12 months. The all-cause mortality in the dofetilide group compared to placebo was 26% versus 28%, respectively (P = NS). Arrhythmic deaths were 17% vs. 18%, respectively (P = NS). Similarly, in the AzimiLide Post Infarct SurVival Evaluation (ALIVE)[39] trial 3717 patients with a recent MI were randomized to receive either azimilide at 75 mg or 100 mg versus placebo. The all-cause mortality in both groups was 11.6%.

It is important to recognize that although the previously mentioned randomized studies with amiodarone, D,L-sotalol, dofetilide, and azimilide did not show a mortality benefit, they demonstrated safety when used in the high-risk, post-MI patient. This is in contrast to the increased mortality seen in the CAST trials.[30,31] This observation has been used to justify development and approval of these drugs for treatment of patients with symptomatic supraventricular arrhythmias.

ICD Versus Control Postinfarction

Four major randomized control trials comparing ICD to placebo in postinfarction populations have been published. The Multicenter Automatic Defibrillator Implantation Trial (MADIT)[40] included patients with a history of MI, an ejection fraction of 35% or less, and nonsustained VT. An electrophysiologic study was required, and only patients with reproducibly induced VT or fibrillation that was not suppressed by procainamide was eligible for randomization to ICD versus "conventional" therapy. Conventional therapy was at the primary physician's discretion. A total of 196 patients were randomized. After an average follow-up of 27 months, the study was terminated when the sequential monitoring design reached a prespecified stopping point. At that time, there were 15 deaths in the defibrillator group and 39 in the conventional therapy group (hazard ratio 0.46; P = 0.009).

A survival benefit with ICD therapy was also seen in the Multicenter Unsustained Tachycardia Trial (MUSTT),[41] but this trial was designed to compare therapy guided by serial electrophysiologic studies versus no therapy. This study enrolled similar patients to those in MADIT except the ejection fraction cut-off was 40% or less. Patients underwent an electrophysiologic study at baseline. If a sustained ventricular arrhythmic that met protocol criteria was induced, they were then randomized to antiarrhythmic therapy guided by serial electrophysiologic studies or to no antiarrhythmic therapy. An ICD could be given after one unsuccessful drug test.

A total of 704 patients were randomized. A 27% reduction in risk of death or cardiac arrest was seen in the electrophysiologic-guided group. However, the reduction in risk was only in those patients who received an ICD. Patients who received drug therapy did slightly worse that the untreated control group.

In contrast to MADIT and MUSTT, the Coronary Artery Bypass Graft Patch Trial (CABG-Patch)[42] did not show a reduction in overall mortality with ICD therapy. This study included patients scheduled for surgical coronary revascularization, a left-ventricular ejection fraction below 36%, and an abnormal signal average ECG. At the time of coronary artery bypass grafting, patients were assigned to ICD implantation or no implantation. After a mean follow-up of 32 months there was no difference in overall mortality (101 in the defibrillator group vs. 95 in the control group; relative risk 1.07; 95% CI 0.81-1.42, P = 0.64). A substudy of the trial showed that although ICD therapy reduced arrhythmic death by 45%, most of the deaths in this patient group were not the result of arrhythmia (71%); therefore, ICD therapy did not reduced overall mortality.[43]

In the Multicenter Automatic Defibrillator Implantation Trial II (MADIT II),[44] the patient population consisted of those with a prior MI and an ejection fraction of 30% or less. Neither nonsustained VT or an inducible arrhythmia was required for study enrollment. A total of 1232 patients were randomized in a 3:2 ratio for ICD versus no ICD. The Kaplan-Meier estimate of survival after 3 years showed a 28% reduction in risk of death in the ICD group.

CONGESTIVE HEART FAILURE

During the 1990s there were significant advances in the medical treatment of congestive heart failure (CHF). The two most significant advances were the use of angiotensin-converting enzyme (ACE) inhibitors and beta blockers. Both classes of medication clearly result in improved overall survival. However, sudden cardiac death remains a major cause of mortality in this group (Table 13-5).

Antiarrhythmic Drug versus Placebo

In the Grupo de Estudio de la Sorbrevida en la Insuficiencia Cardiac en Argentina (GESICA)[45] study, 516 patients with CHF (NYHA class II–IV) and an ejection fraction of 35% or less were randomized to receive either amiodarone or placebo. They were followed for 2 years. The

■ ■ ■

TABLE 13-5 PRIMARY PREVENTION TRIALS IN CONGESTIVE HEART FAILURE

| Trial | Design | RESULTS | | |
		Harm	Neutral	Benefit
GESICA[45]	Amiodarone vs. placebo			X
CHF-STAT[46]	Amiodarone vs. placebo		X	
DIAMOND-CHF[47]	Dofetilide vs. placebo		X	
AMIOVIRT[48]	ICD vs. amiodarone		X	
CAT[9]	ICD vs. placebo		X	
SCD-HeFT[50]	ICD vs. amiodarone vs. placebo	Pending	Pending	Pending

overall mortality was 41.4% in the control arm and 33.5% in the amiodarone group. This represented a risk reduction of 28%. Interestingly, the majority of the patients in this study had nonischemic cardiomyopathy.

The two other studies comparing an antiarrhythmic drug to placebo have had neutral results. In the Survival Trial of Antiarrhythmic Therapy in Congestive Heart Failure (CHF-STAT)[46] 674 patients with CHF, cardiac enlargement, 10 or more VPBs/hr, and an ejection fraction of 40% or less were randomized to receive amiodarone or placebo. After a mean follow-up of 45 months there was no overall mortality benefit. There were 131 deaths in the amiodarone group and 143 in the placebo group. However, a beneficial trend in those patients with nonischemic cardiomyopathies was noted.

In the Danish Investigation of Arrhythmia and Mortality on Dofetilide in patients with Congestive Heart Failure (DIAMOND-CHF)[47] trial, 1518 patients were randomized to receive either dofetilide or placebo. After a follow-up of 18 months there was no mortality benefit derived from dofetilide. The death rates were 41% in the dofetilide group and 42% in the placebo group.

ICD Versus Antiarrhythmic Drug or Placebo

Two small trials have been published evaluating ICD therapy in patients with CHF. The first trial compared amiodarone and ICD therapy. In the Amiodarone Versus Implantable Defibrillators in Patients with Nonischemic Cardiomyopathy and Nonsustained Ventricular Tachycardia Trial (AMIOVIRT),[48] 178 patients with nonischemic dilated cardiomyopathy with an ejection fraction of less than 35% and nonsustained VT were assigned to either amiodarone or ICD therapy. Of these, only 103 patients were randomized because 75 refused randomization. After a mean follow-up of 4 years there was no difference in mortality between two groups (8 deaths in the amiodarone group and 13 in the ICD group, P = NS).

The second trial dealing with primary prevention of sudden death in nonischemic cardiomyopathy was the Cardiomyopathy Trial (CAT).[49] In this study, 104 patients with idiopathic dilated cardiomyopathy and an ejection fraction of 30% or less were randomized to receive an ICD or no therapy. After a mean follow-up of 5.5 years there was no survival benefit associated with the ICD (13 deaths in the ICD group and 17 in the control group; P = NS).

In summary, it is interesting to note the low mortality rates in both ICD studies that enrolled patients with nonischemic dilated cardiomyopathies. This may partially explain the overall neutral effect. However, in patients with nonischemic cardiomyopathies, both GESICA and CHF-STAT showed improved survival. A significantly larger trial, Sudden Cardiac Death in Heart Failure Treatment (SCD-HeFT),[50] comparing amiodarone and the ICD to placebo is ongoing. SCD-HeFT has enrolled more than 2500 patients with NYHA class II–III heart failure symptoms and an ejection fraction 35% or less. Because of the large size of this trial, there will be many patients with both ischemic and nonischemic cardiomyopathies available for analysis. The primary end-point for the trial is total mortality.

CONCLUSIONS

The last 20 years have witnessed a transformation in our approach to the management of ventricular arrhythmias. Treatment approaches now can be based on data from controlled clinical trials. Unfortunately, the efficacy of available antiarrhythmic therapy is still not optimal. Strategies that focus on prevention of coronary artery disease, management of acute ischemic syndromes, and treatment of heart failure remain vital.

REFERENCES

1. Griffith MJ, Linker NJ, Garratt CJ, et al: Relative efficacy and safety of intravenous drugs for termination of sustained ventricular tachycardia. Lancet 1990; 336:670-673.
2. Gorgels APM, van den Dool A, Hofs A, et al: Comparison of procainamide and lidocaine in terminating sustained monomorphic ventricular tachycardia. Am J Cardiol 1996; 78:43-46.
3. Kowey PR, Marinchak RA, Rials SJ, et al: Intravenous amiodarone. J Am Coll Cardiol 1997; 29:1190-1198.
4. Levine JH, Massumi A, Scheinman MM, et al: For The Intravenous Amiodarone Multicenter Trial Group. Intravenous amiodarone for recurrent sustained hypotensive ventricular tachyarrhythmias. J Am Coll Cardiol 1996; 27:67-75.
5. Scheinman MM, Levine JH, Cannom DS, et al: Dose-ranging study of intravenous amiodarone in patients with life-threatening ventricular tachyarrhythmias. Circulation 1995; 92:3264-3272.
6. Kowey PR, Levine JH, Herre JM, et al: Randomized, double-blind comparison of intravenous amiodarone and bretylium in the treatment of patients with recurrent, hemodynamically destabilizing ventricular tachycardia or fibrillation. Circulation 1995; 92:3255-3263.
7. Fogel RI, Herre JM, Kopelman HA, et al:. Long-term follow-up of patients requiring intravenous amiodarone to suppress hemodynamically destabilizing ventricular arrhythmias. Am Heart J 2000; 139:690-695.
8. Eisenberg MS, Mengert TJ: Cardiac resuscitation. N Engl J Med 2001; 344:1304-1313.
9. Kudenchuk PJ, Cobb LA, Copass MK, et al: Amiodarone for resuscitation after out-of-hospital cardiac arrest due to ventricular fibrillation. N Engl J Med 1999; 341:871-878.
10. Dorian P, Cass D, Schwartz B, et al: Amiodarone as compared with lidocaine for shock-resistant ventricular fibrillation. N Engl J Med 2002; 346:884-890.
11. Steinbeck G, Greene L: Management of patients with life-threatening sustained ventricular tachyarrhythmia—The role of guided antiarrhythmic drug therapy. Progr Cardiovasc Dis 1996; 38:419-428.
12. Mitchell LB, Duff HJ, Manyari DE, et al: A randomized clinical trial of the noninvasive and invasive approaches to drug therapy of ventricular tachycardia. N Engl J Med 1987; 317:1681-1687.
13. The CASCADE Investigators: Randomized antiarrhythmic drug therapy in survivors of cardiac arrest. Am J Cardiol 1993; 72:280-287.
14. Mason JW: A comparison of electrophysiologic testing with holter monitoring to predict antiarrhythmic-drug efficacy for ventricular tachyarrhythmias. N Engl J Med 1993; 329:445-451.
15. Mason JW: A comparison of seven antiarrhythmic drugs in patients with ventricular tachyarrhythmias. N Engl J Med 1993; 329:452-458.
16. Priori SG, Aliot E, Blomstrom-Lundqvist C, et al: Task force report on sudden cardiac death of the European Society of Cardiology. Eur Heart J 2001; 22:1374-1450.
17. The Antiarrhythmics Versus Implantable Defibrillators (AVID) Investigators: A comparison of antiarrhythmic drug therapy with implantable defibrillators in patients resuscitated from near fatal ventricular arrhythmias. N Engl J Med 1997; 337:1576-1583.
18. Connolly SJ, Gent M, Roberts RS, et al: Canadian implantable defibrillator study (CIDS): A randomized trial of the implantable cardioverter defibrillator against amiodarone. Circulation 2000; 101:1297-1302.
19. Kuck KH, Cappato R, Siebels J, et al: Randomized comparison of antiarrhythmic drug therapy with implantable defibrillators in patients resuscitated from cardiac arrest: The Cardiac Arrest Study Hamburg (CASH). Circulation 2000; 102:748-754.

20. Connolly SJ, Hallstrom AP, Cappato R, et al: Meta-analysis of the implantable cardioverter defibrillator secondary prevention trials. Eur Heart J 2000; 21:2071-2078.
21. Amiodarone vs Sotalol Study Group: Multicentre randomized trial of sotalol vs amiodarone for chronic malignant ventricular tachyarrhythmias. Eur Heart J 1989; 10:685-694.
22. Steinbeck G, Andresen D, Bach P, et al: A comparison of electrophysiologically guided antiarrhythmic drug therapy with beta-blocker therapy in patients with symptomatic, sustained ventricular tachyarrhythmias. N Engl J Med 1992; 327:987-992.
23. Pacifico A, Hohnloser SH, Williams JH, et al: Prevention of implantable defibrillator shocks by treatment with sotalol. N Engl J Med 1999; 340:1855-1862.
24. Seidl K, Hauer B, Schwick NG, et al: Comparison of metoprolol and sotalol in preventing ventricular tachyarrhythmias after the implantation of a cardioverter/defibrillator. Am J Cardiol 1998; 82:744-748.
25. Boriani G, Lubinski A, Capucci A, et al: A multicentre, double-blind randomized crossover comparative study on the efficacy and safety of dofetilide vs sotalol in patients with inducible sustained ventricular tachycardia and ischaemic heart disease. Eur Heart J 2001; 22:2180-2191.
26. Myerburg, RJ, Mitrani R, Interian A, et al: Interpretation of outcomes of antiarrhythmic clinical trials: Design features and population impact. Circulation 1998; 97:1514-1521.
27. BHAT Investigator Group: A randomized trial of propranolol in patients with acute myocardial infarction. I. Mortality results. JAMA 1982; 247:1707-1714.
28. Yusuf S, Peto R, Lewis J, et al: Beta blockade during and after myocardial infarction: An overview of the randomized trials. Prog Cardiovasc Dis 1985; 27:335-371.
29. Gottlieb SS, McCarter RJ, Vogel RA: Effect of beta-blockade on mortality among high-risk and low-risk patients after myocardial infarction. N Engl J Med 1998; 339:489-497.
30. Echt DS, Liebson PR, Mitchell LB, et al: Mortality and morbidity in patients receiving encainide, flecainide, or placebo: the Cardiac Arrhythmia Suppression Trial. N Engl J Med 1991; 324:781-788.
31. The Cardiac Arrhythmia Suppression Trial II Investigators: Effect of the antiarrhythmic agent moricizine on survival after myocardial infarction. N Engl J Med 1992; 327:227-233.
32. Burkart F, Phisterer ME, Kiowski W, et al: Effect of antiarrhythmic therapy on mortality in survivors of myocardial infarction with asymptomatic complex ventricular arrhythmias: Basel Antiarrhythmic Study of Infarct Survival (BASIS). J Am Coll Cardiol 1990; 16:1711-1718.
33. Pfisterer ME, Kiowski W, Brunner H, et al: Long-term benefit of 1 year amiodarone treatment for persistent complex ventricular arrhythmias after myocardial infarction. Circulation 1993; 87:309-311.
34. Julian DG, Camm AJ, Franglin G, et al: Randomized trial of effect of amiodarone on mortality in patients with left-ventricular dysfunction after recent myocardial infarction: EMIAT. Lancet 1997; 349:667-674.
35. Cairns JA, Connolly SJ, Roberts R, et al: Randomized trial of outcome after myocardial infarction in patients with frequent or repetitive ventricular premature depolarisations: CAMIAT. Lancet 1997; 349:675-582.
36. Julian DG, Prescott RJ, Jackson FS, et al: Controlled trial of sotalol for one year after myocardial infarction. Lancet 1982; 1:1142-1147.
37. Waldo AL, Camm AJ, deRuyter H, et al: Effect of d-sotalol on mortality in patients with left ventricular dysfunction after recent and remote myocardial infarction. Lancet 196; 348:7-12.
38. Kober L, Bloch Thomsen PE, Moller M, et al: Effect of dofetilide in patients with recent myocardial infarction and left ventricular dysfunction: A randomized trial. Lancet 2000; 356:2052-2058.
39. Best of the AHA Scientific Sessions 2001: Highlights from the American Heart Association Scientific Sessions 2001 November 11-14, 2001, Anaheim, CA. Rev Cardiovasc Med 2002; 3:22-48.
40. Moss AJ, Hall JW, Cannom DS, et al: Improved survival with an implanted defibrillator in patients with coronary disease at high risk for ventricular arrhythmia. N Engl J Med 1996; 335: 1933-1940.
41. Bruxton AE, Lee KL, Fisher JD, et al: A randomized study of the prevention of sudden death in patients with coronary artery disease. N Engl J Med 1999; 341:1882-1890.
42. Bigger JT: Prophylactic use of implanted cardiac defibrillators in patients at high risk for ventricular arrhythmias after coronary artery bypass graft surgery. N Engl J Med 1997; 337:1569-1575.
43. Bigger JT, Whang W, Rottman JN, et al: Mechanisms of death in the CABG-Patch trial. A randomized trial of implantable cardiac defibrillator prophylaxis in patients at high risk of death after coronary artery bypass graft surgery. Circulation 1999; 99:1416-1421.
44. Moss AJ, Zareba W, Hall WJ, et al: Prophylactic implantation of a defibrillator in patients with myocardial infarction and reduced ejection fraction. N Engl J Med 2002; 346:877-883.
45. Doval HC, Nul DR. Grancelli HO, et al: Randomized trial of low dose amiodarone in severe congestive heart failure. Lancet 1994; 344:493-498.
46. Singh SN, Fletcher RD, Fisher SG, et al: Amiodarone in patients with congestive heart failure and symptomatic ventricular arrhythmia. N Engl J Med 1995; 333:77-82.
47. Torp-Pedersen C, Moller M, Bloch-Thomsen PE, et al: Dofetilide in patients with congestive heart failure and left ventricular dysfunction. N Engl J Med 1999; 341:857-865.
48. Strickberger SA, Hummel JD, Bartlett TG, et al: Amiodarone versus implantable cardioverter-defibrillator: Randomized trial in patients with nonischemic dilated cardiomyopathy and asymptomatic nonsustained ventricular tachycardia—AMIOVIRT. J Amer Coll Cardiol 2003; 41:1707-1712.
49. Bänsch D, Antz M, Boczor S, et al: Primary prevention of sudden cardiac death in idiopathic dilated cardiomyopathy: The Cardiomyopathy Trial (CAT). Circulation 2002; 105:1453-1458.
50. Wilber DJ, Kall JG, Kapp DE: What can we expect from prophylactic implantable defibrillators? Am J Cardiol 1997; 80(5B): 20F-27F.

■ ▨ ■ c h a p t e r **14**

Drug Therapy for Supraventricular Tachycardia

Sharon C. Reimold

Clinical trials investigating the efficacy of antiarrhythmic therapy in supraventricular tachycardias (SVTs) are numerous. Compared with other investigative disciplines within cardiology, however, most of the randomized trials are small, single-center studies with short duration of follow-up. These studies are difficult to compare and contrast because of variability in enrollment criteria and study endpoints (Table 14-1). Many investigators have enrolled patients with various forms of SVT including atrioventricular nodal reentrant tachycardia, atrioventricular reentrant tachycardia (Wolff-Parkinson-White syndrome), and atrial fibrillation in a single study. The response of a given supraventricular arrhythmia to pharmacologic therapy may be variable; therefore, combining data for arrhythmias of multiple mechanisms may be inappropriate when evaluating overall efficacy. Clinical trials designed to investigate acute termination of supraventricular arrhythmias frequently use dissimilar dosing regimens and examine the likelihood of success at intervals ranging from 1 to 8 hours after antiarrhythmic drug administration. The definition of successful therapy may extend from complete suppression of an arrhythmia to a reduction in the frequency and duration of paroxysms of an arrhythmia. For long-term suppression of these arrhythmias, the duration of follow-up is generally on the order of 3 to 12 months, a small duration given the natural history of these disorders.

Trials examining suppression of paroxysmal arrhythmias most frequently use the randomized crossover design. The duration of the crossover is variable, ranging from 1 to 3 months. These studies often incorporate a dose-finding or dose-titration phase, in which patients are placed on increasing doses of a pharmacologic agent in an attempt to assess the optimal dose for a given patient. Patients who develop significant side effects or who develop worsening arrhythmia during the dose-finding phase generally are excluded from participation in the randomized component of each trial. Thus, the reported efficacy often is based on a selected subset of patients (i.e., patients who are more likely to tolerate a given medication).

Some investigators have chosen to study the impact of antiarrhythmic agents on inducible as opposed to spontaneous arrhythmias. In some supraventricular as well as ventricular arrhythmia trials, there is evidence that termination or suppression of inducible arrhythmia

is predictive of the ambient response to a pharmacologic agent. Although the response of a spontaneous arrhythmia to a pharmacologic agent is the ideal endpoint to evaluate, there are some situations in which it is technically difficult to accrue sufficient patients with spontaneous arrhythmias to study effectively the likelihood of acute termination of that arrhythmia. This difficulty may be related to the duration of spontaneous rhythm disturbance as well as the likelihood of the patient being in a hospital environment at the time of arrhythmia onset.

Despite these limitations, it is useful to examine the available trials of antiarrhythmic therapy in supraventricular arrhythmias. As radiofrequency ablation gains acceptance for the long-term treatment of atrioventricular nodal reentrant and atrioventricular reentrant tachycardias on a worldwide basis, many of these clinical trials will primarily be of historical importance. An underlying tenet of the trials of persistent atrial fibrillation has been the concept that rhythm control is better than rate control. This tenet has been questioned based on results of recent controlled clinical trials.

This chapter focuses on the use of pharmacologic agents for (1) acute termination or heart rate control of SVTs, (2) long-term suppression of SVTs, (3) acute termination of paroxysmal atrial fibrillation, (4) long-term suppression of paroxysmal atrial fibrillation, (5) suppression of recurrent persistent atrial fibrillation, (6) comparison of the strategies of rate control versus rhythm control in atrial fibrillation (7) prevention of supraventricular arrhythmias after cardiac surgery, and (8) control of the ventricular heart rate response in atrial fibrillation.

ACUTE TERMINATION AND HEART RATE CONTROL OF SUPRAVENTRICULAR TACHYCARDIAS

Conventional atrioventricular nodal blocking agents as well as types I and III antiarrhythmic agents have been used for the acute termination of SVTs. These studies have focused on acute conversion rates, the duration of time from drug administration to conversion, and adverse effects. Results from patients with atrioventricular nodal reentrant tachycardia, atrioventricular reentrant

TABLE 14-1 LIMITATIONS IN COMPARING AND CONTRASTING CLINICAL STUDIES OF PHARMACOLOGIC THERAPY IN SUPRAVENTRICULAR TACHYCARDIA

Small number of patients
Combining patients with arrhythmias of varying mechanisms
    Atrioventricular nodal reentrant tachycardia
    Atrioventricular reentrant tachycardia
    Atrial fibrillation/flutter
Dose-finding/titration period
Variable follow-up time for acute and long-term studies
Variable dosing regimens for the same agent
Sporadic nature of paroxysmal arrhythmias
Different definitions of successful therapy (i.e., complete suppression of arrhythmia vs. reduction in
    the frequency and duration of arrhythmia)
Multiple ways of assessing efficacy
    Patient self-reporting
    Electrocardiogram
    Transtelephonic monitoring
    Holter monitoring
Presence of adjunctive atrioventricular nodal blocking agents
Uneven distribution of underlying cardiac diseases
Variable severity of underlying cardiac disorders

tachycardia, atrial fibrillation or flutter, and automatic atrial tachycardia have been pooled in some studies.

Heart Rate Control in Acute Supraventricular Arrhythmias

Esmolol has been compared with placebo in 71 patients with supraventricular arrhythmias (heart rate >120 beats/min) lasting for at least 30 minutes.[1] This study included patients primarily with atrial fibrillation or atrial flutter but also included patients with supraventricular arrhythmias such as automatic atrial tachycardia (n = 6). Patients were randomized to esmolol (50–300 μg/kg/min) or placebo and treated for up to 30 minutes. Efficacy endpoints included conversion to sinus rhythm, decrease in heart rate to less than 100 beats/min, or a 20% decrease in heart rate. Patients not responding to the initial regimen were allowed to cross over to the other regimen. Of the 32 patients randomized to esmolol, 23 patients responded to therapy, whereas only two of 31 patients responded to placebo therapy. Crossovers to esmolol also had a higher likelihood of response (16 of 29) as compared with placebo (1 of 8). Only two patients converted to sinus rhythm. Increasing the esmolol infusion beyond 150 μg/kg/min did not result in any additional increase in therapeutic efficacy. Major side effects included hypotension (n = 8) and diaphoresis (n = 7) in patients treated with esmolol. There was one episode of symptomatic hypotension in a placebo-treated patient.

The Esmolol Multicenter Study Research Group compared the efficacy of esmolol and propranolol for the control of heart rate in supraventricular tachyarrhythmias.[2] Esmolol dosing, inclusion criteria, and endpoints were the same as discussed previously.[1] Atrial fibrillation or flutter was present in 95% of 127 study subjects. Esmolol and propranolol were equally effective in decreasing heart rate or converting the patient to sinus rhythm (66% for esmolol vs. 65% for propranolol). Approximately 75% of patients achieved heart rate control during the 4-hour maintenance infusion or injections for both agents. Hypotension developed in 23 of 64 patients receiving esmolol. Hypotension developed in four patients receiving propranolol. Four patients receiving propranolol also developed nausea.

Acute Termination of Supraventricular Tachyarrhythmias

Intravenous verapamil has been used extensively to terminate supraventricular arrhythmias. Supraventricular arrhythmias (atrioventricular nodal reentry [n = 9], sinus node reentry [n = 2], and atrioventricular reentry [n = 9]) were induced in 20 patients undergoing programmed electrical stimulation.[3] Fifteen of 19 patients converted to sinus rhythm with verapamil (0.075 mg/kg), whereas only 1 of 16 patients converted to sinus rhythm after receiving placebo.

Verapamil has been compared with adenosine in a larger randomized trial using a sequential dose-ranging protocol.[4] Patients had both spontaneous and induced arrhythmias. Pre-excitation was present in 22% of patients. In the first portion of this trial, adenosine was given in sequential doses of 3, 6, 9, and 12 mg (n = 137) or matching placebo was administered (n = 64). Adenosine was significantly more effective than placebo, and its efficacy increased with dose (Fig. 14-1). In the second phase of the study, patients were randomized between adenosine (n = 77, 6 mg followed by 12 mg intravenously) or verapamil (n = 81, 5 mg followed by 7.5 mg intravenously if no response). Efficacy was similar between the two agents if both doses were included (93.4% for adenosine and 90.6% for verapamil). Concomitant digoxin use, evidence of preexcitation in sinus rhythm, and mechanism of arrhythmia initiation did not influence efficacy. Facial flushing, chest pain, and dyspnea were common with adenosine (approximately 40% of patients) but were transient, generally resolving within 2 minutes. Side effects with verapamil were less

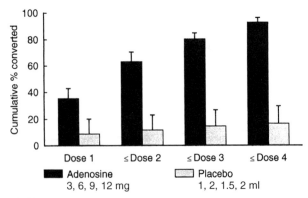

FIGURE 14-1. Cumulative efficacy of adenosine. The bars represent the cumulative percentage (with 95% CI) of eligible patients converting to sinus rhythm after adenosine and placebo. Data on both patients initially assigned to adenosine and those who crossed over to adenosine after four placebo injections are included. Each bar represents the percent converting after completion of that dose and the preceding dose or doses with each agent. Intravenous doses of adenosine were 3, 6, 9, and 12 mg; corresponding volumes of saline injected were 1, 2, 1.5, and 2 mL. Significant differences (P < 0.001) were seen at each dose level. (From DiMarco JP, Miles W, Akhtar M, et al: Adenosine for paroxysmal supraventricular tachycardia: Dose ranging and comparison with verapamil—assessment in placebo-controlled, multicenter trials. Ann Intern Med 1990; 113:104–110.)

common (12.4%) but occasionally lasted longer (hypotension in one patient lasting 20 minutes and facial flushing in one patient lasting 20 minutes).

The central intravenous administration of adenosine has been evaluated in 30 patients (atrioventricular reentrant tachycardia in 18, atrioventricular nodal reentrant tachycardia in 12) undergoing programmed electrical stimulation.[5] Sequential adenosine doses of 3, 6, 9, and 12 mg were administered by the peripheral and central routes. The dose required for central conversion was less (3.8 ± 1.6 mg) than for peripheral conversion (6.3 ± 3.3 mg). The time from drug administration to conversion was also less with central injections (12.7 ± 5.1 seconds vs. 19.2 ± 7.9 seconds). Side effects did not differ between the two arms. This time difference should not influence the clinician's decision regarding route of drug administration. Adenosine triphosphate has been compared with adenosine.[6] Efficacy rates (93% with adenosine and 88% with adenosine triphosphate) and time to conversion were similar between the two agents.

Intravenous diltiazem has been studied by two groups for the termination of paroxysmal SVTs.[7,8] Dougherty and colleagues[7] found that conversion to sinus rhythm was dose dependent. Patients receiving 0.05 mg/kg of diltiazem were much less likely to convert to sinus rhythm than those patients receiving 0.15 mg/kg of diltiazem or higher. Overall efficacy for conversion was 75% (47 of 63) for all doses of diltiazem and 25% (six of 24) for the control group. Hypotension was the most common side effect, occurring in seven (12%) patients receiving diltiazem. In another study, 34 patients with atrioventricular reentrant tachycardia and 20 patients with atrioventricular nodal reentrant tachycardia were treated with intravenous diltiazem after arrhythmia induction.[8] Diltiazem was effective in 24 of 28 (86%) patients, whereas only 5 of 26 (19%) of placebo-treated patients converted to sinus rhythm.

The median time to conversion was 2 minutes after beginning the diltiazem infusion. Propafenone, sotalol, and flecainide also have been used for acute termination of supraventricular arrhythmias. In a group of 20 patients, 15 of 20 patients receiving propafenone (2 mg/kg intravenously) converted to sinus rhythm, but 0 of 11 patients receiving placebo converted to sinus rhythm.[9] Sotalol appears to be equally efficacious (conversion in 30 minutes in 83% of sotalol-treated patients and 16% of placebo-treated patients; n = 43).[10] In another study, sotalol was effective in 67% of patients compared with 14% of control patients.[11]

β-adrenergic blocking agents (esmolol and propranolol) have been shown to reduce the heart rate of patients with SVTs. Acute termination of atrioventricular nodal reentrant tachycardias may be achieved in almost all patients with adenosine or verapamil. Efficacy increases with dosage. The side-effect profiles vary slightly between adenosine and verapamil and may form the basis for choosing one agent versus the other. Intravenous diltiazem as well as type I or III antiarrhythmic agents are effective in terminating supraventricular arrhythmias. In many centers, these agents are not first-line therapy because of cost and concerns regarding side effects.

LONG-TERM SUPPRESSION OF SUPRAVENTRICULAR TACHYCARDIAS

Few randomized trials exist studying pharmacologic therapy for the long-term suppression of SVTs. Those trials that do exist frequently pool patients with atrioventricular nodal reentrant tachycardia and atrioventricular reentrant tachycardia (Wolff-Parkinson-White syndrome) into one group. Because the mechanisms of the arrhythmias are different, this pooling ultimately may influence the results obtained.

The efficacy of verapamil in suppressing SVTs was investigated in a small trial of 12 patients (atrioventricular nodal reentrant tachycardia [n = 7], concealed bypass tract [n = 3], Wolff-Parkinson-White syndrome [n = 2]).[12] Each patient was required to have at least two episodes of arrhythmia per month on no suppressive therapy. After a dose-finding phase, patients entered a 4-month blinded protocol of alternating verapamil and placebo therapy in a randomized fashion. Efficacy was judged by the number of episodes of arrhythmia as well as the duration of arrhythmia by patient report and weekly Holter monitor. Patients had 0.7 ± 0.7 episodes per day on placebo by Holter versus 0.3 ± 0.5 episodes per day taking verapamil (P < 0.05). The average duration of arrhythmia fell dramatically on treatment (67 ± 111 min/day on placebo vs. 1 ± 2 min/day taking verapamil [P < 0.05]). These results suggest a beneficial effect of verapamil on the suppression of these arrhythmias over a relatively short period.

Winniford and colleagues[13] then studied 11 patients with documented supraventricular arrhythmia occurring at least two times per month in the absence of therapy and no evidence of ventricular preexcitation. Patients received digoxin, propranolol, or verapamil for 1 month followed by a 1-week washout period. Efficacy was judged by patient diary as well as weekly Holter monitors. According to the patient diaries, the number of weekly episodes of tachycardia did not vary between agents (digoxin, 2.3 ± 3.1 episodes; propranolol, 1.5 ± 2.3 episodes; verapamil, 2.9 ± 5.7 episodes). The authors did not include a placebo arm in this small study to allow the absolute effect of these atrioventricular nodal blocking agents to be determined.

Clair and associates[14] have studied the influence of oral diltiazem on the prevention of SVT in 17 patients without bypass tracts who experienced arrhythmias at least three times in 6 months. After a dose-ranging study to select the optimal dose of diltiazem (60–90 mg every 6 hours), patients entered a 2-month randomized phase followed by crossover to the other arm. Each randomized phase lasted for 60 days or until the first recurrence of arrhythmia. Endpoints included the duration of time until first recurrence and heart rate during tachycardia. Diltiazem did not significantly prolong the time until first recurrence but did decrease the heart rate during active therapy (average 208 beats/min without therapy to 189 beats/min on diltiazem; P < 0.01). This study was too small to detect anything but a large difference between diltiazem and placebo.

The type IC agents, flecainide and propafenone, have been studied in the suppression of SVT. The Flecainide Supraventricular Tachycardia Study Group enrolled 34 patients with a history of at least one episode of arrhythmia in the month before drug initiation.[15] A dose-ranging trial of flecainide was performed for 3 weeks to determine the maximal tolerated drug dosage for each patient (up to 200 mg twice a day). The next phase consisted of an 8-week randomized, placebo-controlled, crossover study. Patients could cross over after the documentation of four episodes of SVT. Although 51 patients qualified for the study, only 34 were available for the randomized phase. Three of these patients had adverse cardiac effects, including myocardial infarction (n = 1), ventricular fibrillation during programmed electrophysiologic stimulation (n = 1), and incessant SVT after intravenous flecainide (n = 1). Of the patients randomized, the cumulative proportion of patients free of tachycardia at 8 weeks was 0.79 for flecainide and 0.15 for placebo. Twenty-nine of 34 patients had a least one paroxysm while on placebo as compared with eight of 34 with at least one event while taking flecainide. Pritchett and colleagues[16] studied propafenone in a similar protocol in 16 patients with paroxysmal SVT. The time to first recurrence was prolonged in patients receiving propafenone in this trial; data from patients with atrial fibrillation were pooled with those who had SVT.

The UK Propafenone Paroxysmal Supraventricular Tachycardia (PSVT) Study Group has studied the influence of propafenone versus placebo in 52 patients with paroxysmal SVT.[17] The study design included two crossover phases of propafenone 300 mg twice a day versus placebo and propafenone 300 mg three times a day versus placebo. Recurrent arrhythmia was documented by diary and transtelephonic monitor. Twenty-nine of 45 patients completing the first phase of the study were free of arrhythmia and adverse effects while

on propafenone, whereas 11 of 45 were free of events while on placebo. Propafenone was even more effective at the higher dose (31 of 34 patients), but adverse events were more frequent (7 of 34 patients).

Type III antiarrhythmic agents may be effective in suppressing paroxysmal SVT. Azimilide is an investigational agents that blocks I(Kr) and I(Ks). Four small double-blind, randomized, placebo-controlled trials enrolled 193 patients with SVT.[18] These trials used a range of azimilide doses. One primary outcome was the time to first recurrence of the arrhythmia. The time to first recurrence was prolonged in patients taking 100 or 125 mg of azimilide twice a day in comparison with placebo. One case of nonfatal torsades des pointes was noted in this study.

Dofetilide, another type III agent, has been compared to propafenone and placebo in the suppression of SVT.[19] This 6 month, randomized, placebo-controlled trial enrolled 122 patients. These patients received either propafenone (150 mg three times per day), dofetilide (500 mcg once a day), or placebo. At 6 months, the probability of successful suppression of SVT was 54% in the propafenone treatment group, 50% in the dofetilide group, and 6% in the placebo group. No proarrhythmia occurred in the group taking dofetilide; three patients receiving propafenone suffered significant side effects.

Thus, few trials are available investigating the efficacy of pharmacologic therapy in the suppression of paroxysmal SVT. Trials that exist suggest that both atrioventricular nodal blocking agents and type IC antiarrhythmic agents may be effective in reducing the frequency, duration, or heart rate of episodes. Trials investigating calcium channel blockers are small and have shown equivocal results. Most of these studies are of short duration. Prescription of a given agent may depend not only on effectiveness but also on the side-effect profiles and cost. It is unlikely that large-scale trials of these agents will be performed because no long-term suppressive therapy may be needed for the patient with rare episodes, and radiofrequency ablation may be recommended as the most effective therapy to many patients with frequent paroxysms.

ACUTE TERMINATION OF PAROXYSMAL ATRIAL FIBRILLATION

Paroxysmal atrial fibrillation is a difficult clinical entity because the acute episodes may lead to palpitations, dyspnea, lightheadedness, or chest discomfort as well as a variety of other symptoms. Patients with brief episodes may not present for acute medical attention, but patients with more severe symptoms frequently present emergently. Effective, prompt therapy is ideal for alleviating patient symptoms. A summary of the efficacy of these trials is given in Table 14-2.

Digoxin is the primary therapy that has been available to clinicians for several decades. Because of its vagally mediated effects, however, digoxin has the potential for having little effect or a negative effect on the acute termination of atrial fibrillation. One randomized trial investigating digoxin in the conversion of recent-onset atrial fibrillation has been performed.[20]

■ ■ ■

TABLE 14-2 EFFECTIVENESS OF ANTIARRHYTHMIC AGENTS
IN TERMINATING ACUTE ATRIAL FIBRILLATION

Drug 1	Drug 2	Duration of trial (hr)	Drug 1	Drug 2	Value	Reference
			PROPORTION IN NORMAL SINUS RHYTHM			
Digoxin	Placebo	18	9/18	8/18	NS	18
Pirmenol	Placebo	1	12/20	3/20	<0.01	19
Flecainide	Procainamide	1	37/40	25/40	<0.001	20
Flecainide plus digoxin	Digoxin	1	29/51	7/51	<0.001	21
Flecainide	Verapamil	1	14/20	1/20	<0.001	22
Flecainide	Amiodarone	8	20/22	17/19	NS	23
Flecainide	Amiodarone	2	20/34	11/32	NS	24
Flecainide	Propafenone	1	10/20	5/20	<0.05	25
Flecainide	Propafenone	1	18/20	11/20	<0.02	26
Propafenone	Placebo	24	89/98	27/84	<0.001	27
Propafenone	Digoxin plus quinidine	24	25/29	23/29	NS	28
Sotalol	Digoxin plus quinidine	12	17/33	24/28	<0.001	30
Amiodarone	Digoxin plus quinidine	24	31/33	27/29	NS	31
Amiodarone	Digoxin	24	24/26	17/24	NS	32

Falk and colleagues[20] enrolled 36 patients with atrial fibrillation (≤7 days duration) and randomized them to treatment with digoxin or placebo (0.6, 0.4, 0.2, and 0.2 mg at 0, 4, 8, and 14 hours). Patients were monitored for 18 hours for the return of sinus rhythm. Eight of 18 patients receiving placebo and 9 of 18 patients receiving digoxin converted to sinus rhythm within the observation period. The average time to conversion was 5.1 hours with digoxin and 3.3 hours with placebo (P = NS). Thus, in this small trial, there were no significant differences between digoxin and placebo in the conversion of atrial fibrillation to sinus rhythm.

Pirmenol is a type I agent that has been investigated for the acute conversion of atrial fibrillation. In a randomized intravenous protocol, patients receiving pirmenol were more likely to convert to sinus rhythm (12 of 20) in 1 hour than those receiving placebo (3 of 20).[21] No controlled trials exist comparing other type IA agents with placebo.

Flecainide, a type IC agent, has been studied by several groups and compared with other agents as well as to placebo. In comparison to procainamide, patients receiving flecainide were more likely to convert to sinus rhythm within 1 hour of infusion (37 of 40 vs. 25 of 40).[22] The time to conversion was not different between the agents. Oral treatment also has been found to be effective for conversion to sinus rhythm, but the time to conversion is longer (104 minutes vs. 14 minutes in a group of 27 patients).[23] In another trial, flecainide (2 mg/kg) was administered concurrently with digoxin and compared with digoxin monotherapy.[24] Six hours after therapy was initiated, 34 of 51 patients receiving flecainide plus digoxin and 18 of 51 patients receiving digoxin monotherapy were in sinus rhythm.[24] Transient significant hypotension was more common in patients receiving flecainide than in the control group.

In comparison to verapamil, flecainide is more effective in terminating atrial fibrillation (14 of 20 vs. 1 of 20).[25]

Oral loading of flecainide has been compared with amiodarone and placebo therapy. Flecainide was associated with a higher rate of conversion (20 of 22 vs. 10 of 21 in the placebo group), with mean conversion times of 190 ± 147 minutes.[26] Amiodarone was associated with a lower rate of conversion (7 of 19) than flecainide in the first day of therapy. In another trial with similar design but a higher dose of amiodarone (7 mg/kg), flecainide was more effective in the first 2 hours after drug administration, but this superiority was not apparent 8 hours after drug administration (flecainide 68%, amiodarone 59%, placebo 56%).[27] Amiodarone, however, was more effective in acutely controlling the ventricular rate response.

Propafenone is another type IC agent used for the treatment of atrial fibrillation. In two trials comparing propafenone with flecainide, flecainide was more effective (pooled results 28 of 40 converted to normal sinus rhythm with flecainide and 16 of 40 converted to normal sinus rhythm with propafenone).[28,29] Hypotension may be associated with either therapy. In comparison to placebo, propafenone (2 mg/kg followed by a 10 mg/kg per 24-hour infusion) was more likely to result in sinus rhythm (89 of 98 vs. 27 of 84).[30] Termination of arrhythmia was quicker in patients treated with propafenone (2.5 ± 2.8 hours vs. 17.2 ± 7.8 hours for placebo). The efficacy of oral propafenone has been contrasted with digoxin plus quinidine combination therapy and placebo in a group of 87 patients.[31] Although the 12-hour conversion rates were higher in the propafenone group as compared with the other treatment arms, the 48-hour conversion to sinus rhythm was 76% in the placebo group, which was similar to the propafenone group at this time point. Intravenous propafenone and amiodarone have been administered at home for acute conversion of atrial fibrillation.[32] The median time of conversion was shorter for propafenone (10 minutes) than for amiodarone (60 minutes). Termination of the arrhythmia was also more frequent in patients receiving propafenone (88%) than amiodarone (40%).

Acute conversion to sinus rhythm with sotalol (17 of 33) was less effective than digoxin plus quinidine (24 of 28) in an oral-loading trial.[33] Asymptomatic ventricular tachycardia was observed in several patients in both arms of the trial; hypotension or bradycardia developed in nearly half of the patients receiving sotalol (80 mg at 0, 2, 6, and 10 hours).[33]

Intravenous amiodarone is also effective for the acute conversion of atrial fibrillation. Amiodarone was as effective as quinidine (31 of 33 vs. 27 of 29) over a 24-hour period.[34] Twenty-four of 26 patients receiving amiodarone achieved sinus rhythm versus 17 of 24 patients randomized to digoxin monotherapy in another trial.[35] Sotalol, amiodarone, and digoxin have been compared in patients with recent-onset atrial fibrillation.[36] The mean time to conversion to sinus rhythm was significantly shorter in the sotalol (13 hr) and amiodarone (18.1 hr) than in the digoxin arm (26.9 hr).[36] Acute rate control was better in those individuals receiving sotalol.

Dofetilide is a newly approved Class III antiarrhythmic agent used for the conversion of atrial fibrillation and flutter to normal sinus rhythm and maintenance of sinus rhythm over time. It has been compared to amiodarone and placebo in 150 patients.[37] Over a 3-hour period, sinus rhythm was more likely to be restored in the dofetilide arm (35%) than either of the other treatment arms (4% each). Six patients receiving dofetilide had significant ventricular arrhythmias during the study. In another trial, dofetilide was effective in converting 30.3% of patients to sinus rhythm compared with 3.3% of placebo-treated patients.[38] These patients had a duration of atrial fibrillation up to 60 days. Torsades des pointes was noted in two patients receiving dofetilide.[38]

Many studies have focused on the utility of ibutilide fumarate for the acute conversion of atrial fibrillation or the facilitation of direct current cardioversion. In most trials patient rhythm status is classified as either fibrillation or flutter because early data suggested this agent was more efficacious with flutter than with fibrillation. A 90-minute time point for evaluating conversion to sinus rhythm is the endpoint used most frequently. Early studies examined differences between various dosing regimens. Initially the drug was dosed according to weight. Doses of 0.015 and 0.020 mg/kg appeared to be the most effective in terminating atrial fibrillation/flutter, with a 3.6% incidence of polymorphic ventricular tachycardia.[39] Subsequent dosing has been standardized without the need for weight adjustment. In a trial of 266 patients, 47% of 180 patients receiving ibutilide had termination of their arrhythmia, in comparison to 2% of patients taking placebo.[40] No meaningful difference was seen between the use of 1.5 mg and 2.0 mg of ibutilide. Termination of atrial fibrillation (31%) was less likely than flutter (63%). Polymorphic ventricular tachycardia occurred in 15 patients receiving ibutilide.[40] Another multicenter study examined the effects of ibutilide on conversion of atrial fibrillation/flutter ranging from 3 hours to 90 days. Of patients, 35% (73/209) receiving active agent reverted to sinus rhythm within 90 minutes compared to 0/41 placebo patients.[41] Electrical cardioversion may be more successful in patients following administration of ibutilide.

Ibutilide has been compared to procainamide for the reversion of atrial fibrillation and atrial flutter.[42] In 120 patients randomized to ibutilide (1 mg × 2) or procainamide (400 mg IV × 3) ibutilide was clearly superior to procainamide. Thirty-five of 60 ibutilide-treated patients (58.3%) and 11/60 (18.3%) of procainamide-treated patients had successful conversion to sinus rhythm in 90 minutes after starting the protocol. The treatment difference was more apparent in those patients with atrial flutter (76% vs. 14%) than in those with fibrillation (51% vs. 21%). Polymorphic ventricular tachycardia requiring cardioversion occurred in one patient receiving ibutilide. Hypotension was the most common complication of procainamide.

In comparison to DL-sotalol, ibutilide appears to be more effective in the acute conversion of atrial fibrillation or flutter.[43] In a trial of 308 patients randomized to 1 mg ibutilide, 2 mg ibutilide, or 1.5 mg/kg dl-sotalol, atrial flutter was more likely to convert with ibutilide (70% higher dose, 56% lower dose) than with sotalol (19%). The 2-mg dose of ibutilide converted 48% of patients with atrial fibrillation to sinus rhythm. Two patients (of 211) receiving the 2-mg dose of ibutilide had polymorphic ventricular tachycardia.

Although many classes of pharmacologic therapy are useful for the acute termination of arrhythmias, the primary result of antiarrhythmic administration appears to be decreasing the duration of a paroxysm. The American College of Cardiology, American Heart Association, and the European Society of Cardiology have published practice guidelines for the management of atrial fibrillation.[44] Class I recommendations imply that there is evidence for and/or general agreement that the procedure or treatment is useful and effective.[44] Dofetilide, flecainide, propafenone, and ibutilide have been given class I recommendations for pharmacologic conversion of atrial fibrillation of less than 7 days duration. Only dofetilide has received a class I recommendation for the pharmacologic conversion of atrial fibrillation of a longer duration. Depending on the nature of the underlying heart disease and patient symptoms, terminating an episode more quickly may help the patient feel better and decrease the use of medical resources.

ANTIARRHYTHMIC THERAPY FOR THE PREVENTION OF PAROXYSMS OF ATRIAL FIBRILLATION

Episodes of paroxysmal atrial fibrillation occur at varying frequencies but are believed to occur according to a Poisson distribution. Trials investigating the role of antiarrhythmic therapy in the prevention of recurrent paroxysms focus on endpoints such as time to first recurrence of arrhythmia, the frequency of arrhythmia recurrence, or the likelihood of total suppression of the arrhythmia. These trials are difficult to perform and interpret when the frequency of events is uncommon or rare. As a result, most trials focus on patients with frequent symptomatic atrial arrhythmias.

Van Wijk and colleagues[45] studied 49 patients with weekly episodes of paroxysmal atrial fibrillation. These patients were randomized to flecainide 100 mg twice a day or quinidine 500 mg twice a day. Drug dosages were adjusted upward for symptomatic recurrences (flecainide 150 mg twice a day or quinidine 500 mg three times a day), and patients were treated for 3 months followed by a 3-month crossover to the other drug regimen. Recurrences were documented by self-report, electrocardiogram, and monthly 24-hour Holter monitoring. At the maximal dose prescribed during this 3-month period, flecainide totally suppressed atrial fibrillation by Holter in 50% of patients, and quinidine was effective in 32% (P = NS). Of patients, 20% discontinued quinidine because of undesirable side effects, including one patient with prolonged QT. One patient receiving flecainide developed hemodynamically well-tolerated ventricular tachycardia necessitating drug withdrawal. One patient receiving flecainide died; this death was deemed unrelated to drug therapy by the authors.

A comparison of flecainide and quinidine for this purpose was also performed by Lau and coworkers,[46] who randomized 19 patients without structural heart disease to these agents. Trial design included blinded therapy for 8 weeks followed by a crossover phase. Thirteen patients also completed a placebo phase. Transtelephonic monitoring was used to record recurrences in addition to monthly Holter monitors. All patients experienced symptoms during the placebo phase, whereas flecainide resulted in suppression of symptoms in 4 of 19 patients, and quinidine resulted in control of symptoms in 2 of 11 patients. Alternative ways of expressing the efficacy of therapy include a prolongation of the time to first recurrence of arrhythmia (placebo, 2 days; flecainide, 21 days; quinidine 15 days [P < 0.01]), symptomatic duration of arrhythmia (placebo, 1619 ± 616 minutes; flecainide, 975 ± 424 minutes; quinidine, 865 ± 306 minutes), and frequency of arrhythmia (placebo, 25 ± 9 episodes per 8 weeks; flecainide, 14 ± 8 episodes; quinidine, 24 ± 10 episodes). Although both quinidine and flecainide appeared to decrease the duration of therapy and the time to first recurrence, quinidine did not alter the frequency of arrhythmia.

The Flecainide Multicenter Atrial Fibrillation Study Group studied flecainide (n = 122) versus quinidine (n = 117) in patients with symptomatic paroxysmal atrial fibrillation.[47] Patients with significant ventricular arrhythmias, conduction defects, or left-ventricular dysfunction, as well as those with significant noncardiac diseases, were excluded from participating in the study. Patients kept a diary to record characteristics and frequency of attacks on medication. Antiarrhythmic agents were discontinued for development of significant conduction defects, QT prolongation, or drug-related toxicity. These patients had frequent paroxysms of arrhythmia (13.4 per month in the flecainide group and 10.7 per month in the quinidine group). The majority of patients had been treated with antiarrhythmics previously. Approximately 10% of patients in each group (9.8% flecainide and 12.0% quinidine) discontinued therapy because of an unacceptable response. Approximately one fifth of patients (23.8% flecainide and 20.5% quinidine) had total suppression of arrhythmia during a 9-month period. In approximately three fourths of all patient months, there were no symptomatic arrhythmias with both agents. Side effects resulted in discontinuation of therapy in 29.9% of quinidine-treated patients and 18.0% of flecainide-treated patients. There were no deaths in this trial. Thus, both quinidine and flecainide effectively reduced the frequency of paroxysms of atrial fibrillation. Quinidine was more likely to be associated with adverse effects.

The Danish–Norwegian Flecainide Multicenter Study Group administered flecainide (150 mg twice a day) or placebo to 43 patients with paroxysmal atrial fibrillation for 3 months with a crossover period.[48] Entry criteria included a minimum of three symptomatic paroxysms over a 3-month interval on 3 different days lasting less than 72 hours. Flecainide decreased the mean paroxysms per week (0.2 ± 0.4) in comparison to placebo (1.9 ± 12.1) in individuals completing both treatment periods. Complete response was seen in 12 of 24 flecainide-treated patients, with no response in eight patients. Of note, two patients died during the flecainide treatment period, one with pulmonary carcinoma and one while swimming in the North Sea.

Propafenone is another type IC antiarrhythmic agent studied in the treatment of paroxysmal atrial fibrillation. Connolly and Hoffert[49] studied 18 patients with monthly symptomatic episodes of atrial fibrillation. These patients entered a randomized trial with four monthly treatment periods alternating between propafenone and placebo. Early crossovers were permitted on patient request for perceived inefficacy. Patient diaries and transtelephonic monitors were used to document arrhythmia recurrences. Only 12 of 18 patients participated in the crossover study. The other six withdrew because of side effects or inefficacy during the dose-ranging study (n = 5) or because of noncompliance (n = 1). Efficacy was judged by reduction in episodes of atrial fibrillation. During the placebo phase, patients experienced fibrillation on 51% ± 34% of days. This was reduced to 27% ± 34% of days on propafenone. Patients were more likely to cross over prematurely on placebo (45%) than on propafenone (14%). One patient receiving placebo experienced sudden death during the trial.

Pritchett and colleagues[16] investigated propafenone in 17 patients with paroxysmal atrial fibrillation. After a dose-finding phase, patients were randomly assigned to placebo or propafenone for up to 60 days. The observation period began 3 days after the beginning of therapy and continued until the recurrence of arrhythmia or 60 days, the maximal length of the study period. Patients then were treated with the second agent in a similar fashion. Patients were allowed to continue digoxin therapy. Only 9 of 17 patients with paroxysmal atrial fibrillation entered the randomized phase of the study. In these 9 patients, the time to first recurrence of arrhythmia was prolonged with propafenone. Data pooled from patients with SVT as well as atrial fibrillation suggest that the rate of recurrent arrhythmia is approximately 21% that of placebo therapy. Cardiac adverse events included one episode of atrial flutter with a rate of 263 beats/min in one patient and the development of chest discomfort, presyncope, and dyspnea in another patient, both of whom were receiving propafenone in an open-label fashion after completion of the randomized phase.

The Flecainide AF French Study Group enrolled 97 patients with paroxysmal atrial fibrillation into a study of flecainide versus placebo.[50] Patients with heart failure, significant conduction disturbances, or recent amiodarone usage were excluded from participation. Hypertension and lone atrial fibrillation were the most common causes of underlying disease. Of patients, 23% of those treated with flecainide and 24% of those treated with propafenone discontinued therapy because of an inadequate response. At 1 year of therapy, the probability of successful treatment with flecainide was 62% and with propafenone was 47%. One patient with hypertension receiving propafenone died during the study.

Reimold and colleagues[51] have studied propafenone and sotalol in patients with paroxysmal atrial fibrillation (n = 47). In their study, the randomization was stratified according to arrhythmia pattern and left atrial size. The likelihood of any recurrence of atrial fibrillation at 6 months was similar between those patients treated with propafenone (42 ± 10) and sotalol (48 ± 12) (P = NS). Thirty patients with paroxysmal atrial fibrillation received propafenone or placebo in the UK Propafenone PSVT Study Group, a 3-month double-blind, double-crossover study.[17] Patients were less likely to have adverse effects or recurrent atrial fibrillation on propafenone 300 mg twice a day (17 of 30) versus placebo (8 of 30). As the dose of propafenone increased to 300 mg three times a day, the incidence of adverse events increased to 40%. Propafenone has been compared with hydroquinidine in a larger study of 200 patients with a minimum of three recurrences of atrial fibrillation in 6 months.[52] At 6 months after drug initiation, survival of sinus rhythm was 60% for propafenone and 56% for quinidine, suggesting similar efficacy rates.

Thus, these randomized trials investigating antiarrhythmic therapy in the prevention of episodes of paroxysmal atrial fibrillation demonstrate drug efficacy when examining parameters such as frequency of recurrence, time to first recurrence, and duration of episodes. Total suppression of arrhythmia over a long period seems less likely. Because the authors of these studies chose different endpoints and enrolled a heterogeneous group of patients in terms of underlying heart disease, they are difficult to compare. Most trials lasted a brief time relative to the duration of this chronic disease process. Extrapolating from these data to long-term efficacy is extremely difficult because the underlying disease process may not remain stable over time. The ultimate decision to use antiarrhythmic therapy in a given patient should be based on the degree and frequency of symptoms as well as the patient tolerability of the antiarrhythmic agent.

SUPPRESSION OF PERSISTENT ATRIAL FIBRILLATION

Quinidine is a type IA agent that has been available for decades for the maintenance of sinus rhythm. With the advent of direct current cardioversion in the early 1960s, reestablishment of sinus rhythm became possible in a large proportion of patients with sinus rhythm, and the influence of quinidine on the maintenance of sinus rhythm over time could be observed. Coplen and coworkers[53] examined six randomized, controlled trials of quinidine in the maintenance of sinus rhythm. These six trials together enrolled 808 patients. The efficacy of quinidine in maintaining sinus rhythm was evident at 3, 6, and 12 months after cardioversion (Fig. 14-2), with an absolute difference of 24.4% (14.0, 34.8) between quinidine and placebo therapy 12 months after cardioversion. This meta-analysis raised the issue of increased mortality in patients treated with quinidine (1.8%) versus placebo (0.3%).[54] A smaller study (n = 53) evaluated the efficacy of verapamil versus quinidine in the conversion and maintenance of sinus rhythm.[54] There was a higher conversion to sinus rhythm with quinidine; long-term maintenance of sinus rhythm was similar between these agents at 12 and 24 months.

Disopyramide has been compared with placebo in several studies.[55,56] The overall efficacy of disopyramide is similar to quinidine in these studies. Karlson and associates[56] studied 90 patients who were randomized to disopyramide or placebo. At 1 year after cardioversion, 54% of disopyramide and 30% of placebo patients remained in sinus rhythm.[56]

A contemporary comparison between quinidine and sotalol, a type III antiarrhythmic agent, was made by Juul-Moller and colleagues.[57] They studied 183 patients with chronic atrial fibrillation who were cardioverted to normal sinus rhythm. Two hours after conversion, patients were randomized to quinidine (n = 85) or sotalol (n = 98). At 6 months of follow-up, 52% of

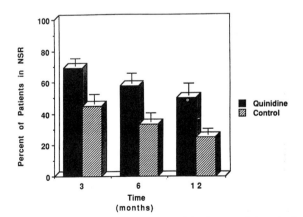

FIGURE 14-2. Proportion of patients remaining in normal sinus rhythm (NSR) at 3, 6, and 12 months after cardioversion was greater at all time intervals in a quinidine-treated group as compared with a control group (P < 0.001). (From Coplen SE, Antman EM, Berlin JA, et al: Efficacy and safety of quinidine therapy for maintenance of sinus rhythm after cardioversion: A meta-analysis of randomized control trials. Circulation 1990; 82: 1106–1116.)

sotalol-treated patients and 48% of quinidine-treated patients remained in sinus rhythm (P = NS). Relapses to atrial fibrillation occurred in 34% of sotalol-treated patients and in 22% of quinidine-treated patients. Adverse effects were more likely in quinidine-treated (50%) than in sotalol-treated (28%) patients. Two patients died during the study, one receiving sotalol (posterolateral myocardial infarction) and one receiving quinidine (cerebral embolism). Ventricular tachycardia and ventricular fibrillation occurred in an additional two patients receiving quinidine; both these episodes occurred during hospital monitoring and had successful outcomes. Propafenone and sotalol were compared by Reimold and colleagues[51] in 53 patients with persistent atrial fibrillation. These agents were equally effective at maintaining sinus rhythm 6 months after starting therapy.

The efficacy of flecainide versus placebo for the maintenance of sinus rhythm was tested by Van Gelder and coworkers[58] in 81 patients with persistent atrial fibrillation. Patients without congestive heart failure or significant angina pectoris, as well as those patients with myocardial infarction within 2 years of enrollment, major conduction defects, or severe systemic disease, were excluded. Sinus rhythm was maintained in 49% of flecainide-treated patients versus 36% of untreated patients 12 months after initiation of therapy. This difference was not significant given the small number of patients in this study. New York Heart Association (NYHA) class and flecainide treatment were predictive of outcome, whereas left atrial size and duration of atrial fibrillation were not predictive of rhythm outcome. Adverse cardiac events related to flecainide included syncope, sinus arrest, high-grade atrioventricular block, rate-related left bundle branch block, and proarrhythmic ventricular premature beats.

Although amiodarone has been shown to improve maintenance of sinus rhythm in patients with persistent atrial fibrillation, there are no randomized trials comparing this agent with placebo. One nonrandomized trial found the 3-year likelihood of staying in sinus rhythm in patients who had failed other therapy to be 53%.[59] Another trial studying a similar group of patients (n = 100) found the actuarial rate of sinus rhythm survival at 3 years to be 70%, a rate far better than results with conventional therapy.[60] The Canadian Trial of Atrial Fibrillation investigated the role of amiodarone in comparison to propafenone and sotalol in the maintenance of sinus rhythm.[61] Patients with paroxysmal and persistent atrial fibrillation were enrolled in this trial. Amiodarone was more effective than propafenone or sotalol after the first month of therapy but was more likely to be discontinued as a result of side effects (18% at 1 year versus 11% of sotalol or propafenone treated patients).[61]

Azimilide has been used to suppress persistent atrial fibrillation. In a dose-finding trial (35–125 mg once a day maintenance dose), doses of 100 and 125 mg/day results in a prolongation of time to recurrent arrhythmia (hazard ratio of 1.34 [1.05,1.72, P < 0.01 for the 100 mg/day dose] and 1.32 [1.07,1.62, P < 0.01 for the 125 mg/day dose]).[62] Lower doses were not effective in suppressing arrhythmia. The presence of heart failure or ischemic heart disease was predictive of an increased treatment

effect. Torsades des pointes was observed in 0.9% of patients receiving active therapy at the 100 and 125 mg/day dose levels.

Dofetilide has been approved in the United States for the suppression of atrial fibrillation. The DIAMOND trial (Danish Investigations of Arrhythmia and Mortality on Dofetilide) examined the role of this agent on all-cause mortality and morbidity in patients (n = 1510) with left-ventricular dysfunction following myocardial infarction.[63] No significant differences in mortality, cardiac mortality, or arrhythmic deaths were seen between the active and placebo-treated groups.[63] The small proportion of patients with atrial fibrillation in this trial (8% of total), were more likely to revert to sinus rhythm if they received dofetilide (25/59 on active agent versus 7/56 on placebo). A dose-finding trial of dofetilide (125, 250, or 500 mcg twice a day) versus placebo in 325 patients investigated the acute conversion of arrhythmia and the 1-year maintenance of sinus rhythm.[37] The probability of maintaining sinus rhythm at 1 year was greater in the 500-mcg dose group (58%) than in the 125-mcg (40%) or the 250-mcg (37%) dose group. All groups were superior to placebo maintenance of sinus rhythm (25%).[37] Pharmacologic conversion rates were higher in the 500-mcg dose group (29.9%) than in all other treatment/placebo groups. Two cases of torsades des pointes and one case of sudden death were noted in the patients treated with dofetilide.

Type IA and IC antiarrhythmic agents and sotalol have been shown to be effective in preventing recurrences of persistent atrial fibrillation in randomized clinical trials. This effectiveness extends over a period ranging from 6 months to 2 years in most patients. Amiodarone may be more effective than these agents, but there are minimal controlled data investigating its efficacy and it has more significant adverse effects. Amiodarone, flecainide, propafenone (alone and in combination with verapamil), quinidine, and sotalol have been given the American College of Cardiology Recommendation Class I based on the available evidence.[44] The decision to use any agent to maintain sinus rhythm must be weighed against the potential side effects of each individual agent, especially because many of these side effects could be serious.

MANAGEMENT OF PERSISTENT ATRIAL FIBRILLATION—RHYTHM CONTROL VERSUS RATE CONTROL

Although many trials have explored the efficacy of antiarrhythmic agents in suppressing atrial fibrillation, there have been limited data investigating whether rhythm control (restoration of sinus rhythm) provides better outcomes in terms of survival than rate control. Outcomes of these two management approaches is being investigated by trials such as the AFFIRM and Pharmacologic Intervention in Atrial Fibrillation (PIAF) trial.[64,65]

Preliminary results were released at the American College of Cardiology's 51st Annual Scientific Session and have been published.[66] The AFFIRM trial enrolled 4060 patients with an average age of 70 years.[66] The primary outcome was all-cause mortality. Of the population, 61% was male. Contributing cardiac etiologies included hypertension in 51% and coronary artery disease in 26%. The majority of patients had normal left-ventricular function. Drug therapy in the rate-control arm included beta blockers, calcium-channel blockers, and digoxin or combination therapy.[66] Although there was a broad selection of antiarrhythmics, the most commonly used agents were amiodarone (39%), sotalol (33%), and propafenone (10%). Therapy was often switched during follow-up. After 5 years, all-cause mortality was 23.8% in the rhythm-control arm as compared to 21.3% in the rate-control arm (P = 0.08) (Fig. 14–3). Warfarin use was higher in the rate-control (approximately 85%) arm than in the rhythm-control (approximately 70%) arm. The rates of secondary endpoints of death, major bleeding, disabling stroke or anoxic encephalopathy, or cardiac arrest were similar in the two groups (32.0% in the rhythm-control arm and 32.7% in the rate-control arm).[66]

A smaller study sponsored by the Rate Control versus Electrical Cardioversion for Persistent Atrial Fibrillation Study Group investigated the strategies of rate and rhythm control when a patient had a first recurrence of atrial fibrillation following cardioversion.[67] The primary endpoint was a composite of death from heart failure, thromboembolic complications, bleeding, need for a pacemaker, or severe adverse effects of antiarrhythmic agents. The primary endpoint occurred in 17.2% of the rate-control group and in 22.6% of the rhythm-control group.[67] This suggests that rhythm control is not superior to rate control in this context.

Taken together, these trials support the concept that either rate of rhythm control represents acceptable strategies in the management of patients with atrial fibrillation. The decision to use either one of these strategies may depend on patient symptoms and presentation.

PREVENTION OF SUPRAVENTRICULAR ARRHYTHMIAS AFTER CARDIAC SURGERY

Supraventricular arrhythmias, most frequently atrial fibrillation, are common complications of coronary artery bypass surgery. Several randomized trials have been performed investigating the role of digoxin, β-adrenergic blocking agents, and calcium channel blocking agents in the prevention of these arrhythmias. Trial design has been variable in terms of the time of initiation of therapy (preoperatively or postoperatively), dosage and choice of agent, and duration and type of monitoring postoperatively as well as the duration of arrhythmias needed for reaching the study endpoint. Trials have also varied according to arrhythmia type included (e.g., SVT, atrial fibrillation, atrial flutter). Twenty-four randomized trials published before 1990 were included in a meta-analysis published in 1991.[68] Three of these trials evaluated the efficacy of verapamil, five evaluated the efficacy of digoxin, and 16 examined various β-adrenergic blocking agents. Verapamil and digoxin were not associated with a reduction in supraventricular arrhythmias (Fig. 14-4). β-adrenergic blocking agents, however, were associated with a profound reduction in the development of these arrhythmias (pooled odds ratio, 0.28 [0.21 to 0.36]; P < 0.0001). This marked reduction in supraventricular arrhythmias was noted regardless of time of drug initiation, exact agent used, and dosage selected (for propranolol). Verapamil, digoxin, and β-adrenergic blocking agents all were associated with a reduction in the ventricular rate during supraventricular arrhythmias. Limitations in interpreting these four

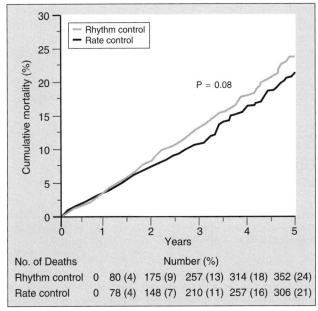

FIGURE 14-3. The cumulative mortality over time is shown for the rhythm- and rate-control arms of the AFFIRM trial. There was no significant difference in the incidence of this endpoint. (From The Atrial Fibrillation Follow-up Investigation of Rhythm Management (AFFIRM) Investigators: A comparison of rate control and rhythm control in patients with atrial fibrillation. N Engl J Med 2002; 347:1825–1833.)

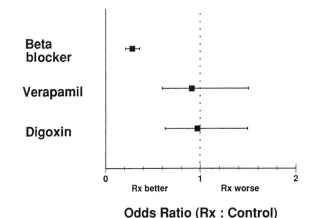

Odds Ratio (Rx : Control)

FIGURE 14-4. Summary odds ratio for the development of supraventricular arrhythmias as estimated by the Mantel-Haenszel method for treatment (Rx) with digoxin, verapamil, or beta blockers. The width of the horizontal lines indicates the 95% confidence intervals for the estimates of the odds ratios shown. (From Andrews TC, Reimold SC, Berlin JA, et al: Prevention of supraventricular arrhythmias after coronary artery bypass surgery: A meta-analysis of randomized control trials. Circulation 1991; 84 (Suppl 3):III-236–III-244.)

studies relate to the type of patient enrolled. Most patients were male, had preserved left-ventricular systolic function, and had been taking β-adrenergic blocking agents preoperatively. Patients enrolled in these studies underwent coronary artery bypass grafting but did not have valvular surgery.

Other studies have focused on the use of type IA, type IC, and type III agents on the incidence of atrial fibrillation after cardiac surgery. Intravenous procainamide has been administered for the prevention of postoperative atrial fibrillation. In one series of 46 patients, procainamide reduced the number of tachycardia episodes (five episodes per 129 patient days at risk vs. 17 episodes in 161 patient days at risk in the control group).[69] The use of procainamide to convert atrial fibrillation to sinus rhythm has been compared with digoxin in 30 patients; conversion to sinus rhythm occurred in 87% of procainamide-treated patients as opposed to 60% of digoxin-treated patients.[70] Conversion to sinus rhythm occurred sooner after the start of treatment with procainamide (40 minutes) than with digoxin (540 minutes).[70] Sotalol, a type III agent, has been used by several investigators to treat postoperative atrial fibrillation. Campbell and colleagues[71] randomized patients to sotalol (n = 22) versus disopyramide plus digoxin (n = 20). Seventeen patients in each group reverted to sinus rhythm within 12 hours. Patients taking disopyramide plus digoxin were more likely to develop recurrent atrial fibrillation than those given sotalol. The efficacy of sotalol versus conventional β-adrenergic blocking agents was studied by Nystrom and colleagues[72] in 101 patients. Postoperative atrial fibrillation was more common in those patients taking conventional β-adrenergic blocking agents (29%) than in those treated with sotalol (10%) (P = 0.028). In a larger series, Suttorp and coworkers[73] studied 300 patients after coronary artery bypass grafting who had been given sotalol versus placebo. SVT was seen in 24 (16%) sotalol-treated patients and in 49 (33%) placebo-treated patients (P < 0.005), consistent with a major benefit of sotalol for the prevention of postcoronary artery bypass surgery atrial arrhythmias.

Propafenone (300 mg twice daily), a type IC agent, was compared with atenolol (50 mg per day) in 207 patients undergoing bypass surgery (n = 198) or valve replacement (n = 9) for arrhythmia prophylaxis.[74] Supraventricular arrhythmias developed in 13 of 105 patients receiving propafenone and 11 of 102 receiving atenolol (P = NS). Propafenone was compared with amiodarone in the acute conversion of atrial fibrillation or flutter.[75] There was a greater likelihood of converting to sinus rhythm 1 hour after treatment initiation in those patients treated with propafenone (45%) than with amiodarone (20%). By 24 hours after the onset of therapy, there was no significant difference in the proportion of patients in sinus rhythm receiving propafenone (68%) than in those receiving amiodarone (83%).

Considerable interest has been developed in the use of amiodarone to prevent postoperative atrial fibrillation. One protocol used amiodarone 600 mg per day for 7 days. The incidence of atrial fibrillation decreased from 53% of the placebo group to 25% in the treated group (n = 125).[76] In another preoperative protocol in which approximately 90% of the patients also received beta blocker therapy, atrial fibrillation was decreased from 38.0% to 22.5%.[77] A less-intense strategy used in the Amiodarone Reduction in Coronary Heart (ARCH) trial (n = 300) demonstrated that use of intravenous amiodarone (1 g/day for the first 2 days postoperatively) had a modest effect on decreasing the development of this arrhythmia (47% to 35%).[78]

In a population of 80 patients undergoing coronary artery bypass surgery or valve replacement who developed atrial fibrillation, oral quinidine was more effective in converting to sinus rhythm than intravenous amiodarone (64% vs. 41%) during the 16-hour study period.[79] Predictors of drug failure during this time period included preoperative atrial fibrillation, longer time from arrhythmia recognition to treatment, mitral valve operations, and concomitant propranolol therapy. This is one of the few studies including a moderate number of patients undergoing valve operations (40 patients). In comparison to placebo, intravenous amiodarone reduced the incidence of atrial fibrillation (5% vs. 21%).

Ibutilide has been compared to placebo for the rapid reversion of atrial fibrillation to sinus rhythm after cardiac surgery.[80] The primary endpoint was the proportion of patients reverting to sinus rhythm within 90 minutes of drug administration. Two 10-minute blinded infusions of placebo or ibutilide at varying doses were given. Atrial fibrillation (n = 201) or atrial flutter (n = 101) was present for 1 hour to 3 days prior to enrollment. Sinus rhythm was achieved in 15% of placebo patients and 40% (0.25 mg), 47% (0.5 mg), and 57% (1 mg) of ibutilide-treated patients. Polymorphic ventricular tachycardia was noted in 1.2% of placebo-treated patients and 1.8% of ibutilide treated patients.

Thus, a variety of antiarrhythmic agents are efficacious in decreasing supraventricular arrhythmias after coronary artery bypass grafting. Of all agents, however, β-adrenergic blocking agents are the most efficacious in decreasing the occurrence and frequency of supraventricular arrhythmias in this setting and should be considered in patients undergoing this operation.

CONTROL OF THE VENTRICULAR RESPONSE IN ATRIAL FIBRILLATION

An important use of atrioventricular nodal blocking agents is to control the ventricular response to atrial fibrillation. Many studies have been performed investigating the relative efficacies of β-adrenergic blocking agents, calcium channel blockers, digoxin, and combinations of these agents on resting and exercise heart rate control as well as exercise tolerance with these agents. Most of these trials do not use a treatment-free arm. The control arm generally consists of patients treated with digoxin. Similarly, most of the treatment arms use combination as opposed to monotherapy; combination therapy generally includes digoxin plus another agent. The combination of nadolol and digoxin therapy has been compared with digoxin in 20 patients with persistent atrial fibrillation whose baseline average heart rates were greater than 80 beats/min.[81] After a nadolol dose titration period, patients taking digoxin underwent a double-blind cross-over of nadolol versus placebo. The resting heart rate decreased from 92 ± 19 beats/min to 73 ± 16 beats/min on nadolol (87 mg/day). Maximal exercise heart rate was diminished by nadolol (126 ± 25 beats/min vs. 175 ± 24 beats/min on placebo) as was maximal exercise time (380 ± 143 seconds vs. 466 ± 143 seconds). Nadolol/digoxin combination therapy and digoxin monotherapy also were compared by another group of investigators in 32 patients.[82] Using a similar trial design, the average heart rate dropped from 78 ± 4 beats/min to 63 ± 3 beats/min on combination therapy with an average daily nadolol dose of 59 ± 16 mg/day. Exercise duration was not different between the two arms of this study, but exercise-related average heart rate dropped from 154 to 120 beats/min.

The rate-controlling effects of labetalol were studied in 10 patients with persistent atrial fibrillation who underwent four phases of treatment with a randomized crossover design (placebo, digoxin, digoxin with half-dose labetalol, and full-dose labetalol).[83] Exercise duration was not reduced with labetalol. Maximal exercise heart rate was reduced with labetalol therapy (156 ± 4 beats/min vs. 177 ± 2 beats/min on placebo). The resting and exercise rate pressure products were decreased in patients receiving labetalol. Digoxin had no effect on peak exercise heart rate compared with placebo.

Pindolol, a β-adrenergic blocking agent with intrinsic sympathomimetic activity, has been combined with digoxin for controlling the heart rate in atrial fibrillation.[84] Twelve patients were treated with pindolol plus digoxin versus digoxin treatment alone or digoxin plus verapamil. The addition of pindolol therapy was useful in decreasing maximal heart rate as well as heart rate variability. The addition of verapamil therapy to digoxin resulted in a minor decrease in heart rate.

Sotalol (80–160 mg/day) has been combined with digoxin as therapy for the control of ventricular response in atrial fibrillation.[85] Twenty patients were randomized to placebo, dl-sotalol 80 mg/day, or dl-sotalol 160 mg/day after a dose-finding period. Digoxin was continued in the sotalol arms. Efficacy was assessed by determining the heart rate at rest as well as the exercise heart rate. Resting heart rate was reduced significantly in patients receiving sotalol (95 ± 4 beats/min at baseline to 79 ± 3 beats/min for sotalol 80 mg/day and 97 ± 4 beats/min to 79 ± 3 beats/min for sotalol 160 mg/day). The maximal heart rate during exercise was not influenced by digoxin therapy but was significantly decreased with both doses of sotalol.

The influence of verapamil, a calcium channel blocker, has been studied by several groups. In 27 patients, the resting heart rate was lower in patients treated with verapamil and digoxin (69 ± 13 beats/min) compared with digoxin alone (87 ± 20 beats/min).[86] The heart rate at the conclusion of 3 minutes of exercise also was decreased in those receiving verapamil (104 ± 14 beats/min vs. 136 ± 23 beats/min). Doses of 240 to 480 mg/day of verapamil were used to achieve this heart rate control. Lewis and colleagues[87] studied the influence of verapamil on 12 patients. Patients entered a double-blind crossover study with a placebo arm (no verapamil) versus verapamil 40 mg three times a day, 80 mg three times a day, or 120 mg three times a day. The resting heart rate was not significantly influenced by the addition of verapamil. The exercise heart rate decreased, especially with the higher doses of verapamil (postexercise digoxin, 147 ± 23 beats/min; verapamil 80 mg three times a day, 127 ± 15 beats/min; verapamil 120 mg three times day, 132 ± 30 beats/min). Exercise duration did not significantly vary between the treatment arms in this study. In another trial, 20 patients were given verapamil/digoxin combination or digoxin.[88] In these patients, exercise capacity and resting and peak exercise heart rates were decreased by verapamil therapy. In these patients, who were either in NYHA functional class II or III, exercise duration increased from 219 ± 77 seconds to 292 ± 71 seconds in those receiving verapamil. Intravenous verapamil (0.075 mg/kg) also has been found to reduce the average ventricular rate from 151 to 118 beats/min as compared to a small change from 144 to 138 beats/min.[89]

Diltiazem, another calcium channel blocker with atrioventricular nodal blocking characteristics, has been compared with propranolol. Twenty-two patients entered a study with three arms: (1) digoxin plus propranolol (20 mg three times a day), (2) digoxin plus oral diltiazem (60 mg three times a day), or (3) digoxin plus diltiazem and propranolol.[90] Resting heart rate and maximal heart rate were more dramatically influenced by the combination of digoxin, diltiazem, and propranolol. Exercise duration was not influenced by these agents. In a trial of 13 patients, Vitale and colleagues[91] noted that diltiazem reduced resting heart rate from 107 ± 19 beats/min to 85 ± 12 beats/min. Maximal exercise heart rate was also blunted by diltiazem (142 ± 13 beats/min vs. 160 ± 14 beats/min during digoxin plus placebo treatment). Diltiazem was associated with a decrease in exercise rate–pressure product but an improvement in exercise capacity.

Intravenous diltiazem has been investigated as an agent to decrease heart rate in hospitalized patients with atrial fibrillation. These trials have enrolled a moderate number of patients. Salerno and coworkers[92] reported on the results of the Diltiazem–Atrial Fibrillation/Flutter Study Group. Patients with atrial fibrillation or flutter at an average heart rate $\pm$ 120 beats/min were randomized to placebo or diltiazem (0.25 mg/kg as a 2-minute infusion) followed by a repeat injection of placebo or diltiazem (0.35 mg/kg) 15 minutes later if efficacy had not been achieved. Efficacy was defined as a decrease in the ventricular rate to less than 100 beats/min or a 20% reduction in heart rate from baseline. Nonresponders randomized to placebo were given the option to receive open-label diltiazem after the randomized phase. Patients were evenly randomized to placebo and diltiazem (113 total patients). At the low dose, 7% of placebo-treated patients and 75% of diltiazem-treated patients responded to therapy. After administration of the higher dose, 12% of the placebo-treated patients and 93% of diltiazem-treated patients reached the efficacy endpoint. The effect of diltiazem on heart rate was evident as early as 2 minutes after the initiation of intravenous therapy. Systolic blood pressure dropped by 8% in patients receiving diltiazem.

The efficacy of intravenous diltiazem in patients with moderate to severe congestive heart failure has been investigated by Goldenberg and associates,[93] who studied 37 patients in a protocol similar to Salerno and colleagues. Of the patients, 95% responded to either the low or high dose of diltiazem, whereas no patient responded to placebo. All placebo-treated patients ultimately received open-label diltiazem, with all patients reaching a therapeutic endpoint. The only significant side effect associated with the diltiazem infusion was hypotension (4 of 37 patients).

An alternative therapy for rate control is clonidine, a centrally acting α_2-agonist that may block sympathetic outflow. This agent was compared with placebo in 20 patients presenting to the emergency department for evaluation of atrial fibrillation.[94] The clonidine was administered as a 0.075-mg dose and was repeated 2 hours later if the heart rate had not decreased by 20%. In the clonidine group, the average heart rate dropped from 135 ± 26 beats/min to 82 ± 10 beats/min. There was a small decrease in heart rate in patients receiving placebo (132 ± 25 beats/min to 117 ± 31 beats/min). Six patients receiving clonidine converted to normal rhythm, whereas only one patient receiving placebo converted to sinus rhythm.

Digoxin has been compared to low-dose amiodarone for rate control in persistent atrial fibrillation.[95] In this small trial of 16 patients, similar reductions in baseline and exercise ventricular rate were seen over a 6-month period. Resting heart rate decreased by approximately 25%. Peak exercise heart rate decreased by approximately 13%. Thus, neither was particularly effective in decreasing the maximal ventricular response with exercise.

Heart rate control in atrial fibrillation may be achieved with a variety of antiarrhythmic agents. β-adrenergic blocking agents are better than digoxin therapy for blunting the exercise-related increase in heart rate. Calcium channel blockers and β-adrenergic blockers may be effective in the emergent control of heart rate. The choice of agent and route of administration depend on the urgency and nature of the clinical situation.

SUMMARY

SVTs continue to be a clinical problem for many patients. The criteria for initiating pharmacologic therapy or considering radiofrequency ablation depend on clinical judgment and patient preference in most instances. Future areas of investigation include the long-term assessment of safety and efficacy of radiofrequency ablation as well as the development of newer, more effective pharmacologic agents for the treatment of these arrhythmias.

REFERENCES

1. Anderson S, Blanski L, Byrd RC, et al: Comparison of the efficacy and safety of esmolol, a short-acting beta blocker, with placebo in the treatment of supraventricular tachyarrhythmia: The Esmolol Versus Placebo Multicenter Study Group: Am Heart J 1986; 111:42–48.
2. Abrams J, Allen J, Allin D, et al: Efficacy and safety of esmolol versus propranolol in the treatment of supraventricular tachyarrhythmias: A multicenter double-blind clinical trial: The Esmolol Multicenter Study Research Group. Am Heart J 1985; 110:913–922.
3. Sung RJ, Elser B, McAllister RG Jr: Intravenous verapamil for termination of re-entrant supraventricular tachycardias: Intracardiac studies correlated with plasma verapamil concentrations. Ann Intern Med 1980; 93:682–689.
4. DiMarco JP, Miles W, Akhtar M, et al: Adenosine for paroxysmal supraventricular tachycardia: Dose ranging and comparison with verapamil: Assessment in placebo-controlled, multicenter trials. The Adenosine for PSVT Study Group. Ann Intern Med 1990; 113:104–110.
5. McIntosh-Yellin NL, Drew BJ, et al: Safety and efficacy of central intravenous bolus administration of adenosine for termination of supraventricular tachycardia. J Am Coll Cardiol 1993; 22:741–745.
6. Rankin AC, Oldroyd KG, Chong E, et al: Adenosine or adenosine triphosphate for supraventricular tachycardias? Comparative double-blind randomized study in patients with spontaneous or inducible arrhythmias. Am Heart J 1990; 119(2 Pt 1):316–323.
7. Dougherty AH, Jackman WM, Naccarelli GV, et al: Acute conversion of paroxysmal supraventricular tachycardia with intravenous diltiazem. IV Diltiazem Study Group. Am J Cardiol 1992; 70:587–592.
8. Huycke EC, Sung RJ, Dias VC, et al: Intravenous diltiazem for termination of reentrant supraventricular tachycardia: A placebo-controlled, randomized, double-blind, multicenter study. J Am Coll Cardiol 1989; 13:538–544.
9. Shen EN, Keung E, Huycke E, et al: Intravenous propafenone for termination of re-entrant supraventricular tachycardia: A placebo-controlled, randomized, double-blind, crossover study. Ann Intern Med 1986; 105:655–661.
10. Jordaens L, Gorgels A, Stroobanmdt R, et al: Efficacy and safety of intravenous sotalol for termination of paroxysmal supraventricular tachycardia: The Sotalol Versus Placebo Multicenter Study Group. Am J Cardiol 1991; 68:35–40.
11. Sung RJ, Tan HL, Karagounis L, et al: Intravenous sotalol for the termination of supraventricular tachycardia and atrial fibrillation and flutter: A multicenter, randomized, double-blind, placebo-controlled study. Am Heart J 1995; 129:739–748.
12. Mauritson DR, Winniford MD, Walker WS, et al: Oral verapamil for paroxysmal supraventricular tachycardia: A long-term, double-blind randomized trial. Ann Intern Med 1982; 96:409–412.
13. Winniford MD, Fulton KL, Hillis LD: Long-term therapy of paroxysmal supraventricular tachycardia: A randomized, double-blind comparison of digoxin, propranolol and verapamil. Am J Cardiol 1984; 54:1138–1139.
14. Clair WK, Wilkinson WE, McCarthy EA, et al: Treatment of paroxysmal supraventricular tachycardia with oral diltiazem. Clin Pharmacol Ther 1992; 51:562–565.
15. Henthorn RW, Waldo AL, Anderson JL, et al: Flecainide acetate prevents recurrence of symptomatic paroxysmal supraventricular tachycardia. Circulation 1991; 83:119–125.
16. Pritchett ELC, McCarthy EA, Wilkinson WE: Propafenone treatment of symptomatic paroxysmal supraventricular arrhythmias. Ann Intern Med 1991; 114:539–544.
17. UK Propafenone PSVT Study Group: A randomized, placebo-controlled trial of propafenone in the prophylaxis of paroxysmal supraventricular tachycardia and paroxysmal atrial fibrillation. Circulation 1995; 91:2550–2557.
18. Page RL, Connolly SJ, Wilkinson WE, et al: Azimilide Supraventricular Arrhythmia Program (ASAP) Investigators. Am Heart J. 2002; 143:643–649.
19. Tendera M, Wnuk-Wojnar AM, Kulakowski P, et al: Efficacy and safety of dofetilide in the prevention of symptomatic episodes of paroxysmal supraventricular tachycardia: A 6-month double-blind comparison with propafenone and placebo. Am Heart J 2001; 142:93–98.
20. Falk RH, Knowlton AA, Bernard SA, et al: Digoxin for converting recent-onset atrial fibrillation to sinus rhythm: A randomized, double-blinded trial. Ann Intern Med 1987; 106:503–506.

21. Toivonen LK, Nieminen MS, Manninen V, et al: Conversion of paroxysmal atrial fibrillation to sinus rhythm by intravenous pirmenol: A placebo controlled study. Br Heart J 1986; 55:176-180.
22. Madrid AH, Marin-Huerta E, Novo ML, et al: Comparison of flecainide and procainamide in cardioversion of atrial fibrillation. Eur Heart J 1993; 14:1127-1131.
23. Crijns HJGM, van Wijk M, van Gilst WH, et al: Acute conversion of atrial fibrillation to sinus rhythm: Clinical efficacy of flecainide acetate: Comparison of two regimens. Eur Heart J 1988; 9:634-638.
24. Donovan KD, Dobb GJ, Coombs LJ, et al: Efficacy of flecainide for the reversion of acute onset atrial fibrillation. Am J Cardiol 1992; 70:50A-55A.
25. Suttorp MJ, Kingma JH, Lie-A-Huen L, et al: Intravenous flecainide versus verapamil for acute conversion of paroxysmal atrial fibrillation or flutter to sinus rhythm. Am J Cardiol 1989; 63:693-696.
26. Capucci A, Lenzi T, Boriani G, et al: Effectiveness of loading oral flecainide for converting recent onset atrial fibrillation to sinus rhythm in patients without organic heart disease or with only systemic hypertension. Am J Cardiol 1992; 70:69-72.
27. Donovan KD, Power BM, Hockings BEF, et al: Intravenous flecainide versus amiodarone for recent-onset atrial fibrillation. Am J Cardiol 1995; 75:693-697.
28. Kondili A, Kastrati A, Popa Y: Comparative evaluation of verapamil, flecainide and propafenone for the acute conversion of atrial fibrillation to sinus rhythm. Wien Klin Wochenschr 1990; 102:510-513.
29. Suttorp MJ, Kingma JH, Jessurun ER, et al: The value of class IC antiarrhythmic drugs for acute conversion of paroxysmal atrial fibrillation or flutter to sinus rhythm. J Am Coll Cardiol 1990; 16:1722-1727.
30. Bellandi F, Cantini F, Pedone T, et al: Effectiveness of intravenous propafenone for conversion of recent-onset atrial fibrillation: A placebo-controlled study. Clin Cardiol 1995; 18:631-634.
31. Capucci A, Boriani G, Rubino I, et al: A controlled study on oral propafenone versus digoxin plus quinidine in converting recent onset atrial fibrillation to sinus rhythm. Int J Cardiol 1994; 43:305-313.
32. Bertini G, Conti A, Fradella G, et al: Propafenone versus amiodarone in field treatment of primary atrial tachydysrhythmias. J Emerg Med 1990; 8:15-20.
33. Halinen MO, Huttunen M, Paakkinen S, et al: Comparison of sotalol with digoxin-quinidine for conversion of acute atrial fibrillation to sinus rhythm (The Sotalol Digoxin-Quinidine Trial). Am J Cardiol 1995; 76:495-498.
34. Negrini M, Gibelli G, De Ponti C: Confronto tra amiodarone e chinidina nella conversione a ritmo sinusale della fibrillazione atriale di recente insorgenza. G Ital Cardiol 1990; 20:207-214.
35. Hou ZY, Chang MS, Chen CY, et al: Acute treatment of recent-onset atrial fibrillation and flutter with a tailored dosing regimen of intravenous amiodarone: A randomized, digoxin-controlled study. Eur Heart J 1995; 16:521-528.
36. Singh S, Zoble RG, Yellen L, et al: Efficacy and safety of oral dofetilide in converting to and maintaining sinus rhythm in patients with chronic atrial fibrillation or atrial flutter: The symptomatic atrial fibrillation investigative research on dofetilide (SAFIRE-D) study. Circulation 2000; 102:2385-2390.
37. Bianconi L, Castro A, Dinelli M, et al: Comparison of intravenously administered dofetilide versus amiodarone in the acute termination of atrial fibrillation and flutter: A multicentre, randomized, double-blind placebo-controlled study. Eur Heart J 2000; 21:1265-1273.
38. Joseph AP, Ward MR: A prospective, randomized controlled trial comparing the efficacy and safety of sotalol, amiodarone, and digoxin for the reversion of new-onset atrial fibrillation. Ann Emerg Med 2000; 36:1-9.
39. Ellenbogen KA, Stambler BS, Wood MA, et al: Efficacy of intravenous ibutilide for rapid termination of atrial fibrillation and atrial flutter: A dose-response study. JACC 1996; 28:130-136.
40. Stambler BS, Wood MA, Ellenbogen KA et al: Efficacy and safety of repeated intravenous doses of ibutilide for rapid conversion of atrial flutter or fibrillation: Ibutilide Repeat Dose Study Investigators. Circulation 1996; 94:1613-1621.
41. Abi-Mansour P, Carberry PA, McCowan RJ, et al: Conversion efficacy and safety of repeated doses of ibutilide in patients with atrial flutter and atrial fibrillation. Am Heart J 1998; 136:632-642.
42. Volgman AS, Carberry PA, Stambler B, et al: Conversion efficacy and safety of intravenous ibutilide compared with intravenous procainamide in patients with atrial flutter or fibrillation. JACC 1998; 31:1414-1419.

43. Vos MA, Golitsyn SR, Stangl K, et al: Superiority of ibutilide (a new class III agent) over DL-sotalol in converting atrial flutter and atrial fibrillation: The Ibutilide/Sotalol Comparator Study Group. Heart 1998; 79:568-575.
44. Fuster V, Ryden LE, Asinger RW, et al: ACC/AHA/ESC guidelines for the management of patients with atrial fibrillation: A report of the American College of Cardiology/American Heart Association Task Force on Practice Guidelines and the European Society of Cardiology Committee for Practice Guidelines and Policy Conferences (Committee to Develop Guidelines for the Management of Patients with Atrial Fibrillation). J Am Coll Cardiol 2001; 38:XX-XXX.
45. Van Wijk LM, den Heijer P, Crijns HJ, et al: Flecainide versus quinidine in the prevention of paroxysms of atrial fibrillation. J Cardiovasc Pharmacol 1989; 13:32-36.
46. Lau CP, Leung, WH, Wong CK: A randomized double-blind crossover study comparing the efficacy and tolerability of flecainide and quinidine in the control of patients with symptomatic paroxysmal atrial fibrillation. Am Heart J 1992; 124:645-650.
47. Naccarelli GV, Dorian P, Hohnloser SH, et al: Prospective comparison of flecainide versus quinidine for the treatment of paroxysmal atrial fibrillation/flutter. Am J Cardiol 1996; 77:53A-59A.
48. Pietersen AH, Helleman H: Usefulness of flecainide for prevention of paroxysmal atrial fibrillation and flutter: Danish-Norwegian Flecainide Multicenter Study Group. Am J Cardiol 1991; 67:713-717.
49. Connolly SJ, Hoffert DL: Usefulness of propafenone for recurrent paroxysmal atrial fibrillation. Am J Cardiol 1989; 63:817-819.
50. Aliot E, Denjoy I: Comparison of the safety and efficacy of flecainide versus propafenone in hospital out-patients with symptomatic paroxysmal atrial fibrillation/flutter. Am J Cardiol 1996; 77: 66A-71A.
51. Reimold SC, Cantillon CO, Friedman PL, et al: Propafenone versus sotalol for suppression of recurrent symptomatic atrial fibrillation. Am J Cardiol 1993; 71:558-563.
52. Richiardi E, Gaita F, Greco C, et al: Propafenone versus idrochinidina nella profilassi farmacologica a lungo termine della fibrillazione atriale. Cardiologia 1992; 37:123-127.
53. Coplen SE, Antman EM, Berlin JA, et al: Efficacy and safety of quinidine therapy for maintenance of sinus rhythm after cardioversion: A meta-analysis of randomized control trials. Circulation 1990; 82:1106-1116.
54. Rasmussen K, Wang H, Fausa D: Comparative efficiency of quinidine and verapamil in the maintenance of sinus rhythm after DC conversion of atrial fibrillation: A controlled clinical trial. Acta Med Scand Suppl 1981; 645:23-28.
55. Lloyd EA, Gersh BJ, Forman R: The efficacy of quinidine and disopyramide in the maintenance of sinus rhythm after electroconversion from atrial fibrillation. S Afr Med J 1984; 65:367-369.
56. Karlson BW, Torstensson I, Abjorn C, et al: Disopyramide in the maintenance of sinus rhythm after electroconversion of atrial fibrillation: A placebo-controlled one-year follow-up study. Eur Heart J 1988; 9:284-290.
57. Juul-Moller S, Edvardsson N, Rehnqvist-Ahlberg N: Sotalol versus quinidine for the maintenance of sinus rhythm after direct current conversion of atrial fibrillation. Circulation 1990; 82:1932-1939.
58. Van Gelder IC, Crijns HJ, Van Gilst WH, et al: Efficacy and safety of flecainide acetate in the maintenance of sinus rhythm after electrical cardioversion of chronic atrial fibrillation or atrial flutter. Am J Cardiol 1989; 64:1317-1321.
59. Gosselink AT, Crijns HJ, Van Gelder IC, et al: Low-dose amiodarone for maintenance of sinus rhythm after cardioversion of atrial fibrillation or flutter. JAMA 1992; 267:3289-3293.
60. Chun SH, Sager PT, Stevenson WG, et al: Long-term efficacy of amiodarone for the maintenance of normal sinus rhythm in patients with refractory atrial fibrillation or flutter. Am J Cardiol 1995; 76:47-50.
61. Roy D, Talajic M, Dorian P, et al: Amiodarone to prevent recurrence of atrial fibrillation. N Engl J Med 2000; 342:913-920.
62. Connolly SJ, Schnell DJ, Page RL, et al: Dose-response relations of azimilide in the management of symptomatic, recurrent, atrial fibrillation. Am J Cardiol 2001; 88:974-979.
63. Kiber L, Bloch Thompson PE, Miller M, et al: Effect of dofetilide in patients with recent myocardial infarction and left ventricular dysfunction: A randomized trial. Lancet 2000; 356:2052-2058.
64. Planning and Steering Committees of the AFFIRM study for the NHLBI AFFIRM investigators: Atrial fibrillation follow-up investigation of rhythm management: The AFFIRM study design. Am J Cardiol 1997; 79:1198-1202.

65. Hohnloser SH, Kuck KH, Lilienthal J: Rhythm or rate control in atrial fibrillation: Pharmacological Intervention in Atrial Fibrillation (PIAF): A randomized trial. Lancet 2000; 356:1789-1794.

66. The Atrial Fibrillation Follow-up Investigation of Rhythm Management (AFFIRM) Investigators: A comparison of rate control and rhythm control in patients with atrial fibrillation. N Engl J Med 2002; 347:1825-1833.

67. Van Gelder IC, Hagens VE, Bosker HA, et al: A comparison of rate control and rhythm control in patients with recurrent persistent atrial fibrillation. N Engl J Med 2002; 347:1834-1840.

68. Andrews TC, Reimold SC, Berlin JA, et al: Prevention of supraventricular arrhythmias after coronary artery bypass surgery: A meta-analysis of randomized control trials. Circulation 1991; 84(suppl III):III-236-III-244.

69. Laub GW, Janeira L, Muralidharan S, et al: Prophylactic procainamide for prevention of atrial fibrillation after coronary artery bypass grafting: A prospective, double-blind, randomized, placebo-controlled pilot study. Crit Care Med 1993; 21:1471-1478.

70. Hjelms E: Procainamide conversion of acute atrial fibrillation after open-heart surgery compared with digoxin treatment. Scand J Thorac Cardiovasc Surg 1992; 26:193-196.

71. Campbell TJ, Gavaghan TP, Morgan JJ: Intravenous sotalol for the treatment of atrial fibrillation and flutter after cardiopulmonary bypass: Comparison with disopyramide and digoxin in a randomized trial. Br Heart J 1985; 54:86-90.

72. Nystrom U, Edvardsson N, Berggren H, et al: Oral sotalol reduces the incidence of atrial fibrillation after coronary artery bypass surgery. Thorac Cardiovasc Surg 1993; 41:34-37.

73. Suttorp MJ, Kingma JH, Peels HO, et al: Effectiveness of sotalol in preventing supraventricular tachyarrhythmias shortly after coronary artery bypass grafting. Am J Cardiol 1991; 68:1163-1169.

74. Merrick AF, Odom NJ, Keenan DJM, et al: Comparison of propafenone to atenolol for the prophylaxis of postcardiotomy supraventricular tachyarrhythmias: A prospective trial. Eur J Cardiothorac Surg 1995; 9:146-149.

75. Di Biasi P, Scrofani R, Paje A, et al: Intravenous amiodarone vs propafenone for atrial fibrillation and flutter after cardiac operation. Eur J Cardiothorac Surg 1995; 9:587-591.

76. Daoud EG, Strickberger SA, Man KC, et al: Preoperative amiodarone as prophylaxis against atrial fibrillation after heart surgery. N Engl J Med 1997; 337:1785-1791.

77. Giri S, White CM, Dunn AM, et al: Oral amiodarone for prevention of atrial fibrillation after open heart surgery: The Atrial Fibrillation Suppression Trial (AFIST): A randomized placebo-controlled trial. Lancet 2001; 357:830-836.

78. Guarnieri T, Nolan S, Gottlieb SO, et al: Intravenous amiodarone for the prevention of atrial fibrillation after open heart surgery: The Amiodarone Reduction in Coronary Heart (ARCH) Trial. J Am Coll Cardiol 1999; 34:343-347.

79. McAlister HF, Luke RA, Whitlock RM, et al: Intravenous amiodarone bolus versus oral quinidine for atrial flutter and fibrillation after cardiac operations. J Thorac Cardiovasc Surg 1990; 99:911-918.

80. VanderLugt JT, Mattioni T, Denker S. et al: Efficacy and safety of ibutilide fumarate for the conversion of atrial arrhythmias after cardiac surgery. Circulation 1999; 100:369-375.

81. DiBianco R, Morganroth J, Freitag JA, et al: Effects of nadolol on the spontaneous and exercise-provoked heart rate of patients with chronic atrial fibrillation receiving stable dosages of digoxin. Am Heart J 1984; 108(4 Pt 2):1121-1127.

82. Zoble RG, Brewington J, Olukotun AY, et al: Comparative effects of nadolol-digoxin combination therapy and digoxin monotherapy for chronic atrial fibrillation. Am J Cardiol 1987; 60:39D-45D.

83. Wong CK, Lau CP, Leung WH, et al: Usefulness of labetalol in chronic atrial fibrillation. Am J Cardiol 1990; 66:1212-1215.

84. James MA, Channer KS, Papouchado M, et al: Improved control of atrial fibrillation with combined pindolol and digoxin therapy. Eur Heart J 1989; 10:83-90.

85. Brodsky M, Saini R, Bellinger R, et al: Comparative effects of the combination of digoxin and DL-sotalol therapy versus digoxin monotherapy for control of ventricular response in chronic atrial fibrillation: DL-Sotalol Atrial Fibrillation Study Group. Am Heart J 1994; 127:572-577.

86. Panidis IP, Morganroth J, Baessler C: Effectiveness and safety of oral verapamil to control exercise-induced tachycardia in patients with atrial fibrillation receiving digitalis. Am J Cardiol 1983; 52:1197-1201.

87. Lewis R, Lakhani M, Moreland TA, et al: A comparison of verapamil and digoxin in the treatment of atrial fibrillation. Eur Heart J 1987; 8:148-153.

88. Lang R, Klein HO, Di Segni E, et al: Verapamil improves exercise capacity in chronic atrial fibrillation: Double-blind crossover study. Am Heart J 1983; 105:820-825.

89. Waxman HL, Myerburg RJ, Appel R, et al: Verapamil for control of ventricular rate in paroxysmal supraventricular tachycardia and atrial fibrillation or flutter: A double-blind randomized cross-over study. Ann Intern Med 1981; 94:1-6.

90. Dahlstrom CG, Edvardsson N, Nasheng C, et al: Effects of diltiazem, propranolol, and their combination in the control of atrial fibrillation. Clin Cardiol 1992; 15:280-284.

91. Vitale P, Auricchio A, De Stefano R, et al: Efficacia del Diltiazem nel controllare la risposta ventricolare e migliorare la capacita di esercizio nella fibrillazione atriale cronica: Studio in doppio cieco, cross-over. Cardiologia 1989; 34:73-81.

92. Salerno DM, Dias VC, Kleiger RE, et al: Efficacy and safety of intravenous diltiazem for treatment of atrial fibrillation and atrial flutter: The Diltiazem-Atrial Fibrillation/Flutter Study Group. Am J Cardiol 1989; 63:1046-1051.

93. Goldenberg IF, Lewis WR, Dias VC, et al: Intravenous diltiazem for the treatment of patients with atrial fibrillation or flutter and moderate to severe congestive heart failure. Am J Cardiol 1994; 74:884-889.

94. Roth A, Kaluski E, Felner S, et al: Clonidine for patients with rapid atrial fibrillation. Ann Intern Med 1992; 116:388-390.

95. Tse HF, Lam YM, Lau CP, et al: Comparison of digoxin versus low-dose amiodarone for ventricular rate control in patients with chronic atrial fibrillation. Clin Exp Pharmacol Physiol 2001; 28:446-450.

■■■chapter **15**

Anticoagulant and Antiplatelet Drug Therapy in Atrial Fibrillation

Daniel E. Singer
Elaine M. Hylek
Margaret C. Fang

Research conducted during the past two decades has established that atrial fibrillation (AF) is a potent risk factor for ischemic stroke and that this risk is largely reversible with long-term anticoagulant therapy. This chapter reviews the randomized trials that have tested anticoagulants and antiplatelet agents in the prevention of stroke in AF and discusses relevant observational studies that have extended our understanding of stroke prevention in AF.

AF occurring in patients with rheumatic heart disease (i.e. "rheumatic AF"), principally mitral stenosis, has been long accepted as a major stroke risk and a strong indication for lifelong anticoagulation. AF results in the loss of coordinated atrial contraction, which, combined with mitral stenosis-induced obstruction of outflow from the left atrium, leads to relative stasis of blood. This presumably promotes the formation of atrial thrombi that become a source of systemic embolism. The clinical studies supporting the efficacy of anticoagulation in preventing embolism in rheumatic AF are methodologically weak.[1] Nonetheless, the frequent occurrence of thromboembolism in young patients with mitral stenosis and AF prompted acceptance of an atrioembolic mechanism and of anticoagulation as the appropriate intervention.

NONRHEUMATIC ATRIAL FIBRILLATION AS A RISK FACTOR FOR STROKE: EPIDEMIOLOGY

There was more controversy about whether nonrheumatic AF, otherwise known as nonvalvular AF, also caused embolic stroke. Nonrheumatic AF is by far the more common category of AF and is predominantly a condition occurring in older individuals and in those with other cardiac illnesses.[2] Stroke in such individuals simply might be a result of older age or associated comorbidities. However, several clinical and autopsy studies appeared to demonstrate a stronger

link between nonrheumatic AF and stroke.[3,4] High-quality epidemiologic studies subsequently provided firm evidence that nonrheumatic AF is an important cause of stroke.[2,5] In particular, the Framingham Heart Study demonstrated that AF increased the risk of stroke fivefold. This increased relative risk occurred across the entire span of the stroke-prone older decades, establishing AF as the most potent common risk factor for stroke. The Framingham Study also established AF as the most common clinically significant cardiac arrhythmia, affecting approximately 6% of persons older than age 65 and 10% of those older than age 80. This has been corroborated further by a more recent assessment in a large health maintenance organization.[6] As a result of this sizable prevalence and strong association with increased stroke risk, 14% of all strokes in the United States can be attributed to AF.[2,7]

RANDOMIZED TRIALS OF ANTITHROMBOTIC THERAPY TO PREVENT STROKE IN NONRHEUMATIC ATRIAL FIBRILLATION

In response to the accumulating epidemiologic evidence implicating AF as a cause of stroke, a set of five roughly contemporaneous randomized trials were begun to assess whether long-term antithrombotic therapy could prevent stroke in nonrheumatic AF.[8-12] These first five studies were all primary prevention trials, where most of the enrolled patients had no prior history of stroke. All five evaluated the efficacy of oral anticoagulants; two trials also evaluated aspirin in a randomized fashion.[8,10] Remarkably, all five trials terminated early because of the demonstrated efficacy of anticoagulation in reducing stroke risk. All except the Canadian Atrial Fibrillation Anticoagulation (CAFA) trial showed a marked reduction in stroke risk with anticoagulation; CAFA was stopped early because the results of the other studies demonstrated efficacy. This chapter reviews the results of these first five primary prevention trials and the findings of a pooled analysis of their results. Following this, the chapter reviews later-generation trials addressing the secondary prevention of stroke, the optimal intensity of anticoagulation, the efficacy of aspirin therapy, and risk stratification in AF.

CLINICAL FEATURES OF RANDOMIZED TRIAL PARTICIPANTS

A recurrent concern in the interpretation of randomized trials is the generalizability of the results. Only a small fraction of apparently eligible patients with AF participated in these trials. As a result, it is of interest to examine the features of the participants. Patients were predominantly elderly, with a mean age of 69 years (Table 15-1). and one-fourth were older than age 75. However, relatively few participants were older than age 80. Although most participants were men, a large number of women were included. Most subjects experienced AF for well over a year. Only 13% had intermittent, or "paroxysmal" AF; the remainder had sustained AF. It is probable that the frailest patients with AF were excluded and that most participants were considered reasonably safe candidates for anticoagulation, although a large number of patients had significant cardiovascular comorbid illnesses. Overall, the subjects in these trials had many of the features characteristic of the general population with AF, although because the most elderly patients were underrepresented, we should be cautious of extrapolating results to this population.

■ ▪ ■

TABLE 15-1   FIRST FIVE TRIALS* IN ATRIAL FIBRILLATION FOR PRIMARY PREVENTION OF STROKE: CLINICAL FEATURES OF SUBJECTS AT ENTRY

Clinical features	%
Age (years), mean	69[†]
Male	73
Race, white	94
Onset of atrial fibrillation >1 year	68
Intermittent atrial fibrillation	13
Associated diagnosis	
Hypertension	46
Diabetes	15
Angina	22
Myocardial infarction	14
Congestive heart failure	20

*The five trials are AFASAK (Atrial Fibrillation, Aspirin, Anticoagulation Study), BAATAF (Boston Area Anticoagulation Trial for Atrial Fibrillation), CAFA (Canadian Atrial Fibrillation Anticoagulation Study), SPAF (Stroke Prevention in Atrial Fibrillation Study), and SPINAF (Veterans Affairs Stroke Prevention in Nonrheumatic Atrial Fibrillation Study).
†Mean
(Adapted from Atrial Fibrillation Investigators: Risk factors for stroke and efficacy of antithrombotic therapy in atrial fibrillation. Arch Intern Med 1994; 154:1449–1457.)

RESULTS OF THE INITIAL FIVE PRIMARY PREVENTION TRIALS

Atrial Fibrillation, Aspirin, Anticoagulation Trial

The Atrial Fibrillation, Aspirin, Anticoagulation Trial (AFASAK,[8] or AFASAK-I) was a three-armed trial randomizing patients to either warfarin (with a target International Normalized Ratio [INR] of 2.8–4.2), aspirin (75 mg/day), or aspirin-placebo (Tables 15-2 and 15-3). Warfarin therapy was not blinded. Patients were identified at two outpatient electrocardiography laboratories used by general practitioners in Denmark. Of 1842 eligible patients, 1007 entered the trial, a very high recruitment fraction. Of patients, 335 were assigned to warfarin, 336 to aspirin, and 336 to placebo. A high percentage (38%) of patients assigned to warfarin withdrew from the study after an average follow-up of less than 1 year. This high percentage of withdrawals could have been a result of the high recruitment fraction because more highly selected samples of patients may have greater medication compliance. AFASAK reported four outcome events in the warfarin group, 20 in the aspirin group, and 21 on placebo, with 90% of these outcomes ischemic strokes. There were two major hemorrhages on warfarin, including one fatal intracerebral bleed. The demonstration of a marked benefit with warfarin coupled with the low rate of major hemorrhage led to the early termination of the trial.

Two additional points about AFASAK are worth noting. First, the comparisons initially reported were not the result of an intention-to-treat analysis. Patients who withdrew from the study, including the 38% assigned to warfarin, were not counted. A subsequent standard intention-to-treat analysis resulted in a P value of approximately 0.05, meeting the usual standard for statistical significance but certainly too large to activate an early termination rule.[13] Table 15-2 presents the estimated intention-to-treat results, with a preventive efficacy of 59% with warfarin therapy. It is also of interest that three of the four patients in the warfarin arm who sustained a thromboembolic event were inadequately anticoagulated at the time of the event.

Boston Area Anticoagulation Trial for Atrial Fibrillation

The Boston Area Anticoagulation Trial for Atrial Fibrillation (BAATAF),[9] and subsequently the Stroke Prevention In Nonvalvular Atrial Fibrillation (SPINAF)[12] and CAFA trials[11], made the fortuitous decision to use a lower-intensity anticoagulation target, adopting the strategy successfully applied by Hull and colleagues in treating deep-vein thrombophlebitis.[14] BAATAF randomized 212 patients to "low-dose" warfarin (target prothrombin time ratio [PTR] 1.2–1.5, roughly equivalent to an INR of 1.5–2.7) and 208 to control (see Table 15-2). Therapy was not blinded. Subjects in the control group could take aspirin, and approximately half did.

■ ▩ ■

TABLE 15-2 OVERVIEW OF THE RANDOMIZED TRIALS OF ANTICOAGULATION VERSUS CONTROL FOR ATRIAL FIBRILLATION*

Features	AFASAK	BAATAF	SPAF-I	CAFA	SPINAF	EAFT
Anticoagulation						
Target INR†	2.8–4.2	1.5–2.7	2.0–4.5	2.0–3.0	1.4–2.8	2.5–4.0
Subjects (n)	335	212	210	187	260	225
Emboli (n)	10	2	6	7	4	20
Annual rate (%)	2.3	0.41	2.3	3.0	0.88	3.9
Control						
Subjects (n)	336	208	211	191	265	214
Emboli (n)	22	13	18	11	19	50
Annual rate (%)	5.6	3.0	7.4	4.6	4.3	12.3
Preventive efficacy (%)	59	86	67	35	79	66
95% CI	(+15, +81)	(+51, +96)	(+27, +85)	(−64, +75)	(+52, +90)	(+43, +80)

*Preventive efficacy is the relative risk reduction and calculated as $(1-RR) \times 100$, where RR is the annual rate in the anticoagulation group divided by the annual rate in the control group. Outcome events for AFASAK, BAATAF, SPAF, and CAFA are ischemic stroke plus systemic embolism. For SPINAF and EAFT, the outcome events shown include only ischemic stroke. The person-years of observation used to calculate incidence rates for AFASAK were obtained from the Atrial Fibrillation Investigators' pooled database.[18] For all studies, the intention-to-treat analysis is presented. Preventive efficacy and 95% CI are reproduced from the original study report for the BAATAF, SPAF, SPINAF, and EAFT trials. For the AFASAK and CAFA studies, where the data presented differ from the study's original report, the preventive efficacy and 95% CI were calculated using the method of Breslow and Day.[68]

†The BAATAF, SPAF, and SPINAF trials used prothrombin time ratios (PTRs) to monitor the intensity of anticoagulation. For comparison purposes, we report the equivalent international normalized ratios (INRs).

INR, international normalized ratio; CI, confidence interval.

BAATAF observed two strokes in the warfarin arm versus 13 strokes in the control, for a preventive efficacy of 86%. There were no other embolic events. There was one presumed subdural hematoma that was fatal in a patient taking warfarin. Otherwise, the rate of serious bleeding was essentially the same in warfarin as in the control group. A secondary analysis, based on a nonrandomized comparison, found no evidence of benefit among control patients who were taking aspirin.[15]

Stroke Prevention in Atrial Fibrillation Trial

The Stroke Prevention in Atrial Fibrillation Trial (SPAF,[10] or SPAF-I) study was a two-tiered trial that assessed antithrombotic therapy in warfarin-eligible ("Group 1") and warfarin-ineligible ("Group 2") patients. Group 1 consisted of 627 patients who were randomly assigned to either warfarin (target PTR of 1.3–1.8, roughly equivalent to an INR of 2.0–4.5), aspirin (325 mg/day), or aspirin-placebo (see Table 15-2). Warfarin therapy was

■ ▩ ■

TABLE 15-3 OVERVIEW OF THE RANDOMIZED TRIALS OF ASPIRIN VERSUS PLACEBO FOR ATRIAL FIBRILLATION*

Features†	AFASAK	SPAF-I, 1	SPAF-I, 2	EAFT	LASAF, 1	LASAF, 2
Aspirin						
Dose (mg)	75/day	325/day	325/day	300/day	125/day	125/every other day
Subjects (n)	336	206	346	404	104	90
Emboli (n)	19	1	25	87	4	1
Annual rate (%)	4.7	0.37	5.5	10.4	2.8	0.7
Control						
Subjects (n)	336	211	357	378	91	91
Emboli (n)	22	18	28	90	3	3
Annual rate (%)	5.6	6.6	6.1	12.6	2.2	2.2
Preventive efficacy (%)	16	94	8	18	−24	70
95% CI	(−54, +54)	(+58, +99)	(−54, +46)	(−9, +38)	(−657, +71)	(−181, +99)

*Outcome events reported for the AFASAK and SPAF trials are ischemic stroke plus systemic embolism. Data for SPAF-I,1 and SPAF-I,2 were estimated from results presented in References 10 and 16. The EAFT and LASAF events are stroke only. The person-years of observation used to calculate incidence rates for AFASAK were obtained from the Atrial Fibrillation Investigators' pooled database.[18] The annual rates of stroke for LASAF were calculated from their reported results.[32] For all studies, the intention-to-treat analysis is presented. Preventive efficacy for the SPAF trials are those reported in Reference 16. The 95% CI for all trials were calculated using the method of Breslow and Day.[68]

†SPAF-I,1 and SPAF-I,2 are the two separate trials of aspirin in the first SPAF study. LASAF,1 and LASAF,2 are the two separate arms of aspirin in the LASAF trial.

CI, confidence interval.

not blinded. Group 2 consisted of 703 patients considered ineligible for warfarin therapy and patients were randomized to either aspirin (325 mg/day) or aspirin-placebo. Reasons for ineligibility included patient/provider preference, being older than age 75 years, and having a high risk of bleeding complications. SPAF estimated that a relatively small fraction of eligible patients (7%) was actually recruited, a finding consistent with other U.S. studies.

SPAF observed that warfarin reduced the risk of ischemic stroke and systemic embolic events by 69%. Of the six patients in the warfarin arm who had strokes, four were not taking warfarin at the time of their stroke. The effectiveness of aspirin was less clear (see Table 15-3). There was a statistically significant overall reduction in risk of stroke and systemic emboli of 42% with aspirin therapy. However, this effect was markedly heterogeneous in its two separately randomized studies of aspirin.[16] Group 1, which included warfarin as a possible therapy, found only one outcome event in the aspirin group versus 18 in the placebo group, for a calculated efficacy of 94%. Group 2, in which patients were ineligible for warfarin, noted 25 events with aspirin versus 28 with placebo, for an efficacy of 8% that was not statistically significant. Among those treated with warfarin, one patient sustained a fatal intracerebral hemorrhage and one sustained a subdural hematoma with full recovery. Two patients in the placebo group had subdural hematomas and fully recovered. They found no increase in major bleeding from other anatomic sites with warfarin.

Canadian Atrial Fibrillation Anticoagulation Trial

CAFA[11] was a double-blind, placebo-controlled trial of low-dose warfarin (target INR 2.0–3.0) in AF (see Table 15-2). After the AFASAK report and a preliminary report of the SPAF trial, the CAFA investigators decided to stop their trial early to allow all patients access to warfarin. CAFA counted events using an "efficacy" analysis where events occurring more than 28 days after stopping therapy would not be counted. The CAFA study did not include apparent lacunar stroke as an endpoint. Table 15-2 includes the one lacunar stroke and presents the intention-to-treat analysis, demonstrating a preventive efficacy of 35% with warfarin therapy. Regardless of approach, however, the CAFA study observed too few events to achieve a statistically significant result. Once again, most of the events in the warfarin arm of the trial occurred among subjects who were not fully anticoagulated. Major bleeding occurred in five patients taking warfarin, including one fatal intracranial hemorrhage, and in one patient taking placebo.

Stroke Prevention In Nonvalvular Atrial Fibrillation

The SPINAF[12] study was the only completed first generation trial to provide a fully blinded assessment of warfarin. As a Department of Veterans Affairs study, it enrolled only men. SPINAF used a 12 hour cutoff to distinguish transient ischemic attacks from strokes, rather than the more usual 24 hour cutoff used by the other studies. In this study, warfarin at low dose (target PTR of 1.2–1.5, roughly equivalent to an INR of 1.4–2.8) reduced the risk of stroke by 79% (see Table 15-2). There was one nonfatal intracerebral hemorrhage in the warfarin treated group versus none in placebo. There were six other major hemorrhages in warfarin versus four in placebo (all gastrointestinal hemorrhages).

POOLED ANALYSIS OF THE EFFICACY OF ANTICOAGULATION

The first five primary prevention trials provided consistent evidence for the striking efficacy of warfarin in AF. Warfarin removed most of the risk of stroke in AF with little increase in major bleeding. These trials also demonstrated the potential advantages of multiple studies of the same intervention.[17] Each of the individual trials had features that could have added controversy to interpretation of the trial's results, such as unblinded use of warfarin, use of aspirin in the control arm, or enrollment solely of men. These potential limitations were addressed by similar results in other trials that did not have the given limitation. Additionally, because of the small number of outcome events observed in the trials because of their early termination, the estimates of warfarin's efficacy were relatively imprecise as demonstrated by wide confidence intervals (CI). Precise estimates of efficacy are particularly important when deciding whether to use a risky and demanding therapy such as warfarin. The presence of five trials allowed pooling of results to provide a much tighter CI describing warfarin's efficacy.

The Atrial Fibrillation Investigators (AFI) performed a pooled analysis of the initial five primary prevention trials.[18] In the process of pooling, some data were recategorized to provide consistent definitions across the trials, and some previously unreported data were included in the analysis. The pooled estimate showed that warfarin dramatically reduced the risk of stroke in AF, with a relative risk reduction (RRR) of 68% (95% CI 50% to 79%). These estimates were calculated based on an intention-to-treat analysis. Because 29% of all strokes counted in the warfarin group occurred among patients not actually taking warfarin at the time of the stroke, it is reasonable to assume that warfarin's true efficacy is even higher. Assuming a relative risk of five, 80% of the stroke risk faced by individuals with AF is attributable to AF itself, and nearly all of this additional risk is reversed by anticoagulation. Across all five primary prevention trials the absolute risk of stroke was reduced by 3.1% per year (4.5% per year in control versus 1.4% in anticoagulated patients). For a cardiovascular prevention trial, this is a sizable effect. As a point of comparison, anticoagulation is approximately five times more effective in preventing strokes in elderly patients than through treating hypertension.[19]

To assess the efficacy of aspirin versus placebo, the AFI subsequently performed a pooled analysis of three trials (AFASAK-I, SPAF-I, and the European Atrial Fibrillation Trial [EAFT])[8,10,20] and showed that aspirin had at best a small effect in the prevention of stroke in AF. As described previously, SPAF-I divided patients into warfarin-eligible (Group 1) and warfarin-ineligible patients (Group 2). The efficacy of aspirin differed dramatically between the two, with an unexpectedly high RRR observed in the Group 1 patients. In the AFI pooled analysis, inclusion of the SPAF-I Group 1 patients resulted in statistically significant heterogeneous effect estimates; as a result, it is not clear that pooling SPAF-I Group 1 with the other three estimates would be meaningful. If the Group 1 patients were included in the pooled analysis, the estimated efficacy of aspirin was 21%, with a 95% CI that reached 0%. If excluded, the pooled estimate of aspirin's efficacy was not statistically significant. Further analysis failed to identify any subgroup of patients where aspirin's effect was enhanced significantly. Thus, the pooled analysis concluded that the efficacy of aspirin in AF is at best small.[21]

The rate of bleeding complications observed in the pooled analyses was low.[18,21] It is probable that patients enrolled in the studies were at low risk for bleeding and were carefully monitored. The annual rate of major bleeding events in warfarin-treated patients in the pooled analysis was 1.3%, compared with 1.0% in the placebo/control arm and 1.0% in the aspirin-treated patients. There were six intracranial hemorrhages in the warfarin-treated patients and two in the controls.

SECONDARY PREVENTION OF STROKE IN ATRIAL FIBRILLATION

European Atrial Fibrillation Trial

The first five trials clearly demonstrated warfarin's efficacy in the primary prevention of stroke in AF. EAFT[20] was designed to evaluate the efficacy of warfarin in secondary prevention. The study enrolled 1007 patients with AF who had suffered a minor stroke or transient ischemic attack (TIA) within the previous 3 months. The structure of the trial was similar to that of SPAF-I.[10] Patients considered eligible for anticoagulation were randomized to oral anticoagulation (INR 2.5–4.0), aspirin at 300 mg/day, or an aspirin-placebo. Anticoagulation was not blinded and the choice of anticoagulant was at the discretion of the participating physician. Acenocoumarol was the most commonly used anticoagulant, but warfarin and fenprocoumon also were used. Patients who were considered ineligible for anticoagulation were randomized to either aspirin at 300 mg/day or placebo. Older age was the primary reason for ineligibility; the mean age of those eligible for warfarin was 71 years; in ineligible patients, it was age 77 years. The annual rate of stroke was much higher in this secondary prevention trial (12% in the placebo arm) compared to that observed in the primary prevention studies (4.5%). Anticoagulation reduced the rate of stroke by 66%, a finding that was virtually identical to the RRR found in the pooled results of the primary prevention trials (see Table 15-2). Oral anticoagulation was also more

effective than aspirin in the prevention of a primary outcome event. Although the rate of stroke in patients taking aspirin was slightly lower than those administered placebo, this difference was not statistically different (see Table 15-3).

THE SPAF II AND SPAF III TRIALS

Once the efficacy of warfarin was demonstrated, further studies attempted to find potentially safer and more convenient therapeutic regimens. The subsequent SPAF trials[22,23] tested the efficacy of aspirin versus warfarin and assessed a low-intensity regimen of anticoagulant therapy.

Stroke Prevention in Atrial Fibrillation II

SPAF-I[10] raised the possibility that aspirin might be comparable to warfarin in efficacy. SPAF-II[22] was an extension of SPAF-I, limiting the comparison to warfarin at PTR 1.3–1.8 (subsequently converted to a target of INR 2.0–4.5) and aspirin at 325 mg/day. SPAF-II consisted of two parallel trials in which patients were divided into two analysis groups (age ≤ 75 years and age > 75 years) and separately randomized. This was motivated by SPAF-I's finding that aspirin appeared to have a differential effect depending on age, with the younger patients receiving a greater benefit.

Warfarin appeared to be modestly more effective than aspirin in preventing ischemic stroke in both age-groups. However, there was an unusually high annual rate (1.8%) of intracranial hemorrhage among patients older than age 75. When the intracranial hemorrhages were added to the ischemic strokes, the aggregate rates of stroke with residual deficit were very similar in both the aspirin and warfarin groups: about 1.5% per year in the younger group and about 4.5% per year in the older group. This latter rate of adverse events was more than double that seen in the warfarin arms of the earlier primary prevention trials.

Problems in the design and the execution of SPAF-II appear to weaken its conclusions. Inclusion of SPAF-I Group 1's anomalous findings regarding aspirin likely resulted in an overestimate of aspirin's efficacy in SPAF-II, particularly in patients 75 years and younger. In addition, many of the events occurring in the warfarin groups occurred in patients who were not actually taking warfarin. Accounting for these considerations, the findings of SPAF-II are consistent with warfarin being substantially more effective than aspirin in preventing stroke in AF.

The increased rate of intracranial bleeding among the elderly observed in SPAF-II clearly was concerning. However, the upper bound of SPAF-II's INR target, 4.5, was the highest of any trial in AF, and there was a suggestion that increased anticoagulant intensity was associated with intracranial bleeding. In the pooled analysis of the primary prevention trials, the rate of intracranial hemorrhage among those older than age 75 was only 0.3% per year, and the secondary prevention trial EAFT reported no intracranial hemorrhages. Nonetheless, SPAF-II highlighted the need to monitor carefully the rate of intracranial hemorrhage, particularly as warfarin use was extended to more elderly patients.

Stroke Prevention in Atrial Fibrillation III

SPAF-III was crafted in response to the findings of the SPAF-II trial. It included both a randomized trial[23] and an observational cohort study of low-risk patients.[24] The randomized trial tested whether low-intensity fixed-dose warfarin combined with aspirin was comparably effective to adjusted-dose warfarin in high-risk patients with AF. The combination of low-intensity warfarin with aspirin was aimed at three goals: prevention of thromboembolism, reduction of bleeding risk, and reduced burden of INR monitoring. Patients were classified as having either high or low risk of thromboembolism based on the findings of SPAF-II. The four specific factors denoting high-risk were as follows: (1) having impaired left-ventricular function, (2) having systolic blood pressure greater than 160 mm Hg, (3) having a prior stroke, TIA, or systemic embolism, and (4) being both female and older than 75 years. Patients with none of these high-risk features were felt to have a low rate of stroke and therefore were considered to be adequately treated with aspirin.

The randomized trial of SPAF-III enrolled 1044 high-risk patients and randomized them to either adjusted-dose warfarin (target INR 2.0–3.0) or to low-intensity fixed-dose warfarin combined with aspirin at 325 mg/day. In the low-intensity arm, patients were prescribed warfarin for a target INR of 1.2 to 1.5. Therapy was unblinded, with the mean INR in the adjusted-dose arm being 2.4 and 1.3 in the low-intensity arm.

The SPAF-III randomized trial was stopped well before its planned termination date when the rate of primary events in the low-intensity warfarin arm was noted to be significantly higher than that in the adjusted-dose warfarin group. There were 11 strokes in the adjusted-dose arm for a rate of 1.9% per year, compared with 43 strokes and one systemic embolism in the combination therapy arm for a rate of 7.9% per year. After adjusting for baseline blood pressure, the RRR of adjusted-dose versus fixed combination therapy was 74% (95% CI 50% to 87%). The rate of intracranial bleeding was not statistically different: 0.5% per year in the adjusted-dose arm compared to 0.9% per year in the combination arm. SPAF-III clearly demonstrated that low-intensity warfarin combined with aspirin was ineffective in patients with AF who had a significant annual risk of stroke. Indeed, the RRR observed in SPAF-III with adjusted-dose warfarin versus combination therapy was actually slightly higher than the RRR of adjusted-dose warfarin versus no antithrombotic therapy.

MORE RECENT TRIALS

A number of more recent trials continued the search for more optimal means of stroke prevention. Several of these studies were underpowered as a result of early termination and small sample sizes. As a consequence, these trials generated indeterminate results.

The **AFASAK-II**[25] study randomized 677 patients with chronic nonvalvular atrial fibrillation to one of four treatment arms: low-dose warfarin (1.25 mg/day), low-dose warfarin in combination with aspirin (300 mg/day), aspirin alone, and adjusted-dose warfarin with a goal INR of 2.0 to 3.0. The primary outcome was stroke (either ischemic or hemorrhagic) or systemic thromboembolism.

This trial was stopped prematurely because of results from the SPAF-III trial, which indicated that low-dose warfarin combined with aspirin was significantly less effective than adjusted-dose warfarin. In addition, other studies demonstrated that the risk of stroke increased sharply with INRs of less than 2.0.[26,27] There was no significant difference in outcomes between the four groups. Although this study was underpowered as a result of its early termination, there was a trend toward a lower stroke rate in the adjusted-dose warfarin group after 1 year compared to the low-dose warfarin plus aspirin group (2.8% vs. 7.2%). There was a significantly higher rate of bleeding complications in the adjusted-dose warfarin group (41.1% over 3 years vs. 30.0% with aspirin and 24.4% with combination therapy), although this difference was the result of minor bleeding events.

The **Minidose Warfarin in Nonrheumatic AF**[28] study randomized 303 patients to fixed low-dose warfarin (1.25 mg/day) or adjusted-dose warfarin (target INR 2.0–3.0) to evaluate the efficacy of low-dose warfarin in the prevention of ischemic stroke and systemic embolism. Like the AFASAK-II trial, this study was terminated early because of the results of SPAF-III. Although underpowered to detect a statistically significant difference in the primary endpoints, the annual rate of ischemic strokes was higher in the low-dose warfarin group (3.7% vs. 0%).

The **Primary Prevention of Arterial Thromboembolism in nonrheumatic AF (PATAF)**[29] study was designed to evaluate the efficacy of different anticoagulant intensities and aspirin, specifically recruiting patients seen in general practice. The 394 subjects eligible for standard anticoagulation were randomized to low-dose coumarin (either fenprocoumon or acenocoumarol) at a target INR of 1.1 to 1.6, adjusted-dose coumarin (INR 2.5–3.5), or aspirin (150 mg/day). The 335 subjects ineligible for standard anticoagulation were randomized to either low-dose coumarin or aspirin. Of note, ineligibility criteria for standard anticoagulation included age 78 years or older. This study reported a low annual stroke rate in all groups: 1% per year in each arm of the anticoagulant-eligible group. In the anticoagulant-ineligible group, there was a 4% annual stroke rate in the low-intensity group and 5% in the aspirin group. These results contrast with previous studies demonstrating the inefficacy of low-dose anticoagulation and aspirin. However, it must be noted that 40% of the participants were categorized as having "lone AF" (or AF without cardiac comorbidity) and therefore were likely to be at low risk for stroke.

The **Japanese Nonvalvular Atrial Fibrillation-Embolism Secondary Prevention**[30] study group sought to identify the optimal intensity of oral anticoagulation for the secondary prevention of stroke in AF. The study randomized 115 patients who had an AF-related stroke or TIA within 1 to 6 months to standard-intensity warfarin (INR 2.2–3.5) or low-intensity warfarin (INR 1.5–2.1). This study was terminated early because of a higher rate of major hemorrhagic complications in the standard-intensity warfarin group (6.6% per year vs. 0% in the low-intensity group). Three of the six major hemorrhagic complications were intracranial hemorrhages. The rate of stroke events in both groups was low (1.1% per year in the standard-intensity group and 1.7% per year in the low-intensity group). Although definitive conclusions cannot be drawn from this relatively small study, it cautioned that elderly patients may have a higher risk of bleeding complications and might benefit from a lower target intensity anticoagulation.

The **Studio Italiano Fibrillazione Atriale (SIFA)**[31] trial was another secondary prevention study, this time comparing warfarin to indobufen, a reversible inhibitor of platelet cyclooxygenase. The study randomized 916 patients to either adjusted-dose warfarin (target INR 2.0–3.5) or indobufen (200 mg BID). Patients were eligible if they had a stroke/TIA within 15 days of study entry. During the follow-up period of 1 year, 23 subjects (5%) in the indobufen group experienced a stroke compared with 18 (4%) in the warfarin group. The difference between the two was not statistically significant. Further investigation is warranted to assess whether indobufen is a viable alternative to warfarin.

The **LASAF**[32] trial compared two different dosing strategies of aspirin with placebo. It randomized 285 subjects with AF to aspirin 125 mg/day, 125 mg every other day, or placebo, excluding those with a history of prior angina, myocardial infarction or TIAs. The measured outcomes were overall mortality, stroke, systemic embolism, and myocardial infarction. The inclusion phase of the study was terminated early because of the published results of other studies that failed to demonstrate the efficacy of aspirin. The rates of stroke in the two aspirin groups were not statistically different from placebo, and there were extremely wide CIs (see Table 15-3).

META-ANALYSES OF ORAL ANTICOAGULANTS AND OF ASPIRIN VERSUS NO ANTITHROMBOTIC THERAPY

Several meta-analyses[33,34] have attempted to calculate a more precise estimate of the effect of antithrombotic therapy on stroke risk in AF. Hart and colleagues[33] analyzed the findings of sixteen randomized trials published between 1989 and 1999. They calculated that adjusted-dose warfarin reduced the relative risk of stroke, both ischemic and hemorrhagic, by 62% (95% CI 48% to 72%), with an absolute risk reduction for all

strokes of 2.7% per year for primary prevention and 8.4% per year for secondary prevention. All-cause mortality decreased in patients receiving warfarin (RRR 26%, 95% CI 4% to 43%). The relative risk of major extracranial hemorrhages in patients receiving warfarin was 2.4 (95% CI 1.2 to 4.6). The rate of intracranial hemorrhages was low, with only six events in the warfarin-treated arms compared with three in the placebo.

The meta-analysis also analyzed the results of six trials comparing aspirin and placebo, including two that were AF subgroups of larger stroke prevention trials.[35,36] It found that aspirin reduced the incidence of stroke by 22%, although with a wide 95% CI ranging from 2% to 38%. All-cause mortality was not significantly reduced (RRR 16%, 95% CI −5% to 33%). Similar to the AFI pooled analysis, the meta-analysis concluded that aspirin appears to have a modest protective effect on stroke risk in AF when compared to placebo but is not as effective as warfarin.

ASPIRIN COMPARED DIRECTLY WITH WARFARIN

Aspirin was compared to adjusted-dose warfarin in several trials,[8,20,22,23] both alone and in combination with low-intensity warfarin. AFASAK-I[8] and EAFT[20] both showed that warfarin had greater efficacy than aspirin alone (RRR of primary events 48% and 40%, respectively). Although SPAF-II[22] observed fewer outcome events in the warfarin group than in the aspirin group, the difference was not statistically significant. Other trials, including AFASAK-II[25] and PATAF,[29] were underpowered to directly compare warfarin and aspirin. With regard to aspirin in combination with low-dose warfarin, SPAF-III[23] showed that combination therapy was less effective than adjusted-dose warfarin in high-risk AF patients. A meta-analysis of the five studies comparing adjusted-dose warfarin with aspirin alone showed that warfarin reduced overall stroke risk by 36% (95% CI 14% to 52%) compared with aspirin and by 46% (95% CI 27% to 60%) when considering only ischemic stroke.[33] Taken together, these results indicate that adjusted-dose warfarin is superior to aspirin in the prevention of stroke in AF, either singly or in combination with low-dose warfarin.

RISK STRATIFICATION IN ATRIAL FIBRILLATION

An important aspect of the AFI pooled analysis was the identification of the following independent clinical risk factors for stroke with AF: (1) prior stroke or TIA, relative risk (RR) of 2.5; (2) age, RR of 1.4 per decade; (3) hypertension, RR of 1.6; and (4) diabetes, RR of 1.7. Coronary heart disease and congestive heart failure were significant risk factors on univariate analysis but did not add significantly to the prediction of stroke once the other risk factors were included in the multivariable model. Moderate to severe left-ventricular dysfunction on echocardiogram also was found to increase stroke risk, although this feature was not included in multivariable models including clinical risk factors.[37] For subjects younger than age 65 with none of the other three clinical risk factors, the annual risk of stroke was 1% regardless of whether they received warfarin. For the vast majority of subjects in the trials who had at least one of the risk factors and/or were aged 65 years or older, the annual untreated risk of stroke ranged from 3.5% to 8.1%. This annual risk was reduced in all categories to approximately 1.5% with anticoagulant treatment. These results indicate that only the youngest patients with AF at the lowest risk of stroke may forego anticoagulation safely (Table 15-4).

A second risk-stratification scheme was proposed by the SPAF investigators, who performed a pooled analysis of 2012 patients assigned to aspirin in the three SPAF studies.[38] This analysis differed in some respects from the AFI pooled analysis. First, SPAF patients were all assigned to aspirin or aspirin plus low-dose warfarin. Second, subjects younger than 60 years with "lone" AF (i.e., without associated cardiovascular disease) were excluded from the analysis. This study found that prior stroke/TIA, hypertension, female sex, and increasing age were associated with stroke on multivariable analysis. Diabetes was associated with a greater risk of disabling or fatal stroke. Because the high risk of stroke with prior stroke/TIA had been documented previously,[18,20,23] the SPAF investigators restricted the analysis to patients without prior history of stroke/TIA and developed a risk-stratification scheme for the primary prevention of AF related stroke. Patients without prior stroke/TIA

were separated into three risk categories (see Table 15-4). High-risk patients were considered to be women older than 75 years, those with a history of hypertension and older than 75, and patients of any age with a systolic blood pressure higher than 160 mm Hg. Moderate-risk patients were those aged 75 or younger with a history of hypertension or diabetes. Patients were considered at low-risk for ischemic stroke if they had no high- or moderate-risk characteristics. Patients with a prior history of stroke or TIA were at high risk of future stroke even when taking aspirin, with a 13.0% annual ischemic stroke rate noted in the 159 patients with prior stroke/TIA.

A secondary analysis of the pooled SPAF studies subsequently assessed stroke risk in subjects with intermittent (i.e., "paroxysmal") AF who were taking aspirin.[39] Of the total 2012 SPAF participants, 23% were classified as having intermittent AF. The analysis determined that subjects with intermittent AF shared similar stroke rates and risk factors for stroke compared with those with sustained AF and recommended that the same risk-stratification scheme should be used in both categories. Similarly, the AFI pooled analysis found that the type of AF (intermittent vs. sustained) had no discernible effect on stroke rate.[18]

These risk-stratification schemes have been incorporated into several AF guidelines.[40,41] One widely used guideline was published by the Sixth Consensus Conference on Antithrombotic Therapy of the American College of Chest Physicians (ACCP).[40] These recommendations were based on expert consensus and took

TABLE 15-4 ANNUAL RATES OF ISCHEMIC STROKE IN ATRIAL FIBRILLATION BY RISK GROUP FROM THE ATRIAL FIBRILLATION INVESTIGATORS (AFI) POOLED ANALYSIS AND SPAF INVESTIGATORS POOLED ANALYSIS*

| | AFI POOLED ANALYSIS | | SPAF INVESTIGATORS | |
| | Control | Warfarin | Aspirin | |
AFI risk category[†]	Annual rate (95% CI)	Annual rate (95% CI)	SPAF risk category[‡]	Annual rate (95% CI)
Age < 65 years			Primary prevention	
No risk factors	1.0 (0.3–3.1)	1.0 (0.3–3.0)	Low risk	0.9 (0.6–1.6)
≥1 risk factor	4.9 (3.0–8.1)	1.7 (0.8–3.9)		
Age 65–75 years			Moderate risk	2.6 (1.9–3.6)
No risk factors	4.3 (2.7–7.1)	1.1 (0.4–2.8)		
≥1 risk factor	5.7 (3.9–8.3)	1.7 (0.9–3.4)	High risk	7.1 (5.4–9.5)
Age >75 years				
No risk factors	3.5 (1.6–7.7)	1.7 (0.5–5.2)	Secondary prevention (prior stroke or transient ischemic attack)	13 (7.8, 18)
≥1 risk factor	8.1 (4.7–14)	1.2 (0.3–5.0)		

*For the SPAF pooled analysis, subjects aged <60 years with "lone AF" (i.e., no associated cardiovascular disease) were excluded. Of the 2012 subjects included, 1722 participants were assigned aspirin alone; 290 were assigned aspirin plus low-dose warfarin.
[†]AFI risk factors include history of hypertension, diabetes, and prior stroke or transient ischemic attack (TIA).
[‡]SPAF primary prevention risk factors: High-risk factors include women older than 75 years, age over 75 years plus history of hypertension, and systolic blood pressure >160 mm Hg. Moderate risk factors are history of hypertension plus age ≤ 75 years, and diabetes. Low risk subjects are those without high or moderate risk factors. Primary prevention refers to patients without a history of prior stroke or TIA. 95% CI for annual stroke rate in secondary prevention calculated from data provided in reference 38.
(Adapted from Atrial Fibrillation Investigators: Risk factors for stroke and efficacy of antithrombotic therapy in atrial fibrillation. Arch Intern Med 1994; 154:1449–1457; and Hart R, Pearce L, McBride R, et al: Factors associated with ischemic stroke during aspirin therapy in atrial fibrillation: Analysis of 2012 participants in the SPAF I–III clinical trials. Stroke 1999; 30:1223–1229.)
CI, confidence interval.

into account both the AFI and SPAF risk-stratification schemes. AF patients were divided into three risk groups based on clinical factors. High-risk factors were identified as prior stroke/TIA/systemic embolism, being older than age 75, history of hypertension, prosthetic heart valve, rheumatic mitral valvular disease, and poor left-ventricular systolic function. For these high-risk patients, adjusted-dose warfarin was recommended. Patients younger than age 65 years with no clinical or echocardiographic evidence of cardiovascular disease were considered low-risk, and aspirin was recommended. Because the baseline risk of stroke in patients with moderate-risk features (age 65 to 75, diabetes, coronary artery disease) is low, the absolute impact of warfarin versus aspirin is similar in these patients, and use of either was deemed acceptable. Patients with multiple moderate-risk features should be viewed as having higher risk.

Prospective validation of these risk criteria is needed to better apply their use to clinical practice. As part of the SPAF-III trial, an observational cohort of 892 "low-risk" AF patients was assigned aspirin (325 mg/day) and was prospectively followed to assess rates of embolic events.[24] Patients not meeting criteria for low risk included those with impaired left-ventricular function, systolic blood pressure greater than 160 mm Hg, prior stroke/TIA, and women older than age 75 years. A 2.2% annual primary event rate was observed over the mean follow-up period of 2 years. In another study, the AFI, SPAF, and ACCP risk-stratification schemes were applied to a longitudinal cohort of AF patients who had participated in SPAF-III.[42] Although all schemes were able to classify patients by stroke risk, the differentiation was crude and varied among the three. This variation also was noted in another study, which examined the agreement between the schemes using data from 13,559 patients with AF enrolled in a large health maintenance organization. There was a nearly threefold difference in the proportion of patients who would be categorized as low risk.[43] Clearly, risk-stratification schemes with better discrimination are required.

IDENTIFYING THE OPTIMAL RANGE OF ANTICOAGULANT INTENSITY IN ATRIAL FIBRILLATION

Numerous studies have demonstrated that higher INR levels are associated with increased risks of major hemorrhage.[44-47] To optimize therapy, physicians need to know the lowest intensity of anticoagulation that is still effective in preventing stroke in AF. The lowest target intensity of anticoagulation in the randomized trials that was still fully effective was a PTR of 1.2 to 1.5 (roughly equivalent to an INR of 2.0–3.0), and the SPAF-III results indicated that INR values just slightly higher than 1.0 were not effective in AF.

It is difficult to define the lowest effective INR from the completed randomized trials. Although a large percentage of the strokes occurring in the anticoagulation arms of the trials occurred in patients who had either

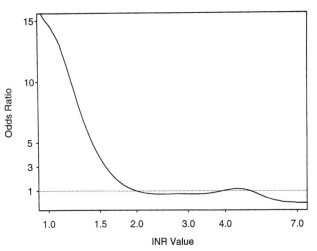

FIGURE 15-1. The relative odds (odds ratio) for stroke according to the International Normalized Ratio (INR) value among patients with atrial fibrillation (AF) taking warfarin. This figure was generated from a case-control study comparing patients with AF who sustained a stroke while taking warfarin (*cases*) with patients with AF without stroke while taking warfarin (*controls*). (Modified with permission from Hylek E, Skates S, Sheehan M, et al: An analysis of the lowest effective intensity of prophylactic anticoagulation for patients with nonrheumatic atrial fibrillation. N Engl J Med 1996; 335(8): 540–546. Copyright ©1996 Massachusetts Medical Society. All rights reserved.)

discontinued their therapy or had very low INR values,[48] the total number of events was too low to precisely describe the risk of stroke at INR levels below 2.0. Studies from clinical practice provide rich alternative sources of information. One case-control study based at a large general hospital assembled 74 consecutive cases of ischemic stroke in patients with AF who were taking warfarin.[26] These cases were compared to 222 patients with AF who had not had a stroke while anticoagulated and were followed at the hospital's anticoagulant therapy unit. The relative odds for stroke increased rapidly as the INR level decreased below 2.0 (Fig. 15-1). For example, the relative odds for stroke at an INR of 1.8 was 1.5 and was 2.5 at an INR of 1.6. At an INR of 1.3 the relative odds for stroke became 6.0. These values for relative odds were estimated from a logistic regression model that adjusted for the effects of other determinants of stroke in AF including prior stroke.

INR levels above 2.0 do not appear to increase the stroke-preventive efficacy of warfarin in AF. In contrast, the risk of intracranial hemorrhage increases rapidly above INR levels of 4.0 to 5.0.[46,47] SPAF-II was the only study to report an unusually high rate of intracranial hemorrhages with warfarin therapy in AF. This may have been related in part to the larger proportion of very elderly participants and the higher range of the target INR (up to 4.5). These studies support an INR of 2.5 (range of 2.0–3.0) as the appropriate target for AF.[40] There continues to be interest in using modestly lower targets among elderly patients as a tactic to minimize major hemorrhage, although it is likely such lower INR targets will increase the risk of ischemic stroke.[41]

TRANSLATION OF RANDOMIZED TRIAL FINDINGS INTO CLINICAL PRACTICE

The results of the randomized trials of anticoagulation in AF were dramatic, demonstrating striking efficacy and low complication rates. Nonetheless, long-term anticoagulation poses substantial burdens for both patient and physician. Patients who may be asymptomatic are required to have regular INR monitoring and must be alert to the effects of new medications, changes in diet, or intercurrent illnesses. They also must face the increased risk of hemorrhage posed by taking anticoagulants. For physicians, close monitoring of INR values and the need to respond rapidly to abnormal INR levels can be burdensome. Many elderly patients with AF have moderate contraindications to anticoagulation such as increased fall risk that may dampen physician enthusiasm for anticoagulation. Preventive practices are often slowly assimilated into routine care despite demonstrated efficacy in clinical trials. One might expect adoption of anticoagulation in AF to proceed even more slowly given its inconvenience and risk. Despite this, there is now evidence for a clear increase in the use of anticoagulants for AF following the reports of the randomized trials.[49-51] Roughly 10% of patients with AF received anticoagulants before the first randomized trials, but this figure increased sharply to 33% in 1993 after publication of the first five trials.[50] This proportion appears to have increased since then. A recent study from a large health maintenance organization reported that 55% of its nonvalvular AF patients received warfarin.[52] One can conclude that the randomized trials have changed physician behavior but that more physician education and support, such as that provided through anticoagulation clinics, will be needed to increase further the numbers of patients with AF who are anticoagulated safely.

FUTURE RESEARCH

AF is the most common clinically significant arrhythmia, and its prevalence is increasing as the population of elderly patients grows. It has been estimated that the number of patients with AF is likely to increase 2.5-fold by the year 2050.[6] There are at least three general areas for future research in stroke prevention in AF. The first is to optimize the application of randomized clinical trial data into usual clinical practice. Continued monitoring of actual clinical practice is crucial for the appropriate targeting of quality improvement initiatives. Anticoagulation clinics have been demonstrated to provide better control of INR levels, the single most important determinant of outcome among patients who are anticoagulated.[53,54] New dosing algorithms and novel technologies such as self-testing apparatus also have been investigated.[55-57] Quality control programs should include systems to track the percentage of patients with AF who are being anticoagulated, the INR control for such patients, and the bleeding and thromboembolism rates experienced by anticoagulated patients.

A second area of research should focus on refining current risk-stratification methods and should investigate new determinants of risk among patients with AF. Current stroke risk stratification in AF is crude and dictated by simple clinical features. More sophisticated hematologic measures, imaging approaches, and transesophageal echocardiography may allow physicians to better determine which patients receive the greatest benefit from therapy.[58-61] Further research also is required to better identify those patients who are at disproportionate risk of anticoagulant-associated complications.[62]

Finally, we should continue the search for safer and less intrusive alternatives to current methods of anticoagulation.[63] There has been great interest in whether restoring the heart to sinus rhythm would reduce the need for anticoagulation. The AFFIRM (Atrial Fibrillation Follow-Up Investigation of Rhythm Management) trial[64] randomized 4060 patients with AF to a strategy of either rate-control or pharmacologic restoration of sinus rhythm, with the primary outcome being mortality. All patients were aged 65 years or older and/or had additional risk factors for stroke. All patients in the rate-control arm were required to take warfarin therapy. Patients randomized to the rhythm-control arm could discontinue warfarin after at least 4 weeks of continuous sinus rhythm maintenance. After a mean follow-up of 3.5 years, there were no significant differences in overall mortality or ischemic stroke; both groups had an annual stroke rate of about 1%. It must be noted that most patients (85% of the rate-control arm and 70% of the rhythm-control arm) continued taking anticoagulation throughout the trial. However, ischemic strokes were seen primarily in patients not taking warfarin or whose INRs were less than 2.0. Of the 80 patients in the rhythm-control arm who developed ischemic stroke, 61 events occurred after discontinuation of warfarin or at subtherapeutic INRs, and 55 of the 80 patients were in sinus rhythm at the time of the stroke. Thus, the results of this trial suggest that a strategy of sinus-rhythm restoration using antiarrhythmic medications does not obviate the need for anticoagulation, possibly because patients did not remain continuously out of AF. It remains to be seen if other strategies to restore sinus rhythm, such as radiofrequency or surgical ablation, are effective in reducing stroke risk.[65,66]

There has been interest in other, more convenient modes of anticoagulation. One such agent is the oral direct thrombin inhibitor ximelagatran.[67] The SPORTIF-III (Stroke Prevention Using an Oral Thrombin Inhibitor in Atrial Fibrillation) trial was conducted to assess the efficacy and safety of ximelagatran in patients with nonvalvular AF (Late-Breaking Clinical Trials, American College of Cardiology 52nd Annual Scientific Session, 2003). The study randomized 3407 patients with AF and at least one additional risk factor for stroke. Patients were randomized to either adjusted-dose warfarin or fixed-dose ximelagatran. Preliminary reports indicate that ximelagatran may be as effective and safe as adjusted-dose warfarin for the prevention of stroke and systemic embolism. We await the full analysis of the SPORTIF-III trial results and its companion North American trial, SPORTIF-V, to begin to determine ximelagatran's role in preventing stroke in AF.

REFERENCES

1. Szekely P: Systemic embolism and anticoagulant prophylaxis in rheumatic heart disease. BMJ 1964; 1:209-212.
2. Wolf PA, Abbott RD, Kannel WB: Atrial fibrillation: A major contributor to stroke in the elderly. The Framingham Study. Arch Intern Med 1987; 147(9):1561-1464.
3. Fisher C: Reducing risks of cerebral embolism. Geriatrics 1979; 34:59-61.
4. Hinton RC, Kistler JP, Fallon JT, et al: Influence of etiology of atrial fibrillation on incidence of systemic embolism. Am J Cardiol 1977; 40(4):509-513.
5. Friedman G, Loveland D, Ehrlich SJ: Relationship of stroke to other cardiovascular disease. Circulation 1968; 38:533-541.
6. Go AS, Hylek EM, Phillips KA, et al: Prevalence of diagnosed atrial fibrillation in adults: National implications for rhythm management and stroke prevention: The Anticoagulation and Risk Factors In Atrial Fibrillation (ATRIA) Study. JAMA 2001; 285(18):2370-2375.
7. Wolf PA, Abbott RD, Kannel WB: Atrial fibrillation as an independent risk factor for stroke: The Framingham Study. Stroke 1991; 22(8):983-988.
8. Petersen P, Boysen G, Godtfredsen J, et al: Placebo-controlled, randomised trial of warfarin and aspirin for prevention of thromboembolic complications in chronic atrial fibrillation. Lancet 1989; 1:175-178.
9. The Boston Area Anticoagulation Trial for Atrial Fibrillation Investigators: The effect of low-dose warfarin on the risk of stroke in patients with nonrheumatic atrial fibrillation. N Engl J Med 1990; 323(22):1505-1511.
10. Stroke Prevention in Atrial Fibrillation Investigators: Stroke Prevention in Atrial Fibrillation study: Final results. Circulation 1991; 84:527-539.
11. Connolly S, Laupacis A, Gent M, et al: Canadian atrial fibrillation anticoagulation (CAFA) study. J Am Coll Cardiol 1991; 18:349-355.
12. Ezekowitz M, Bridgers S, James K, et al: Warfarin in the prevention of stroke associated with nonrheumatic atrial fibrillation. N Engl J Med 1992; 327:1406-1412.
13. Petersen P, Boysen G, Godtfredsen J, et al: Warfarin to prevent thromboembolism in chronic atrial fibrillation [Letter]. Lancet 1989; 1:670.
14. Hull R, Hirsh J, Jay R, et al: Different intensities of oral anticoagulant therapy in the treatment of proximal vein thrombosis. N Engl J Med 1982; 307(27):1676-1681.
15. Singer DE, Hughes RA, Gress DR, et al: The effect of aspirin on the risk of stroke in patients with nonrheumatic atrial fibrillation: The BAATAF Study. Am Heart J 1992; 124(6):1567-1573.
16. Stroke Prevention in Atrial Fibrillation Investigators: A differential effect of aspirin on prevention of stroke in atrial fibrillation: J Stroke Cerebrovasc Dis 1993; 3:181-188.
17. Singer DE: Problems with stopping rules in the trials of risky therapies: The case of warfarin to prevent stroke in atrial fibrillation. Clin Res 1993; 41(3):482-486.
18. Atrial Fibrillation Investigators: Risk factors for stroke and efficacy of antithrombotic therapy in atrial fibrillation: Analysis of pooled data from five randomized controlled trials. Arch Intern Med 1994; 154(13):1449-1457.
19. Mulrow C, Cornell J, Herrera C, et al: Hypertension in the elderly: Implications and generalizability of randomized trials. JAMA 1994; 272:1932-1938.
20. EAFT (European Atrial Fibrillation Trial) Study Group: Secondary prevention in non-rheumatic atrial fibrillation after transient ischaemic attack or minor stroke. Lancet 1993; 342(8882): 1255-1262.
21. Atrial Fibrillation Investigators: The efficacy of aspirin in patients with atrial fibrillation: Analysis of pooled data from three randomized trials. Arch Intern Med 1997; 157:1237-1240.
22. Stroke Prevention in Atrial Fibrillation Investigators: Warfarin versus aspirin for prevention of thromboembolism in atrial fibrillation: Stroke Prevention in Atrial Fibrillation II Study. Lancet 1994; 343(8899):687-691.
23. Stroke Prevention in Atrial Fibrillation Investigators: Adjusted-dose warfarin versus low-intensity, fixed-dose warfarin plus aspirin for high-risk patients with atrial fibrillation: Stroke Prevention in Atrial Fibrillation III randomised clinical trial. Lancet 1996; 348(9028): 633-638.
24. Stroke Prevention in Atrial Fibrillation Investigators: Patients with nonvalvular atrial fibrillation at low risk of stroke during treatment with aspirin. JAMA 1998; 279(16):1273-1277.
25. Gullov A, Keofoed B, Petersen P, et al: Fixed mini-dose warfarin and aspirin alone and in combination versus adjusted-dose warfarin for stroke prevention in atrial fibrillation: Second Copenhagen Atrial Fibrillation, Aspirin, and Anticoagulation Study. Arch Intern Med 1998; 158:1513-1521.
26. Hylek E, Skates S, Sheehan M, et al: An analysis of the lowest effective intensity of prophylactic anticoagulation for patients with nonrheumatic atrial fibrillation. N Engl J Med 1996; 335(8):540-546.
27. European Atrial Fibrillation Trial Study Group: Optimal oral anticoagulant therapy in patients with nonrheumatic atrial fibrillation and recent cerebral ischemia. N Engl J Med 1995; 333:5-10.
28. Pengo V, Zasso A, Barbero F, et al: Effectiveness of fixed minidose warfarin in the prevention of thromboembolism and vascular death in nonrheumatic atrial fibrillation. Am J Cardiol 1998; 82(4):433-437.
29. Hellemons B, Langenberg M, Lodder J, et al: Primary prevention of arterial thromboembolism in non-rheumatic atrial fibrillation in primary care: Randomised controlled trial comparing two intensities of coumarin with aspirin. Br Med J 1999; 3:958-964.
30. Yamaguchi T: Optimal intensity of warfarin therapy for secondary prevention of stroke in patients with nonvalvular atrial fibrillation: A multicenter, prospective, randomized trial. Stroke 2000; 31:817-821.
31. Morocutti C, Amabile G, Fattapposta F, et al: Indobufen versus warfarin in the secondary prevention of major vascular events in nonrheumatic atrial fibrillation: SIFA (Studio Italiano Fibrillazione Atriale) Investigators. Stroke 1997; 28(5):1015-1021.
32. Posada I, Barriales V: Alternate-day dosing of aspirin in atrial fibrillation. Am Heart J 1999; 138:137-143.
33. Hart R, Benavente O, McBride R, et al: Antithrombotic therapy to prevent stroke in patients with atrial fibrillation: A meta-analysis. Ann Intern Med 1999; 131:492-501.
34. Segal J, McNamara R, Miller M, et al: Prevention of thromboembolism in atrial fibrillation: A meta-analysis of trials of anticoagulants and antiplatelet drugs. J Gen Intern Med 2000; 15:56-67.
35. Diener H, Cunha L, Forbes C, et al: European Stroke Prevention Study 2: Dipyridamole and acetylsalicylic acid in the secondary prevention of stroke. J Neurol Sci 1996; 143(1):1-13.
36. Benavente O, Hart R, Koudstaal P, et al: Antiplatelet therapy for preventing stroke in patients with nonvalvular atrial fibrillation and no previous history of stroke or transient ischemic attacks. The Cochrane Database of Systematic Reviews 2002.
37. Atrial Fibrillation Investigators: Echocardiographic predictors of stroke in patients with atrial fibrillation. Arch Intern Med 1998; 158:1316-1320.
38. Hart R, Pearce L, McBride R, et al: Factors associated with ischemic stroke during aspirin therapy in atrial fibrillation: Analysis of 2012 participants in the SPAF I-III clinical trials. Stroke 1999; 30:1223-1229.
39. Hart R, Pearce L, Rothbart R, et al: Stroke with intermittent atrial fibrillation: Incidence and predictors during aspirin therapy. J Am Coll Cardiol 2000; 35:183-187.
40. Albers GW, Dalen JE, Laupacis A, et al: Antithrombotic therapy in atrial fibrillation. Chest 2001; 119(1):194S-206S.
41. ACC/AHA/ESC guidelines for the management of patients with atrial fibrillation: Executive summary. A Report of the American College of Cardiology/American Heart Association Task Force on Practice Guidelines and the European Society of Cardiology Committee for Practice Guidelines and Policy Conferences (Committee to Develop Guidelines for the Management of Patients With Atrial Fibrillation): developed in collaboration with the North American Society of Pacing and Electrophysiology. J Am Coll Cardiol 2001; 38(4):1231-1266.
42. Pearce L, Hart R, Halperin J: Assessment of three schemes for stratifying stroke risk in patients with nonvalvular atrial fibrillation. Am J Med 2000; 109(1):45-51.
43. Go A, Hylek E, Phillips KA, et al: Implications of stroke risk criteria on the anticoagulation decision in nonvalvular atrial fibrillation: The Anticoagulation and Risk Factors in Atrial Fibrillation (ATRIA) study. Circulation 2000; 102(1):11-13.
44. Landefeld C, Rosenblatt M, Goldman L: Bleeding in outpatients treated with warfarin: Relation to the prothrombin time and important remediable lesions. Am J Med 1989; 87:153-159.
45. Fihn S, McDonell M, Martin D, et al: Risk factors for complications of chronic anticoagulation. Ann Intern Med 1993; 118:511-520.

46. Hylek E, Singer D: Risk factors for intracranial hemorrhage in outpatients taking warfarin. Ann Intern Med 1994; 120(11): 897–902.

47. Cannegieter S, Rosendaal F, Wintzen A, et al: Optimal oral anticoagulant therapy in patients with mechanical heart valves. N Engl J Med 1995; 333:11–17.

48. Atrial Fibrillation Investigators: Atrial Fibrillation: Risk factors for embolization and efficacy of anti-thrombotic therapy. Arch Intern Med 1994; 154:1449–1457.

49. Gottlieb LK, Salem-Schatz S: Anticoagulation in atrial fibrillation. Does efficacy in clinical trials translate into effectiveness in practice? Arch Intern Med 1994; 154(17):1945–1953.

50. Stafford R, Singer D: National patterns of warfarin use in atrial fibrillation. Arch Intern Med 1996; 156(22):2537–2541.

51. Smith N, Psaty B, Furberg C, et al: Temporal trends in the use of anticoagulants among older adults with atrial fibrillation. Arch Intern Med 1999; 159:1574–1578.

52. Go A, Hylek E, Borowsky L, et al: Warfarin use among ambulatory patients with nonvalvular atrial fibrillation: The Anticoagulation and Risk Factors in Atrial Fibrillation (ATRIA) study. Ann Intern Med 1999; 131:927–934.

53. Chiquette E, Amato M, Bussey H: Comparison of an anticoagulation clinic with usual medical care. Arch Intern Med 1998; 158:1641–1647.

54. Fitzmaurice D, Hobbs R, Murray E, et al: Oral anticoagulation management in primary care with the use of computerized decision support and near-patient testing. Arch Intern Med 2000; 160: 2343–2348.

55. Ansell J, Patel N, Ostrovsky D, et al: Long-term patient self-management of oral anticoagulation. Arch Intern Med 1995; 155: 2185–2189.

56. Arnsten JH, Gelfand JM, Singer DE: Determinants of compliance with anticoagulation: A case-control study. Am J Med 1997; 103(1): 11–17.

57. Ansell J, Hirsch J, Dalen JE, et al: Managing oral anticoagulant therapy. Chest 2001; 119:22S–38S.

58. Stollberger C, Chnupa P, Kronik G, et al: Transesophageal echocardiography to assess embolic risk in patients with atrial fibrillation. Ann Intern Med 1998; 128(8):630–638.

59. Stroke Prevention in Atrial Fibrillation Investigators Committee on Echocardiography: Transesophageal echocardiographic correlates of thromboembolism in high-risk patients with nonvalvular atrial fibrillation. Ann Intern Med 1998; 128:639–647.

60. Loebstein R, Yonath H, Peleg D, et al: Interindividual variability in sensitivity to warfarin—Nature or nurture? Clin Pharmacol Ther 2001; 70(2):159–164.

61. Higashi M, Veenstra D, Kondo L, et al: Association between CYP2C9 genetic variants and anticoagulation-related outcomes during warfarin therapy. JAMA 2002; 287(13):1690–1698.

62. Hylek EM, Regan S, Go AS, et al: Clinical predictors of prolonged delay in return of the international normalized ratio to within the therapeutic range after excessive anticoagulation with warfarin. Ann Intern Med 2001; 135:393–400.

63. Weitz J, Hirsch J: New anticoagulant drugs. Chest 2001; 119(1): 95S–107S.

64. AFFIRM Investigators: A comparison of rate control and rhythm control in patients with atrial fibrillation. N Engl J Med 2002; 347(23):1825–1833.

65. Haissaguerre M, Jais P, Shah DC, et al: Spontaneous initiation of atrial fibrillation by ectopic beats originating in the pulmonary veins. N Engl J Med 1998; 339:659–666.

66. Cox JL, Ad N, Palazzo T: Impact of the maze procedure on the stroke rate in patients with atrial fibrillation. J Thorac Cardiovasc Surg 1999; 118(5):833–840.

67. Heit J, Colwell C, Francis C, et al: Comparison of the oral direct thrombin inhibitor ximelagatran with enoxaparin as prophylaxis against venous thromboembolism after total knee replacement. Arch Intern Med 2001; 161:2215–2221.

68. Breslow NE, Day NE: Statistical methods in cancer research. *In* The Analysis of Case-Control Studies, Vol 1. Lyon, International Agency for Research on Cancer, 1980, p 134.

■ ■ ■ c h a p t e r 16

Arrhythmia Ablation

Kyoko Soejima
William G. Stevenson

In the last 20 years many cardiac arrhythmias have become curable, initially with cardiac surgery for elimination of conduction over accessory atrioventricular (AV) connections in the Wolff-Parkinson-White (WPW) syndrome or ventricular resections for recurrent ventricular tachycardia (VT) from a prior myocardial infarction. In 1982, Gallagher and colleagues and Gonzalez and colleagues developed a method of percutaneous catheter ablation using direct current (DC) shocks applied through an electrode catheter.[1,2] Ablation of the AV junction to intentionally produce heart block was achieved. The method was effective, but high-voltage shocks caused barotrauma with a risk of cardiac perforation and required general anesthesia.

Little more than a decade ago, a technique using radiofrequency (RF) energy for ablation was adapted for delivery through electrode catheters and was adopted rapidly and widely.[3] High-frequency (200–750 K Hz) sinusoidal current is applied to the tip electrode of the ablation catheter, and an adhesive grounding pad is placed on the patient's skin. Application of RF energy is associated with no or a small amount of discomfort; general anesthesia is not required. The thermal injury causes discrete lesions, typically 3 to 7 mm in diameter, characterized by coagulation necrosis and desiccation.

The success and risks of the procedure are determined by a variety of factors including a number of specific technical aspects. Because the lesions created are relatively small, precise targeting of the tissue causing the arrhythmia is required for success. This need for precision has led to careful study and better understanding of a variety of ventricular and supraventricular arrhythmias. The coagulation necrosis at the center of the lesion is surrounded by a region of edema and reversibly injured tissue.[4-7] With healing, recovery of tissue in the periphery occasionally results in recurrence of the arrhythmia, despite apparent acute procedural success. Ablation of large areas, or to create lines of block to interrupt a large reentry circuit, presently is achieved by repeated RF energy applications as the catheter is moved from point to point over the target. With healing of these lesions, gaps in the ablation line occur and are probably common but do not always allow conduction sufficient to support the arrhythmia.[8,9] The efficacy and risks of catheter ablation have been largely defined by single-center series and a small number of uncontrolled multicenter trials.

The patients studied generally have been drawn from those referred to tertiary centers and likely were selected for frequent and symptomatic arrhythmias. For ablation of supraventricular tachycardias (SVTs) long-term outcome usually has been assessed based on absence of symptomatic recurrences, which is a clinically relevant endpoint but subject to patient reporting bias.

SUPRAVENTRICULAR TACHYCARDIAS

Initial catheter ablation procedures targeted the AV junction and subsequently accessory AV pathways and the slow AV nodal pathway for AV nodal reentry tachycardia (AVNRT)[1,10-12] (Table 16-1). Subsequently, ablation approaches have been developed for focal atrial tachycardias, atrial flutter, and atrial fibrillation. Calkins and coworkers reported a prospective, multicenter clinical trial evaluating the safety and efficacy of catheter ablation for supraventricular arrhythmias.[13] A total of 1050 patients, with a mean age of 37 ± 18 years (range 8 months to 90 years) undergoing ablation for AVNRT (373 patients), ablation of an accessory AV pathway causing AV reentry tachycardia (500 patients), ablation of the AV junction (121 patients) to control a rapid ventricular response usually resulting from atrial fibrillation, or ablation of more than one type of SVT (56 patients) enrolled in this study. The ablation procedure was initially successful in 996 (95%) of patients. The probability of procedural success was highest for ablation of the AV junction (100%), and although lower ($P < 0.001$), still better than 90%, for patients with an accessory pathway (93%), or AV nodal reentry (97%). Separate logistic regression model univariate predictors ($P < 0.05$) of ablation success included the following: ablation for AV nodal reentry (OR 2.23), ablation of the AV junction, and ablation at an experienced center with 40 or more patients enrolled in the study. During a median follow-up of 6.3 months, arrhythmia recurrences were observed in 56 patients (6%)—31 of 500 (6.2%) with accessory pathways, 16 of 373 (4%) with AVNRT, and 2 of 121 (1.7%) after AV junction ablation. The median time to recurrence was 35 days (0–244 days). The likelihood of recurrence was greater for patients with multiple accessory pathways or a pathway in the right free wall or posteroseptal location. Major complications occurred in

■ ▢ ■

TABLE 16-1   CONSIDERATIONS FOR CATHETER ABLATION OF PAROXYSMAL SUPRAVENTRICULAR TACHYCARDIAS

WPW evident in sinus rhythm + any symptoms of tachyarrhythmia

Electrophysiology study with potential catheter ablation warranted because of possible risk of rapid response to atrial fibrillation.
Exception: known low risk for rapid response to atrial fibrillation from a prior EP study or prior episode of atrial fibrillation.

Asymptomatic WPW

Need for EP study/ablation controversial because of low risk of sudden death.

Paroxysmal SVT with no preexcitation during sinus rhythm

Most likely cause is AV nodal reentry.
Second most common cause is AV reentry with concealed accessory pathway.
Catheter ablation success >95% with 3% risk of complications.
Catheter ablation is a reasonable alternative to antiarrhythmic drug therapy for patients with symptomatic tachycardia and is preferred for those
    with drug refractory arrhythmia or severe symptoms during their arrhythmia.

WPW, Wolff-Parkinson-White syndrome; EP, electrophysiology; SVT, supraventricular tachycardia; AV, atrioventricular.

32 patients (3%), including unintended complete AV block (n = 10), cardiac perforation with tamponade (n = 6), and thromboembolism (n = 4, including two strokes). There were three periprocedural deaths for a procedure mortality of 0.3%. Procedural complications were predicted by the presence of structural heart disease (OR 2.02) and the presence of more than one ablation target, such as two accessory pathways or an accessory pathway and AV nodal reentry (OR 8.56).

Atrioventricular Nodal Reentrant Tachycardia

AV nodal reentry is the most common form of paroxysmal SVT in adults (Fig. 16-1), accounting for 50% of paroxysmal SVTs. A female predominance is observed in most series, with 70% in one large multicenter trial being women.[14] The AV node is a lobulated structure, with a compact portion that joins the His bundle and superior and inferior extensions.[15] Some patients also have a leftward extension. In patients with AV nodal reentry these extensions create the potential for two functionally distinct pathways for propagation through the AV node. The faster of the two pathways typically is located in the superior (cranial) aspect of the septum, close to the compact portion of the AV node. The slower pathway is most likely an extension of the AV node, extending inferiorly along the tricuspid annulus, between the annulus and the coronary sinus (Fig. 16-2). In typical AV nodal reentry the reentry wavefront propagates through the slow pathway to the compact AV node and then retrogradely to the atrium through the fast pathway; therefore it is designated "slow-fast AV nodal reentry."

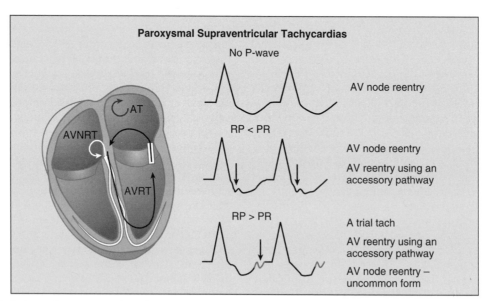

FIGURE 16-1. Mechanisms of supraventricular tachycardia and typical electrocardiographic findings are shown for atrioventricular nodal reentrant tachycardia (AVNRT), atrial tachycardia (AT), and atrioventricular reciprocating tachycardia (AVRT) using an accessory pathway. If no P-wave is observed on the surface electrocardiogram (ECG) because of simultaneous atrial and ventricular depolarization, the tachycardia is most likely AVNRT. In tachycardias with a P-wave following the QRS with an RP interval that is shorter than the PR interval, the mechanism is most likely either AVNRT or AVRT. If the PR interval during tachycardia is shorter than RP, the rhythm is most likely AVRT or AT. Exceptions to all of these situations occur, however; assessment of the spontaneous tachycardia from the ECG is useful for estimating likely efficacy and risk of catheter ablation.

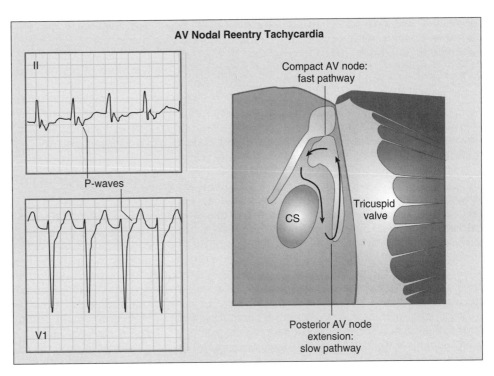

AV Nodal Reentry Tachycardia

FIGURE 16-2. The likely reentry circuit of atrioventricular nodal reentry tachycardia (AVNRT) is shown. The AV node is a lobulated structure that includes an inferior extension along the tricuspid valve annulus that serves as the slow AV nodal pathway. The reentry wave circulates down the slow pathway, then back to the atrium over the fast pathway, but the route is not clearly defined. Separation of the slow and fast pathway portions of the AV node allows ablation of the slow pathway to be performed with preservation of the fast pathway and AV node conduction to the ventricle. As the atrium and ventricles are activated simultaneously during tachycardia, the P-wave is usually right after the QRS or buried in the QRS.

Fast Pathway Ablation

Initial ablation approaches, prior to identification of the location of the slow AV nodal pathway, targeted the fast pathway. In a single-center series of 39 patients, AVNRT was abolished in 33 (85%) of patients, but 8% of patients developed high-degree heart block requiring permanent pacemaker placement.[16] Successful ablation typically produced first-degree AV block because remaining antegrade conduction occurred over the slow AV nodal pathway. The high incidence of AV block was likely the result of the proximity of the fast AV nodal pathway to the compact AV node and bundle of His.

Slow Pathway Ablation

In contrast, ablation of the slow pathway can be achieved at locations inferior to and at a greater distance from the compact AV node (see Fig. 16-2). The risk of heart block is much less and residual AV conduction is usually normal, with no PR interval prolongation. Ablation of the slow AV nodal pathway can be guided by the anatomic position using the coronary sinus and His bundle recording sites as landmarks for reference, or it can target specific types of electrograms in that region that may indicate the AV nodal slow pathway.[11,17] Anatomic variations exist that can complicate the procedure. Monitoring fast pathway conduction during ablation is important to avoid inadvertent heart block.[18]

Jazayeri and colleagues compared the safety and efficacy of selective fast versus slow pathway ablation using RF energy in 49 patients.[19] First, 16 patients underwent a fast pathway ablation. The slow AV nodal pathway was targeted initially in the remaining 33 patients. Fast pathway ablation was successful in all 16 patients and in three patients who failed slow pathway ablation; however, four of these 19 patients developed complete AV block. In the remaining 15 patients, the conduction time through the AV node was prolonged, as indicated by an increase in AH interval from a mean of 89 msec to 138 msec following the ablation. Slow pathway ablation was attempted in 33 patients and in another two who had uncommon forms of AVNRT inducible after successful fast pathway ablation. Of these 35 patients, 32 had no AVNRT inducible after ablation. No patients developed AV block. During 6.5 ± 3.0 months of follow-up, no patients had recurrent tachycardia. They concluded that although both fast and slow pathways can be selectively ablated for control of AVNRT, slow pathway ablation, by obviating the risk of AV block appears to be safer and should be considered as the first approach.

Kalbfleisch and colleagues compared slow pathway ablation guided by the anatomic approach with that guided by electrogram mapping.[20] The approach was randomly assigned in 50 consecutive patients either to anatomic or an electrogram mapping approach for targeting the slow pathway. If the initial approach was ineffective after 12 RF lesions, the alternative approach was used. Success was defined as inability to induce AVNRT both before and during an infusion of isoproterenol sufficient to increase the sinus rate to 120 to 140 beats/min. The anatomic approach was effective in 84% of patients, and the electrogram mapping approach was effective in all patients (P = 0.1). The four patients with an ineffective anatomic approach had a successful outcome with the electrogram-guided approach. There were no significant differences between the two methods with respect to the time required for ablation (anatomic and electrogram; 28 ± 21 vs. 31 ± 31 minutes, $P = 0.07$), fluoroscopic time (27 ± 20 vs. 27 ± 18 minutes, $P = 0.09$), or mean number of RF applications (6.3 ± 3.9 vs. 7.2 ± 8.0, $P = 0.06$). No patient developed high-degree heart block. Mean follow-up was 8 ± 1 months. One patient who had slow pathway ablation guided by electrograms had a recurrence of AVNRT after 1 week of the procedure; a second ablation procedure was successful with no further episodes during 8 months of follow-up. This study demonstrated that the anatomic and electrogram mapping approaches for ablation of the slow pathway are comparable in efficacy and procedure duration. The electrogram approach was uniformly effective in eliminating the AVNRT, and a majority of the effective target sites were located within the areas that would have been targeted in the anatomic approach.

Other single-center series also have been reported. Jackman and coworkers reported slow pathway ablation in 80 patients with AVNRT using the electrogram mapping approach.[21] Ablation guided by an electrogram approach abolished or modified slow pathway conduction in 78 patients, eliminating AVNRT without affecting normal AV nodal conduction. In the single patient without slow pathway potentials, application of RF current to the proximal coronary sinus ablated the fast pathway and AVNRT. Atrioventricular block occurred in one patient (1.3%). AVNRT did not recur during a mean ($\pm$ SD) follow-up of 15.5 ± 11.3 months. Electrophysiologic study 4.3 ± 3.3 months after ablation in 32 patients demonstrated normal AV nodal conduction without AVNRT.

In the multicenter trial reported by Calkins and coworkers 373 patients had AVNRT ablation targeting the slow AV nodal pathway. The procedure was acutely successful in 97%. Heart block requiring pacemaker placement occurred in 1.3% of patients. During a median follow-up of 6.3 months, 357 patients (95.4%) were free of symptomatic recurrences.

In summary, catheter ablation targeting the AV node slow pathway is highly effective for eliminating AVNRT. The major complication is heart block, which occurs in 1% to 2% of patients.

Accessory Atrioventricular Pathways

Accessory pathways are a common cause of paroxysmal SVT, occurring in approximately 0.1 to 3.1 in 1000 people.[22] When the accessory pathway allows conduction from atrium to ventricle, the electrocardiographic pattern of the WPW syndrome with ventricular preexcitation usually is present on the sinus rhythm electrocardiogram (ECG) (Fig. 16-3). The most common tachycardia caused by accessory pathways is AV reentry tachycardia (AVRT) (Figs. 16-1 and 16-3). The reentry excitation wavefront propagates over the AV node to the ventricles, then retrogradely to the atrium over the accessory pathway. Thus, preexcitation is absent during tachycardia and the QRS is narrow or has the appearance of left or right bundle branch block if conduction occurs with aberrancy. Much less commonly, AV reentry revolves in the opposite direction, causing a preexcited tachycardia, electrocardiographically indistinguishable from VT. Rapid conduction from atrium to ventricle during atrial fibrillation is possible in about 25% of accessory pathways, potentially causing syncope or precipitating ventricular fibrillation.[23] Because of this concern, electrophysiologic study with potential catheter ablation is considered for patients with symptomatic WPW syndrome.

FIGURE 16-3. Accessory pathway and atrioventricular reciprocating tachycardia (AVRT) mechanism is shown. During sinus rhythm, if the accessory pathway has antegrade conduction, the QRS morphology is the result of the fusion between the conduction over the AV node and accessory pathway, producing a short PR interval and slurring of the initial portion of the QRS. The most common tachycardia associated with this syndrome is orthodromic AV reentry, in which antegrade conduction occurs over the AV node and retrograde conduction back to the atrium occurs over the accessory pathway. Ablation targets the accessory pathway.

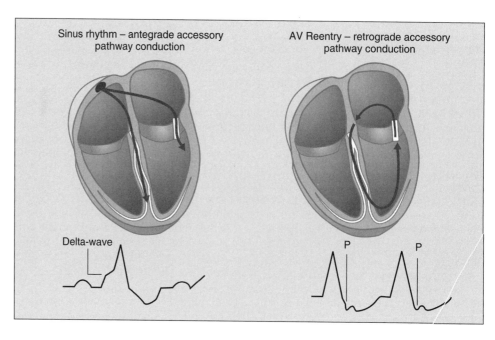

A significant number of accessory pathways are "concealed." They allow conduction only from ventricle to atrium. Preexcitation is absent during sinus rhythm and there is no risk of rapid preexcited tachycardia during atrial fibrillation, but AV reentry tachycardia occurs.

Catheter ablation requires precise localization of the accessory pathway around the tricuspid or mitral annulus. The location of the pathway and presence or absence of multiple accessory pathways is a determinant of the likelihood of success. Large single-center series have been reported. Jackman and colleagues reported a single-center series of 166 patients.[24] Ablation eliminated accessory pathway conduction in 99% of patients. During a mean follow-up of 8.0 ± 5.4 months, preexcitation or AVRT recurred in 15 patients (9%). All underwent a second, successful ablation. A late electrophysiologic study was performed at 3.1 ± 1.9 months in 75 patients and confirmed absence of accessory pathway conduction in all. Significant complications occurred in three patients (1.8 %), including AV block, pericarditis, and cardiac tamponade after RF application in a small branch of coronary sinus. Kuch and colleagues reported a single-center series of 105 patients with overall success of 89% and a 3% risk of significant complications.[25]

In the multicenter study reported by Calkins and coworkers, ablation was performed in 500 patients with accessory pathways.[14] The procedure was acutely successful in 465 patients (93%). Procedural complications were not described for the different arrhythmia subgroups but as noted was 3% for patients having all types of SVT ablation and included complete heart block in five, stroke in one, and one death as a result of left-main coronary artery dissection. During a median follow-up of 6.3 months, recurrence of accessory pathway conduction was detected in 31 patients (7.8%). Success depended on accessory pathway location, being 95% for pathways spanning the mitral annulus in the left free wall location, 90% for right free wall accessory pathways, and 88% for posteroseptal pathways.

Procedural failure is sometimes related to location of the pathway deep to the endocardium. Use of saline-irrigated RF ablation catheters that make deeper lesions was evaluated by Yamane and coworkers.[26] In 301 consecutive patients, ablation with a conventional RF catheter failed to eliminate accessory pathway conduction in 18 of 314 accessory pathways in 18 patients (5.7%), six of which were located in the left free wall, five in the middle/posterior-septal space, and seven inside the coronary sinus (CS) or its tributaries. Irrigated-tip catheter ablation subsequently was performed with temperature control mode (50 °C), a moderate saline flow rate (17 ml/min), and a power limit of 50 W (outside CS) or 20 to 30 W (inside CS) at sites where the pathway appeared to be located but had not been interrupted by conventional ablation. Seventeen of the 18 resistant accessory pathways (94%) were ablated successfully with a median of three RF applications using irrigated-tip catheters. A significant increase in power delivery was achieved

(20.3 ± 11.5 vs. 36.5 ± 8.2 W; P < 0.01) with irrigated-tip catheters, irrespective of the accessory pathway location, particularly inside the CS or its tributaries. No serious complications occurred. This particular catheter is under investigational study in the United States.

Macroreentrant Atrial Tachycardia (Atrial Flutter)

Common (Isthmus-Dependent) Atrial Flutter

With the advent of catheter ablation, the term atrial flutter has been increasingly applied to those atrial tachycardias that are the result of relatively large atrial reentry circuits. Several different types of these macroreentrant atrial tachycardias have been defined. The most common type results from reentry in the right atrium around the tricuspid annulus (Fig. 16-4). The excitation wave revolves up the septum, across the roof of the atrium, down the free wall, and then through an isthmus defined by the inferior vena cava orifice and the inferior (diaphragmatic) portion of the tricuspid annulus. The circuit also may revolve in the opposite direction. This type of circuit gives rise to the most common type of flutter, with characteristic "saw-tooth-shaped" P-waves in ECG leads II, III, and AVF. It commonly is referred to as isthmus dependent because ablation that interrupts conduction in the isthmus between the tricuspid annulus and inferior vena cava abolishes the arrhythmia.

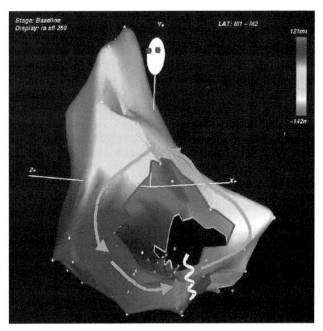

FIGURE 16-4. Activation map of typical counterclockwise atrial flutter is shown. The right atrium is viewed from the left anterior oblique projection. The central hole is the region of the tricuspid valve. The activation sequence is indicated by colors; progressing from red (earliest), yellow, green, blue, and purple (latest). The activation wavefront propagates up the septum and over the roof and goes down the right lateral free wall of the right atrium. The isthmus between the tricuspid valve annulus and inferior vena cava is targeted for ablation.

Atrial flutter is often resistant to pharmacologic suppression. Natale and colleagues compared antiarrhythmic therapy to catheter ablation in a single-center, randomized trial of patients with suspected isthmus dependent atrial flutter.[27] A total of 61 patients who had at least two symptomatic episodes of atrial flutter in the last 4 months were prospectively randomized to either pharmacologic antiarrhythmic therapy (30 patients) or to first-line RF catheter ablation (31 patients). Antiarrhythmic drugs were selected by the treating physician. In the ablation-treated group, RF ablation of isthmus-dependent flutter was successful in all 31 patients; five patients also had an uncommon type of macroreentrant atrial flutter. Procedural complications were a hematoma at the site of the venous puncture in one patient and chest discomfort that persisted for about 2 weeks after the procedure, possibly as a result of pericarditis, in another patient. Arrhythmia recurrences were assessed largely by reported symptoms and ECG at routine follow-up. After a mean follow-up of 21 months, 80% of patients who had RF ablation were free of recurrent atrial flutter ($P < 0.01$). In contrast, only 36% of patients in the drug therapy group were in sinus rhythm ($P < 0.01$), despite trials of an average of 3.4 ± 1.1 different antiarrhythmic drugs to attempt to maintain sinus rhythm. Two patients crossed over to atrial flutter ablation, and one patient required AV node ablation and pacemaker implantation as a result of the inability to maintain normal sinus rhythm and to achieve adequate rate control. Of the 11 patients who continued to receive drug therapy, rather than rate-controlling medications, to maintain sinus rhythm, 8 were treated with amiodarone, 1 with propafenone and atenolol, and 2 with procainamide and digoxin. More patients in the drug treatment group were rehospitalized (63 vs. 22%, $P < 0.001$) and developed atrial fibrillation (53 % vs. 29%, $P < 0.05$). Sense of well being and function in daily life, assessed by Quality of Life Enjoyment and Satisfaction Questionnaire (Endicott), improved after ablation but did not change significantly in the patients taking drugs for atrial flutter. By the end of the follow-up period, 53% (16 of 30 patients) in the drug treatment group were receiving only rate-controlling agents because of failure of antiarrhythmic drugs to maintain sinus rhythm.

Because ablation of the common atrial flutter isthmus requires a line of RF lesions, recovery of conduction through the isthmus during healing is a concern. Several groups have defined specific electrophysiologic markers indicating complete conduction block in this isthmus, which serve as valuable endpoints for ablation. Ablation that achieves conduction block is associated with a low risk of recurrent atrial flutter.[28,29]

Creation of a line of block through the flutter isthmus is also likely to be facilitated by ablation methods that create larger lesions. Cooling the ablation electrode by irrigation has been shown to prevent both overheating of the electrode-tissue interface and impedance rise during RF delivery, allowing greater power delivery and larger and deeper lesions.[30] Jais

and colleagues compared the safety and efficacy of an irrigated-tip catheter (presently investigational in the United States) with that of conventional RF catheters in a prospective and randomized study of 60 patients.[31] The end point was bidirectional isthmus block, and patients crossed over to the other ablation catheter if block was not achieved after 21 RF applications. Complete bidirectional isthmus block was achieved for all patients. Four patients crossed over from conventional to irrigated-tip catheters. The number of applications (5 ± 3 vs. 13 ± 10, $P = 0.001$), procedure duration (27 ± 16 vs. 53 ± 41 minutes, $P = 0.0008$), and fluoroscopic time (9 ± 6 vs. 18 ± 14 minutes, $P = 0.01$) were significantly lower in the irrigated-tip catheter group. No significant side effects occurred in either group. Coronary angiograms performed after ablation in the first 30 patients revealed no detectable injury to the underlying right coronary artery. Although saline irrigation of the RF electrode can increase the size of ablation lesions, coronary artery damage and cardiac perforation were not seen in these patients.

Atrial Flutter in Patients Treated for Atrial Fibrillation

Atrial flutter can occur for the first time during antiarrhythmic drug therapy for atrial fibrillation. Tai and coworkers administered chronic amiodarone or propafenone therapy to 136 patients with atrial fibrillation. Of these, 15 (11%) developed isthmus-dependent atrial flutter. All underwent acutely successful ablation, and antiarrhythmic drug therapy for atrial fibrillation was continued. During a follow-up period of 12.3 ± 4.2 months, 14 of 15 (93%) remained in sinus rhythm on drug therapy; one patient had recurrent atrial fibrillation. Nabar and coworkers performed ablation for isthmus-dependent atrial flutter in 16 patients in whom flutter developed during antiarrhythmic drug therapy for atrial fibrillation.[32] They then discontinued the antiarrhythmic drug. Atrial flutter recurred in nine patients (12%), and atrial fibrillation recurred in 86% of patients within 4 ± 2 months.

Nonisthmus-Dependent Atrial Flutter

Atrial macroreentry circuits that do not use the cavotricuspid isthmus are less frequent than isthmus-dependent flutter. Most are related to areas of atrial scar that create conduction block such that a reentry wavefront can circulate around the area of block. Atrial incisions placed at the time of repair of congenital heart disease are the most common cause, giving rise to "*lesion macroreentrant atrial tachycardia.*" The electrocardiographic appearance is variable, and the distinction of "nonisthmus"-dependent macroreentrant atrial tachycardias from isthmus-dependent atrial flutter usually requires catheter mapping at invasive electrophysiologic study. Multiple reentry circuits often are present in these patients. Isthmus-dependent flutter often coexists with nonisthmus-dependent mechanisms.

Surgical incisions in the right atrium for repair of atrial septal defects are probably the most common cause.[33-36] The incision often is placed in the lateral right atrium. The most common type of reentry circuit circulates around the incision and can be interrupted with a line of ablation lesions extending from the inferior margin of the scar to the inferior vena cava or from the superior margin of the scar to the superior vena cava. Some of these tachycardias use a narrow channel of conduction between regions of dense scar in the lateral right atrium.

In six recent series encompassing 134 patients, predominantly young adults, ablation abolished arrhythmia recurrences in 50% to 88% of patients during average follow-up periods of up to 2 years.[33,34-38] Complications of diaphragmatic paralysis resulting from phrenic nerve injury and possible thromboembolism after conversion from atrial flutter have occurred.

Lesion-related reentry also can occur as a result of gaps in incisional or ablation lines created for atrial maze procedures.[39,40] Stable macroreentry circuits occasionally occur in the left atrium but are much less common than right atrial circuits.[41,42] Catheter mapping and ablation can be effective but are often difficult.

Atrial Flutter Ablation Conclusions

Catheter ablation of atrial flutter is highly effective for abolishing isthmus-dependent flutter. However, a substantial number of patients subsequently develop atrial fibrillation, likely indicating that the atrial disease predisposing to flutter also predisposes to fibrillation. Paydak and colleagues[43] reported that 28 of 110 patients with atrial flutter treated with ablation developed atrial fibrillation during 20.1 ± 9.2 months of follow-up. A history of spontaneous atrial fibrillation (relative risk 3.9, 95% confidence intervals 1.8–8.8, P = 0.001) and left-ventricular ejection fraction (LVEF) of less than 50% (relative risk 3.8, 95% CI 1.7–8.5, P = 0.001) were significant and independent predictors of subsequent atrial fibrillation.

In summary, ablation for common, isthmus-dependent flutter abolishes this arrhythmia in approximately 90% of patients, but atrial fibrillation emerges in a substantial number of patients during follow-up, with an increasing incidence in patients with heart disease. Ablation is also effective for abolishing atrial flutter when it complicates drug therapy for atrial fibrillation but does not allow withdrawal of the antiarrhythmic drug if sinus rhythm is the goal because atrial fibrillation will recur in the majority of patients. Nonisthmus-dependent flutter is encountered less frequently and is particularly a problem in patients with prior atrial surgery. Ablation can be effective, but efficacy has not been well defined.

Atrial Fibrillation

Two types of ablation procedures have been developed for atrial fibrillation. The first is designed to control heart rate during persistent atrial fibrillation either by creation of heart block and implantation of a permanent pacemaker or by modification of the AV node to impair conduction. The second group of procedures aims to restore sinus rhythm by ablating triggers that initiate atrial fibrillation or creating lines of block in the atrium in a manner that prevents atrial reentry, commonly referred to as an "atrial maze procedure." Catheter-based atrial maze procedures are still evolving and face significant technical challenges.

AV Node Ablation and Pacemaker Implantation for Heart Rate Control

The Ablate and Pace Trial (APT) prospectively assessed the effects of catheter ablation of the AV node and permanent pacemaker implantation for medically refractory atrial fibrillation in 156 patients—70 patients with chronic atrial fibrillation, 31 patients with recurrent episodes of atrial fibrillation lasting more than 72 hours or requiring electrical cardioversion, and 55 with shorter self-terminating episodes of paroxysmal atrial fibrillation.[44] Patients with atrial fibrillation were deemed candidates for catheter ablation if, in the opinion of the investigator, medical therapy did not control symptoms or produced intolerable adverse effects. All patients underwent AV junction ablation and pacemaker implantation. Quality of life and symptoms were assessed by questionnaires prior to and at 3 and 12 months after the procedure. There was no concurrent control group. The procedure was successfully performed in all patients. Complications early after the procedure occurred in seven patients; most were related to pacemaker implantation (including ventricular lead dislodgment requiring reoperation in two, stroke, hemopneumothorax, femoral vein thrombosis, pacemaker pocket hematomas, and transient hypotension). Late complications occurred in eight patients (including stroke in four, pacer lead problems requiring revision in two, and nonsustained VT in one patient, respectively). During a follow-up of 12 months, significant improvements in quality-of-life scores were noted for all eight subscales of the Health Status Questionnaire for the overall rating of the Quality of Life Index, the Health and Function subscales; arrhythmia-related symptoms were reduced. The mean LVEF improved from 0.50 ± 0.20 at baseline to 0.54 ± 0.2 at 3 months (P = 0.03). Compared to baseline, there was no significant change in treadmill exercise duration (10.0 ± 4.3 vs. 11.1 ± 4.2, 11.6 ± 3.6 min) or VO$_2$ ax (1467 ± 681 vs. 1538 ± 736, 1629 ± 739 l/min) at 3 and 12 months. Thus, this approach was associated with improved quality of life and left-ventricular (LV) function in this selected population of highly symptomatic patients with atrial fibrillation refractory to medical therapy. During follow-up 13 patients died within 3 months following the ablation; 5 died suddenly (2 of these were monitored to be ventricular fibrillation).

Brignole and colleagues reported a multicenter, randomized, 6-month evaluation of the clinical effects of AV junction ablation and DDDR mode-switching pacemaker versus pharmacologic treatment in 43 patients with recurrent paroxysmal atrial fibrillation who had three or more episodes in the previous 6 months not controlled with antiarrhythmic drugs.[45] Before completion of the study, three patients in the drug group withdrew because of severe symptoms and one patient crossed over to AV junctional ablation and pacemaker implantation. In one patient, ablation of AV junction could not be achieved. At the end of the 6 months, the ablation/pacemaker group (31 patients) had lower (better) scores in the Living with Heart Failure Questionnaire (-51%, P = 0.0006), palpitations (-71%, P = 0.0000), effort dyspnea (-36%, P = 0.04), exercise intolerance score (-46%, P = 0.001), and easy fatigue (-51%, P = 0.02). At the end of the study, palpitations were no longer present in 81% of the ablation/pacemaker group and in 11% of the drug group (P = 0.0000). They concluded that in patients with paroxysmal atrial fibrillation not controlled by pharmacologic therapy, ablation and pacemaker implantation is highly effective and superior to drug therapy in controlling symptoms and improving quality of life.

Sudden death after AV junction ablation is an important concern, initially recognized as an anecdotal observation. Scheinman and coworkers observed the polymorphic VT torsades de pointes in one out of 47 patients and one sudden death early after AV junction ablation.[46] It has been hypothesized that the sudden decrease in heart rate may lead to QT prolongation and an increased risk of torsades de pointes. In a retrospective analysis Brugada and colleagues performed AV junction ablation in 100 consecutive patients and observed torsades de pointes or sudden death in 6 patients.[47] In a second consecutive series of 135 patients they implemented a strategy of pacing at a rate of 90 beats/min for 1 to 3 months after ablation. None of the 135 patients experienced torsades des pointes or sudden death during 12 months of follow-up.

The safety of AV junction ablation was assessed in a single-center, retrospective series by Ozcan et al.[48] Of 350 patients, 78 died during a mean follow-up of 36 ± 26 months. Previous myocardial infarction (P < 0.001), a history of congestive heart failure (P = 0.02), and treatment with cardiac drugs (digoxin; calcium-channel blockers; beta blockers; angiotensin-converting enzyme inhibitors; nitrates; diuretics; and antiarrhythmic agents including propafenone, sotalol, amiodarone, and mexiletine) after ablation (P = 0.03) were independent predictors of death. Observed survival among patients without these three risk factors was similar to expected survival in control and age- and sex-matched members of the Minnesota population.

Thus, control of the ventricular rate by ablation of the AV node and permanent pacing does not appear to adversely affect long-term survival. Further study, however, is warranted because there is increasing recognition that the activation sequence produced by right-ventricular (RV) pacing, which resembles left bundle branch block, may have an adverse impact on cardiac contractility in some patients with depressed ventricular function.[49]

AV Node Modification for Rate Control

Partial ablation of the AV node sufficient to slow the rate in atrial fibrillation but not to the degree that complete heart block is produced has been tested as a method for control of the ventricular rate during atrial fibrillation by Williamson and colleagues.[50] This method has the potential advantage that permanent pacing may not be required and ventricular activation is still over the His bundle and Purkinje system. In 19 consecutive patients with atrial fibrillation and uncontrolled ventricular rates refractory to drug therapy, RF application starting from the posterior septum or midseptal right atrium and moving progressively more superiorly, closer to the compact AV node, was performed until the heart rate during isoproterenol infusion was reduced to an average of 120 beats/min. Successful control of the ventricular rate without pathologic AV block was achieved in 14 (74%) patients, but persistent heart block requiring pacemaker implantation occurred in 4 patients (21%). Although the ventricular response remained irregular with the approach, the 14 patients with rate control achieved by modification without heart block had resolution of the symptom during the follow-up of 8 ± 2 months. One patient with dilated cardiomyopathy died suddenly 5 months after a successful procedure. Thus, the technique is feasible, but it has not achieved widespread use, because of the limitations noted above.

Knight and colleagues compared the cost effectiveness between these two methods.[51] On the basis of the long-term follow-up of patients who underwent each procedure, it was assumed that 31% of patients selected for the modification procedure would require a permanent pacemaker for inadvertent AV block or because of AV nodal ablation after a failed modification procedure and that the recurrence rate after AV node ablation would be 2%. The annual charges during follow-up were predicted and adjusted for recurrences and the need for additional procedures. The adjusted total charges at 1 year of follow-up were significantly lower for the modification procedure ($19,389 ± $2002 vs. $28,485 ± $2023, P < 0.001). After 10 years of follow-up, the cumulative, adjusted charges for modification were $20,016 (42%) less than for AV node ablation.

Catheter Ablation to Restore Sinus Rhythm

Haissagurre and coworkers demonstrated that some episodes of atrial fibrillation are initiated by a rapidly firing atrial focus, which serves as the trigger for atrial fibrillation.[52] They demonstrated that ablation of such a focus can prevent atrial fibrillation and that the foci frequently are located in sleeves of atrial myocardium that extend along the pulmonary veins from the left atrium. Approaches to ablation of these muscular sleeves to electrically isolate the pulmonary veins from the left atrium have been reported in single-center series. Ablation in the left atrium introduces concerns of embolism from thrombus formation on either catheters or ablation lesions and of narrowing of the pulmonary vein orifice with stenoses as the RF lesions heal.

Aiming at isolating each pulmonary vein from the left atrium, Pappone and coworkers reported an anatomic approach in which a series of RF lesions is placed in the left atrium circumferentially around each of the four ostia of the pulmonary veins.[53] In a single-center series he reported 26 patients, 12 with permanent and 14 with paroxysmal atrial fibrillation. The mean age of the patient population was 48 ± 8, and 19 (73%) were men. Underlying heart disease, including hypertension (15%), valvular heart disease (4%), and coronary artery disease (12%), was present in 31% of patients. Recurrence of atrial fibrillation during follow-up was assessed from Holter monitoring performed on symptom recurrence or routinely at 1 week and every month for 6 months or longer. During 9 ± 3 months of follow up, 85% patients remained free of atrial fibrillation—62% of whom were not receiving any antiarrhythmic medications and 23% of whom were receiving previously ineffective antiarrhythmic agents. One patient had hemopericardium requiring pericardiocentesis. Two patients had mild pericardial effusion managed medically. No thromboembolic events or pulmonary vein stenoses were reported.

Papone and coworkers subsequently reported a larger series of 251 consecutive patients with paroxysmal (179 patients) or permanent (72 patients) atrial fibrillation.[54] Cardiac tamponade occurred in 2 patients (0.8%) and no pulmonary vein stenoses were detected by transesophageal echocardiography. During a follow-up of 10.4 ± 4.5 months, 152 patients with paroxysmal AF (85%) and 49 with permanent AF (68%) had no symptomatic atrial fibrillation.

Oral and coworkers reported segmental pulmonary vein isolation guided by targeting electrical potentials felt to be markers for the sleeves of myocardium extending from the atrium along the vein.[55] In a series of 70 patients (average age of 53 ± 11 years, 57 male) 5 had some underlying heart disease, with paroxysmal (58 patients) or persistent atrial fibrillation (12 patients). Electrical isolation of all targeted pulmonary veins was achieved in 59 patients. One of 70 patients suffered an embolus with unilateral quadrantanopsia early after the procedure. Among 70 patients, 15 (21%) were treated with antiarrhythmic agents (Class I or III) for incomplete isolation of the targeted pulmonary vein or history of persistent atrial fibrillation or recurrence of atrial fibrillation during the 24-hour observation period after the procedure. If there was no recurrence of atrial fibrillation after 1 month, antiarrhythmic agents were discontinued. At 5 months of follow-up, 70% of patients with a history of frequent paroxysmal atrial fibrillation and 22% of those with persistent atrial fibrillation were free from atrial fibrillation. In total, 83% of patients with paroxysmal atrial fibrillation were either free of symptomatic atrial fibrillation or had significant improvement in symptoms.

Oral and coworkers also reported in an extension of the initial series that early recurrence of atrial fibrillation after ablation is not always indicative of failure of the procedure.[56] Of 110 consecutive patients followed for a mean of 208 ± 125 days, symptomatic atrial fibrillation recurred in 45%. The first recurrence atrial fibrillation was within 2 weeks of the procedure in 35%, 2 to 4 weeks after ablation in 7%, and at 1 to 2 months in 3%. The mean time to first recurrence was 3.7 ± 3.5 days. However, despite initial early recurrences, during continued follow-up 31% of these patients became free from recurrent episodes of atrial fibrillation without antiarrhythmic drug therapy. In comparison, among the 71 patients who did not have the recurrence, 85% remained free from recurrent episodes of atrial fibrillation without antiarrhythmic drug therapy. Initial irritation from the ablation procedure followed by healing may contribute to the early arrhythmias after the procedure.

Atrial Fibrillation Ablation Conclusions

Relatively small studies and case series indicate that catheter ablation of the AV junction with placement of a permanent pacemaker effectively controls rapid rates in atrial fibrillation. Although sudden death from VT has been observed after this procedure, with attention to adequate pacing rate this risk is small and a case-controlled study found no decrease in survival. In patients with LV dysfunction, RV apical pacing may have an adverse hemodynamic effect; the use of biventricular pacing (RV and LV) is under investigation for this group of patients. Ablation that seeks to isolate pulmonary vein triggers is feasible and effective for some patients, based on single-center series with relatively short follow-ups. Patients with paroxysmal atrial fibrillation have better outcomes than those with persistent atrial fibrillation. Risks and long-term outcomes and optimal approaches are still being defined.

VENTRICULAR TACHYCARDIA

VTs can be broadly classified as monomorphic, with each QRS resembling the preceding and following QRS, and polymorphic, with a continually changing QRS morphology from beat to beat (Table 16-2). Monomorphic VTs have repetitive ventricular activation from a stable arrhythmogenic substrate that potentially can be targeted for ablation. In contrast, polymorphic VTs lack a defined target; rarely, a trigger for polymorphic VT can be targeted for ablation.[57]

Catheter ablation methods for several different types of monomorphic VT have been developed and reported largely, in single-center series. Catheter ablation of VT is generally more difficult than ablation of the common SVTs. The efficacy and risk of complications vary with the type of tachycardia and underlying heart disease. In general these monomorphic VTs fall into two broad groups, idiopathic VT and VT associated with heart disease, such as prior myocardial infarction.

Idiopathic Ventricular Tachycardia

Idiopathic VT occurs in the absence of structural heart disease. Most have a focal origin, amenable to ablation if the focus is on the endocardial surface. The most common location is at the RV or LV outflow tract, giving rise to VT that has a left bundle branch block, inferior axis configuration. In single-center series ablation abolishes VT in approximately 85% of patients.[58-62] Failures occur when the tachycardia cannot be reproducibly induced to allow localization in the electrophysiology laboratory or when the focus is deep to the endocardium or in the epicardium. Complications are infrequent, but cardiac perforation and tamponade can occur.

■ ■ ■

TABLE 16-2   CONSIDERATIONS FOR CATHETER ABLATION OF VENTRICULAR TACHYCARDIA

Structural heart disease (prior myocardial infarction or cardiomyopathy)

ICD is generally first-line therapy if any of the following are present: depressed ventricular function, cardiac arrest, or severe symptoms.
Catheter ablation typically is reserved for frequent ICD shocks or incessant VT.
Ablation markedly reduces ICD therapies in >70% of patients, but 20 to 50% of patients will have at least one recurrence of VT.
Major complications occur in 1% to 3% (stroke, myocardial infarction, tamponade).
Present methods allow ablation even if multiple VTs are present or VT is hemodynamically unstable and not tolerated.

Idiopathic VT not resulting from structural heart disease

Origin is most commonly from RV outflow tract, LV outflow tract, or fascicles of the LV Purkinje system.
Indications for ablation include: recurrent symptomatic VT; ineffective drug therapy (including recurrent arrhythmia or intolerable side effects);
   incessant VT (even if asymptomatic) because of its potential for causing tachycardia induced cardiomyopathy.
Efficacy of ablation is 83% to 90%.
Complications occur in 1% to 3%, including vascular complication and pericardial effusion.

ICD, implantable cardioverter defibrillator; VT, ventricular tachycardia; RV, right ventricular; LV, left ventricular.

Ventricular Tachycardia Associated with Heart Disease

VT associated with heart disease is most commonly the result of reentry involving areas of ventricular scar.[64-67] Myocardial infarction is the most common cause, but scar-related VTs also occur as a result of arrhythmogenic RV dysplasia, sarcoidosis, Chagas' disease, and other non-ischemic cardiomyopathies.

VT resulting from prior myocardial infarction has been most extensively studied. The infarct regions causing these VTs are typically large, often extending over more than 20 square centimeters, and the reentry circuits can be large.[68-71] Circuits can consist of multiple loops or a single loop. RF ablation lesions are substantially smaller, typically 5 to 10 mm in diameter, than these reentry circuits. Ablation has been guided by mapping methods that sought to identify a narrow, critical portion of the reentry circuit where a limited number of RF lesions could interrupt reentry.[70,72-75] De Chillou and colleagues performed detailed catheter mapping in a selected group of 21 patients who had stable, tolerated VT that allowed mapping in the electrophysiology laboratory. Maps of VT demonstrated large reentry circuits (31 ± 7 mm [ranging from 18 to 41 mm] long and 16 ± 8 mm [ranging from 6 to 36 mm] wide). Circuits that were adjacent to the mitral annulus had an isthmus oriented parallel to the plane of the mitral annulus.[76] Linear ablation performed across the most accessible part of the isthmus prevented the recurrence of VT in 90% of patients with a follow-up of 16 ± 8 months.

Feasibility also has been shown in other single-center case series of patients who were largely referred for ablation because of difficult-to-control, recurrent episodes of sustained VT. These studies also identified obstacles to ablation. More than one QRS morphology of monomorphic VT is usually inducible, indicating the potential presence of multiple reentry circuits. Some circuits are deep to the endocardium, where they cannot be easily located or ablated. Induced VTs are often unstable in the electrophysiology laboratory, producing hemodynamic collapse or changing from one morphology of VT to another, impeding attempts to locate the reentry circuit during the arrhythmia. Tachycardias that are induced in the elec-

trophysiology laboratory that have not been previously documented to occur spontaneously are referred to by some laboratories as "nonclinical tachycardias" and are not targeted for ablation. In many patients, however, spontaneous VTs are terminated by an implanted defibrillator or medical personnel before an ECG is obtained, preventing adequate definition of the "clinical tachycardia" prior to the procedure.

Gonska and coworkers reported RF catheter ablation targeting a single "clinical" VT in a single-center series of 72 patients.[77] The targeted tachycardia was no longer inducible at the end of the procedure in 74% of patients. During a mean follow-up of 24 ± 13 months 60% of the group were free from recurrent tachycardia. In three separate series Stevenson, Rothman, Strickberger, and their coworkers targeted multiple tachycardias for ablation in patients with recurrent episodes of sustained monomorphic tachycardia.[78-80] Average LVEF ranged from 0.22 to 0.33; amiodarone therapy had been ineffective in 14% to 76% of patients. During the ablation procedure an average of 3.6 to 4.7 different VTs were inducible per patient. Ablation abolished all inducible monomorphic tachycardias in 33% of patients; tachycardias were inducible but modified in 45% or patients, and the procedure failed to abolish targeted, inducible tachycardias in 22% of patients. During mean follow-ups ranging from 12 to 18 months, 66% of patients remained free of sustained VT and 24% suffered one or more recurrences. Sudden death occurred in 2.8% of patients (the majority of patients in all three series had implantable defibrillators).

Of the 180 patients reported in these four series, the procedure mortality was 1% and complications occurred in 10% of patients, including AV block from ablation of part of the conduction system, vascular complications from arterial access, and pericardial effusion without tamponade.[79-80] During follow-up of 12 to 18 months death from heart failure occurred in approximately 10% of patients. Heart failure is not unexpected given the antecedent history of heart failure and depressed ventricular function in this patient population. However, damage to adjacent contracting myocardium outside the infarct or injury to the aortic or mitral valves are procedural complications that could exacerbate heart failure.

Cooled Radiofrequency Energy for Ventricular Tachycardia

Catheter ablation with a saline-irrigated catheter that produces larger lesions than conventional RF in animal models has been evaluated in a multicenter trial.[14] Patients with recurrent episodes of monomorphic VT associated with heart disease were enrolled; 82% had prior myocardial infarction. Patients were required to have a "stable" VT that allowed mapping in the electrophysiology laboratory. Initially patients were randomized to continue antiarrhythmic drug therapy or to catheter ablation. However, some ablation as "compassionate use" for patients without drug options was allowed. Results have been published only for the 146 patients in the catheter ablation cohort. These patients had a mean age of 65 ± 12.6 years and an LVEF of 31% ± 13%; 82% had prior myocardial infarction. The mean number of VT episodes in 2 months prior to enrollment was 25 ± 31. An implantable cardioverter defibrillator was present in 106 patients. Catheter ablation was acutely successful, eliminating all mappable VTs in 106 patients (75%). At the end of the procedure 59 patients (41%) had no VT of any type (mappable or unmappable) inducible after ablation. The difficulty of these procedures is indicated by average procedure duration of 4.8 hours and fluoroscopy time of 56 minutes. Procedure mortality was 2.7%. Major complications occurred in 12 patients (8%), including four strokes (2.7%), four pericardial tamponades (2.7%), two complete heart blocks (1.4), one myocardial infarction, and one aortic valve injury. Mean follow-up was 243 days, during which 66 patients (46%) patients developed one or more episodes of a sustained ventricular arrhythmia. The mean time to VT recurrence was 24 days. During follow-up, at a mean of 243 days 26 patients died, including 16 from heart failure and four with sudden death.

Unstable Ventricular Tachycardia

It is common for VTs to be unstable for extensive mapping because of hemodynamic intolerance, frequent termination to other VTs or inability to reliably initiate VT. Of 40 consecutive patients referred for ablation to Soejima and coworkers,[69] 33 had multiple different VTs and 80% had at least one unstable VT inducible. Only seven (20%) had stable VT as their only inducible VT; 33% had only unstable VTs inducible and 47% had both stable and unstable VTs inducible. Relatively small single-center series have demonstrated feasibility of ablation approaches for these patients.

Substrate Mapping

Identification of the VT substrate during stable sinus rhythm is often possible and can allow ablation to be performed during hemodynamically stable sinus rhythm. Areas of myocardial scar causing VT contain regions of dense, unexcitable fibrosis that create regions of conduction block and surviving regions of myocardium that create a potential path for reentry. The electrograms recorded have an abnormally low amplitude (typically less than 1.5 mV in the left ventricle) and often a fractionated appearance with multiple rapid components.[81] A mapping system that allows reconstruction of ventricular anatomy with superimposed color coding of electrogram amplitude allows creation of ventricular "Voltage maps" in which the areas of scar of infarction appear as discrete low amplitude regions. Marchlinski and coworkers targeted these regions for ablation in 16 patients with drug refractory, unstable monomorphic VT; nine had coronary artery disease and seven had nonischemic cardiomyopathy.[81] One to nine lines of RF lesions (8 to 87 lesions, median 55) averaging 3.9 cm in length, were placed across the borders of low-amplitude areas. All inducible VTs were abolished in seven patients (44%); the induced VTs were modified to faster or different VTs in five patients, and three patients continued to have a slow VT inducible. Complications occurred in one patient (stroke). During a follow-up (3 to 36 months) 75% patients were free of VT. Although the follow-up period was relatively short, only 50% patients had follow-up longer than 3 months; a marked reduction in VT episodes was observed.

Soejima and coworkers used the same mapping system in a series of 40 consecutive patients with recurrent VT after myocardial infarction.[69] Unstable VTs were present in 33 patients, 20 of whom also had at least one stable VT. After substrate mapping during sinus rhythm, potential reentry circuit isthmus sites in low voltage regions were identified by pacing at the sites and comparing the paced QRS morphology with that of VT and analysis of conduction delay, or by inducing VT for brief assessment of the site during tachycardia followed by immediate termination of the VT. A VT isthmus was identified in 63% of patients and for 60% of the unstable VTs. A line of RF lesions averaging 4.3 cm in length created by a mean of 18 RF applications abolished all VTs in 18 of 25 (72%) of patients who had an isthmus identified. Minor complications related to vascular access occurred in four patients. During follow-up of 350 days, 47% of patients were free of any VT, including 19 of the 33 patients with unstable VTs. For the entire group, a marked reduction in VT episodes detected by implantable cardioverter defibrillators (ICDs) from a mean of 11.9 to 0.4 episodes per month was observed. Although voltage maps identify the infarct area, the best method of designing placement of ablation lesions in these areas still is being investigated.

Noncontact Mapping

Another approach to guiding ablation for unstable tachycardias utilizes mapping systems that record from multiple sites simultaneously, potentially allowing reconstruction of electrical activation from a single beat of tachycardia. Schilling and colleagues reported the feasibility of the noncontact catheter mapping system for guiding ablation of VT.[82] This system, approved for use in the right atrium, consists of a balloon electrode array placed in the ventricle that allows mathematic reconstruction of 3360 "virtual electrograms" from a single beat of tachycardia. In a series of 24 patients with prior myocardial infarction referred for ablation of VT, sites of initial endocardial activation that are often near exit sites in reentry circuits were identified for 80 of 81 VTs in 22 patients. In addition, diastolic electrical activity, potentially marking the reentry circuit isthmus, was found in 67% of VTs. Complication included vascular complications, cardiogenic shock after VF, hemothorax, and one stroke. During follow up of 1.5 years, 64% of patients had no recurrence.

Strickberger reported the use of this system for guiding ablation of VT in 15 patients with a total of 21 VTs, 12 of which were unstable.[83] Fifteen out of 19 targeted VTs were successfully ablated. Complications occurred in five patients, including femoral pseudoaneurysm, cerebrovascular event, cardiogenic shock after ventricular fibrillation, and hemothorax.

Cost Effectiveness of Ventricular Tachycardia Ablation

Calkins and colleagues evaluated the cost-effectiveness of catheter ablation therapy compared to amiodarone therapy for VT in patients with structural heart disease.[84] Incremental cost effectiveness of ablation relative to amiodarone over 5 years after treatment initiation was estimated using data from the randomized trial reported by Calkins and coworkers, the literature, and a consensus panel. Costs were from 1998 national Medicare reimbursement schedules. Quality-of-life weights were estimated using an established preference measurement technique. In a hypothetic cohort, 5-year costs were higher for patients undergoing ablation compared with amiodarone therapy. Ablation also produced a greater increase in quality of life. This yielded a cost-effectiveness ratio of $20,923 per quality-adjusted life year (QALY) gained for ablation compared with amiodarone. Results were relatively insensitive to assumptions about ablation success and durability. If VT ablation was used in patients with preserved LV function after their first VT episode, the incremental cost-effectiveness ratio was $6028 per QALY gained. From a societal perspective, catheter ablation appears to be a cost-effective alternative to amiodarone for treating patients with VT.

Conclusions—Catheter Ablation of VT

Single-center studies have established catheter ablation as an important option for patients with recurrent idiopathic VT. In patients with heart disease and VT who are at risk for sudden death from arrhythmia, ICDs are first-line therapy. Only one multicenter trial evaluating catheter ablation of VT has been published. This trial and single-center series support use of catheter ablation as an important therapy for preventing or reducing recurrences of symptomatic VT in patients with ICDs,[80,85] avoiding antiarrhythmic drug toxicities and the potential adverse impact of many drugs, particularly amiodarone, on defibrillation threshold. In some patient populations the risk of sudden death may be acceptably low, such that successful ablation may be adequate as sole therapy.[77] Techniques and technology are continuing to evolve.

REFERENCES

1. Gallagher JJ, Svenson RH, Kasell JH, et al: Catheter technique for closed-chest ablation of the atrioventricular conduction system. N Engl J Med 1982; 306:194-200.
2. Gonzalez R, Scheinman M, Margaretten W, et al: Closed-chest electrode-catheter technique for His bundle ablation in dogs. Am J Physiol 1981; 241:H283-287.
3. Huang SK, Bharati S, Graham AR, et al: Closed chest catheter desiccation of the atrioventricular junction using radiofrequency energy: A new method of catheter ablation. J Am Coll Cardiol 1987; 9:349-358.
4. Huang SK, Graham AR, Lee MA, et al: Comparison of catheter ablation using radiofrequency versus direct current energy: Biophysical, electrophysiologic and pathologic observations. J Am Coll Cardiol 1991; 18:1091-1097.
5. Bartlett TG, Mitchell R, Friedman PL, et al: Histologic evolution of radiofrequency lesions in an old human myocardial infarct causing ventricular tachycardia. J Cardiovasc Electrophysiol 1995; 6:625-629.
6. Saul JP, Hulse JE, Papagiannis J, et al: Late enlargement of radiofrequency lesions in infant lambs: Implications for ablation procedures in small children. Circulation 1994; 90:492-499.
7. Delacretaz E, Stevenson WG, Winters GL, et al: Ablation of ventricular tachycardia with a saline-cooled radiofrequency catheter: Anatomic and histologic characteristics of the lesions in humans. J Cardiovasc Electrophysiol 1999; 10:860-865.
8. Thomas SP, Wallace EM, Ross DL: The effect of a residual isthmus of surviving tissue on conduction after linear ablation in atrial myocardium. J Interv Card Electrophysiol 2000; 4:273-281.
9. Mitchell MA, McRury ID, Everett TH, et al: Morphological and physiological characteristics of discontinuous linear atrial ablations during atrial pacing and atrial fibrillation. J Cardiovasc Electrophysiol 1999; 10:378-386.
10. Scheinman MM, Morady F, Hess DS, et al: Catheter-induced ablation of the atrioventricular junction to control refractory supraventricular arrhythmias. JAMA 1982; 248:851-855.
11. Jackman WM, Wang XZ, Friday KJ, et al: Catheter ablation of atrioventricular junction using radiofrequency current in 17 patients: Comparison of standard and large-tip catheter electrodes. Circulation 1991; 83:1562-1576.
12. Lesh MD, Van Hare GF, Schamp DJ, et al: Curative percutaneous catheter ablation using radiofrequency energy for accessory pathways in all locations: Results in 100 consecutive patients. J Am Coll Cardiol 1992; 19:1303-1309.
13. Calkins H, Yong P, Miller JM, et al: Catheter ablation of accessory pathways, atrioventricular nodal reentrant tachycardia, and the atrioventricular junction: Final results of a prospective, multicenter clinical trial—The Atakr Multicenter Investigators Group. Circulation 1999; 99:262-270.
14. Calkins H, Epstein A, Packer D, et al: Catheter ablation of ventricular tachycardia in patients with structural heart disease using cooled radiofrequency energy: Results of a prospective multicenter study—Cooled RF Multi Center Investigators Group. J Am Coll Cardiol 2000; 35:1905-1914.
15. Inoue S, Becker AE: Posterior extensions of the human compact atrioventricular node: A neglected anatomic feature of potential clinical significance. Circulation 1998; 97:188-193.
16. Lee MA, Morady F, Kadish A, et al: Catheter modification of the atrioventricular junction with radiofrequency energy for control of atrioventricular nodal reentry tachycardia. Circulation 1991; 83:827-835.
17. Jazayeri MR, Hempe SL, Sra JS, et al: Selective transcatheter ablation of the fast and slow pathways using radiofrequency energy in patients with atrioventricular nodal reentrant tachycardia. Circulation 1992; 85:1318-1328.
18. Jentzer JH, Goyal R, Williamson BD, et al: Analysis of junctional ectopy during radiofrequency ablation of the slow pathway in patients with atrioventricular nodal reentrant tachycardia. Circulation 1994; 90:2820-2826.
19. Jazayeri MR, Deshpande S, Dhala A, et al: Transcatheter mapping and radiofrequency ablation of cardiac arrhythmias. Curr Probl Cardiol 1994; 19:287-395.
20. Kalbfleisch SJ, Strickberger SA, Williamson B, et al: Randomized comparison of anatomic and electrogram mapping approaches to

ablation of the slow pathway of atrioventricular node reentrant tachycardia. J Am Coll Cardiol 1994; 23:716-723.

21. Jackman WM, Beckman KJ, McClelland JH, et al. Treatment of supraventricular tachycardia due to atrioventricular nodal reentry, by radiofrequency catheter ablation of slow-pathway conduction. N Engl J Med 1992; 327:313-318.

22. Mandel WJ LM, Fink B, Obayashi K: Comparative electrophysiologic features of the WPW syndrome in the pediatric and adult patient. Am J Cardiol 1974; 33:155.

23. Klein GJ, Bashore TM, Sellers TD, et al: Ventricular fibrillation in the Wolff-Parkinson-White syndrome. N Engl J Med 1979; 301:1080-1085.

24. Jackman WM, Wang XZ, Friday KJ, et al: Catheter ablation of accessory atrioventricular pathways (Wolff-Parkinson-White syndrome) by radiofrequency current. N Engl J Med 1991; 324:1605-1611.

25. Kuck KH, Schluter M, Geiger M, et al: Radiofrequency current catheter ablation of accessory atrioventricular pathways. Lancet 1991; 337:1557-1561.

26. Yamane T, Jais P, Shah DC, et al: Efficacy and safety of an irrigated-tip catheter for the ablation of accessory pathways resistant to conventional radiofrequency ablation. Circulation 2000; 102:2565-2568.

27. Natale A, Newby KH, Pisano E, et al: Prospective randomized comparison of antiarrhythmic therapy versus first-line radiofrequency ablation in patients with atrial flutter. J Am Coll Cardiol 2000; 35:1898-1904.

28. Anselme F, Savoure A, Cribier A, et al: Catheter ablation of typical atrial flutter: A randomized comparison of 2 methods for determining complete bidirectional isthmus block. Circulation 2001; 103:1434-1439.

29. Shah DC, Takahashi A, Jais P, et al: Tracking dynamic conduction recovery across the cavotricuspid isthmus. J Am Coll Cardiol 2000; 35:1478-1484.

30. Nakagawa H, Yamanashi WS, Pitha JV, et al: Comparison of in vivo tissue temperature profile and lesion geometry for radiofrequency ablation with a saline-irrigated electrode versus temperature control in a canine thigh muscle preparation. Circulation 1995; 91:2264-2273.

31. Jais P, Haissaguerre M, Shah DC, et al: Successful irrigated-tip catheter ablation of atrial flutter resistant to conventional radiofrequency ablation. Circulation 1998; 98:835-838.

32. Nabar A, Rodriguez LM, Timmermans C, et al: Radiofrequency ablation of "class IC atrial flutter" in patients with resistant atrial fibrillation. Am J Cardiol 1999; 83:785-787, A10.

33. Akar JG, Kok LC, Haines DE, et al: Coexistence of type I atrial flutter and intra-atrial re-entrant tachycardia in patients with surgically corrected congenital heart disease. J Am Coll Cardiol 2001; 38:377-384.

34. Chan DP, Van Hare GF, Mackall JA, et al: Importance of atrial flutter isthmus in postoperative intra-atrial reentrant tachycardia. Circulation 2000; 102:1283-1289.

35. Delacretaz E, Ganz LI, Soejima K, et al: Multi atrial maco-re-entry circuits in adults with repaired congenital heart disease: Entrainment mapping combined with three-dimensional electroanatomic mapping. J Am Coll Cardiol 2001; 37:1665-1676.

36. Hebe J, Hansen P, Ouyang F, et al: Radiofrequency catheter ablation of tachycardia in patients with congenital heart disease. Pediatr Cardiol 2000; 21:557-575.

37. Nakagawa H, Shah N, Matsudaira K, et al: Characterization of reentrant circuit in macroreentrant right atrial tachycardia after surgical repair of congenital heart disease: Isolated channels between scars allow "focal" ablation. Circulation 2001; 103:699-709.

38. Triedman JK, Bergau DM, Saul JP, et al: Efficacy of radiofrequency ablation for control of intraatrial reentrant tachycardia in patients with congenital heart disease. J Am Coll Cardiol 1997; 30:1032-1038.

39. Duru F, Hindricks G, Kottkamp H: Atypical left atrial flutter after intraoperative radiofrequency ablation of chronic atrial fibrillation: Successful ablation using three-dimensional electroanatomic mapping. J Cardiovasc Electrophysiol 2001; 12:602-605.

40. Thomas SP, Nunn GR, Nicholson IA, et al: Mechanism, localization and cure of atrial arrhythmias occurring after a new intraoperative endocardial radiofrequency ablation procedure for atrial fibrillation. J Am Coll Cardiol 2000; 35:442-450.

41. Jais P, Shah DC, Haissaguerre M, et al: Mapping and ablation of left atrial flutters. Circulation 2000; 101:2928-2934.

42. Tai CT, Lin YK, Chen SA: Atypical atrial flutter involving the isthmus between the right pulmonary veins and fossa ovalis. Pacing Clin Electrophysiol 2001; 24:384-387.

43. Paydak H, Kall JG, Burke MC, et al: Atrial fibrillation after radiofrequency ablation of type I atrial flutter: Time to onset, determinants, and clinical course. Circulation 1998; 98:315-322.

44. Kay GN, Ellenbogen KA, Giudici M, et al: The Ablate and Pace Trial: A prospective study of catheter ablation of the AV conduction system and permanent pacemaker implantation for treatment of atrial fibrillation: APT Investigators. J Interv Card Electrophysiol 1998; 2:121-135.

45. Brignole M, Gianfranchi L, Menozzi C, et al: Assessment of atrioventricular junction ablation and DDDR mode-switching pacemaker versus pharmacological treatment in patients with severely symptomatic paroxysmal atrial fibrillation: A randomized controlled study. Circulation 1997; 96:2617-2624.

46. Rosenquvist M, Lee MA, Moulinier L, et al: Long-term follow-up of patients after transcatheter direct current ablation of the atrioventricular junction. J Am Coll Cardiol 1990; 16:1467-1474.

47. Geelen P, Brugada J, Andries E, et al: Ventricular fibrillation and sudden death after radiofrequency catheter ablation of the atrioventricular junction. Pacing Clin Electrophysiol 1997; 20:343-348.

48. Ozcan C, Jahangir A, Friedman PA, et al: Sudden death after radiofrequency ablation of the atrioventricular node in patients with atrial fibrillation. J Am Coll Cardiol 2002; 40:105-110.

49. Blanc JJ, Etienne Y, Gilard M, et al: Evaluation of different ventricular pacing sites in patients with severe heart failure: Results of an acute hemodynamic study. Circulation 1997; 96:3273-3277.

50. Williamson BD, Man KC, Daoud E, et al: Radiofrequency catheter modification of atrioventricular conduction to control the ventricular rate during atrial fibrillation. N Engl J Med 1994; 331:910-917.

51. Knight BP, Weiss R, Bahu M, et al: Cost comparison of radiofrequency modification and ablation of the atrioventricular junction in patients with chronic atrial fibrillation. Circulation 1997; 96:1532-1536.

52. Haissaguerre M, Jais P, Shah DC, et al: Spontaneous initiation of atrial fibrillation by ectopic beats originating in the pulmonary veins. N Engl J Med 1998; 339:659-666.

53. Pappone C, Rosanio S, Oreto G, et al: Circumferential radiofrequency ablation of pulmonary vein ostia: A new anatomic approach for curing atrial fibrillation. Circulation 2000; 102:2619-2628.

54. Pappone C, Oreto G, Rosanio S, et al. Atrial electroanatomic remodeling after circumferential radiofrequency pulmonary vein ablation: efficacy of an anatomic approach in a large cohort of patients with atrial fibrillation. *Circulation*. 2001; 104:2539-44.

55. Oral H, Knight BP, Tada H, et al: Pulmonary vein isolation for paroxysmal and persistent atrial fibrillation. Circulation 2002; 105:1077-1081.

56. Oral H, Knight BP, Ozaydin M, et al: Clinical significance of early recurrences of atrial fibrillation after pulmonary vein isolation. J Am Coll Cardiol 2002; 40:100-104.

57. Haissaguerre M, Shah DC, Jais P, et al. Role of Purkinje conducting system in triggering of idiopathic ventricular fibrillation. Lancet 2002; 359:677-678.

58. O'Connor BK, Case CL, Sokoloski MC, et al: Radiofrequency catheter ablation of right ventricular outflow tachycardia in children and adolescents. J Am Coll Cardiol 1996; 27:869-874.

59. Movsowitz C, Schwartzman D, Callans DJ, et al: Idiopathic right ventricular outflow tract tachycardia: Narrowing the anatomic location for successful ablation. Am Heart J 1996; 131:930-936.

60. Rodriguez LM, Smeets JL, Timmermans C, et al: Predictors for successful ablation of right- and left-sided idiopathic ventricular tachycardia. Am J Cardiol 1997; 79:309-314.

61. Coggins DL, Lee RJ, Sweeney J, et al: Radiofrequency catheter ablation as a cure for idiopathic tachycardia of both left and right ventricular origin. J Am Coll Cardiol 1994; 23:1333-1341.

62. Lee SH, Chen SA, Tai CT, et al: Electropharmacologic characteristics and radiofrequency catheter ablation of sustained ventricular tachycardia in patients without structural heart disease. Cardiology 1996; 87:33-41.

63. Wen MS, Taniguchi Y, Yeh SJ, et al: Determinants of tachycardia recurrences after radiofrequency ablation of idiopathic ventricular tachycardia. Am J Cardiol 1998; 81:500-503.

64. de Bakker JM, Coronel R, Tasseron S, et al: Ventricular tachycardia in the infarcted, Langendorff-perfused human heart: Role of the

arrangement of surviving cardiac fibers. J Am Coll Cardiol 1990; 15:1594-1607.

65. de Bakker JM, van Capelle FJ, Janse MJ, et al: Reentry as a cause of ventricular tachycardia in patients with chronic ischemic heart disease: Electrophysiologic and anatomic correlation. Circulation 1988; 77:589-606.

66. Pogwizd SM HR, Saffitz JE, et al: Reentrant and focal mechanisms underlying ventricular tachycardia in the human heart. Circulation 1991; 86:1872-1887.

67. Delacretaz E, Stevenson WG, Ellison KE, et al: Mapping and radiofrequency catheter ablation of the three types of sustained monomorphic ventricular tachycardia in nonischemic heart disease. J Cardiovasc Electrophysiol 2000; 11:11-17.

68. Marchlinski FE, Callans DJ, Gottlieb CD, et al: Linear ablation lesions for control of unmappable ventricular tachycardia in patients with ischemic and nonischemic cardiomyopathy. Circulation 2000; 101:1288-1296.

69. Soejima K, Suzuki M, Maisel WH, et al: Catheter ablation in patients with multiple and unstable ventricular tachycardias after myocardial infarction: Short ablation lines guided by reentry circuit isthmuses and sinus rhythm mapping. Circulation 2001; 104:664-669.

70. Stevenson WG, Friedman PL, Sager PT, et al: Exploring postinfarction reentrant ventricular tachycardia with entrainment mapping. J Am Coll Cardiol 1997; 29:1180-1189.

71. de Bakker JM, van Capelle FJ, Janse MJ, et al: Macroreentry in the infarcted human heart: The mechanism of ventricular tachycardias with a "focal" activation pattern. J Am Coll Cardiol 1991; 18:1005-1014.

72. Bogun F, Bahu M, Knight BP, et al: Response to pacing at sites of isolated diastolic potentials during ventricular tachycardia in patients with previous myocardial infarction. J Am Coll Cardiol 1997; 30:505-513.

73. Bogun F, Bahu M, Knight BP, et al: Comparison of effective and ineffective target sites that demonstrate concealed entrainment in patients with coronary artery disease undergoing radiofrequency ablation of ventricular tachycardia. Circulation 1997; 95:183-190.

74. Kocovic DZ, Harada T, Friedman PL, et al: Characteristics of electrograms recorded at reentry circuit sites and bystanders during ventricular tachycardia after myocardial infarction. J Am Coll Cardiol 1999; 34:381-388.

75. El-Shalakany A, Hadjis T, Papageorgiou P, et al: Entrainment/mapping criteria for the prediction of termination of ventricular tachycardia by single radiofrequency lesion in patients with coronary artery disease. Circulation 1999; 99:2283-2289.

76. de Chillou C, Lacroix D, Klug D, et al: Isthmus characteristics of reentrant ventricular tachycardia after myocardial infarction. Circulation 2002; 105:726-731.

77. Gonska BD, Cao K, Schaumann A, et al: Catheter ablation of ventricular tachycardia in 136 patients with coronary artery disease: Results and long-term follow-up. J Am Coll Cardiol 1994; 24: 1506-1514.

78. Stevenson WG, Friedman PL, Kocovic D, et al: Radiofrequency catheter ablation of ventricular tachycardia after myocardial infarction. Circulation 1998; 98:308-314.

79. Rothman SA, Hsia HH, Cossu SF, et al: Radiofrequency catheter ablation of postinfarction ventricular tachycardia: Long-term success and the significance of inducible nonclinical arrhythmias. Circulation 1997; 96:3499-3508.

80. Strickberger SA, Man KC, Daoud EG, et al: A prospective evaluation of catheter ablation of ventricular tachycardia as adjuvant therapy in patients with coronary artery disease and an implantable cardioverter-defibrillator. Circulation 1997; 96:1525-1531.

81. Marchlinski FE, Callans DJ, Gottlieb CD, et al: Linear ablation lesions for control of unmappable ventricular tachycardia in patients with ischemic and nonischemic cardiomyopathy. Circulation 2000; 101:1288-1296.

82. Schilling RJ, Peters NS, Davies DW: Mapping and ablation of ventricular tachycardia with the aid of a non-contact mapping system. Heart 1999; 81:570-575.

83. Strickberger SA, Knight BP, Michaud GF, et al: Mapping and ablation of ventricular tachycardia guided by virtual electrograms using a noncontact, computerized mapping system. J Am Coll Cardiol 2000; 35:414-421.

84. Calkins H, Bigger JT, Jr., Ackerman SJ, et al: Cost-effectiveness of catheter ablation in patients with ventricular tachycardia. Circulation 2000; 101:280-288.

85. Stevenson WG, Friedman PL, Sweeney MO: Catheter ablation as an adjunct to ICD therapy. Circulation 1997; 96:1378-1380.

chapter 17

Implantable Cardioverter-Defibrillators and Cardiac Resynchronization Therapy

Michael O. Sweeney

Sudden cardiac death is the leading cause of mortality in the United States. It is estimated that 200,000 to 400,000 sudden deaths occur annually.[1] The vast majority of these deaths occur among patients with symptomatic heart failure associated with reduced left-ventricular (LV) function. In the Framingham study, the sudden death rate for patients with heart failure was nine times the general age-adjusted population rate.[2] The annual incidence of sudden death is expected to increase coincident with the increasing incidence of heart failure. There are 4 million to 5 million people living with chronic heart failure, and an additional 400,000 are newly diagnosed yearly.[3-5] The increasing incidence of heart failure is primarily the result of the advancing age of the population with coronary artery disease, which is now the principal cause of heart failure associated with reduced ventricular function.[2]

Mortality resulting from progressive heart failure associated with reduced LV function has declined. In the Framingham study total mortality was 24% and 55% within 4 years of developing symptomatic heart failure for women and men, respectively.[2] These statistics approximate well the natural history of heart failure because the subject population was untreated by contemporary standards. Recognition of the beneficial effects of angiotensin-converting enzyme (ACE) inhibitors, diuretics, digoxin, and beta blockade has yielded substantial reductions in mortality resulting from progressive pump failure. However, despite these improvements in medical therapy, symptomatic heart failure still confers a 20% to 25% risk of premature death in the first 2.5 years after diagnosis. At least 50% of these premature deaths are sudden and attributable to ventricular tachycardia (VT) or ventricular fibrillation (VF). This proportionate contribution of sudden death to total mortality in heart failure associated with reduced LV function has not changed substantially between the Framingham data and the modern era.[2]

IMPLANTABLE CARDIOVERTER DEFIBRILLATORS FOR PREVENTION OF SUDDEN DEATH ASSOCIATED WITH REDUCED LEFT-VENTRICULAR SYSTOLIC FUNCTION

Trials of Secondary Prevention

Three multinational trials comparing implantable cardioverter defibrillator (ICD) therapy and drug therapy in 2024 survivors of life-threatening ventricular arrhythmia were completed in the 1990s (Table 17-1 and Fig. 17-1).

Antiarrhythmics Versus Implantable Defibrillator

The Antiarrhythmics Versus Implantable Defibrillator (AVID) trial was a multicenter, randomized comparison of drug therapy (amiodarone or sotalol) versus ICD therapy in survivors of cardiac arrest as a result of VF, sustained VT with syncope, or hemodynamically unstable sustained VT with left-ventricular ejection fraction (LVEF) of less than 40%.[6] The study was initiated in 1993 and prematurely terminated in 1997 when a significant difference in the primary outcome (total mortality) was revealed. A total of 1016 patients were enrolled, of which 507 were randomized to ICD and 509 were randomized to drug therapy. The majority of patients in both groups had chronic coronary disease (81%). The mean LVEF was 31% to 32%, and a slight majority of patients in both groups (55% to 60%) had mild to moderate heart failure symptoms (New York Heart Association [NYHA] Class II or III). Patients with NYHA Class IV heart failure were excluded from the study. Approximately two thirds of patients were taking ACE inhibitors, and half were taking diuretics and digoxin. The vast majority (96%) of patients randomized to drug therapy were taking amiodarone at hospital discharge. The mean daily maintenance dose of amiodarone at 3 years follow-up was 259 mg. Sotalol was given infrequently because of concerns about exacerbation of heart failure

TABLE 17-1   RANDOMIZED TRIALS OF IMPLANTABLE CARDIOVERTER DEFIBRILLATORS FOR SECONDARY PREVENTION OF SUDDEN DEATH

	AVID	CIDS	CASH
Target population	VT/VF	VT/VF	VF
Treatment	ICD vs. drug (amiodarone/sotalol)	ICD vs. amiodarone	ICD vs. amiodarone vs. metoprolol*
Patients enrolled	1016	659	349
Arrhythmia qualifier	VF, syncopal VT, or poorly tolerated VT + LVEF <40%	VF, syncopal VT, VT >150 beats/min + LVEF <35%, syncope + inducible VT	VF requiring defibrillation
LVEF (%) qualifier	Yes (see "Arrhythmia qualifier")	Yes (see "Arrhythmia qualifier")	None
CHF qualifier	None	None	None
No CHF	42	~50	~27
NYHA II (%)	48	~38	57
NYHA III (%)	10	~10 (including IV)	16
NYHA IV (%)	Excluded	~10 (including III)	Excluded
Revascularization (%)	37	~30	~20
Mean LVEF (%)	31–32	33–34	>45
ACE inhibitors (%)	~66	Not reported	Not reported
Beta blockers (%)	~42% ICD vs. 17% drug group	54% ICD vs. 23% amiodarone group	1/3 randomized to metoprolol alone
Outcome	*Survival advantage in ICD group*	*Trend toward survival advantage in ICD group*	*Survival advantage in ICD group*
Total mortality rate	11% ICD vs. 18% drug at 1 year (RR 32%)	8.3%/yr ICD vs. 10.2%/yr amiodarone (RR 19.7%, P = 0.14)	12.1% ICD vs. 19.6% amiodarone/metoprolol at 2 years (RR 37%)
Sudden death rate	5% ICD vs. 11% drug (unadjusted)	3.0%/yr ICD vs. 4.5%/yr amiodarone (RR 32%, P = 0.09)	2% ICD vs. 11% to 12% amiodarone/metoprolol
Comments	96% of drug group received empiric amiodarone; 40% to 45% had no CHF symptoms	Fewer patients had symptomatic CHF vs. AVID	

*Propafenone arm stopped in 1992 due to excess mortality (all sudden deaths).
AVID, Antiarrythmics versus Implantable Defibrillator Trial; CIDS, Canadian Implantable Defibrillator Study; CASH, Cardiac Arrest Study Hamburg; VT, ventricular tachycardia; VF, ventricular fibrillation; LVEF, left-ventricular ejection fraction; CHF, congestive heart failure; NYHA, New York Heart Association functional class; ACE, angiotensin-converting enzyme; ICD, implantable cardioverter defibrillator; RR, risk reduction.

or demonstration of inadequate suppression of ambient or induced ventricular arrhythmia.

ICD therapy was associated with a significant reduction in mortality compared to drug therapy. The 1-year survival rate was 89% in the ICD group and 82% in the drug group. This differential yielded a significant 32% reduction in mortality that was maintained throughout at least 3

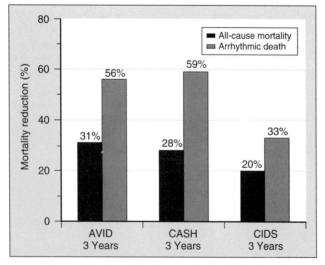

FIGURE 17-1. Mortality reduction associated with implantable cardioverter defibrillator (ICD) therapy for secondary prevention of sudden cardiac death.

years of follow-up. A subsequent analysis confirmed that the mortality benefit of ICD therapy was attributable to reduction in sudden deaths versus antiarrhythmic drugs.[7]

There were several methodologic limitations to this study. There was no control group, which was perceived to be unethical among patients who had survived life-threatening ventricular arrhythmia. The treatment crossover rates were substantial (ICD to drug therapy 26%, drug therapy to ICD 19%) but did not compromise statistical power. There were several important baseline differences between the treatment groups. Significantly fewer patients in the drug therapy group were taking beta blockers (17% vs. 42%). There were nearly twice as many patients with NYHA Class III heart failure symptoms in the drug therapy group (12% vs. 7%).

Cardiac Arrest Study of Hamburg

The Cardiac Arrest Study of Hamburg (CASH) was a multicenter, open-label, randomized comparison of drug therapy (propafenone, amiodarone, metoprolol) versus ICD therapy in survivors of cardiac arrest resulting from VF requiring defibrillation.[8] The study was initiated in 1987 and terminated in 1997 after 349 patients were enrolled. The propafenone arm was stopped in March 1992 when an interim analysis (mean follow-up 11 months) revealed excess mortality compared with ICD therapy. There were 11 sudden deaths in the propafenone arm and none in the ICD arm, with a corresponding total mortality of 29% and 11%, respectively. The majority of patients had chronic coronary disease (approximately 75%).

After a 2-year minimum average follow-up, total mortality was 12.1% in the ICD group versus 19.6% in the amiodarone and metoprolol groups (combined). This yielded a significant 37% total mortality risk reduction in the ICD group versus amiodarone/metoprolol group (P = 0.047). It is interesting that there was no significant difference in mortality among patients treated with amiodarone or metoprolol. The treatment cross-over rate was low and equivalent (ICD to amiodarone/metoprolol 6%, amiodarone/metoprolol to ICD 6%).

There were several interesting characteristics of the CASH study population. LV was generally well preserved (mean ejection fraction > 44%). Sustained monomorphic VT was induced at baseline electrophysiology study in only 30% of patients. Of patients, 50% had no inducible ventricular arrhythmia and 20% had inducible polymorphic VT or VF. These observations suggest a powerful role for ischemic triggers of VF in the study population and may account for the beneficial mortality effect of stand-alone beta blocker therapy.

Canadian Implantable Defibrillator Study

The Canadian Implantable Defibrillator Study (CIDS) was a multicenter, randomized comparison of empiric amiodarone versus ICD therapy in patients with cardiac arrest requiring defibrillation, sustained VT with syncope, VT of more than 150 beats/min with near syncope and LVEF of 35% or less, or unmonitored syncope and either inducible VT or spontaneous VT on monitor.[9] The study was initiated in 1990 and completed in 1997. A total of 659 patients were enrolled, of which 328 were randomized to ICD and 331 were randomized to amiodarone. The majority of patients in both groups had chronic coronary disease (76% to 77%). The mean LVEF was 33% to 34%, and approximately 50% of patients in both groups had symptomatic heart failure. Amiodarone was administered as 1200 mg/day for 1 week, then 400 mg/day for 10 weeks, with a target maintenance dose of 300 mg/day.

After an average follow-up of 4 years (at least 1 year in all patients), total mortality was 27% in the ICD group versus 33% in the amiodarone group. This yielded a 19.7% total mortality risk reduction in the ICD group versus amiodarone group, which did not reach statistical significance (P = 0.09). The treatment cross-over rates at 5 years were substantial (ICD to amiodarone 30%, amiodarone to ICD 16%).

Trials of Primary Prevention

Survival from out-of-hospital cardiac arrest remains abysmal; it is estimated that less than 20% of victims will leave the hospital alive.[10] The principal reason for this dismal statistic is unavailability of, or delayed time to, successful defibrillation. Prevention, or at least effective treatment, of the first episode of cardiac arrest is thus critically important. Accordingly, attention has focused on identification and treatment of patients at risk for sudden death as a result of ventricular arrhythmias

(Table 17-2 and Fig. 17-2). As noted previously, the majority of such patients had symptomatic heart failure associated with reduced LV function.

Multicenter Automatic Defibrillator Trial

The Multicenter Automatic Defibrillator Trial (MADIT) was the first study to randomly compare prophylactic ICD therapy and antiarrhythmic drug therapy among patients at high risk for sudden cardiac death.[11] Patients with chronic coronary disease; LVEF of 35% or less; spontaneous nonsustained VT; and inducible, nonsuppressible sustained monomorphic VT were randomized to prophylactic ICD or conventional medical therapy. The study was initiated in 1990 and prematurely terminated in 1996 when a significant difference in the primary outcome (total mortality) was discovered. A total of 196 patients were enrolled, of which 95 were randomized to ICD therapy and 101 to drug therapy. Approximately two thirds of patients had mild to moderately symptomatic heart failure (NYHA Class II or III), and the mean LVEF was 25% to 27%. Approximately 50% of patients were receiving conventional heart failure therapy (ACE inhibitors, digoxin, and diuretics). Amiodarone was the most commonly used antiarrhythmic drug in the conventional therapy group (80% at hospital discharge). However, 11% of patients were receiving Class IA drugs and 9% were receiving no specific antiarrhythmic therapy.

ICD therapy conferred a dramatic reduction in total mortality compared to conventional medical therapy. The 1-year survival was 84% in the ICD group versus 66% in the conventional therapy group. This differential was maintained throughout at least 3 years of follow-up and was associated with a hazard ratio of 0.46 (P = 0.009), indicating a powerful relative survival benefit for the ICD-treated patients.

There were numerous methodologic limitations of MADIT.[12] The number of patients screened for enrollment was not reported. No information regarding the numbers of eligible patients with no inducible VT or inducible VT suppressed by antiarrhythmic drug therapy was reported. These issues raised questions about referral and enrollment bias. An overall small percentage of patients were receiving beta blockers, and there were important differences between groups (16% and 29% in the conventional therapy versus ICD therapy groups, respectively). Heart failure therapy appears to have been underused, as described earlier. The use of Class IA drugs, although common in the era when the study was initiated, later was recognized to be hazardous in the study population. Finally, a substantial portion of patients in the conventional medical therapy group were not receiving any antiarrhythmic drug at hospital discharge (9%) or last follow-up (28%). This was particularly problematic because persistently inducible sustained monomorphic VT despite antiarrhythmic drug therapy predicts a very high risk of cardiac arrest or sudden death (up to 34% and 50% at 1 and 2 years, respectively) in this setting.[13]

Despite these limitations, MADIT was a landmark study that fully realized the concept of risk stratification.

■ ▪ ■

TABLE 17-2   RANDOMIZED TRIALS OF IMPLANTABLE CARDIOVERTER DEFIBRILLATORS FOR PRIMARY PREVENTION OF SUDDEN DEATH IN CORONARY ARTERY DISEASE

	MADIT	CABG-Patch	MUSTT	MADIT-II
Target population	Postmyocardial infarction	Postcoronary artery bypass grafting	Nonsustained VT	Postmyocardial infarction
Treatment	ICD versus best-available drug therapy	ICD versus control	ICD versus EPS-guided drug therapy or no therapy	ICD versus no ICD
Patients enrolled	196	900	704	1232
Arrhythmia qualifier	Spontaneous NSVT + inducible, nonsuppressible VT/VF	None (abnormal signal-averaged electrocardiogram)	Spontaneous NSVT + inducible VT/VF	None
LVEF (%) qualifier	≤35	<36	None	≤30
CHF qualifier	None	None	None	None
NYHA II–III (%)	~65	70–75	70–75	~60
NYHA IV (%)	Excluded	Excluded	Excluded	~5
Revascularization (%)	~75	100	56	~93
Mean LVEF (%)	26	27	30	23
ACE inhibitors (%)	~50	~50	~75	~70
Beta blockers (%)	~29% ICD vs. 16% drug group	24% ICD vs. 17% control	51% ICD vs. 29% non-ICD	~70 in all patients
Outcome	*Survival advantage in ICD group*	*No difference in survival*	*Survival advantage in ICD group*	*Survival advantage in ICD group*
Total mortality rate	16% ICD vs. 34% drug at 1 year (hazard ratio 0.46)	27% ICD vs. 24% control at 4 years	24% ICD vs. 48% no treatment vs. 55% drug treatment at 5 years	14% ICD vs. 20% non-ICD at 1 year (hazard ratio 0.69)
Sudden death rate	3% ICD vs. 13% non-ICD	Not reported*	9% ICD vs. 37% non-ICD at 5 years	Not reported*
Comments	Drug therapy: 80% amiodarone, 11% Class IA, 9% no antiarrhythmic drug at discharge	Amiodarone 4% in both groups; Class IA drugs 17% ICD vs. 12% control	Most patients randomized to drug therapy were taking Class IA agents	Drug therapy: 10% to 13% amiodarone in both groups, <3% Class IA

*Not reported indicates data have not been published.

MADIT, Multicenter Automatic Defibrillator Trial; CABG-Patch, Coronary Artery Bypass Graft Patch Trial; MUSTT, Multicenter Unsustained Tachycardia Trial; MADIT-II, Multicenter Automatic Defibrillator Trial II; VT, ventricular tachycardia; ICD, implantable cardioverter defibrillator; EPS, electrophysiology study; NSVT, nonsustained ventricular tachycardia; VF, ventricular fibrillation; LVEF, left-ventricular ejection fraction; CHF, congestive heart failure; NYHA, New York Heart Association Functional Class; ACE, angiotensin-converting enzyme.

Namely, that effective therapy (ICDs) based on the result (drug-unresponsive sustained VT) of a diagnostic test (programmed ventricular stimulation) directed at a specific pathophysiologic substrate (scar-related reentry resulting from prior myocardial infarction) identified by nonspecific clinical markers (coronary disease, reduced

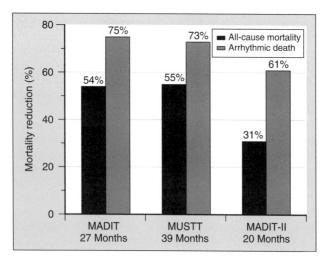

FIGURE 17-2. Mortality reduction associated with implantable cardioverter defibrillator (ICD) therapy for primary prevention of sudden cardiac death.

ventricular function, and nonsustained VT) could alter individual patient outcome.

Coronary Artery Bypass Graft-Patch

The Coronary Artery Bypass Graft (CABG)-Patch trial randomly compared prophylactic ICD therapy to no antiarrhythmic therapy among patients with chronic coronary artery disease, LVEF of less than 36%, and abnormal signal-averaged electrocardiogram (ECG).[14] Epicardial systems were implanted at the time of coronary bypass surgery among patients randomized to ICD therapy. The study began in 1990 and was terminated in 1997 when statistical analysis suggested that no significant difference in the primary outcome (total mortality) would ever be observed between randomized groups. The baseline clinical characteristics of the study population were remarkably similar to MADIT. By design, all patients had coronary artery disease and the mean LVEF was reduced severely (27%). Most patients had mild to moderately symptomatic heart failure (71% to 74% NYHA Class II or III, combined). Approximately half of the patients were taking ACE inhibitors and diuretics; nearly two thirds were taking digoxin. Like MADIT, a relatively small overall percentage of patients were taking beta blockers, but, in distinction, use was greater in the control group versus ICD group (24% vs. 17%).

Multicenter Automatic Defibrillator Trial and Coronary Artery Bypass Graft-Patch: Overview of Results

The divergent results of MADIT and CABG-Patch have been incompletely reconciled. The patient groups had similar baseline demographic characteristics recognized as predictive of a high mortality risk. Correspondingly, total mortality in CABG-Patch was substantial (although less than MADIT); the 4-year mortality was 24% in the control group and 27% in the ICD group. Patients were dying at significant rates in CABG-Patch. These deaths, the majority (>70%) of which were classified as cardiac, were not prevented by ICD therapy. One possible explanation is that the arrhythmia qualifiers were very different. VT induced by electrophysiologic testing (MADIT) is a more powerful predictor of arrhythmia recurrence than a positive signal-averaged ECG (CABG-Patch). Another possibility is that somehow a lower risk population was enrolled in CABG-Patch versus MADIT. A high proportion of patients with noninducible VT and low arrhythmic risk may have offset the benefit of ICD therapy in CABG-Patch. To address this issue, a subset of the CABG-Patch population underwent electrophysiologic testing after the main study results were reported.[15] There were no important demographic differences between the electrophysiology study subset and the remainder of the main study population. VT or VF was induced in 43% of patients. This result refutes the hypothesis that a lower risk population was enrolled in CABG-Patch. Rather, this suggests that the CABG-Patch study population had sufficient substrate for spontaneous VT, as in MADIT, but that surgical revascularization "unlinked" this arrhythmic substrate from arrhythmic outcome (sudden death).

Multicenter Unsustained Tachycardia Trial

The Multicenter Unsustained Tachycardia Trial (MUSTT)[16] was designed to test the hypothesis that antiarrhythmic therapy guided by electrophysiologic testing would reduce sudden death and cardiac arrest among patients with coronary artery disease, nonsustained VT, and reduced LV function. Patients with sustained monomorphic VT induced with any method of stimulation or sustained polymorphic VT or VF induced with one or two extrastimuli were randomized to antiarrhythmic drug therapy guided by electrophysiology testing or no antiarrhythmic therapy. Other cardiac medications were not controlled. Patients with inducible VT that was suppressed or rendered hemodynamically stable by drug therapy were discharged on that drug. Patients with persistently inducible VT could receive ICDs. Patients with no inducible VT were followed in a registry.

A total of 2202 patients were enrolled; of these, 767 patients (35%) had inducible VT and 704 were randomized. Baseline clinical characteristics in the two groups (electrophysiologically guided therapy and no antiarrhythmic therapy) were similar. The mean LVEF was 29% to 30%. Most patients had no mild heart failure symptoms (NYHA Class II or II, 74% to 76%). No patients with NYHA Class IV heart failure symptoms were enrolled. The majority of patients were taking ACE inhibitors (72% to 77%), whereas about half were taking diuretics (58%) and digoxin (52% to 53%). At the last follow-up, 66% of the patients in the electrophysiologically guided group had ICDs and 34% were taking antiarrhythmic drugs. Of the no antiarrhythmic therapy group, 3% had crossed over to ICD and 10% were taking antiarrhythmic drugs, for which atrial fibrillation was the indication in approximately 50%.

Sudden death and cardiac arrest from arrhythmia were lowest in the ICD group and equivalently highest in the no antiarrhythmic treatment and drug treatment groups. The 5-year sudden death and cardiac arrest rate in the ICD group was 9% versus 32% and 37% in the no antiarrhythmic and drug treatment groups, respectively. Virtually all of the reduction in sudden death and cardiac arrest rates in the electrophysiologically guided therapy group was because of the use of ICDs. Although there was a survival benefit in the ICD group attributable to this reduction in sudden death and cardiac arrest, total mortality remained substantial. The 5-year total mortality in the ICD group was 24% versus 48% and 55% in the no antiarrhythmic and drug treatment groups, respectively.

There are several obvious criticisms of this study. Most patients randomized to drug therapy were receiving Class IA agents, reflective of the era in which the study began (1989). It is unknown whether increased use Class III agents (amiodarone) would have modified outcome in the drug treatment group. Significantly fewer patients in the electrophysiologically guided therapy group were taking beta blockers (29% vs. 51%, P = 0.001), which may have influenced arrhythmia event rates.

Despite these limitations, this large, randomized study produced striking reinforcement of previous observations made on weaker scientific grounds. Patients with nonsustained VT, chronic coronary artery disease, reduced LV function, and inducible sustained VT are at very high risk for sudden death and cardiac arrest. This risk is not significantly modified by antiarrhythmic drug therapy guided by electrophysiologic testing. ICD therapy reduces sudden death and cardiac arrest and improves survival in these patients.

Multicenter Automatic Defibrillator Implantation Trial II

The Multicenter Automatic Defibrillator Implantation Trial (MADIT) II tested the hypothesis that prophylactic ICD therapy (in the absence of spontaneous or ventricular arrhythmia) in patients with prior myocardial infarction and LVEF of less than 30% would improve survival compared to conventional medical therapy.[17] A total of 1232 patients were randomized to prophylactic ICD therapy or no ICD therapy over 4 years. The study was terminated early when an interim analysis revealed a significant mortality difference between treatment arms favoring ICD therapy. During an average follow-up of 20 months, the mortality rates were 19.8% in the conventional therapy group versus 14.2% in the ICD group. The hazard ratio for the risk of death from any cause in the ICD group as compared to the conventional therapy group was 0.69 (95% confidence interval, 0.51–0.93, P = 0.016), corresponding to a 31% reduction in total mortality. The majority of patients had symptomatic heart failure and were taking ACE inhibitors (68%), beta blockers (70%), and statins (67%).

Trials of ICDs for Prevention of Sudden Cardiac Death in Nonischemic Dilated Cardiomyopathy

The benefit of ICD therapy for primary and secondary prevention of sudden cardiac death among appropriately selected patients with ischemic cardiomyopathy is now well established (Table 17-3). Much less is known about the mortality benefit, if any, among patients with nonischemic dilated cardiomyopathy. Such patients were included in trials of secondary prevention such as AVID and CIDS but comprised less than 20% of the enrollment population. A subgroup analysis of nonischemic dilated cardiomyopathy in AVID showed a survival benefit despite low mortality rates in the ICD arm (11% after 2 years). The reduction in mortality was to the result of the higher mortality rates in the control arm (18% after 2 years).[18]

Sudden Cardiac Death in Heart Failure Trial

One ongoing trial of ICDs for primary prevention of sudden death in patients with and without coronary artery disease is the Sudden Cardiac Death in Heart Failure Trial (SCD-HeFT). This trial has completed enrollment of 2500 patients with mild to moderately symptomatic heart failure (NYHA Class II or III) and LVEF of less than 36%. Patients are randomized to prophylactic ICD therapy, amiodarone therapy, or placebo. This is the first and only primary prevention study that specifically targets patients with symptomatic heart failure. Similar to MADIT II, there is no arrhythmia qualifier and prior history of sustained VT or VF is an exclusion criterion. The primary endpoint is total mortality. Secondary endpoints include arrhythmic and nonarrhythmic mortality, incidence of spontaneous ventricular arrhythmias, quality-of-life, and cost-effectiveness. Approximately 40% to 50% of enrolled patients have nonischemic dilated cardiomyopathy, and the study is in the follow-up phase.

Amiodarone Cardioverter Trial and German Cardiomyopathy Trial

Two small, prospective, randomized clinical trials have failed to show a mortality benefit from prophylactic ICD therapy in nonischemic dilated cardiomyopathy. The Amiodarone Cardioverter Trial (AMIOVIRT) randomized 103 patients with nonischemic dilated cardiomyopathy, asymptomatic nonsustained VT, LVEF of less than 35%, and mild to moderately symptomatic heart failure to ICD or amiodarone.[19] There were no differences in baseline clinical characteristics between the treatment arms. Over a mean follow-up of 21 months, there was no significant mortality difference between the groups. The trial was stopped prematurely when it became evident that there was no possibility of survival advantage in either treatment group. The German Cardiomyopathy Trial (CAT) randomized 104 patients with nonischemic dilated cardiomyopathy of less than 9 months duration, LVEF of less than 30%, and mild to moderately symptomatic heart failure to ICD or no ICD therapy.[20] There

■ ■ ■

TABLE 17-3   RANDOMIZED TRIALS OF IMPLANTABLE CARDIOVERTER DEFIBRILLATORS FOR PRIMARY PREVENTION OF SUDDEN DEATH IN NONISCHEMIC DILATED CARDIOMYOPATHY

	SCD-HeFT*	AMIOVIRT	CAT
Target population	Symptomatic congestive heart failure	NDCMP	Recent-onset NDCMP (<9 months)
Treatment	ICD versus amiodarone/placebo	ICD versus amiodarone	ICD versus control
Patients enrolled	2500	103	104
Arrhythmia qualifier	None	NSVT	None
LVEF (%) qualifier	≤36	<35	<30
CHF qualifier	NYHA II-III	NYHA I-III	NYHA II or III
Revascularization (%)	Not reported	0	0
Mean LVEF (%)	Not reported†	22	24
ACE inhibitors (%)	Not reported†	Not reported†	~95
Beta-blockers (%)	Not reported†	Not reported†	24% ICD vs. 17% control
Outcome	*Enrollment complete; ongoing*	*No difference in survival*	*No difference in survival*
Total mortality rate	Not reported†	8% at 1 years in both groups	8% ICD vs. 4% control at 1 year
Sudden death rate	Not reported†	Not reported	0% sudden deaths in either group
Comments	Approximately 50% NDCMP	Study terminated due to low event rate in either group	Study terminated due to low event rate in either group

*SCD-HeFT also enrolled patients with coronary artery disease.
†Not reported-indicates data have not been published.
SCD-HeFT, Sudden Cardiac Death in Heart Failure Trial; AMIOVIRT, Amiodarone Cardioverter Trial; CAT, German Cardiomyopathy Trial; NDCMP, nonischemic dilated cardiomyopathy; ICD, implantable cardioverter defibrillator; NSVT, nonsustained ventricular tachycardia; LVEF, left-ventricular ejection fraction; CHF, congestive heart failure; NYHA, New York Heart Association functional class; ACE, angiotensin-converting enzyme.

were no differences in baseline clinical characteristics between the treatment arms. More than 90% of patients were taking ACE inhibitors and diuretics; less than 5% were taking beta blockers. The overall 1-year mortality rate for all patients was only 5.6% and markedly below the assumed value of 30%. There was no difference in survival between ICD and no ICD groups, and the trial was stopped because of futility after 1 year. An important qualification to the interpretation of these neutral results is that requiring recent-onset nonischemic dilated cardiomyopathy might have biased enrollment in favor of patients who experienced spontaneous improvement in LV function over the course of the study. Prior studies of patients with nonischemic dilated cardiomyopathy and moderately symptomatic heart failure have reported 1-year mortality rates in the range of 15% to 50%, of which half are presumed to be the result of VT or VF. Data supporting or refuting this possibility were not provided in the primary publication.

Implantable Cardioverter Defibrillators for Primary and Secondary Prevention of Sudden Death Associated with Reduced Left-Ventricular Systolic Function: Summary of Evidence from Clinical Trials

The results of large-scale randomized treatment trials in patients with reduced LV function and VF or hemodynamically unstable sustained uniform VT that occurs spontaneously or can be induced consistently demonstrate a survival advantage associated with ICD therapy compared to antiarrhythmic drugs. Accordingly, ICD therapy can be recommended as first-line treatment for the prevention of sudden cardiac death in this setting. However, despite the stunning outcome of MADIT II, most authorities are not recommending prophylactic ICD therapy for all patients with coronary artery disease and reduced LVEF in the absence of any ambient or provocable ventricular arrhythmia pending further clinical trial data.

Implantable Cardioverter Defibrillator Therapy: The Sickest Patients Benefit The Most

Although the results of these diverse clinical trials encourage enthusiastic generalization to all patients regarding the relative mortality benefit of device versus drug therapy, the optimal application of ICD therapy is unsettled. The ICD is highly effective at terminating potentially life-threatening ventricular tachyarrhythmias and reducing sudden death rates, in most studies to 1% and 5% at 1 and 3 years, respectively. This effect is consistent across diverse patient populations. However, despite the near elimination of sudden cardiac death resulting from ventricular tachyarrhythmias, the total mortality benefit conferred by ICD therapy varies across populations in a predictable manner and may not be proportionate to the reduction in sudden death. Total mortality may not proportionately reflect a reduction in

sudden death from the powerful influence of other clinical factors that constrain survival in the majority of patients with ventricular tachyarrhythmias.

It is interesting that the sickest patients appear to derive the greatest mortality benefit from ICD therapy. Post-hoc analysis of three secondary prevention trials consistently demonstrates that the mortality benefit of ICD therapy is almost entirely confined to patients with the most severely depressed LV systolic function and more advanced symptomatic heart failure. Among patients in the AVID trial with LVEF of 35% or more, average 2-year survival was 83% and was not significantly different between device and drug treatment.[21] However, there was a significant survival advantage among AVID patients with reduced ejection fraction (20% to 34%) treated with ICDs (82% vs. 72% at 2 years). This difference persisted among patients with LVEF of less than 20%, although it did not reach statistical significance, probably because of the extremely small size of this group.[21] Concordant results were reported in subanalyses of CIDS and MADIT primary data. The study population of CIDS was retrospectively divided into four quartiles of risk based on multivariate predictors of mortality in the amiodarone group (advanced age, reduced ejection fraction, and poor NYHA functional class). ICD therapy was associated with a 50% relative risk reduction of death compared to amiodarone in the highest risk quartile but conferred no benefit in the three lower risk quartiles.[22] The CIDS data show that the subgroup of patients that receive virtually all the benefit of ICD therapy have two or more of the following characteristics: age older than 70 years, LVEF of less than 35%, or NYHA III or IV. ICDs had a very small effect on survival compared to amiodarone in the remainder of the study population. Similarly, the MADIT population was partitioned into high- and low-risk subsets for three risk factors: LVEF, QRSd duration, and symptomatic heart failure requiring therapy. ICD therapy was associated with a significant reduction in mortality in high-risk subsets with ejection fraction of less than 26%, QRS duration of more than 120 ms, and history of symptomatic heart failure. ICD therapy was associated with a progressive reduction in the risk of death at each increased level of mortality risk. Patients with all three risk factors had the highest mortality risk and achieved the largest mortality reduction from ICD therapy. The magnitude of risk reduction in this subgroup was 80%.[23]

These studies consistently demonstrate that the sickest patients benefit the most from ICD therapy relative to medical therapy. However, a lower bound for this beneficial effect likely exists. Patients with severely reduced LV function and highly symptomatic heart failure in whom, for example, cardiac transplantation is being considered are considerably more problematic. The majority of these patients are at equivalently high risk for recurrent life-threatening ventricular tachyarrhythmias and nonarrhythmic cardiac death resulting from progressive heart failure. Mortality generally increases with increasing NYHA functional class; however, the proportion of sudden deaths may decline, presumably because progressive pump failure dominates the clinical picture.[24,25] The proportion of total deaths that are sudden may vary between 50% and 80% among patients with Class II symptoms and 5% and 30% among patients with Class IV symptoms. Such patients either have been systematically excluded from clinical trials of sudden death prevention or enrolled in very small numbers.

Can the results of ICD trials for primary and secondary prevention of sudden cardiac death be extrapolated to the heart failure population? It is crucial to recognize that none of these trials specified heart failure as a requisite for entry, although the majority of patients had mild to moderate heart failure symptoms (NYHA Class II or III) associated with reduced LV function. Furthermore, substantial portions of patients were not receiving optimal medical therapy for LV dysfunction. It is unlikely that a clinical trial of conventional ICD therapy will be done in patients with severe LV dysfunction and advanced symptomatic heart failure; however, such patients are the target of clinical trials with cardiac resynchronization therapy (CRT) combined with defibrillation (CRTD).

Implantable Cardioverter Defibrillators for Prevention of Sudden Death and Treatment of Heart Failure Associated with Reduced Left-Ventricular Systolic Function

CRT is an effective adjunctive treatment for moderate to severely symptomatic heart failure associated with depressed LV function and ventricular dyssynchrony.[26-28] The incidence of ventricular dyssynchrony (usually left bundle branch block or other interventricular conduction delay) as designated by prolonged QRS duration of more than 120 ms among patients with chronic congestive heart failure and reduced systolic function is in the range of 35% to 50%. The aggregate experience with CRT among clinical trials involving more than 2000 patients demonstrates a consistent clinical benefit. The magnitude of the benefits is modest and concordant. These include about a one-step improvement in NYHA class, a 10-point improvement in quality-of-life measures, a 1 to 2 ml/kg/min improvement in peak VO_2, a 50 to 70-meter improvement in 6-minute hall walk, and a trend toward reduced heart failure hospitalizations. Despite impressive technical hurdles, CRT has been hybridized successfully with conventional ICD therapy delivery systems and implanted successfully in humans.

Trials of Cardiac Resynchronization Therapy/Defibrillation for Prevention of Sudden Death and Treatment of Heart Failure (Table 17-4)

CONTAK CD and MIRACLE ICD

Two studies of CRTD involving 945 patients have been reported. The study populations were similar to trials of CRT (without defibrillation capability) except there was conventional indication for ICD therapy. CONTAK CD showed a significant improvement in NYHA Class, 6-minute hall walk, peak VO_2, and standardized quality of life. Post-hoc analysis showed that the greatest benefit was observed in the patients with the most advanced heart failure. However, the primary goal of a 25% reduction in heart failure, as measured by a composite outcome of death, heart failure hospitalization, worsening heart failure requiring other interventions, and ventricular arrhythmias, was not met. Patients receiving CRTD had a 21% reduction in this composite endpoint (P = 0.17). However, the study probably was underpowered to detect significant differences in this composite endpoint, particularly because 80% of the patients were NYHA I or II after 6 months of CRTD. MIRACLE ICD showed a reduction in NYHA class and

■ ▪ ■

TABLE 17-4   RANDOMIZED TRIALS OF CARDIAC RESYNCHRONIZATION THERAPY WITH DEFIBRILLATION FOR PRIMARY AND SECONDARY PREVENTION OF SUDDEN DEATH AND TREATMENT OF CONGESTIVE HEART FAILURE

	MIRACLE ICD	CONTAK CD
Target population	CHF + QRSd prolongation + ICD	CHF + QRSd prolongation + ICD
Treatment	ICD vs. CRTD	ICD vs. CRTD
Patients enrolled	364	581
Arrhythmia qualifier	ICD indication	ICD indication
LVEF (%) qualifier	≤35	<35
CHF qualifier (NYHA Class)	II–IV	II–IV
QRS duration qualifier (ms)	>120	>130
Improvement in NYHA Class	65% decreased 1 class vs. 50% control	23% decreased 1 class, 11.6% decreased 2 classes vs. control
Improvement in 6 min. hall walk (m)	No difference	35 overall; 47 Class IV
Improvement in QOL	7.2 ± 2.0	6
Improvement in VO_2 (ml/kg/min)	1.1	0.9 overall; 1.8 Class IV
Total mortality rate	Not reported	Not reported
Sudden death rate	Not reported	Not reported
Comments	Single blind	Double blind

*Not reported indicates data have not been published.

CHF, congestive heart failure; ICD, implantable cardioverter defibrillator; CRTD, cardiac resynchronization therapy with defibrillation; LVEF, left-ventricular ejection fraction; NYHA, New York Heart Association; QOL, Minnesota Living with Heart Failure Quality of Life; VO_2, oxygen uptake determination.

improvement in quality of life but not 6-minute hall walk. It is important to note that there are no data on the effect of CRTD on mortality and limited data on whether the clinical benefits of CRT or CRTD are sustainable for more than 12 months.

REFERENCES

1. Gillium RF: Sudden coronary death in the United States. Circulation 1989; 79:756-765.
2. Kannel WB, Plehn JF, Cupples A: Cardiac failure and sudden death in the Framingham study. Am Heart J 1988; 115:869-875.
3. Schocken DD, Arrieta MI, Leaverton PE, et al: Prevalence and mortality of congestive heart failure in the United States. J Am Coll Cardiol 1992; 20:301-306.
4. Ho KKL, Anderson KM, Kannel WB, et al: Survival after the onset of congestive heart failure in the Framingham Heart Study subjects. Circulation 1993; 88:107-115.
5. Massie BM, Shah NB: Evolving trends in the epidemiologic factors of heart failure. Am Heart J 1997; 133:703-712.
6. The Antiarrhythmics versus Implantable Defibrillator (AVID) Investigators: A comparison of antiarrhythmic-drug therapy with implantable defibrillators in patients resuscitated from near-fatal ventricular arrhythmias. N Engl J Med 1997; 337:1576-1583.
7. The AVID Investigators: Causes of death in the antiarrhythmics versus implantable defibrillators (AVID) trial. J Am Coll Cardiol 1999; 34:1552-1559.
8. Kuck KH, Cappato R, Siebels J, et al: Randomized comparison of antiarrhythmia drug therapy with implantable defibrillators in patients resuscitated from cardiac arrest: The Cardiac Arrest Study Hamburg (CASH). Circulation 2000; 102:748-754.
9. Connolly SJ, Gent M, Roberts RS, et al: Canadian implantable defibrillator study (CIDS): A randomized trial of the implantable cardioverter defibrillator against amiodarone. Circulation 2000; 101: 1297-1302.
10. Moss AJ: Sudden cardiac death and national health. Pacing Clin Electrophysiol 1993; 16:2190-2191.
11. Moss AJ, Hall WJ, Cannom DS, et al: Improved survival with an implanted defibrillator in patients with coronary disease at high risk for ventricular arrhythmia. N Engl J Med 1996; 335: 1993-1940.
12. Friedman PL, Stevenson WG: Unsustained ventricular tachycardia—to treat or not to treat. N Engl J Med 1996; 335:1984-1985.
13. Wilber DJ, Olshansky B, Moran JF, et al: Electrophysiological testing and nonsustained ventricular tachycardia: Use and limitations among patients with coronary artery disease and impaired ventricular function. Circulation 1990; 82:350-358.
14. Bigger JT: Prophylactic use of implanted cardiac defibrillators in patients at high risk for ventricular arrhythmias after coronary artery bypass graft surgery. N Engl J Med 1997; 337:1569-1575.
15. Bigger JT, Rottman JN, Whang W, et al: CABG surgery unlinked the arrhythmic substrate from arrhythmia outcomes in the CABG-Patch Trial. Circulation 199; 100 (Suppl I):I-367. Abstract.
16. Buxton AE, Lee KL, Fisher JD, et al: A randomized study of the prevention of sudden death among patients with coronary artery disease. N Engl J Med 1999; 341:1882-1890.
17. Moss AJ, Zareba W, Hall WJ, et al: Prophylactic implantation of a defibrillator in patients with myocardial infarction and reduced ejection fraction. N Engl J Med 2002; 346(12):877-883.
18. Ehlert FA, Cannom DS, Renfroe EG, et al: Comparison of dilated cardiomyopathy and coronary artery disease in patients with life-threatening ventricular arrhythmias: Differences in presentation and outcome in the (AVID) registry. Am Heart J 2001; 142(5): 816-822.
19. Strickberger AS: Amiodarone vs. implantable defibrillator in patients with nonischemic cardiomyopathy and asymptomatic nonsustained ventricular tachycardia. Circulation 2000; 102:2794. Abstract.
20. Bansch D, Antz M, Boczor S, et al: Primary prevention of sudden cardiac death in idiopathic dilated cardiomyopathy: The Cardiomyopathy Trial (CAT). Circulation 2002; 105:1453-1458.
21. Domanski MJ, Sakseena S, Epstein AE, et al: Relative effectiveness of the implantable cardioverter-defibrillator and antiarrhythmia drugs among patients with varying degrees of left ventricular dysfunction who have survived malignant ventricular arrhythmias. J Am Coll Cardiol 199; 34:1090-1095.
22. Sheldon R, Connolly S, Krahn A, et al: Indentification of patients most likely to benefit from implantable cardioverter-defibrillator therapy: The Canadian Implantable Defibrillators Study. Circulation 2000; 101:1660-1664.
23. Moss AJ, Fadl Y, Zareba W, et al: Survival benefit with an implanted defibrillator in relation to mortality risk in chronic coronary artery disease. Am J Cardiol 2001; 88:516-520.
24. Uretsky B, Sheahan G: Primary prevention of sudden cardiac death in heart failure: Will the result be shocking? J Am Coll Cardiol 1997; 30:1589-1597.
25. MERIT-HF Study Group: Effect of metoprolol CR/XL in chronic heart failure: Metoprolol CR/XL randomized intervention trial in congestive heart failure (MERIT-HF). Lancet 1999; 353:2001-2007.
26. Abraham WT, Fisher WG, Smith AL, et al: Cardiac resynchronization in chronic heart failure. N Engl J Med 2002; 346(24): 1845-1853.
27. Cazeau S, Leclerq C, Lavergne T, et al: Effects of multisite biventricular pacing in patients with heart failure and intraventricular conduction delay. N Engl J Med 2001; 344:873-880.
28. Auricchio A, Stellbrink C, Sack S, et al: Long-term benefit as a result of pacing resynchronization in congestive heart failure: Results of the PATH-CHF Trial. Circulation 2000; 102:II-693A.

Pacing

Elizabeth McNeill
Charles R. Kerr
Stanley Tung
John A. Yeung-Lai-Wah

The indications for permanent pacing in conduction disease such as acquired atrioventricular (AV) block, chronic bifascicular block and trifascicular block, and symptomatic sinus node dysfunction are well established.[1] However, the accumulation of new clinical evidence from randomized trials and the development of clinical consensus has lead to recent changes in the recommendations for pacing in more specific conditions.[2]

This chapter will review three areas of clinical interest, namely the treatment of patients with congestive heart failure (CHF), atrial tachyarrhythmias (AT), and neurocardiogenic syncope, in which new or revised roles for pacing have been advocated primarily on the basis of trial data. The important issue of the effect of pacing on morbidity and mortality will also be addressed by a discussion of the current trial data investigating the effects of pacing mode on survival.

BIVENTRICULAR PACING FOR HEMODYNAMIC IMPROVEMENT IN CONGESTIVE HEART FAILURE

Pacing, for hemodynamic purposes, was initially introduced as a class IIb indication in specific patients with dilated cardiomyopathy (DCM). A limited role for simple dual chamber (DDD) pacing was proposed[3,4]; however, benefit was restricted to patients with adequate AV optimization.[5-7] Biventricular (BiV) pacing has now been proposed as a class IIa indication for patients in medically refractory, symptomatic New York Heart Association (NYHA) class III–IV heart failure with idiopathic or ischemic dilated cardiomyopathy, prolonged QRS interval (≥130 msec), left-ventricular (LV) end-diastolic diameter ≥55 mm, and ejection fraction ≤35%.

Since the initial success of atrial-synchronized BiV or cardiac resynchronization therapy (CRT) in 1994,[8] a number of early acute or short-term studies have shown that BiV or LV pacing alone improves symptoms and indices of systolic function in patients with severe DCM (either ischemic or idiopathic) and a major left-sided intraventricular conduction disorder such as left bundle branch block.[8-16] In these patients, marked delay in intraventricular activation leads to severe intraventricular dyssynchrony.[17-19] CRT corrects this by epicardially pacing an area of late activation in the left ventricle via a lead advanced through the coronary sinus[20,21] while simultaneously stimulating the right-ventricular (RV) apex. Because the left ventricle is able to complete contraction and begin relaxation earlier, diastolic filling time is increased. A reduction in LV cavity size may result in reverse LV modeling and correlate with improved LV function.[22,23] Improvement in septal motion, transmitral blood flow, and preloading of the left ventricle occurs. Doppler studies have also shown that CRT restores normal mitral valve timing and reduces or eliminates mitral regurgitation.[7,24-26] Acutely this effect may be related to an increase in transmitral pressure gradient, independent from geometric changes in the left ventricle.[22,27,28]

Short-Term Studies

Short-term studies have shown acute improvements in invasive hemodynamic parameters of LV function. These improvements include increased arterial pulse pressure and LV dP/dT and decreased arteriovenous oxygen saturation[29-32] without an increase in metabolic demand,[33,34] which correlate with improved cardiac index, systolic function, isovolumetric contraction, and pulmonary wedge pressure.[9,13,35] Both ventricular stimulation site and the atrioventricular delay (AV delay optimization), which modulates the preload, appear to contribute to the improvement.[29,36,37] RV pacing is inferior to, and in some cases detrimental when compared with, BiV or LV pacing.[37,38] Of interest, nonrandomized acute studies also showed that LV pacing was comparable[39] and potentially superior to BiV pacing.[11,15,38]

Long-Term Studies

Long-term benefits of BiV pacing (improvement in heart failure symptoms, exercise capacity, quality of life, and systolic function) generally parallel the acute hemodynamic effects. CRT also has significant neurohormonal effects,[40-43] including an improvement in heart rate variability indices.[44,45] The clinical trials in which the impact of CRT has been assessed in patients with heart failure are summarized in Table 18-1. Most of the trials to date have shown improvements in the end-points. Two trials are worthy of special attention, namely the MUSTIC (MUltisite STimulation in Cardiomyopathy) studies, which were the first properly randomized trials of CRT, and the MIRACLE (Multicentre InSync Randomized Clinical Evaluation) trial, which was the first moderately sized parallel group study with medium-term follow-up.

The MUSTIC studies[45-51] (see Table 18-1) were the first randomized studies comparing BiV pacing with no pacing in patients with NYHA class III heart failure and intraventricular conduction delay. A CRT device was used in which the LV lead was placed in a branch of the coronary sinus. The implantation success rate was 92% (attempted in 64 patients), and the LV lead was functional in 88% of patients at the end of the crossover phase.

Patients underwent a 6-month single-blind randomized crossover phase during which atrio-BiV (active) pacing was compared with ventricular-inhibited pacing (inactive group) at a base rate of 40 bpm, each for a 3-month period. Of patients, 85% preferred BiV pacing. Statistically significant improvements were achieved in the quality-of-life score (P < 0.001), peak VO$_2$ (P < 0.02), exercise time (P < 0.001), and oxygen pulse (P < 0.01). There were also improvements in submaximal measures of exercise capacity including the 6-minute walk distance (6MWD) (P = 0.001); anaerobic threshold (AT) (P = 0.02) minute ventilation (VE)/ventilated carbon dioxide (VCO$_2$) (P = 0.03); and normalization of the VE/VCO$_2$ slope (P = 0.002), which is a measure of ventilatory drive.[50] During the first randomization period, there were significantly fewer hospitalizations for heart failure (P < 0.05).

A second study group had persistent atrial fibrillation (AF) (>3 months) with a slow ventricular rate or had undergone previous AV node ablation. Patients were implanted with a BiV-VVIR pacemaker generator, which was programmed to RV mode for a 10-week stabilization period. They then underwent a randomized crossover comparison of 3 months each of BiV and RV-VVIR pacing. In this group, 86.5% preferred BiV-VVIR pacing. Significant improvements were seen in measures of peak exercise (oxygen consumption and duration of exercise) and submaximal exercise (anaerobic threshold and ventilatory efficiency).[48]

A 12-month intrapatient long-term comparison of patients programmed at the end of the crossover phase recently revealed a significant sustained benefit from BiV pacing in exercise tolerance and quality of life, with reductions in mitral regurgitation (MR) and improved ejection fraction in both groups, although the magnitude of improvements was less in the AF group.[49] LV dimensions were also significantly reduced in the sinus rhythm (SR) group, especially in patients with idiopathic DCM. The increase in peak VO$_2$ at 12 months correlated with the decrease in end-systolic dimensons.[51]

A significant decrease in QRS width in the SR group (8% to 14%) and the AF group (14% to 24%) occurred during BiV pacing, although there was no incremental reduction in the paced QRS duration over time. Equally, the duration of spontaneous QRS remained unchanged over time.

A substudy of 22 patients revealed a significant improvement in the heart rate variability, which correlated with the baseline intrinsic QRS duration but was not related to clinical efficacy assessed by the 6MW distance.[45]

The MIRACLE trial[52-55] (see Table 18-1) was the first moderately large trial to assess whether CRT produces clinical benefit in patients with CHF and an intraventricular conduction delay. Successfully implanted patients (92%) were randomly assigned to CRT (n = 228) or to a control group (no pacing, n = 225) for 6 months.

The CRT group showed statistically significant improvements in NYHA class, 6MWD, and quality-of-life score (P < 0.001, P = 0.005, P = 0.001, respectively). This improvement commenced 1 month after treatment and persisted for more than 6 months. Patients (n = 67) who received 12 months of CRT maintained improvement in all these parameters (P < 0.001).[56] At 6 months follow-up there was also a reduction in LV end-diastolic and end-systolic volumes, in the area of mitral regurgitation and in QRS duration (median change only 20 msec) and an increase in left-ventricular ejection fraction (LVEF) and myocardial performance index (all P < 0.001 compared with the unpaced control group). The LV mass was reduced (P < 0.01), and there were significant improvements in maximal exercise performance measured by the peak VO$_2$ and total exercise time (P = 0.009 and P = 0.001, respectively).[54,55]

In summary, these studies appear to support a beneficial effect from CRT on the functional status and quality of life of selected patients with severe heart failure and intraventricular conduction delay. Notably the degree of QRS reduction does not necessarily parallel the clinical response to CRT. The major limitation is that the CRT groups were predominantly compared with nonpaced patients, thus discounting the potential benefit of merely increasing the heart rate from pacing. Moreover the duration of follow-up was also relatively short, and data on long-term improvement in survival and functional status are still lacking. The benefit to patients in AF is also unresolved.[57,58]

Biventricular Internal Cardioverter Defibrillator Pacing Versus Univentricular Internal Cardioverter Defibrillator Pacing

Specific trials evaluating the efficacy of combining an internal cardioverter defibrillator (ICD) with CRT are listed in Table 18-2. The question of whether ICD therapies are reduced by this treatment modality is debatable.[61,72,73] Therefore, the impact of combined therapy on arrhythmic profile and mortality needs further analysis.[74,75]

TABLE 18-1 TRIALS ASSESSING CARDIAC RESYNCHRONIZATION THERAPY IN PATIENTS WITH HEART FAILURE*

Study and design	N (mean age)	CRT vs.	Follow-up months	BASELINE NYHA class	LVEF, %	LVEDD, mm	QRS, msec	Primary endpoints	Outcome	References
Insync observational longitudinal	103 (67)	Control	12	III-IV	<35 (22)	>60 (72)	>150 (178)	NYHA class, QOLS, 6MWD	Improvement in all primary endpoints LVEF improved and QRS duration reduced	59,60
Brompton and Harefield crossover single blind, 3 months per arm	12 SR 8 AF (60)	No pacing (SR) or VVIR—60bpm (AF)	3	III-IV	NA	(62)	(163 in SR) (183 in AF)	Mean heart rate, ventricular ectopy; sustained VT (>30 sec)	No change in mean heart rate, reduction in ventricular ectopy; reduction in salvo counts in SR group	61
Bordeaux series	47 (68)	Control	8	II-IV	NA (20)	NA	≥140 (197)	NA	Improvement in NYHA class, reduction in MR	62
MUSTIC Group 1-SR Crossover double blind, 3 month per arm	67 (63)	Control	6-12	III	<35 (22)	>60 (73)	>150 (176)	6MWD (<450 m at inclusion)	Improvement in 6MWD; see text	45,46,49-51
MUSTIC Group II-AF Crossover double blind, 3 months per arm	64 (65)	VVIR pacing	6-12	III	<35 (26)	>60 (68)	>200 with RV pacing (206)	6MWD	See text	47,48
MIRACLE parallel arm double blind	453 (64)	Control	6	III-IV	≤35 (21)	≥55 (69)	≥130 (165)	NYHA class, QOLS, 6MWD (≤450 m at inclusion)	Improvement in all primary (and secondary) endpoints	52-56
VIGOR-CHF crossover, double blind active washout, 6 weeks per arm	73	Control	–	II-IV	≤30	NA	>120, PR >160	Peak VO$_2$ AT	Trial abandoned in favor of transvenous approach	63,22
PATH-CHFII crossover double blind, 3 months per arm	89 (61)	Control	6	II-IV	≤30	NA	≥120 (158)	Peak VO$_2$, peak VO$_2$ AT (VO$_2$max ≤ 18 ml/kg/min at inclusion) 6MWD	Improvement in all endpoints for patients with QRS >150 msec; nonsignificant benefit for patients with QRS 120-150 msec	64
VecTor crossover double blind, 6 months per arm	EN	Control	6	II-IV	≤35	≥54	≥140	QOLS, 6MWD	Not reported	

*Mean values when available recorded in parentheses.
NYHA., New York Heart Association; LVEF, left-ventricular ejection fraction; LVEDD, left-ventricular end diastolic dimension; NA, not applicable; VT, ventricular tachycardia; SR, sinus rhythm; MR, mitral regurgitation; VO$_2$, oxygen uptake; AT, anaerobic threshold; QOLS, quality of life score (Minnesota); 6MWD, six minute walk distance; EN, enrolling.

■■ ■

TABLE 18-2   TRIALS COMBINING ICD THERAPY WITH CARDIAC RESYNCHRONIZATION THERAPY*

| Study and design | N (mean age) | ICD-CRT vs. | Follow-up months | BASELINE | | | | Primary endpoints | Outcome | References |
				NYHA class	LVEF, %	LVEDD, mm	QRS, msec			
VENTAK-CHF cross-over double blind, active washout, 6 weeks per arm	215	Control	NA	II–IV	≤35	NA	>120	Peak VO₂ AT	Converted to CONTAK-CD	63
CONTACT-CD parallel arm double blind, 3 months	581 (66)	Control	6	II–IV	≤35 (21)	NA	>120 (158)	Combined morbidity and mortality	Primary endpoint not met. Improved QOL in NYHA class III–IV patients with no RBBB	65
INSYNC/ MIRACLE-ICD double blind	362	Control	6	II–IV	≤35	≤55	≥130	QOLS, NYHA class, 6MWD	Improved QOLS, NYHA class. (Class II NYHA patients n = 215, not yet analyzed)	66,67
INSYNC III prospective nonran-domized	189	–	6	III–IV	≤35	≥55	≥130	NYHA class, 6MWD safety and efficacy of device, V-V delays	Device safety confirmed. Significant improvement in endpoints	68
BELIEVE Pilot double blind	74	LV pacing	12	II–IV	≤35	≥55	≥130	Echo indices-including LVEF, LV and LA dimen-sions and Doppler parameters	Not reported	
CART-HF double blind	EN	Control	6	II–IV	≤35	NA	>120	LVESV from MUGA	Not reported	

*Mean values when available recorded in parentheses.
NYHA, New York Heart Association; LVEF, left-ventricular ejection fraction; LVEDD, left-ventricular end diastolic dimension; NA, not applicable; VO₂, oxygen uptake; AT, anaerobic threshold; QOLS, quality of life score (Minnesota); 6MWD, six-minute walk distance; RBBB, right bundle branch block; echo, echocardiography; LV, left ventricle; LA, left atrium; LVESV, Left-ventricular End Systolic Volume; MUGA, multiple gated acquisition scan; EN, enrolling.

Biventricular Versus Univentricular Pacing

The completed and ongoing studies assessing the relative merits of single-site LV pacing or RV pacing versus BiV pacing are summarized in Table 18-3.

Mortality

Data on the long-term survival of patients with end-stage heart failure following BiV pacing are scarce. An improvement in survival with CRT has been suggested from observational studies[76] and meta-analysis of randomized controlled studies.[77] The InSync Study, the Insync Italian registry,[78,79] the MUSTIC,[80] and the Pacing Therapies for Congestive Heart Failure II (PATH CHF II) studies[64] reported improved survival rates; however, the latter two studies were underpowered to detect a statistically significant difference in mortality.

This encouraging effect has fueled three ongoing prospective studies to evaluate the impact of CRT on survival in patients with NYHA class II–IV heart failure, reduced ejection fraction, and wide QRS complex.

The COMPANION (Comparison of Medical Therapy, Pacing and Defibrillation in Heart Failure) trial had a combined primary endpoint of 1-year all-cause mortality and hospitalization (including administration of an intravenous agent for heart failure exacerbation). The secondary endpoints were cardiac morbidity, exercise performance, and total survival.

Patients with DCM (LV end-diastolic dimension [EDD] >60 mm, NYHA class III–IV functional class, LVEF <35%, QRS duration >120 msec, PR >150 msec) and no preexisting indication for an ICD or pacemaker were enrolled into this open-label, three-arm trial comparing optimal medical therapy alone (OPT), optimal medical therapy with CRT (OPT-CRT), and optimal medical therapy with CRT and an ICD (OPT-CRT-D). The trial was terminated prematurely, following the enrollment of 1520 patients, because of the superior efficacy of the primary endpoint in both CRT arms of the study.

■ ■ ■

TABLE 18-3   TRIALS COMPARING SINGLE LV OR RV PACING TO BIVENTRICULAR PACING*

Study and design	N (mean age)	CRT vs.	Follow-up months	BASELINE NYHA class	LVEF, %	LVEDD, mm	QRS, msec	Primary endpoints	Outcome	References
PATH-CHFI crossover, single blind, 4 weeks	42 (60)	'Best' Uni-V pacing	6	III-IV	<35 (23)	NA	>120 (175)	Peak VO$_2$ VO$_2$AT 6MWD	Improved functional capacity and QOL with CRT and Uni-V pacing	29–31, 69–71
BELIEVE (see Table18-2)										
RD-CHF crossover, single blind	EN	RV pacing	6	III-IV	NA	NA	NA	SVT and ventricular arrhythmia NYHA class, QOLS	Not reported	
PAVE† single blind	EN	RV pacing	6	I-III	NA	NA	NA	6MWD; <450 m at inclusion	Not reported	

*Mean values when available recorded in parentheses.
†Only the PAVE trial does not specifically require patients who have chronic heart failure.
NYHA, New York Heart Association; LVEF, left-ventricular ejection fraction; LVEDD, left-ventricular end diastolic dimension; NA, not applicable; VO$_2$, oxygen uptake; AT, anaerobic threshold; QOLS, quality of life score (Minnesota); 6MWD, six-minute walk distance; SVT, supraventricular tachycardia; EN, enrolling.

There was an 18.6% reduction in the primary endpoints in the OPT-CRT arm (P = 0.015) and a 19.2% reduction in the OPT-CRT-D arm (P = 0.005). Although the result implied that ICD therapy conferred no additional benefit over CRT alone, total mortality in the OPT-CRT-D arm was reduced by 43.4% (P = 0.002). Total mortality in this arm was 11% compared with 19% in the OPT arm and 15% in the OPT-CRT arm (23.9% reduction, P = 0.12).

The rate of the combined endpoint of time to mortality or heart failure hospitalization was reduced by 34.5% in the OPT-CRT arm (P < 0.001) and by 38.3% in the OPT-CRT-D arm (P < 0.001). Subgroup analyses revealed similar treatment effects, although final analyses and adjudication of the endpoint data are pending.[81-83]

Ongoing Trials

The PACMAN (Pacing for Cardiomyopathies) trial is a randomized, parallel, single-blind study of more than 300 patients with CHF, with and without an indication for ICD. The primary endpoint is improvement in functional capacity (6 MWD). Secondary endpoints include NYHA class, quality-of-life scores (QOLS), mortality and morbidity, hospitalization, and incidence of ventricular arrhythmias.

The CARE-HF (Cardiac Resynchronization in Heart Failure) study has a composite primary endpoint of all-cause mortality or unplanned cardiovascular hospitalization. It plans to randomize 800 patients to optimal medical therapy with or without CRT. Patients in sinus rhythm with NYHA class III-IV heart failure on optimal drug treatment, LVEF of 35% or less, LV dyssynchrony defined by QRS duration of 150 msec or more (or > 120 msec if echo criteria met), and LV EDD of 30 mm/m

(height) or more will be included. Recruitment should be completed this year and the study will be reported in 2004.[84]

The PERFECT (Pacing Efficiently by Resynchronization for Efficacy in CHF Therapy) study, currently in the planning stages, intends to randomize patients requiring ventricular pacing who have heart failure or major LV dysfunction to either standard RV pacing or CRT. The proposed combined primary endpoint is one of mortality and morbidity. One hypothesis is that conventional RV pacing may induce dyssynchrony if previously absent.[85-87]

The theory that RV pacing may be detrimental was also tested in the DAVID (Dual Chamber and VVI Implantation Defibrillator) trial. Its composite endpoint was time to death or first hospitalization with heart failure. Patients (n = 506) with LV dysfunction (LVEF ≤ 40%) and ischemic heart disease (>80% of patients) on pharmacologic therapy (96%) received an ICD dual-chamber pacemaker. They had a primary or secondary indication for ICD therapy but no indication for antibradycardia pacing.

Patients were randomized to ventricular-only backup pacing at a lower rate of 40 bpm (VVI-40; n = 256) or dual-chamber rate-responsive pacing at a lower rate of 70 bpm (DDDR-70; n = 250). Because the atrioventricular interval most commonly was programmed at 180 ms in the latter group, intrinsic conduction was generally not permitted. Indeed ventricular pacing occurred 60% of the time in the DDDR-70 group compared with 1% in the VVI-40 group.

The trial was terminated early because of a trend toward worse outcome in the DDDR-70 group (P < 0.03). This effect was evident during the index hospitalization. One-year survival free of the composite endpoint was

83.9% in the VVI-40 group compared with 73.3% in the DDDR-70 group. The components of the composite endpoint also trended toward an improvement in the VVI-40 group: mortality was 6.5% in the VVI-40 group versus 10.1% in the DDDR-70 group (relative hazard ratio 1.61, P = 0.15), and hospitalization for congestive heart failure was 13.3% in the VVI-40 group and 22.6% and DDDR-70 group.

At 18-month follow-up the DDDR-70 group had approximately 60% higher relative probability of death or hospitalization for new or worsened CHF compared with the VVI-40 group.

It was postulated that single-chamber pacing in patients with intrinsically normal distal conduction generates conduction delay, which results in mechanical dyssynchrony and chamber dysfunction. This effect may be more poorly tolerated in the population of study patients with coronary heart disease whose energy supply demand probably already was compromised.[88-90]

Responders

Although the prevalence of potential candidates for CRT has been evaluated according to the selection criteria of completed trials,[91-93] the identification of patients who may benefit from CRT remains undetermined.[94,95]

The current purported indicators of a positive response to CRT are primarily determined by the inclusion/exclusion criteria of the MIRACLE trial. They are NYHA class III and IV heart failure despite optimal standard medical therapy; LVEF less than 35%; LVEDD greater than 55–60 mm; and QRS duration ≥130 msec. The outcome of CRT may also be related to the underlying cause of heart failure[51,96] and the presence of MR may be predictive of a positive response.[101]

Although QRS duration has been shown in several studies to be of strong prognostic significance,[15,30,97-100] some groups have found no correlation between baseline QRS duration or reduction in QRS duration and clinical response to CRT.[53,62,101,102] Reports of narrower BiV-paced complexes in responders compared with nonresponders may suggest that more effective global synchronization of activation times is associated with benefit.[103]

Although ventricular asynchrony was initially diagnosed on the basis of QRS duration of more than 150 msec, it now appears that QRS width does not necessarily correlate with the presence of mechanical interventricular or intra-LV dyssynchrony.[62] As a result, newer techniques are being proposed to more effectively determine dyssynchrony. These include tissue Doppler imaging with tissue tracking, which directly measures synchrony of LV segment contraction[55,104-111]; contrast variability imaging[112]; magnetic resonance imaging[6,113-115]; equilibrium radionuclide angiography[116]; and specific echocardiographic parameters,[117,118] some of which are under evaluation in the **CARE-HF** trial.[84] These techniques may aid optimal programming of CRT[119] and help in the identification of responders.[71,108,120,121]

In summary, BiV pacing shows promise in improving hemodynamic parameters and symptoms in some patients with heart failure. Further studies are still required to identify both the long-term effects of the therapy and the patients who may benefit.

PACING FOR PREVENTION AND TERMINATION OF ATRIAL TACHYCARDIAS

The prevention of symptomatic, drug-refractory, recurrent AF in patients with coexisting sinus node dysfunction is now a class IIb indication for "prevention and termination of tachyarrhythmias by pacing."[2] Pacing therapy may increase the efficacy of pharmacologic treatment of atrial tachycardias by preventing their pathophysiologic triggers or perpetuators, thereby modifying the electrophysiologic conditions that initiate and sustain them.

Pacing Mode

A reduced incidence of AF with atrial-based pacing was initially reported in retrospective studies of patients with sick sinus syndrome.[122-127] Selection bias was a major limitation of these studies. Subsequent prospective randomized trials were designed to evaluate the impact of the pacing mode on the development of chronic atrial tachycardias.

The Danish trial randomized 225 patients with sick sinus syndrome and normal AV conduction to atrial or ventricular single-chamber pacing. The incidence of intermittent or chronic AF was lower in patients receiving atrial pacing systems. This effect was observed only 3 years after initiation of therapy.[87,128-131]

The PASE (Pacemaker Selection in the Elderly) trial was a software randomized trial comparing VVIR pacing with DDDR pacing in 407 patients with sick sinus syndrome, AV block, and other indications for permanent pacing. In the sick sinus group (175 patients) there was a trend toward a higher incidence of AF in patients receiving single-chamber ventricular pacing devices.[132]

Patients with sick sinus syndrome were software randomized to DDDR or VVIR pacing in the Pac-A-Tach (Pacemaker Atrial Tachycardia) trial. There was no significant difference in AF recurrence between the two groups.[133] There were high crossover rates to DDDR pacing in both of these studies (26% to 40%) as a result of pacemaker syndrome and atrial tachycardias.

In the CTOPP (Canadian Trial of Physiologic Pacing) symptomatic patients with AV node disease (52%) and SN disease (35%) were randomized to either a ventricular (VVIR) pacemaker (n = 1474) or a physiologic (AAI[R] or DDD[R]) pacemaker (n = 1094) using hardware randomization. CTOPP therefore avoided the high crossover rates of software randomized VVI/DDD comparison trials. The principal analysis follow-up at 3 years found a significant relative risk reduction of 18% in the development of AF with physiologic pacing that began 2 years after permanent pacemaker implantation and persisted at the extended mean follow-up of 6 years (20.1%).[134,135]

The primary endpoint of the PA[3] (Atrial Pacing Periablation for Prevention of Atrial Fibrillation) trial was time to first recurrence of AF as detected by the atrial high rate diagnostics in the Medtronic Thera DR device.[136-138] Three months before planned AV node ablation, patients with paroxysmal AF (PAF) were randomized to atrial pacing (DDIR lower rate 70 bpm) (n = 49) or no pacing therapy (DDI rate 30 bpm) (n = 48). There was no significant difference between the two groups in either the primary endpoint or in the number of episodes and rate of PAF. The interval between the first and second episodes of PAF was also similar. The atrial premature beat (APB) frequency was suppressed. Although patients were being paced 70% of the time before AF onset, it was suggested that a higher base rate or more aggressive rate-responsive therapy could have altered the outcome.[139]

In the MOST (Mode Selection Trial) patients with sick node dysfunction (n = 2010) were randomized to dual (n = 1014) or single-chamber (ventricular) pacing (n = 996). The median follow-up was 33.1 months. There was a significant reduction in both the incidence of atrial fibrillation and the progression to chronic AF after randomization in the dual-chamber group. This group also had an improvement in quality-of-life scores. Thirty-one percent of patients crossed over to the dual-chamber group secondary to symptoms of pacemaker syndrome.[140,141]

The recently presented UK PACE (United Kingdom Pacing and Cardiovascular Events) trial was designed to evaluate the efficacy and cost utility of dual-chamber pacing (DDDR) versus single-chamber pacing (VVI) in elderly patients with high-grade AV block.

No difference was found in all-cause mortality, heart failure, or myocardial infarction between the VVI, VVIR, and DDDR arms of the study, suggesting that pacemaker selection is not associated with differences in clinical outcome. Comparisons, however, between DDDR versus VVI pacing revealed an increase in stroke or transient ischemic attack (hazard ratio HR 1.58, P = 0.035), although there was no difference when VVI and VVIR combined pacing and VVIR pacing alone was compared with DDDR pacing (HR1.28, P = 0.20 and HR 0.98, P = 0.93, respectively).[142,143] A published analysis of the full results, including the effect of pacing mode on AF, is pending. Finally, the ongoing STOP AF trial (The Systematic Trial Of Pacing to Prevent AF) aims to compare the effect of DDD versus VVI pacing on the development of chronic atrial fibrillation.[144]

In summary, these trials support physiologic pacing (atrial or dual chamber) in reducing the development of AF and permanent AF compared with ventricular pacing in patients with standard indications for pacing. The PA[3] study, however, suggested that atrial-based pacing does not reduce AF when atrial pacing is the primary treatment strategy.

Pacing Site

In an attempt to suppress or prevent AF, alternative sites of stimulation have been evaluated. Biatrial stimulation; dual-site atrial stimulation; and pacing at Bachmann's bundle, the interatrial septum, and coronary sinus have all been proposed as optimal pacing methods to prevent atrial tachycardias.

Biatrial Pacing

Biatrial pacing utilizes simultaneous pacing from the high right atrium and mid or distal coronary sinus.[145] Although biatrial pacing may shorten interatrial conduction resulting in a reduction in p-wave duration, conflicting trial data exists regarding its clinical efficacy in maintaining sinus rhythm.[146] The feasibility of the technique and its beneficial effect have been reported in both single-center series and randomized trials using endocardial and epicardial approaches,[147-149] including studies of patients following cardiovascular surgery.[150-158] Specifically, however, the SYNBIPACE (Biatrial Synchronous Pacing for Atrial Arrhythmia Suppression) study reported only a trend toward an increase in the AF-free interval with biatrial pacing in patients with a p-wave duration of 120 msec or more, two or more episodes of AF in a 3-month period, and a standard indication for pacing.[159]

Dual-Site Right-Atrial Pacing

Dual-site right-atrial pacing is defined as simultaneous pacing from the high right atrium and coronary sinus os. Although controversial,[160] combining this mode of pacing with antiarrhythmic therapy in patients with bradycardia and atrial tachycardias previously refractory to antiarrhythmic drugs, may be efficacious in the prevention of atrial tachycardias.[161-164] A 2002 study suggests that this benefit may extend further to include patients with drug-refractory atrial tachycardias unrelated to spontaneous or drug-induced bradycardia.[165] The initial degree of intraatrial conduction delay (p-wave duration of >120 msec) may be a factor in determining benefit.[166-168]

The DAPPAF (Dual Site Atrial Pacing in Paroxysmal Atrial Fibrillation) trial was a prospective randomized cross-over study utilizing dual-site atrial pacing, single-site high right atrial pacing, and support pacing (VVI/DVI at 50 bpm). The endpoints were time to first recurrence of AF, the need for cardioversion, and the development of permanent AF. There were fewer electrical cardioversions in the dual-site group, but the arrhythmia-free interval was not modified by pacing mode.[169,170]

Other Novel Right-Atrial Pacing Sites

Single-site pacing at Bachmann's bundle, right posterior interatrial septum, distal coronary sinus, or triangle of Koch may be more effective than pacing from the right-atrial appendage in suppressing atrial tachycardias and slowing the progression of paroxysmal to permanent atrial fibrillation.[171-178] Indeed, acute data have shown that pacing at Bachmann's bundle, right posterior interatrial septum, and distal coronary sinus was more successful than biatrial and dual-site pacing in suppressing atrial tachycardias.[179]

Atrial septal pacing is also safe and feasible over long-term study,[180] although there may be higher risks of lead dislodgment and far-field R-wave sensing, particularly at the lower atrial septal sites.[181] Most studies have assessed patients with paroxysmal. AF in whom pacing was indicated to prevent bradycardia[182-184]; however, a reduction in the propensity to chronic AF has also been found in observational studies of patients without bradycardia utilizing septal pacing in combination with antiarrhythmic therapy.[176,185]

Pacing Algorithms

PAF can be facilitated and perpetuated by various factors such as prolongation of intra-atrial conduction times, increased dispersion of atrial refractoriness, and shortening of the atrial refractory period. Atrial pacing is believed to reduce intra-atrial conduction delay by eliminating short-long sequences that can initiate AF. Overdrive atrial pacing also prevents APBs and junctional escape beats, which can initiate intra-atrial reentry. Therefore pacing algorithms have been designed based on these considerations to reduce vulnerability to AF.

Overdrive Pacing

Because the efficacy for AF prevention may relate to the percentage of atrial pacing, different algorithms have been developed to allow continuous atrial pacing (CAP) while monitoring the intrinsic atrial rate. The algorithms are well tolerated by patients because they do not elevate the mean heart rate significantly.[139,186]

The efficacy of conventional overdrive pacing using the dynamic atrial overdrive (DAO) algorithm (St. Jude Medical), which individually tailors atrial pacing at different levels of activity and circadian rhythm, was assessed in the ADOPT-ALL (Atrial Dynamic Overdrive Pacing Trial-ALL) study. Patients with persistent or paroxysmal AF and sinus node dysfunction received a DDDR pacemaker that was randomized to DAO off (n = 158) and DAO on (n = 130). This AF suppression algorithm significantly reduced the mean number of AF episodes and the burden of atrial tachycardias as well as the number of electrocardioversions required when compared with DDDR pacing alone.[187,188]

A recent study randomized patients with PAT (n = 100) to DDD pacing (Inos 2 CLS pacemaker) with or without DAO for a crossover period of 6 months. The AT burden was reduced by 26% (P = 0.066) in patients with DAO programmed on. This effect was most beneficial in a subgroup analysis of patients with more than 80% atrial pacing in the DDD mode (45% reduction) and in patients with a base rate of 65 to 75 bpm (43% reduction).[189] Other investigators assessing constant atrial capture and continuous overdrive algorithms[179,190,191] have found mixed results.

Trials of Specific Pacing Algorithms

CAP is achieved by two algorithms in the Medtronic AT 500 device, namely atrial pacing preference (APP), which monitors the beat-by-beat spontaneous atrial activity (updating the atrial pacing interval to be slightly faster than the intrinsic rate), and atrial rate stabilization (ARS), which responds to the post atrial ectopic interval and applies successive paced beats coupled with an autoadaptive rate decay. Additionally the post mode switch overdrive facility (PMOP) effects high-rate overdrive pacing at a programmable value after cessation of an AT. PMOP was devised to address the phenomenon of early reinitiation of AT attributed to electrical remodeling. In conjunction with ARS the mean number of AT episodes was reduced in a prospective randomized study of patients with dual-chamber ICDs[193]; however, a high recurrence of AT/AF was found by other investigators despite PMOP.[194]

The ASPECT (Atrial septal lead placement and atrial pacing algorithms for prevention of paroxysmal atrial fibrillation) trial evaluated the effect of combining these three algorithms in two groups of patients using atrial septal pacing (n = 69) or nonseptal pacing (n = 51). To date, the results have only been presented in abstract form. After a 1-month monitoring period with DDDR pacing at 60 bpm, patients were randomized to 3 months of the atrial prevention pacing algorithms (PPA) programmed on or off in a crossover fashion. Preliminary subgroup analysis revealed a reduction in AT burden in patients with nonseptal lead placement and a high frequency of APBs (>2481/day) during the monitoring period.[195,196]

In the ATTEST (Atrial Therapy Efficacy and Safety) trial (n = 370) Medtronic AT500 devices were implanted in patients with paroxysmal or persistent AF and bradycardia. Patients were randomized to on or off programming of the previously described PPAs, as well as to two antitachycardia pacing therapies, for a period of 3 months. The majority of patients had an improvement in symptoms; however, there was no reduction in the frequency or burden of AT.[197]

Other algorithms devised to prevent initiation of AT resulting from inhomogeneous distribution of atrial refractoriness include algorithms reacting to APBs, which apply a single-paced beat with a coupling interval equal to the mean of the preceding beats or with a pacing rate acceleration for a programmable time (ELA Post-Extrasystolic Pause Suppression; Vitatron Post-PAC-Response; Vitatron PAC Suppression; ELA Acceleration on PAC). Limited data suggest that patients with frequent AT episodes may benefit from algorithms reacting to APBs.[198]

AT may be triggered by an atrial rate decrease in susceptible patients.[199] The Post-Exercise Response algorithm was therefore devised by Vitatron to maintain a higher pacing rate as soon as the sensor input for rate response detects that exercise has stopped. This algorithm was evaluated in the Atrial Fibrillation Therapy trial. Vitatron Selection DDDRP cardiac stimulators were implanted in 97 patients with drug-refractory PAF. Four programmable PPAs, including the previously mentioned algorithm to prevent AT induction during sinus rate decay, were randomized to on or off. There was a reduction in AF burden and increased duration of sinus rhythm in the total group, although this was less pronounced in the patients with a pacemaker indication (n = 38), suggesting that standard pacing already offered AF prevention in this group.[200]

Pacing Algorithms and Dual-Site Pacing

The PIPAF (Dual site pacing versus monosite pacing in prevention of atrial fibrillation) study randomized patients with PAF to dual-site right-atrial pacing (n = 47) or high right atrial pacing (n = 44). Using a crossover design, DDD pacing with or without sinus rhythm overdrive algorithm (SRO) was successively evaluated in two 6-month periods. SRO resulted in a significant increase in atrial pacing in both groups. There was no significant reduction in AF recurrences.[201,202]

NIPP-AF (New indication for preventive pacing in AF) studied patients with PAF, refractory to treatment with sotalol, who had no bradycardic indication for pacing. The patients continued sotalol and were randomized in a crossover fashion for 12-week periods to either dual-site RA pacing with consistent atrial pacing algorithm or dual-chamber pacing at a backup rate of 30 bpm. The final phase utilized conventional single-site adaptive overdrive pacing. Dual-site RA pacing with continuous sinus overdrive significantly reduced the time to AF recurrence. Although the AF burden was reduced, there was no improvement in symptoms.[203]

In summary, although dual-site right-atrial pacing, biatrial pacing, and pacing at novel sites may reduce the AF burden in selected patients with drug-refractory paroxysmal AF, it remains to be proved whether these pacing modalities will have any long-term beneficial effects on the incidence of AF. Despite the safety of preventive pacing algorithms,[186] further studies are needed to assess their true clinical impact because their effects on AF burden to date have been limited and heterogeneous.[148,182,190,192-194,204] Ultimately the subgroups of patients who may benefit from all these therapies remain to be identified.

(A discussion of antitachycardia pace termination methods is not within the scope of this chapter.)

VASOVAGAL SYNCOPE

The previous requirement for temporary pacing to prove efficacy in neurocardiogenic vasovagal syncope (VVS) with significant cardioinhibitory component was removed from the 1998 pacemaker guidelines.[1] The 2002 updated guidelines support permanent pacing as a class IIa indication in patients with significantly symptomatic and recurrent neurocardiogenic syncope associated with bradycardia documented spontaneously or at the time of tilt-table testing.[2] Vasovagal syncope is a common disorder of autonomic cardiovascular regulation that results in significant morbidity.[206,207]

Pacing has been advocated for cardioinhibitory forms of VVS defined as a hemodynamic collapse pattern, occurring during tilt testing, which involves a decrease in heart rate before or simultaneously with a fall in arterial pressure and may result in asystole.[208,209] Correlation between tilt-induced bradycardia and bradycardias during clinical VVS is poor. In addition, there is only limited evidence from chronic monitoring studies to support occurrence of bradycardia and asystole in patients with frequent syncope.[210-214] The profound vasodila-

tion that occurs with cardioinhibition is not addressed by pacing.[215-217] However, the rate of fall in arterial pressure may be reduced by pacing and[209,218] translate into a longer prodrome. This in turn could result in prolongation of consciousness, which may avoid injury.[219]

Single-chamber ventricular pacing was ineffective in early small studies in improving symptoms of VVS, if a cardioinhibitory response prevailed, because the accompanying peripheral vasodilation was believed to be aggravated by the absence of an atrial contribution.[220,221] To date three randomized nonblinded trials now support pacing to reduce syncope in specific patients with VVS. Pacing was less effective in reducing symptoms such as presyncope and lightheadedness.

VPS 1 (Vasovagal Pacemaker Study) was the first randomized trial of permanent pacing for the prevention of VVS. This pilot study was terminated early because an interim analysis revealed a marked treatment effect. Recurrent syncope was reproduced in 54 patients by tilt test. They had a relative bradycardia (<60 beats/min) and were randomized to receive no pacemaker or a pacemaker with a rate drop response (RDR) function programmed on. There was an 85.4% risk reduction in syncope at the termination of the study (although syncope still occurred in 22% of patients during a 2-month follow-up period). In the treatment group and control group the time to first syncopal episode was 112 days and 54 days, respectively.[222] The VASIS (Vasovagal Syncope International Study) randomized 47 patients with tilt-positive cardioinhibitory syncope and more than three episodes of syncope over the preceding 2 years to receive a DDI pacemaker programmed to 80 bpm (n = 19) with rate hysteresis of 45 bpm or no pacemaker (n = 23).

Syncope recurred in one patient (5%) in the pacemaker arm after 15 months and in 14 patients (60%) in the no pacemaker arm after a median of 5 months. The highly significant difference (P = 0.0006) between the two groups confirmed that active therapy (DDI with rate hysteresis) has the ability to reduce the interval to first recurrence of syncope in this limited select group of patients. The benefit of pacing was maintained for 5 or more years.[223]

A similarly symptomatic, although older, patient group to VPS I, was enrolled in the SYDIT (Syncope Diagnosis and Treatment) Study. This randomized study compared the effects of beta blockade with atenolol (n = 47) and permanent dual-chamber cardiac pacing with RDR function (n = 46). The study was terminated after an interim analysis revealed a highly significant reduction in recurrence of VVS to 4.3% in the pacemaker arm after a median of 390 days (P = 0.004), compared with 26% in the pharmacologic arm after a median of 135 days.[224] Because bias in assessment of outcome and potential "placebo" effect confounded these unblinded studies, the results of the VPS II (second Vasovagal Pacemaker Study) were eagerly awaited. This was the first double-blinded randomized trial in patients with recurrent syncope (six or more episodes) who had a positive tilt-table test. All patients received a pacemaker, which was randomized to the DDD mode with RDR (n = 48) or the ODO mode (n = 52).

The primary endpoint was recurrence of syncope. Intention-to-treat analysis of the first phase of the study revealed a trend toward a lower cumulative risk of having syncope in the DDD pacemaker group. The relative risk reduction was not significant at 28.7% (P one sided = 0.153). The results were similar using an on-treatment analysis. The study was insufficiently powered to draw a definitive conclusion because there was a lower than expected event rate in the control and a smaller treatment effect observed.[225]

Sensing and Pacing Modes

The major issues in the development of effective pacing strategies for VVS are how to detect the onset of syncope and how to pace during the episode. Rate hysteresis (RH),[208,223] rate drop,[222,226,227] and rate-smoothing sensors[228] have been used in studies to detect transient heart rate drops. Although the clinical results were comparable, none of the studies compared the pacing modes directly. One small, randomized clinical trial suggested that RDR was superior to RH in preventing syncope.[229] This therefore indirectly suggested that the entire pacemaker effect was not caused by placebo alone. The role of pacing above any possible placebo effect was also addressed in a small three-way randomized crossover study of highly symptomatic children (n = 12), in which pacemakers were programmed to no pacing, ventricular pacing with RH, or DDD pacing with RDR. DDD pacing was superior to ventricular pacing in preventing syncope, although both pacing modes were more effective than no pacing.[230]

The ability of the RDR algorithm to reduce syncopal relapses is currently being evaluated in the multicenter, prospective, double-blind SYNPACE (Vasovagal, Syncope and Pacing) trial. Patients with syncope (more than six episodes, including one following positive head-up tilt-testing [HUTT]) and positive HUTT with an asystolic or mixed response are being implanted with a pacemaker randomized to RDR programmed on or off. The primary clinical endpoint of the trial is syncope.[231]

Novel "syncope sensors" such as minute volume sensing in combination with heart rate change may offer earlier detection of imminent VVS than heart rate alone.[232] Many other sensors are under evaluation (including QT intervals; core temperature; RV pressure transduction [dP/dt]; and online ventricular lead-measured endocardial acceleration, which assesses indices of contractility), which may help to predict occurrence of syncope.[233-237]

The INOS 2 CLS (closed loop) pacemaker detects changes in myocardial contraction dynamics, which may precede a fall in heart rate in incipient VVS,[238] through RV intracardiac impedance measurements. The information is subsequently transferred into individual pacing rates adequate for the patient's circulatory demand. Encouraging preliminary results were obtained in uncontrolled nonrandomized studies using this pacemaker.[239,240] The ongoing INVASY (INotropy controlled pacing in VAsovagal SYncope) trial is randomizing patients with recurrent VVS and significant bradycardia during HUTT to DDD-CLS pacing or backup DDI to evaluate whether DDD pacing with this closed-loop stimulation is able to prevent syncopal recurrences.[241,242]

In summary, the majority of syncopal episodes in VVS are not associated with symptomatic bradycardia. Moreover the hemodynamic response to HUTT does not necessarily predict either the hemodynamic response during spontaneous syncope or the response to pacemaker insertion.[208,243]

As a result, because the therapeutic mechanism of dual-chamber pacing in VVS is undefined and may in fact include a significant placebo effect, it is recommended that this treatment be reserved for older, highly symptomatic patients who are at greater risk of sustaining injury.[244] A clearer role for this treatment modality may emerge following the publication of VPS II, SynPace, and long-term observational studies.[245]

PACING MODE AND SURVIVAL

Several prospective clinical trials have evaluated the role of physiologic pacing in preventing death and stroke. These trials have generally shown no benefit in preventing death or stroke by physiologic pacing but have shown a reduction in development of AF.

The development of atrial-based pacing permitted the preservation of AV synchrony (physiologic pacing).[246] As physiologic pacing became more widespread, many retrospective, nonrandomized trials suggested that physiologic pacing reduced death, stroke, and AF.[122-124,247,248]

One small prospective, randomized study compared single-chamber atrial pacing to single-chamber ventricular pacing in patients with sick sinus syndrome.[86] It showed a reduction in stroke with atrial pacing. An extension of the study to 5.5 years also demonstrated a reduction in death and AF, although few patients completed this follow-up period.[87] Other small studies reported conflicting results.[132,133]

The previously discussed CTOPP was the first large, randomized study designed to evaluate the potential benefit of physiologic pacing (DDD[R], AAI [R]) compared with ventricular pacing (VVI [R]). The primary endpoint was a combination of cardiovascular death and stroke. At the end of the initial 3-year follow-up phase, there was no difference in the primary endpoint or in overall mortality and hospitalization for heart failure. However, there was a significant, modest reduction in AF with physiologic pacing (relative risk reduction 18.0%).[134]

Because of the potential translation of the short-term reduction in AF to long-term reduction in the primary endpoints, the study was continued for a further 3 years. At 6 years there continued to be no significant reduction in the primary outcome of cardiovascular death or stroke, but it reinforced the reduction in the development of AF, which was now highly significant.[135]

In the MOST study, patients with sinus node disease were implanted with dual-chamber pacemakers and then randomized to physiologic versus ventricular pacing.[140,141] Physiologic pacing did not impart any improvement in the primary outcomes of total mortality, cardiovascular mortality, or nonfatal stroke. However, there was a reduction in the development of AF similar to CTOPP.

The UKPACE trial compared physiologic with ventricular pacing in elderly patients with complete AV block. An increase in stroke and transient ischemic attack was found in the DDDR group compared with the VVI group. This difference was not present when combined VVI and VVIR pacing and VVIR pacing alone was compared with DDDR pacing. All-cause mortality, heart failure, and myocardial infarction also did not differ between the three groups.[142,143]

In summary, the results from large prospective studies suggest no benefit from physiologic pacing in reducing mortality. They do show a significant reduction in AF, however.

SUMMARY

Clinical evidence from randomized trials has generated new recommendations for a role for pacing in CHF, AT, and VVS. CRT has a beneficial effect on the functional status and quality of life of selected patients with CHF. Ongoing and future trials should more precisely measure its long-term clinical benefits and specifically assess survival. The efficacies of combination therapy with ICD and comparative stimulation sites are being evaluated. Further studies will also help to define the economic impact of the treatment and those patients who should derive greatest benefit.

Physiologic pacing is associated with a reduction in AT; however, trial data do not support a reduction in mortality. The alternative sites of atrial stimulation and pacing algorithms currently under review may also reduce the incidence of AT, although to date, the short-term effects have been equivocal.

Finally, pacing may reduce recurrence of syncope in highly symptomatic patients with VVS. A clearer role for this modality may emerge following further study.

REFERENCES

1. Gregoratos G, Cheitlin MD, Conill A, et al: ACC/AHA guidelines for implantation of cardiac pacemakers and antiarrhythmia devices: Executive summary—a report of the American College of Cardiology/American Heart Association Taskforce on Practice Guidelines (Committee on Pacemaker Implantation). Circulation 1998; 97:1325-1335.
2. Gregoratos G, Abrams J, Epstein AE, et al: ACC/AHA/NASPE 2002 Guideline update for the implantation of cardiac pacemakers and antiarrhythmia devices: A report of the American College of Cardiology/American Heart Association task Force on Practice Guidelines (ACC/AHA/NASPE committee to update the 1998 practice guidelines). Circulation 2002; 106:2145-2161.
3. Hochleitner M, Hortnagl H, Ng CK, et al: Usefulness of physiologic dual-chamber pacing in drug resistant idiopathic dilated cardiomyopathy. Am J Cardiol 1990; 66:198-202.
4. Hochleitner M, Hortnagl H, Hortnagl H, et al: Long term efficacy of physiologic dual chamber pacing in the treatment of end-stage idiopathic dilated cardiomyopathy. Am J Cardiol 1992; 70: 1320-1325.
5. Linde C, Gadler F, Edner M, et al: Results of atrioventricular synchronous pacing with optimized delay in patients with severe congestive heart failure. Am J Cardiol 1995; 75:919-923.
6. Gold MR, Feliciano Z, Gottlieb SS, et al: Dual chamber pacing with a short atrioventricular delay in congestive heart failure: A randomized study. J Am Coll Cardiol 1995; 26:967-973.
7. Nishimura RA, Hayes DL, Holmes DR Jr, et al: Mechanism of hemodynamic improvement by dual chamber pacing for severe left ventricular dysfunction: An acute Doppler and catheterization hemodynamic study. J Am Coll Cardiol 1995; 25:281-288.
8. Cazeau S, Ritter P, Bakdach S, et al: Four chamber pacing in dilated cardiomyopathy. Pacing Clin Electrophysiol 1994; 17:1974-1979.
9. Foster AH, Gold MR, McLaughlin JS: Acute hemodynamic effects of atrio-biventricular pacing in humans. Ann Thorac Surg 1995; 59:294-300.
10. Cazeau S, Ritter P, Lazarus A, et al: Multisite pacing for end-stage heart failure: Early experience. Pacing Clin Electrophysiol 1996; 19:1748-1757.
11. Blanc JJ, Etienne Y, Gilard M, et al: Evaluation of different ventricular pacing sites in patients with severe heart failure: Results of an acute hemodynamic study. Circulation 1997; 96:3273-3277.
12. Auricchio A, Salo RW: Acute hemodynamic improvement by pacing in patients with severe congestive heart failure. Pacing Clin Electrophysiol 1997; 20:313-324.
13. Leclercq C, Cazeau S, Le Breton H, et al: Acute hemodynamic effects of biventricular DDD pacing in patients with end-stage heart failure. J Am Coll Cardiol 1998; 32:1825-1831.
14. Saxon LA, Kerwin WF, Cahalan MK, et al: Acute effects of intraoperative multisite ventricular pacing on left ventricular function and activation/contraction sequence in patients with depressed ventricular function. J Cardiovasc Electrophysiol 1998; 9:13-21.
15. Kass DA, Chen CH, Curry C, et al: Improved left ventricular mechanics from acute VDD pacing in patients with dilated cardiomyopathy and ventricular conduction delay. Circulation 1999; 99:1567-73.
16. Etienne Y, Mansourati J, Gilard M, et al: Evaluation of left ventricular based pacing in patients with congestive heart failure and atrial fibrillation. Am J Cardiol 1999; 83:1138-1140.
17. Grines CL, Bashore TM, Boudoulas H, et al: Functional abnormalities in isolated left bundle branch block: The effect of interventricular asynchrony. Circulation 1989; 79:845-853.
18. Xiao HB, Brecker SJ, Gibson DG: Effects of abnormal activation on the time course of the left ventricular pressure pulse in dilated cardiomyopathy. Br Heart J 1992; 68:403-407.
19. Xiao HB, Lee CH, Gibson DG: Effect of left bundle branch block on diastolic function in dilated cardiomyopathy. Br Heart J 1991; 66:443-447.
20. Ritter P, Bakdach M, Bourgeois Y, et al: Implanting techniques for definitive left ventricular pacing (Abstract 531). Pacing Clin Electrophysiol 1996; 19(II):698.
21. Gras D, Cebron JP, Brunel P, et al: Optimal stimulation of the left ventricle. J Cardiovasc Electrophysiol 2002; 13(Suppl):S57-62.
22. Saxon LA, De Marco T, Schafer J, et al: Effects of long-term biventricular stimulation for resynchronization on echocardiographic measures of remodeling. Circulation 2002; 105:1304-1310.
23. Aurricchio A, Spinell JC, Trautmann SI, et al: Effect of cardiac resynchronisation therapy on ventricular remodeling. J Card Fail 2002; 8(6Suppl):S549-555.
24. Panidis IP, Ross J, Munley B, et al: Diastolic mitral regurgitation in patients with atrioventricular conduction abnormalities: A common finding by Doppler echocardiography. J Am Coll Cardiol 1986; 7:768-774.
25. Etienne Y, Mansourati J, Touiza A, et al: Evaluation of left ventricular function and mitral regurgitation during left ventricular-based pacing in patients with heart failure. Eur J Heart Fail 2001; 3:441-447.
26. Alonso C, Rotter P, Le Breton H, et al: Effects of biventricular pacing in drug refractory congestive heart failure (Cardiostim). Arch Maladies 1998; 91(III):246.
27. Breithardt OA, Sinha AM, Schwammenthal E, et al: Acute effects of cardiac resynchronization on functional mitral regurgitation in advanced systolic heart failure. J Am Coll Cardiol 2003; 41: 765-770.
28. Stellbrink C, Breithardt OA, Franke A, et al: Impact of cardiac resynchronization therapy using hemodynamically optimized pacing on left ventricular remodeling in patients with congestive cardiac failure and ventricular conduction disturbances. J Am Coll Cardiol 2001; 38:1957-1965.
29. Auricchio A, Stellbrink C, Block M, et al: Effect of pacing chamber and atrioventricular delay on acute systolic function of paced patients with congestive heart failure: The Pacing Therapies for Congestive Heart Failure Study Group—The Guidant Congestive Heart Failure Research Group. Circulation 1999; 99:2993-3001.

30. Auricchio A, Stellbrink C, Sack S, et al: The Pacing Therapies for Congestive Heart Failure (PATH-CHF) study: Rationale, design, and endpoints of a prospective randomized multicenter study. Am J Cardiol 1999; 83:130D-135D.

31. Auricchio A, Stellbrink C, Stephan S, et al: Long term benefit as a result of pacing resynchronization in congestive heart failure: Results of the PATH-CHF trial.(Abstract 3352). Circulation 2000; 102(Suppl II):II-693.42

32. Nelson GS, Berger RD, Fetics BJ, et al: Left ventricular or biventricular pacing improves cardiac function at diminished energy cost in patients with dilated cardiomyopathy and left bundle-branch block. Circulation 2000; 102:3053-3059.

33. Ukkonen H, Beanlands RSB, Burwash IG, et al: Effect of cardiac resynchronization on myocardial efficiency and regional oxidative metabolism. Circulation 2003; 107:28-31.

34. Nielsen JC, Bottcher M, Jensen HK, et al: Regional myocardial perfusion during chronic biventricular pacing and after acute change or the pacing mode in patients with congestive heart failure and bundle branch block treated with an atrioventricular sequential biventricular pacemaker. Eur J Heart Fail 2002; 5:179-186

35. Garrigue S, Bordachar P, Reuter S, et al: Comparison of permanent left ventricular and biventricular pacing on patients with heart failure and chronic atrial fibrillation: Prospective hemodynamic study. Heart 2002; 87:529-534.

36. Nelson GS, Curry CC, Wyman BT, et al: Predictors of systolic augmentation from left ventricular pre-excitation in patients with dilated cardiomyopathy and intraventricular conduction delay. Circulation 2000; 101:2703-2709.

37. Burkhoff D, Sagawa K: Influence of pacing site on canine left ventricular force-interval relationship. Am J Physiol 1986; 250:H 414-418.

38. Blanc JJ, Benditt DG, Gilard M, et al: A method for permanent transvenous left ventricular pacing. Pacing Clin Electrophysiol 1998; 21:2021-2024.

39. Bordachar P, Garrigue S, Reuter S, et al: Hemodynamic assessment of right, left, and biventricular pacing by peak endocardial acceleration and echocardiography in patients with end-stage heart failure. Pacing Clin Electrophysiol 2000; 23:1726-1730.

40. Saxon L, DeMarco T, Chatterjee K, et al: Chronic biventricular pacing decreases serum norepinephrine in dilated heart failure patients with the greatest sympathetic activation at baseline (Abstract 519). Pacing Clin Electrophysiol 1999; 22(II):830.

41. Hamdan MH, Zagrodzky JD, Joglar JA, et al: Biventricular pacing decreases sympathetic activity compared with right ventricular pacing in patients with depressed ejection fraction. Circulation 2000; 102:1027-1032.

42. Auricchio A: Pacing therapy reduces heart rate and increases heart rate variability in CHF patients. J Cardiac Failure 1999; 5(Suppl 1):44.

43. Hamdan MH, Barbera S, Kowal RC, et al: Effects of resynchronization therapy on sympathetic activity in patients with depressed ejection fraction and intraventricular conduction delay due to ischemic or idiopathic dilated cardiomyopathy. Am J Cardiol 2002; 89:1047-1051.

44. Livanis EG, Flevari P, Theodorakis GN, et al: Effect of biventricular pacing on heart rate variability in patients with chronic heart failure. Eur J Heart Fail 2003; 5:175-178.

45. Alonso C, Ritter P, Leclerq C, et al: Effects of cardiac resynchronization therapy on heart rate variability in patients with chronic systolic heart failure and intraventricular conduction delay. Am J Cardiol 2003; 91:1144-1147.

46. Cazeau S, Leclercq C, Lavergne T, et al: Effects of multisite biventricular pacing in patients with heart failure and intraventricular conduction delay. N Engl J Med 2001; 344:873-880.

47. Daubert JC, Linde C, Cazeau S, et al: Clinical effects of biventricular pacing in patients with severe heart failure and chronic atrial fibrillation: Results from the multisite stimulation in cardiomyopathy—MUSTIC study—Group II (Abstract 3349). Circulation 2000; 102(Suppl II):II-693.

48. Varma C, Sharma S, Firoozi S, et al: Biventricular pacing improves measures of exercise in patients with atrial fibrillation and heart failure (Abstract 1138-110). J Am Coll Cardiol 2002; 39(Suppl A):108A.

49. Linde C, Leclercq C, Rex S, et al: Long-term benefits of biventricular pacing in congestive heart failure: Results from the MUstic STimulation In Cardiomyopathy (MUSTIC) Study. J Am Coll Cardiol 2002; 40:111-118.

50. Varma C, Sharma S, Firoozi S, et al: Atrioventricular pacing improves exercise capacity in patients with heart failure and intraventricular conduction delay. J Am Coll Cardiol 2003; 41:582-588

51. Duncan A, Wait D, Gibson D, et al: Left ventricular remodeling and hemodynamic effects of multisite biventricular pacing in patients with left ventricular systolic dysfunction and activation disturbances in sinus rhythm: Sub-study of the MUSTIC (Multisite Stimulation in Cardiomyopathies) trial. Eur Heart J 2003; 24: 430-441.

52. Abraham WT: Rationale and design of a randomized clinical trial to assess the safety and efficacy of cardiac resynchronization therapy in patients with advanced heart failure: The Multicentre InSync Randomized Clinical Evaluation (MIRACLE). J Card Fail 2000; 6:369-380.

53. Abraham WT, Fisher WG, Smith AL, et al: Cardiac resynchronization in chronic heart failure. N Engl J Med 2002; 346: 1845-1853.

54. St John Sutton MG, Plappert T, Abraham WT, et al: Effect of cardiac resynchronization therapy on left ventricular size and function in chronic heart failure. Circulation 2003; 107:1985-1990.

55. Popovic ZB, Grimm RA, Perlic G, et al: Noninvasive assessment of cardiac resynchronization therapy for congestive heart failure using myocardial strain and left ventricular peak power as parameters of myocardial synchrony and function. J Cardiovasc Electrophysiol 2002; 13:1203-1208.

56. Abraham WT, Fisher W, Smith A, et al: Long term improvement in functional status, quality of life and exercise capacity with cardiac resynchronization therapy: The MIRACLE trial experience (Abstract 1111-1139). J Am Coll Cardiol 2002; 39(Suppl A):159A.

57. Leclercq C, Victor F, Alonso C, et al: Comparative effects of permanent biventricular pacing for refractory heart failure in patients with stable sinus rhythm or chronic atrial fibrillation. Am J Cardiol 2000; 85:1154-1156.

58. Leon AR, Greenberg JM, Kanuru N, et al: Cardiac resynchronization in patients with congestive heart failure and chronic atrial fibrillation: Effect of upgrading to biventricular pacing after chronic right ventricular pacing. J Am Coll Cardiol 2002; 39:1258-1263.

59. Gras D, Mabo P, Tang T, et al: Multisite pacing as a supplemental treatment of congestive heart failure: Preliminary results of the Medtronic Inc. InSync Study. Pacing Clin Electrophysiol 1998; 21:2249-2255.

60. Gras D, Leclercq C, Tang ASL, et al: Cardiac resynchronization therapy in advanced heart failure the multicenter Insync clinical study. Eur J Heart Failure 2002; 4:311-320.

61. Walker S, Levy TM, Rex S, et al: Usefulness of suppression of ventricular arrhythmia by biventricular pacing in severe congestive cardiac failure. Am J Cardiol 2000; 86:231-233.

62. Reuter S, Garrigue S, Bordachar P, et al: Intermediate-term results of biventricular pacing in heart failure: Correlation between clinical and hemodynamic data. Pacing Clin Electrophysiol 2000; 23:1713-1717.

63. Saxon LA, Boehmer JP, Hummel J, et al: Biventricular pacing in patients with congestive heart failure: Two prospective randomized trials—The VIGOR CHF and VENTAK CHF Investigators. Am J Cardiol 1999; 83:120D-123D.

64. Auricchio A, Stellbrink C, Butter C, et al: Clinical efficacy of cardiac resynchronization therapy in heart failure patients stratified by severity of ventricular conduction delay: Results of the PATH-CHF II. (Abstract 103). Pacing Clin Electrophysiol 2002; 25(II):548.

65. Thackray S, Coletta A, Jones P, et al: Clinical trials update: Highlights of the Scientific Sessions of Heart Failure, a meeting of the working group on Heart Failure of the European Society of Cardiology. CONTAK-CD, CHRISTMAS, OPTIME-CHF. Eur J Heart Failure 2001; 3:491-494.

66. Young JB, Abraham WT: Results of the MIRACLE ICD Trial: Presented at the American College of Cardiology 51st Annual Scientific Sessions; March 17-20, 2002; Atlanta GA. J Am Coll Cardiol 2002; 40:1-18.

67. Abraham WT, Young J, Kocovic D, et al: Cardiac resynchronization therapy benefits patients: Combined results of the MIRACLE and MIRACLE ICD trials. (Abstract 144). Pacing Clin Electrophysiol 2002; 25 (II):558.

68. Mortensen P, Sogaard P, Mansour H, et al: European study on the safety and efficacy of sequential biventricular pacing (Abstract 685). Pacing and Clin Electrophysiol 2002; 25(II):694.

69. Auricchio A, Stellbrink C, Sack S, et al: Long-term clinical effect of hemodynamically optimized cardiac resynchronization therapy in patients with heart failure and ventricular conduction delay. J Am Coll Cardiol 2002; 39:2026-2033.

70. Auricchio A, Ding J, Spinelli J, et al: Cardiac resynchronization therapy restores optimal atrioventricular mechanical timing in heart failure patients with ventricular conduction delay. J Am Coll Cardiol 2002; 39:1163-1169.

71. Breithardt OA, Stellbrink C, Kramer AP, et al: Echocardiographic quantification of left ventricular asynchrony predicts an acute hemodynamic benefit of cardiac resynchronization therapy. J Am Coll Cardiol 2002; 40:536-545.

72. Higgins SL, Yong P, Sheck D, et al: Biventricular pacing diminishes the need for implantable cardioverter defibrillator therapy: Ventak CHF Investigators. J Am Coll Cardiol 2000; 36:824-827.

73. Kuehlkamp V, Doernberger V, Suchalla R, et al: Does biventricular pacing affect the incidence of ventricular tachyarrhythmias? (Abstract 3675). Circulation 2000; 102 (Suppl II):II-761.

74. Gasparini M, Lunati M, Bocchiardo M, et al: Cardiac resynchronization therapy and implantable cardioverter defibrillator therapy: Preliminary results from the InSync implantable cardioverter defibrillator Italian registry. Pacing Clin Electrophysiol 2003; 26:148-151.

75. Kuhlkamp V: Initial experience with an implantable cardioverter-defibrillator incorporating cardiac resynchronization therapy. J Am Coll Cardiol 2002; 39:790-797.

76. Molhoek SG, Bax JJ, van Herven L, et al: Effectiveness of resynchronization therapy in patients with end-stage heart failure. Am J Cardiol 2002; 90:379-383.

77. Bradley DJ, Bradley EA, Baughman Kl, et al: Cardiac resynchronization therapy and death from progressive heart failure: A meta-analysis of randomized controlled trials. JAMA 2003; 289:730-740.

78. Gras D, Ritter P, Lazarus, et al: Long term outcome of advanced heart failure patients with cardiac resynchronization therapy (Abstract 423). Pacing Clin Electrophysiol 2000; 23(II):658.

79. Zardini M, Tritto M, Bargiggia G, et al: The InSync Italian Registry: Analysis of clinical outcome and considerations on the selection of candidates to left ventricular resynchronization. Eur Heart J 2000; 2(Suppl J):J16-J22.

80. Daubert C, Linde C, Cazeau S, et al: Mortality in patients included in the MUSTIC study: Long term data (>2 years) follow up (Abstract 142). Pacing Clin Electrophysiol 2002; 25 (II):558.

81. Bristow MR, Feldman AM, Saxon LA. Heart failure management using implantable devices for ventricular resynchronization: Comparison of Medical Therapy, Pacing, and Defibrillation in Chronic Heart Failure (COMPANION) trial—COMPANION Steering Committee and COMPANION Clinical Investigators. J Card Fail 2000; 6:276-285.

82. Salukhe TV, Francis DP, Sutton R: Comparison of medical therapy, pacing and defibrillation in heart failure (COMPANION) trial terminated early: Combined biventricular pacemaker-defibrillators reduce all-cause mortality and hospitalization. Int J Cardiol 2003; 87:119-120.

83. Results of the Comparison of medical therapy, pacing and defibrillation therapies in heart failure trial (COMPANION). Presented at the American College of Cardiology Annual Scientific Sessions, 2003 Late-Breaking Clinical Trials.

84. Cleland JG, Daubert JC, Erdmann E, et al: The CARE-HF study (CARdiac REsynchronization in Heart Failure study): Rationale, design and end-points. Eur J Heart Fail 2001; 3:481-489.

85. Pavia SP, Perez-Lugones A, Lam C, et al: Symptomatic deterioration post dual chamber cardioverter–defibrillator implantation: A retrospective, observational study (Abstract 1029-127). J Am Coll Cardiol 2001; 37(Suppl A):89 A.

86. Andersen HR, Thuesen L, Bagger JP, et al: Prospective randomized trial of atrial versus ventricular pacing in sick-sinus syndrome. Lancet 1994; 344:1523-1528.

87. Andersen HR, Nielsen JC, Thomsen PE, et al: Long-term follow-up of patients from a randomized trial of atrial versus ventricular pacing for sick-sinus syndrome. Lancet 1997; 350:1210-1216.

88. Wilkoff BL: Should all patients receive dual chamber pacing ICDs? The rationale for the DAVID Trial. Curr Control Trials Cardiovasc Med 2001; 2:215-217.

89. Wilkoff BL, Cook JR, Epstein AE, et al: Dual-chamber pacing or ventricular back-up pacing in patients with an implantable defibrillator: The Dual Chamber and VVI Implantable Defibrillator (DAVID) Trial. JAMA 2003; 288:3115-3123.

90. Kass DA: Pathophysiology of physiologic pacing: Advantages of leaving well enough alone. JAMA 2003; 288:3159-3161.

91. Galizio NO, Pesce R, Valero E, et al: Which patients may benefit from biventricular pacing? Pacing Clin Electrophysiol 2003; 26:158-161.

92. Grimm W, Sharkova J, Funck R, et al: How many patients with dilated cardiomyopathy may potentially benefit from cardiac resynchronization therapy? Pacing Clin Electrophysiol 2003; 26:155-157.

93. Erdogan A, Rueckleben S, Tillmanns HH, et al: Proportion of candidates for cardiac resynchronization therapy. Pacing Clin Electrophysiol 2003; 26:152-154.

94. Thackery SDR, Owen E, Witte K, et al: The prevalence of heart failure in the permanently paced population. (Abstract). Eur J Heart Failure 2001; 3:S112.

95. De Sutter J, De Bondt P, Van de Wiele C, et al: Prevalence of potential candidates for biventricular pacing among patients with known coronary artery disease: A prospective registry from a single center. Pacing Clin Electrophysiol 2000; 23:1718-1721.

96. Gasparini M, Mantica M, Galimberti P, et al: Is the outcome of cardiac resynchronization therapy related to underlying etiology? Pacing Clin Electrophysiol 2003; 26:175-180.

97. Wilensky RL, Yudelman P, Cohen AI, et al: Serial electrocardiographic changes in idiopathic dilated cardiomyopathy confirmed at necropsy. Am J Cardiol 1998; 62:276-283.

98. Shamin W, Francis DP, Yousufuddin M, et al: Intraventricular conduction delay: A prognostic marker in chronic heart failure. Intern J Cardiol 1999; 70:171-178.

99. Xiao HB, Roy C, Fujimoto S, et al: Natural history of abnormal conduction and its relation to prognosis in patients with dilated cardiomyopathy. Intern J Cardiol 1996; 53:163-170.

100. Gasparini M, Mantica M, Galimberti P, et al: Beneficial effects of biventricular pacing in patients with a "narrow" QRS. Pacing Clin Electrophysiol 2003; 26:169-174.

101. Farwell D, Patel NR, Hall A, et al: How many people with heart failure are appropriate for biventricular resynchronization? Eur Heart J 2000; 21:1246-1250.

102. Reuter S, Garrigue S, Barold SS, et al: Comparison of characteristics in responders versus nonresponders with biventricular pacing for drug-resistant congestive heart failure. Am J Cardiol 2002; 89:346-350.

103. Alonso C, Leclercq C, Victor F, et al: Electrocardiographic predictive factors of long-term clinical improvement with multisite biventricular pacing in advanced heart failure. Am J Cardiol 1999; 84:1417-1421.

104. Ansalone G, Giannantoni P, Ricci R, et al: Doppler myocardial imaging in patients with heart failure receiving biventricular pacing treatment. Am Heart J 2001; 142:881-896.

105. Ansalone G, Giannantoni P, Ricci R, et al: Doppler myocardial imaging to evaluate the effectiveness of pacing sites in patients receiving biventricular pacing. J Am Coll Cardiol 2002; 39:489-499.

106. Yu CM, Chau E, Sanderson JE, et al: Tissue Doppler echocardiographic evidence of reverse remodeling and improved synchronicity by simultaneously delaying regional contraction after biventricular pacing therapy in heart failure. Circulation 2002; 105:438-445.

107. Anselme F, Savoure A, Schuster I, et al: Is QRS duration a good predictor of right to left ventricular asynchrony? Comparison with conventional Doppler and tissue Doppler imaging criteria (Abstract 22). Pacing Clin Electrophysiol 2002; 25 (II):528.

108. Sogaard P, Egeblad H, Kim WY, et al: Tissue Doppler imaging predicts improved systolic performance and reversed left ventricular remodeling during long-term cardiac resynchronization therapy. J Am Coll Cardiol 2002:40:723-730

109. Pan C, Hoffmann R, Kuhl H, et al: Tissue tracking allows rapid and accurate visual evaluation of left ventricular function. Eur J Echocardiogr 2001; 2:197-202

110. Sogaard P, Kim WY, Jensen HK, et al: Impact of acute biventricular pacing on left ventricular performance and volumes in patients with severe heart failure: A tissue Doppler and three-dimensional echocardiographic study. Cardiology 2001; 96:173-182.

111. Yu CM, Fung WH, Lin H, et al: Predictors of left ventricular reverse remodeling after cardiac resynchronization therapy for

heart failure to idiopathic dilated or ischemic cardiomyopathy. Am J Cardiol 2002; 91:684–688.

112. Kawaguchi M, Murbayashi T, Fetics B, et al: Quantitation of basal dyssynchrony and acute resynchronization from left or biventricular pacing by novel echo-contrast variability imaging. J Am Coll Cardiol 2002; 39:2052–2058.

113. Earls JP, Ho VB, Foo TK, et al: Cardiac MRI: Recent progress and continued challenges. J Magn Reson Imaging 2002; 16,111–127.

114. Wyman BT, Hunter WC, Prinzen FW, et al: Mapping propagation of mechanical activation in the paced heart with MRI tagging. Am J Physiol 1999; 276:H881–891.

115. Prinzen FW, Hunter WC, Wyman BT, et al: Mapping of regional myocardial strain and work during ventricular pacing: Experimental study using magnetic resonance imaging tagging. J Am Coll Cardiol 1999; 33:1735–1742.

116. Faucier L, Marie O, Casset-Senon D: Ventricular dyssynchrony and risk markers of ventricular arrhythmias in nonischemic dilated cardiomyopathy: A study with phase analysis of angioscintigraphy. Pacing Clin Electrophysiol 2003; 26:352–356.

117. Cazeau S, Gras D, Lazarus A, et al: Multisite stimulation for correction of cardiac asynchrony. Heart 2000; 84:579–581.

118. Cazeau S, Bordachar P, Jauvert G, et al: Echocardiographic modeling of cardiac dyssynchrony before and during multisite stimulation: A prospective study. Pacing Clin Electrophysiol 2003; 26: 137–143.

119. Sogaard P, Egeblad H, Pedersen AK, et al: Sequential versus simultaneous biventricular resynchronization for severe heart failure: Evaluation by Tissue Doppler Imaging. Circulation 2002; 106: 2078–2084.

120. Abraham WT: Cardiac resynchronization therapy for heart failure: Biventricular pacing and beyond. Curr Opin Cardiol 2002; 17:346–352.

121. Pitzalis MV, Iacoviello M, Romito R, et al: Cardiac resynchronization therapy tailored by echocardiographic evaluation of ventricular asynchrony. J Am Coll Cardiol 2002; 40:1615–1622.

122. Rosenqvist M, Brandt J, Schuller H: Long-term pacing in sinus node disease: Effects of stimulation mode on cardiovascular morbidity and mortality. Am Heart J 1988; 116:16–22.

123. Hesselson AB, Parsonnet V, Berstein AD, et al: Deleterious effects of long-term single-chamber pacing in patients with sick sinus syndrome: The hidden benefits of dual chamber pacing. J Am Coll Cardiol 1992; 19:1542–1549.

124. Connolly SJ, Kerr C, Gent M, et al: Dual chamber pacing versus ventricular pacing: Critical appraisal of the literature. Circulation 1996; 94:578–583.

125. Sgarbossa EB, Pinski SL, Maloney JD, et al: Chronic atrial fibrillation and stroke in paced patients with sick sinus syndrome: Relevance of clinical characteristics and pacing modalities. Circulation 1993; 88:1045–1053.

126. Santini M, Alexidou G, Ansalone G, et al: Relation of prognosis in sick sinus syndrome to age, conduction defects and modes of permanent cardiac pacing. Am J Cardiol 1990; 65:729–735.

127. Stangl K, Seitz K, Wirtzfeld A, et al: Differences between atrial single chamber pacing (AAI) and ventricular single chamber pacing (VVI) with respect to prognosis and antiarrhythmic effect in patients with sick sinus syndrome. Pacing Clin Electrophysiol 1990; 13:2080–2085.

128. Andersen HR, Thuesen L, Bagger JP, et al: Prospective randomized trial of atrial versus ventricular pacing in sick-sinus syndrome. Lancet 1994; 344:1523–1528.

129. Andersen HR, Nielsen JC, Thomsen PE, et al: Arterial thromboembolism in patients with sick sinus syndrome: Prediction from pacing mode, atrial fibrillation, and echocardiographic findings. Heart 1999; 81:412–418.

130. Nielsen JC, Andersen HR, Thomsen PE, et al: Heart failure and echocardiographic changes during long-term follow-up of patients with sick sinus syndrome randomized to single-chamber atrial or ventricular pacing. Circulation 1998; 97:987–995.

131. Andersen HR, Nielsen JC, Thomsen PE, et al: Atrioventricular conduction during long-term follow-up of patients with sick sinus syndrome. Circulation 1998; 98:1315–1321.

132. Lamas GA, Orav EJ, Stambler BS, et al: Quality of life and clinical outcomes in elderly patients treated with ventricular pacing outcomes in elderly patients treated with ventricular pacing as compared with dual-chamber pacing: Pacemaker Selection in the Elderly Investigators. N Engl J Med 1998; 338:1097–1104.

133. Wharton JM, Sorrentino RA, Campbell P, et al: The PAC-A-TACH Investigators: Effect of pacing modality on atrial tachyarrhythmia recurrence in the tachycardia-bradycardia syndrome: Preliminary results of the pacemaker atrial tachycardia trial (Abstract 2601). Circulation 1998; 98 (Suppl I):I-494.

134. Connolly SJ, Kerr CR, Gent M, et al: Effects of physiologic pacing versus ventricular pacing on the risk of stroke and death due to cardiovascular causes: Canadian Trial of Physiologic Pacing Investigators. N Engl J Med 2000; 342:1385–1391.

135. Kerr CR, Connolly SJ, Roberts RS, et al: Effect of pacing mode on cardiovascular death and stroke: The Canadian trial of Physiologic pacing: Long term follow up. (Abstract 122). Pacing Clin Electrophysiol 2002; 25(II):553.

136. Gillis AM, Connolly SJ, Dubuc M, et al: for the PA3 Investigators: Comparison of DDDR versus VDD pacing post total AV node ablation for the prevention of atrial fibrillation (Abstract 404). Pacing Clin Electrophysiol 1999; 22(II):801.

137. Gillis AM, Wyse DG, Connolly SJ, et al: Atrial pacing periablation for prevention of paroxysmal atrial fibrillation. Circulation 1999; 99:2553–2558.

138. Hill MS, Dinsmoor DA, Kleckner K, et al: Impact of atrial pacing on atrial fibrillation onsets in the PA3 trial (Abstract 3740). Circulation 1998; 98(Suppl I):I-711.

139. Ricci A, Puglisi A, Neja CP, et al: Consistent atrial pacing: Can this new algorithm suppress recurrent atrial fibrillation? (Abstract 710). Pacing Clin Electrophysiol 1997; 20(II):227.

140. Lamas GA, Lee K, Sweeney M, et al: The Mode Selection Trial (MOST) in sinus node dysfunction: Design, rationale, and baseline characteristics of the first 1000 patients. Am Heart J 2000; 140:541–551.

141. Lamas GA, Lee KL, Sweeney MO, et al: Mode Selection Trial in sinus-node dysfunction: Ventricular pacing or dual chamber pacing for sinus-node dysfunction. N Engl J Med 2002; 346:1854–1862.

142. Toff WD, Skehan JD, De Bono DP, et al: The United Kingdom pacing and cardiovascular events (UKPACE) trial: United Kingdom Pacing and Cardiovascular Events. Heart 1997; 78:221–223.

143. Results of the United Kingdom Pacing and Cardiovascular Events (UKPACE) trial. Presented at the American College of Cardiology Annual Scientific Sessions, 2003 Late-Breaking Clinical Trials.

144. Charles RG, McComb JM: Systematic trial of pacing to prevent atrial fibrillation (STOP-AF). (Editorial) Heart 1997; 78:221–223.

145. Daubert C, Leclercq C, Le Breton H, et al: Permanent left atrial pacing with a specifically designed coronary sinus lead. Pacing Clin Electrophysiol 1997; 20:2755–2764.

146. Levy T, Walker S, Rochelle J, et al: Evaluation of biatrial pacing, right atrial pacing, and no pacing in patients with drug refractory atrial fibrillation. Am J Cardiol 1999; 84:426–434.

147. Daubert JC, Mabo P, Berder V, et al: Atrial tachyarrhythmias associated with high degree interatrial conduction block: Prevention by permanent atrial resynchronization. Eur J Card Pacing Electrophysiology 1994; 4:35–44.

148. D'Allonnes R, Pavin D, Leclercq C, et al: Long term effects of biatrial synchronous pacing to prevent drug-refractory atrial tachyarrhythmia: A nine-year experience. J Cardiovasc Electrophysiol 2000; 11:1081–1091.

149. Mirza I, James S, Holt P: Biatrial pacing for paroxysmal atrial fibrillation: A randomized prospective study into the suppression of paroxysmal atrial fibrillation using biatrial pacing. J Am Coll Cardiol 2002; 40:457–463.

150. Daoud EG, Dabir R, Archambeau M, et al: Randomized, double-blind trial of simultaneous right and left atrial epicardial pacing for prevention of post-open heart surgery atrial fibrillation. Circulation 2000; 102:761–765.

151. Fan K, Lee KL, Chiu CS, et al: Effects of biatrial pacing in prevention of postoperative atrial fibrillation after coronary artery bypass surgery. Circulation 2000; 102:755–760.

152. Gerstenfeld EP, Hill MR, French SN, et al: Evaluation of right atrial and biatrial temporary pacing for the prevention of atrial fibrillation after coronary artery bypass surgery. J Am Coll Cardiol 1999; 33:1981–1988.

153. Goette A, Mittag J, Friedl A, et al: Effectiveness of atrial pacing in preventing atrial fibrillation after coronary bypass surgery (Abstract 7). Pacing Clin Electrophysiol 1999; 23(II):700.

154. Greenberg MD, Katz NM, Iuliano S, et al: Atrial pacing for the prevention of atrial fibrillation after cardiovascular surgery. J Am Coll Cardiol 2000; 35:1416–1422.

155. Kurz DJ, Naegeli B, Kunz M, et al: Epicardial, biatrial synchronous pacing for prevention of atrial fibrillation after cardiac surgery. Pacing Clin Electrophysiol 1999; 22:721-726.

156. Levy T, Fotopoulos G, Walker S, et al: Randomized controlled study investigating the effect of biatrial pacing in prevention of atrial fibrillation after coronary artery bypass grafting. Circulation 2000; 102:1382-1387.

157. Orr W, Tsui S, Stafford P, et al: Synchronized bi-atrial pacing after coronary by-pass surgery (Abstract 219). Pacing Clin Electrophysiol 1999; 22(II):755.

158. Crystal E, Connolly SJ, Sleik K, et al: Interventions on prevention of postoperative atrial fibrillation in patients undergoing heart surgery: A meta-analysis. Circulation 2002; 106:75-80.

159. Mabo P, Daubert C, Bouchour A: Biatrial synchronous pacing for atrial arrhythmia prevention: The SYNBIAPACE study (Abstract 221). Pacing Clin Electrophysiol 1999; 22(II):755.

160. Levy T, Walker S, Rex S, et al: No incremental benefit of multisite atrial pacing compared with right atrial pacing in patients with drug refractory paroxysmal atrial fibrillation. Heart 2001; 85:48-52.

161. Saksena S, Prakash A, Hill M, et al: Prevention of recurrent atrial fibrillation with chronic dual-site right atrial pacing. J Am Coll Cardiol 1996; 28:687-694.

162. Prakash A, Saksena S, Hill M, et al: Acute effects of dual-site right atrial pacing in patients with spontaneous and inducible atrial flutter and fibrillation. J Am Coll Cardiol 1997; 29:1007-1014.

163. Delfaut P, Saksena S, Prakash A, et al: Long-term outcome of patients with drug-refractory atrial flutter and fibrillation after single- and dual-site right atrial pacing for arrhythmia prevention. J Am Coll Cardiol 1998; 32:1900-1908.

164. Lau CP, Tse HF, Yu CM, et al: Effect of dual site right atrial pacing on burden of atrial fibrillation in patients with drug-refractory atrial fibrillation (Abstract 1004-1175). J Am Coll Cardiol 2000; 35(Suppl A):109A.

165. Boccadamo R, Di Belardino N, Mammucari A, et al: Dual site right atrial pacing in the prevention of symptomatic atrial fibrillation refractory to drug therapy and unrelated to sinus bradycardia. J Interv Card Electrophysiol 2002; 6:141-147.

166. Friedman PA, Hill MR, Hammill SC, et al: Randomized prospective pilot study of long-term dual-site atrial pacing for prevention of atrial fibrillation. Mayo Clin Proc 1998; 73:848-854.

167. Leclercq JF, De Sisti A, Fiorello P, et al: Is dual site better than single site atrial pacing in the prevention of atrial fibrillation? Pacing Clin Electrophysiol 2000; 23:2101-2107.

168. Prakash A, Saksena S, Krol R, et al: Dual site pacing is effective for atrial fibrillation in patients with and without atrial conduction delay (Abstract 1063-1132). J Am Coll Cardiol 2001; 37(Suppl A):95A.

169. Fitts SM, Hill MR, Mehra R, et al: Design and implementation of the dual site atrial pacing to prevent atrial fibrillation (DAPPAF) clinical trial: DAPPAF Phase 1 Investigators. J Interv Card Electrophysiol 1998; 2:139-144.

170. Saksena S, Prakash A, Ziegler P, et al: Results from late-breaking clinical trials sessions at ACC 2001: The Dual Site Atrial Pacing for Prevention of Atrial Fibrillation (DAPPAF) trial: Improved suppression of recurrent atrial fibrillation with dual site atrial pacing and antiarrhythmic drug therapy. J Am Coll Cardiol 2001; 38:598-599.

171. Padeletti L, Porciani MC, Michelucci A, et al: Interatrial septum pacing: A new approach to prevent recurrent atrial fibrillation. J Interv Card Electrophysiol 1999; 3:35-43.

172. Bennett DH: Comparison of the acute effects of pacing the atrial septum, right atrial appendage, coronary sinus os, and the latter two sites simultaneously on the duration of atrial activation. Heart 2000; 84:193-196.

173. Padeletti L, Capucci A, Boriani G, et al: Prevention of paroxysmal atrial fibrillation in patients with sinus bradycardia by interatrial septal pacing at the triangle of Koch: Results of a randomized prospective multicenter trial (Abstract 3460). Circulation 2000; 102(Suppl II):II-715.

174. Bailin SJ, Adler S, Giudici M: Prevention of chronic atrial fibrillation by pacing in the region of Bachmann's bundle: Results of a multicenter randomized trial. J Cardiovasc Electrophysiol 2001; 12:912-917.

175. Bailin SJ, Giudici MC, Solinger B, et al: Pacing from Bachmann's bundle prevents chronic atrial fibrillation: Final results from a prospective randomized trial (Abstract 227). Pacing Clin Electrophysiol 2001; 24(II):595.

176. Kale M, Bennett DH: Atrial septal pacing in the prevention of atrial fibrillation refractory to antiarrhythmic drugs. Inter J Cardiol 2002; 82:167-175.

177. Becker R, Senges JC, Bauer A, et al: Suppression of atrial fibrillation by multisite and septal pacing in a novel experimental model. Cardiovasc Res 2002; 54:476-481.

178. Padeletti L, Pieragnoli P, Ciapetti C, et al: Randomized crossover comparison of right atrial appendage pacing versus interatrial septum pacing for prevention of paroxysmal atrial fibrillation in patients with sinus bradycardia. Am Heart J 2001; 142: 1047-1055.

179. Yu WC, Tsai CF, Hsieh MH, et al: Prevention of the initiation of atrial fibrillation: Mechanism and efficacy of different atrial pacing modes. Pacing Clin Electrophysiol 2000; 23:373-379.

180. Padeletti I, Pieragnoli P, Ciapetti C, et al: Prevention of paroxysmal atrial fibrillation by permanent septal pacing: Long term follow up. Eur Heart J Suppl 2001; 3(Suppl P):2-6.

181. Israel CW: Conflicting issues in permanent right atrial lead positioning. Pacing Clin Electrophysiol 2000; 23:1581-1584.

182. Boriani G, Biffi M, Padeletti L, et al: Effects of consistent atrial pacing and atrial rate stabilization-two pacing algorithms to suppress recurrent paroxysmal atrial fibrillation an brady-tachy syndrome. Eur Heart J Suppl 2001; 3(Suppl P):7-15.

183. Spencer WH 3rd, Zhu DW, Markowitz T, et al: Atrial septal pacing: A method for pacing atria simultaneously. Pacing Clin Electrophysiol 1997; 20:2739-2745.

184. Katsivas A, Manolis AG, Lazaris E, et al: Atrial septal pacing to synchronize atrial depolarization in patients with delayed interatrial conduction. Pacing Clin Electrophysiol 1998; 21:2220-2225.

185. Manolis AG, Katsivas AG, Vassilopoulos C, et al: Prevention of atrial fibrillation by inter-atrial septum pacing guided by electrophysiological testing in patients with delayed interatrial conduction. Europace 2002; 4:165-174.

186. Lam CT, Lau CP, Leung SK, et al: Efficacy and tolerability of continuous overdrive atrial pacing in atrial fibrillation. Europace 2000; 2:286-291.

187. Beinhauer A, Vock P, Nobis H, et al: AF suppression by atrial dynamic overdrive pacing in the ADOPT-ALL trial: Program and abstracts of the XXIII Congress of the European Society of Cardiology; September 1-5, 2001: Stockholm, Sweden. Abstract P2965.

188. Carlson MD, Gold MR, Ip J, et al: Dynamic atrial overdrive pacing decreases symptomatic atrial arrhythmia burden in patients with sinus node dysfunction (Abstract 1825). Circulation 2001; 104(Suppl II):II-383.

189. Konz KH, Brachmann J, Attuel P, et al: Prevention of atrial fibrillation by atrial overdrive pacing: Final results of a randomized crossover study (Abstract 1017-1011) J Am Coll Card 2003; 87A.

190. Israel CW, Hugl B, Unterberg C, et al: Pace-termination and pacing for prevention of atrial tachyarrhythmias: Results from a multicenter study with an implantable device for atrial therapy. J Cardiovasc Electrophysiol 2001; 12:1121-1128.

191. Saksena S, Prakash A, Ziegler P, et al: Improved suppression of recurrent atrial fibrillation with dual-site right atrial pacing and antiarrhythmic drug therapy. J Am Coll Card 2002; 40: 1140-1150.

192. Funck RC, Adamec R, Lurje L, et al: Atrial overdriving is beneficial in patients with atrial arrhythmias: First results of the PROVE study. Pacing Clin Electrophysiol 2000; 23:1891-1893.

193. Saksena S, Sulke N, Manda V, et al: Reduction in frequency of atrial tachyarrhythmia episodes using novel prevention algorithms of an atrial pacemaker defibrillator (Abstract 115). Pacing Clin Electrophysiol 2000; 23(II):581.

194. Israel CW, Hugl B, Unterberg-Buchwald C, et al: Performance of a new implantable DDDRP device incorporating preventative and antitachycardia pacing modalities: Results of the international prospective AT500 verification study (Abstract) Pacing Clin Electrophysiol 2001; 24:554.

195. Padeletti L, Purerfellner H, Adler S, et al: Atrial septal lead replacement and atrial pacing algorithms for prevention of paroxysmal atrial fibrillation: ASPECT study results (Abstract 659) Pacing Clin Electrophysiol 2002; 25(II):687

196. Harvey M, Holbrook R, Young M, et al: Combined atrial pacing prevention algorithms reduce atrial tachyarrhythmia burden in bradycardia patients with frequent premature atrial contractions and standard atrial lead placement: ASPECT trial results (Abstract 1017-1015) J Am Coll Cardiol 2003; 88A.

197. Lee MA, Weachter R, Pollak S, et al: Can preventative and anti-tachycardia pacing reduce the frequency and burden of atrial tachyarrhythmias? The ATTEST study results (Abstract 74) Pacing Clin Electrophysiol 2002; 25(II):541.

198. Murgatroyd FD, Nitzsche R, Slade AK, et al: A new pacing algorithm for overdrive suppression of atrial fibrillation. Pacing Clin Electrophysiol 1994; 17:1966-1973

199. Coumel P: Paroxysmal atrial fibrillation: A disorder of autonomic tone? Eur Heart J 1994; 15(Suppl A):9-16.

200. Camm J: AF therapy study: Preventative pacing for paroxysmal atrial fibrillation (Abstract 125) Pacing and Clin Electrophysiol 2002; 25(II):554.

201. Anselme F, Saoudi N, Cribier A: Pacing in prevention of atrial fibrillation: The PIPAF studies. J Interv Card Electrophysiol 2000; 4:177-184.

202. Seidl K, Cazeau S, Gaita F, et al: Dual site pacing versus mono-site pacing in prevention of atrial fibrillation (Abstract 184) Pacing Clin Electrophysiol 2002; 25(II):568.

203. Lau CP, Tse HF, Yu CM, et al: For the New Indication for Preventive Pacing in Atrial Fibrillation (NIPP-AF) Investigators: Dual site atrial pacing for atrial fibrillation in patients without bradycardia. Am J Cardiol 2001; 88:371-375.

204. Ricci R, Santini M, Puglisi A, et al: Impact of consistent atrial pacing algorithm on premature atrial complex number and paroxysmal atrial fibrillation recurrences in brady-tachy syndrome: A randomized prospective cross over study. J Interv Card Electrophysiol 2001; 5:33-44.

205. Israel CW, Lawo T, Lemke B, et al: Atrial pacing in the prevention of paroxysmal atrial fibrillation: First results of a new combined algorithm. Pacing Clin Electrophysiol 2000; 23:1888-1890.

206. Linzer M, Pontinen M, Gold DT, et al: Impairment of physical and psychosocial function in recurrent syncope. J Clin Epidemiol 1991; 44:1037-1043.

207. Rose MS, Koshman ML, Spreng S, et al: The relationship between health-related quality of life and frequency of spells in patients with syncope. J Clin Epidemiol 2000; 53:1209-1216.

208. Petersen ME, Chamberlain-Webber R, Fitzpatrick AP, et al: Permanent pacing for cardioinhibitory malignant vasovagal syndrome. Br Heart J 1994; 71:274-281.

209. Fitzpatrick A, Theodorakis G, Ahmed R, et al: Dual chamber pacing aborts vasovagal syncope induced by head-up 60 degrees tilt. Pacing Clin Electrophysiol 1991; 14:13-19.

210. Sheldon R, Garred J, Wilson W, et al: Heart periods during syncope: Holter analysis of patients with neurally mediated syncope (Abstract 16). Pacing Clin Electrophysiol 1998; 21(II):793.

211. Menozzi C, Brignole M, Lolli G, et al: Follow-up of asystolic episodes in patients with cardioinhibitory, neurally mediated syncope and VVI pacemaker. Am J Cardiol 1993; 72:1152-1155.

212. Krahn AD, Klein GJ, Yee R, et al: Randomized assessment of syncope trial: Conventional diagnostic testing versus a prolonged monitoring strategy. Circulation 2001; 104:46-51.

213. Moya A, Brignole M, Mendozzi C, et al: Mechanism of syncope in patients with isolated syncope and in patients with tilt-positive syncope. Circulation 2001; 104:1261-1267.

214. Krahn AD, Klein GJ, Fitzpatrick A, et al: Predicting the outcome of patients with unexplained syncope undergoing prolonged monitoring. Pacing Clin Electrophysiol 2002; 25:37-41.

215. Sra JS, Akhtar M: Cardiac pacing during neurocardiogenic (vasovagal) syncope. J Cardiovasc Electrophysiol 1995; 6:751-760.

216. Sra JS, Jazayeri MR, Avitall B, et al: Comparison of cardiac pacing with drug therapy in the treatment of neurocardiogenic (vasovagal) syncope with bradycardia or asystole. N Engl J Med 1993; 328:1085-1090.

217. El-Bedawi KM, Wahbha MA, Hainsworth R: Cardiac pacing does not improve orthostatic tolerance in patients with vasovagal syncope. Clin Auton Res 1994; 4:233-237.

218. Samoil D, Grubb BP, Brewster P, et al: Comparison of single and dual chamber pacing techniques in the prevention of upright tilt induced vasovagal syncope. Eur J Card Pacing Electrophysiol 1993; 3:36-41.

219. Sutton R: How and when to pace in vasovagal syncope. J Cardiovasc Electrophysiol 2002; 13(Suppl):S14-16.

220. Fitzpatrick A, Travill CM, Vardas PE, et al: Recurrent symptoms after ventricular pacing in unexplained syncope. Pacing Clin Electrophysiol 1994; 13:619-629.

221. Raviele A, Menozzi C, Brignole M, et al: Value of head-up tilt testing potentiated with sublingual nitroglycerin to assess the origin of unexplained syncope. Am J Cardiol 1995; 76:267-272.

222. Connolly SJ, Sheldon R, Roberts RS, et al: The North American Vasovagal Pacemaker Study (VPS): A randomized trial of permanent cardiac pacing for the prevention of vasovagal syncope. J Am Coll Cardiol 1999; 33:16-20.

223. Sutton R, Brignole M, Menozzi C, et al: Dual-chamber pacing in the treatment of neurally mediated tilt-positive cardioinhibitory syncope: Pacemaker versus no therapy: A multicenter randomized study. The Vasovagal Syncope International Study (VASIS) Investigators. Circulation 2000; 102:294-299.

224. Mahanonda N, Bhuripanyo K, Kangkagate C, et al: Randomized double-blind, placebo-controlled trial of oral atenolol in patients with unexplained syncope and positive upright tilt table test results. Am Heart J 1995; 130:1250-1253.

225. Results of the Second Vasovagal Pacemaker Study (VPSII). Presented by Stuart J. Connolly at the North American Society of Pacing and Electrophysiology 23rd Annual Scientific Sessions, May 11, 2002 Late-breaking clinical trials.

226. Benditt DG, Sutton R, Gammage MD, et al: Clinical experience with Thera DR rate-drop response pacing algorithm in carotid sinus syndrome and vasovagal syncope: The International Rate-Drop Investigators Group. Pacing Clin Electrophysiol 1997; 20: 832-839.

227. Ammirati F, Colivicchi F, Santini M, et al: Permanent cardiac pacing versus medical treatment for the prevention of recurrent vasovagal syncope. Circulation 2001; 104:52-57.

228. Sheldon R, Koshman ML, Wilson W, et al: Effect of dual-chamber pacing with automatic rate-drop sensing on recurrent neurally mediated syncope. Am J Cardiol 1998; 81:158-162.

229. Ammirati F, Colivicchi F, Toscano S, et al: DDD pacing with rate drop response function versus DDI with rate drop hysteresis pacing for cardioinhibitory vasovagal syncope. Pacing Clin Electrophysiol 1998; 21:2178-2181.

230. McLeod KA, Wilson N, Hewitt J, et al: Cardiac pacing for severe childhood neurally mediated syncope with reflex anoxic seizures. Heart 1999; 82:721-725.

231. Raviele A, Giada F, Sutton R, et al: The Vasovagal Syncope and Pacing (Synpace) trial: Rationale and study design. Europace 2001; 3:336-341.

232. Kurbaan AS, Erickson M, Petersen ME, et al: Respiratory changes in vasovagal syncope. J Cardiovasc Electrophysiol 2000; 11: 607-611.

233. Brignole M, Menozzi C, Corbucci G, et al: Detecting incipient vasovagal syncope: Intraventricular acceleration. Pacing Clin Electrophysiol 1997; 20:801-805.

234. Clementy J, Kobeissi A, Garrigue S, et al: Validation by serial standardized testing of a new rate-responsive pacemaker sensor based on variations in myocardial contractility. Europace 2001; 3:124-131.

235. Mangin L, Kobeissi A, Lelouche D, et al: Simultaneous analysis of heart rate variability and myocardial contractility during head-up tilt in patients with vasovagal syncope. J Cardiovasc Electrophysiol 2001; 12:639-644.

236. Binggeli C, Duru F, Corti R, et al: Autonomic nervous system-controlled cardiac pacing: A comparison between intracardiac impedance signal and muscle sympathetic nerve activity. Pacing Clin Electrophysiol 2000; 23:1632-1637.

237. Osswald S, Cron T, Gradel C, et al: Closed-loop stimulation using intracardiac impedance as a sensor principle: Correlation of right ventricular dp/dtmax and intracardiac impedance during dobutamine stress test. Pacing Clin Electrophysiol 2000; 23: 1502-1508.

238. Deharo JC, Peyre JP, Ritter PH, et al: A sensor-based evaluation of heart contractility in patients with head-up tilt induced syncope. Pacing Clin Electrophysiol 1998; 21:223-226.

239. Griesbach L, Huber T, Knote B, et al: Therapy of malignant vasovagal syncope with closed loop pacemaker stimulation. (Abstract 882-885) J Am Coll Card 2003; 139A.

240. Occhetta E, Bortnik M, Vassanelli C: The DDDR closed loop stimulation for the prevention of vasovagal syncope: Results from the INVASY prospective feasibility registry. Europace 2003; 5:153-162.

241. Occhetta E, Bortnik M, Pedrigi C, et al: Vasovagal syncope: To pace or not to pace? Europace 2000:(Suppl D):241.

242. Occhetta E, Bortnik M, Audoglio R, et al: Sincope vasovagale e sti-molazione CLS: Risultati preliminari dello studio "INVASY". G Ital Aritmol Cardiostimol 2002; 5(Suppl 2):19-22.
243. Raj SR, Koshman ML, Sheldon RS, et al: Five year follow-up of patients with dual chamber pacemakers for vasovagal syncope (Abstract 274). Can J Cardiol 2002; 18:186B.
244. Sheldon R: Role of pacing in the treatment of vasovagal syncope. Am J Cardiol 1999; 84:26Q-32Q.
245. Raj SR, Sheldon RS: Role of pacemakers in treating neurocardio-genic syncope. Curr Opin Cardiol 2003; 18:47-52.

246. Kristensson BE, Arnman K, Smedgard P, et al: Physiological pacing versus single-rate ventricular pacing: A double blind cross-over study. Pacing Clin Electrophysiol 1985; 8:73-84.
247. Menozzi C, Brignole M, Moracchini PV, et al: Intrapatient compari-son between chronic VVIR and DDD pacing in patients affected by high degree AV block without heart failure. Pacing Clin Elec-trophysiol 1990; 13:1816-1822.
248. Lamas GA, Paschos CL, Mormand SLT, et al: Permanent pacemaker selection and subsequent survival in elderly Medicare pacemaker recipients. Circulation 1995; 91:1063-1069.

■ ■ ■ c h a p t e r **19**

Drugs Blocking the Renin-Angiotensin-Aldosterone System

Gary S. Francis
W.H. Wilson Tang

INTRODUCTION

The renin-angiotensin-aldosterone system (RAAS) likely evolved more than 600 million years ago, about the time of the transformation of species from saltwater to land.[1] The development of this very important system presumably offered an evolutionary advantage by allowing organisms to conserve sodium and water, thus expanding circulating volume and thereby protecting circulatory homeostasis. Although the sympathetic nervous system (SNS) likely evolved around the same time, the principal function of RAAS is somewhat different. The RAAS basically operates to stabilize bodily fluids and other electrolytes during periods of stress, such as deprivation of saltwater and electrolytes, relative hypovolemia, and inadequate renal perfusion.[2] It is a system that is slower to react than the SNS, and the RAAS appears to have both a circulating and an important tissue-bound component.[3,4] However, the SNS and the RAAS are highly integrated, and this interaction is of great importance in the pathogenesis of heart failure.[5-7]

It has long been recognized by the pharmaceutical industry and academic pharmacologists that inhibition of the RAAS might be useful for the treatment and modification of various disease states. Such drugs are now widely used to treat hypertension and heart failure.[8] The introduction of angiotensin-converting enzyme (ACE) inhibitors and angiotensin-II receptor blockers (ARBs) has revolutionized the management of patients with cardiovascular diseases. Not only do such agents reduce blood pressure and offset the retention of salt and water,[9] but they also appear to have cardiac, renal, and vascular protective properties leading to an astounding array of potential benefits.[10,11] The purpose of this chapter is to review the results of the most important clinical trials whereby drugs designed to block the RAAS were compared with placebo or active controls.

DRUGS THAT SUPPRESS THE RENIN-ANGIOTENSIN-ALDOSTERONE SYSTEM

The RAAS is part of a complex homeostatic feedback loop in which the juxtaglomerular cells of the kidney in response to hypotension or diminished delivery of sodium to the macula densa secrete the enzyme renin (Fig. 19-1). Renin circulates in the blood and cleaves angiotensinogen, a very large circulating α_2-globulin molecule synthesized by the liver. This interaction between renin and angiotensinogen generates a very small decapeptide, angiotensin I. Although angiotensin I has no intrinsic hemodynamic effects, it is converted quickly by kininase-2 or ACE to the octapeptide, angiotensin II (A-II). Angiotensin II is a very hemodynamically potent peptide, with a vast spectrum of biologic activity including cell growth and organ remodeling (Fig. 19-2). It likely had a very primitive and highly conserved role in inflammation and response to organ injury. Recently, a second enzyme, ACE2, that converts angiotensin I to angiotensin 1-9 has been described.[12] Although angiotensin 1-9 has no known intrinsic effects, it can be converted to angiotensin 1-7, which is a known vasodilator. The physiologic significance of ACE2 in heart failure is unknown, but its discovery underscores how our knowledge of the RAAS continues to grow. The RAAS is complex well beyond our original, overly simplistic understanding. Its clinical importance lies in our ability to pharmacologically block it, resulting in very consistent clinical benefits.

Current guidelines recommend ACE inhibitors for the primary therapy for all patients with systolic heart failure and ARBs in those patients intolerant to ACE inhibitors.[13] Although further investigation is needed, ACE inhibitors and ARBs are also likely to be beneficial in the treatment of heart failure with preserved left-ventricular (LV) function (or so-called "diastolic heart failure"). Importantly, ACE inhibitors have emerged as

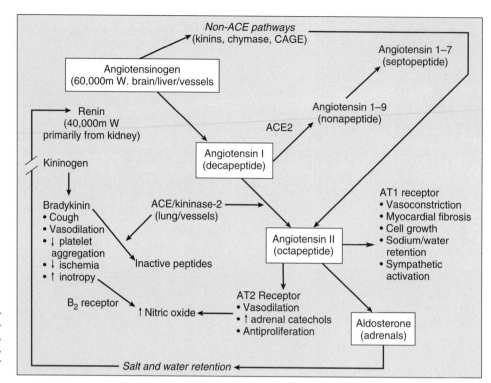

FIGURE 19-1. The renin-angiotensin-aldosterone system (RAAS). mW, molecular weight; AT, angiotensin; ACE, angiotensin-converting enzyme CAGE, chymostatin-sensitive angiotensin II-generating enzyme.

"cardioprotective" and "vasculoprotective" in patients without heart failure who harbor cardiovascular risk factors. It is possible that ARBs and other drugs that block the RAAS will be similarly effective. This has already been shown for use of ARBs for patients with proteinuria, where renal protection occurs.[14,15] To date, however, we have insufficient data to say that ACE inhibitors and ARBs are equivalent. ACE inhibitors, ARBs, and aldosterone receptor antagonists will be described separately, although in clinical practice they are sometimes used in various combinations.

Angiotensin-Converting Enzyme Inhibitors

ACE inhibitors were developed in the late 1960s and early 1970s in the Squibb laboratories as part of a program to synthesize innovative antihypertensive drugs.[16] The prototype ACE inhibitor that evolved from this highly creative effort was captopril. There are now at least a dozen ACE inhibitors, all with somewhat different pharmacokinetic and pharmacodynamic properties (Table 19-1).[17] The use of these agents results in a modest reduction in blood pressure, accompanied by a variable reduction in cardiac filling pressures and heart rate and a small but consistent improvement in cardiac index.[18] However, the ability of these drugs to prevent progression of heart failure and vascular and renal disease is perhaps more closely tied to their long-term ability to prevent the growth, proliferative, and proinflammatory effects of A-II on various organs. The importance of their hemodynamic properties has come under challenge.[19]

The mechanism of action whereby ACE inhibitors benefit patients with hypertension, heart failure, and vascular diseases is still widely debated.[11] Although there is an acute hemodynamic response to these drugs, the long-term benefits are likely uncoupled to some extent from their short-term hemodynamic effects.[20] The neurohormonal hypothesis suggests that blocking RAAS offers a "cardioprotective" benefit that may be in the form of reduced LV and vascular remodeling, thereby resulting in fewer clinical events.[21] Favorable effects on the heart, vasculature, and mesangium, although poorly understood, may be related to their ability to attenuate the long-term growth and inflammatory properties of A-II—that is, there is less cellular hypertrophy and fibrosis in response to injury with ACE inhibitors. This concept supports the observation that the beneficial clinical effects of taking ACE inhibitors may not be observed for several months or even years. A reduction in left-ventricular remodeling and hypertrophy,[22] vascular remodeling,[23] thrombosis,[24] sudden cardiac death,[25] and other cardiovascular events has been a very consistent feature of all clinical trials with ACE inhibitors (Table 19-2). Whether these are dose-dependent effects is still debatable because there are limited data indicating any significant impact of ACE inhibitor dose on the degrees of neurohormonal suppression.[26,27] There is also uncertainty whether these benefits are to the result of "tissue ACE" effects or whether these are class effects common to all ACE inhibitors.

ACE inhibitors block kininase II, a ubiquitous enzyme that degrades bradykinin and converts angiotensin I to A-II (see Fig. 19-1). ACE inhibitors are associated with incremental changes in local tissue levels of bradykinin.[28] Numerous experimental studies have suggested that increased bradykinin may be associated with antigrowth and anti-inflammatory properties.[29-31] Unfortunately, local

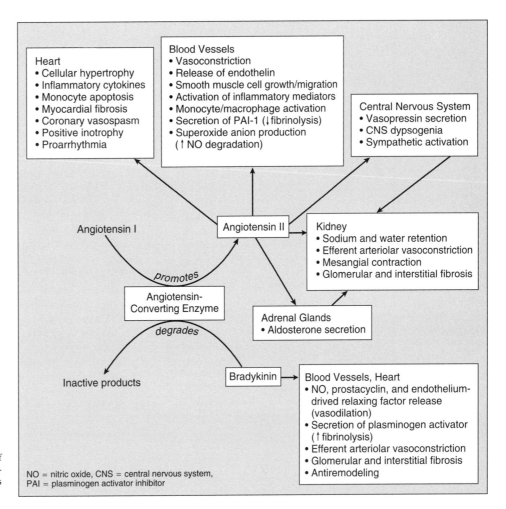

FIGURE 19-2. Biologic activities of angiotensin-II. PAI-1, platelet activator inhibitor-1; CNS, central nervous system; NO, nitric oxide.

NO = nitric oxide, CNS = central nervous system, PAI = plasminogen activator inhibitor

■ ■ ■

TABLE 19-1   SUMMARY OF DRUGS BLOCKING THE RENIN-ANGIOTENSIN-ALDOSTERONE SYSTEM

Drug	Trade name in the U.S.	HF indication	Post-MI indication	Dosing
Angiotensin-converting enzyme inhibitors				
Benazepril	Lotensin	No	No	5–40 mg qd
Captopril	Capoten	Yes	No	6.25–150 mg tid
Enalapril	Vasotec	Yes	No	2.5–20 mg bid
Fosinopril	Monopril	Yes	No	10–80 mg qd
Lisinopril	Prinivil, Zestril	Yes	No	5–20 mg qd
Moexipril	Univasc	No	No	7.5–60 mg qd
Perindopril	Aceon	No	No	2–16 mg qd
Quinapril	Accupril	Yes	No	5–20 mg bid
Ramipril	Altace	Yes	Yes	2.5–20 mg qd
Trandolapril	Mavik	No	Yes	1–4 mg qd
Zofenopril	Bifril	NA	NA	7.5–60 mg qd
Angiotensin-II receptor blockers				
Candesartan	Atacand	No	No	8–32 mg qd/bid
Eprosartan	Teveten	No	No	400–800 mg qd
Irbesartan	Avapro	No	No	150–300 qd
Losartan	Cozaar	No	No	50–100 mg qd/bid
Telmisartan	Micardis	No	No	40–80 qd
Valsartan	Diovan	Yes	No	80–320 mg qd
Olmesartan	Benicar	No	No	20–40 mg qd
Aldosterone antagonists				
Spironolactone	Aldactone	Yes	No	25–50 mg qd
Eplerenone	Inspra	Yes (post-MI only)	Yes	25–50 mg qd

HF, heart failure; MI, myocardial infarction; qd, once daily; tid, three times daily; bid, twice daily; NA, not available.

TABLE 19-2 SUMMARY OF MORTALITY TRIALS OF DRUGS BLOCKING THE RENIN-ANGIOTENSIN-ALDOSTERONE SYSTEM

Trial [reference]	Year published	HF stage	Study population	Comparison and target dose	Sample size	Withdrawal at end of study (%)	Duration (months)	% ischemics	All-cause mortality	Annualized mortality[a]	Absolute mortality reduction
Angiotensin-converting enzyme inhibitors											
CONSENSUS [116, 117]	1987	C–D	NYHA IV	Enalapril 20 mg bid / Placebo	127 / 126	17 / 14	12	73	46 (36%) / 66 (52%)	36%	18% RRR 31%
V-HeFT II [102]	1991	C	NYHA II–III LVEF <45%	Enalapril 10 mg bid / Hydralazine 75 mg qid + isosorbide dinitrate 40 mg qid	403 / 401	22 / Hyd 29 + ISDN 31	24	53	132 (18%) / 153 (25%)	13%	7% RRR 28%
SOLVD-T [90]	1991	C	NYHA II–III LVEF ≤35%	Enalapril 10 mg bid / Placebo	1285 / 1284	33 / 42	41	71	42 (35%) / 510 (40%)	10%	4.5% RRR 16%
SOLVD-P [91]	1992	B	NYHA I LVEF ≤35%	Enalapril 10 mg bid / Placebo	2111 / 2117	24 / 27	37	83	313 (15%) / 334 (16%)	5%	RRR 9%
SAVE [89]	1992	C	Post-MI LVEF ≤40%	Captopril 50 mg tid / Placebo	1115 / 1116	30 / 27	42	100	228 (20%) / 275 (25%)	6%	4.2% RRR 19%
AIRE [103]	1993	C	Post-MI NYHA II–III	Ramipril 5 mg bid / Placebo	1004 / 982	35 / 32	15	100	170 (17%) / 222 (23%)	16%	5.6% RRR 27%
TRACE [104]	1995	C	Post-MI LVEF ≤35%	Trandolapril / Placebo	876 / 873	37 / 36	48	100	304 (35%) / 369 (42%)	24%	7.6% RRR 22%
NETWORK [119]	1998	C	NYHA II–IV	Enalapril 2.5 mg bid / Enalapril 5 mg bid / Enalapril 10 mg bid	506 / 510 / 516	20 / 19 / 26	6	71	21 (4%) / 17 (3%) / 15 (3%)	7%	6% NS
ATLAS [109]	1999	C	NYHA II–III LVEF ≤30%	Lisinopril 5 mg qd / Lisinopril 35 mg qd	1596 / 1568	31 / 27	48	65	717 (45%) / 666 (43%)	11%	2% NS
HOPE [88]	2000	A–B	NYHA I LVEF >50%	Ramipril 2.5 mg qd / Placebo	4645 / 4652	33 / 31	60	80	482 (10%) / 569 (12%)	2%	2% RRR 16%
EUROPA [70]	2003	A–B	NYHA I	Perindopril 8 mg qd / Placebo	6110 / 6108	19 / 16	50	100	375 (6%) / 420 (7%)	1.5%	1% RRR 11%
Angiotensin-II receptor blockers											
ELITE-I [56]	1997	C	NYHA II–IV LVEF ≤40%	Losartan 50 mg qd / Captopril 25 mg tid	352 / 370	18 / 30	12	68	17 (5%) / 32 (9%)	7%	4% RRR 46%

Trial [ref]	Year		Inclusion criteria	Treatment	N				Events n (%)	Annualized mortality*	RRR
RESOLVD [113]	1999	C	NYHA II–IV LVEF ≤40%	Candesartan 4–16 mg qd	327	NR	11	72	20 (6%)	8%	−3% NS
				Enalapril 10 mg bid	109				4 (4%)		
				Candesartan 4–8 mg qd + Enalapril 10 mg bid	332				29 (9%)		
ELITE-II [54]	2000	C	NYHA II–IV LVEF ≤40%	Losartan 50 mg qd	1578	10	18	80	280 (18%)	11%	−2% NS
				Captopril 25 mg tid	1574	15			250 (16%)		
Val-HeFT [55]	2001	C	NYHA II–IV LVEF ≤40%	Valsartan 160 mg bid	2511	10	23	57	495 (20%)	10%	−1% NS
				Placebo	2499	7			484 (19%)		
LIFE [100]	2002	B	LVH LVEF >40%	Losartan 100 mg qd	4605	2	48	16	383 (8%)	2%	1% RRR 12%
				Atenolol 100 mg qd	4588	2			431 (9%)		
OPTIMAAL [112]	2002	C	Post-MI NYHA II–III	Losartan 50 mg qd	5477	17	18	100	499 (18%)	6%	−2% NS
				Captopril 50 mg tid		23			447 (16%)		
CHARM [114]	2003	C	NYHA II–III	Candesartan 32 mg qd	3803	23	38	53	886 (23%)	8%	2% RRR 9%
				Placebo	3796	19			945 (25%)		
Aldosterone antagonists											
RALES [77]	1999	C–D	NYHA III–IV LVEF ≤35%	Spironolactone 25 mg qd	822	26	24	55	284 (35%)	20%	RRR 30%
				Placebo	841	24			386 (46%)		
EPHESUS [81]	2003	C	Post-MI NYHA II–III	Eplerenone 50 mg qd	3319	15	16	100	478 (14%)	14%	3% RRR 15%
				Placebo	3313	19			554 (17%)		
Vasopeptidase inhibitors											
OVERTURE [84]	2002	C	NYHA II–IV LVEF ≤0%	Omapatrilat 40 mg qd	2886	27	15	56	477 (16%)	14%	2% NS
				Enalapril 10 mg bid	2884	25			509 (18%)		

*Annualized mortality = (total mortality/duration) for ACE-inhibitor–treated group.

HF, heart failure; NYHA, New York Heart Association functional class; RRR, relative risk reduction; LVEF, left-ventricular ejection fraction; Hyd, hydralazine; ISDN, isosorbide dinitrate; MI, myocardial infarction; NS, not statistically significant;

concentration of bradykinin in various tissues is not easily measured. Although the role of ACE inhibitor–induced bradykinin in protecting the heart and vasculature in patients treated with ACE inhibitors is now widely assumed, there are undoubtedly other mechanisms whereby ACE inhibitors improve clinical outcomes, and probably not all are related to this aspect of their activity.[32] Adverse effects of ACE inhibitors may also derive from increased bradykinin. The dry, unproductive cough that necessitates stoppage of ACE inhibitors in 5% to 7% of patients treated with ACE inhibitors may be related to increased bradykinin activity in the upper respiratory tract. Likewise, angioedema, which occurs in 1% to 2% of patients treated with ACE inhibitors, may be related to bradykinin release and can occur with ARBs.

There is considerable interest in the concept that the use of aspirin may offset the benefits of ACE inhibitors.[33-35] However, virtually all aspirin/ACE inhibitor interaction studies have been retrospective, small, and observational in nature. There are no large, prospective, randomized, controlled trials investigating the interaction between aspirin and ACE inhibitors. Until such data are available, the combination of aspirin and ACE inhibitors will likely continue to be widely used.[36,37]

It is apparent that the initiation of ACE inhibitors in patients with heart failure can lead to transient or occasionally severe renal impairment.[38,39] Nevertheless, the development of modest renal insufficiency should not necessarily preclude the use of ACE inhibitors.[40] A 20% increment in serum creatinine is common. There is a long-recognized concept that A-II normally protects intraglomerular hydraulic pressure in heart failure and dehydration through its vasoconstrictor effects on renal efferent arteriolar tone. When ACE inhibitors are used, there is a transient reduction in efferent glomerular arteriolar tone, leading to a decrease in intraglomerular hydraulic pressure. Reduced intraglomerular hydraulic pressure is associated with a transient reduction in glomerular filtration rates.[41] This commonly leads to a 10% to 20% increase in serum creatinine and blood urea nitrogen.[42] The use of ACE inhibitors in patients who have been vigorously diuresed or who are volume deplete may magnify this effect, which also can be accompanied by striking, transient hypotension.[43] It is therefore advisable not to use ACE inhibitors in the face of severe intravascular volume depletion. It is also important to remember that modest changes in renal function from ACE inhibitors are reversible and are not the result of any structural changes within the kidney.[44] These biochemical changes can often be reversed by temporary reduction of diuretic dose or careful volume expansion.[45] Severe renal function impairment may occur when ACE inhibitors are used in patients with severe, bilateral renal artery stenosis or cardiogenic shock.[46] The modest increase in serum potassium that usually accompanies the use of ACE inhibitors is typically viewed as a beneficial effect.[47] Severe hyperkalemia may occasionally occur when ACE inhibitors are combined with nonsteroidal anti-inflammatory agents or aldosterone receptor antagonists,[48] particularly in patients with baseline renal function impairment, underlying diabetes mellitus,[49] or severe dehydration.

The concept of tissue ACE as an important factor in the pathophysiology of cardiac and vascular dysfunction is still evolving.[3] There has been a long-standing debate as to the importance of "tissue" ACE inhibitors versus "nontissue" ACE inhibitors. Several ACE inhibitors including quinapril and ramipril are known to penetrate tissue more readily. However, whether tissue activity has any influence on clinical outcomes such as mortality and hospitalization rate has remained unproved.[50] Nevertheless, the beneficial effects of ACE inhibitors exceed those attributable to blood pressure reduction alone. ACE inhibitors may exert an important part of their effects via direct tissue action. The clinical importance of tissue-binding affinity of ACE inhibitors is not fully established.

Angiotensin-II Receptor Blockers

Angiotensin-II receptor blockers were developed in the early 1990s when it became widely recognized that ACE inhibitors were associated with incomplete blockade of the RAAS and were sometimes poorly tolerated by patients. It became clear that alternative pathways generate A-II and that ACE inhibitors therefore did not continuously suppress A-II and aldosterone. There are currently half a dozen ARBs in the market (see Table 19-1). These drugs are now widely used to treat hypertension, and valsartan is approved to treat patients with heart failure who do not tolerate ACE inhibitors.

The first ARB to be developed was losartan, which was widely studied and was found to be an excellent antihypertensive agent that was better tolerated than ACE inhibitors. Not unexpectedly, there has since been widespread interest in the use of ARBs in the treatment of patients with heart failure.[51-53] Because ACE inhibitors have become the cornerstone of treatment for heart failure, placebo-controlled trials using ARBs are not possible. Only comparison trials using ARBs and ACE inhibitors and "add-on" trials with a combination of ARB-ACE inhibitor have been performed (see Table 19-2).[54,55] In general, there appears to be no marked difference in clinical outcomes between these two classes of RAAS drugs in patients with hypertension and heart failure, although the database for ACE inhibitors is much larger. However, equivalency or noninferiority of the two classes of drugs (which requires enormous sample size) has not yet been proved. Both classes of drugs can impair renal function to the same extent.[56] One fact that has consistently emerged from this multitude of clinical trials is that ARBs are better tolerated than ACE inhibitors. The incidence of cough is lower, and there may be less angioedema. In the SPICE (Study of Patients Intolerant of Converting Enzyme Inhibitors) trial, candesartan was tolerated in 83% of patients following a 12-week treatment protocol similar to that of placebo in patients with systolic heart failure who were previously intolerant to ACE inhibitors.[57] Patients-intolerant to ACE inhibitors can be treated with ARBs, and results from the Valsartan in Heart Failure Trial (Val-HeFT)[55] and Candesartan in Heart failure: Assessment of Reduction in Mortality and morbidity (CHARM)[58] studies have supported this strategy. The soon to be completed Valsartan in Acute Myocardial Infarction Trial (VALIANT) study,[59] and the Prevention of Events with Angiotensin Converting Enzyme Inhibition trial (PEACE),[60] should further enlighten us with regard to head-to-head comparison with ACE inhibitors (Table 19-3).

The combination of ACE inhibitor and ARB to treat hypertension and heart failure has not yet been widely studied. In the Val-HeFT, the combination of valsartan and an ACE inhibitor reduced hospitalization rate in patients with heart failure, but no further improvement in survival was derived.[55] More data will be available soon from the VALIANT trial that bear on the combined use of ACE inhibitors and ARBs.[59] Interestingly, all-cause mortality was also similar between those treated with candesartan versus placebo when added to standard regimen of ACE inhibitors and beta-blockers in the CHARM-Added study (30% vs. 32%, P = 0.89).[61] However, the same CHARM-Added study demonstrated that the addition of candesartan to standard ACE inhibitor and beta-blocker therapy leads to a further clinically important reduction in a predefined composite endpoint of cardiovascular death or heart failure hospitalization in patients with systolic heart failure (38% vs. 42%, P = 0.01).[61]

There is little information regarding the use of ARBs to reduce coronary events or cardiovascular risk. Mechanistic studies in small groups of patients have demonstrated the effects of ARBs in improving hemodynamics and exercise tolerance,[62-65] reducing microalbuminuria and improving endothelial dysfunction in people with diabetes,[15,66-68] reducing inflammation,[69] and reversing left-ventricular hypertrophy (LVH).[70] The CHARM-Preserved study also explored the role of ARBs in patients with heart failure and preserved LV function, but found neither the composite endpoint nor cardiovascular death were reduced by candesartan; only the number of investigator-reported admissions for heart failure was significantly reduced (230 vs. 279, P = 0.017).[71]

Although it is possible that combining ARBs with ACE inhibitors may provide incremental benefit in patients with heart failure, concern regarding overaggressive neurohormonal suppression has been raised in a post-hoc analysis, which indicated that "triple therapy" with an ACE inhibitor plus valsartan plus beta blocker in a subset of 1610 patients was associated with an unfavorable outcome and a higher mortality rate. However, this "triple therapy" concern has not been confirmed in the CHARM dataset.[55,61] For now, ARBs are considered to be the drug of choice for patients intolerant to ACE inhibitors.[13] One possible exception is angioedema, in which there may be crossover of this serious side effect between the two classes of drugs. If this occurs with either agent, the other should not be used.[72]

Aldosterone Receptor Antagonists

It is now more widely recognized that inhibition of aldosterone is effective therapy for both hypertension and heart failure.[73,74] Spironolactone, a nonspecific aldosterone receptor antagonist that has been available since the 1950s as treatment for hypertension, refractory edema, and hyperaldosteronism, has become mainstream treatment for patients with New York Heart Association (NYHA) class IV and some class III patients. The long-term use of spironolactone is associated with rather substantial side effects, including painful gynecomastia and hyperkalemia.[75] In patients with advanced heart failure, there is a dose-dependent improvement in LV structure and function as well as exercise tolerance when treated with spironolactone.[76]

The Randomized Aldosterone Evaluation Study (RALES) revived interest in aldosterone antagonism by providing rather striking findings that spironolactone, when used in modest doses of 12.5 to 25 mg/day in patients with advanced heart failure and preserved renal function, was associated with 30% improvement in mortality.[77]

■ ■ ■

TABLE 19-3   SUMMARY OF UPCOMING LARGE-SCALE CLINICAL TRIALS OF DRUGS SUPPRESSING RAAS

Trial	HF stage	Sample size	Design of trial comparison	Estimated follow-up
PEACE [71]	A–B	8,000	Trandolapril vs. placebo in at-risk patients	5 years
ONTARGET [96]	A–B	23,400	Telmisartan vs. ramipril vs. combination in patients at-risk population	5.5 years
TRANSCEND [96]	A–B	5,000	Telmisartan vs. placebo in ACE inhibitor-intolerant	5.5 years
VALIANT [59]	C	14,500	Valsartan vs. captopril vs. placebo in post-MI patients with ejection fraction ≤35%	6 years
HEAAL	C	3,240	Losartan (50 mg/day) vs. losartan (150 mg/day) in patients with heart failure	4 years
I-PRESERVE	C	3,600	Irbesartan vs. placebo over ACE inhibitor/beta blocker therapy in patients with heart failure and preserved left-ventricular function	3 years

ACE, angiotensin-converting enzyme.

Sudden death, although always a "soft" endpoint, was also remarkably reduced. This has spurred renewed interest in the development of better-tolerated and more selective aldosterone receptor antagonists. Aldosterone receptors are present on some epithelial surfaces but are primarily in cell nuclei. These nuclear receptors subserve a host of genomic and nongenomic-related biologic and pharmacologic effects (Fig. 19-3). A new, highly selective aldosterone receptor antagonist (SARA), eplerenone, is being investigated in patients with hypertension. It is about 1000 times more selective than spironolactone for the aldosterone receptor. Preliminary data have suggested eplerenone has important antihypertensive properties.[78,79] Its ability to inhibit remodeling and promote regression of LVH is at least as impressive as enalapril. The combination of enalapril and eplerenone has potent synergistic ability to reverse myocardial hypertrophy.[80] As with spironolactone, hyperkalemia can occur with this drug. Recent data from the Eplerenone Neurohormonal Efficacy and Survival Study (EPHESUS) further demonstrated the benefits of aldosterone antagonism in patients with less advanced heart failure. In the EPHESUS study, in which 6200 patients experienced clinical heart failure 3 to 10 days post-myocardial infarction (LV ejection fraction <40%), addition of eplerenone to patients receiving standard aggressive medical therapy for heart failure provided significant morbidity and mortality benefits.[81] A large National Heart, Lung, and Blood Institute (NHLBI) sponsored trial of aldosterone receptor antagonists in treating diastolic heart failure is currently in the planning stages. It is anticipated that newer and even more specific aldosterone receptor antagonists or aldosterone synthesis inhibitors will emerge, and these may also have a prominent role in preventing chronic cardiovascular diseases. However, the exact place of eplerenone or any new SARAs in heart failure therapy will in large

part be determined by its cost and whether or not future studies will be able to demonstrate a clinical benefit of this agent over generic spironolactone or other currently available treatments.

Vasopeptidase Inhibitors

Counter-regulatory peptides such as atrial natriuretic factor (ANF or ANP) and B-type natriuretic peptide (BNP) are released from the atrium and ventricles of the heart into the circulation where they are associated with vasorelaxant and antigrowth properties. These activities are mediated by membrane receptors coupled to cyclic GMP. The stimulus for the release of ANP and BNP is primarily heightened cardiac wall stress. These counter-regulatory peptides are normally degraded by neutralendopeptidases (NEP) that are found on endothelial cells and on the brush border of the kidney. ANP and BNP are also deactivated by C-type receptors, also present in large concentration in the kidneys. It is now widely recognized that inhibition of NEP by specific molecules is associated with enhanced and prolonged counter-regulatory peptide activity, including vasodilation, natriuresis, and antigrowth/remodeling in the heart and vasculature. Omapatrilat is a combined ACE/NEP inhibitor that is designed to lower blood pressure and improve cardiac function through inhibition of ANP and BNP degradation.[82,83] Such drugs would seemingly be effective as antihypertensive agents and as therapy for patients with heart failure.[82] However, preliminary results of the clinical trial (Omapatrilat versus Enalapril Randomized Trial of Utility in Reducing Events Study, OVERTURE) indicate that omapatrilat, when added to conventional therapy, provides no incremental benefit in patients with systolic heart failure.[84] At this time it is unclear if dual ACE/NEP inhibition will emerge as an

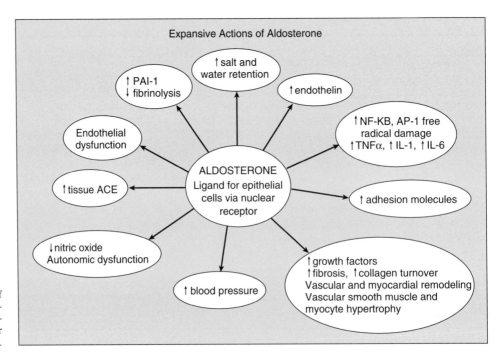

FIGURE 19-3. Biologic activities of aldosterone. PAI-1, platelet activator inhibitor-1; ACE, angiotensin-converting enzyme; TNFα, tumor necrosis factor alpha; IL, interleukin.

important therapeutic modality in heart failure or hypertension.

Other Cardiovascular Drugs That Interact with the Renin-Angiotensin-Aldosterone System

Although beta blockers are widely understood to inhibit the sympathetic nervous system, they also have important effects on the RAAS. Release of renin in the kidney is modulated in part through β-adrenergic receptors. Therefore, beta blockade is associated with an attenuation of RAAS stimulation.[85,86] It is possible, although not certain, that some of the benefits of beta blockers in patients with heart failure are mediated through this mechanism. Digitalis also inhibits the RAAS. This appears to be a direct and indirect property of the drug.[87] In contrast, diuretics stimulate the RAAS by promoting volume contraction and by reducing the delivery of sodium to the macula densa of the kidney. Both acute and chronic diuretic uses are associated with renin release. It is therefore logical to consider renin a potential therapeutic target, and several compounds that directly inhibit renin release or binding to renin receptors are currently in the drug development pipeline.

DRUGS SUPPRESSING THE RAAS IN THE SPECTRUM OF HEART FAILURE

The latest American College of Cardiology/American Heart Association guidelines in the management of patients with heart failure categorize patients with heart failure according to four stages. It is logical to now consider treatment according to these stages, with particular reference to inhibition of the RAAS.

Treating Patients with Stage A Heart Failure

Patients with stage A heart failure do not yet have signs and symptoms of heart failure or structural heart disease but are clearly at risk of developing heart failure.[13] The Heart Outcomes Prevention Evaluation (HOPE) trial was a landmark randomized controlled trial that evaluated the effects of ramipril, an ACE inhibitor, in a high-risk population without heart failure.[88] The rationale for HOPE was based on previous observations from the Survival and Ventricular Enlargement Study (SAVE)[89] and the Studies of Left-ventricular Dysfunction (SOLVD)[90,91] that ACE inhibitors reduce acute coronary events. In the HOPE trial, a total of 9297 high-risk patients (age 55 years or older) with evidence of cardiovascular disease or diabetes mellitus plus one other cardiovascular risk factor were randomly assigned to receive ramipril 10 mg/day or placebo. Patients with known systolic dysfunction or heart failure were excluded. The trial was a 2 × 2 factorial design structured to evaluate the benefits of both ramipril and vitamin E. The effects of vitamin E were neutral. However, ramipril significantly reduced overall mortality, myocardial infarction, and stroke in

this broad range of high-risk patients. For the first time, prospective data from HOPE demonstrated that an ACE inhibitor prevents the development of cardiovascular events including heart failure and diabetes mellitus. Complications related to diabetes were also reduced.[92] The magnitude of benefit from HOPE was at least as large as that observed in secondary prevention trials for myocardial infarction.

Recently, the European Trial on Reduction of Cardiac Events with Perindopril in Stable Coronary Artery Disease (EUROPA) study randomized 12,218 patients (without clinical evidence of heart failure) with previous myocardial infarction (64%), angiographic evidence of coronary artery disease (61%), coronary revascularization (55%), or a positive stress test only (5%) to receive either perindopril or placebo. Perindopril was found to reduce the combined frequency of cardiovascular death, myocardial infarction and cardiac risk within 4.2 years by 20% and to reduce non-fatal myocardial infarction by 22%.[93] Together with the HOPE data, this is strong evidence that patients at risk for developing heart failure should be given consideration for initiating ACE inhibitor therapy.

The mechanism whereby patients in HOPE demonstrated such a remarkable reduction in cardiovascular events is not entirely clear, and the impact of very modest blood pressure reduction is debatable.[19] Other studies including the Perindopril Protection Against Recurrent Stroke Study (PROGRESS)[94] and the Reduction of Endpoints in NIDDM with Angiotensin II Antagonist Losartan Study (RENAAL)[14] have also demonstrated the usefulness of RAAS blockade in patients with high-risk cardiovascular diseases but not overt heart failure. Similar to ramipril, losartan has been shown to reduce the incidence of diabetes mellitus.

Irrespective of the importance of blood pressure reduction as a mechanism of efficacy of ACE inhibitors, aggressive blood pressure lowering should remain a primary objective in the treatment of these patients. However, mean blood pressure reduction as reported in these studies can be misleading. In a substudy of HOPE, systolic and diastolic ambulatory blood pressures fell much more over 24 hours in the ramipril group, especially at night when the drug was given. These changes are greater than those reported for the whole group in the *New England Journal of Medicine* manuscript.[88,95] Studies with somewhat similar design to HOPE and EUROPA (such as PEACE[60]) are currently ongoing, and may provide additional enlightenment regarding the role of blood pressure reduction versus direct tissue effects of ACE inhibitors in these high-risk patients.

A number of trials using ARBs in this population are also in progress.[96] The largest, the Ongoing Telmisartan Alone or in Combination with Ramipril Global Endpoint Trial (ONTARGET), is a trial comparing telmisartan 80 mg per day versus ramipril 10 mg per day using a 2 × 2 factorial design. ONTARGET intends to enroll 23,400 patients and is expected to last for 5.5 years. The study intends to explore the possibility that the effects of ACE inhibitors are incomplete and allow for escape from A-II suppression, thus limiting their cardioprotective effects. The study is also designed to investigate whether the combination of ACE inhibitor plus ARB eliminates this escape phenomenon. The primary endpoint of ONTARGET includes a composite outcome of cardiovascular death, acute myocardial infarction, stroke, and hospitalization for heart failure. There are large numbers of secondary outcomes in ONTARGET. A parallel study (Telmisartan Randomized Assessment Study in ACE inhibitor Intolerant Subjects with Cardiovascular Disease, TRANSCEND) will explore the role of ARBs in ACE inhibitor–intolerant patients.

Treating Patients with Stage B Heart Failure

Patients with Stage B heart failure differ from Stage A patients in that they have structural heart disease (LVH or reduced LV function) but are without any signs and symptoms of heart failure.[13] They are presumably at greater risk than patients in Stage A. Often they have experienced a previous myocardial infarction but are clinically without signs or symptoms.

Patients with Stage B were part of the SOLVD prevention trial, in which the use of enalapril was associated with reversal of LV remodeling.[97] Moreover, patients with asymptomatic LV dysfunction randomly allocated to enalapril were hospitalized less often than those allocated to placebo.[91] These data suggest that there is benefit in treating minimally symptomatic or even asymptomatic patients with structural heart disease who are at risk of developing overt heart failure (Stage B). Such therapy not only may reverse the underlying structural abnormality but may forestall the onset of symptomatic heart failure.

Many studies have been done with ACE inhibitors in patients with Stage B heart failure. Regression of structural heart disease is used as a surrogate marker in these studies. For example, regression of LVH, as in HOPE,[22] RACE (Ramipril Cardioprotective Evaluation Study),[98] PRESERVE (Prospective Randomized Enalapril Study Evaluating Regression of Ventricular Enlargement Study),[99] LIFE (Losartan Intervention For Endpoint Reduction in Hypertension Study),[100] and 4E (Eplerenone, Enalapril, and Eplerenone/Enalapril Combination Therapy in Patients with Left-ventricular Hypertrophy Study),[80] and reversal of LV remodeling in SOLVD[101] were the surrogate targets of investigation. It has not been conclusively proved that improvement in these surrogate endpoints antedate survival benefit, but substantial data support this concept. The LIFE study was particularly impressive in this regard because patients had to have LVH by electrocardiographic criteria to enter the trial.[100] LVH by electrocardiographic criteria is generally more stringent than echocardiographic criteria. Nevertheless, in LIFE there was a highly statistically significant regression of LVH in patients randomly assigned to losartan compared to atenolol despite equivalent blood pressure reduction. These data support the concept that inhibition of RAAS is associated with a consistent reduction in LVH. This concept will be further supported by the ongoing Telmisartan Effectiveness on Left-ventricular Mass Reduction (TELMAR) study, which is comparing the effect of telmisartan with metoprolol succinate on regression of LVH, measured by magnetic resonance imaging. It is worth noting that in the 4E study, although both enalapril and eplerenone are associated with equivalent regression of LVH over 6 months as measured by magnetic resonance imaging, the combination of enalapril plus eplerenone produces significantly more LVH regression than either agent used alone.[80]

Several important ongoing trials including PEACE[60] also include Stage B patients and will test the concept that early introduction of RAAS blocking therapy in patients destined to develop heart failure can prevent the onset of symptoms and delay the progression of disease.

Treating Patients with Stage C Heart Failure

Patients with overt heart failure make up the primary patient population in most of the clinical trials to date. The hypothesis that inhibition of RAAS favorably alters the natural history of systolic heart failure has been thoroughly tested.

Angiotensin-Converting Enzyme Inhibitors

In SOLVD treatment[90] and V-HeFT II,[102] enalapril 10 mg twice daily demonstrated benefit over placebo (SOLVD treatment) or a combination of hydralazine and isosorbide dinitrate (Veterans Administration Cooperative Vasodilator-Heart Failure Trial, V-HeFT-II). In SAVE,[92] AIRE (Acute Infarction Ramipril Efficacy Study),[103] and TRACE (Trandolapril Cardiac Evaluation)[104] studies, captopril, ramipril, and trandolapril were found to prolong survival in patients who experienced symptomatic heart failure or cardiac dysfunction following acute myocardial infarction, respectively. These five trials offer substantial evidence that RAAS blockade with ACE inhibitors should be the cornerstone of treatment of patients with systolic heart failure.[105]

There has been some uncertainty regarding when to introduce ACE inhibitors following acute myocardial infarction. In general, these agents should be introduced when there is clinical and hemodynamic stability, usually on day 2 or 3 after infarction. Although it is true that very early introduction of ACE inhibitors in patients with large anterior myocardial infarction may lead to more substantial inhibition of LV remodeling with subsequent morbidity and mortality benefits,[106,107] there is a modest but finite risk of hypotension in early postinfarction use of ACE inhibitors. Recent post-hoc analysis from CAPRICORN (Carvedilol Post-Infarct Survival Controlled Evaluation Study) also suggests that carvedilol provides the maximal benefit in patients with postinfarction heart failure when added at least 48 hours after the ACE inhibitor has been initiated.[108]

The ATLAS (Assessment of Treatment with Lisinopril And Survival) trial was a large, randomized, controlled study comparing low-dose versus high-dose lisinopril in patients with heart failure.[109] In this trial, 3164 patients with NYHA II–IV heart failure and left-ventricular ejection fraction (LVEF) of 30% or less were randomly allocated to either low-dose lisinopril (2.5 to 5 mg daily) or high-dose lisinopril (32.5 to 35 mg daily). There was no significant difference in time to death between the two groups. However, the combined endpoint of time to death plus all-cause hospitalization marginally favored the high-dose group. On balance, the results of ATLAS indicate that there is no striking difference between the two doses of lisinopril. The relative benefits of high-dose versus conventional-dose ACE inhibitor therapy are small, although some clinicians favor the up-titration of ACE inhibitors to doses higher than the doses used in the large trials.

Angiotensin-II Receptor Blockers

Evidence of morbidity and mortality benefits with ARBs in patients with Stage C heart failure are also accumulating. There have been two large randomized controlled trials evaluating the effects of losartan in elderly patients with heart failure. The Evaluation of Losartan in the Elderly Study (ELITE-I) was primarily designed to examine the influence of losartan versus captopril on renal function.[56] Both drugs are associated with a modest but equivalent increase in serum creatinine and blood urea nitrogen. Although ELITE-I was not powered to study the influence of these drugs on mortality, there was a striking reduction in all-cause mortality, particularly the incidence of sudden death, in patients assigned to losartan.[110] This prompted the initiation of the much larger Losartan Heart Failure Survival Study (ELITE-II), a study designed to compare losartan versus captopril in elderly patients with systolic heart failure.[54] Although the study was not powered for equivalency, there was no obvious advantage of losartan over captopril. If anything, there was a slight trend for captopril to have a more favorable effect on mortality. ELITE-II has been criticized for using a modest dose of losartan, and therefore another randomized controlled trial similar to ELITE-II (Heart Failure Endpoint Evaluation with the Angiotensin II Antagonist Losartan Study, HEAAL) will be initiated soon in Europe using a higher dose of losartan.

Losartan has also been studied in the setting of heart failure following acute myocardial infarction. In the European OPTIMAAL trial (Optimal trial in Myocardial Infarction with Angiotensin II Antagonist Losartan), 5477 patients were randomly assigned to losartan (25 to 50 mg once daily) versus captopril (25 to 50 mg three times a day).[111] Results of this trial demonstrated no significant difference between therapies. Captopril had a more favorable trend on mortality, similar to ELITE-II (16.4% vs. 18.2% respectively, P = 0.069).[112] It is important to note that there was no significant interaction between beta blockers and ARBs, as suggested in a post-hoc analysis from ELITE. Although ARBs are better tolerated, ACE inhibitors should remain the first-choice treatment in patients with heart failure after acute myocardial infarction.

The Randomized Evaluation of Strategies for Left-ventricular Dysfunction (RESOLVD) pilot study investigated the effects of candesartan (an ARB) alone, enalapril alone, or their combination on exercise tolerance, ventricular function, quality of life, neurohormones, and tolerability in 768 patients with systolic heart failure.[113] Candesartan was as effective, safe, and well tolerated as enalapril. The combination of candesartan and enalapril was more beneficial in preventing LV remodeling than either one alone. Death, heart failure hospitalization, or any hospitalization was not significantly different among the three groups over 43 weeks of follow-up. To further investigate candesartan as a potentially useful drug for heart failure, the CHARM study was conducted and recently reported.[114] In CHARM, 7601 patients were randomly assigned candesartan (n = 3803, titrated to 32 mg once daily) or matching placebo (n = 3796). The patients were allocated into one of three different studies: (1) CHARM-Added—depressed LV systolic function (LVEF ≤40%) treated with ACE inhibitors[61]; (2) CHARM-Alternative—depressed LV systolic function and intolerance to ACE inhibitors[58]; (3) CHARM-Preserved—preserved LV function not treated with ACE inhibitors.[71] Overall, a median follow-up was 37.7 months; 886 (23%) patients in the candesartan and 945 (25%) in the placebo group died (covariate adjusted Hazard ratio 0.90, P = 0.032), with fewer cardiovascular deaths (covariate adjusted Hazard ratio 0.87, P = 0.006) and heart failure hospitalizations (20% vs. 24%, P < 0.0001) in the candesartan group. The primary endpoint of cardiovascular mortality and hospitalization for heart failure was achieved in the first two studies but not in CHARM-Preserved study.

The Val-HeFT study randomized 5010 patients with heart failure (NYHA II–IV) to receive valsartan 160 mg twice daily or placebo.[55] Valsartan or placebo was prescribed as "add-on" to standard therapy (diuretics, ACE inhibitors). The primary endpoints were mortality and a combined endpoint of morbidity and mortality, defined as the incidence of cardiac arrest with resuscitation, hospitalization for heart failure, or receipt of intravenous inotropic or vasodilator therapy for at least 4 hours. The overall mortality was similar in the two groups, indicating that valsartan added to ACE inhibitor did not improve survival. However, there were fewer patients hospitalized for heart failure in the group treated with a combination of valsartan and ACE inhibitor. Treatment with valsartan plus ACE inhibitor also resulted in significant improvement in NYHA class, ejection fraction, signs and symptoms of heart failure, quality of life, and neurohormones.

The VALIANT trial is a multicenter, double-blind, active control study comparing the efficacy and safety of long-term treatment of valsartan, captopril, or the combination of the two in high-risk patients following myocardial infarction.[59] This 14,500 patient trial is designed with three arms, giving equal statistical consideration to survival comparisons of captopril versus valsartan as well as the captopril–valsartan combination.

Aldosterone Receptor Antagonists

According to the latest guidelines, aldosterone receptor antagonists are usually reserved for patients with advanced heart failure (Stages C to D).[13] The RALES trial was done in patients with relatively advanced heart failure (NYHA IV, or NYHA III with previous Class IV symptoms).[77] It enrolled 1663 patients with heart failure (LVEF ≤ 35%) who were being treated with loop diuretics; ACE inhibitors; and in most cases, digoxin. In RALES, 822 patients were randomly assigned to spironolactone 12.5 to 25 mg daily, and 841 patients received placebo. The primary endpoint was all-cause mortality. There was an astounding 30% reduction in the risk of death among patients in the spironolactone group. Both sudden death and death from progressive heart failure were substantially reduced. In addition, spironolactone was associated with significant improvement in heart failure symptoms. The incidence of serious hyperkalemia was minimal with this small dose of spironolactone. In a RALES substudy, higher baseline serum levels of collagen synthesis markers were associated with worse outcomes and were decreased during spironolactone therapy.[115] Eplerenone has been studied in a Phase III multicenter, double-blind, placebo-controlled trial (EPHESUS)[81] in which eplerenone 25 to 50 mg daily is being compared with placebo plus standard therapy in 6644 patients with heart failure following acute myocardial infarction. The addition of eplerenone to optimal medical therapy (75% beta blocker users) reduced total all-cause mortality by 15% and reduced cardiovascular-related deaths and hospitalizations by 13%.[81] It is interesting that patients have already been optimally treated (ACE inhibitor/ARB plus beta blocker, statin, aspirin, and reperfusion) had a further 26% reduction in all-cause mortality when eplerenone was added.

Treating Patients with Stage D Heart Failure

The Stage D group includes patients with advanced heart failure requiring specialized interventions such as mechanical assist devices, continuous inotropic therapy, or heart transplantation. Such patients are generally considered in the end stages of heart failure and may even be in a hospice environment.

Although patients from the Cooperative North Scandinavian Enalapril Survival Study (CONSENSUS)[116,117] and RALES[77] were not all Stage D patients, it is clear that patients in these two studies suffered from very advanced heart failure. CONSENSUS, the seminal ACE inhibitors study, was prematurely stopped by the Data and Safety Monitoring board when there was an astonishingly obvious mortality benefit demonstrated with the use of enalapril. This study, along with the U.S. captopril heart failure program,[118] provided strong evidence that ACE inhibitors were safe and beneficial in the treatment of advanced heart failure. Blockade of the RAAS is indicated in patients with Stage D heart failure, although these patients seldom undergo investigation in randomized controlled trials. There is a greater risk of hypotension and renal insufficiency in patients with Stage D heart failure.

CONCLUSIONS

Drugs suppressing the RAAS have evolved as the cornerstone of treatment for patients with cardiovascular diseases. Their safety and effectiveness have exceeded by far our greatest expectations. Inhibition of the RAAS is associated with a substantially favorable biologic profile. Effects of RAAS inhibition are also consistently associated with improvement in clinical outcomes in patients with heart failure, hypertension, and cardiac risk factors. The mechanisms whereby inhibition of RAAS improves clinical out-

comes are still not entirely clear but are undoubtedly multifactorial. Despite our incomplete knowledge about these drugs, they have emerged as a dominant force in the management of patients with cardiovascular diseases.

The transformation from small observational studies to large-scale multicenter clinical trials began with the initiation of the study of drugs suppressing RAAS. Not only did we gain precious knowledge from the results of such important studies, but the trial methodologies have become increasingly more sophisticated in attempt to address important scientific questions. Nevertheless, many uncertainties remain. For example, is tissue penetrance of these drugs vitally important? What are the optimal doses of ACE inhibitors and ARBs? What is the timing and sequence of drug initiation? The large trials also underscore the notion that hypertension and heart failure are part of the same continuum. Drugs that improve hypertension always seem to benefit the patients with heart failure.

The use of drugs to suppress the RAAS is a prime example of the coming together of basic scientists and clinical investigators to develop therapy for a common and serious cardiovascular threat. This integrative strategy has provided a model in which future drug development for cardiovascular disease can evolve. It is a case of common and serious cardiovascular disorders driving the quest for mechanistic data, ultimately providing for testable hypotheses in large clinical trials. It is of some comfort to now see at least 30 years of highly collaborative research being translated into better patient care. We can now look forward to studies of pharmacogenomics and a better understanding as to why some patients respond more favorably than others.

Postscript

The VALIANT trial was presented at the American Heart Association Scientific Sessions in 2003. During a mean follow-up of 24.7 months, mortality in the VALIANT trial was 19.9% in the valsartan group, 19.5% in the captopril group; and 19.3% in the combined valsartan-captopril group.[120] These findings confirm the role of ARBs as an alternative to ACE inhibitors in treating patients with heart failure. However, in light of the CHARM results, the exact role of ARBs-ACE inhibitor combination in heart failure remains controversial.

REFERENCES

1. Harris P: Evolution and the cardiac patient. Cardiovasc Res 1983; 17:313-319, 373-378, 437-445.
2. Harris P: Congestive cardiac failure: Central role of the arterial blood pressure. Br Heart J 1987; 58:190-203.
3. Dzau VJ, Bernstein K, Celermajer D, et al: Pathophysiologic and therapeutic importance of tissue ACE: A Consensus Report. Cardiovasc Drugs Ther 2002; 16:149-160.
4. Dostal DE, Baker KM: The cardiac renin-angiotensin system-conceptual, or a regulator of cardiac function? Circ Res 1999; 1999.
5. Francis GS: The relationship of the sympathetic nervous system and the renin-angiotensin system in congestive heart failure. Am Heart J 1989; 118:642-648.
6. Francis GS, Cohn JN, Johnson G, et al: Plasma norepinephrine, plasma renin activity, and congestive heart failure: Relations to survival and the effects of therapy in V-HeFT II. Circulation 1993; 87:VI40-VI48.

7. Liu JL, Zucker IH: Regulation of sympathetic nerve activity in heart failure: A role for nitric oxide and angiotensin II. Circ Res 1999; 84:417–423.

8. Unger T: The role of the renin-angiotensin system in the development of cardiovascular disease. Am J Cardiol 2002; 89:3A-9A; discussion 10A.

9. Cadnapaphornchai MA, Gurevich AK, Weinberger HD, et al: Pathophysiology of sodium and water retention in heart failure. Cardiology 2001; 96:122–131.

10. Borghi C, Ambrosioni E: Evidence-based medicine and ACE inhibition. J Cardiovasc Pharmacol 1998; 32:S24–35.

11. Brunner-La Rocca HP, Vaddadi G, Esler MD: Recent insight into therapy of congestive heart failure: Focus on ACE inhibition and angiotensin-II antagonism. J Am Coll Cardiol 1999; 33:1163–1173.

12. Crackower MA, Sarao R, Oudit GY, et al: Angiotensin-converting enzyme 2 is an essential regulator of heart function. Nature 2002; 417:822–828.

13. Hunt SA, Baker DW, Chin MH, et al: ACC/AHA guidelines for the evaluation and management of chronic heart failure in the adult: Executive summary: A report of the American College of Cardiology/American Heart Association Task Force on Practice Guidelines (Committee to revise the 1995 Guidelines for the Evaluation and Management of Heart Failure). J Am Coll Cardiol 2001; 38:2101–2113.

14. Brenner BM, Cooper ME, de Zeeuw D, et al: Effects of losartan on renal and cardiovascular outcomes in patients with type 2 diabetes and nephropathy. N Engl J Med 2001; 345:861–869.

15. Parving HH, Lehnert H, Brochner-Mortensen J, et al: The effect of irbesartan on the development of diabetic nephropathy in patients with type 2 diabetes. N Engl J Med 2001; 345:870–878.

16. Opie LH, Kowolik H: The discovery of captopril: From large animals to small molecules. Cardiovasc Res 1995; 30:18–25.

17. Song JC, White CM: Clinical pharmacokinetics and selective pharmacodynamics of new angiotensin converting enzyme inhibitors: An update. Clin Pharmacokinet 2002; 41:207–224.

18. Brown NJ, Vaughan DE: Angiotensin-converting enzyme inhibitors. Circulation 1998; 97:1411–1420.

19. Sleight P, Yusuf S, Pogue J, et al: Blood-pressure reduction and cardiovascular risk in HOPE study. Lancet 2001; 358:2130–2131.

20. Thavarajah S, Mansoor GA: Are clinical endpoint benefits of angiotensin converting enzyme inhibitors independent of their blood pressure effects? Curr Hypertens Rep 2002; 4:290–297.

21. Packer M: The neurohormonal hypothesis: A theory to explain the mechanism of disease progression in heart failure. J Am Coll Cardiol 1992; 20:24–254.

22. Mathew J, Sleight P, Lonn E, et al: Reduction of cardiovascular risk by regression of electrocardiographic markers of left ventricular hypertrophy by the angiotensin-converting enzyme inhibitor ramipril. Circulation 2001; 104:1615–1621.

23. Lonn E: Angiotensin-converting enzyme inhibitors and angiotensin receptor blockers in atherosclerosis. Curr Atheroscler Rep 2002; 4:363–372.

24. Vaughan DE: The renin-angiotensin system and fibrinolysis. Am J Cardiol 1997; 79:12–16.

25. Domanski MJ, Exner DV, Borkowf CB, et al: Effect of angiotensin converting enzyme inhibition on sudden cardiac death in patients following acute myocardial infarction: A meta-analysis of randomized clinical trials. J Am Coll Cardiol 1999; 33:598–604.

26. Pacher R, Stanek B, Globits S, et al: Effects of two different enalapril dosages on clinical, haemodynamic and neurohumoral response of patients with severe congestive heart failure. Eur Heart J 1996; 17:1223–1232.

27. Tang WH, Vagelos RH, Yee YG, et al: Neurohormonal and clinical responses to high-versus low-dose enalapril therapy in chronic heart failure. J Am Coll Cardiol 2002; 39:70–78.

28. Gainer JV, Morrow JD, Loveland A, et al: Effect of bradykinin-receptor blockade on the response to angiotensin-converting-enzyme inhibitor in normotensive and hypertensive subjects. N Engl J Med 1998; 339:1285–1292.

29. Witherow FN, Helmy A, Webb DJ, et al: Bradykinin contributes to the vasodilator effects of chronic angiotensin-converting enzyme inhibition in patients with heart failure. Circulation 2001; 104:2177–2181.

30. Nikolaidis LA, Doverspike A, Huerbin R, et al: Angiotensin-converting enzyme inhibitors improve coronary flow reserve in dilated cardiomyopathy by a bradykinin-mediated, nitric oxide-dependent mechanism. Circulation 2002; 105:2785–2790.

31. Vapaatalo H, Mervaala E: Clinically important factors influencing endothelial function. Med Sci Monit 2001; 7:1075–1085.

32. Tschope C, Schultheiss HP, Walther T: Multiple interactions between the renin-angiotensin and the kallikrein-kinin systems: Role of ACE inhibition and AT1 receptor blockade. J Cardiovasc Pharmacol 2002; 39:478–487.

33. Takkouche B, Etminan M, Caamano F, et al: Interaction between aspirin and ACE Inhibitors: Resolving discrepancies using a meta-analysis. Drug Saf 2002; 25:373–378.

34. Peterson JG, Topol EJ, Sapp SK, et al: Evaluation of the effects of aspirin combined with angiotensin-converting enzyme inhibitors in patients with coronary artery disease. Am J Med 2000; 109:371–377.

35. Moskowitz R: The angiotensin-converting enzyme inhibitor and aspirin interaction in congestive heart failure: Fear or reality? Curr Cardiol Rep 2001; 3:247–253.

36. Olson KL: Combined aspirin/ACE inhibitor treatment for CHF. Ann Pharmacother 2001; 35:1653–1658.

37. Ahmed A: Interaction between aspirin and angiotensin-converting enzyme inhibitors: Should they be used together in older adults with heart failure? J Am Geriatr Soc 2002; 50:1293–1296.

38. Schoolwerth AC, Sica DA, Ballermann BJ, et al: Renal considerations in angiotensin converting enzyme inhibitor therapy: A statement for healthcare professionals from the Council on the Kidney in Cardiovascular Disease and the Council for High Blood Pressure Research of the American Heart Association. Circulation 2001; 104:1985–1991.

39. Knight EL, Glynn RJ, McIntyre KM, et al: Predictors of decreased renal function in patients with heart failure during angiotensin-converting enzyme inhibitor therapy: Results from the studies of left ventricular dysfunction (SOLVD). Am Heart J 1999; 138:849–855.

40. Frances CD, Noguchi H, Massie BM, et al: Are we inhibited? Renal insufficiency should not preclude the use of ACE inhibitors for patients with myocardial infarction and depressed left ventricular function. Arch Intern Med 2000; 160:2645–2650.

41. Suki WN: Renal hemodynamic consequences of angiotensin-converting enzyme inhibition in congestive heart failure. Arch Intern Med 1989; 149:669–673.

42. Ahmed A: Use of angiotensin-converting enzyme inhibitors in patients with heart failure and renal insufficiency: How concerned should we be by the rise in serum creatinine? J Am Geriatr Soc 2002; 50:1297–1300.

43. Mandal AK, Markert RJ, Saklayen MG, et al: Diuretics potentiate angiotensin converting enzyme inhibitor-induced acute renal failure. Clin Nephrol 1994; 42:170–174.

44. Wynckel A, Ebikili B, Melin JP, et al: Long-term follow-up of acute renal failure caused by angiotensin converting enzyme inhibitors. Am J Hypertens 1998; 11:1080–1086.

45. Bakris GL, Weir MR: Angiotensin-converting enzyme inhibitor-associated elevations in serum creatinine: Is this a cause for concern? Arch Intern Med 2000; 160:685–693.

46. Kumar A, Asim M, Davison AM: Taking precautions with ACE inhibitors: A theoretical risk exists in patients with unilateral renal artery stenosis. BMJ 1998; 316:1921.

47. Reardon LC, Macpherson DS: Hyperkalemia in outpatients using angiotensin-converting enzyme inhibitors. How much should we worry? Arch Intern Med 1998; 158:26–32.

48. Schepkens H, Vanholder R, Billiouw JM, et al: Life-threatening hyperkalemia during combined therapy with angiotensin-converting enzyme inhibitors and spironolactone: an analysis of 25 cases. Am J Med 2001; 110:438–441.

49. Ahuja TS, Freeman D Jr, Mahnken JD, et al: Predictors of the development of hyperkalemia in patients using angiotensin-converting enzyme inhibitors. Am J Nephrol 2000; 20:268–272.

50. Dzau VJ, Bernstein K, Celermajer D, et al: The relevance of tissue angiotensin-converting enzyme: manifestations in mechanistic and endpoint data. Am J Cardiol 2001; 88:1L–20L.

51. Burnier M: Angiotensin II type 1 receptor blockers. Circulation 2001; 103:904–912.

52. Jamali AH, Tang WH, Khot UN, et al: The role of angiotensin receptor blockers in the management of chronic heart failure. Arch Intern Med 2001; 161:667–672.

53. Pitt B: Clinical trials of angiotensin receptor blockers in heart failure: What do we know and what will we learn? Am J Hypertens 2002; 15:22S–27S.

54. Pitt B, Poole-Wilson PA, Segal R, et al: Effect of losartan compared with captopril on mortality in patients with symptomatic heart failure: Randomised trial: The Losartan Heart Failure Survival Study ELITE II. Lancet 2000; 355:1582–1587.

55. Cohn JN, Tognoni G: A randomized trial of the angiotensin-receptor blocker valsartan in chronic heart failure. N Engl J Med 2001; 345:1667–1675.

56. Pitt B, Segal R, Martinez FA, et al: Randomised trial of losartan versus captopril in patients over 65 with heart failure (Evaluation of Losartan in the Elderly Study, ELITE). Lancet 1997; 349: 747–752.

57. Granger CB, Ertl G, Kuch J, et al: Randomized trial of candesartan cilexetil in the treatment of patients with congestive heart failure and a history of intolerance to angiotensin-converting enzyme inhibitors. Am Heart J 2000; 139:609–617.

58. Granger CB, McMurray JJ, Yusuf S, et al: Effects of candesartan in patients with chronic heart failure and reduced left-ventricular systolic function intolerant to angiotensin-converting-enzyme inhibitors: The CHARM-Alternative trial. Lancet 2003; 362:772–776.

59. Pfeffer MA, McMurray J, Leizorovicz A, et al: Valsartan in acute myocardial infarction trial (VALIANT): Rationale and design. Am Heart J 2000; 140:727–750.

60. Pfeffer MA, Domanski M, Rosenberg Y, et al: Prevention of events with angiotensin-converting enzyme inhibition (the PEACE study design): Prevention of events with angiotensin-converting enzyme inhibition. Am J Cardiol 1998; 82:25H–30H.

61. McMurray JJ, Ostergren J, Swedberg K, et al: Effects of candesartan in patients with chronic heart failure and reduced left-ventricular systolic function taking angiotensin-converting-enzyme inhibitors: The CHARM-Added trial. Lancet 2003; 362:767–771.

62. Havranek EP, Thomas I, Smith WB, et al: Dose-related beneficial long-term hemodynamic and clinical efficacy of irbesartan in heart failure. J Am Coll Cardiol 1999; 33:1174–1181.

63. Lang RM, Elkayam U, Yellen LG, et al: Comparative effects of losartan and enalapril on exercise capacity and clinical status in patients with heart failure: The Losartan Pilot Exercise Study Investigators. J Am Coll Cardiol 1997; 30:983–991.

64. Riegger GA, Bouzo H, Petr P, et al: Improvement in exercise tolerance and symptoms of congestive heart failure during treatment with candesartan cilexetil: Symptom, Tolerability, Response to Exercise Trial of Candesartan Cilexetil in Heart Failure (STRETCH) Investigators. Circulation 1999; 100:2224–2230.

65. Parker AB, Azevedo ER, Baird MG, et al: ARCTIC: Assessment of haemodynamic response in patients with congestive heart failure to telmisartan: A multicentre dose-ranging study in Canada. Am Heart J 1999; 138:843–848.

66. Tan KC, Chow WS, Ai VH, et al: Effects of angiotensin II receptor antagonist on endothelial vasomotor function and urinary albumin excretion in type 2 diabetic patients with microalbuminuria. Diabetes Metab Res Rev 2002; 18:71–76.

67. Viberti G, Wheeldon NM: Microalbuminuria reduction with valsartan in patients with type 2 diabetes mellitus: a blood pressure-independent effect. Circulation 2002; 106:672–678.

68. Mogensen CE, Neldam S, Tikkanen I, et al: Randomised controlled trial of dual blockade of renin-angiotensin system in patients with hypertension, microalbuminuria, and non-insulin dependent diabetes: The candesartan and lisinopril microalbuminuria (CALM) study. BMJ 2000; 321:1440–1444.

69. Kramer C, Sunkomat J, Witte J, et al: Angiotensin II receptor-independent antiinflammatory and antiaggregatory properties of losartan: Role of the active metabolite EXP3179. Circ Res 2002; 90:770–776.

70. Thurmann PA, Kenedi P, Schmidt A, et al: Influence of the angiotensin II antagonist valsartan on left ventricular hypertrophy in patients with essential hypertension. Circulation 1998; 98:2037–2042.

71. Yusuf S, Pfeffer MA, Swedberg K, et al: Effects of candesartan in patients with chronic heart failure and preserved left-ventricular ejection fraction: The CHARM-Preserved Trial. Lancet 2003; 777–781.

72. Howes LG, Tran D: Can angiotensin receptor antagonists be used safely in patients with previous ACE inhibitor-induced angioedema? Drug Saf 2002; 25:73–76.

73. Rocha R, Williams GH: Rationale for the use of aldosterone antagonists in congestive heart failure. Drugs 2002; 62:723–731.

74. Palmieri EA, Biondi B, Fazio S: Aldosterone receptor blockade in the management of heart failure. Heart Fail Rev 2002; 7:205–219.

75. Soberman J, Chafin CC, Weber KT: Aldosterone antagonists in congestive heart failure. Curr Opin Investig Drugs 2002; 3:1024–1028.

76. Cicoira M, Zanolla L, Rossi A, et al: Long-term, dose-dependent effects of spironolactone on left ventricular function and exercise tolerance in patients with chronic heart failure. J Am Coll Cardiol 2002; 40:304–310.

77. Pitt B, Zannad F, Remme WJ, et al: The effect of spironolactone on morbidity and mortality in patients with severe heart failure: Randomized Aldactone Evaluation Study Investigators. N Engl J Med 1999; 341:709–717.

78. Krum H, Nolly H, Workman D, et al: Efficacy of eplerenone added to renin-angiotensin blockade in hypertensive patients. Hypertension 2002; 40:117–123.

79. Weinberger MH, Roniker B, Krause SL, et al: Eplerenone, a selective aldosterone blocker, in mild-to-moderate hypertension. Am J Hypertens 2002; 15:709–716.

80. Pitt B, Reichek N, Willenbrock R, et al: Effects of eplerenone, enalapril, and eplerenone/enalapril in patients with essential hypertension and left ventricular hypertrophy: The 4E-left ventricular hypertrophy study. Circulation 2003; 108:1831–1838.

81. Pitt B, Remme W, Zannad F, et al: Eplerenone, a selective aldosterone blocker, in patients with left ventricular dysfunction after myocardial infarction. N Engl J Med 2003; 348:1309–1321.

82. McClean DR, Ikram H, Mehta S, et al: Vasopeptidase inhibition with omapatrilat in chronic heart failure: acute and long-term hemodynamic and neurohumoral effects. J Am Coll Cardiol 2002; 39:2034–2041.

83. McClean DR, Ikram H, Garlick AH, et al: The clinical, cardiac, renal, arterial and neurohormonal effects of omapatrilat, a vasopeptidase inhibitor, in patients with chronic heart failure. J Am Coll Cardiol 2000; 36:479–486.

84. Packer M, Califf RM, Konstam MA, et al: Comparison of omapatrilat and enalapril in patients with chronic heart failure: The Omapatrilat Versus Enalapril Randomized Trial of Utility in Reducing Events (OVERTURE). Circulation 2002; 106:920–926.

85. Dendorfer A, Raasch W, Tempel K, et al: Interactions between the renin-angiotensin system (RAS) and the sympathetic system. Basic Res Cardiol 1998; 93:24–29.

86. Akers WS, Cross A, Speth R, et al: Renin-angiotensin system and sympathetic nervous system in cardiac pressure-overload hypertrophy. Am J Physiol Heart Circ Physiol 2000; 279:H2797–2806.

87. Gheorghiade M: Neurohumoral effects of digoxin: A target for further investigation. Cardiologia 1996; 41:967–972.

88. Yusuf S, Sleight P, Pogue J, et al: Effects of an angiotensin-converting-enzyme inhibitor, ramipril, on cardiovascular events in high-risk patients: The Heart Outcomes Prevention Evaluation Study Investigators. N Engl J Med 2000; 342:145–153.

89. Pfeffer MA, Braunwald E, Moye LA, et al: Effect of captopril on mortality and morbidity in patients with left ventricular dysfunction after myocardial infarction: Results of the survival and ventricular enlargement trial: The SAVE Investigators. N Engl J Med 1992; 327:669–677.

90. The SOLVD Investigators: Effect of enalapril on survival in patients with reduced left ventricular ejection fractions and congestive heart failure. N Engl J Med 1991; 325:293–302.

91. The SOLVD Investigators: Effect of enalapril on mortality and the development of heart failure in asymptomatic patients with reduced left ventricular ejection fractions. N Engl J Med 1992; 327:685–691.

92. Heart Outcomes Prevention Evaluation Study Investigators: Effects of ramipril on cardiovascular and microvascular outcomes in people with diabetes mellitus: Results of the HOPE study and MICRO-HOPE substudy. Lancet 2000; 355:253–259.

93. The EURopean trial On reduction of cardiac events with Perindopril in stable coronary Artery disease Investigators: Efficacy of perindopril in reduction of cardiovascular events among patients with stable coronary artery disease: Randomised, double-blind, placebo-controlled, multicentre trial (the EUROPA study). Lancet 2003; 362:782–788.

94. PROGRESS Collaborative Group: Randomised trial of a perindopril-based blood-pressure-lowering regimen among 6,105 individuals

with previous stroke or transient ischaemic attack. Lancet 2001; 358:1033-1041.

95. Svensson P, de Faire U, Sleight P, et al: Comparative effects of ramipril on ambulatory and office blood pressures: A HOPE Substudy. Hypertension 2001; 38:E28-32.

96. Yusuf S: From the HOPE to the ONTARGET and the TRANSCEND studies: challenges in improving prognosis. Am J Cardiol 2002; 89:18A-25A; discussion 25A-26A.

97. Konstam MA, Kronenberg MW, Rousseau MF, et al: Effects of the angiotensin converting enzyme inhibitor enalapril on the long-term progression of left ventricular dilatation in patients with asymptomatic systolic dysfunction: SOLVD (Studies of Left Ventricular Dysfunction) Investigators. Circulation 1993; 88:2277-2283.

98. Agabiti-Rosei E, Ambrosioni E, Dal Palu C, et al: ACE inhibitor ramipril is more effective than the beta-blocker atenolol in reducing left ventricular mass in hypertension. Results of the RACE (ramipril cardioprotective evaluation) study on behalf of the RACE study group. J Hypertens 1995; 13:1325-1334.

99. Devereux RB, Palmieri V, Sharpe N, et al: Effects of once-daily angiotensin-converting enzyme inhibition and calcium channel blockade-based antihypertensive treatment regimens on left ventricular hypertrophy and diastolic filling in hypertension: the prospective randomized enalapril study evaluating regression of ventricular enlargement (PRESERVE) trial. Circulation 2001; 104:1248-1254.

100. Dahlof B, Devereux RB, Kjeldsen SE, et al: Cardiovascular morbidity and mortality in the Losartan Intervention For Endpoint reduction in hypertension study (LIFE): A randomised trial against atenolol. Lancet 2002; 359:995-1003.

101. Greenberg B, Quinones MA, Koilpillai C, et al: Effects of long-term enalapril therapy on cardiac structure and function in patients with left ventricular dysfunction: Results of the SOLVD echocardiography substudy. Circulation 1995; 91:2573-2581.

102. Cohn JN, Johnson G, Ziesche S, et al: A comparison of enalapril with hydralazine-isosorbide dinitrate in the treatment of chronic congestive heart failure. N Engl J Med 1991; 325:303-310.

103. Effect of ramipril on mortality and morbidity of survivors of acute myocardial infarction with clinical evidence of heart failure: The Acute Infarction Ramipril Efficacy (AIRE) Study Investigators. Lancet 1993; 342:821-828.

104. Kober L, Torp-Pedersen C, Carlsen JE, et al: A clinical trial of the angiotensin-converting-enzyme inhibitor trandolapril in patients with left ventricular dysfunction after myocardial infarction: Trandolapril Cardiac Evaluation (TRACE) Study Group. N Engl J Med 1995; 333:1670-1676.

105. Sleight P: Angiotensin II and trials of cardiovascular outcomes. Am J Cardiol 2002; 89:11A-16A.

106. de Kam PJ, Voors AA, van den Berg MP, et al: Effect of very early angiotensin-converting enzyme inhibition on left ventricular dilation after myocardial infarction in patients receiving thrombolysis: Results of a meta-analysis of 845 patients. FAMIS, CAPTIN and CATS Investigators. J Am Coll Cardiol 2000; 36:2047-2053.

107. Indications for ACE inhibitors in the early treatment of acute myocardial infarction: systematic overview of individual data from 100,000 patients in randomized trials: ACE Inhibitor Myocardial Infarction Collaborative Group. Circulation 1998; 97:2202-2212.

108. Otterstad J, Ford I: The effect of carvedilol in patients with impaired left ventricular systolic function following an acute myocardial infarction: How do the treatment effects on total mortality and recurrent myocardial infarction in CAPRICORN compare with previous beta-blocker trials? Eur J Heart Fail 2002; 4:501.

109. Packer M, Poole-Wilson PA, Armstrong PW, et al: Comparative effects of low and high doses of the angiotensin-converting enzyme inhibitor, lisinopril, on morbidity and mortality in chronic heart failure. ATLAS Study Group. Circulation 1999; 100:2312-2318.

110. Brooksby P, Robinson PJ, Segal R, et al: Effects of losartan and captopril on QT dispersion in elderly patients with heart failure: ELITE study group. Lancet 1999; 354:395-396.

111. Dickstein K, Kjekshus J: Comparison of the effects of losartan and captopril on mortality in patients after acute myocardial infarction: The OPTIMAAL trial design. Optimal Therapy in Myocardial Infarction with the Angiotensin II Antagonist Losartan. Am J Cardiol 1999; 83:477-481.

112. Dickstein K, Kjekshus J, and the OPTIMAAL Steering Committee, for the OPTIMAAL Study Group: Effects of losartan and captopril on mortality and morbidity in high-risk patients after acute myocardial infarction: the OPTIMAAL randomised trial. Lancet 2002; 360:752-760.

113. McKelvie RS, Yusuf S, Pericak D, et al: Comparison of candesartan, enalapril, and their combination in congestive heart failure: Randomized evaluation of strategies for left ventricular dysfunction (RESOLVD) pilot study: The RESOLVD Pilot Study Investigators. Circulation 1999; 100:1056-1064.

114. Pfeffer MA, Swedberg K, Granger CB, et al: Effects of candesartan on mortality and morbidity in patients with chronic heart failure: The CHARM-Overall programme. Lancet 2003; 362:759-766.

115. Zannad F, Alla F, Dousset B, et al: Limitation of excessive extracellular matrix turnover may contribute to survival benefit of spironolactone therapy in patients with congestive heart failure: Insights from the randomized aldactone evaluation study (RALES). RALES Investigators. Circulation 2000; 102:2700-2706.

116. The CONSENSUS Trial Study Group: Effects of enalapril on mortality in severe congestive heart failure: Results of the Cooperative North Scandinavian Enalapril Survival Study (CONSENSUS). N Engl J Med 1987; 316:1429-1435.

117. Swedberg K, Kjekshus J, Snapinn S: Long-term survival in severe heart failure in patients treated with enalapril: Ten year follow-up of CONSENSUS I. Eur Heart J 1999; 20:136-139.

118. Captopril Multicenter Research Group: A placebo-controlled trial of captopril in refractory chronic congestive heart failure. J Am Coll Cardiol 1983; 2:755-763.

119. The NETWORK Investigators: Clinical outcome with enalapril in symptomatic chronic heart failure: a dose comparison. Eur Heart J 1998; 19:481-489.

120. Pfeffer MA, McMurray JJ, Velazquez EJ, et al: Valsartan, captopril, or both in myocardial infarction complicated by heart failure, left ventricular dysfunction, or both. N Engl J Med 2003; 349:1893-1996.

Beta Blockers

Eric J. Eichhorn

Heart failure is a syndrome of progressive right-ventricular and left-ventricular (LV) dysfunction and symptoms resulting from a process of pathologic ventricular remodeling.[1] This pathologic remodeling process is a result of biologic alterations in the myocytes and interstitium of the heart with progressive loss of myocytes and contractile units resulting from cell death. The signals driving this pathologic process are load[1,2] and neurohormonal activation.[1,3-6] Medical therapy directed at either reducing neurohormonal effects (angiotensin-converting enzyme [ACE] inhibitors, beta blockers, aldosterone antagonists) or reducing load without concomitant neurohormonal activation (nitrates, natriuretic peptide agonists, diuretics) may be effective treatments for patients with heart failure.

PATHOPHYSIOLOGY OF HEART FAILURE PROGRESSION

Bioenergetic and Phenotypic Changes in the Failing Heart

To understand the rationale for use of a beta blocker to treat heart failure, it is important to understand the mechanism by which the heart progressively fails. The pathophysiology of heart failure is depicted in Figure 20-1.[1] Heart failure initiates as a result of an insult to the heart muscle. In the United States, approximately 70% of heart failure cases are a result of ischemic heart disease and myocardial infarction.[7] In the African-American community, long-standing hypertension is a major cause of heart failure.[8] Heart failure also may result from genetic or idiopathic causes or from valvular disease or myocarditis. Damage to the myocardium results in an increase in loading conditions in the heart, and this leads to tissue-level activation of neurohormonal pathways (natruretic peptides,[9] tumor necrosis factor-alpha [TNF-α][10] angiotensin II[11,12]) as a result of atrial and ventricular stretch. The reduction in stroke volume as a result of loss of contractile units from the initial injury results in the following: (1) poor renal perfusion, which leads to renin-angiotensin activation systemically[1] and (2) resetting of baroreceptors, causing deinhibition of sympathetic drive and activation of the adrenergic nervous system.[4] These key neurohormonal pathways cross-activate each other as renin is released in response to

$\beta1$ stimulation from the adrenergic nervous system[13] and norepinephrine is released in response to presynaptic AT1 stimulation from angiotensin.[14] Nonosmotic release of vasopressin (AVP) is accomplished by both β-adrenergic[15] and angiotensin-II[16] receptor mechanisms in the neurohypophysis.

Short-term effects of this neurohormonal activation are salt and water reabsorption in the kidney producing an increase in preload in the heart and increasing stroke volume by a Starling mechanism. Contractility and heart rate are increased by norepinephrine, angiotensin II, and perhaps endothelin stimulation. These short-term adaptations are acute responses that maintain circulation.

Longer term compensation occurs by increasing the number of contractile elements.[1] This process of developing new contractile elements accounts for the primary process of hypertrophy and ventricular remodeling, which is a major cause of heart failure progression.[1,17,18] Angiotensin II,[11,12,19] norepinephrine,[20-25] endothelins,[26] cardiotrophins,[27,28] cytokines,[29,30] neuropeptide Y,[23] and other hormones such as insulinlike growth factor[31] may all activate downstream pathways in the heart, which promotes growth and hypertrophy in the failing myocyte. Norepinephrine may produce a growth response via the α-receptor by activating protein kinase C and inositol 1,4,5-triphosphate (IP$_3$), which may produce mitogen-activated protein (MAP) kinase activation[21,22] or may activate cyclic adenosine monophosphate (cAMP) response elements (cAMP response element binding [CREB]) by a protein kinase A pathway.[24] Norepinephrine may also produce a growth response via the β-receptors by activation of downstream cAMP response elements[26] and may produce calcium overload, which may activate the calmodulin-calcineurin-CAM kinase pathways.[32-34] Although the exact mechanisms of downstream growth activation are not elucidated, it is clear that inhibition of the β-adrenergic pathways in patients with heart failure has the potential to reverse this pathologic growth process.[35,36]

Within the myocyte, the remodeling process begins as contractile units are added in series rather than in parallel.[37] Thus, the failing myocyte thickens slightly and elongates significantly. This results directly in a large increase in chamber radius with only a modest increase in wall thickness. By LaPlace's law, wall stress is increased by this architecture, leading to high preload and afterload. The increase in afterload (end-systolic wall stress) impairs LV emptying (performance),[38] and the increase in preload

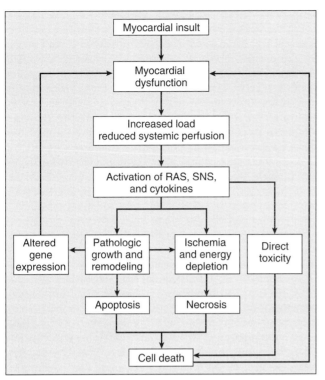

FIGURE 20-1. Relationship of neurohormonal activation and production of cardiac myocyte loss as a result of apoptosis and necrosis and altered gene expression. Cell loss and altered gene expression results in more myocardial dysfunction, and a vicious cycle is established. (From Eichhorn EJ, Bristow MR: Medical therapy can improve the biologic properties of the chronically failing heart: A new era in the treatment of heart failure. Circulation 1996; 94:2285–2296. Reprinted with permission of the American Heart Association.)

(diastolic wall stress) results in stress on the mitral subvalvular apparatus and annulus, leading to functional mitral insufficiency.[17,39,40] These changes in architecture lead to a change in shape in the left ventricle from elliptical to more spherical or globular in shape.

Both neurohormonal activation and calcium overload as a result of activation of the downstream β-adrenergic pathway results in a change in contractile proteins and calcium regulatory proteins within the myocyte, which recapitulates a fetal-like phenotype.[1,41,42] There may be downregulation of cardiac α-actin and α-myosin heavy chain and an upregulation in the more fetal-like, slower β-myosin heavy chain. Even minor downregulation of α-myosin heavy chain may lead to significant impairment of ventricular function.[43] There may also be downregulation of calcium regulatory proteins such as sarcoplasmic reticulum calcium ATPase (adenosine 5′ triphosphate) (smooth endoplasmic reticulum C^{++} antiporter [SERCA]), leading to diastolic calcium overload.[42,44]

Activation of matrix metalloproteases may result from aldosterone[45–47] and TNF-α[48] activation within the interstitium. This activation may produce dissolution of the normal interstitial framework that anchors the myocytes.[47,49] Without this framework, the myocytes contract less efficiently and the increase in myocyte slippage produces an increase in ventricular volumes, a change in shape of the ventricle, and a reduction in the force of contraction.[17,49] Because myocytes die as a

result of apoptosis and necrosis, an augmentation of collagen synthesis is produced by fibroblasts stimulated by aldosterone and angiotensin II.[45,46] This process produces replacement fibrosis, which is inelastic, increases chamber stiffness, and produces no contractile force.

A major problem in heart failure is the relative energy depletion and ischemia that may result from neurohormonal activation, load, and the biologic changes that follow.[1,50,51] The relative ischemia exacerbates the vicious cycle of heart failure. Relative ischemia may occur in the dilated failing heart for several reasons: (1) Elevated heart rate and high wall stress or load in the dilated heart produces an increase in myocardial oxygen consumption (oxygen demand). (2) Change in interstitial and myocyte architecture produces an increase in intercapillary distance as a result of hypertrophy and interstitial collagen deposition, which impairs diffusion of oxygen.[52,53] This leads to a reduction in the vascularity to myocyte ratio. (3) Reduced blood pressure as a result of a low stroke volume and elevated ventricular diastolic pressures leads to a reduction in transmyocardial (epicardial to endocardial) driving pressure for oxygenated blood. This may lead to endocardial underperfusion. Positron emission tomography has shown evidence of a mismatch in viability and perfusion in regions of heart tissue in patients with dilated cardiomyopathy.[54] This mismatch is most pronounced in ventricles with high wall stress. (4) Histologic evidence of mitochondrial changes have been noted, although the significance of these changes is unclear.[55] (5) Creatine phosphokinase, a key enzyme for transport of high-energy phosphates from the mitochondria to the cytosol, may be downregulated in heart failure.[56,57] (6) High ATP concentrations may exert allosteric effects on calcium ion exchangers and ion pumps in the myocyte, enhancing both contraction force and relaxation.[58,59] A reduction in ATP would thus result in a reduction in calcium flux producing a diminished contractile force and slower relaxation. (7) The increase in adrenergic activity in the failing heart may lead to an increase in free fatty acid utilization.[60-62] This fuel is less efficient than glucose at producing ATP when oxygen is limited.[60,61,63] Changes in the phenotype of the failing heart produced by neurohormonal activation and energetic/metabolic shifts may result in a shift in the phenotype of contractile proteins and calcium transient proteins to slower and less contractile isoforms.[1,41,42,64-68] These isoforms slow ATP utilization and may be energy "sparing," but they are not necessarily energy efficient. For all of these reasons, the failing heart is energy starved, poorly contractile, inefficient, and relatively ischemic.

β-Adrenergic Desensitization in the Failing Heart

Another problem in heart failure is the alteration in β-adrenergic pathway. In response to adrenergic activity at the cell surface, the neurotransmitter norepinephrine is released and both α- and β-adrenergic receptors are activated. Release of norepinephrine can be modulated locally by presynaptic α2 receptors (inhibitory)[69] and presynaptic angiotensin II,[14,70,71] β2 receptors[72,73] and bradykinin receptors (facilitory).[71,74] Thus, ACE inhibitors and angiotensin receptor blockers will initially reduce adrenergic activity in part by inhibiting norepinephrine release.[14,70,71] Postsynaptic norepinephrine from the adrenergic nervous system stimulates β-receptors and elevated circulating epinephrine stimulates β2 receptors. The signals from these β-adrenergic receptors are transduced and amplified by G-stimulatory guanine nucleotide binding proteins-adenylate cyclase complex (Gs).[75] The alpha-subunit of these Gs proteins may directly open L-type calcium channels in the sarcolemma and allow calcium influx.[76] The adenylate cyclase activity in this complex produces cAMP from ATP. cAMP increases the activity of protein kinases, which phosphorylate several intracellular proteins.[77] Sarcolemmal protein phosphorylation and ryanodine receptor/Ca^{2+} release channel phosphorylation results in both L-channel Ca^{2+} influx and Ca^{2+} release from the sarcoplasmic reticulum respectively.[77] Phospholamban, a protein located within the sarcoplasmic reticulum, is likewise phosphorylated, resulting in its deactivation and deinhibition of sarcoplasmic reticulum calcium ATPase (SERCA 2) activity.[78] These events cause increased cytosolic Ca^{2+} flux, producing calcium overload.[79] In addition, the inhibitory subunit of troponin and myosin-binding protein C are phosphorylated.[80] Phosphorylation of these intracellular proteins results in positive chronotropic, inotropic, and lusitropic effects.

Long-term adrenergic activation from heart failure produces a desensitization of this pathway, which includes the following: (1) downregulation and perhaps some uncoupling of β1 receptors to adenylate cyclase activity,[81] (2) uncoupling of β2 receptors to adenylate cyclase,[81] (3) upregulation of the Gi (inhibitory G-protein),[82] and (4) upregulation of β-adrenergic receptor kinase.[83] These changes serve to reduce downstream production of cAMP.[84] The reduction in cAMP produces less phosphorylation of phospholamban,[85] leading to more inhibition of SERCA2, and this in turn may produce more ventricular dysfunction and cardiomyopathy.[86] The clinical significance of β-receptor desensitization is a reduction in myocardial reserve and exercise tolerance in times of stress or physical activity.[87]

TRIALS OF THE EFFECTS OF BETA BLOCKADE ON VENTRICULAR FUNCTION, REMODELING, ENERGETICS, AND EXERCISE TOLERANCE

Ventricular Function and Remodeling

In 1975 a group of Swedish investigators administered a beta blocker to a woman with refractory heart failure and tachycardia.[88] The aim of this novel approach was to slow the heart rate enough to allow improved diastolic filling, thereby reducing her filling pressures. They noted that over time, the patient improved her ventricular function, and two subsequent case series demonstrated that long-term therapy with beta blockade produced improvement in shortening fraction and symptoms, and withdrawal resulted in deterioration.[89,90] This concept was counterintuitive because a negative inotrope was felt to be contraindicated in a heart failure patient. These early case

series were met with significant skepticism. Two subsequent studies of 1-month duration, a period too short to demonstrate improvement with beta blockers, were negative, and this served to augment worldwide cynicism about the utility of this therapy.[91,92] It was 10 more years until a placebo-controlled study in the United States found significant improvement in exercise tolerance with metoprolol[93] and a study from Utah suggested possible long-term benefit.[94] These promising studies opened the door for more investigation, although persistent skepticism for a counterintuitive therapy remained strong. Over the ensuing 5 to 10 years, multiple small mechanistic studies in Europe and the United States found consistent improvement in left-ventricular ejection fraction (LVEF) and symptoms with beta blockade.[95-108]

Four studies mechanistically examined whether the improvement in LVEF was as a result of improvement in contractility or an alteration in loading conditions.[106-109] Using relatively load-independent indices[106-108] and isolated myocyte preparations,[109] these studies found that ventricular function improved as a result of an increase in chamber and myocyte performance and contractility, which appeared by 3 months of therapy. One study examined the time course of ventricular function changes using serial echocardiograms and found that the initial effect of beta blocker therapy on the first day of therapy was a reduction in LVEF (Fig. 20-2).[35] This was felt to be a result of pharmacologic withdrawal of adrenergic support to the failing ventricle and supported the concept of starting beta blockers at very low dose to minimize adrenergic withdrawal. By 1 month of metoprolol therapy in this study, ejection fraction was similar to baseline. However, by 3 months, ejection fraction had improved significantly over baseline and LV chamber dimensions were reduced. This very late effect was felt to be a biologic effect of adrenergic withdrawal on the myocyte.[1]

This same study examined late changes in LV architecture with beta blocker therapy added to background ACE inhibitors. The authors found a reduction in LV mass and an increase in the length to radius dimensions after

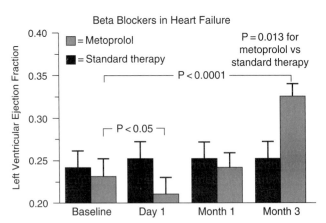

FIGURE 20-2. Changes in left-ventricular ejection fraction at baseline, day 1, month 1, and month 3 are shown for the metoprolol and standard therapy groups. Ejection fraction decreased at 1 day and increased only after 1 month of therapy. In the standard therapy group, the ejection fraction did not change. (From Hall SA, Cigarroa CG, Marcoux L, et al: Time course of improvement in left ventricular function, mass, and geometry in patients with congestive heart failure treated with β-adrenergic blockade. J Am Coll Cardiol 1995; 25:1154–1161.)

18 months of metoprolol therapy.[35] This meant that the combination of beta blockers and ACE inhibitors not only attenuated pathologic remodeling but in many cases reversed this process. Hypertrophy was reduced and the ventricular chamber went from spherical to more elliptical in shape. The reduction in ventricular chamber size and change in shape to elliptical may be the reason why functional mitral insufficiency is reduced in patients receiving beta blockers.[36] These findings were confirmed by a study of carvedilol showing reverse remodeling after 12 months of therapy.[36]

Energetics

It is important that the improvement in ventricular performance in the patient with an ischemic, energy-depleted ventricle not come at the cost of an increase in myocardial oxygen consumption, which can lead to further energy depletion.[51,57] This may lead to calcium overload, arrhythmias, and cell injury/death. This may lead to an increase in patient mortality. Although agents that act pharmacologically may improve ventricular function acutely, they also may increase myocardial oxygen consumption in a dose-related or function-related manner.[110] By contrast, beta blockers improve ventricular function by biologic and energetic changes rather than by pharmacologic stimulation.[1,42] This results in a reduction in arrhythmias, cell death, and prolongation of survival of patients. Two studies of energetics in patients with heart failure taking beta blockers demonstrated a trend toward reduction in myocardial oxygen consumption despite an increase in mechanical work of the ventricle.[106,107] This means that myocardial mechanical efficiency is improving with beta blocker therapy. One of these studies suggested a link between adrenergic stimulation and substrate utilization and further suggested that some of the improvement in mechanical efficiency might have been a result of a shift in substrate utilization from free fatty acids, an inefficient fuel in the face of ischemia, to glucose, a more oxygen-efficient fuel.[106] Other reasons for improved efficiency may be a result of reduced calcium overload,[111] phenotypic changes in intracellular proteins to more efficient isoforms (see later in this chapter),[42] reductions in functional mitral insufficiency,[36] reductions in heat generation, and a reduction in load allowing more efficient use of contractile force.[38]

Exercise Tolerance

The ability to exercise is dependent on many different conditions including the ability of the heart to respond to adrenergic drive and peripheral adaptations. A direct linear relationship has been shown between β-receptor density and VO_2 max, suggesting that β-receptor desensitization may play a contributory role in the reduced exercise tolerance found in patients with heart failure.[87] Because beta blockers work by competitively inhibiting adrenergic activity at the receptor, it is no surprise that beta blockers have shown little or no ability to improve maximal exercise tolerance despite consistently showing improvement in symptomatology. Nonselective beta blockers that block all adrenergic effects on the myocyte have shown no ability to improve exercise

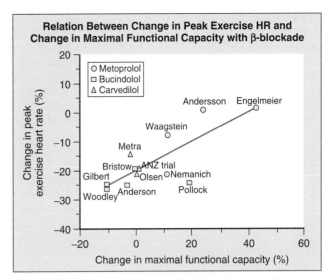

FIGURE 20-3. Relationship between the change in maximal functional capacity (%) and change in peak exercise heart rate (%) for multiple beta blocker trials with the selective agent metoprolol (*circles*) or the nonselective agents bucindolol (*squares*) and carvedilol (*triangles*). Only the selective agents have improvement in functional capacity. (From Metra M, Nodari S, D'Aloia A, et al: Effects of neurohormonal antagonism on symptoms and quality-of-life in heart failure. Eur Heart J 1998; 19 (Suppl B): B25–35.)

tolerance,[112-118] whereas β1-selective agents, which allow some transmission of adrenergic effects via the β2 receptor, have shown modest improvement (Fig. 20-3).[93,119]

CELLULAR AND MOLECULAR EFFECTS OF BETA BLOCKADE

Long-term therapy with beta-blocking agents produce improvements in systolic function, energetics, and a reversal of the pathologic remodeling process.[1,35,36,106-109] The improvement in energetics may be a result of several factors: (1) a reduction in heart rate, a major determinant of myocardial oxygen consumption; (2) a reduction in systolic and diastolic wall stress, another major determinant of myocardial oxygen consumption[120]; (3) a shift in substrate utilization from free fatty acids to glucose, a more efficient fuel in the face of myocardial ischemia[60-62,106]; and (4) a shift in phenotype of the failing heart to more energy-efficient isoforms.[41-43] The amount of heart rate reduction provided by beta blockers is dependent on their pharmacologic properties including beta-selectivity (i.e., β1 or β2 selective vs. nonselective), amount of intrinsic sympathomimetic activity, and degree of inverse agonism (the ability of a beta blocker to inactivate active state receptors).[121-123] By Holter recording, nonselective agents tend to reduce maximal heart rate the most, whereas agents with strong inverse agonism tend to reduce minimal heart rate the most. Agents with intrinsic sympathomimetic activity tend to raise minimal heart rates, especially nocturnal heart rates while patients are sleeping.[124] Partial agonists should never be used in heart failure because they increase mortality.[124] The reduction in systolic and diastolic wall stress is a result of the reverse remodeling process with a large reduction in the radius of the failing heart. By LaPlace's law, such a reduction in radius will reduce wall stress or load of the heart significantly. As load is reduced, the heart ejects more blood with the same contractile force and the same or reduced energy consumption.[120] Because heart rate and wall stress are major determinants of myocardial oxygen consumption,[120] a reduction in heart rate and wall stress will produce a large decrease in ischemia and energy depletion.

Because adrenergic effects on the heart increase free fatty acid utilization,[62] beta blockade tends to shift substrate utilization toward glucose,[106] a more oxygen-efficient fuel. Fatty acids and glucose provide a majority of substrate for energy production in the heart. As mentioned, patients with heart failure have an ischemic, energy-depleted ventricle, even if they do not have coronary artery disease.[51,54] Although there are many reasons for ischemia and energy depletion in the failing ventricle, one primary reason is a shift in substrate utilization from glucose to free fatty acids, which is partially driven by the adrenergic activation of heart failure.[62,106] Catecholamines and hyperadrenergic states clearly force free fatty acid utilization by the heart. Under aerobic conditions and at normal workloads, the heart generates ATP by oxidation of free fatty acids whereas glucose is less important. However, free fatty acids produce approximately 5.6 ATPs per molecule of O_2 consumed as compared to glucose, which produces 6.3 ATPs per molecule of O_2 consumed.[63] Thus, in the presence of ischemia, glucose is a much more oxygen-efficient substrate for the heart to use. This is exemplified by the addition of glucose and insulin to an ischemic hypertrophied rat heart, which produces improved energetics, an increase in developed pressure, and a reduction in end-diastolic pressure.[125] Much of the increase in diastolic pressure with ischemia may be mediated by rigor-mediated mechanisms as a result of disordered high-energy phosphate metabolism, which can be corrected by insulin and glucose.[126] The use of beta blockers helps to shift substrate utilization more to glucose, thus improving oxygen efficiency and improving diastolic function.[106]

As the heart fails, there is energy depletion, calcium overload, and a change in the phenotype of several important proteins controlling contraction, relaxation, and load.[1,41,42] These phenotypic changes allow the heart to "downregulate" energy expenditure by slowing ATP expenditure for contraction, calcium reuptake, and potassium extrusion. Some of these changes include an upregulation in gene expression of natriuretic peptides and β-myosin heavy chain and downregulation in the expression of SR-calcium ATPase, α-myosin heavy chain, creatine phosphokinase, and genes encoding outward potassium (K^+) currents (I_{to}).[1,41,42,127,128] These shifts in gene expression recapitulate embryonic or neonatal patterns and have been termed activation of a "fetal" program.[1,41,42,50] Angiotensin-II,[11,12,19] endothelin-1,[26] and adrenergic stimulation[20-25,42] have been shown to be potent inducers of the fetal/hypertrophy gene program in model systems. In addition, the prolongation of action potentials by downregulation of I_{to} can increase Ca^{2+} influx through L-type Ca^{2+} channels in the sarcolemma, thereby elevating intracellular calcium levels.[127] This may lead to activation of several hypertrophy-signaling pathways including mitogen-activated protein kinases

(MAPK); protein kinase C; and most importantly, the calcineurin pathway.[32-34] Activation of these hypertrophic pathways may lead to further shifts in phenotype and activation of a fetal-like genetic program.

The downregulation of α-myosin heavy chain and upregulation of the more fetal-like, slower β-myosin heavy chain results in less utilization of ATP[41-43] but may not be as efficient as the adult isoform (because less mechanical work is performed). In addition, in the failing heart there may be downregulation of SR-calcium ATPase (SERCA 2a).[41,42,44] Impairment in the normal phospholamban-SERCA 2a relationship by either overexpressing phospholamban (a protein that inhibits SERCA-2a when activated) or by inhibiting SERCA-2a will result in contractile deficiency and progressive heart failure.[44,85,86] Thus a reduction in SERCA-2a will produce more calcium overload and diastolic dysfunction. Creatine phosphokinase is an enzyme-controlling transfer of ATP from the mitochondria to the cytosol.[128] Downregulation of this enzyme would produce a deficit in high-energy phosphate in the cytosol. Use of beta blockade reverses or partially reverses some of these alterations.[42] After beta blockade, there is upregulation of the faster adult α-myosin heavy chain; downregulation of the slower, more fetal-like β-myosin heavy chain; and upregulation of SERCA-2a in patients who have improvement in ventricular function. Patients who have no improvement in ventricular function do not have a reversal in phenotype to the faster, higher energy-consuming adult isoforms. Thus, part of the explanation for improved ventricular function in heart failure patients taking beta blockers may be the reversal in phenotype. Furthermore, although an upregulation in creatine phosphokinase and I_{to} with beta blockers has never been shown, if beta blockers were to improve outward potassium current, it could lead to less Ca^{2+} overload, less activation of hypertrophic pathways such as calcineurin, and less risk of dangerous arrhythmias. Because beta blockers reduce sudden death in clinical trials, this is a possible contributing mechanism.

Use of beta blockade in a canine model of heart failure results in a reduction in apoptosis both in the border zone of myocardial injury and in remote areas of myocardium.[129] The reduction in cell death, shift in molecular phenotype, and improvement in energetics of the failing heart produces a biologic benefit that may take 1 to 3 months to appear clinically.[35]

RELATIONSHIP OF VIABILITY TO BIOLOGIC IMPROVEMENT

If the benefit of beta blockade on ventricular function is modulated biologically,[1] then the corollary to this hypothesis would be that the degree of improvement would be related to the amount of viable myocardium present when beta blockers are initiated. One study demonstrated a greater amount of hemodynamic improvement in patients with less fibrosis on endomyocardial biopsy.[130] A recent study of contractile reserve in response to intravenous dobutamine prior to beta blockade, a surrogate measure of myocardial viability, demonstrated a linear relationship between contractile reserve and improvement in LVEF after 3 months of therapy with bucindolol.[131] Univariate regression analysis revealed contractile reserve, systolic blood pressure, and LV end-systolic volume to be predictors of improvement in LVEF after beta blockade. However, only contractile reserve was an independent predictor by multivariate analysis. The patients in this study who had no contractile reserve were more likely to have jugular venous distention and peripheral edema than patients with contractile reserve. These data suggest that beta blocker therapy should be initiated as early as possible when contractile reserve is most preserved. Because there is a disconnection between pathologic ventricular remodeling and development of symptoms,[132] the choice of when to start a beta blocker should be more a function of the status of ventricular performance and size rather than presence of symptoms. Patients may have severe pathologic remodeling of the ventricle with little symptomatology. If beta blocker therapy is delayed as a result of a lack of severe symptoms, it will result in the loss of more myocytes (contractile units) through necrosis and apoptosis, the production of more fibrosis, and a lesser eventual response to beta blockade. Because the use of a beta blocker balances the biologic improvement in ejection fraction (from improvement in phenotype and energetics) versus the pharmacologic worsening of ejection fraction (from adrenergic withdrawal), the net effect will depend on viability.[131] Patients with more viability will have a net effect producing improvement in ejection fraction. By contrast, those with little viability will have a net no change or worsening of ejection fraction. Because there may be a relation between improvement in ejection fraction and a reduction in mortality,[133] it is imperative to treat early.

EARLY CLINICAL TRIALS WITH BETA BLOCKADE

From 1975 to the mid 1990s there were multiple small mechanistic trials examining the effect of β-blockade on LV function, exercise tolerance, and symptoms.[88-109] These small pilot trials were generally favorable showing improvement in LV function and symptoms. However, improvement in exercise tolerance was either marginally better or no better after beta blocker therapy.

The first multicenter trial of beta blockade was the Metoprolol in Dilated Cardiomyopathy (MDC) trial.[119] This study randomized 383 patients with heart failure as a result of idiopathic causes to metoprolol or placebo. The primary endpoint of this pilot trial was death or need for transplantation. There were 34% (95% CI -6 to 62%, P = 0.058) fewer endpoints in the metoprolol than placebo group. The primary effect appeared to be metoprolol's ability to reduce the need for transplantation (19 vs. 2 patients). These data suggested that metoprolol prevented pump failure progression and was a pivotal pilot study that formed the basis of subsequent, larger, multicenter trials. In addition, this study demonstrated a modest improvement in exercise tolerance and an improvement in ejection fraction with metoprolol tartrate.

Three larger studies were performed to examine the clinical effects of beta blockade and were pivotal to establishing a rationale for larger mortality studies: Cardiac Insufficiency Bisoprolol (CIBIS) trial,[134] the U.S. Carvedilol program,[114-117,135] and the Australia–New Zealand Carvedilol study.[118,136] The Cardiac Insufficiency Bisoprolol (CIBIS) trial[134] randomized 641 patients with heart failure to the β1 selective agent, bisoprolol, or placebo and found a 20% reduction in mortality (RR = 0.80, CI 0.56-1.15, P = 0.22). However, this did not reach statistical significance because the trial was underpowered. A post-hoc analysis of a subgroup of patients in this study who had echocardiograms performed at baseline and 5 months of therapy found a relationship between the change in LVEF and outcome.[133] Patients randomized to bisoprolol who had improvement in ejection fraction had a reduction in mortality compared to placebo patients. By contrast, there was a small group of patients randomized to bisoprolol who had a reduction in ejection fraction, and these patients had no protective effect of bisoprolol on survival. These data again suggest earlier intervention, whereas patients who have viability can reverse remodel (improve ejection fraction). This may be critical to successful treatment with beta blockade.

The U.S. Carvedilol program was a series of four trials designed to examine the effect of carvedilol, a nonselective beta blocker with α1 blocking properties, on exercise tolerance and progression of disease in patients with mild,[116] moderate,[114,115] and severe[117] heart failure. The four carvedilol studies had a single Data and Safety Monitoring board watching the effect of carvedilol on patient safety as a combined analysis. In this program, carvedilol reduced mortality in 1094 patients entered by 65% (relative reduction [RR] = 0.35, 95% CI 0.20-0.61, P < 0.001).[135] However, these data were not viewed as conclusive as a result of the small number of events, short follow-up, and open-label run-in period prior to randomization, which may have biased the results. Although the individual studies failed to show improvement in exercise tolerance, which was the primary endpoint of the largest two trials, they did find improvement in ejection fraction.[114,115] One of the studies, the MOCHA trial,[114] which was a dose-ranging study, did show a dose-related improvement in LVEF. Although the number of events was small, MOCHA did show a dose-related trend toward reducing mortality with carvedilol and an overall mortality benefit in the cohort as a whole. These data suggest that the adrenergic nervous system plays an active role in the downhill course of patients with heart failure and that complete (but reversible) blockade of receptors may be more beneficial than partial blockade.

The Australia–New Zealand Heart Failure Research Collaborative Group examined the effects of carvedilol on submaximal exercise and morbidity/mortality in 415 patients with mild to moderate heart failure as a result of ischemic heart disease.[118,136] Submaximal exercise tolerance did not increase with carvedilol compared to placebo. However, as in the U.S. Carvedilol studies, LVEF improved. After 19 months of therapy, the frequency of episodes of worsening heart failure was similar in the carvedilol and placebo groups (RR = 1.12, 95% CI 0.82-1.53, P = NS), but the rate of death or hospital admission was lower in the carvedilol group (RR = 0.74, 95% CI 0.57-0.95, P = 0.02). Although all cause mortality was reduced by 14%, this was not statistically significant (RR = 0.76, 95% CI 0.42–1.36, P = NS).

BETA BLOCKER MORTALITY STUDIES

Four large-scale mortality studies with beta blockade have demonstrated a survival benefit of this therapy when added to ACE inhibitors.[137-140] The second Cardiac Insufficiency BISoprolol (CIBIS-2) trial[137] and the MEtoprolol Randomized Intervention Trial in Heart Failure (MERIT-HF)[138] were large-scale prospective studies of the effect of a β-1-selective agent in patients with mild to moderate heart failure. The CIBIS-2 study examined the effect of bisoprolol in patients with ambulatory NYHA class III and IV heart failure. The low placebo mortality (13% annual mortality) in this study suggests that the patients in CIBIS-2 may have been more moderate in severity with few class IV patients. The MERIT-HF trial randomized patients with mild to moderate heart failure (NYHA class II–IV) and an ejection fraction of ≤0.35 (or ≤0.40 with impaired exercise tolerance). The mild annual placebo mortality in this study (11%) suggests that this study was done primarily in patients with mild to moderate heart failure. Both of these studies were terminated prematurely by their respective Data and Safety Monitoring Committees for a strong mortality benefit of beta blockade (Fig. 20-4). Beta blockers in both of these studies reduced mortality by 34% when added to ACE inhibitors as compared to use of ACE inhibitors alone. In both of these trials, the Kaplan-Meier curves in the placebo and active treatment groups are superimposable for approximately 3 months before they diverge. This "lag" in effect is the time it takes for biologic benefit to begin. The CIBIS-2 trial demonstrated a 44% reduction in sudden death (P = 0.0011), a 26% reduction in pump failure death (P = 0.17), a 36% reduction in heart failure hospitalization (P = 0.0001), and a 20% reduction

in all cause hospitalization (P = 0.0006). The MERIT-HF study demonstrated a 41% reduction in sudden death (P = 0.0002), a 49% reduction in pump failure death (P = 0.0023), a 35% reduction in heart failure hospitalization (P = 0.00001), and an 18% reduction in all-cause hospitalization (P = 0.005). Thus, the results of these two trials were very complementary. Subgroup analysis in CIBIS-2 and MERIT-HF by heart rate, gender, age, etiology of heart failure, history of prior myocardial infarction, and presence of diabetes consistently demonstrated a benefit or a trend toward benefit for active therapy across all strata. The only subgroups not showing a clear benefit in these studies were patients with atrial fibrillation in a post-hoc analysis of the CIBIS-2 study[141] and NYHA class IV patients in both studies in which the sample of patients from these studies were too small to be meaningful.[137,138]

The CarvedilOl ProspEctive RaNdomIzed CUmulative Survival Trial (COPERNICUS) was a trial examining a more advanced heart failure population.[140] Entry criteria for this trial required the patient to have symptoms at rest or at a low level of exertion and a LVEF of 0.25 or below. However, exclusion criteria included patients who had significant peripheral or pulmonary edema or recent decompensation. Because the presence of edema and jugular venous distension are more likely to occur in patients with no contractile reserve,[131] this exclusion may have selected for highly symptomatic patients with contractile reserve. This possibility is supported by the finding that the mean systolic blood pressure in this trial at entry was 123 mm Hg, a rather high pressure for advanced heart failure. Like the CIBIS-2 and MERIT-HF trials, this study demonstrated a 35% reduction in death (95% CI 19% to 48%, P = 0.0014 adjusted for interim analyses) with carvedilol. The annual placebo mortality in this trial was 18.5%, which was higher than the 11.0% annual mortality in MERIT-HF and 13.2% in CIBIS-2, suggesting a more advanced heart failure population.

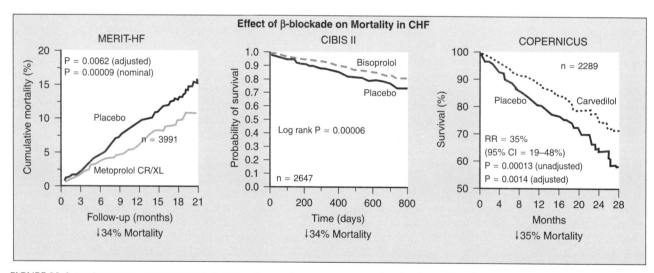

FIGURE 20-4. Kaplan-Meier analysis of the probability of survival among patients in the placebo and beta blocker groups in the CIBIS-2, MERIT-HF, and COPERNICUS trials. (From CIBIS-II Investigators and Committees: The Cardiac Insufficiency Bisoprolol Study II (CIBIS-II): A randomised trial. Lancet 1999; 353:9–13; MERIT-HF Group: Effect of metoprolol CR/XL in chronic heart failure: Metoprolol CR/XL randomised intervention trial in congestive heart failure (MERIT-HF). Lancet 1999; 353:2001–2007; and Packer M, Coats AJS, Fowler MB, et al: Effect of carvedilol on survival in severe chronic heart failure. N Engl J Med 2001; 344:1651–1658.)

A post-hoc analysis of the MERIT-HF trial excluding NYHA class II patients or patients with a LVEF of more than 0.25 was performed to examine a "COPERNICUS"-like population.[142] The annual placebo mortality was 19.1% in this analysis, and there was a 39% reduction (95% CI 11% to 58% reduction, P = 0.0086) in mortality with metoprolol CR/XL. The data from the COPERNICUS trial[140] and post-hoc analysis of MERIT-HF[142] extend the spectrum of patients eligible to get beta blockade to patients with low ejection fraction and moderate to severe symptoms. However, these data do not establish the benefit of beta blockade for either class IV patients or patients who cannot reach compensation (i.e., patients who are more likely to have exhausted contractile reserve).

Another post-hoc analysis of MERIT-HF examined the patients who were unable to achieve a higher dose of metoprolol CR/XL in the trial.[143] The most common reason for inability to achieve a target dose was bradycardia with low-dose beta blockade. In the patients who ended up on low-dose versus high-dose, there were similar reductions in heart rate in the two groups and similar effects on survival. These data suggest that some patients may be more susceptible to bradycardia with beta blockade, and in these patients, if a significant reduction in heart rate is achieved, there should be a survival benefit. However, the data do not suggest that lower dose beta blockade is just as effective as high-dose beta blockade in the general population.

The Beta-blocker Evaluation of Survival Trial (BEST) examined the effect of a nonselective beta blocker with sympatholytic effects on survival in patients with moderate to advanced heart failure (NYHA classes III–IV) and a LVEF of 0.35 or less.[139] This study also uniquely stratified patients in each site based on gender, ejection fraction (>vs. ≤0.20); presence or absence of coronary artery disease; and importantly, race (black vs. nonblack). BEST was prematurely terminated after CIBIS-II and MERIT-HF concluded by the Data and Safety Monitoring Committee based on "the totality of evidence regarding the usefulness of beta blocker treatment derived from BEST and other studies." The BEST study found a 10% reduction in mortality (95% CI -2% to 22% reduction, P = 0.10 unadjusted) with bucindolol. Bucindolol reduced cardiovascular mortality by 14% (95% CI 1% to 26% reduction, P = 0.04) and reduced all-cause hospitalization by 8% (P = 0.08). The reason for the lesser effect of bucindolol, as compared to metoprolol CR/XL, carvedilol, and bisoprolol can be found in the subgroup analyses. Patients who were NYHA class III had a benefit from therapy, but patients who were NYHA class IV had no evidence of benefit (hazard ratio = 1.10, 95% CI 0.76-1.60),[139] albeit there were small numbers of events. The black patients also had no benefit from therapy (hazard ratio = 1.17, 95% CI 0.89-1.54, P = 0.27),[139] whereas nonblack patients appeared to benefit (hazard ratio = 0.82, 95% CI 0.70-0.96, P = 0.013). Bucindolol is unique as compared to bisoprolol, metoprolol CR/XL, and carvedilol because it has moderate sympatholytic effects that the other drugs do not have. This sympatholytic effect was most pronounced in black and NYHA class IV patients, those who did poorly on therapy.[131,144] Sympatholysis may be deleterious in heart failure patients because it irreversibly inhibits sympathetic support as opposed to beta blockade, which is reversible in the face of increased sympathetic support (i.e.,beta agonists can compete with beta blockers at the β-adrenergic receptor for occupancy as neurotransmitters are released during stress). This irreversible loss of support may be most noticeable in patients who have the most advanced disease and least contractile reserve. These are the patients who are most dependent on sympathetic support to maintain circulation. In BEST, the NYHA class IV patients and the black patients had the most advanced disease at entry,[139,144] the highest baseline plasma norepinephrine, the largest reduction in norepinephrine in response to bucindolol, and a trend toward an adverse effect of bucindolol on survival. Other beta-blocking agents, such as carvedilol and metoprolol CR/XL, do not have sympatholytic effects and appear to have benefits in blacks and patients with more advanced heart failure.[137,138,140,145]

The BEST trial raises the issue of possible genetic differences in response to cardiovascular therapy. Although African-American populations have not been shown to have a different allele frequency for ACE genotype from European populations,[146] serum ACE activity for the same genotype varies by race.[147] In addition, the allele frequency of the M235T angiotensinogen gene is very different in blacks and whites in the United States.[146] Because both ACE inhibitors and beta blockers may have salutary effects by inhibition of the renin-angiotensin system,[148] genetic differences between the races may alter response to therapy. Several polymorphisms of the β1 receptor have been reported with a serine to glycine substitution at amino acid 49 or an Arg substitution at position 389.[149,150] The Arg substitution, especially if combined with an alpha2Cdel322–325, results in increased synaptic norepinephrine release (alpha2C polymorphism) and enhanced receptor function (β1 receptor polymorphism), which may predispose to heart failure.[151] This combination of polymorphisms have been identified in African American patients but have yet to be demonstrated in nonblack patients.[151] Differences in allele frequency may exist between blacks and whites, producing differing effects in response to beta blockade. Differences in access to medical care for races[152,153] have been reported but are not likely to account for the findings in this trial as a result of site vigilance with regard to all patients. Although the MERIT-HF,[138] CIBIS-II,[137] U.S. Carvedilol,[135,145] and COPERNICUS[140] studies had few black patients and few events in these patients, based on the consistency of response and magnitude of benefit of this therapy in these studies, beta blockade should not be withheld from black patients based on the isolated results of BEST.

LEFT-VENTRICULAR DYSFUNCTION AFTER MYOCARDIAL INFARCTION

The CArvedilol Post InfaRct SurvIval COntRol in LV DysfunctioN (CAPRICORN) study, in patients with LV dysfunction, was performed to assess the effect of beta blockers in patients with mild or no symptoms and LV dysfunction after myocardial infarction.[154] This trial randomized 1959 patients taking an ACE inhibitor after myocardial infarction and an LVEF of 0.40 or less to carvedilol (n = 975) or placebo (n = 984). The primary endpoint was originally all-cause mortality, but as a result of a low event rate was changed midtrial to a combination of all-cause mortality or a cardiovascular hospital admission. Although the primary endpoint failed to reach statistical significance with a hazard ratio of 0.92 (95% CI 0.80–1.07, P = 0.296), the original primary endpoint of all-cause mortality did reach conventional statistical significance with a hazard ratio of 0.77 (95% CI 0.60–0.98, P = 0.031). Cardiovascular mortality was reduced by 25% (P = 0.024) primarily as a result of a 26% reduction in sudden death (P = 0.098). Although this study randomized patients with milder symptoms of heart failure than other large mortality studies,[137-140] the patients were all post-myocardial infarction where the benefit of beta blockade has been well established in patients who have not had ejection fraction quantitated.[155-157]

PHARMACOLOGIC PROPERTIES OF BETA BLOCKERS

Beta blockers are not alike.[121,122,158] They differ significantly in their pharmacologic properties of selectivity,[121,122,158] lipophilicity,[159,160] sympathomimetic activity,[124,161] alpha blockade, inverse agonism,[121-123] and ancillary properties.[121,122,158] These characteristics will result in differing tolerabilities to beta blocker titration and in some cases different outcomes in heart failure patients.[121,122,124,139] For this reason, they cannot be assumed to be equivalent for the treatment of heart failure. This concept is most apparent when comparing the results of the BEST study[139] with MERIT-HF,[138] CIBIS II,[137] and COPERNICUS.[140] BEST had a much smaller effect size (which was not statistically significant) as compared to the other trials in which beta blockers produced large reductions in mortality.

There are three generations of beta blockers.[121,158] The first-generation agents, such as propranolol and timolol, are nonselective agents with no ancillary properties. Second-generation agents, such as metoprolol, bisoprolol, and betaxolol, are β1 selective agents with no ancillary properties. Third-generation agents, such as bucindolol, labetolol, carvedilol, and nebivolol, are agents with the ancillary properties of vasodilation. The vasodilation produced by carvedilol is mediated through α1 blockade, whereas the vasodilation produced by nebivolol is achieved by nitric oxide (NO) release (via iNOS).[162,163] Bucindolol has mild direct vasodilatory properties, which may be mediated by a cyclic guanosine monophosphate (cGMP)-dependant mechanism.[121,158,162] Carvedilol and a metabolite have significant antioxidant properties,[164,165] and both carvedilol and bucindolol have unique receptor regulatory properties that contribute to their antiadrenergic profile.[121,158,162] Additionally, these agents differ with regard to "inverse agonism," which is the ability of a beta blocker to inactivate active state receptors and eliminate basal levels of intracellular cAMP production (even in the absence of agonist occupancy).[121-123] Compounds with high degrees of inverse agonism, such as propranolol, would be expected to produce more substantial negative chronotropic and inotropic effects and thus be tolerated less well, whereas agents such as bucindolol with little inverse agonism are very well tolerated.

β1-selective agents (such as metoprolol and bisoprolol) or agents that have mild vasodilation and low inverse agonism (such as carvedilol or bucindolol) are very well tolerated in patients with heart failure, whereas agents with more inverse agonism, no β-selectivity, and no vasodilation (such as propranolol) are less well tolerated in patients with heart failure.[121,122,166] Agents that have too much inverse agonism (which can cause bradycardia), are nonselective (which can result in too much negative inotropism) and that have either no vasodilation or excessive vasodilation (which can cause hypotension) are tolerated less well.[167] Large clinical trials of second-generation (metoprolol CR/XL in MERIT-HF and bisoprolol in CIBIS II) and third-generation agents (carvedilol in COPERNICUS, CAPRICORN, US Carvedilol, Australia–New Zealand trials and bucindolol in BEST) have demonstrated good tolerability of these agents in a spectrum of heart failure patients.

Beta blockers also differ in lipophilicity.[121,159,160] Hydrophilic agents such as atenolol do not cross the blood–brain barrier, whereas lipophilic agents such as metoprolol will cross the blood–brain barrier. Some animal data suggest that agents that are lipophilic raise the ventricular fibrillation threshold more as a result of central effects,[160] although this has not been tested in humans and one small trial has suggested a benefit of the nonlipophilic compound, atenolol.[168]

Beta blockers differ in receptor modulation.[121,169] Second-generation agents such as metoprolol upregulate β-receptors,[95,96] whereas third-generation agents such as carvedilol and bucindolol do not. In the cell-surface membrane carvedilol, through "tight binding" renders the β-adrenergic receptor pharmacologically unrecognizable.[121,169,170] Bucindolol, however, produces a true decrease in β-receptor density that is distinct from that produced by agonists.[169] The clinical relevance of these findings is unclear.

Some beta blockers, such as xamoterol, pindolol, or celiprolol, have a large amount of intrinsic sympathomimetic activity (i.e., are partial agonists).[124,161] These agents block exercise heart rate effects but increase resting heart rate over baseline during sleep.[124] One trial with xamoterol, an agent with moderate sympathomimetic activity, resulted in a significant increase in mortality (HR = 2.54; 95% CI 1.04–6.18; P = 0.02).[124] Thus, agents with partial agonist activity should not be used to treat patients with heart failure.

Finally, beta blockers differ in their effects on norepinephrine release. As mentioned, bucindolol reduces plasma norepinephrine as compared to metoprolol, bisoprolol, and carvedilol, which do not.[139,171,172] This may have lead to a smaller beneficial beta blocker mortality effect with bucindolol as compared to these other compounds in the large clinical trials.

Based on these large differences in pharmacologic properties of beta blockers, and based on the differing results of clinical trials with different agents, it is very clear that beta blockade is not a class effect. Furthermore, agents that have been proved in large, prospective clinical trials should be used to treat patients with heart failure.

TRIALS OF BETA BLOCKER WITHDRAWAL

Beta blocker therapy should continue indefinitely in patients with heart failure.[173] Several studies have examined the effect of beta blocker withdrawal in patients with cardiovascular disease.[90,96,174-176] In the face of high levels of adrenergic stimulation present in patients with heart failure,[3-6] beta blocker withdrawal may result in sudden death or a progressive reduction in the biologic benefit achieved with the beta-blocking agent. Patients who have received an improvement in LVEF with beta blocker therapy will often return to the pretherapy ejection fraction or even lower several months after withdrawal. This results in worsening symptomatology and hastened death. If a beta blocker must be electively stopped, slow downtitration is strongly preferred over immediate cessation. In addition, fluid overload and/or low output syndrome in a patient taking beta blockade can often be handled by adjustment of diuretics, natriuretic peptide infusions, nitrates, and/or low-dose phosphodiesterase inhibitor (milrinone) support until compensation is reached. This usually does not necessitate beta blocker cessation unless cardiogenic shock is present. Practical guidelines for beta blocker uptitration and treatment of decompensation are published.[122]

REFERENCES

1. Eichhorn EJ, Bristow MR: Medical therapy can improve the biologic properties of the chronically failing heart: A new era in the treatment of heart failure. Circulation 1996; 94:2285-2296.
2. Zafeiridis A, Jeevanandam V, Houser SR, et al: Regression of cellular hypertrophy after left ventricular assist device support. Circulation 1998; 98:656-662.
3. Packer M, Lee WH, Kessler PD, et al: Role of neurohormonal mechanisms in determining survival in patients with severe chronic heart failure. Circulation 1987; 75(Suppl IV):IV-80-92.
4. Leimbach WN, Wallin BG, Victor RG, et al: Direct evidence from intraneural recordings for increased central sympathetic outflow in patients with heart failure. Circulation 1986; 73:913-919.
5. Cohn JN, Levine TB, Olivari MT, et al: Plasma norepinephrine as a guide to prognosis in patients with chronic congestive heart failure. N Engl J Med 1984; 311:819-823.
6. Hasking GJ, Esler MD, Jennings GL, et al: Norepinephine spillover to plasma in patients with congestive heart failure. Evidence of increased overall and cardiorenal sympathetic nervous activity. Circulation 1986; 73:615-621.
7. Gheorghiade M, Bonow RO: Chronic heart failure in the United States: A manifestation of coronary artery disease. Circulation 1998; 97:282-289.
8. Philbin EF, Weil HF, Francis CA, et al: Race-related differences among patients with left ventricular dysfunction: Observations from a biracial angiographic cohort. J Card Failure 2000; 6:187-193.
9. Edwards BS, Zimmerran RS, Schwab TR, et al: Atrial stretch, not pressure, is the principal determinant controlling the acute release of atrial natriuretic factor. Circ Res 1988; 62:191-195.
10. Kapadia SR, Oral H, Lee J, et al: Hemodynamic regulation of tumor necrosis factor-α gene and protein expression in adult feline myocardium. Circ Res 1997; 81:187-195.
11. Sadoshima J, Xu Y, Slayter HS, et al: Autocrine release of angiotensin II mediates stretch-induced hypertrophy of cardiac myocytes in vitro. Cell 1993; 75:977-984.
12. Sadoshima J, Izumo S: Molecular characterization of angiotensin II-induced hypertrophy of cardiac myocytes and hyperplasia of cardiac fibroblasts: Critical role of the AT1 receptor subtype. Circ Res 1993; 73:413-423.
13. McLeod AA, Brown JE, Kuhn C, et al: Differentiation of hemodynamic, humoral and metabolic responses to β1- and β2-adrenergic stimulation in man using atenolol and propranolol. Circulation 1983; 67:1076-1084.
14. Bristow, MR, Abraham WT: Anti-adrenergic effects of angiotensin converting enzyme inhibitors. Eur Heart J 1995; 16:37-41.
15. Schrier RW, Bichet DG: Osmotic and nonosmotic control of vasopressin release and the pathogenesis of impaired water excretion in adrenal, thyroid, and edematous disorders. J Lab Clin Med 1981; 98:1-15.
16. Bonjour JP, Malvin RL: Stimulation of ADH release by the renin-angiotensin system. Am J Physiol 1970; 218:1555-1559.
17. Sabbah HN, Goldstein S: Ventricular remodeling: consequences and therapy. Eur Heart J 1993; 14(Suppl C):24-29.
18. Cohn, JN: Structural basis for heart failure: Ventricular remodeling and its pharmacological inhibition. Circulation 1995; 91:2504-2507.
19. Sadoshima J, Qiu Z, Morgan JP, et al: Angiotensin II and other hypertrophic stimuli mediated by G protein-coupled receptors activate tyrosine kinase, mitogen-activated protein kinase, and 90-kD S6 kinase in cardiac myocytes: The critical role of Ca2+-dependent signaling. Circ Res 1995; 76:1-15.
20. Meidell RS, Sen A, Henderson SA, et al: Alpha 1-adrenergic stimulation of rat myocardial cells increases protein synthesis. Am J Physiol 1986; 251:H1076-H1084.
21. Yamazaki T, Komuro I, Zou Y, et al: Norepinephrine induces the raf-1 kinase/mitogen-activated protein kinase cascade through both a1- and β-adrenoceptors. Circulation 1997; 95:1260-1268.
22. Mier K, Kemken D, Katus HA, et al: Adrenergic activation of cardiac phospholipase D: Role of alpha(1)-adrenoceptor subtypes. Cardiovasc Res 2002; 54:133-139.
23. Zeng C, Zhou Y, Liu G, et al: The signal transduction pathway causing the synergistic hypertrophic effects of neuropeptide Y and norepinephrine on primary cardiomyocyte. Neuropeptides 2001; 35:211-218.
24. Lin RZ, Chen J, Hu ZW, et al: Phosphorylation of the cAMP response element-binding protein and activation of transcription by alpha1 adrenergic receptors. J Biol Chem 1998; 273:30033-30338.
25. Hajjar RJ, Muller FU, Schmitz W, et al: Molecular aspects of adrenergic signal transduction in cardiac failure. J Mol Med 1998; 76:747-755.
26. Shubeita HE, McDonough, PM, Harris AN, et al: Endothelin induction of inositol phospholipid hydrolysis, sarcomere assembly, and cardiac gene expression in ventricular myocytes: A paracrine mechanism for myocardial cell hypertrophy. J Biol Chem 1990:265:20555-20562.
27. Pennica D, King KL, Shaw KJ, et al: Expression cloning of cardiotrophin 1, a cytokine that induces cardiac myocyte hypertrophy. Proc Natl Acad Sci U S A 1995; 92:1142-1146.
28. Wollert KC, Taga T, Saito M, et al: Cardiotrophin-1 activates a distinct form of cardiac muscle cell hypertrophy: Assembly of sarcomeric units in series via gp130/ leukemia inhibitory factor receptor-dependent pathways. J Biol Chem 1996; 271:9535-9545.
29. Mann DL: The effect of tumor necrosis factor-alpha on cardiac structure and function: a tale of two cytokines. J Cardiac Failure 1996; 2(Suppl): S165-S172.
30. Yokoyama T, Nakano M, Bednarczyk JL, et al: Tumor necrosis factor-a provokes a hypertrophic growth response in adult cardiac myocytes. Circulation 1997; 95:1247-1252.
31. Duerr RL, Huang S, Miraliakbar HR, et al: Insulin-like growth factor-1 enhances ventricular hypertrophy and function during the onset of experimental cardiac failure. J Clin Invest 1995; 95:619-627.
32. Molkentin JD, Lu J-R, Antos CL, et al: A calcineurin-dependent transcriptional pathway for cardiac hypertrophy. Cell 1998; 93:1-14.
33. Olson EN, Williams RS: Calcineurin signaling and muscle remodeling. Cell 2000; 101:689-692.
34. Passier R, Zeng H, Frey N, et al: CaM kinase signaling induces cardiac hypertrophy and activates the MEF2 transcription factor in vivo. J Clin Invest 2000; 105:1395-1406.
35. Hall SA, Cigarroa CG, Marcoux L, et al: Time course of improvement in left ventricular function, mass, and geometry in patients with congestive heart failure treated with β-adrenergic blockade. J Am Coll Cardiol 1995; 25:1154-1161.
36. Lowes BD, Gill EA, Abraham WT, et al: Effects of carvedilol on left ventricular mass, chamber geometry, and mitral regurgitation in chronic heart failure. Am J Cardiol 1999; 83:1201-1205.
37. Gerdes AM, Kellerman SE, Moore JA, et al: Structural remodeling of cardiac myocytes in patients with ischemic cardiomyopathy. Circulation 1992; 86:426-430.
38. Borrow KM, Green LH, Grossman W, et al: Left ventricular end-systolic stress-shortening and stress-length relations in humans: normal values and sensitivity to inotropic state. Am J Cardiol 1982; 50:1301-1308.

39. Kono T, Sabbah HN, Rosman H, et al: Left ventricular shape is the primary determinant of functional mitral regurgitation in heart failure. J Am Coll Cardiol 1992; 20:1594-1598.

40. Yiu SF, Enriquez-Sarano M, Tribouilloy C, et al: Determinants of the degree of functional mitral regurgitation in patients with systolic left ventricular dysfunction: A quantitative clinical study. Circulation 2000; 102:1400-1406.

41. Lowes BD, Minobe W, Abraham WT, et al: Changes in gene expression in the intact human heart: Downregulation of a-myosin heavy chain in hypertrophied, failing ventricular myocardium. J Clin Invest 1997; 100:2315-2324.

42. Lowes BD, Gilbert EM, Abraham WT, et al: Myocardial gene expression in dilated cardiomyopathy treated with beta-blocking agents. New Engl J Med 2002; 346:1357-1365.

43. Herron TJ, McDonald KS: Small amounts of α-myosin heavy chain isoform expression significantly increase power output of rat cardiac myocyte fragments. Circ Res 2002; 90:1150-1152.

44. Arai M, Alpert NR, MacLennan DH, et al: Alterations in sarcoplasmic reticulum gene expression in human heart failure. Circ Res 1993; 72:463-469.

45. Zannad F, Alla F, Dousset B, et al: Limitation of excessive extracellular matrix turnover may contribute to survival benefit of spironolactone therapy in patients with congestive heart failure: Insights from the randomized aldactone evaluation study (RALES). Circulation 2000; 102:2700-2706.

46. Brilla CG, Zhou G, Matsubara L, et al: Collagen metabolism in cultured adult rat cardiac fibroblasts: Response to angiotensin II and aldosterone. J Mol Cell Cardiol 1994; 26:809-820.

47. Weber KT, Anversa P, Armstrong PW, et al: Remodeling and reparation of the cardiovascular system. J Am Coll Cardiol 1992; 20:3-16.

48. Bradham WS, Moe G, Wendt KA, et al: TNF-alpha and myocardial matrix metalloproteinases in heart failure: Relationship to LV remodeling. Am J Physiol Heart Circ Physiol 2002; 282:H1288-295.

49. D'Armiento J: Matrix metalloproteinase disruption of the extracellular matrix and cardiac dysfunction. Trends Cardiovasc Med 2002; 12:97-101.

50. Katz A: The cardiomyopathy of overload: An unnatural growth response in the hypertrophied heart. Ann of Int. Med.1994; 121:363-371.

51. Katz AM: Cellular mechanisms in congestive heart failure. Am J Cardiol 1988; 62:3A-8A.

52. Sabbah HN, Sharov VG, Lesch M, et al: Progression of heart failure: A role for interstitial fibrosis. Mol Cell Biochem 1995; 147:29-34.

53. Engelmann GL, Vitullo JC, Gerrity RG: Morphometric analysis of cardiac hypertrophy during development, maturation, and senescence in spontaneously hypertensive rats. Circ Res 1987; 60:487-494.

54. van den Heuvel AF, van Veldhuisen DJ, van der Wall EE, et al: Regional myocardial blood flow reserve impairment and metabolic changes suggesting myocardial ischemia in patients with idiopathic dilated cardiomyopathy. J Am Coll Cardiol 2000; 35:19-28.

55. Sabbah HN, Sharov V, Riddle JM, et al: Mitochondrial abnormalities in myocardium of dogs with chronic heart failure. J Mol Cell Cardiol 1992; 24:1333-1347.

56. Ingwall JS, Kramer MF, Fifer MA, et al: The creatine kinase system in normal and depressed human myocardium. N Engl J Med 1985; 313:1050-1054.

57. Neubauer S, Horn M, Naumann A, et al: Impairment of energy metabolism in intact residual myocardium of rat hearts with chronic myocardial infarction. J Clin Invest 1995; 95:1092-1100.

58. Kameyama M, Hescheler J, Hofmann F, et al: Modulation of Ca current during the phosphorylation cycle in guinea pig heart. Pflugers Arch 1986; 407:123-128.

59. Smith J, Coronado R, Meissner G: Single channel measurements of the calcium release channel from sarcoplasmic reticulum: Activation by calcium and ATP and modulation by magnesium. J Gen Physiol 1986; 88:573-588.

60. Vik-Mo H, Mjos OD: Influence of free fatty acids on myocardial oxygen consumption and ischemic injury. Am J Cardiol 1981; 48:361-365.

61. Kjekshus JK, Mjos OD: Effect on inhibition of lipolysis on myocardial oxygen consumption in the presence of isoproterenol. J Clin Invest 1972; 51:1767-1776.

62. Simonsen S, Kjekshus JK: The effect of free fatty acids on myocardial oxygen consumption during atrial pacing and catecholamine infusion in man. Circulation 1978; 58:484-491.

63. Apstein CS: Increased glycolytic substrate protection improves ischemic cardiac dysfunction and reduces injury. Am Heart J 2000; 139:S107-S114.

64. Rupp H, Wahl R, Hansen M: Influence of diet and carnitine palmitoyltransferase I inhibition on myosin and sarcoplasmic reticulum. J Appl Physiol 1992; 72:352-360.

65. Zarain-Herzberg A, Rupp H, et al: Modification of sarcoplasmic reticulum gene expression in pressure overload cardiac hypertrophy by etomoxir. FASEB J 1996; 10:1303-1309.

66. Depre C, Young ME, Ying J, et al: Streptozotocin-induced changes in cardiac gene expression in the absence of severe contractile dysfunction. J Mol Cell Cardiol 2000; 32:985-996.

67. Taegtmeyer H: Genetics of energetics: Transcriptional responses in cardiac metabolism. Ann Biomed Engineering 2000; 28:871-876.

68. Arai M, Alpert NR, MacLennan DH, et al: Alterations in sarcoplasmic reticulum gene expression in human heart failure. Circ Res 1993; 72:463-469.

69. Parker JD, Newton GE, Landzberg JS, et al: Functional significance of presynaptic alpha-adrenergic receptors in failing and nonfailing human left ventricle. Circulation 1995; 92:1793-1800.

70. Gilbert EM, Sandoval A, Larrabee P, et al: Lisinopril lowers cardiac adrenergic drive and increases β-receptor density in the failing human heart. Circulation 1993; 88:472-480.

71. Wolfrum RD, Buttner C, Schafer U, et al: Effect of ACE-inhibitor-ramiprilat and AT1-receptor antagonist candesartan on cardiac norepinephrine release: Comparison between ischemic and nonischemic conditions. J Cardiovasc Pharmacol 2002; 40:641-646.

72. Newton GE, Azevedo ER, Parker JD: Inotropic and sympathetic responses to the intracoronary infusion of a beta2-receptor agonist: A human in vivo study. Circulation 1999; 99:2402-2407.

73. Azevedo ER, Kubo T, Mak S, et al: Nonselective versus selective beta-adrenergic receptor blockade in congestive heart failure: Differential effects on sympathetic activity. Circulation 2001; 104:2194-199.

74. Chulak C, Couture R, Foucart S: Modulatory effect of bradykinin on noradrenaline release in isolated atria from normal and B2 knockout transgenic mice. Eur J Pharmacol 1998; 346:167-174.

75. Bristow MR, Port JD, Sandoval AB, et al: β-Adrenergic receptor pathways in the failing human heart. Heart Failure 1989; 5:77-90.

76. Yatani A, Brown AM: Rapid β-adrenergic modulation of cardiac calcium channel currents by a fast G protein pathway. Science 1989; 245:71-74.

77. Keef KD, Huymer JR, Zhong J: Regulation of cardiac and smooth muscle Ca(2+) channels (Ca(V)1.2a,b) by protein kinases. Am J Physiol Cell Physiol 2001; 281:C1743-756.

78. Frank K, Kranias EG: Phospholamban and cardiac contractility. Ann Med 2000; 32:572-578.

79. Schmidt U, Hajjar RJ, Helm PA, et al: Contribution of abnormal sarcoplasmic reticulum ATPase activity to systolic and diastolic dysfunction in human heart failure. J Mol Cell Cardiol 1998; 30:1929-1937.

80. Turnbull L, Hoh JF, Ludowyke RI, et al: Troponin I phosphorylation enhances crossbridge kinetics during beta-adrenergic stimulation in rat cardiac tissue. J Physiol 2002; 542:911-920.

81. Bristow MR, Ginsburg R, Umans V, et al: β1- And β2-adrenergic-receptor subpopulations in nonfailing and failing human ventricular myocardium: Coupling of both receptor subtypes to muscle contraction and selective β1-receptor down-regulation in heart failure. Circ Res 1986; 59:297-309.

82. Feldman AM, Cates AE, Veazey WB, et al: Increase of the 40,000-mol wt pertussis toxin substrate (G protein) in the failing human heart. J Clin Invest 1988; 82:189-197.

83. Akhter SA, Eckhart AD, Rockman HA, et al: In vivo inhibition of elevated myocardial beta-adrenergic receptor kinase activity in hybrid transgenic mice restores normal beta-adrenergic signaling and function. Circulation 1999; 100:648-653.

84. Danielsen W, v der Leyen H, Meyer W, et al: Basal and isoprenaline-stimulated camp content in failing versus nonfailing human cardiac preparations. J Cardiovasc Pharmacol 1989; 14:171-173.

85. Schwinger RH, Munch G, Bolck B, et al: Reduced Ca(2+)-sensitivity of SERCA 2a in failing human myocardium due to reduced serin-16 phospholamban phosphorylation. J Mol Cell Cardiol 1999; 31:479-491.

86. Dash R, Kadambi V, Schmidt AG, et al: Interactions between phospholamban and beta-adrenergic drive may lead to cardiomyopathy and early mortality. Circulation 2001; 103:889-896.

87. White M, Yanowitz F, Gilbert EM, et al: Role of beta-adrenergic receptor downregulation in the peak exercise response in patients with heart failure due to idiopathic dilated cardiomyopathy. Am J Cardiol 1995:76:1271-1276.

88. Waagstein F, Hjalmarson A, Varnauskas E, et al: Effect of chronic β-adrenergic receptor blockade in congestive cardiomyopathy. Br Heart J 1975;37:1022-1036.

89. Swedberg K, Hjalmarson A, Waagstein F, et al: Beneficial effects of long-term beta-blockade in congestive cardiomyopathy. Br Heart J 1980;44:117-133.

90. Swedberg K, Hjalmarson A, Waagstein F, et al: Adverse effects of beta-blockade withdrawal in patients with congestive cardiomyopathy. Br Heart J 1980;44:134-142.

91. Ikram H, Fitzpatrick D: Double blind trial of chronic oral beta blockade in congestive cardiomyopathy. Lancet 1981; 2:490-493.

92. Currie PJ, Kelly KJ, McKenzie A, et al: Oral beta-adrenergic blockade with metoprolol in chronic severe dilated cardiomyopathy. J Am Coll Cardiol 1984; 3:203-209.

93. Engelmeier RS, O'Connell JB, Walsh R, et al: Improvement in symptoms and exercise tolerance by metoprolol in patients with dilated cardiomyopathy: A double-blind, randomized, placebo-controlled trial. Circulation 1985; 72:536-546.

94. Anderson JL, Lutz JR, Gilbert EM, et al: A randomized trial of low-dose beta-blockade therapy for idiopathic dilated cardiomyopathy. Am J Cardiol 1985; 55:471-475.

95. Heilbrunn SM, Shah P, Bristow MR, et al: Increased β-receptor density and improved hemodynamic response to catecholamine stimulation during long-term metoprolol therapy in heart failure from dilated cardiomyopathy. Circulation 1989; 79:483-490.

96. Waagstein F, Caidahl K, Wallentin I, et al: Long term β-blockade in dilated cardiomyopathy: Effects of short- and long term metoprolol treatment followed by withdrawal and readministration of metoprolol. Circulation 1989; 80:551-563.

97. Gilbert EM, Anderson JL, Deitchman D, et al: Chronic β-blocker-vasodilator therapy improves cardiac function in idiopathic dilated cardiomyopathy: A double-blind, randomized study of bucindolol versus placebo. Am J Med 1990; 88:223-229.

98. Woodley SL, Gilbert EM, Anderson JL, et al: β-Blockade with bucindolol in heart failure due to ischemic vs idiopathic dilated cardiomyopathy. Circulation 1991; 84:2426-2441.

99. Andersson B, Blomstrom-Lundqvist C, Hedner T, et al: Exercise hemodynamics and myocardial metabolism during long-term beta-adrenergic blockade in severe heart failure. J Am Coll Cardiol 1991; 18:1059-1066.

100. Paolisso G, Gambardella A, Marrazzo G, et al: Metabolic and cardiovascular benefits deriving from β-adrenergic blockade in chronic congestive heart failure. Am Heart J 1992; 123:103-110.

101. Bristow MR, O'Connell JB, Gilbert EM, et al: Dose-response of chronic β-blocker treatment in heart failure from either idiopathic dilated or ischemic cardiomyopathy. Circulation 1994; 89:1632-1642.

102. Metra M, Nardi M, Giubbini R, et al: Effects of short- and long-term carvedilol administration on rest and exercise hemodynamic variables, exercise capacity and clinical conditions in patients with idiopathic dilated cardiomyopathy. J Am Coll Cardiol 1994; 24:1678-1687.

103. Fisher ML, Gottlieb SS, Plotnick GD, et al: Beneficial effects of metoprolol in heart failure associated with coronary artery disease: A randomized trial. J Am Coll Cardiol 1994; 23:943-950.

104. Olsen SL, Gilbert EM, Renlund DG, et al: Carvedilol improves left ventricular function and symptoms in chronic heart failure: A double-blind randomized study. J Am Coll Cardiol 1995; 25:1225-1231.

105. Krum H, Sackner-Bernstein J, Goldsmith RL, et al: Double-blind, placebo-controlled study of the long-term efficacy of carvedilol in patients with severe chronic heart failure. Circulation 1995; 92:1499-1506.

106. Eichhorn EJ, Heesch CM, Barnett JH, et al: Effect of metoprolol on myocardial function and energetics in patients with non-ischemic dilated cardiomyopathy: A randomized, double-blind, placebo-controlled study. J Am Coll Cardiol 1994; 24:1310-1320.

107. Eichhorn EJ, Bedotto JB, Malloy CR, et al: Effect of beta-adrenergic blockade on myocardial function and energetics in congestive heart failure: Improvements in hemodynamic, contractile, and diastolic performance with bucindolol. Circulation 1990; 82: 473-483.

108. Wisenbaugh T, Katz I, Davis J, et al: Long-term (3 month) effects of a new beta-blocker (nebivolol) on cardiac perform-ance in dilated cardiomyopathy. J Am Coll Cardiol 1993; 21: 1094-1100.

109. Tsutsui H, Spinale FG, Nagatsu M, et al: Effects of chronic β-adrenergic blockade on the left ventricular and cardiocyte abnormalities of chronic canine mitral regurgitation. J Clin Invest 1994; 93:2639-2648.

110. Takaoka H, Takeuchi M, Hata K, et al: Beneficial effects of a Ca^{2+} sensitizer, MCI-154, on the myocardial oxygen consumption-cardiac output relation in patients with left ventricular dysfunction after myocardial infarction: Comparison with dobutamine and phosphodiesterase inhibitor. Am Heart J 1997; 133:283-289.

111. Gwathmey JK, Kim CS, Hajjar RJ, et al: Cellular and molecular remodeling in a heart failure model treated with the beta-blocker carteolol. Am J Physiol 1999; 276: H1678-690.

112. Metra M, Nodari S, D'Aloia A, et al: Effects of neurohormonal antagonism on symptoms and quality-of-life in heart failure. Eur Heart J 1998; 19(Suppl B): B25-35.

113. Gilbert EM, Abraham WT, Olsen S, et al: Comparative hemodynamic, left ventricular functional, and antiadrenergic effects of chronic treatment with metoprolol versus carvedilol in the failing heart. Circulation 1996; 94:2817-2825.

114. Bristow MR, Gilbert EM, Abraham WT, et al: Carvedilol produces dose-related improvements in left ventricular function and survival in subjects with chronic heart failure. Circulation 1996; 94:2807-2816.

115. Packer M, Colucci WS, Sackner-Bernstein JD, et al: Double-blind, placebo-controlled study of the effects of carvedilol in patients with moderate to severe heart failure: The PRECISE trial. Circulation 1996; 94:2793-2799.

116. Colucci WS, Packer M, Bristow MR, et al: Carvedilol inhibits clinical progression in patients with mild symptoms of heart failure. Circulation 1996; 94:2800-2806.

117. Cohn JN, Fowler MB, Bristow MR, et al: Safety and efficacy of carvedilol in severe heart failure: The U.S. Carvedilol Heart Failure Study Group. J Card Fail 1997; 3:173-179.

118. Australia-New Zealand Heart Failure Research Collaborative Group: Effects of carvedilol, a vasodilator-β-blocker, in patients with congestive heart failure as a result of ischemic heart disease. Circulation 1995; 92:212-218.

119. Waagstein F, Bristow MR, Swedberg K, et al: Beneficial effects of metoprolol in idiopathic dilated cardiomyopathy. Lancet 1993; 342:1441-1446.

120. Hasenfuss G, Holubarsch C, Heiss HW, et al: Myocardial energetics in patients with dilated cardiomyopathy: Influence of nitroprusside and enoximone. Circulation 1989; 80:51-64.

121. Bristow MR: β-adrenergic receptor blockade in chronic heart failure. Circulation 2000; 101:558-569.

122. Eichhorn EJ, Bristow MR: Practical guidelines for initiation of β-adrenergic blockade in patients with chronic heart failure. Am J Cardiol 1997; 79:794-798.

123. Chidiac P, Herbert TE, Valiquette M, et al: Inverse agonist activity of β-adrenergic antagonists. Mol Pharmacol 1993; 45:490-499.

124. The Xamoterol in Severe Heart Failure Study Group: Xamoterol in severe heart failure. Lancet 1990; 336:1-6.

125. Cunningham MJ, Apstein CS, Weinberg EO, et al: Influence of glucose and insulin on the exaggerated diastolic and systolic dysfunction of hypertrophied rat hearts during hypoxia. Circ Res 1990; 66:406-415.

126. Varma N, Eberli FR, Apstein CS: Left ventricular diastolic dysfunction during demand ischemia: Rigor underlies increased stiffness without calcium-mediated tension: Amelioration by glycolytic substrate. J Am Coll Cardiol 2001; 37:2144-2153.

127. Kaprielian R, Wickenden AD, Kassiri Z, et al: Relationship between K^+ channel down-regulation and [Ca2+]i in rat ventricular myocytes following myocardial infarction. J Physiol 1999; 517:229-245.

128. Ingwall JS, Kramer MF, Fifer MA, et al: The creatine kinase system in normal and depressed human myocardium. N Engl J Med 1985; 313:1050-1054.

129. Sabbah HN, Sharov VG, Gupta RC, et al: Chronic therapy with metoprolol attenuates cardiomyocyte apoptosis in dogs with heart failure. J Am Coll Cardiol 2000; 36:1698-1705.

130. Yamada T, Fukunami M, Ohmori M, et al: Which subgroup of patients with dilated cardiomyopathy would benefit from long-term beta-blocker therapy? A histologic viewpoint. J Am Coll Cardiol 1993; 21:628-633.

131. Eichhorn EJ, Grayburn PA, Mayer S, et al: Myocardial contractile reserve by dobutamine stress echocardiography predicts improvement in ejection fraction with β-blockade in patients with heart failure: The BEST trial. Circulation 2003; 108:2336-2341.

132. Cohn JN, Johnson GR, Shabetai R, et al: Ejection fraction, peak exercise oxygen consumption, cardiothoracic ratio, ventricular arrhythmias, and plasma norepinephrine as determinants of prognosis in heart failure. Circulation 1993; 87(suppl VI):VI-5-VI-16.

133. Lechat P, Escolano S, Golmard JL, et al: Prognostic value of bisoprolol-induced hemodynamic effects in heart failure during the Cardiac Insufficiency BIsoprolol Study (CIBIS). Circulation 1997; 96:2197-2205.

134. CIBIS Investigators and Committees: A Randomized trial of beta-blockade in heart failure: The Cardiac Insufficiency Bisoprolol Study (CIBIS). Circulation 1994; 90:1765-1773.

135. Packer M, Bristow MR, Cohn JN, et al: Effect of carvedilol on morbidity and mortality in chronic heart failure. N Engl J Med 1996; 334:1349-1355.

136. Australia/New Zealand Heart Failure Research Collaborative Group: Randomised, placebo-controlled trial of carvedilol in patients with congestive heart failure due to ischaemic heart disease. Lancet 1997; 349:375-380.

137. CIBIS-II Investigators and Committees: The Cardiac Insufficiency Bisoprolol Study II (CIBIS-II): A randomised trial. Lancet 1999; 353:9-13.

138. MERIT-HF Group: Effect of metoprolol CR/XL in chronic heart failure: Metoprolol CR/XL randomised intervention trial in congestive heart failure (MERIT-HF). Lancet 1999; 353:2001-2007.

139. The Beta-Blocker Evaluation of Survival Trial Investigators: A trial of the beta-blocker bucindolol in patients with advanced chronic heart failure. N Engl J Med 2001; 344:1659-1667.

140. Packer M, Coats AJS, Fowler MB, et al: Effect of carvedilol on survival in severe chronic heart failure. N Engl J Med 2001; 344:1651-1658.

141. Lechat P, Hulot JS, Escolano S, et al: Heart rate and cardiac rhythm relationships with bisoprolol benefit in chronic heart failure in CIBIS II Trial. Circulation 2001; 103:1428-1433.

142. Goldstein S, Fagerberg B, Hjalmarson A, et al: Metoprolol controlled release/extended release in patients with severe heart failure: Analysis of the experience in the MERIT-HF study. J Am Coll Cardiol 2001; 38:932-938.

143. Wikstrand J, Hjalmarson A, Waagstein F, et al: Dose of metoprolol CR/XL and clinical outcomes in patients with heart failure: Analysis of the experience in metoprolol CR/XL randomized intervention trial in chronic heart failure (MERIT-HF). J Am Coll Cardiol 2002; 40:491-498.

144. Eichhorn EJ, Domanski M, Adams K, et al: Hemodynamic, myocardial functional and neurohormonal responses to β-blockade in black vs non-black patients in BEST. Circulation 2000; 102 (Suppl II): II-778. Abstract

145. Yancy CW, Fowler MB, Colucci WS, et al: Race and the response to adrenergic blockade with carvedilol in patients with chronic heart failure. N Engl J Med 2001; 344:1358-1365.

146. Rotimi C, Puras A, Cooper R, et al: Polymorphisms of renin-angiotensin genes among Nigerians, Jamaicans, and African Americans. Hypertension 1996; 27:558-563.

147. Bloem LJ, Manatunga AK, Pratt JH: Racial difference in the relationship of an angiotensin I-converting enzyme gene polymorphism to serum angiotensin I-converting enzyme activity. Hypertension 1996; 27:62-66.

148. Eichhorn EJ, McGhie AI, Bedotto JB, et al: Effects of bucindolol on neurohormonal activation in congestive heart failure. Am J Cardiol 1991; 67:67-73.

149. Mason DA, Moore JD, Green SA, et al: A gain-of-function polymorphism in a G-protein coupling domain of the human beta1-adrenergic receptor. J Biol Chem 1999; 274:12670-12674.

150. Rathz DA, Brown KM, Kramer LA, et al: Amino acid 49 polymorphisms of the human beta1-adrenergic receptor affect agonist promoted trafficking. J Cardiovasc Pharmacol 2002; 39: 155-160.

151. Small KM, Wagoner LE, Levin AM, et al: Synergistic polymorphisms of beta1- and alpha2c-adrenergic receptors and the risk of congestive heart failure. N Engl J Med 2002; 347:1135-1142.

152. Ayanian JZ, Weissman JS, Chasan-Taber S, et al: Quality of care by race and gender for congestive heart failure and pneumonia. Med Care 1999; 37:1260-1269.

153. Jha AK, Shlipak MG, Hosmer W, et al: Racial differences in mortality among men hospitalized in the Veterans Affairs Health Care system. JAMA 2001; 285:297-303.

154. Dargie HJ: Effect of carvedilol on outcome after myocardial infarction in patients with left-ventricular dysfunction: The CAPRICORN randomised trial. Lancet 2001; 357:1385-1390.

155. Hjalmarson A, Elmfeldt D, Herlitz J, et al: Effect on mortality of metoprolol in acute myocardial infarction: A double-blind randomised trial. Lancet 1981; 823-827.

156. Timolol-induced reduction in mortality and reinfarction in patients surviving acute myocardial infarction. N Engl J Med 1981; 304:801-807.

157. Chadda K, Goldstein S, Byington R, et al: Effect of propranolol after acute myocardial infarction in patients with congestive heart failure. Circulation 1986; 73:503-510.

158. Bristow MR: Pathophysiologic and pharmacologic rationales for clinical management of chronic heart failure with beta-blocking agents. Am J Cardiol 1993; 71:12C-22C.

159. Hjarlmason A: Empiric therapy with β-blockers. PACE Pacing Clin Electrophysiol 1994; 17:460-466.

160. Ablad B, Bjuro T, Bjorkman J-A, et al: Role of central nervous beta-adrenoceptors in the prevention of ventricular fibrillation through augmentation of cardiac vagal tone. J Am Coll Cardiol 1991; 17 (Suppl A):165A. Abstract.

161. Shanes JG, Wolfkiel C, Ghali J, et al: Acute hemodynamic effects of pindolol and propranolol in patients with dilated cardiomyopathy: Relevance of intrinsic sympathomimetic activity. Am Heart J 1988; 116:1268-1275.

162. Hershberger RE, Wynn JR, Sundberg L, et al: Mechanism of action of bucindolol in human ventricular myocardium. J Cardio Pharm 1990, 15:959-967.

163. Broeders MA, Doevendans PA, Bekkers BC, et al: Nebivolol: A third-generation beta-blocker that augments vascular nitric oxide release: Endothelial beta(2)-adrenergic receptor-mediated nitric oxide production. Circulation 2000; 102:677-684.

164. Yue T-L, Mckenna PJ, Lysko PG, et al: SB211475, a metabolite of carvedilol, a novel antihypertensive agent, is a potent antioxidant. Eur J Pharmacol 1994; 251:237-243.

165. Kukin ML, Kalman J, Charney RH, et al: Prospective, randomized comparison of effect of long-term treatment with metoprolol or carvedilol on symptoms, exercise, ejection fraction, and oxidative stress in heart failure. Circulation.1999; 99:2645-2651.

166. Haber HL, Simek CL, Gimple LW, et al: Why do patients with congestive heart failure tolerate the initiation of beta-blocker therapy? Circulation 1993; 88:1610-1619.

167. Talwar KK, Bhargava B, Upasani PT, et al: Hemodynamic predictors of early intolerance and long-term effects of propranolol in dilated cardiomyopathy. J Cardiac Failure 1996; 2:273-277.

168. Sturm B, Pacher R, Strametz-Juranek J, et al: Effect of beta 1 blockade with atenolol on progression of heart failure in patients pretreated with high-dose enalapril. Eur J Heart Fail 2000; 2:407-412.

169. Asano K, Zisman LS, Yoshikawa T, et al: Bucindolol, a nonselective β1- and β2-adrenergic receptor antagonist, decreases β-adrenergic receptor density in cultured embryonic chick cardiac myocyte membranes. J Cardiovasc Pharmacol 2001; 37:678-691.

170. Yoshikawa T, Port JD, Asano K, et al: Cardiac adrenergic receptor effects of carvedilol. Eur Heart J 1996; 17(Suppl B):8-16.

171. Lowes BD, Gilbert EM, Lindenfeld JA, et al: Differential effects of β-blocking agents on adrenergic activity. Circulation 2000; 102 (Suppl II): II-628-II-629.

172. Bristow MR, Zelis R, Nuzzo R, et al: Baseline and three month change in systemic venous norepinephrine as predictors of clinical outcomes in the BEST trial. J Am Coll Cardiol 2001; 37:281A. Abstract

173. Eichhorn EJ: Beta-blocker withdrawal: The Song of Orpheus. Am Heart J 1999; 138:387-389.

174. Morimoto S, Shimizu K, Yamada K, et al: Can beta-blocker therapy be withdrawn from patients with dilated cardiomyopathy? Am Heart J 1999; 138:456-459.

175. Nattel S, Rangno RE, Van Loon G: Mechanism of propranolol withdrawal phenomena. Circulation 1979; 59:1158-1164.

176. Miller RR, Olson HG, Amsterdam EA, et al: Propranolol-withdrawal rebound phenomenon: Exacerbation of coronary events after abrupt cessation of antianginal therapy. N Engl J Med 1975; 293:416-418.

Heart Transplantation and Mechanical Cardiac Support

Lynne Warner Stevenson

The development of donor organ replacement and mechanical support therapies for the expanding population of patients with end-stage heart failure has created new scientific, ethical, and policy challenges. Experiences rather than experimentation continue to dominate progress, although the landmark randomized trial of left-ventricular assist devices (LVADs) has demonstrated that one randomized controlled trial could be done (Table 21-1). The dramatic nature of many of these procedures and the desperation of patients facing imminent death move new therapies out of the controlled trial template that has established beneficial therapies for mild–moderate stages of heart failure. Future advances in the field will be propelled both by modifications of trial design and refinement of registries designed to reshape the application of technology that has passed the initial clinical trials.

CARDIAC TRANSPLANTATION: EARLY PHASE

Cardiac transplantation developed as a surgical therapy for heart disease. After experimental heterotopic cardiac transplantation in puppies in 1905, the first and third human heart transplants were performed by Christiaan Barnard in South Africa in 1967. The first human heart transplant in the United States was performed in Brooklyn on a neonate who died on the same day. The second heart transplant patient in the United States lived for 15 days after the procedure was performed in January 1968 by Norman Shumway. Because of the challenge of controlling graft rejection, transplantation in general encompassed a broad range of scientific research prior to human application, whereas the procedure itself was technically straightforward. Once performed, the initial success led to excitement and introduction at 54 centers by 1970. Unlike most previous surgical procedures, however, the complexity of postoperative follow-up was extensive as a result of the immunosuppression and infections, requiring extensive commitment and expertise, which were not available at most sites. Thus the enthusiasm waned rapidly as national 1-year survival for 90 recipients reached only 25%.

Subsequent progress in heart transplantation occurred painstakingly at Stanford University and the Medical College of Virginia, who reported ongoing animal experiments and clinical outcomes to a small audience. The development of the endomyocardial biopsy improved the ability to detect and treat rejection before physical findings and low electrocardiographic voltage heralded imminent hemodynamic compromise. By 1980, 1-year survival had improved to more than 60%, with 5-year survival approximately 40%.[1] With many new developments, the increasing success of the experiment thrust it into a realm where the distinction between experimental and therapeutic blurred. The local decisions of the California and Arizona Medicare intermediaries to reimburse transplantation brought the issue to national attention. In January 1980, the U.S. National Institutes of Health recommended that Medicare pay for heart transplants performed at Stanford, the University of Arizona, and other centers that met comparable standards, for patients who fit the Stanford selection criteria. This was adopted on an interim basis in the face of multiple concerns regarding the selection criteria and process.

CARDIAC TRANSPLANTATION: VALIDATION PHASE

In June 1980, the U.S. Department of Health and Human Services announced that new technologies would be evaluated on the basis of social consequences before financing wide distribution. Heart transplantation was declared as the prototype of an aggressive procedure requiring technology assessment. One of the goals was definition of the statutory requirement for "reasonable and necessary" medical care in this setting. The Health Care Financing Administration awarded the contract for the National Heart Transplantation Study to The Battelle Human Affairs Research Centers in 1981.

Patient Population

The definition of cardiac transplantation as "standard medical therapy" was based on this study, which

■ ■ ■

TABLE 21-1 DEVELOPMENT OF PROCEDURES FOR ADVANCED HEART FAILURE

Percutaneous devices

Southey tubes to drain peripheral edema
Atrioventricular interval pacing
Implantable cardioverter defibrillators (trials in subset*)
Biventricular pacing*
External counterpulsation

Surgical procedures

Thyroidectomy
Pericardiectomy
Valvular reconstruction/replacement
Coronary revascularization (trials in subset + ongoing*)
Aneurysmectomy
Ventricular reduction surgery
Surgical ventricular restoration (ongoing*)
Cardiac transplantation
    Orthotopic
    Heterotopic
Ventricular assist devices
    Postcardiotomy
    Bridge to recovery from fulminant myocarditis
    Bridge to transplantation
    Destination therapy* (completed)

*Relevant randomized trials.

accepted 6 of 12 applying centers who would receive reimbursement for 15 cardiac transplants each but would provide information about consecutive patients undergoing transplantation since 1975. Data ultimately included 441 patients undergoing transplantation at the major centers since human heart transplantation began in 1968, with detailed information on 152 patients alive during the study period.[2] The results continued to improve during the study period, in part because of increasing experience with the new immunosuppressive agent cyclosporine, which decreased the severity of rejection episodes and infection-related complications.

As for many landmark studies, the population to which the results are generalized is increasingly disparate from the original validation trial. The mean age of recipients at that time was 42 years, 73% of patients were living with spouses, and 52% of patients had attended college. More than half of patients had idiopathic cardiomyopathy as their diagnosis, and the average duration of disease was 5 years. Few patients had any of the potential relative contraindications to transplantation, in part because of the Battelle-directed compliance with original exclusion criteria, which specified cardiac cachexia and significant cardiac-related renal dysfunction, which characterize many recipients now.

Patient Survival

The Battelle study faced the fundamental challenge of determining the impact of cardiac transplantation on survival with severe heart failure. When therapies are introduced to rescue patients from the brink of death, it is difficult to step out of the circular reasoning: The patient was selected for the procedure because otherwise he would have died; if he lived it is because the

procedure saved his life. Comparison to patients not eligible for the procedure could be biased in either direction. If ineligibility related to contraindications, the same factors could worsen survival compared to eligible patients with or without the procedure. Conversely, patients ineligible because of a milder degree of illness could survive longer than sicker patients subjected to a major procedure. Cardiac transplantation offers a unique random element of donor availability, creating a variable length of time to observe natural history prior to transplantation. For the early period of cardiac transplantation, mortality for patients after selection was 90% within 3 months if transplantation was not performed.[1] By the conclusion of the Battelle study in 1984, the average length of survival for patients listed but not transplanted was 45 days. Although subject to the biases listed previously, the qualitative difference between this figure and the mean survival time of 705 days after transplantation provided convincing evidence of a survival benefit for cardiac transplantation. Almost 25% of transplant recipients were projected to live 10 years based on the results during this study.

Based on these data and the previous experiences, cardiac transplantation came to be known as a procedure for patients with "less than 6 months to live." Despite the introduction of multiple clinical and biochemical factors predicting outcome in heart failure, reliable identification of patients with less than 6 months to live remains difficult. The proliferation of transplant centers and the sophistication of the patient population seeking therapies have increased the demand for cardiac transplantation at the same time as optimal medical management of advanced heart failure has improved both quality of life and survival without transplantation. Patients surviving out of the hospital for 6 months on the transplant list may not have appreciable increase in survival over the next year with cardiac transplantation.[3] Thus the original survival benefits attributed to cardiac transplantation have been diluted by the curve of downshifting risks, as discussed in the next section.

Patient Function and Quality of Life

The Battelle National Study of Heart Transplantation assessed quality of life in both objective and subjective domains. Objective information included an increase in patient employment from 8% at the time of evaluation to 32% at last follow-up after transplantation, although 55% had been employed during the year prior to transplantation. This was lower than the 49% reported for the parallel study of kidney transplant recipients, compared to 29% for patients on chronic dialysis. Many of the heart transplant patients reported restrictions based on employers and insurance security rather than functional limitation.

Without a control group of similar patients surviving without transplantation, the benefit on quality of life was difficult to place into perspective during the Battelle study (Table 21-2). Comparisons can be made to other chronic conditions. Quantitated measures of functional impairment according to the Karnofsky Index showed heart transplant recipients to have Total Sickness Impact Profiles midway between the limitations of patients on

TABLE 21-2   QUALITY OF LIFE FOR TRANSPLANT RECIPIENTS*

	Ability to work (%)	Working at 1 year (%)	Sickness impact score	Well-being	Life satisfaction
Heart transplant	58	34	9.6	11.11	5.11
Kidney transplant	74	49	5.5	11.83	5.66
Home hemodialysis	59	37	9.5	11.12	5.19
In-center hemodialysis	37	19	13.9	10.77	5.11

*For the "Sickness impact score," higher numbers are worse. For "Well-being" and "Life satisfaction," higher numbers are better. General population scores at the time were 10.9 for Well-being and 5.45 for Life satisfaction.
(Modified from Evans RW, Broida JH: National Heart Transplantation Study. Seattle, Washington: Battelle Human Affairs Research Centers, 1985.)

dialysis and those with renal transplants, who were the best.[2] A subsequent study done prospectively within a single center compared the improvements occurring in quality-of-life measurements for evaluated patients surviving transplantation and those surviving without listing for transplantation. Both groups of survivors at a mean of 40 months showed similar improvement from baseline quality of life as assessed by the Multiple Affect Adjective Checklist, the Psychosocial Adjustment to Illness Scale, and the Heart Failure Functional Inventory, although they remained dysfunctional.[4]

More recent data have measured peak oxygen consumption and 6-minute walk distance as objective measures of exercise capacity.[5] In the absence of a randomized trial, the control group was difficult to establish. The cohorts chosen for comparison were from ambulatory patients stable at 1 month after evaluation who subsequently underwent transplantation or had been evaluated during the same time and were found to be ineligible for cardiac transplantation. More transplant recipients were alive for exercise testing after 6 months, and the LV ejection fraction had improved from 15% to 60% after transplantation (from 15% to 20% without transplantation). However, the functional capacity was similar between survivors of the two groups, with peak oxygen consumption 17 ml/kg/min after transplantation and 19 ml/kg/min undergoing medical therapy, representing about 60% of predicted values.[5] Patients after heart transplantation perceived that exercise was more often limited by fatigue, compared to shortness of breath for survivors remaining on medical therapy.[4]

There is no way to subtract the impact of life changes resulting from recognition of imminent mortality, implications of donor harvesting, and survival through unique adversity. Functional limitations are perceived differently by transplant recipients and patients without such a history. Despite objective differences in functional capacity, subjective measures of well-being, psychologic effect, and life satisfaction from the Battelle report were virtually equivalent as perceived by heart transplant recipients, renal transplant recipients, and the normal population (see Table 21-2).

On the basis of the Battelle National Heart Transplant Study released in 1984, cardiac transplantation was considered standard therapy for patients meeting criteria for indications and contraindications as were applied during that test period. Medicare and other insurers have routinely provided reimbursement for the procedure at centers selected by meeting minimum standards for procedure volume and survival.

CARDIAC TRANSPLANTATION: RANDOMIZED CONTROLLED TRIALS OF THERAPY

Once the procedure itself was accepted as standard therapy, interest shifted toward the refinement of therapies for immunosuppression and complications of cardiac transplantation. Multiple aspects of heart transplantation provide challenges to the development of a basis of evidence derived from performance of large randomized clinical trials. The majority of rigorous trials completed have addressed issues at the periphery of management.

Complex therapy and surveillance strategies evolved simultaneously at multiple institutions, leading to marked variation in practice patterns. Rejection and infection are appropriate intermediate endpoints for trials, but the diagnosis of rejection itself has been difficult to standardize on endomyocardial biopsy, despite multiple consensus proceedings for definitions to be used in the trials.[6] Interventions targeted to rejection then trigger other changes in therapy for which there is limited consensus. Regional differences may affect the intensity of immunosuppression, with fewer episodes of rejection occurring in centers presumed to have greater genetic homogeneity of donors and recipients. The tapering, pulsing, and weaning of corticosteroid therapy provide a prime example. Perhaps the dominant feature of new immunosuppressive therapies, however, has been the spillover from renal transplantation. Most new immunosuppressive drugs for transplantation have been tested first in the renal population.[7,8] Once the drug is approved, use rapidly translates into other organ system transplantation, contaminating equipoise for randomized trials.

Immunosuppressive agents can influence endpoints of rejection, infection, and resultant mortality. The largest recent trial completed was the trial comparing mycophenolate mofetil, an inhibitor of the de novo path of purine synthesis, to the traditional agent azathioprine, both in addition to cyclosporine and corticosteroids. After a relatively high rate of drug discontinuation, the drug was associated with a slightly[9] lower incidence of severe rejection but slightly higher rate of infection. The ongoing randomized trial of rapamycin suggests decreased rejection with an increased incidence of renal dysfunction. These trials are complicated by the disparity between randomization and continued treatment because multiple events lead to discontinuation of one immunosuppressive agent in favor of another. Trials comparing different formulations of the same agent have been easier to perform and interpret but are not pivotal.

Hypertension is a common complication affecting a majority of patients after cardiac transplantation. After multiple small comparisons of agents, a multicenter trial was organized with 11 centers, enrolling 116 patients in a prospective randomized trial of diltiazem versus lisinopril.[10] Both therapies were found to be safe, although 19% had the drug withdrawn for minor side effects. Used as monotherapy, both were effective in fewer than 50% of patients.

With such daunting challenges of standardizing protocols at multiple sites, the majority of published trials for therapies in cardiac transplantation have been performed in single centers. Patient numbers are provided either by high center volume or enrollment extending over many years and thus may not always be applicable to programs or eras with different populations and protocols for therapy and surveillance.

A major nonfatal endpoint of cardiac transplantation is the development of accelerated graft vasculopathy. Diltiazem was suggested in an early single-center study to decrease vasculopathy[11] and is also useful to decrease cyclosporin metabolism and thus cost. A randomized study in 97 patients in a single center demonstrated that the lipid-lowering agent pravastatin decreased the rate of luminal thickening during the first and subsequent years after transplantation[12] (Fig. 21-1); these results subsequently were confirmed in other studies. Unexpectedly, lipid-lowering therapies also have decreased incidence of severe rejection, attributed to immunomodulatory effects on T-cell populations, which may contribute to early survival benefit.

When procedures are limited and the experience is divided among a large number of centers, careful scrutiny and collection of data is crucial to advance the field. The majority of information regarding therapies in cardiac transplantation has derived from the Cardiac Transplant Research Database. Originated and supported by the team at University of Alabama at Birmingham, the database currently includes almost 10,000 patients for whom meticulous follow-up information is maintained and checked, with complete enrollment from the dedicated sites without external financial support. This collaborative work, with unprecedented inclusion of all participating investigators in analysis and authorship, has already generated 17 published full publications and 36 abstracts. Among the major contributions are the recipient and donor risk factors for early and late mortality after transplantation; the determinants and competing risks for fatal rejection, infection, and malignancy; and the interventions and outcomes with transplant graft vasculopathy.[13,14]

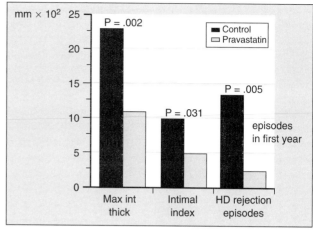

FIGURE 21-1. Impact of pravastatin therapy 20 mg daily begun within 2 weeks of cardiac transplantation in a randomized trial of 97 patients. Significant decreases were seen during the first year on serial angiography in the increase of maximal intimal thickness (max int thick) and intimal index. Although total rejection episodes were not significantly decreased, rejection accompanied by hemodynamic (HD) compromise occurred less often on pravastatin treatment. (Data from Kobashigawa J, Katznelson S, Laks H, et al: Effect of pravastatin on serum cholesterol, rejection, survival, and coronary vasculopathy after cardiac transplantation. N Engl J Med 1995;333:621–627.)

Larger numbers are available through the International Heart Transplant Registry, which includes 53,000 patients and 223 current centers throughout the world.[15] This database demonstrates the feasibility of collaboration across countries for the collection of basic demographic information and risk factors of donor and recipient for subsequent mortality after transplantation. The personnel resources required to enter detailed data preclude mandated entry and analysis of treatment regimens and critical intermediate endpoints such as rejection and vasculopathy. Like other large surgical databases, however, this information is critical to provide variables for case-mix adjustment and benchmarks of changing outcomes in an evolving field.

CARDIAC TRANSPLANTATION: DEFINING A BROADER POPULATION

Although cardiac transplantation has been performed in 53,000 patients over a period spanning more than 25 years, many more patients have been encompassed within its sphere of influence. The possibility of cardiac transplantation drew many potential candidates from the obscurity to which they had been consigned without hope. The majority of patients seen were ineligible for cardiac transplantation but in need of some other therapy as a "consolation prize." As the waiting list grew, more robust therapy needed to be developed to keep candidates alive during the longer wait. As these patients became concentrated at transplant centers, the prevalence of advanced heart failure and the potential impact of alternative approaches became increasingly recognized.[16] "Patients referred for cardiac transplantation" became a new population descriptor.[17]

INTRODUCTION OF MECHANICAL ASSIST DEVICES FOR "BRIDGE TO TRANSPLANT"

Mechanical cardiac assist devices were introduced into the clinical setting for postcardiotomy or acute cardiogenic shock. The intra-aortic balloon pump was used clinically in 1967. Attempts by Norman to define this experience led to the definition of cardiogenic shock that was used through the early trials of LVADs: cardiac output of less than 2 L/min/m^2, systolic blood pressure of less than 90 mm Hg, left or right atrial pressures of more than 20 mm Hg, systemic vascular resistance of more than 2100 dynes-sec-cm-5, and urine output less than 20 ml/hr.[18]

Setbacks in the development of a permanent artificial heart shifted attention to shorter-term support as a laboratory for new mechanical devices. In 1978, the first patient was bridged for 5 days to cardiac transplantation by a pneumatically driven ventricular assist device at the Texas Heart Institute. A multicenter experience with bridging to transplantation was reported in 34 patients,[19] in whom marked improvement in renal and hepatic function was seen early after support.

Duration of use for devices implanted for short-term support was stretched by unpredictable organ availability. The feasibility of implantable investigational devices was quickly demonstrated. The improvement in perfusion, organ function, and rehabilitation for patients awaiting transplant on mechanical devices was often a dramatic before-and-after comparison after failure of inotropic infusions and the confining intra-aortic balloon pump support that limited not only ambulation but even the sitting position. Approval for the devices was based largely on the perception of improved outcome from the desperate situation. A cohort study was done of 108 patients with cardiac index less than 2 L/min/m^2 or systolic blood pressure of 80 mm Hg or less and pulmonary capillary wedge pressure *of* 20 mm Hg or more.[20] The implantable LVAD was used in 75 patients, who were compared to 33 patients who had no obvious contraindications to device placement but did not receive devices because of logistic reasons. Survival to transplant was 71% with the assist device versus 36% without, and survival after 1 year for transplant recipients was 91% for those transplanted with a ventricular assist device support versus 67% for those who were not, although the former had a longer waiting time before transplantation. This comparison was obviously limited by the nonrandom nature of the logistic reasons but contributed to the momentum for approval of LVADs for bridge to transplantation (Fig. 21-2). Approval was obtained first for pneumatically powered devices in 1994 and subsequently in 1998 for the electrically powered portable device that allowed potential discharge home to await transplantation.

As the waiting time out of hospital increased even for patients with ventricular assist devices, greater experience accumulated regarding longer term support. A growing

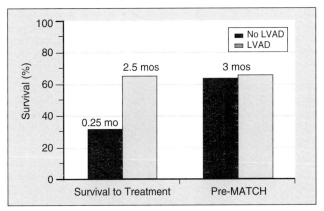

FIGURE 21-2. Bar graphs demonstrating percent survival with and without left-ventricular assist devices. The first pair of bars indicates survival to undergo transplantation for transplant candidates meeting criteria for hemodynamic decompensation. The first bar represents patients who did not receive implantable left-ventricular assist devices although eligible, and the second bar indicates patients who received device support, with significantly better survival.[20] Median time to death or transplant is shown above the bars. The second pair of bars indicates 3-month survival with and without left-ventricular assist devices for 21 patients randomized during a pilot phase (Pre-MATCH) of the REMATCH trial.[32] There is no significant difference between early survival for the randomized patients, thus justifying the performance of the larger randomized REMATCH trial.

number of survivors had exceeded a year of support prior to transplantation. Because transplantation is limited to only 3000 recipients worldwide each year, the inevitable question arose as to whether these devices could provide not only a "bridge" to transplantation but also a "destination" for patients unable to undergo transplantation.[21] These considerations represented a return to the original itinerary for device development after the detour provided by the bridging indication.

EVALUATION OF MECHANICAL SUPPORT FOR END-STAGE HEART FAILURE

Precedents with Cardiac Transplantation

Cardiac transplantation was approved as best therapy in 1984, based on the systematic scrutiny of patients undergoing transplantation and assumptions regarding their outcomes without transplantation. The acceptance of transplantation is sometimes cited as an example within the "breakthrough" realm of therapies, similar to penicillin, for which the early experience is so dramatic that equipoise cannot be found for a randomized trial that includes a control arm without therapy (Fig. 21-3). Transplantation can also be considered, however, to have acceptance under the "grandfather clause." At the time, there had been no therapies demonstrated in a controlled trial to improve survival in heart failure. The Vasodilator in Heart Failure Trial, demonstrating favorable impact of the hydralazine combination, was not published until 1986.[22] The trial demonstrating the benefit of angiotensin-converting enzyme (ACE) inhibitors for advanced heart failure was published the next year.[23] During the same era, controlled trials of inotropic therapy consistently demonstrated worse outcome, despite the appealing

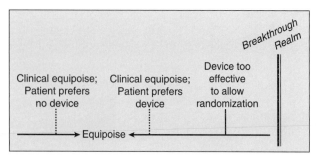

FIGURE 21-3. Line depicting the dynamic interaction between equipoise and efficacy of a new therapy after initial investigation.[27] It is conceivable but uncommon that the early experience could be so positive that the scientific and regulatory community consider it to be "breakthrough" in nature when compared to the known history of the condition. More commonly, the scientific community but not the regulatory bodies may be sufficiently convinced of benefit that they cannot find a position of equipoise from which to perform randomized trials, in which case the gap for regulatory approval may be filled by careful continued investigation without a controlled group, analogous to the Battelle study of transplantation.[2] Preferences of patients consenting to consider new therapies generally lie to the right of equipoise, exerting tension on the equipoise of physicians. The asymmetry of the line to the right of equipoise reflects the weight of initial enthusiasm necessary to drive further development.

rationale for this approach.[24,25] Not until after the acceptance of cardiac transplantation was the template of the randomized clinical trial refined into the gold standard for validation of new therapies for heart failure.

Implementation of mechanical support devices bypassed this scrutiny because it was initially perceived as a preliminary surgical procedure in preparation for transplantation. The experience gained with the devices in transplant candidates contributed to the confidence with which to pursue longer term support. However, the enthusiasm engendered by this favorable short-to-intermediate–term experience with devices threatened the equipoise required to embark on a randomized trial for longer term support. The comparison of survival to transplant with an LVAD to survival of a simultaneous cohort without the device (see Fig. 21-2) was sufficient evidence for some to feel that a randomized trial for destination therapy was not ethical. During the design and implementation of the randomized controlled trial of mechanical support as destination therapy for end-stage disease, critical challenges arose to the application of this "gold standard" approach, as derived from trials of medical therapy in less severe heart failure.

Fundamental Differences Between Testing for Drugs and Devices

The target population for surgical implantation of mechanical support devices must have disease of sufficient severity to warrant intervention that carries cost, inconvenience, and major irreducible risk.[26] Benefits must be proportionately large to be meaningful to an individual, not just to a population at risk. The temporal relationship between cause and effect is transparent for the support devices, compared to drug therapies in which both benefits and risks are often masked or mimicked by the natural history of heart failure. The rapidity

and transparency of cause and effect focus close attention for both patient and physician on the expected and realized early outcomes. Even if it were ethically feasible to perform sham surgery or to insert the device without activating it, even if it were practically feasible to mimic the sounds and sensations of device function, the clinical effects of the device would usually reveal the treatment. One could debate the utility of a circulatory assist device whose function was not rapidly apparent in a patient with critical hemodynamic compromise. Thus the high-risk population with potential front-loaded benefit complicates traditional trial design.[27]

Because the patient and physician cannot generally be blinded to treatment arm, the randomized controlled design does not serve to eliminate the physician observer bias for outcome measurement in trials of mechanical support devices. Of perhaps more concern, the patient is fully aware of the treatment received. This is a major difference between device trials and drug trials, in which patients on placebo often assume that they have after all received the active therapy. Even when equipoise can truly be said to exist for physicians based on previous clinical information,[28] patients who perceive that they have "lost" through randomization have incurred an additional psychic cost that influences the outcome of the patient and the study. Such issues have arisen in drug development for acquired immunodeficiency syndrome.[29] Another unmeasurable component is the potential compromise of the therapeutic relationship when the patient receives a therapy that has not been selected by the physician and when the patient perceives that a better therapy has been withheld. When the therapy being tested is available elsewhere outside of the trial, patients may leave to "cross over," understandably considering their own survival before trial validity.[30]

Both drugs and devices undergo extensive testing and refinement prior to human experimentation. Compared to the development of new drugs, however, device innovation remains more incremental during clinical testing. Before and after clinical approval and marketing, these devices have undergone multiple sequential modifications of components such as drivelines, controllers, valves, connectors, and power systems. Whether advantageous or deleterious, these changes can potentially confound interpretation of results extending over the period of the trial. Although drug development could benefit from more supervised evolution of initiation and titration protocols, these generally remain fixed during a trial unless altered by major adverse findings.

THE RANDOMIZED EVALUATION OF MECHANICAL ASSISTANCE FOR THE TREATMENT OF CONGESTIVE HEART FAILURE STUDY

Evolution of Patient Population

Sick Enough but Not Too Sick

As plans were being made in 1994 for the eventual Randomized Evaluation of Mechanical Assistance for the

Treatment of Congestive Heart Failure (REMATCH) study, a major challenge was selection of the patient population. Who was sick enough to benefit but well enough to survive the operation?[31] The previous data were based on patients who were awaiting transplantation, in whom follow-up was short, or who had major contraindications to transplantation. Although destination therapy was aimed at patients ineligible for transplantation, many transplant contraindications would also limit survival with mechanical support devices. Furthermore, to allow adequate time for follow-up, patients enrolled had to remain ineligible for transplantation. The transplant ineligibility criteria usually involved having chronic renal dysfunction, having end-organ damage from diabetes; or, most commonly, being older than age 65 years (Table 21-3). Older patients were generally not accepted for transplantation during the era of the study, although the chronologic age restriction to transplantation has increasingly been removed.

Reasonable Versus Optimal Medical Management

The initial concept was that patients would not be eligible until all possible attempts had been made to adjust medical therapies at expert institutions. During the small pilot trial of 21 patients, rigorous "gatekeeping" was practiced by heart failure specialists at the coordinating center in communication with heart failure specialists at the investigating site. Experiences during this time suggested that such efforts could delay randomization until patients had died or deteriorated to a status inappropriate for surgery. Furthermore, if extended efforts at stabilization at the investigating site had already been unsuccessful, randomization was to device or despair. The outcomes for these 21 patients in the pilot trial confirmed their dismal fate. The lack of significant difference in survival between LVAD and medical

■ ■ ■

TABLE 21-3 INCLUSION CRITERIA FOR REMATCH TRIAL

Severity of disease

1. New York Heart Association Class IV symptoms for 60–90* days
2. Attempted therapy with angiotensin-converting enzyme inhibitors, diuretics, and digoxin
3. Left-ventricular ejection fraction ≤25%
4. A. Peak oxygen consumption of ≤12–14* ml/kg/min with achievement of respiratory exchange ratio of ≥1.1
   or
   B. Demonstrated dependence on inotropic infusions
5. Ineligibility for cardiac transplantation as a result of the following:
   A. Age >65 years
   B. Insulin-dependent diabetes mellitus with noncardiac end-organ damage
   C. Chronic renal failure with serum creatinine concentration ≥2.5 mg/dl for at least 90 days before randomization
   D. Other irreversible contraindications not felt to compromise operative outcome or long-term survival

*Modified during trial
Modified from Rose EA GA, Moskowitz AJ, Heitjan DF, et al: Long-term Use of a left-ventricular assist device for end-stage heart failure. N Engl J Med 2001; 345:1435–1443.

management patients in this trial was felt to reflect the unexpected severity of illness in the recipients.[32] This pilot result did, however, strengthen the position of equipoise regarding randomization in the REMATCH trial (see Fig. 21-2).

For the formal REMATCH trial, an attempt was made to move the eligibility for randomization slightly earlier in the natural history of escalating disease and therapies (see Table 21-3). Patients were considered eligible if they fulfilled the first three criteria at the time of randomization and were receiving "reasonable" therapy with attempted ACE inhibitor and diuretic use, without necessarily having undergone therapy with other vasoactive agents or therapy adjusted to hemodynamic goals. Patients undergoing reasonable therapy would then be randomized to the LVAD or the institution of "optimal medical management (OM²)" to be provided by cardiologists certified for expertise in heart failure management. In addition to offering a more optimistic therapy for the control arm, it was felt that this would better anticipate the eventual application of trial results. As the trial progressed, however, it became clear that the entry point for the trial had really not moved and that the patients and referring physicians willing to consider enrollment had generally already exhausted current therapies.

Unprecedented Severity of Heart Failure

The sample size was calculated based on a 2-year mortality of 75% in the medical therapy arm, with a 33% reduction in mortality with the LVAD. As the trial proceeded, enrollment was slow and the entry criteria were further relaxed to allow class IV symptoms for only 60 of 90 days and peak VO_2 up to 14 ml/kg/min. Although half of study enrollment occurred after this change, only three patients fell outside the initial criteria.

The final population in REMATCH was the most compromised patient population studied in any heart failure trial (Table 21-4). The blood pressure and serum creatinine levels were higher and serum sodium was lower than any trial demonstrating benefit of therapy for heart failure. Intravenous inotropic infusions were being administered at the time of randomization in 91 (71%) of the 129 randomized patients. Despite this pharmacologic support, their mean systolic blood pressure was 99 mm Hg and serum sodium was 134 mEq/L. Optimal medical management offered little beyond the therapies at baseline. Overall use of ACE inhibitors was 53% initially, with all others having unsuccessful previous therapy with ACE inhibitors. Re-institution was attempted in some, with utilization increased to 63% by 1 month early after randomization and subsequent decline to 45% because patients with circulatory compromise failed to tolerate inhibition of their neurohormonal compensatory mechanisms. Attempts to wean intravenous inotropic therapy were unsuccessful, largely as a result of recurrent hypotension and renal dysfunction. Survival for the group undergoing optimal medical management overall was 25% at 1 year. Survival with medical management of the subgroup of patients initially receiving intravenous inotropic therapy was 22% at 1 year.

TABLE 21-4   ADVANCED HEART FAILURE TRIAL POPULATIONS* AND EARLY MORTALITY† ON MEDICAL THERAPY

	Consensus	Promise	Rales	Copernicus	REMATCH—oral medical therapy	REMATCH—medical therapy + IV Inotropic therapy
# patients in group	126	527	841	1113	15	46
Age (years)	63	64	65	64	67	67
LVEF (%)	NA	21	25	20	17	17
SBP (mm Hg)	125	115	122	125	107	99
Na (mEq/liter)	137	139	NA	137	137	134
Creatinine (mg/dl)	1.5	1.5	1.2	1.5	1.7	1.8
6-month mortality (%)	29	20	13	9	39	61

*Populations are those receiving angiotensin-converting enzyme inhibitor therapy (Consensus) with placebo for other therapies studied.
†Survival for other trials estimated from published survival curves.
LVEF, left-ventricular ejection fraction; SBP, systolic blood pressure; Na, sodium.

Benefit of Left-ventricular Assist Device in REMATCH

Left-Ventricular Assist Devices and Survival

The LVADs were associated with a dramatic improvement in survival at 1 year, from 25% to 52%.[33] Two-year survival was increased almost fourfold but was still only 23% in the LVAD group, as reported in the original analysis. The difference in survival was best seen in the patients initially undergoing intravenous inotropic therapy (Fig. 21-4). Despite their greater compromise preoperatively, this group had outcomes with LVAD that were comparable to those patients with less severe compromise at randomization. At the time of randomization, only 38 (29%) of the patients were on oral therapy alone, without intravenous inotropic therapy. In this group there was no difference in survival at 6 months between LVAD and medical therapy. Survival at 1 year was better with the LVAD for patients receiving oral therapy, but the difference was not significant in this small cohort.

The major cause of death was LV failure in the medical management group. After LVAD, sepsis and device failure were the most common causes of death. There were no device failures within the first 12 months, but the probability of device failure was 35% by 24 months, and 10 devices were replaced.

The REMATCH trial demonstrated not only the benefit of the LVAD but also the wisdom of including a control group for this first trial of destination therapy. Although it was anticipated that the LVAD arm would have 50% survival at 2 years (33% better survival than a control group with 75% mortality),[31] the actual LVAD mortality itself was in the range of 75% at 2 years.[33] Without the actual assessment of the control group, in which there were virtually no survivors, it would not have been possible to make the case for the benefit of the LVAD.

Quality of Life with Left-Ventricular Assist Devices

Improved quality of life was seen in LVAD survivors. The Minnesota Living with Heart Failure scores at baseline were 75, worse than in any previous heart failure trial. The scores improved to 41 in the 23 patients of the LVAD group studied at 1 year and to 58 in the 6 medical management groups surviving to be studied.[33] From this estimate, LVAD conferred a quality of life similar to that for NYHA class III heart failure in patients with initial severity of illness worse than the usual NYHA class IV patients (Fig. 21-5). Patients' assessment of physical functional and role emotional items on the Short-Form 36 also improved. Patients with the LVAD had 88 total hospital days compared to 24 for the medical management group. However, the median number of days spent alive out of the hospital was 340 with the LVAD, more than three times as high as the 106 days with medical management.[33] The extension of life with the ventricular assist device thus did provide meaningful life outside the hospital.

From Device Trials into Practice

Applying Results from REMATCH

The completion of the REMATCH trial represented a landmark in the rigorous evaluation of a surgical therapy for end-stage heart failure. The demonstration of benefit with only 129 randomized patients reflects the dramatic natural history of the disease at that stage and the impact of the therapy. However, this small number of patients limits

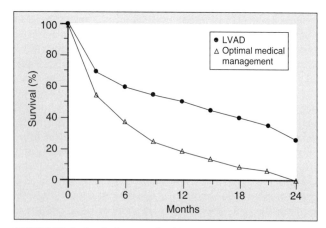

FIGURE 21-4. Survival curves for 91 patients receiving intravenous inotropic therapy at the time of randomization in REMATCH (Randomized Evaluation of Mechanical Assistance in Therapy of Congestive Heart Failure). LVAD, left-ventricular assist device.

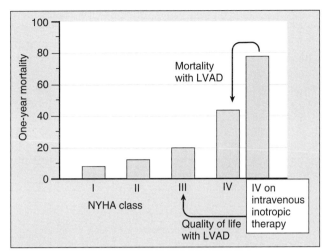

FIGURE 21-5. Conceptualization of the benefit of left-ventricular assist device placement on 1-year mortality as estimated for New York Heart Association (NYHA) classes of symptoms, reducing mortality from a level beyond class IV for patients receiving intravenous inotropic therapy in REMATCH to that observed for class IV patients in previous trials. Benefit of the assist device for quality of life is estimated to return patients to a level consistent with NYHA class III.

generalization to a larger population. Most patients in each group died within 2 years, leaving only 1 year of data from which to seek subgroups with different expected benefit. The criteria for eligibility into REMATCH were relatively broad, applying to many patients with advanced heart failure. However, the patient population actually randomized, as demonstrated in the patient profile, was much more severely compromised than required for enrollment and certainly was more compromised than many patients labeled as having class IV heart failure for trials of medical therapy. The trial does not provide enough information through which individuals likely to benefit from current LVAD technology could be identified outside of centers already experienced in the iterative procedure by which other therapies are adjusted and ultimately found to be ineffective.

Furthermore, the technology and supporting care have changed considerably even since the end of the study 1 year ago. Prophylaxis regimens for infection and design modifications to reduce drive-line infections and valvular incompetence were introduced during the latter part of the trial. These factors should improve LVAD outcomes over those observed in the trial. Medical therapy has also advanced, however, during the same period. No new therapies for heart failure of this severity have recently been introduced or even advanced to full-scale investigation. However, the broader penetrance of therapies such as beta blockers for earlier stages of disease and biventricular pacing for patients with marked QRS prolongation may change the clinical profile of patients who ultimately deteriorate to be considered for replacement therapies.

The Curves of Downshifting Risk

The implementation of new therapies evolves rapidly after introduction. For medications, the testing has often been in relatively healthier heart failure populations, from which results are extended into patients with more severe clinical disease. For surgical approaches, however, the trend of development is often in the other direction. Uncertain risk limits initial application to patients who are clearly at very high risk without therapy, the "all would have died" group. There is an early excitement phase during which inexperienced centers join the gold rush only to find that success is hard to duplicate. Some centers will withdraw, whereas others will persevere and prevail if the initial promise of the procedure is realized.

Once survival has been recognized outside the trial, patients with less severe disease may also be considered. These patients have lower risk of early operative complications. The promise of better performance statistics provides incentive for programs to pursue the healthier candidates, who are likely to do well after surgery. However, these patients may also have relatively good survival without the new procedure.[17] This can be depicted as the curves of downshifting risk (Fig. 21-6), as has previously been described for new surgical therapies, particularly transplantation[34] and, more recently, cardiomyoplasty. It is important to step back to review the overall goal, which is not to maximize absolute survival after the intervention but to maximize outcomes for all. It is the magnitude of the difference between the outcomes with and without the procedure that should drive the intervention.

FUTURE TRIALS FOR DEVICES IN END-STAGE HEART DISEASE

Increasing partnership between the design engineers, investigators, and industry focuses attention on the goals that are parallel and those that diverge. Once a device has passed bench testing into patients, the results are keenly observed, regardless of whether this initial clinical experience is labeled as "feasibility" or "safety." It is

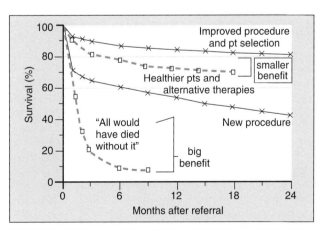

FIGURE 21-6. Concept of "downshifting risk" during evolution of surgical therapies for advanced heart failure. Survival with procedure is shown in solid lines; survival without procedure is in dashed lines. Initially tried only in patients facing imminent death, procedures found to be successful may then be extended more electively to patients with less severe disease. Such patients may have better operative survival but less benefit at a time when the natural history of the disease is also more favorable.

the hope of the sponsor that such experience will be of such unprecedented success that investigators cannot find a stand of equipoise regarding a subsequent randomized trial. It is certainly possible to envision such a case, in which the new development would move rapidly into the "breakthrough realm" (Fig. 21-3).[27] The scientific community could become convinced of efficacy before the regulatory agencies were prepared for approval, a gap that might need to be bridged by continued investigation at limited sites with a reference group of historical controls only. For the majority of cases, however, the early experience showing promise is not sufficient to establish efficacy. Clinical trials thus require more rigorous design for further testing.

The REMATCH trial will not be repeated. The survival shown for the device arm will be the benchmark against which modifications of current LVADs and new devices will be tested. Although the randomized, double-blind, controlled trial template from drug therapies remains a "gold standard" against which to judge investigation of other therapies, the increasing appreciation of unique aspects of device surgery for end-stage heart failure does warrant careful consideration of potential variations in this design of randomized trials. The spectre of imminent death may lead to modifications in the course of the trial after randomization, such as potential "compassionate use" or one-way crossover to the device in the event that certain signposts of impending endpoints are reached. Models for randomized trials in which patients could be informed and allowed some option to select their preferred therapy might provide more information on patients not desiring therapy as well as those who do and those who consent to randomization.

VITAL ROLE OF REGISTRIES

Regardless of the specific trials performed, the controlled data obtained will be very limited in comparison to the actual utilization of devices found effective. Some of the factors of cost, maintenance, and transparent effects that limit the extent of rigorous trials for devices before approval actually facilitate the ability to learn about them afterward. To obtain heart donors for transplantation, institutions must submit data to the United Network of Organ Sharing registry. The precedent for registering all implanted devices such as valves and defibrillators carries over for the new devices once approved. The requirement for continued quality control can be extended into baseline characterization of recipients and fundamental outcomes such as death and device malfunctions for approved mechanical support devices. This is under way through a contract between the International Society for Heart and Lung Transplantation and the same United Network of Organ Sharing team. In contrast to pharmaceutical therapies, which are easier to study before approval and harder to track afterward, the weight of evidence for various mechanical cardiac devices, through required registry documentation, may be heavier with postapproval experience than with preapproval trials.

The role of registries in progress with mechanical support devices will be complemented by the eventual coalescence of registries of advanced heart failure from which device candidates will become eligible. There is currently an industry-sponsored voluntary registry for heart failure hospitalization and a new one beginning for the burgeoning heart failure/pacing device population. Because these types of data, together with the device registry, will likely constitute the core of progress in this field, it is critical that support, interpretation, and extension be supervised and controlled independently from commercial incentive.

REFERENCES

1. Jamieson S, Oyer P, Reitz B, et al: Cardiac transplantation at Stanford. J Heart Transplant 1982; 1:86-92.
2. Evans RW, Broida JH: National Heart Transplantation Study. Seattle, Washington: Battelle Human Affairs Research Centers, 1985.
3. Stevenson LW, Hamilton MA, Tillisch IH, et al: Decreasing survival benefit from cardiac transplantation for outpatients as the waiting list lengthens. J Am Coll Cardiol 1991; 18:919-925.
4. Walden JA, Stevenson LW, Dracup K, et al: Extended comparison of quality of life between stable heart failure patients and heart transplant recipients. J Heart Lung Transplant 1994; 13:1109-1118.
5. Stevenson LW, Sietsema K, Tillisch JH, et al: Exercise capacity for survivors of cardiac transplantation or sustained medical therapy for stable heart failure. Circulation 1990; 81:78-85.
6. Winters GL, McManus BM: Consistencies and controversies in the application of the International Society for Heart and Lung Transplantation working formulation for heart transplant biopsy specimens: Rapamycin Cardiac Rejection Treatment Trial Pathologists. J Heart Lung Transplant 1996; 15:728-735.
7. Busque S, Shoker A, Landsberg D, et al: Canadian multicentre trial of tacrolimus/azathioprine/steroids versus tacrolimus/mycophenolate mofetil/steroids versus neoral/mycophenolate mofetil/steroids in renal transplantation. Transplant Proc 2001; 33:1266-1267.
8. A randomized clinical trial of cyclosporine in cadaveric renal transplantation: Analysis at three years. The Canadian Multicentre Transplant Study Group. N Engl J Med 1986; 314:1219-1225.
9. Kobashigawa J, Miller L, Renlund D, et al: A randomized active-controlled trial of mycophenolate mofetil in heart transplant recipients: Mycophenolate Mofetil Investigators. Transplantation 1998; 66:507-515.
10. Brozena SC, Johnson MR, Ventura H, et al: Effectiveness and safety of diltiazem or lisinopril in treatment of hypertension after heart transplantation: Results of a prospective, randomized multicenter trial. J Am Coll Cardiol 1996; 27:1707-1712.
11. Schroeder JS, Gao SZ, Alderman EL, et al: A preliminary study of diltiazem in the prevention of coronary artery disease in heart-transplant recipients. N Engl J Med 1993; 328:164-170.
12. Kobashigawa J, Katznelson S, Laks H, et al: Effect of pravastatin on serum cholesterol, rejection, survival, and coronary vasculopathy after cardiac transplantation. N Engl J Med 1995; 333:621-627.
13. Bourge RC, Naftel DC, Costanzo-Nordin MR, et al: Pretransplantation risk factors for death after heart transplantation: A multiinstitutional study. The Transplant Cardiologists Research Database Group. J Heart Lung Transplant 1993; 12:549-562.
14. Rodeheffer RJ, Naftel DC, Stevenson LW, et al: Secular trends in cardiac transplant recipient and donor management in the United States, 1990 to 1994: A multi-institutional study. Cardiac Transplant Research Database Group. Circulation 1996; 94:2883-2889.
15. Hosenpud JD, Bennett LE, Keck BM, et al: The Registry of the International Society for Heart and Lung Transplantation: seventeenth official report-2000. J Heart Lung Transplant 2000; 19:909-931.
16. Stevenson LW, Dracup KA, Tillisch JH: Efficacy of medical therapy tailored for severe congestive heart failure in patients transferred for urgent cardiac transplantation. Am J Cardiol 1989; 63:461-464.
17. Stevenson WG, Stevenson LW, Middlekauff HR, et al: Improving survival for patients with advanced heart failure: A study of 737 consecutive patients. J Am Coll Cardiol 1995; 26:1417-1423.

18. Norman JC, Colley DA, Igo S: Prognostic indices for survival during post-cardiotomy intra-aortic balloon pumping. J Thorac Cardiovasc Surg 1977; 74:709-713.
19. Frazier OH, Rose EA, Macmanus Q, et al: Multicenter clinical evaluation of the HeartMate 1000 IP left ventricular assist device. Ann Thorac Surg 1992; 53:1080-1090.
20. Frazier OH, Rose EA, McCarthy P, et al: Improved mortality and rehabilitation of transplant candidates treated with a long-term implantable left ventricular assist system. Ann Surg 1995; 222:327-336; discussion 336-338.
21. Oz MC, Argenziano M, Catanese KA, et al: Bridge experience with long-term implantable left ventricular assist devices: Are they an alternative to transplantation? Circulation 1997; 95:1844-1852.
22. Cohn JN, Archibald DG, Ziesche S, et al: Effect of vasodilator therapy on mortality in chronic congestive heart failure: Results of a Veterans Administration Cooperative Study. N Engl J Med 1986; 314:1547-1552.
23. Effects of enalapril on mortality in severe congestive heart failure: Results of the Cooperative North Scandinavian Enalapril Survival Study (CONSENSUS): The CONSENSUS Trial Study Group. N Engl J Med 1987; 316:1429-1435.
24. Packer M, Carver JR, Rodeheffer RJ, et al: Effect of oral milrinone on mortality in severe chronic heart failure: The PROMISE Study Research Group [see comments]. N Engl J Med 1991; 325:1468-1475.
25. Cohn JN, Goldstein SO, Greenberg BH, et al: A dose-dependent increase in mortality with vesnarinone among patients with severe heart failure: Vesnarinone Trial Investigators [see comments]. N Engl J Med 1998; 339:1810-1816.
26. Stevenson LW, Couper G, Natterson B, et al: Target heart failure populations for newer therapies. Circulation 1995; 92:II174-181.
27. Stevenson LW, Kormos RL: Mechanical Cardiac Support 2000: Current applications and future trial design. J Am Coll Cardiol 2001; 37:340-370.
28. Freedman B: Equipoise and the ethics of clinical research. N Engl J Med 1987; 317:141-145.
29. Hellman S, Hellman DS: Of mice but not men: Problems of the randomized clinical trial. N Engl J Med 1991; 324:1585-1589.
30. Volberding PA, Lagakos SW, Koch MA, et al: Zidovudine in asymptomatic human immunodeficiency virus infection: A controlled trial in persons with fewer than 500 CD4-positive cells per cubic millimeter. The AIDS Clinical Trials Group of the National Institute of Allergy and Infectious Diseases. N Engl J Med 1990; 322:941-949.
31. Rose EA, Moskowitz AJ, Packer M, et al: The REMATCH trial: rationale, design, and end points: Randomized Evaluation of Mechanical Assistance for the Treatment of Congestive Heart Failure. Ann Thorac Surg 1999; 67:723-730.
32. Moskowitz AJ, Sollano JA, Heitjan DF, et al: Left ventricular assist devices as long-term therapy for severe heart failure: Pilot study results demonstrate feasibility of randomized trial [abstract]. Circulation 1999; 100:I-514.
33. Rose EA GA, Moskowitz AJ, Heitjan DF, et al: Long-term use of a left ventricular assist device for end-stage heart failure. N Engl J Med 2001; 345:1435-1443.
34. Stevenson L: When is heart failure a surgical disease? In Rose EA SL (ed). Management of End-Stage Heart Disease. Philadelphia-New York: Lippincott-Raven, 1998;129-146.

■ ■ ■ c h a p t e r **22**

Cholesterol Reduction

Richard E. Scranton
J. Michael Gaziano

Cholesterol lowering is one of the greatest success stories in cardiovascular disease prevention and an excellent example of how clinical trial research builds upon and complements other types of empirical investigation. Knowledge of the role played by cholesterol in the development of cardiovascular disease (CVD) derives from basic laboratory research, observational studies, and large-scale clinical trials. Findings from the former two types of studies motivated the development of pharmacologic interventions, the efficacy, safety, and cost-effectiveness of which have been now extensively tested in large trials of diverse populations. Although early trials were largely restricted to middle-aged men, the cardioprotective benefits of cholesterol reduction have in recent years also been demonstrated in elderly individuals and women.

This chapter begins with a brief summary of the observational data on the relationship between cholesterol levels and coronary heart disease (CHD), followed by a review of clinical trials of cholesterol lowering and CHD in secondary and primary prevention settings, including recent trial data on cholesterol lowering in women and elderly individuals. Recent trial data demonstrating reductions in ischemic stroke with cholesterol lowering also are summarized, and because consideration of any intervention must include a careful balancing of potential benefits and risks, nonvascular mortality outcomes are discussed in detail. Finally, the cost efficacy of lipid-lowering therapy is considered.

CORONARY HEART DISEASE

Observational Epidemiology

Numerous human observational studies have left little doubt that elevated cholesterol levels increase the risk of CHD.[1] Observational research indicates a linear relationship, with a 20% increase in risk of CHD for each 10% increase in serum cholesterol.[2] This dose-response effect occurs at all levels of baseline cholesterol[3] and is apparent in both men and women, blacks and whites, and individuals with and without prior cardiovascular disease.

However, estimates from prospective observational data may underestimate the true risk associated with lipoprotein abnormalities because the relationship is generally based on a single measure of total cholesterol.[2] The underestimation results from two forms of bias. First, regression dilution bias, which arises from assay inaccuracies and random fluctuation of cholesterol levels over time in any given subject, introduces random misclassification that tends to underestimate the size of the true association. Second, surrogate dilution bias results from the less-than-perfect correlation between low-density lipoprotein (LDL) cholesterol and total cholesterol levels. Because LDL cholesterol tends to be a stronger predictor of CHD than total cholesterol, the use of the latter tends to underestimate the association. Indeed, studies that avoid these biases by using repeated measures of LDL cholesterol show an approximate 27% increase in risk of CHD for each 10% increase in serum cholesterol.[4]

The consistency of the observational data strongly supported a cause-and-effect relationship between cholesterol and CHD. Numerous pharmaceutical agents were subsequently developed to reduce cholesterol. As a result, large, randomized clinical trials were needed to confirm the anticipated benefits of lowering cholesterol and to assess the potential risks and costs of these new therapies. The earliest trials were conducted among people with preexisting CHD to determine whether cholesterol lowering improved surrogate indicators of future risk of cardiac events. Subsequent secondary prevention studies evaluated whether cholesterol lowering reduced future clinical cardiovascular events and mortality in patients with a history of CVD and in acute coronary syndromes. In the late 1990s and early 2000s, primary prevention trials sought to determine whether cholesterol lowering would prove beneficial to initially healthy individuals. Several recent large secondary and primary trials included sufficient numbers of women and elderly individuals to determine the benefits of cholesterol lowering in these groups.

SECONDARY PREVENTION TRIALS

Angiographic Trials Utilizing Intermediate Endpoints

Angiographic trials show that cholesterol reduction promotes regression or decreases progression of atherosclerotic plaques. The findings are consistent whether cholesterol lowering is accomplished by changes in exercise and diet or by the addition of pharmacologic agents. Most of these trials were too small and too short in duration to demonstrate a significant difference in coronary events between patients receiving cholesterol-lowering intervention and controls.[5] When data from these studies were pooled, however, patients assigned to active treatment experienced a 26% reduction in total mortality and a 39% reduction in nonfatal myocardial infarction (MI).[5]

Although early angiographic trials provided evidence that cholesterol lowering reduced the size and progression of atherosclerotic plaques, change in visible lesions appeared to be small and could not account for the degree of reduction in CHD events found in observational studies and in subsequent secondary prevention studies that utilized clinical endpoints. Thus, reduction of coronary artery disease (CAD) events by cholesterol lowering likely involves other mechanisms beyond the regression of angiographically visible plaques. With recent advances in pathophysiologic research and imaging techniques, it has become clear that such mechanisms include the regression and stabilization of smaller lesions[6,7] and improvements in the vascular architecture, endothelial function,[8,9] and the inflammatory milieu.[10]

The information gained from the early angiographic studies provided further impetus to conduct large, randomized clinical trials sufficiently powered to show a reduction in CHD events as a result of cholesterol-lowering interventions.

Trials Utilizing Hard Clinical Endpoints

Prestatin Trials

Prior to the availability of 3-hydroxy-3-methylglutaryl coenzyme A (HMG-CoA) reductase inhibitors (statins), numerous cholesterol-lowering interventions were studied. Although cholesterol reduction was modest, these trials clearly demonstrated the ability of cholesterol-lowering drugs to reduce CHD events. For instance, the Coronary Drug Project randomized 8341 men aged 30 to 64 years with a history of MI to one of four therapies.[11] The estrogen and dextrothyroxine treatment arms were discontinued prior to the study end because of increased mortality. Niacin and clofibrate lowered cholesterol by 10% and 6%, respectively, but neither treatment produced a significant reduction in cardiovascular mortality. The modest amount of cholesterol lowering in this trial and similar trials likely explains why such interventions failed to reduce cardiovascular mortality. One exception is the 5-year, open-label Stockholm Ischemic Heart Disease Secondary Prevention trial, which found that a combination of clofibrate and nicotinic acid reduced cholesterol by 13% and ischemic cardiovascular mortality by 36% (P < 0.01).[12] Prestatin studies set the stage for later investigations of more potent lipid-lowering therapies.

Statin-Era Trials

Rather than provide a complete review of the voluminous literature in this area, only the largest of the statin-era trials are discussed; these are listed in Table 22-1.

Except as noted, all trials utilized a randomized, double-blind, placebo-controlled design.

Scandinavian Simvastatin Survival Study Trial

The Scandinavian Simvastatin Survival Study (4S) trial[13] adds to the now-irrefutable evidence that secondary prevention with lipid-lowering therapy provides major clinical benefit. In this group of 4444 men and women with a baseline total cholesterol of 5.5 mmol/L or higher and a history of MI or angina pectoris, a 38% LDL cholesterol reduction with simvastatin in the treated group was associated with a 42% reduction, relative to the control group, in cardiac death (P < 0.0001), a 30% reduction in all-cause mortality (P = 0.003), and a 34% reduction in major coronary events (defined as coronary death or nonfatal MI). This is the first randomized trial of lipid therapy that showed a significant reduction in all-cause mortality.

Subgroup analyses of 4S data show that women and men derived similar benefit from lipid therapy with respect to major coronary events, as did users and nonusers of acetylsalicylic acid, beta blockers, and calcium channel antagonists. A modest treatment advantage existed for subjects younger than 60 years (39% risk reduction vs. 29% for those ≥60 years), for those with hypertension (37% vs. 32%), and for never-smokers (41% vs. 31% for current and former smokers). Subjects with diabetes, who comprised 5% of the total sample, achieved striking reductions in major coronary events (55% vs. 32% for those subjects without diabetes).

Cholesterol and Recurrent Events Trial

The Cholesterol and Recurrent Events (CARE) trial was designed to assess the efficacy of pravastatin therapy among post-MI patients with typical cholesterol levels.[14] Entry criteria included total cholesterol less than 240 mg/dL, LDL cholesterol 115 to 174 mg/dL, and fasting triglycerides less than 350 mg/dL at least 5 weeks following MI. At baseline, cholesterol averaged 209 mg/dL, triglycerides 155 mg/dL, LDL cholesterol 139 mg/dL, and high-density lipoprotein (HDL) cholesterol 39 mg/dL. More than half of these patients had prior percutaneous transluminal coronary angioplasty (PTCA) or coronary artery bypass graft (CABG). The primary endpoint, CHD death or nonfatal MI, was reduced 24% by treatment; fatal MI was reduced by 37%; and revascularization by 27%. Subgroup analyses showed patients with hypertension, diabetes, prior revascularization procedures, and low left-ventricular ejection fraction (LVEF) fared as well as their respective counterparts without these features. Modest treatment advantages existed among subjects older than 60 years, those with prior Q-wave MIs, and those with HDL cholesterol levels of 37 mg/dL or less. Treatment advantages were also found for women (46% risk reduction vs. 20% for men [P = NS]), and for current smokers (33% vs. 22% for ex-smokers or nonsmokers). Individuals with the highest baseline LDL cholesterol levels experienced greater risk reductions (3% risk *increase* for those with LDL cholesterol <125 mg/dL, 26% risk reduction when LDL cholesterol 125 to

TABLE 22-1 RECENT LARGE-SCALE RANDOMIZED TRIALS OF CHOLESTEROL LOWERING IN THE SECONDARY PREVENTION OF CARDIOVASCULAR DISEASE

Study	Baseline LDL cholesterol	Study population	Intervention	Duration (yr)	% LDL reduction	CVD event reduction: Relative risk (95% confidence interval)	Overall mortality: Relative risk (95% confidence interval)
4S,[13] 1994	187 mg/dL	4444 men and women; mean age 59 yr	Simvastatin, titration	5.4	35	0.58 (0.46–0.73)	0.70 (0.58–0.85)
CARE,[14] 1996	139 mg/dL	4159 men and women; mean age 59 yr	Pravastatin, 40 mg	5.0	28	0.76 (0.64–0.91)	0.91 (0.74–1.12)
LIPID,[15] 1998	150 mg/dL	9014 men and women age 31–75 yr	Pravastatin, 40 mg	6.1	25	0.76 (0.65–0.88)	0.78 (0.69–0.87)
VA-HIT,[16]1999	112 mg/dL	2531 men age <74 yr	Gemfibrozil, 1200 mg	5.1	–	0.78 (0.65–0.93)	0.89 (0.73–1.08)
HPS,[17] 2002	132 mg/dL	20,526 men and women age 40–80 yr	Simvastatin, 40 mg	5.5	29	0.83 (0.75–0.91)	0.87 (0.81–0.94)
PROSPER,[18] 2002	147 mg/dL	5804 men and women age 70–82 yr	Pravastatin, 40 mg	3.2	34	0.85 (0.74–0.97)	–
GREACE,[19] 2002	180 mg/dL	1600 men and women; mean age 58 yr	Atorvastatin, 10–80 mg	3.0	46	0.49 (0.27–0.73)	0.57 (0.39–0.78)
ASCOT,[20] 2003	133 mg/dL	19,342 men and women age 40–79 yr	Atorvastatin, 10 mg	3.3	29	0.64 (0.50–0.83)	0.87 (0.71–1.06)

ASCOT, Anglo-Scandinavian Cardiac Outcomes Trial-Lipid Lowering Arm; CARE, Coronary Events After Myocardial Infarction in Patients with Average Cholesterol Levels; 4S, Scandinavian Simvastatin Survival Study; GREACE, Greek Atorvastatin and Coronary-Heart-Disease Evaluation; HPS, Heart Protection Study; LIPID, Long-Term Intervention with Pravastatin in Ischemic Disease; PROSPER, Prospective Study of Pravastatin in the Elderly at Risk; VA-HIT, Veterans Affairs High-Density Lipoprotein Intervention Trial.

150 mg/dL, and 35% reduction when LDL cholesterol >150 to 175 mg/dL). The apparent increase in CHD risk among those with the lowest cholesterol should be interpreted with some caution, as the results of this subgroup analysis may be misleading. Subsequent larger studies designed specifically to evaluate patients with lower initial LDL cholesterol levels have found significant risk reductions in this group.

Long-Term Intervention with Pravastatin in Ischemic Disease Trial

The purpose of the Long-term Intervention with Pravastatin in Ischemic Disease (LIPID) trial was to determine whether pravastatin therapy reduced CHD death among patients with a history of MI or unstable angina and initial cholesterol levels ranging from 155 to 271 mg/dL.[15] This study randomized 9014 patients aged 31 to 75 years to pravastatin (40 mg/day) or placebo; the mean duration of treatment was 6.1 years. Pravastatin was associated with a 24% reduction in CHD mortality (P < 0.001) and a 22% reduction in total mortality (P < 0.001). All types of cardiovascular outcomes were reduced in the pravastatin treatment group; these outcomes included MI (risk reduction of 29%; P < 0.001), CHD death or nonfatal MI (risk reduction of 24%; P < 0.001), stroke (risk reduction of 20%; P = 0.48), and coronary revascularization (risk reduction of 20%; P < 0.001).

Heart Protection Study

In the Heart Protection Study (HPS), 20,536 British men and women aged 40 to 80 years, with total cholesterol levels of at least 135 mg/dL and a history of coronary disease, other occlusive arterial disease, or diabetes, were randomized to simvastatin 40 mg/day or to placebo.[21] During 5 years of follow-up, those assigned to simvastatin experienced a reduction in total mortality of 12% (P = 0.0003) and a reduction in CHD mortality of 18% (P < 0.001), as compared with those assigned to placebo. The simvastatin group also experienced significant reductions in nonfatal MI (3.5% vs. 5.6%) and nonfatal stroke (3.6% vs. 4.9%). The proportional reduction in major vascular events was similar across all subgroups, including those without prior CHD but with cerebrovascular disease, peripheral artery disease, or diabetes. Notably, statins conferred equal cardiovascular benefit across a range of total, LDL, and HDL cholesterol, and triglyceride levels. Also, women and those 70 years or older at study entry benefited from statin therapy (see following sections).

Pravastatin in Elderly Individuals at Risk of Vascular Disease Study

The Pravastatin in Elderly Individuals at Risk of Vascular Disease (PROSPER) study randomized 5804 men and women aged 70 to 82 years with a history of, or risk factors for, vascular disease to pravastatin or placebo for a mean of 3.2 years.[18] Of participants, 43% had prior vascular disease. Baseline cholesterol levels ranged from 155 to 328 mg/dL. The composite outcome of coronary death, nonfatal MI, and fatal or nonfatal stroke was significantly reduced in the pravastatin arm (RR = 0.85, 95% CI 0.74-0.97). Coronary events were reduced by 19% (RR = 0.81, 95% CI 0.69-0.94), but there was no reduction in stroke events (RR = 1.03, 95% CI 0.81-1.21) or all-cause mortality (RR = 0.97, 95% CI 0.83-1.14).

Prevention of Coronary and Stroke Events with Atorvastatin in Hypertensive Patients Who Have Average or Lower-Than-Average Cholesterol Concentrations, in the Anglo-Scandinavian Cardiac Outcomes Trial

In the Anglo-Scandinavian Cardiac Outcomes Trial (ASCOT-LLA) study, 19,342 hypertensive patients aged 40 to 79 years were randomly assigned to receive atorvastatin (10 mg/day) or placebo.[20] The primary outcome was a combined endpoint of nonfatal MI, including "silent" MI, and fatal CHD. Men and women with treated or untreated hypertension with total cholesterol levels of 250 mg/dL or less were eligible. Individuals were required to have at least three additional cardiovascular risk factors but were excluded if they had a previous MI, current angina, heart failure, or a cerebrovascular event within the previous 3 months. After a mean treatment duration of 3.3 years, 100 primary events had occurred in the atorvastatin group versus 154 events in the placebo group (RR = 0.64, 95% CI 0.50-0.83). Fatal and nonfatal strokes were reduced (RR = 0.73, 95% CI 0.56-0.96), as were total cardiovascular events (RR = 0.79, 95% CI 0.69-0.90), and total coronary events (RR = 0.71, 95% CI 0.59-0.86). Benefits of treatment emerged after 1 year of follow-up. No significant difference in total mortality existed between the treatment and placebo groups.

Greek Atorvastatin and Coronary-Heart-Disease Evaluation Study

The Greek Atorvastatin and Coronary-Heart-Disease Evaluation (GREACE) study, a 3-year open-label trial of atorvastatin (10–80 mg/day, mean 24 mg/day) versus usual care in 1600 patients with established CHD, found a significant reduction in subsequent CHD events for atorvastatin therapy.[19] Overall mortality, coronary mortality, and nonfatal MI were all significantly reduced in the atorvastatin-treated group. LDL cholesterol levels were reduced 46% in the atorvastatin group and 5% in the usual-care group. Only 14% of usual-care patients were receiving lipid-lowering therapy.

Veterans Affairs High-Density Lipoprotein Cholesterol Intervention Trial

One of the few recent trials to utilize a nonstatin pharmacologic intervention, the Veterans Affairs High-Density Lipoprotein Cholesterol Intervention Trial (VA-HIT) enrolled 2531 men with coronary artery disease whose primary lipid abnormality was a low HDL cholesterol level (i.e., entry criteria were HDL cholesterol level of ≤40 mg/dL and LDL cholesterol level ≤140 mg/dL).[16] Subjects were randomized to gemfibrozil (1200 mg/day) or placebo and followed for a median of 5.1 years. As compared with those assigned to placebo, subjects randomized to gemfibrozil experienced a 22% reduction in the primary endpoint of coronary death or nonfatal MI and a 24% reduction in the secondary endpoint of coronary death, nonfatal MI, and stroke (P < 0.001). Although no significant changes in LDL cholesterol levels were observed over the course of follow-up, HDL cholesterol levels increased and triglyceride levels decreased. This study was the first to provide convincing evidence that raising HDL cholesterol levels results in a reduction in the risk of cardiovascular events.

Meta-analyses of Secondary Prevention Trials

The majority of available meta-analyses report summary estimates combined across secondary and primary prevention trials. However, most endpoints in such combined analyses are from secondary prevention settings.

A comprehensive overview[4,22] of 28 trials of cholesterol reduction from the prestatin era, including 6 multiple-intervention trials with a cholesterol-lowering arm, indicate that a 10% reduction in serum cholesterol results in highly significant reductions of 10% for CHD death and 18% for coronary events. When the duration of treatment is at least 5 years, the estimated event rate reductions are consistent with what would be expected based on prospective observational data. Specifically, a 10% reduction in cholesterol was associated with a 25% reduction in coronary events (95% CI 15%–35%) among those treated for 5 years or more.[22]

The magnitude of cholesterol reduction in prestatin trials was relatively modest (6–10 mg/dL), and these trials were underpowered to detect a benefit on total mortality. Meta-analyses of these trials, however, consistently show a trend toward lower total mortality in the range of what would be anticipated given the modest reduction in CHD mortality.[23-25] In a comprehensive overview,[22,26] the summary estimate of reduction in total mortality was 4% (95% CI 10% reduction to 2% increase). Such data are compatible with the expected 6% overall decline in mortality anticipated with a 10% decline in CHD death, assuming no excess risk of nonvascular death.

Gould and colleagues[27] conducted a meta-analysis in 1998 of all published trials of cholesterol lowering and cardiovascular risk that had treatment durations of at least 2 years. They included 43 trials, including 8 statin trials (4S,[13] CARE,[14] WOSCOPS,[28] AFCAPS/TexCAPS,[29] plus 4 small atheroma trials with relatively few deaths[30-33]) in their analysis. It was estimated that for every 10-percentage-point reduction in cholesterol, CHD mortality would be reduced by 15% and total mortality by 15%. The slope of the relationship between cholesterol reduction and CHD mortality was similar for statin and nonstatin therapy. That is, for a given change in cholesterol level, there was a certain change in CHD mortality, regardless of whether that cholesterol change was produced by a statin or by a nonstatin. Statins reduce CHD mortality to a greater extent because of their more potent cholesterol effects as compared with nonstatins.

In a 1999 meta-analysis of five large statin trials—three secondary prevention trials (4S,[13] CARE,[14] LIPID[15]) and

two primary prevention trials (West of Scotland Coronary Prevention Study,[28] Air Force/Texas Coronary Atherosclerosis Prevention Study[29])—that enrolled 30,817 participants and had treatment durations ranging from 4.9 to 6.1 years (mean of 5.4 years), statin therapy was associated with a 20% reduction in total cholesterol, a 28% reduction in LDL cholesterol, a 13% reduction in triglycerides, and a 5% increase in HDL cholesterol.[34] Statins reduced total mortality by 21% (95% CI 14%–28%) and major coronary events by 31% (26%–36%). The risk reduction in major coronary events was virtually identical for women (29%; 95% CI 13%–42%) and men (31%; 95% CI 26%–35%), as well as for persons aged 65 years and older (32%; 95% CI 23%–39%) and persons younger than 65 years (31%; 95% CI 24%–36%).

Trials in Acute Coronary Ischemia

Several randomized controlled trials have examined the use of statin therapy in acute coronary syndromes. The Myocardial Ischemia Reduction with Aggressive Cholesterol Lowering (MIRACL) study,[35] the Pravastatin Turkish trial,[36,37] the Fluvastatin on Risk Diminishing after Acute Myocardial Infarction (FLORIDA) study,[37] and the Lipid-Coronary Artery Disease (L-CAD)[38] study were not sufficiently powered to determine whether early initiation of statin therapy reduced mortality or reinfarction rates. Nevertheless, three of these trials showed that early initiation of statin therapy reduced subsequent ischemia, whereas one trial—the FLORIDA study—demonstrated neither benefit nor harm. Larger trials are under way to confirm these findings and to determine the effect of statins on mortality. These trials include the Aggrastat and Zocor (A-to-Z) trial,[37] the Pravastatin or Atorvastatin Evaluation and Infection Trial (PROVE IT), Thrombolysis in Myocardial Infarction Grade 22 (TIMI 22), and Pravastatin Acute Coronary Trial (PACT).[37] An overview of the available designs is provided in Table 22-2.

PRIMARY PREVENTION TRIALS

Findings from randomized trials in primary prevention settings are consistent with human observational evidence. Several multifactorial primary prevention trials utilized a dietary intervention to lower cholesterol.[39-43] Although these trials tended to show lower rates of CHD among those in the active treatment group, the magnitude of the benefit cannot be ascribed fully to the cholesterol reduction component, given the simultaneous modification of other risk factors. There are eight large-scale primary prevention trials of cholesterol lowering alone (or that contain a distinct cholesterol-lowering arm), including one dietary[44] and seven pharmacologic trials (Table 22-3).[29,45-51] These trials are discussed in the following sections.

Los Angeles Veterans Affairs Cooperative Study

The earliest trial was the Los Angeles Veterans Affairs Cooperative Study (LA VA) cooperative study, which

TABLE 22-2   ONGOING CHOLESTEROL LOWERING TRIALS IN ACUTE CORONARY SYNDROMES

Trial	Patient characteristic	Drug	Initiation of statin	Randomization period	Switch to open-label Tx	Primary endpoints	Sample size	Duration of study
A-to-Z	ACS	Simvastatin (40 mg/day for 30 days then 80 mg/day) vs. usual care for 120 days	120 hr after hospitalization	120 hr to 120 days	Simvastatin, 80 mg/day vs. 20 mg/day	CV death, reinfarction, hosp for ACS, stroke	About 4500	FU until 970 primary events occur
PROVE IT	ACS	Atorvastatin, 80 mg/day vs. pravastatin 40 mg/day for 2 yr	≤10 days after hospitalization	2 yr	No switch	Death, hospitalization for MI or UA, CABG or PCI, stroke	About 4000	2 yr

A-to-Z, Aggrastat and Zocor Trial; ACS, acute coronary syndrome (MI or UA); CABG, coronary artery bypass grafting; CV, cardiovascular; FU, follow-up; MI, myocardial infarction; PCI, percutaneous coronary intervention; PROVE IT, Pravastatin or Atorvastatin Evaluation and Infection Therapy Trial; Tx, treatment; UA, unstable angina.
From Wright RS, Murphy JG, Bybee KA, et al: Statin lipid-lowering therapy for acute myocardial infarction and unstable angina: Efficacy and mechanism of benefit. Mayo Clin Proc 2002; 77:1085–1092.

randomized 846 subjects to a low-fat diet or no dietary change.[44] Mean cholesterol reduction was 12.7% among those in the diet-modification arm. After a mean follow-up of 7 years, the risk of fatal and nonfatal CHD events was reduced.

Colestipol Trial

During the Colestipol Trial[50]—the first large-scale primary prevention trial of a pharmacologic agent—investigators randomized 2278 subjects to the resin colestipol or placebo. Mean cholesterol level was reduced by 9.8% in the active treatment group compared with subjects in the placebo group. After a mean follow-up of 2 years, the treatment group showed reductions in CHD events and deaths and a trend toward a lower total mortality rate.

World Health Organization Clofibrate Trial

The investigators of the World Health Organization (WHO) Clofibrate Trial randomized 10,621 subjects to clofibrate or placebo and followed them for an average of 5.3 years.[45,48,53] Treatment with clofibrate was associated with an 8.5% reduction in total cholesterol and a 25% reduction in the risk of nonfatal MI. There was no reduction, however, in CHD mortality. Subjects assigned to clofibrate tended to have higher rates of non-CHD and total death compared with those assigned to placebo.

Helsinki Heart Study

In the Helsinki Heart Study, 4081 subjects were randomized to either gemfibrozil or placebo and followed for an average of 5 years.[46] The mean reduction in total

TABLE 22-3   RANDOMIZED TRIALS OF CHOLESTEROL LOWERING IN THE PRIMARY PREVENTION OF CARDIOVASCULAR DISEASE

Study	Study population	Intervention	Major findings associated with active treatment
LA VA,[44] 1969	846 middle-aged men	Diet	Reduced risks of fatal and nonfatal CHD events
Colestipol trial,[50] 1978	2278 middle-aged men and women	Colestipol	Reduced risks of fatal and nonfatal CHD events; trend toward lower rates of total death
LRC-CPPT,[49] 1984	3806 middle-aged men	Cholestyramine	Reduced risk of nonfatal MI and incident CHD
World Health Organization Clofibrate Trial,[45,48,53] 1984	10,621 middle-aged men	Clofibrate	Reduced risk of nonfatal MI; no reduction in fatal CHD; trend toward increased risk from non CHD and total deaths
Helsinki Heart Study,[46] 1987	4081 men age 40-55 yr	Gemfibrozil	Reduced risks of CHD events and fatal CHD; trend toward lower total deaths
WOSCOPS,[28] 1995	6595 men age 45-64 yr	Pravastatin	Reduced risks of total CHD events, revascularization, CHD death, and fatal CHD
AFCAPS/TexCAPS,[29] 1998	6605 men and women age 45-73 yr	Lovastatin	Reduce risks of MI, unstable angina, coronary revascularization, total coronary events, and total cardiovascular events
Antihypertensive and Lipid-Lowering Treatment to Prevent Heart Attack Trial (ALLHAT-LLT),[51] 2002	10,355 men and women age 55 yr and older	Pravastatin	Did not reduce all-cause mortality or CHD events as compared with the usual-care group

AFCAPS/TexCAPS, Air Force/Texas Coronary Atherosclerosis Prevention Study; WOSCOPS, West of Scotland Coronary Prevention Study Group; LRC-CPPT, Lipid Research Clinics Coronary Primary Prevention Trial; LA VA, Los Angeles Veterans Affairs Cooperative Study.

cholesterol of 9.9% resulted in a clear reduction in non-fatal MI (34%) and incident CHD (37%) among those allocated to gemfibrozil.

The Lipid Research Clinics Coronary Primary Prevention Trial

Investigators from the Lipid Research Clinics Coronary Primary Prevention Trial (LRC-CPPT) randomized 3806 subjects to cholestyramine or placebo, with a 9% reduction in total cholesterol among those assigned to the active treatment group.[49] After a mean follow-up of 7.4 years, cholestyramine was associated with a 19% reduction in risk of a CHD event; a 24% reduction in fatal CHD; and 20% to 25% reductions in risk of a positive stress test, angina, or bypass surgery. The risk of total death was not significantly reduced (7%).

West of Scotland Coronary Prevention Study

In the West of Scotland Coronary Prevention Study (WOSCOPS), 6595 hyperlipidemic men aged 45 to 64 years were randomized to pravastatin (40 mg/day) or placebo.[28] Pravastatin lowered total cholesterol levels by 20% and LDL cholesterol levels by 26%—approximately twice the amount observed in previous primary prevention trials. After 4.9 years of follow-up, there were clear reductions in CHD events, defined as nonfatal MI or CHD death (31%, 95% CI 17%–43%). Considering each component of the composite endpoint separately, the risk reduction associated with pravastatin was 31% (95% CI 15%–45%) for nonfatal MI and 28% (−10%–52%) for CHD death. There was also a borderline significant 22% reduction in total mortality in the pravastatin group (95% CI 0%–40%).

Air Force/Texas Coronary Atherosclerosis Prevention Study

In the Air Force/Texas Coronary Atherosclerosis Prevention Study (AFCAPS/TexCAPS), a large-scale trial of lovastatin (20–40 mg/day) among men aged 45 to 73 years and postmenopausal women aged 55 to 73 years who had modest elevations in LDL cholesterol and below-average HDL cholesterol, lovastatin reduced LDL cholesterol by 25% and increased HDL cholesterol by 6%.[29] Compared with subjects assigned placebo, those assigned to lovastatin experienced large reductions in MI risk (relative risk, 0.60; 95% CI 0.43-0.83), unstable angina (RR = 0.68; 95% CI 0.49-0.95), coronary revascularization (RR = 0.67; 95% CI 0.52-0.85), total coronary events (RR = 0.75; 95% CI 0.61-0.92), and total cardiovascular events (RR = 0.75; 95% CI 0.62-0.91).

Antihypertensive and Lipid-Lowering Treatment to Prevent Heart Attack Trial

The Antihypertensive and Lipid-Lowering Treatment to Prevent Heart Attack Trial (ALLHAT-LLT), a recent non-blind randomized trial, was a substudy of a larger trial on drug therapy for hypertension. In this study, 10,355 men and women aged 55 years and older with moderate hypercholesterolemia, hypertension, and at least one other coronary risk factor were randomly assigned to pravastatin (40 mg/day) or to usual care and followed for an average of 4.8 years.[51] Entry criteria included LDL cholesterol levels of 120 to 189 mg/dL for persons without known CHD and 100 to 129 mg/dL for the roughly 14% of participants with preexisting CHD. All-cause mortality, the primary outcome, did not differ between the pravastatin and usual care groups (14.9% vs. 15.3%), nor did CHD event rates (9.3% vs. 10.4%). The nonsignificant findings may be because of various methodologic limitations. At 4 years, only 84% of patients in the pravastatin group were taking statins, compared with 17% of usual-care patients, and the lack of adherence to assigned therapy increased during the trial. Moreover, the use of an open-label design raises the possibility that subjects assigned to usual care may have been more motivated to undertake lifestyle changes to reduce cardiovascular risk because they knew that they were not receiving a statin, thus diminishing any potential treatment effect. In the pravastatin group, total and LDL cholesterol levels were reduced by 17% and 28%, respectively, compared with 8% and 11%, respectively, in the usual-care group. However, changes in LDL cholesterol over time were measured only in a poorly defined subset of patients; if this subset was composed of only the most compliant individuals, then true LDL cholesterol differences between the treatment groups may have been smaller than reported. Finally, although the target sample size was 20,000, only half that number of patients were ultimately enrolled, reducing the power to detect any true treatment differences.

Meta-analysis of Primary Prevention Trials

A recent meta-analysis of the data from four large primary prevention trials (Helsinki Heart Study, LRC-CPPT, WOSCOPS, and AFCAPS/TexCAPS) found that cholesterol-lowering treatment reduced CHD by 30%.[54] Both CHD events and CHD mortality were significantly reduced (summary OR = 0.70, 95% CI 0.62-0.79; and summary OR = 0.71, 95% CI 0.56-0.91, respectively), but total mortality was not (summary OR = 0.94, 95% CI 0.81-1.09). These findings remained essentially unchanged when the analysis was restricted to the statin trials.

Most primary prevention trials of cholesterol lowering are underpowered to assess fully the balance of benefits and risks. The lack of a significant reduction in total mortality in these trials is likely a result of the low absolute baseline risk of the study populations and the relatively short follow-up periods. In WOSCOPS,[28] which enrolled higher-risk individuals, total mortality was reduced by 22%. This reduction is in accord with our knowledge of the effects of cholesterol reduction and the expected event rate in this population. Larger studies of longer duration will be necessary to describe fully the benefits of lipid lowering among individuals at minimal baseline risk for CHD.

Even if reductions in total mortality are ultimately determined to be only modest in primary prevention settings, the public health benefits of cholesterol lowering are still likely to outweigh the risks. This conclusion is illustrated by data from the LRC-CPPT trial.[49] Although there was no clear benefit in terms of total mortality (68 deaths among treated subjects vs. 71 deaths among untreated subjects—a nonsignificant reduction of 4.3%), 206 fewer nonfatal CHD events occurred among treated subjects (906 vs. 1112). The reduction in morbidity is likely to have substantial public health benefits in terms of quality of life and productivity.

CHOLESTEROL REDUCTION IN THE ELDERLY

In contrast to early trials, recent statin trials have included large numbers of older people. In this section, findings from relevant secondary prevention trials are summarized first. Table 22-4 provides risk estimates according to age-group. Among the approximately 2300 participants aged 60 years or older in the 4S trial, those assigned to receive simvastatin were 29% less likely (95% CI 14%–40%) to have a major coronary event than those assigned to placebo.[13] Among their younger counterparts, there was a 39% (95% CI 27%–49%) risk reduction associated with simvastatin treatment.[13] In the CARE trial, more than half of the 4159 participants, who ranged from 21 to 75 years of age, were at least 60 years old.[55] Among those 60 years

or older, pravastatin led to a 27% (95% CI 9%–36%) reduction in the risk of major coronary events, compared with a 20% (95% CI 4%–33%) risk reduction for those younger than 60 years. In LIPID,[15] pravastatin therapy was associated with a reduction in risk of major coronary events in all age-groups studied; for those 55 years and older, 55 to 64 years, 65 to 69 years, and 70 years and older, the reductions in risk were 32% (95% CI 12%–48%), 20% (95% CI 3%–34%), 28% (11%–41%), and 15% (−8%–33%), respectively. In the HPS, which enrolled 5806 participants aged 70 to 80 years, the proportional reduction in the rate of major vascular events associated with simvastatin was approximately 25%, irrespective of baseline age.[21] Among the 1263 participants between the ages of 80 and 85 years by study end, the reduction in event rates in the simvastatin group as compared with the placebo group was significant (23.1% vs. 32.3%, P = 0.0002). As discussed previously, the PROSPER trial, which was designed specifically to evaluate the role of lipid-lowering therapy in the elderly (i.e., persons aged 70 to 82 years at baseline), found that pravastatin therapy was associated with a significant 15% reduction in major vascular events.[18]

Although data are limited, primary prevention trials also suggest that older individuals derive benefit from statin therapy. In AFCAPS/TexCAPS, which enrolled men aged 45 to 73 years and postmenopausal women aged 55 to 73 years, benefit was apparent in men older than the

TABLE 22-4   RANDOMIZED TRIALS OF CHOLESTEROL LOWERING AND CARDIOVASCULAR EVENTS: GENDER- AND AGE-SPECIFIC RESULTS

Study	CVD outcome	Women RR (95% CI)	Men RR (95% CI)	Older age RR (95% CI)	Younger age RR (95% CI)
4S	Fatal or nonfatal MI	0.65 (0.47–0.91)	0.66 (0.58–0.76)	≥60 yr 0.71 (0.60–0.86)	≤60 yr 0.61 (0.51–0.73)
CARE	Fatal or nonfatal MI, CABG, PTCA	0.54 (0.38–0.78)	0.80 (0.70–0.92)	≥60 yr 0.73 (0.62–0.88)	≤60 yr 0.80 (0.67–0.96)
WOSCOPS	Fatal or nonfatal MI	—	—	≥55 yr 0.73 (0.57–0.92)	≤55 yr 0.60 (0.44–0.84)
LIPID	Fatal or nonfatal MI	0.89 (0.67–1.18)	0.74 (0.65–0.83)	≥70 yr 0.85 (0.88–1.08) 65–69 yr 0.72 (0.59–0.89)	≤55 yr 0.68 (0.52–0.88) 55–64 yr 0.80 (0.66–0.97)
VA HIT	Fatal or nonfatal MI	—	—	≥66 yr 0.74 (0.60–0.93)	≤66 yr 0.78 (0.61–0.99)
AFCAPS/ TexCAPS	Fatal or nonfatal MI, unstable angina, sudden death	0.54 (0.22–1.35)	0.63 (0.50–0.81)	—	—
HPS*	Fatal or nonfatal MI, stroke, coronary or noncoronary revascularization	0.88 (0.81–0.96)	0.84 (0.81–0.88)	≥65–<70 yr 0.83 (0.78–0.90) ≥70 yr 0.87 (0.82–0.93)	<65 yr 0.84 (0.80–0.89)
PROSPER	Fatal or nonfatal MI, stroke	0.96 (0.79–1.18)	0.77 (0.65–0.92)	—	—
ASCOT	Fatal or nonfatal MI	1.10 (0.57–2.12)	0.59 (0.44–0.77)	≥60 yr 0.64 (0.47–0.86)	≤60 yr 0.66 (0.41–1.06)

*Relative risks and confidence intervals are estimates derived from reference 17.
AFCAPS/TexCAPS, Air Force/Texas Coronary Atherosclerosis Prevention Study[29,52]; ASCOT, Anglo-Scandinavian Cardiac Outcomes Trial–Lipid Lowering Arm[20]; CARE, Coronary Events After Myocardial Infarction in Patients with Average Cholesterol Levels[14]; CI, confidence interval; 4S, Scandinavian Simvastatin Survival Study[13]; HPS, Heart Protection Study[17]; LIPID, Long-Term Intervention with Pravastatin in Ischemic Disease[15]; PROSPER, Prospective Study of Pravastatin in the Elderly at Risk[18]; RR, relative risk; VA-HIT, Veterans Affairs High Density Lipoprotein Intervention Trial[16]; WOSCOPS, West of Scotland Coronary Prevention Study Group.[28]

median age of 57 years and in women older than the median age of 62 years.[29] In WOSCOPS, although subjects younger than 55 years of age (40%, 95% CI 16%–56%) experienced a larger reduction in risk associated with pravastatin than older participants, pravastatin treatment was also associated with a significant reduction in risk among those 55 to 64 years (27%, 95% CI 8%–43%).[28]

Taken in the aggregate, available evidence provides support for the use of lipid-lowering therapies in elderly individuals, particularly those with established CHD. As discussed in the following sections, the National Cholesterol Education Program (NCEP) recommends screening for all adults older than 20 years.[56]

CHOLESTEROL REDUCTION IN WOMEN

Observational data suggest that cholesterol is a potent risk factor for heart disease in women as well as men. The magnitude of the relative risk associated with elevated cholesterol levels appears to be similar for both genders. Randomized data on cholesterol lowering are derived from predominantly male populations, particularly in primary prevention. However, recent statin trials include increased numbers of women,[17,13-15,28,29] and these studies generally indicate that cardiovascular risk reductions among women are comparable to those in men. Table 22-4 provides gender-specific data on the benefits of cholesterol-lowering therapy.

STROKE

Although an elevated cholesterol level is a clear risk factor for CHD, its role as a precursor to stroke is less certain.[57] Some observational studies suggest that cholesterol level is positively associated with the risk of stroke—ischemic stroke in particular[58]—but other studies have failed to find this association.[59,60] An overview of 45 prospective observational studies that included 450,000 individuals and 13,000 strokes, however, demonstrated an independent association between baseline blood cholesterol and stroke risk.[61]

One difficulty in assessing the association between cholesterol and risk of stroke is that the relationship may differ by the cause of cerebrovascular events. The Multiple Risk Factor Intervention trial screening data showed a positive association between cholesterol level and

ischemic stroke but an inverse relationship for hemorrhagic stroke.[58] These findings are compatible with those of other observational studies of populations with low blood cholesterol levels.[62,63] They are also compatible with studies of Japanese populations that have adopted Western eating habits, either in Japan or after migration to the United States.[62,64-66] The Japanese typically consume less animal fat and have lower blood cholesterol levels than their U.S. counterparts. They also have a higher incidence of stroke, which is primarily hemorrhagic rather than ischemic, but a lower incidence of CHD. With the adoption of Western eating habits, their blood cholesterol levels rise and the incidence of CHD and ischemic stroke increases while the proportion of stroke attributable to hemorrhage decreases. These findings raise the possibility that detecting any benefits of cholesterol lowering on risks of stroke from randomized trials would require far larger samples and reliable classification by ischemic or hemorrhagic cause.

Early randomized trials demonstrating that cholesterol lowering decreases risk of CHD[13,14,28,29,67] were not designed to evaluate stroke or had too few cerebrovascular end points. Overviews of randomized trials that provided data on stroke outcomes prior to the large-scale statin trials revealed no reduction in stroke among those treated with cholesterol-lowering agents compared with placebo.[68,69] These trials contained a mixture of populations with and without CAD. In an overview of trials that collectively enrolled more than 36,000 individuals,[68] the mean reduction in cholesterol level in the treated group as compared with the control group ranged from 6% to 23% (Table 22-4, left-hand column). Those assigned to treatment experienced no significant reduction in total strokes (RR = 1.0; 95% CI 0.8-1.2) or fatal strokes (RR = 1.1; 95% CI 0.8-1.6). There were no clear differences in treatment effects between primary and secondary prevention trials. Insufficient cholesterol lowering and inadequate sample sizes are plausible explanations for the inability to detect reductions in stroke in these early trials.

Subsequent trials of statins, which produce larger reductions of cholesterol than other lipid-lowering agents,[13-15,29,47] provide stronger evidence on the role of cholesterol reduction in the prevention of stroke. In an overview of randomized statin trials that included 29,000 subjects who were followed for a mean of 3.3 years, a substantial reduction in risk of ischemic stroke occurred in the active treatment group (Table 22-5, right-hand column).[70] The average reductions in total and LDL

TABLE 22-5 OVERVIEW OF PRE-STATIN AND STATIN TRIALS ON STROKE REDUCTION

Endpoint	Overview of prestatin trials[68]	Overview of statin trials[70]
	RR (95% CI)	RR (95% CI)
Total stroke	1.0 (0.8-1.2)	0.71 (0.59-0.86)
Primary prevention trials	1.0 (0.8-1.3)	0.80 (0.54-1.16)
Secondary prevention trials	1.0 (0.7-1.3)	0.68 (0.55-0.85)
Stroke death	1.1 (0.8-1.6)	1.17 (0.69-1.97)
Primary prevention trials	1.5 (0.9-2.6)	0.86 (0.29-2.56)
Secondary prevention trials	0.9 (0.6-1.4)	1.28 (0.71-2.32)

CI, confidence interval; RR, relative risk

cholesterol were large—22% and 30%, respectively. A total of 454 strokes occurred during follow-up. Subjects assigned to statin drugs experienced a nearly 30% reduction in risk of total stroke (RR = 0.71; 95% CI 0.59-0.86) but no apparent reduction in risk of fatal stroke. A subsequent meta-analysis of 28 randomized trials of various cholesterol-lowering agents that collectively enrolled 49,477 patients in the intervention group and 56,636 patients in the control group found that the risk ratio for total stroke associated with statin therapy was 0.76 (95% CI 0.62-0.92).[71] This risk ratio differed significantly from the pooled estimates for all other cholesterol-lowering interventions (pooled RR = 1.02; 95% CI 0.91-1.15). Pooled estimates for fibrates, resins, and dietary interventions suggested that these interventions did not affect stroke incidence. Warshafsky and colleagues[72] conducted a meta-analysis that included the eight statin trials used in the prior analysis along with five additional statin trials and found a 30% reduction in stroke (95% CI 8%-38%). Straus and colleagues[73,74] later added two additional statin trials[35,75] that had more stroke endpoints (455) than the prior 13 trials combined (405); they found that statins reduced the risk of stroke by 25% (95% CI 14%-35%). Law and colleagues[76] recently evaluated the effect of decreasing LDL cholesterol concentration on thromboembolic, hemorrhagic, fatal, and nonfatal stroke. They included data from 9 cohort studies and 58 randomized trials. Stroke risk was reduced by approximately 20% for every 1.0 mmol/L reduction in LDL cholesterol (P < 0.0001). The protective effect was greater for individuals with known vascular disease.

There are several possible explanations for the discrepancy between the reduced stroke rates observed in statin trials and the mostly null findings from earlier cholesterol-lowering trials and observational studies. Large reductions in cholesterol level may be necessary to provide a detectable reduction in ischemic strokes. Another explanation may relate to the fact that much of the statin data are from trials among persons with a history of CHD. Statins may prevent stroke secondary to reducing risk of MI. Stroke risk is increased following MI and may be attributable to the formation of mural thrombi that can produce embolic strokes. This explanation is supported by the analysis by Law and colleagues,[76] in which LDL cholesterol reduction was associated with a reduction in thromboembolic stroke events but not hemorrhagic strokes. This difference accounted for the greater-than-expected reduction in stroke events among individuals with known vascular disease. The greater reductions in coronary disease achieved with the statins may, therefore, result in prevention of stroke. Although less likely, it remains possible that statins reduce stroke by a mechanism unrelated to the lipid-lowering effect. Additional randomized trial data are required to clarify the role of lipid-lowering agents in secondary stroke prevention.

NONVASCULAR MORTALITY

Questions have been raised regarding the increased risk of nonvascular deaths observed in some trials.[77,78] This is of particular importance in primary prevention, in which benefits could be offset by any potential risks of nonvascular mortality because of lower baseline risks of CHD. The hypothesis that a potential hazard is associated with lowering cholesterol is based primarily on two facts: (1) observational data have raised the possibility of an association between low serum cholesterol and increased risk of nonvascular mortality, and (2) some randomized trials, especially in primary prevention settings, have failed to show significant reductions in total mortality despite showing clear reductions in risk of CHD. However, currently available evidence does not support the hypothesis that cholesterol reduction increases nonvascular mortality overall or mortality because of any specific cause.[79] First, unlike the association between cholesterol and risk of CHD, randomized trial data do not reinforce concerns raised by observational data. Observational studies suggest that individuals with the lowest cholesterol levels in any given population are at increased risk of nonvascular death. These very low levels of cholesterol have never been achieved in randomized trials. It has been postulated that rapid reductions in blood cholesterol observed in randomized trials may lead to nonvascular events[80]; however, it is highly unlikely that subjects in observational studies with the lowest cholesterol achieved these levels by a rapid decrease. Thus, data from observational studies and randomized trials address two causally distinct hypotheses.

Second, although individuals with very low cholesterol levels have higher rates of nonvascular mortality,[2] it is unclear whether low cholesterol is a marker for or a cause of these increased nonvascular mortality rates. In observational studies, the increase in nonvascular deaths associated with lower cholesterol levels may be the result of the existence of subclinical disease. This is suggested by the attenuation of the relationship if deaths within the first 5 years are excluded.[2]

Third, in contrast with the cholesterol-CHD relationship, evidence for a dose-response relationship between low cholesterol and nonvascular mortality is quite limited. In a meta-analysis, Gordon analyzed data by the extent of cholesterol reduction (11 studies with cholesterol reductions ≥12% vs. 11 studies with reductions <12%).[81] As expected, greater reduction in cholesterol resulted in a greater reduction in CHD incidence (31% vs. 11%) and mortality (27% vs. 2%). In contrast, a greater reduction in cholesterol was not associated with an increase in nonvascular mortality (11% vs. 30%). These results are supported by data from the 4S trial, in which drug therapy resulted in a 25% reduction in total cholesterol (larger than the reduction in any previous trial), yet no increase in nonvascular deaths occurred (46 in the treatment group vs. 49 in the placebo group).[13] Similarly, no increases in nonvascular mortality occurred in other individual large-scale statin trials[13-15,29,47] or in an overview of completed statin trials (RR = 0.93, 95% CI 0.75-1.14).[70]

Fourth, there is no consistent association with any specific nonvascular cause of death,[22,26] and apparent increases in cause-specific mortality are confined to relatively few studies. The trend for increased cancer incidence following cholesterol-lowering therapy is primarily accounted for by the WHO Clofibrate trial[45,48,53] and the LA VA study,[44] in which cholesterol reductions were

9% and 13%, respectively. In both cases, the differences in mortality from cancer in the intervention and control groups, which, if real, might have been expected to persist or even become more accentuated owing to the long latency period of cancer, were in fact diminished with extended follow-up. A recent overview of large-scale statin trials demonstrated no increase in fatal or nonfatal cancer risk.[82] The Helsinki Heart Study[46] of gemfibrozil and the LRC-CPPT[49] (cholestyramine) each found an apparent excess of trauma deaths among the active treatment group as compared with the placebo group. (Helsinki Heart Study: 15 vs. 4; LRC-CPPT: 11 vs. 4). The net cholesterol reductions in these trials were 9% and 10%, respectively. A meta-analysis that included 19 trials (8 primary prevention and 11 secondary prevention) reported an odds ratio of nonillness mortality in the treated groups relative to control groups of 1.18 (95% CI 0.91–1.52).[83] When the analysis was limited to statin trials, the odds ratio dropped to 0.84 (95% CI 0.50–1.41). These findings raise the possibility that increases in cancer or trauma death may be intervention specific and not related to cholesterol reduction perse or, equally as plausible, may be simply the result of chance.

In summary, the potential for confounding by the presence of subclinical disease, the lack of a dose-response or threshold effect, the lack of a consistent effect for any specific cause of death, the appearance of adverse effects in just a few trials, along with the lack of evidence from basic research, all argue against a causal relationship between lower cholesterol and nonvascular causes of death.

COST EFFECTIVENESS OF CHOLESTEROL REDUCTION

CHD is the leading cause of death and the leading source of health care expenditures in the United States. In 1998 alone, the overall cost of CHD exceeded $274 billion spent in medical spending and lost productivity.[84] Lipid-lowering therapy reduces CHD mortality and health care utilization. In determining the cost-effectiveness of an intervention, estimates are calculated as the ratio of net costs to the gain in life expectancy and are usually presented as the cost per quality-adjusted life-year. Interventions with an incremental cost-effectiveness ratio of less than $40,000 per quality-adjusted life-year are comparable to other chronic interventions, such as hypertension management and hemodialysis. Cost-effectiveness ratios of less than $20,000 are very favorable. On the other hand, ratios exceeding $40,000 are unacceptable to most providers.

Secondary Prevention

Individuals with known CHD are at considerably higher risk of subsequent cardiovascular events and death than are those without underlying CHD and thus tend to have more favorable costs per year of life saved. Kupersmith and colleagues[85] have reviewed studies of the cost-effectiveness of cholesterol reduction. Early cost-effectiveness analyses of cholesterol reduction in sec-

ondary prevention showed that interventions were very costly (generally >$40,000 per year of life saved), largely because available drugs such as cholestyramine were relatively ineffective as compared with statin drugs.[86,87] Goldman and colleagues[88] conducted the first comprehensive statin analysis to estimate costs for secondary and primary prevention. These investigators used the well-known CHD policy model, which assumes that data from observational studies and randomized trials can be applied broadly to estimate risk of coronary events and mortality. For secondary prevention among those with cholesterol levels of 250 mg/dL or greater, cost-effectiveness ratios were generally favorable (i.e., <$40,000) for lovastatin at doses of 20 and 40 mg. The relationship between cost per year and age was U-shaped; that is, the costs tended to be highest for younger and older individuals and lowest for middle-aged persons. For those with lower cholesterol levels, ratios were generally favorable at a dose of 20 mg. The costs per year were even more favorable when estimated using the 40% reduction in drug costs expected when generic versions of statins become available.

Using data from the 4S trial and a modified Markov model, Johannesson and colleagues[89] estimated the cost per life-year gained for simvastatin therapy. The estimates were based on actual experience in a randomized trial of simvastatin rather than on extrapolation of possible effects from observational data, as is the CHD policy model. Event costs, provided by the Swedish Institute for Health Services, ranged from $653 for chest pain admission to $80,178 for cardiac transplantation. The price of simvastatin was estimated at $604 per year of treatment. The direct cost per life-year saved was $5400 for men and $10,500 for women. As expected, costs decreased as baseline cholesterol levels increased. For example, the direct cost per life-year saved was $11,400 for a man with baseline total cholesterol of 213 mg/dL and $6700 for a man with a cholesterol level of 309 mg/dL. In contrast with the CHD policy model estimates, the relationship between direct cost per life-year saved and age was not U-shaped. Rather, direct costs fell with increasing age. This key difference in findings between the two models may reflect their differing assumptions.

In the 4S analysis, the estimated indirect costs included estimates for lost productivity, which were based on work status data collected at 6-month intervals during the course of the trial.[89] The indirect cost per life-year saved was $1600 for men and $5100 for women. Indirect costs were higher for older persons than for their younger counterparts because older persons tended to work at a much lower frequency. The use of lost productivity tends to value working individuals more than those who do not work and thus has not been included in most models. The overall incremental costs of treatment in all groups analyzed were attractive by most standards; direct costs were well below $20,000.

Primary Prevention

Using data from LRC-CPPT (cholestyramine), Weinstein and Stason[86] estimated a cost of $237,400 per year of life saved. Oster and Epstein[87] estimated the cost-effectiveness of the same intervention at $99,500 to $1.7 million, depending on age and other risk factors. The CHD policy model provided estimates for lovastatin,[88] finding that favorable costs per life-year were largely confined to middle-aged men with multiple coronary risk factors. Analyses that take into account indirect gains in wages and labor productivity find greater cost-effectiveness of lipid-lowering therapies.[84]

Early cholesterol-lowering trials yielded only modest reductions in cholesterol, and the cost-effectiveness of treatment was favorable only for those populations at highest cardiovascular risk. Subsequent trials using statins find that such therapy is cost-effective at lower thresholds of baseline cardiovascular risk. The cost efficacy of statin treatment (cost <$50,000 per year of life saved) has now been shown for those whose annual CHD risk exceeds 1%.[84] This group includes all patients with known CHD or CHD equivalents (e.g., diabetes mellitus), irrespective of age and gender, as well as many individuals without CHD but with several coronary risk factors.

Cost Effectiveness in the Elderly

Determining the cost of cholesterol-lowering treatment among elderly individuals is a pressing concern as that population is rapidly increasing. Between 1990 and 2000, the number of persons aged 65 and older in the United States jumped 12%, to approximately 35 million.[90] A cost-effectiveness model of statin use in older patients with a history of MI found that there was a 75% chance that the incremental cost of statin therapy would be less than $39,800 per quality-adjusted life-year as compared with usual care.[91] Future cost-effectiveness models using information from the most recent trials and taking into account the lower cost of generic statins will likely find that treatment of elderly individuals without a history of MI but with multiple CHD risk factors are cost-effective as well.

Cost Effectiveness in Women

Although cholesterol lowering in women and men appears to have comparable relative benefits, the fact that women are at lower absolute risk of CHD than similarly aged men affects the assessment of cholesterol reduction in primary prevention in two ways. First, even modest risks may have a larger impact in offsetting the more modest absolute benefits in women. Second, the cost-effectiveness of any given intervention may be reduced in women. If all other risk factors are equivalent, to save one life from CHD requires that more women than men be treated, which increases the cost per life saved among women. However, the cost-effectiveness of treatment will likely improve in both genders as generic versions of statins become available. Moreover, findings from recent trials showing that statins may reduce fracture risk and that postmenopausal hormone therapy does not prevent CHD (see Chapter 27) are likely to strengthen the case for aggressive lipid lowering in women.

GUIDELINES

To reduce the prevalence of elevated cholesterol levels in the United States, the NCEP issued its first Adult Treatment Panel (ATP) report in 1988,[92] a second report in 1993,[93] and a third report in 2001.[56] The NCEP focuses on LDL cholesterol as the primary target of therapy. As before, the most recent guidelines recommend aggressively lowering LDL cholesterol for individuals with established CHD, but a new emphasis is the treatment approach that also targets LDL cholesterol levels among persons with multiple risk factors. In addition, the threshold for a low HDL cholesterol has been raised from 35 to 40 mg/dL.

The NCEP cholesterol-lowering goals are based on an individual's predicted level of CHD risk, irrespective of age or gender (Table 22-6). For persons with CHD,

■ ▦ ■

TABLE 22-6   NATIONAL CHOLESTEROL EDUCATION PROGRAM ADULT TREATMENT PANEL III GUIDELINES

Risk profile	LDL goal (mg/dL)	LDL threshold for initiating diet therapy (mg/dL)	LDL threshold for initiating drug therapy (mg/dL)
History of CHD or CHD equivalent* (calculated[†] 10-yr risk >20%)	<100	≥100	≥130 (100–129: drug optional)
No CHD history, presence of ≥2 risk factors and calculated 10-yr risk ≤20%	<130	≥130	10-yr risk 10%–20%: ≥130 10-yr risk<10%: ≥160
No CHD history, presence of 0 or 1 risk factors	<160	≥160	≥190 (160–189: LDL lowering drug optional)

From Expert Panel on detection, evaluation, and treatment of high blood cholesterol in adults: Summary of the second report of the National Cholesterol Education Program (NCEP) Expert Panel on detection, evaluation, and treatment of high blood cholesterol in adults (Adult Treatment Panel III). JAMA 2001; 285:2486–2496.
CHD, coronary heart disease, LDL, low-density lipoprotein cholesterol.
*CHD risk equivalents: diabetes, clinical atherosclerotic disease (peripheral arterial disease, abdominal aortic aneurysm, and symptomatic carotid artery disease), multiple risk factors that confer a 10-year risk of CHD greater than 20%.
†Calculated using Framingham risk scoring (provided in appendix of Adult Treatment Panel III Guidelines[56]).
Risk factors include age (men ≥45 years, women ≥55 years), cigarette smoking, hypertension (blood pressure ≥140/90 mm Hg or on antihypertensive medication), and low high-density lipoprotein cholesterol level (<40 mg/dL), and family history of premature heart disease (CHD in male first-degree relative <55 years; CHD in female first-degree relative <65 years).

CHD risk equivalents such as diabetes and other forms of atherosclerotic disease (e.g., peripheral artery disease, abdominal aortic aneurysm, symptomatic carotid artery disease), or multiple risk factors that confer a 10-year risk of CHD that exceeds 20%, the target LDL cholesterol level is less than 100 mg/dL. One could argue for drug therapy in all such individuals regardless of their baseline LDL cholesterol level because they are likely to benefit from maximal cholesterol reduction. For persons with no history of CHD and only one other cardiovascular risk factor besides elevated LDL cholesterol (e.g., cigarette smoking, hypertension, low HDL cholesterol, family history of premature CHD), the NCEP recommends that LDL cholesterol not exceed 160 mg/dL. For those without a history of CHD but with two other risk factors and a calculated 10-year CHD risk of 20% or less, the goal is an LDL cholesterol level less than 130 mg/dL. Initiation of drug therapy is based on the calculated 10-year risk for developing CHD. For those with a 10-year risk of 10% to less than 20%, drug therapy should be started if baseline LDL cholesterol levels are 130 mg/dL or greater. However, if the 10-year CHD risk is less than 10%, then drug therapy should be started when LDL cholesterol levels are 190 mg/dL or greater.

For primary prevention, the NCEP recommends a multifaceted lifestyle approach to reduce LDL cholesterol. The key features are a reduction of saturated fats to less than 7% of total calories and cholesterol intake of less than 200 mg/day. Moderate physical exercise, along with consideration of a referral to a dietician, is suggested. For patients who find it difficult to understand amounts based on a percentage of calories, it may be helpful to translate these guidelines into grams of fat, protein, and other dietary constituents, the reporting of which is now mandated on labels of all foods sold in the United States. If after 6 weeks the target LDL cholesterol level is not achieved, then reinforcement of the low-saturated-fat/low-cholesterol diet and the addition of plant sterols (2 g/day) and fiber (2 g/day) is suggested. If after an additional 6 weeks the target LDL level is still not achieved, then drug therapy may be initiated. The choice of drug and initial dose is based on the type of dyslipidemia and percent reduction required, with the aim of using the lowest possible dose necessary to reach the target LDL cholesterol level. Effectiveness of treatment should be evaluated after 6 weeks, with titration of therapy if required.

SUMMARY

The totality of the evidence supports the judgment of a causal relationship between elevated serum cholesterol and risk of CHD. Basic laboratory research provided plausible biologic mechanisms for the relationship. Prospective observational studies revealed a clear monotonic association between elevated cholesterol and CHD. Large-scale randomized controlled trials of lipid-lowering agents confirmed this association and quantified the benefits of such therapy in both secondary and primary prevention settings, men and women, and younger and older populations. Recent statin trials also provide strong

evidence that lowering cholesterol leads to a reduced incidence of thromboembolic stroke. Concerns over potential adverse effects of cholesterol-lowering treatment have been alleviated with recent data showing that statins do not increase nonvascular mortality or any specific cause of nonvascular death.

Although mean age-adjusted serum cholesterol levels steadily fell in the United States from the mid-1960s to the mid-1980s,[94] cholesterol levels declined only slightly from 1988 to 2000.[95] Currently, an estimated 50% of adults in the United States have total cholesterol levels of 200 mg/dL or higher, and 18% have levels of 240 mg/dL or higher,[95] suggesting that millions of Americans who meet guidelines for lipid-lowering therapy are not receiving such treatment, and many who are being treated are not optimally controlled. A renewed commitment to implementing population-based strategies—both behavioral and pharmacologic—to prevent and treat dyslipidemia as a means of reducing CHD is warranted. In addition, future investigations should examine whether setting stricter thresholds for cholesterol lowering than those given by current NCEP guidelines will yield further cardiovascular benefits.

REFERENCES

1. Consensus Conference: Lowering blood cholesterol to prevent heart disease. JAMA 1985; 253:2080–2086.
2. LaRosa JC, Hunninghake D, Bush D, et al: The cholesterol facts: A summary of the evidence relating dietary fats, serum cholesterol, and coronary heart disease: A joint statement by the American Heart Association and the National Heart, Lung, and Blood Institute: AHA Medical/Scientific Statement, AHA, and NHLBI 1990:1721–1733.
3. Chen Z, Peto R, Collins R, et al: Serum cholesterol concentration and coronary heart disease in population with low cholesterol concentrations. BMJ 1991; 303:276–282.
4. Law MR, Wald NJ, Wu T, et al: Systematic underestimation of association between serum cholesterol concentration and ischaemic heart disease in observational studies: data from the BUPA study. BMJ 1994; 308:363–366.
5. Waters D, Pedersen TR: Review of cholesterol-lowering therapy: Coronary angiographic and events trials. Am J Med 1996; 101:4A34S–4A38S.
6. Stulc T, Ceska R: Cholesterol lowering and the vessel wall: New insights and future perspectives. Physiol Res 2001; 50:461–471.
7. Lee RT: Plaque stabilization: The role of lipid lowering. Int J Cardiol 2000; 74(Suppl 1):S11–S15.
8. Libby P, Aikawa M, Kinlay S, et al: Lipid lowering improves endothelial functions. Int J Cardiol 2000; 74(Suppl 1):S3–S10.
9. Krone W, Muller-Wieland D: Lipid lowering therapy and stabilization of atherosclerotic plaques. Thromb Haemost 1999; 82(Suppl 1):60–61.
10. Scott J: The pathogenesis of atherosclerosis and new opportunities for treatment and prevention. J Neural Transm Suppl 2002; 63:1–17.
11. Clofibrate and niacin in coronary heart disease. JAMA 1975; 231:360–381.
12. Carlson LA, Rosenhamer G: Reduction of mortality in the Stockholm Ischaemic Heart Disease Secondary Prevention Study by combined treatment with clofibrate and nicotinic acid. Acta Med Scand 1988; 223:405–418.
13. Randomised trial of cholesterol lowering in 4444 patients with coronary heart disease: The Scandinavian Simvastatin Survival Study (4S). Lancet 1994; 344:1383–1389.
14. Sacks FM, Pfeffer MA, Moye LA, et al: The effect of pravastatin on coronary events after myocardial infarction in patients with average cholesterol levels: Cholesterol and Recurrent Events Trial investigators. N Engl J Med 1996; 335:1001–1009.

15. Prevention of cardiovascular events and death with pravastatin in patients with coronary heart disease and a broad range of initial cholesterol levels: The Long-Term Intervention with Pravastatin in Ischaemic Disease (LIPID) Study Group. N Engl J Med 1998; 339:1349-1357.

16. Rubins HB, Robins SJ, Collins D, et al: Gemfibrozil for the secondary prevention of coronary heart disease in men with low levels of high-density lipoprotein cholesterol: Veterans Affairs High-Density Lipoprotein Cholesterol Intervention Trial Study Group. N Engl J Med 1999; 341:410-418.

17. MRC/BHF Heart Protection Study of cholesterol lowering with simvastatin in 20,536 high-risk individuals: A randomised placebo-controlled trial. Lancet 2002; 360:7-22.

18. Shepherd J, Blauw GJ, Murphy MB, et al: Pravastatin in Elderly Individuals at Risk of Vascular Disease (PROSPER): A randomised controlled trial. Lancet 2002; 360:1623-1630.

19. Mikhailidis DP, Wierzbicki AS: The Greek Atorvastatin and Coronary-heart-disease Evaluation (GREACE) study. Curr Med Res Opin 2002; 18:215-219.

20. Sever P, Daholf, B, Poulter NR, et al: Prevention of coronary and stroke events with atorvastatin in hypertensive patients who have average or lower-than-average cholesterol concentrations, in the Anglo-Scandinavian Cardiac Outcomes Trial: Lipid Lowering Arm (ASCOT-LLA): A multicentre randomised controlled trial. Lancet 2003; 361:1149-1158.

21. MRC/BHF Heart Protection Study of antioxidant vitamin supplementation in 20,536 high-risk individuals: A randomised placebo-controlled trial. Lancet 2002; 360:23-33.

22. Law MR, Wald NJ, Thompson SG: By how much and how quickly does reduction in serum cholesterol concentration lower risk of ischaemic heart disease? BMJ 1994; 308:367-372.

23. Holme I: An analysis of randomized trials evaluating the effect of cholesterol reduction on total mortality and coronary heart disease incidence. Circulation 1990; 82:1916-1924.

24. Rossouw JE, Lewis B, Rifkind BM: The value of lowering cholesterol after myocardial infarction. N Engl J Med 1990; 323:1112-1119.

25. Ravnskov U: Cholesterol lowering trials in coronary heart disease: Frequency of citation and outcome. BMJ 1992; 305:15-19.

26. Peto R, Yusuf S, Collins R: Cholesterol-lowering trials: Results in their epidemiologic context [abstract]. Circulation 1985; 72:451.

27. Gould AL, Rossouw JE, Santanello NC, et al: Cholesterol reduction yields clinical benefit: Impact of statin trials. Circulation 1998; 97:946-952.

28. Shepherd J, Cobbe SM, Ford I, et al: Prevention of coronary heart disease with pravastatin in men with hypercholesterolemia: West of Scotland Coronary Prevention Study Group. N Engl J Med 1995; 333:1301-1307.

29. Downs JR, Clearfield M, Weis S, et al: Primary prevention of acute coronary events with lovastatin in men and women with average cholesterol levels: Results of AFCAPS/TexCAPS. Air Force/Texas Coronary Atherosclerosis Prevention Study. JAMA 1998; 279:1615-1622.

30. Blankenhorn DH, Azen SP, Kramsch DM, et al: Coronary angiographic changes with lovastatin therapy. The Monitored Atherosclerosis Regression Study (MARS). The MARS Research Group. Ann Intern Med 1993; 119:969-976.

31. Waters D, Higginson L, Gladstone P, et al: Effects of monotherapy with an HMG-CoA reductase inhibitor on the progression of coronary atherosclerosis as assessed by serial quantitative arteriography: The Canadian Coronary Atherosclerosis Intervention Trial. Circulation 1994; 89:959-968.

32. Effect of simvastatin on coronary atheroma: The Multicentre Anti-Atheroma Study (MAAS). Lancet 1994; 344:633-638.

33. Byington RP, Jukema JW, Salonen JT, et al: Reduction in cardiovascular events during pravastatin therapy: Pooled analysis of clinical events of the Pravastatin Atherosclerosis Intervention Program. Circulation 1995; 92:2419-2425.

34. LaRosa JC, He J, Vupputuri S: Effect of statins on risk of coronary disease: A meta-analysis of randomized controlled trials. JAMA 1999; 282:2340-2346.

35. Schwartz GG, Olsson AG, Ezekowitz MD, et al: Effects of atorvastatin on early recurrent ischemic events in acute coronary syndromes: The MIRACL study: A randomized controlled trial. JAMA 2001; 285:1711-1718.

36. Kayicioglu M, Can L, Kultursay H, et al: Early use of pravastatin in patients with acute myocardial infarction undergoing coronary angioplasty. Acta Cardiol 2002; 57:295-302.

37. Wright RS, Murphy JG, Bybee KA, et al: Statin lipid-lowering therapy for acute myocardial infarction and unstable angina: Efficacy and mechanism of benefit. Mayo Clin Proc 2002; 77:1085-1092.

38. Arntz HR, Agrawal R, Wunderlich W, et al: Beneficial effects of pravastatin (+/− cholestyramine/niacin) initiated immediately after a coronary event (the randomized Lipid-Coronary Artery Disease [L-CAD] Study). Am J Cardiol 2000; 86:1293-1298.

39. Wilhelmsen L, Berglund G, Elmfeldt D, et al: The multifactor primary prevention trial in Goteborg, Sweden. Eur Heart J 1986; 7:279-288.

40. Multiple Risk Factor Intervention Trial: Risk factor changes and mortality results: Multiple Risk Factor Intervention Trial Research Group. JAMA 1997; 277:582-594.

41. Multiple Risk Factor Intervention Trial: Risk factor changes and mortality results: Multiple Risk Factor Intervention Trial Research Group. JAMA 1982; 248:1465-1477.

42. Miettinen TA, Huttunen JK, Naukkarinen V, et al: Multifactorial primary prevention of cardiovascular diseases in middle-aged men: Risk factor changes, incidence, and mortality. JAMA 1985; 254:2097-2102.

43. Hjermann I, Velve Byre K, Holme I, et al: Effect of diet and smoking intervention on the incidence of coronary heart disease. Report from the Oslo Study Group of a randomised trial in healthy men. Lancet 1981; 2:1303-1310.

44. Dayton S, Pearce ML, Goldman H, et al: Controlled trial of a diet high in unsaturated fat for prevention of atherosclerotic complications. Lancet 1968; 2:1060-1062.

45. Heady JA, Morris JN, Oliver MF: WHO clofibrate/cholesterol trial: Clarifications. Lancet 1992; 340:1405-1406.

46. Frick MH, Elo O, Haapa K, et al: Helsinki Heart Study: Primary-prevention trial with gemfibrozil in middle-aged men with dyslipidemia. Safety of treatment, changes in risk factors, and incidence of coronary heart disease. N Engl J Med 1987; 317:1237-1245.

47. Shepherd J: The West of Scotland Coronary Prevention Study: A trial of cholesterol reduction in Scottish men. Am J Cardiol 1995; 76:113C-117C.

48. A co-operative trial in the primary prevention of ischaemic heart disease using clofibrate: Report from the Committee of Principal Investigators. Br Heart J 1978; 40:1069-1118.

49. The Lipid Research Clinics Coronary Primary Prevention Trial results. I. Reduction in incidence of coronary heart disease. JAMA 1984; 251:351-364.

50. Dorr AE, Gundersen K, Schneider JC Jr, et al: Colestipol hydrochloride in hypercholesterolemic patients: Effect on serum cholesterol and mortality. J Chronic Dis 1978; 31:5-14.

51. Major outcomes in moderately hypercholesterolemic, hypertensive patients randomized to pravastatin vs usual care. JAMA 2002; 288:2998-3007.

52. Clearfield M, Downs JR, Weis S, et al: Air Force/Texas Coronary Atherosclerosis Prevention Study (AFCAPS/TexCAPS): Efficacy and tolerability of long-term treatment with lovastatin in women. J Womens Health Gend Based Med 2001; 10:971-981.

53. WHO cooperative trial on primary prevention of ischaemic heart disease with clofibrate to lower serum cholesterol: Final mortality follow-up. Report of the Committee of Principal Investigators. Lancet 1984; 2:600-604.

54. Pignone M, Phillips C, Mulrow C: Use of lipid-lowering drugs for primary prevention of coronary heart disease: meta-analysis of randomised trials. BMJ 2000; 321:983-986.

55. Pfeffer MA, Sacks FM, Moye LA, et al: Cholesterol and recurrent events: A secondary prevention trial for normolipidemic patients: CARE Investigators. Am J Cardiol 1995; 76:98C-106C.

56. Executive Summary of the third report of the National Cholesterol Education Program (NCEP) expert panel on detection, evaluation, and treatment of high blood cholesterol in adults (Adult Treatment Panel III). JAMA 2001; 285:2486-2497.

57. Wolf PA, Kannel WB, Verter J: Current status of risk factors for stroke. Neurol Clin 1983; 1:317-343.

58. Iso H, Jacobs DR Jr, Wentworth D, et al: Serum cholesterol levels and six-year mortality from stroke in 350,977 men screened for the multiple risk factor intervention trial. N Engl J Med 1989; 320:904-910.

59. Smith GD, Shipley MJ, Marmot MG, et al: Plasma cholesterol concentration and mortality: The Whitehall Study. JAMA 1992; 267:70-76.

60. Serum cholesterol levels and stroke mortality. N Engl J Med 1989; 321:1339-1341.

61. Cholesterol, diastolic blood pressure, and stroke: 13,000 strokes in 450,000 people in 45 prospective cohorts. Prospective studies collaboration. Lancet 1995; 346:1647-1653.

62. Kagan A, Popper JS, Rhoads GG: Factors related to stroke incidence in Hawaii Japanese men: The Honolulu Heart Study. Stroke 1980; 11:14–21.

63. Tanaka H, Ueda Y, Hayashi M, et al: Risk factors for cerebral hemorrhage and cerebral infarction in a Japanese rural community. Stroke 1982; 13:62–73.

64. Blackburn H, Jacobs DR Jr: The ongoing natural experiment of cardiovascular diseases in Japan. Circulation 1989; 79:718–720.

65. Shimamoto T, Komachi Y, Inada H, et al: Trends for coronary heart disease and stroke and their risk factors in Japan. Circulation 1989; 79:503–515.

66. Robertson TL, Kato H, Gordon T, et al: Epidemiologic studies of coronary heart disease and stroke in Japanese men living in Japan, Hawaii and California: Coronary heart disease risk factors in Japan and Hawaii. Am J Cardiol 1977; 39:244–249.

67. Baseline serum cholesterol and treatment effect in the Scandinavian Simvastatin Survival Study (4S). Lancet 1995; 345:1274–1275.

68. Hebert PR, Gaziano JM, Hennekens CH: An overview of trials of cholesterol lowering and risk of stroke. Arch Intern Med 1995; 155:50–55.

69. Atkins D, Psaty BM, Koepsell TD, et al: Cholesterol reduction and the risk for stroke in men: A meta-analysis of randomized, controlled trials. Ann Intern Med 1993; 119:136–145.

70. Hebert PR, Gaziano JM, Chan KS, et al: Cholesterol lowering with statin drugs, risk of stroke, and total mortality. An overview of randomized trials. JAMA 1997; 278:313–321.

71. Bucher HC, Griffith LE, Guyatt GH: Effect of HMGcoA reductase inhibitors on stroke: A meta-analysis of randomized, controlled trials. Ann Intern Med 1998; 128:89–95.

72. Warshafsky S, Packard D, Marks SJ, et al: Efficacy of 3-hydroxy-3-methylglutaryl coenzyme A reductase inhibitors for prevention of stroke. J Gen Intern Med 1999; 14:763–774.

73. Straus SE, Majumdar SR, McAlister FA: New evidence for stroke prevention: Clinical applications. JAMA 2002; 288:1396–1398.

74. Straus SE, Majumdar SR, McAlister FA: New evidence for stroke prevention: Scientific review. JAMA 2002; 288:1388–1395.

75. White HD, Simes RJ, Anderson NE, et al: Pravastatin therapy and the risk of stroke. N Engl J Med 2000; 343:317–326.

76. Law MR, Wald NJ, Rudnicka AR: Quantifying effect of statins on low density lipoprotein cholesterol, ischaemic heart disease, and stroke: Systematic review and meta-analysis. BMJ 2003; 326:1423.

77. Davey Smith G, Pekkanen J: Should there be a moratorium on the use of cholesterol lowering drugs? BMJ 1992; 304:431–434.

78. Oliver MF: Might treatment of hypercholesterolaemia increase non-cardiac mortality? Lancet 1991; 337:1529–1531.

79. Gaziano JM, Hebert PR, Hennekens CH: Cholesterol reduction: Weighing the benefits and risks. Ann Intern Med 1996; 124:914–918.

80. Engelberg H: Low serum cholesterol and suicide. Lancet 1992; 339:727–729.

81. Gordon D: Cholesterol Lowering and total morality: Lowering Cholesterol in High-Risk Individuals. New York, Marcel Dekker: 1995, pp 33–48.

82. Bjerre LM, LeLorier J: Do statins cause cancer? A meta-analysis of large randomized clinical trials. Am J Med 2001; 110:716–723.

83. Muldoon MF, Manuck SB, Mendelsohn AB, et al: Cholesterol reduction and non-illness mortality: Meta-analysis of randomised clinical trials. BMJ 2001; 322:11–5.

84. Hay JW, Yu WM, Ashraf T: Pharmacoeconomics of lipid-lowering agents for primary and secondary prevention of coronary artery disease. Pharmacoeconomics 1999; 15:47–74.

85. Kupersmith J, Holmes-Rovner M, et al: Cost-effectiveness analysis in heart disease. II. Preventive therapies. Prog Cardiovasc Dis 1995; 37:243–271.

86. Weinstein MC, Stason WB: Cost-effectiveness of interventions to prevent or treat coronary heart disease. Annu Rev Public Health 1985; 6:41–63.

87. Oster G, Epstein AM: Cost-effectiveness of antihyperlipidemic therapy in the prevention of coronary heart disease: The case of cholestyramine. JAMA 1987; 258:2381–2387.

88. Goldman L, Weinstein MC, Goldman PA, et al: Cost-effectiveness of HMG-CoA reductase inhibition for primary and secondary prevention of coronary heart disease. JAMA 1991; 265:1145–1151.

89. Johannesson M, Jonsson B, Kjekshus J, et al: Cost effectiveness of simvastatin treatment to lower cholesterol levels in patients with coronary heart disease: Scandinavian Simvastatin Survival Study Group. N Engl J Med 1997; 336:332–336.

90. Census 2000. Vol. 2002: U.S. Census Bureau, 2000.

91. Ganz DA, Kuntz KM, Jacobson GA, et al: Cost-effectiveness of 3-hydroxy-3-methylglutaryl coenzyme A reductase inhibitor therapy in older patients with myocardial infarction. Ann Intern Med 2000; 132:780–787.

92. The Expert Panel: Report of the National Cholesterol Education Program Expert Panel on detection, evaluation, and treatment of high blood pressure in adults. Arch Intern Med 1988; 148:36–69.

93. Summary of the second report of the National Cholesterol Education Program (NCEP) Expert Panel on detection, evaluation, and treatment of high blood cholesterol in adults (Adult Treatment Panel II). JAMA 1993; 269:3015–3023.

94. National Center for Health Statistics, National Heart L, and Blood Institute Collaborative Lipid Group: Trends in serum cholesterol levels among US adults aged 20 to 74 years: Data from the National Health and Nutrition Examination Surveys, 1960 to 1980. JAMA 1987; 257:937–942.

95. Ford ES, Mokdad AH, Giles WH, et al: Serum total cholesterol concentrations and awareness, treatment, and control of hypercholesterolemia among US adults. Circulation 2003; 107:2185–2189.

Blood Pressure Reduction

Paul K. Whelton
Jiang He

Estimates of the prevalence of high blood pressure (BP), as well as the awareness, treatment, and control of hypertension, are available for many countries and ethnic groups.[1,2] The prevalence of hypertension varies substantially depending on geographic setting, characteristics of the survey sample, criteria for diagnosis, and BP measurement methods. Studies have consistently identified a high prevalence of hypertension in economically developed countries, and high BP is being noted with increasing frequency in the economically developing world. In contrast, surveys of isolated populations have consistently identified a low average level of BP and little if any hypertension. Recognizing this, studies in both isolated and economically developed populations have identified a similar pattern for relationships between BP and environmental factors such as diet and exercise. In addition, migration studies have demonstrated that persons from low BP populations are prone to experience a progressively higher BP and increased risk of developing hypertension as they move from their natural environment to a setting where environmental exposures favor a high prevalence of hypertension.[3,4] In aggregate, these studies indicate that hypertension is not an inevitable consequence of life. However, most humans have a strong genetic predisposition to develop hypertension when exposed to the unfavorable environment found in economically developed societies.

PREVALENCE OF HYPERTENSION

Results from the most recent U.S. national survey indicate that 24% of the adult, noninstitutionalized population of the United States, representing 43,186,000 persons, meet the criteria for diagnosis of hypertension proposed by the Joint National Committee for Detection, Evaluation and Treatment of Hypertension (average systolic BP [SBP] ≥140 mm Hg, or average diastolic BP [DBP] ≥90 mm Hg, or treatment with antihypertensive medication).[5] An additional 7.1%, representing 12,744,000 persons who did not meet the criteria for diagnosis at the time of the survey, had

been told by a "doctor or other health care professional" that they had hypertension. The prevalence of hypertension rose progressively with increasing age, from the second to the seventh decade of life. Hypertension was noted in less than 10% of those aged 18 to 29 years but occurred in approximately 60% to 70% of their counterparts in the sixth and seventh decades of life. During the second half of life, much of the age-related increase in prevalence of hypertension was the result of a progressive rise in SBP. DBP rose until about the fifth decade but declined in succeeding years. As a result, much of the hypertension in later years was attributable to an isolated elevation of SBP. In addition to age, prevalence varied by race and gender. The age-adjusted prevalence of hypertension in non-Hispanic blacks was almost 50% higher than the corresponding prevalence in non-Hispanic whites and Mexican Americans. Men had a higher prevalence of hypertension during the first half of life, but the reverse was true after the sixth decade. The magnitude of the sex-associated differences in prevalence was, however, much smaller than the previously described associations for age and race. Overall, approximately two thirds of those with hypertension were aware of their diagnosis (69%), 53% were being treated with antihypertensive medications, and 24% had a SBP of less than 140 mm Hg and a DBP of less than 90 mm Hg while being treated with antihypertensive medications.

Blood Pressure-Associated Risk of Cardiovascular and Renal Disease

Epidemiologic studies have repeatedly demonstrated that high BP is an important, independent predictor of cardiovascular disease (CVD) risk.[6,7] MacMahon and colleagues conducted a pooled analysis of nine prospective cohort studies in which 418,343 adults, aged 25 to 84 years, were followed for an average of 10 years to study the relationship between baseline BP and subsequent occurrence of coronary heart disease (CHD) and stroke.[8] At the outset, none of the study participants had clinical evidence of CHD or stroke. The authors' findings were corrected for the regression dilution bias, which occurs when studying variables that can only be measured in an imprecise manner. The difference between the highest (105 mm Hg) and lowest (76 mm Hg) category of mean usual DBP at entry was only about 30 mm Hg. Even so, the risk of CHD and stroke was about fivefold and tenfold higher, respectively, for those at the higher compared to the lower end of this BP range. A 5 to 6 mm Hg difference in DBP at entry was associated with a 20% to 25% difference in the corresponding risk of CHD and a 35% to 40% difference in the risk of stroke. The relationship between BP and renal disease in observational studies has been equally impressive.[9] In a 16-year follow-up of 332,544 men who were screened for possible participation in the Multiple Risk Factor Intervention Trial (MRFIT), hypertension appeared to be the underlying cause in almost half (49%) of the 814 instances where end-stage renal disease (ESRD) occurred during follow-up.[10] Among those who survived the first 10 years of follow-up without suffering from ESRD, the relative risks of eventually developing the condition were 2.8-, 5.0-, 8.4-, and 12.4-fold higher for those with hypertension of stage 1, 2, 3, or 4 at baseline, compared to their counterparts without hypertension. The risk of ESRD was highest for those with both a high level of systolic as well as DBP at baseline, but much of the risk was the result of the effects of a high SBP.

Taking both prevalence and corresponding risk into account, the approximately 5% of the population with stage 2 to 4 hypertension (SBP ≥160 mm Hg or DBP ≥100 mm Hg) account for about one fourth of the excess BP-related CHD risk; the approximately 20% with phase I hypertension (SBP 140-159 mm Hg or DBP 90-99 mm Hg) account for more than 40% of the population excess risk. Much of the remaining BP-related excess in risk (≥20%) occurs in the approximately 25% who have a high normal BP (SBP 130-139 mm Hg or DBP 80-89 mm Hg).[11] Although stroke and ESRD are somewhat more BP-dependant diseases, the overall pattern for BP-related population excess risk for these two complications appears to be quite similar.

In aggregate, the previously mentioned epidemiologic data provide a strong scientific basis for interest in detection, treatment, and control of hypertension, both in the individual patient and in the community as a whole. The data also underscore the potential for risk reduction following application of effective treatment in those with less severe hypertension. Not only is the risk of serious outcomes such as CHD, stroke, and ESRD twofold to threefold higher in those with stage I hypertension compared to their counterparts with an optimal level of BP (<120 mm Hg systolic and <80 mm Hg diastolic), but stage I hypertensives account for nearly half of the BP-related excess in risk of these outcomes in the general population. Finally, the data indicate the importance of concurrent efforts aimed at prevention of hypertension.[11] Although not the focus of this chapter, primary prevention of hypertension complements and extends the risk reduction goals of treating established hypertension. Furthermore, it provides a potential means to interrupt and reduce the need for the continuing costly and only modestly successful cycle of detecting and treating hypertensive patients.

ANTIHYPERTENSIVE DRUG TREATMENT TRIALS

Over the past four decades, numerous antihypertensive drug treatment trials have been conducted to determine whether BP reduction decreases the risk of CVD. During the 1950s and early 1960s, several nonrandomized, historically controlled trials were conducted in patients with malignant hypertension.[12-14] Although the antihypertensive drugs used in these trials were crude by current standards, their effect on all-cause mortality was so impressive that the value of treatment in this context was rapidly demonstrated and accepted by the medical community. Over the next decade, the value of antihypertensive drug therapy was documented in patients with severe (stages 3-4) but nonmalignant hypertension.[15-17] In each of these trials, treatment benefits were apparent within months of initiating antihypertensive drug therapy and were primarily to the result of a substantial reduction in the frequency of hypertensive complications such as hemorrhagic stroke, congestive heart failure, and uremia.

Despite their value, the trials of the 1950s and 1960s contributed little to our knowledge of the effect of antihypertensive drug therapy on CHD, ischemic stroke, and other BP-related atherosclerotic complications. Such information came from larger and more prolonged trials that subsequently were conducted in patients with less severe hypertension.[18-35] Most of these trials used a diuretic as first-step therapy, but in a few instances beta blockers were the drugs of first choice. In the vast majority of these trials active therapy resulted in a statistically significant and impressive reduction in the incidence of fatal and nonfatal stroke. However, the impact of antihypertensive drug therapy on CHD was less striking and, with a few exceptions,[25,26,33] the risk reduction in individual trials was not statistically significant. This lead to uncertainty regarding the effects of antihypertensive drug treatment on CHD. In large part, however, this lack of statistical significance probably reflected a lack of statistical power to detect moderate reductions in CHD event rates in the individual trials. To overcome this problem, results from individual drug treatment trials have been pooled to obtain a more reliable estimate of the effect of antihypertensive treatment on clinical outcomes.[36-39]

Characteristics of Participants in 17 Trials of Diuretic or Beta Blocker Treatment

Using standard methods,[37] we pooled the results from 17 major randomized, controlled trials in which the effects of first-step diuretic or beta blocker drug therapy versus placebo or usual care on clinical outcomes had been evaluated.[16-35] Characteristics of the 47,653 trial participants who were enrolled in these trials as well as important elements of the study design used in each trial are summarized in Table 23-1. The number of participants enrolled in individual trials ranged from less than 100 to more than 17,000, with a median sample size of 840 participants per trial. An elevated DBP was the

TABLE 23-1 CHARACTERISTICS OF PARTICIPANTS AND STUDY DESIGN FOR 17 RANDOMIZED TRIALS OF ANTIHYPERTENSIVE DRUG THERAPY

Trial and year	Sample size	Entry DBP (mm Hg)	Entry SBP (mm Hg)	Mean age (years)	Males (%)	Mean follow-up (years)	Blinding	Main drug type(s)*	Mean DBP reduction (mm Hg)†	Mean SBP reduction (mm Hg)†
Wolff and Lindeman, 1966[16]	87	100–130	—	49	32	1.4	Double	A	20	—
Veterans Administration, 1967[17]	143	115–129	—	51	100	1.5	Double	D + A + V	27	43
Veterans Administration, 1970[18]	380	90–114	—	51	100	3.3	Double	D + A + V	19	31
Carter, 1970[19]	97	≥110	—	—	57	4	Open	D	—	—
Barraclough et al, 1973[20]	116	100–120	—	56	43	2	Single	D/M	13	—
Hypertension Stroke Study, 1974[21]	452	90–115	140–220	59	41	2.3	Double	D	12	25
USPHS Study, 1977[22]	389	90–114	—	44	80	7	Double	D + A	10	18
VA-NHLBI Study, 1977[23,24]	1012	85–105	—	38	81	1.5	Double	D	7	—
HDFP, 1979[25,26]	10,940	≥90	—	51	55	5	Open	D	6	—
Oslo Study, 1980[27]	785	90–109	—	45	100	5.5	Open	D	10	—
Australian National Study, 1980[29]	3427	95–109	<200	50	63	4	Single	D	6	—
MRC Study (younger), 1985[30]	17,354	90–109	<200	52	52	5	Single	BB/D	6	—
EWPHE Study, 1985[31]	840	90–119	160–239	72	30	4.7	Double	D	8	20
Coope and Warrender, 1986[32]	884	105–120	<280	69	31	4.4	Open	BB	11	18
SHEP Study, 1991[33]	4736	<90	160–219	72	43	4.5	Double	D + BB	4	12
STOP-Hypertension Study, 1991[34]	1627	90–120	180–230	76	37	2.1	Double	BB/D	8	20
MRC Study (older), 1992[35]	4396	<115	160–209	70	42	5.8	Single	BB/D	7	14
Mean or total	47,653	—	—	56	52	4.7	—	—	6.5	16

*A, alkaloid; D, diuretic; V, vasodilator; M, methyldopa; BB, beta blocker.
†The difference in mean blood pressure was based on data from those who attended follow-up for blood pressure measurement. DBP, diastolic blood pressure; SBP, systolic blood pressure.

primary inclusion criterion in most studies, but in some trials participants were required to have both a high systolic and DBP at entry.[21,31,32,34,35] One trial enrolled only patients with isolated systolic hypertension.[33] In five trials, participation was restricted to participants with "mild" to "moderate" diastolic hypertension (DBP 90–110 mm Hg),[23,24,27-30,33] and in four more enrollment was confined to those with a DBP of 115 mm Hg or less.[18,21,22,35] In the Hypertension Detection and Follow-up Program (HDFP), trial results were reported separately for participants within three strata of DBP at entry (DBP <110 mm Hg, DBP 110–115 mm Hg and DBP >115 mm Hg).[25,26]

The mean age (weighted by sample size) of the participants in the 17 trials was 56 years, but the average age in individual trials varied from 38 to 76 years. Five trials with 12,483 participants were conducted exclusively in individuals who were older than 60 years of age at entry.[31-35] Men and women were represented in approximately equal numbers. In most trials, the participants were followed for 4 to 5 years. However, in the U.S. Public Health Service trial and MRC trial in older adults a longer period of follow-up was used, and in four small trials the participants were followed for less than 4 years.[16,17,20,23,24] Treatment was double-blind in nine of the trials, single-blind in four, and open in the remaining four. Diuretics were used as first-step drug therapy in 12 of the 17 trials. Exceptions to this rule were the Wolff and Lindeman trial,[16] in which reserpine was the active therapy; the two MRC trials,[30,35] in which the participants were randomly assigned to active treatment with either a beta blocker or a diuretic; the STOP-Hypertension trial,[34] in which either a diuretic (hydrochlorothiazide plus the potassium-sparing agent amiloride) or a beta blocker (atenolol or pindolol) could be used as first-step therapy; and the atenolol trial in the elderly.[32] In most of the trials, the goal in the active treatment group was to achieve and maintain a DBP ≤90 mm Hg. With the exception of the HDFP trial, in which the control group was assigned to receive usual care, antihypertensive drug therapy was not recommended as a routine treatment for participants in the control group. However, about one fourth of the participants randomized to control therapy received antihypertensive drug therapy at some stage during their follow-up.

The mean reduction in BP during follow-up for those assigned to active treatment compared to their counterparts in the corresponding control group ranged from 4 to 27 mm Hg, with an overall average net reduction of 6.5 mm Hg (weighted by sample size). However, the true overall net reduction in BP may have been closer to about 5 to 6 mm Hg because BP measurements were only obtained in those who continued to participate in the follow-up examinations. Information on SBP during follow-up was available for 9 of the 17 trials. In these studies, the overall weighted average net reduction in SBP was about 16 mm Hg. For both SBP and DBP, the observed reduction was greater in trials in which the participants had a higher level of BP at entry.

Efficacy of Treatment with Diuretics or Beta Blockers

Overall, 934 CHD events occurred in the participants who were assigned to active treatment and 1104 in those who were allocated to control (Table 23-2). When results from the 17 trials were pooled, a highly significant reduction in the odds of total CHD (P < 0.001) and fatal CHD (P = 0.006) was observed among the participants allocated to active treatment. The reduction in total CHD was 16% (95% confidence interval [CI]: 8% to 23%) as was the reduction in fatal CHD (95% CI: 5% to 26%). As shown in Fig. 23-1, antihypertensive drug treatment was associated with a reduction in total CHD in 13 of the 17 trials. However, the reduction was statistically significant in only two of the trials.[25,26,33] In the HDFP trial, total CHD was reduced by 21% (95% CI: 7% to 33%),[25,26] and in the SHEP trial, total CHD was reduced by 28% (95% CI: 6% to 44%).[33]

A total of 525 strokes occurred in participants who were allocated to active treatment, and 768 occurred in those who were assigned to control (Table 23-2). Compared to control, those in active treatment experienced a 38% reduction in the odds of total stroke (95% CI: 31 to 45%; P < 0.001) and a 40% reduction in the odds of fatal stroke (95% CI: 26 to 51%; P < 0.001). In 14 of the 17 trials, the odds of total stroke was reduced for those assigned to active treatment compared to control and in 9 of the trials the reduction was statistically significant (Fig. 23-2).

■ ■ ■

TABLE 23-2 REDUCTION IN RISK FOR CORONARY HEART DISEASE, STROKE, CARDIOVASCULAR DISEASE, AND ALL-CAUSE MORTALITY: RESULTS FROM 17 RANDOMIZED TRIALS WITH 23,847 ACTIVE TREATMENT AND 23,806 CONTROL PARTICIPANTS

	NUMBER OF EVENTS		% Risk reduction (95% CI)*	P value
	Active	Control		
Total coronary heart disease	934	1104	16 (8 to 23)	<0.001
Fatal coronary heart disease	470	560	16 (5 to 26)	0.006
Total stroke	525	835	38 (31 to 45)	<0.001
Fatal stroke	140	234	40 (26 to 51)	<0.001
Cardiovascular disease deaths	768	964	21 (13 to 28)	<0.001
All-cause deaths	1435	1634	13 (6 to 19)	<0.001

*Risk reduction = 1 − odds ratio; CI, confidence interval.

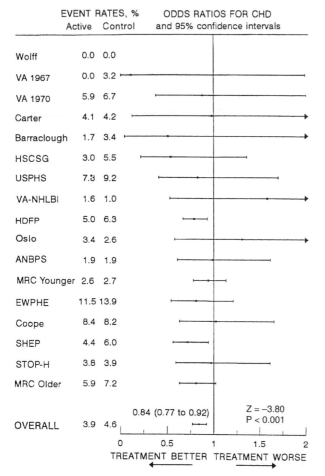

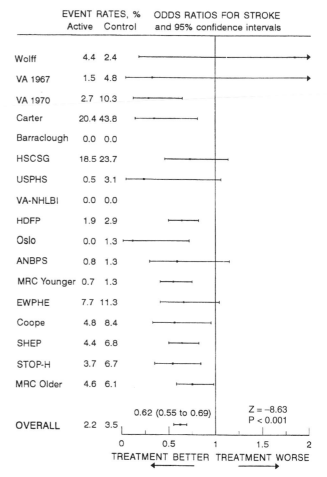

FIGURE 23-1. Odds ratios and 95% confidence intervals for total (fatal and nonfatal) coronary heart disease related to antihypertensive drug treatment. Results from 17 individual randomized, controlled trials and for a pooled estimate of their findings.

FIGURE 23-2. Odds ratios and 95% confidence intervals for total (fatal and nonfatal) stroke related to antihypertensive drug treatment. Results from 17 individual randomized, controlled trials and for a pooled estimate of their findings.

Although the proportional reduction in CHD was less than half that noted for stroke, the absolute reduction in CHD and stroke was less discrepant, given the greater frequency of CHD. Specifically, the absolute reduction in total (fatal) CHD was 7 (4) events/1000 persons, respectively, whereas the corresponding absolute reduction in total (fatal) stroke was 13 (4) events/1000 persons.

Temporal trends from the 17 trials indicated that most of the reduction in stroke risk was achieved within the first year of initiating antihypertensive drug treatment. In contrast, the reduction in CVD risk following institution of lipid-lowering drug therapy is not usually manifest for 2 to 3 years. However, the results of our meta-analysis and others indicate that only about two thirds of the expected reduction in CHD has been achieved in trials of diuretic or beta blocker drug therapy. This shortfall in risk reduction may simply reflect the effect of random variation. In our meta-analysis, the upper band of the 95% CI for reduction in the risk of total (fatal) CHD was 23% (26%). Alternatively, it may indicate that a longer period of treatment is necessary to completely reverse the atherosclerotic changes induced by a prolonged elevation of BP.[40-42] A third possibility is that first-step therapy with diuretic or

beta blocker drugs may have produced cardiotoxic side effects that diminished, but did not eliminate, the beneficial effects of reducing BP.

Overall, 768 deaths from CVD occurred in the participants who were allocated to active treatment and 964 deaths occurred in their counterparts who were allocated to control (Table 23-2). The overall reduction in CVD mortality for active treatment compared to control was 21% (95% CI: 12% to 28%; P < 0.001). In 6 of the 17 trials, the reduction in CVD mortality was statistically significant (Fig. 23-3). Noncardiovascular disease mortality was evenly distributed between the treatment and control groups (667 vs. 670). All-cause mortality was reduced by 13% (95% CI: 6 to 19%, P < 0.001) in those allocated to active compared to control treatment (Table 23-2, Fig. 23-4).

Reduction in Coronary Heart Disease and Stroke by Baseline Level of Blood Pressure and Age

Reduction in CHD and stroke risk by baseline level of DBP is presented in Table 23-3. The reduction in risk for CHD was greater in those with a higher

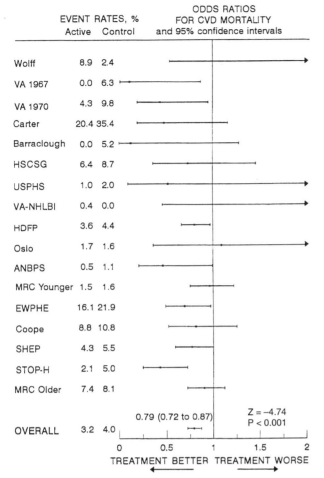

FIGURE 23-3. Odds ratios and 95% confidence intervals for cardiovascular disease mortality related to antihypertensive drug treatment. Results from 17 individual randomized, controlled trials and for a pooled estimate of their findings.

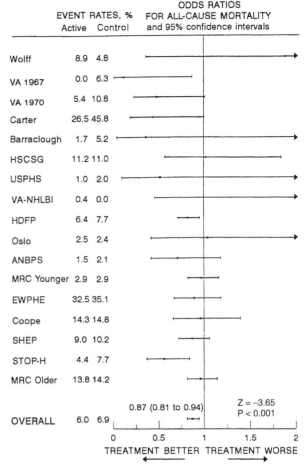

FIGURE 23-4. Odds ratios and 95% confidence intervals for all-cause mortality related to antihypertensive drug treatment. Results from 17 individual randomized, controlled trials and for a pooled estimate of their findings.

level of BP at entry, although the differences between the three BP strata were not statistically significant. The proportional reductions in risk for participants with an entry DBP of less than 110 mm Hg, 110 to 115 mm Hg, and more than 115 mm Hg were 14% (95% CI: 4% to 23%), 17% (95% CI: 1% to 31%), and 21% (95% CI: 1% to 37%), respectively. The absolute reduction in risk was even greater in participants with a higher level of BP at entry as a result of the higher event rate in this group; there were 5, 12, and 15 events/1000 persons for participants with an entry DBP <110, ≤115, and >115 mm Hg, respectively. The proportional reduction in risk for stroke did not differ significantly by level of DBP at entry. However, there was an impressive relationship between absolute reduction in risk and BP at entry because of the higher stroke event rate in those with a higher level of BP; 9, 19, and 35 events/1000 persons in participants with an entry DBP of less than 110, 110 to 115, and more than 115 mm Hg, respectively.

Comparison of the results from 5 trials conducted exclusively in older participants[31-35] with the corresponding findings from the remaining 12 trials identified a similar reduction in relative risk (Table 23-4).

However, the reduction in absolute risk was greater in the trials conducted in older participants. For CHD (fatal and nonfatal), the relative reduction in risk was 19% (95% CI: 7% to 30%) for the trials conducted exclusively in older participants and 14% (95% CI: 4% to 23%) for the remaining 12 trials. The corresponding reductions in absolute risk were 13 and 5 events/1000 persons, respectively. For fatal and nonfatal stroke, the proportional reduction in risk was 34% (95% CI: 24% to 44%) for the 5 trials conducted in older participants and 42% (95% CI: 32% to 51%) for the remaining 12 trials. The corresponding absolute reductions in risk were 23 and none events/1000 persons, respectively.

Comparison of Risk Reduction During Diuretic and Beta Blocker Treatment

The effects of first-step therapy with a diuretic compared to a beta receptor blocker have been explored in four randomized, controlled trials.[30,35,43,44] In the first MRC trial, diuretic treatment yielded a statistically significant 54% (95% CI: 24% to 72%) reduction in the odds of

TABLE 23-3 RISK REDUCTION IN CORONARY HEART DISEASE AND STROKE, BY BLOOD PRESSURE AT TRIAL ENTRY

Participants' entry diastolic blood pressure,* mm Hg (number of trials)	ACTIVE TREATMENT			CONTROL TREATMENT			% RISK REDUCTION, (95% CONFIDENCE INTERVAL)		P VALUE	
	Number of fatal events	Total number of events	Number of participants	Number of fatal events	Total number of events	Number of participants	Fatal events	Total events	Fatal events	Total events
Coronary heart disease										
All <110 (n = 6)	264	572	17,603	291	660	17,536	10 (−7 to 24)	14 (4 to 23)	0.2	0.01
Some ≥110, all ≤115 (n = 5)	124	222	3,843	152	265	3,826	19 (−3 to 36)	17 (1 to 31)	0.09	0.04
Some or all >115 (n = 8)	82	140	2,401	117	179	2,444	29 (5 to 46)	21 (1 to 37)	0.02	0.04
Stroke										
All <110 (n = 6)	50	237	17,603	83	386	17,536	39 (15 to 57)	39 (28 to 48)	0.004	<0.001
Some ≥110, all ≤115 (n = 5)	52	175	3,843	71	248	3,826	27 (−4 to 49)	32 (17 to 44)	0.08	<0.001
Some or all >115 (n = 8)	38	113	2,401	80	201	2,444	52 (30 to 67)	45 (30 to 56)	<0.001	<0.001

*Hypertension Detection and Follow-up Program had three entry diastolic blood pressure strata.

TABLE 23-4 RISK REDUCTION IN CORONARY HEART DISEASE AND STROKE, BY AGE

Participants' age (number of trials)	ACTIVE TREATMENT			CONTROL TREATMENT			% RISK REDUCTION, (95% CONFIDENCE INTERVAL)		P VALUE	
	Number of fatal events	Total number of events	Number of par-ticipants	Number of fatal events	Total number of events	Number of par-ticipants	Fatal events	Total events	Fatal events	Total events
Coronary Heart Disease										
Some or all <60 years (n = 12)	262	588	17,652	281	674	17,518	7 (−10 to 22)	14 (4 to 23)	0.3	0.01
All ≥60 years (n = 5)	208	346	6,195	279	430	6,288	25 (10 to 37)	19 (7 to 30)	0.002	0.004
Stroke										
Some or all <60 years (n = 12)	62	237	17,652	114	397	17,518	46 (27 to 60)	42 (32 to 51)	<0.001	<0.001
All ≥60 years (n = 5)	78	288	6,195	120	438	6,288	34 (12 to 50)	34 (24 to 44)	0.004	<0.001

stroke (fatal and nonfatal) compared to treatment with a beta blocker.[30] There was a similar, albeit nonsignificant, trend in the second MRC trial conducted in the elderly. However, in a pooled estimate of the results from all four trials, diuretics were only associated with a nonsignificant 13% (CI: −8% to 30%) reduction in stroke risk compared to treatment with beta blockers (Fig. 23-5). The MRC trial in older adults identified a statistically significant 40% (95% CI: 14% to 58%) reduction in the odds of CHD for diuretic compared to beta blocker treatment.[35] Again, however, the pooled estimate identified a nonsignificant difference of 4% (95% CI: −11% to 17%) between the treatment effect with diuretics and beta blockers.

Efficacy of Treatment with Newer Classes of Antihypertensive Drug Therapy

Other classes of antihypertensive drug therapy, including angiotensin-converting enzyme (ACE) inhibitors, angiotensin II AT1-receptor blockers (ARB), calcium channel blockers (CCB), and alpha$_1$-receptor blockers have been shown to be effective in lowering BP and are well tolerated.[45] Many have indications for treatment of illnesses such as angina pectoris and prostatic hypertrophy that are common in patients with hypertension, making them useful complements to diuretics and beta blockers.[45,46] In addition, theoretic advantages compared to diuretics and beta blockers have been proposed.[47]

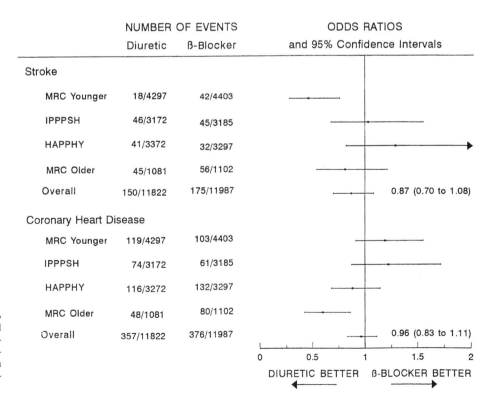

FIGURE 23-5. Odds ratios and 95% confidence intervals for stroke and coronary heart disease in four randomized, controlled trials comparing predominantly diuretic with predominantly beta blocker first-step therapy of hypertension.

Use of these newer classes of antihypertensive drug therapy has become increasingly popular in recent years.[48] At least three quantitative overviews of clinical events experience from randomized controlled trials of BP lowering with ACE inhibitors and CCB have been published.[49-51] Some of the most important findings from these reviews are summarized in the following sections.

The Blood Pressure Lowering Treatment Trialists' (BPLTT) Collaboration conducted a prospective pooling of experience from 74,696 participants in 15 randomized controlled clinical trials.[49] The mean age of those studied was 62 years, and approximately half (53%) were male. Six of the trials provided experience from comparisons of active treatment with placebo.[52-57], eight provided information from comparisons of first-step therapy with different drug classes.[58-66]), and three provided comparisons of different levels of intensity of BP lowering.[66-68]

ACE inhibitors were compared to placebo in four trials (12,124 study participants) with differences in SBP/DBP that ranged from 3/1 mm Hg to 6/4 mm Hg.[52-55] There was no evidence for heterogeneity in trial results, but one of the four studies (Heart Outcomes Prevention Evaluation; HOPE) provided 88% of the clinical event experience and was designed as a drug comparison (ACE inhibitors vs. placebo) rather than a BP reduction trial.[52] In this pooled analysis, ACE inhibitors reduced the risk of stroke and CHD compared to placebo by 30% (95% CI: 15% to 43%) and 20% (95% CI: 11% to 28%), respectively (Fig. 23-6). In a comparison (Perindopril Protection Against Recurrent Stroke Study; PROGRESS), which was published subsequent to the BPLTT analysis, 2916 hypertensive and 3189 nonhypertensive patients with a history of stroke or transient ischemic attack were randomly assigned to the ACE inhibitor perindopril (alone or in combination with the diuretic indapamide) or placebo.[69] Over 4 years of follow-up those assigned to ACE inhibitors versus placebo experienced an average reduction in SBP/DBP of 9/4 mm and a corresponding relative reduction in risk of 28% (95% CI: 17% to 38%) and 26% (95% CI: 16% to 34%) for stroke and major vascular events, respectively. The reductions in both SBP/DBP (12/5 mm Hg) and stroke risk (43%; 95% CI: 30% to 54%) were greater for those who were treated with a combination of ACE inhibitors and diuretic therapy. The reduction in risk of stroke was similar for those who were and were not hypertensive.

The BPLTT Collaborators compared CCB to placebo in a pooled analysis of two trials with 5520 study participants.[56,57] There was no evidence of heterogeneity in trial results, but the larger trial[57] was conducted in patients with isolated systolic hypertension and contributed disproportionately to sample size (4695 study participants), average reduction in SBP/DBP (9/5 mm Hg), and percent of major cardiovascular events (88%). Compared to placebo, CCB therapy reduced the risk of stroke and CHD by 39% (95% CI: 15% to 56%) and 21% (95% CI: −6% to 41%), respectively (Fig. 23-6).

ACE inhibitors were compared to diuretic or beta blocker therapy by the BPLTT Collaboration in a pooled analysis of experience from three trials, with 16,161 study participants,[58-60] but the largest of the three exhibited a baseline difference in BP suggesting some nonran-

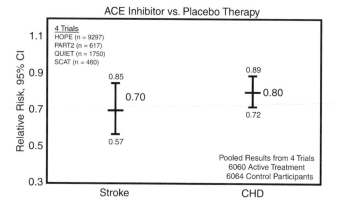

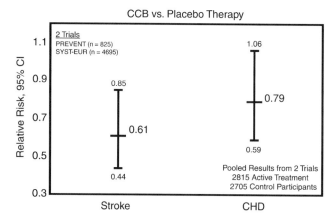

FIGURE 23-6. Relative risks and 95% confidence intervals for stroke and coronary heart disease in four randomized, controlled trials of angiotensin-converting enzyme (ACE) inhibitor therapy versus placebo and two randomized, controlled trials of calcium channel blocker (CCB) therapy versus placebo in first step therapy of hypertension. (Adapted from data presented in Blood Pressure Lowering Treatment Trialists' Collaboration: Effects of ACE inhibitors, calcium antagonists, and other blood-pressure-lowering drugs: results of prospectively designed overviews of randomised trials. Lancet 2000; 355:1955–1964.)

dom allocation of the treatments.[58] Inclusion or exclusion of the larger trial did not materially effect the overall finding that there was no significant difference in reduction of stroke or CHD risk with either of the active treatments. In an analysis confined to the two smaller trials (5176 study participants) the relative reduction in risk of stroke and CHD for ACE inhibitor compared to beta blocker therapy was 8% (95% CI: −9% to 22%) and −2% (95% CI: −20% to 14%), respectively.[59,60] In the more recently published Losartin Intervention For Endpoint reduction (LIFE) trial (n = 9,193), the ARB losartin was compared to the beta blocker atenolol in a randomized controlled trial in 55- to 80-year-old patients with hypertension (SBP/DBP = 160–200/9–115 mm Hg at baseline) and left-ventricular hypertrophy by electrocardiography.[70] After an average of 4.8 years of follow-up, those assigned to losartin compared to atenolol experienced a relative reduction in risk of 25% (95% CI: 11% to 37%) and −7% (95% CI: −31% to 12%) for stroke and CHD, respectively.

The BPLTT Collaborators compared CCB to diuretic or beta blocker therapy in a pooled analysis of experience from five trials with 23,454 study participants,[59,61-65] yielding a relative reduction in risk of stroke and CHD of 13% (95% CI: 2% to 23%) and −12% (95% CI: −26% to 0%), respectively. The pattern was similar for studies that used dihydropyridine (three trials) and nondihydropyridine therapy (two trials).

The BPLTT Collaborators compared ACE inhibitors to CCB based on experience from two trials, with 4871 study participants,[59,66] but one of the two contributed 93% of the major cardiovascular events. Overall, treatment with ACE inhibitors yielded a significant 19% reduction in the relative risk of CHD (95% CI: 3% to 32%) compared to CCB, but there was significant heterogeneity (P = 0.04) between the results from both trials. The corresponding reduction in relative risk of stroke was −2% (95% CI: −21% to 15%).

A second meta-analysis by Pahor and colleagues was focused on a comparison of CCB versus other first-step active therapies (diuretics, beta blockers, ACE inhibitors, or clonidine). Nine randomized, controlled clinical trials (27,743 participants; 12,699 assigned to a CCB and 15,044 to other first-step agents) with durations of follow-up varying from 2 to 7 years were included in the analysis.[59,61-66,72-74] Average reductions in SBP/DBP were almost identical in the two groups. Those assigned to CCB had a 26% higher risk of acute myocardial infarction (95% CI: 11% to 43%), a 25% higher risk of congestive heart failure (95% CI: 7% to 46%), and a 10% higher risk of major cardiovascular events (95% CI: 2% to 18%) but a marginally nonsignificant 10% reduction in stroke risk (95% CI: −20% to 2%).

A third meta-analysis by Staessen and colleagues compared the efficacy of "old" drugs (diuretics or beta blockers) versus "new" drugs (CCB, ACE inhibitors, or alpha₁-receptor blockers) in nine randomized controlled trials of antihypertensive therapy.[58-65,74,75] The authors reported an overall similarity in efficacy between the two groups ("old" and "new" drugs) but noted a 13.5% reduction in risk of stroke (95% CI: 1.3% to 24.2%) and a 19.2% higher risk of myocardial infarction (95% CI: 3.5% to 37.2%) for those assigned to CCB compared to diuretics or beta blockers. The authors felt that much of this difference could be explained on the basis of small but potentially important differences in average BP between the two groups.

Overall, the three meta-analyses provide evidence that treatment with any of the major classes of antihypertensive drug therapy (diuretics, beta blockers, ACE inhibitors, and CCB) reduces cardiovascular risk. However, there was insufficient statistical power to determine whether individual classes of drug therapy provide special protection from the CVD complications of hypertension.[76]

The Antihypertensive and Lipid-Lowering Treatment to Prevent Heart Attack Trial

The Antihypertensive and Lipid-Lowering Treatment to Prevent Heart Attack Trial (ALLHAT) is by far the largest and most comprehensive trial of the efficacy of different first-step drug therapies of hypertension. ALLHAT was a randomized, double-blind, practice-based clinical trial sponsored by the National Heart, Lung, and Blood Institute to determine whether first-step antihypertensive drug therapy with newer and more expensive drugs such as ACE inhibitors, CCB, or alpha₁-receptor blockers provides additional benefits compared to corresponding treatment with low-dose diuretics.[77] A total of 42,418 men and women aged 55 years or older with stage I hypertension and at least one other major risk factor for CVD were assigned at random to treatment with a low-dose diuretic (chlorthalidone), CCB (amlodipine), ACE inhibitors (lisinopril), or alpha₁-receptor blocker (doxazosin). The doxazosin versus diuretic comparison was terminated early after a median of 3.3 years of follow-up because of a 25% excess of CVD in the 9067 study participants assigned to the alpha₁-receptor blocker compared to their 15,268 counterparts assigned to diuretic, including more than a twofold (relative risk: 2.04 and 95% CI: 1.79 to 2.32) increase in congestive heart failure (Fig. 23-7).[75] Those assigned to CCB (n = 9048) or ACE inhibitors (n = 9054) were compared to their counterparts assigned to diuretic (n = 15,255) for up to 8 years (median = 4.9 years). Mean SBP was approximately 2 and 1 mm Hg lower in the diuretic group compared to the ACE inhibitor and CCB groups, respectively, and SBP/DBP was controlled to less than 140/90 mm Hg in 68%, 66%, and 61% in the diuretic, CCB, and ACE inhibitors groups, respectively, at the 5-year follow-up visit.[78] As expected, serum potassium was slightly lower, and serum cholesterol and fasting serum glucose were slightly higher in the diuretic group compared to either the CCB or ACE inhibitors groups. There was no difference between either of the CCB or ACE inhibitors groups versus diuretic for fatal or nonfatal coronary heart disease or for all-cause mortality (Fig. 23-7). Compared to the diuretic group, the CCB group experienced a 38% higher rate of heart failure (95% CI: 25% to 52%), and the ACE inhibitor group had a 15% higher rate of stroke (95% CI: 2% to 30%), a 19% higher rate of heart failure (95% CI: 7% to 31%), an 11% higher rate of angina pectoris (95% CI: 3% to 20%), and a 10% higher rate of coronary revascularizations (95% CI: 0% to 21%). These treatment patterns were noted in a variety of important subgroups defined by age, sex, race, and presence or absence of diabetes, with the relative benefit of diuretics compared to ACE inhibitors for prevention of stroke being significantly (P = 0.01) greater in blacks (1.4; 95% CI: 1.17% to 1.68%) compared to whites (1.00; 95% CI: 0.85% to 1.17%). These results argue strongly for the superiority of low-dose diuretics compared to CCB, ACE inhibitors or alpha₁-receptor blockers in preventing CVD complications during first-step drug therapy of hypertension. A CCB or ACE inhibitor is an acceptable alternative choice for initial drug therapy of hypertension where another therapeutic indication dictates their choice or in the unusual circumstance that a diuretic is contraindicated. A majority of patients require more than one antihypertensive medication to control their BP. In this instance, the combination of a low-dose diuretic with either a CCB or ACE inhibitor is the logical choice. Other agents should probably be reserved for use as second- or third-step agents until trials demonstrate their equivalence or superiority to diuretics, CCB, or ACE inhibitors.

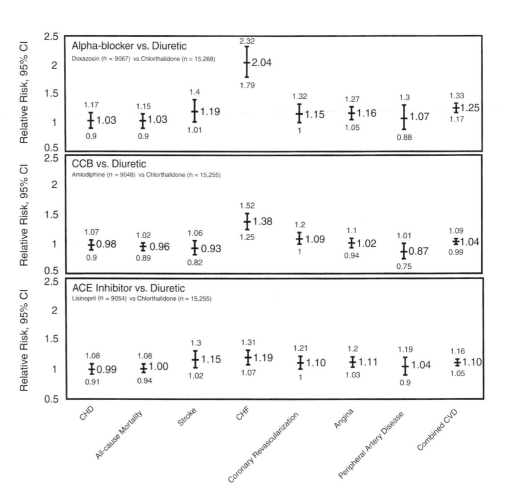

FIGURE 23-7. Relative risks and 95% confidence intervals (CI) for coronary heart disease (CHD), all-cause mortality, stroke, heart failure, coronary revascularization, angina, peripheral artery disease, and combined cardiovascular disease (fatal and nonfatal CHD, stroke, heart failure, coronary revascularization, angina, and peripheral artery disease) in the Antihypertensive and Lipid-Lowering Treatment to Prevent Heart Attack Trial. (Adapted from data published in The ALLHAT Officers and Coordinators for the ALLHAT Collaborative Research Group: Major cardiovascular events in hypertensive patients randomized to doxazosin vs chlorthalidone: The Antihypertensive and Lipid-Lowering Treatment to Prevent Heart Attack Trial (ALLHAT). JAMA 2000; 283:1967–1975; and The ALLHAT Officers and Coordinators for the ALLHAT Investigative Research Group: Major outcomes in high-risk hypertensive patients randomized to angiotensin-converting enzyme inhibitor or calcium channel blocker vs diuretic: The Antihypertensive and Lipid Lowering Treatment to Prevent Heart Attack Trial (ALLHAT). JAMA 2002; 288:2981–2997.)

Other Trials Comparing Different Regimens of Antihypertensive Drug Therapy

The Second Australian National Blood Pressure Study (ANBP2) reported an 11% reduction in CVD events (95% CI: 0% to 21%) for ACE inhibitor- versus diuretic-based treatment during an average of 4.1 years of treatment in 6083 participants aged 65 to 84 years.[79] In contrast to ALLHAT, which was double-blinded, the ANBP2 was an open-label trial. In addition, it had much less statistical power than ALLHAT for the comparison of ACE inhibitor and diuretic therapy, with less than one-fourth as many CVD events and less than one-tenth the number of heart failure events. In contrast to ALLHAT, in which consistent results were noted across all the major demographic subgroups, there was a nonsignificant interaction of treatment effect by gender in ANBP2 with an ACE inhibitor versus diuretic relative risk of 0.83 in men and 1.00 in women. The Controlled Onset Verapamil Investigation of Cardiovascular End Points (CONVINCE) trial was a double-blinded comparison of treatment with a nondihydropiridine CCB with either low-dose diuretic (hydrochlorothiazide) or a beta blocker (atenolol) in 16,602 hypertensive patients aged 55 years or older with at least one additional risk factor for CVD.[80] The trial was stopped prematurely, for commercial reasons, after a mean of 3 years, but the results were consistent with ALLHAT. Several other studies,

including the European/North American SCOPE trial (angiotensin II receptor blocker versus placebo) have been reported in preliminary form at national/international meetings and appear to have generated findings that are consistent with previously mentioned experience. The Blood Pressure Lowering Treatment Trialists' Collaboration published an updated meta-analysis based on experience in 162,341 participants in 29 randomized, controlled trials.[81] The main difference from their report published in 2000 was greater emphasis on the importance of BP reduction, *per se*, in all major outcomes except heart failure. Older agents (diuretics or beta blockers) seemed to provide a drug-specific advantage in preventing heart failure compared to CCB or ACE inhibitors. Psaty et al.[82] also published a recent meta-analysis based on experience in 192,478 participants in 42 randomized, controlled trials. Based on their results, these authors recommend the use of low-dose diuretics as first-step agents for treatment of hypertension. One ongoing study (The Anglo-Scandinavian Cardiac Outcomes Trial; ASCOT) is worthy of special mention.[83] In this trial, beta blocker or diuretic therapy is being compared with calcium antagonist or an ACE inhibitor treatment in 19,342 adults who have hypertension and at least three other risk factors for CVD. As with ALLHAT, the main outcome measure is nonfatal myocardial infarction and fatal CHD.

Nonclinical Endpoints

All of the previously mentioned trials have been designed to compare the efficacy of treatment on clinical endpoints. Many more have been designed on nonclinical endpoints such as change in renal function, left-ventricular hypertrophy, and vessel wall thickness. A review of these trials is beyond the scope of this chapter, but in general the results to date have been consistent with findings in the trials with clinical endpoints.

Optimal Goal for Reduction of Blood Pressure

Observational epidemiologic studies typically have demonstrated a direct relationship between level of BP and risk of subsequent cardiovascular or renal disease.[6-10] However, a J-shaped relationship between BP and CVD has been noted in nonconcurrent prospective analyses of some cohorts who have been treated with antihypertensive drug therapy.[84] Several groups of investigators have demonstrated that treated hypertensives have a higher risk of CVD compared to suitably matched normotensives.[85-88] One explanation for this finding is insufficient lowering of BP; an alternative possibility is that excessive lowering of BP triggered ischemia and infarction in the coronary and cerebral circulations. Clinical trials in which participants are randomly assigned to different intensities of BP lowering provide the best opportunity to determine which of these two possibilities are most likely to explain the findings. Experience from three such trials has been pooled by the Blood Pressure Lowering Treatment Trialists' Collaboration.[49] The relative reductions in risk of stroke and CHD for those assigned to a more versus less intensive BP reduction regimen were

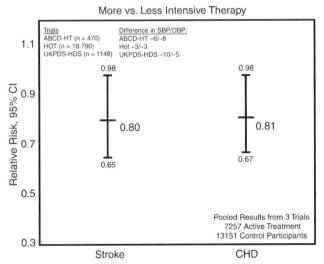

FIGURE 23-8. Relative risks and 95% confidence intervals (CI) for stroke and coronary heart disease in three randomized, controlled trials of more intensive versus less intensive blood pressure reduction. (Adapted from data presented in Blood Pressure Lowering Treatment Trialists' Collaboration: Effects of ACE inhibitors, calcium antagonists, and other blood-pressure-lowering drugs: results of prospectively designed overviews of randomised trials. Lancet 2000;355:1955-1964.)

20% (95% CI: 10% to 63%) and 19% (95% CI: 2% to 33%), respectively (Fig. 23-8). The African-American Study of Kidney Disease and Hypertension (AASK) was designed to investigate whether treatment to a mean arterial BP (MAP) of 92 mm Hg or less would reduce the rate of decline in renal function compared to achievement of a more traditional MAP goal of 102 to 107 mm Hg in approximately 1200 African-American adults with BP-related renal insufficiency.[89,90] An average difference in SBP/DBP during follow-up of 13/7 mm Hg was noted. Proteinuria was significantly less in those assigned to the lower BP, but there was no significant difference in renal function or occurrence of clinical events.

Management of Hypertension in Special Populations

Special considerations are warranted in the management of hypertension in women, minorities, older persons, and those with comorbidity. ACE inhibitors and ARBs should be used with caution in women of childbearing age and specifically should be avoided during pregnancy because of their potential to induce fetal defects. Diuretics and CCBs are more effective than beta blockers, ACE inhibitors, or ARBs in lowering BP in African-Americans, and ACE inhibitor-induced angioedema, albeit rare, is two to four times more common in African-Americans compared to whites. Diuretics and CCBs are highly effective in lowering BP and preventing BP-related CVD complications in older persons with hypertension. Initial drug doses should be lower in older persons than in younger persons, but standard doses and multiple drugs usually are required to obtain the desired level of BP during long-term therapy. Only limited trial experience is available for treatment of the very old, but results to date suggest BP lowering in those 80 years or older reduces the risk of CVD, especially stroke. The presence of comorbidity is often a factor in choice of antihypertensive drug class. For instance, beta blockers or CCBs should normally be a part of the regimen in patients with hypertension and stable angina pectoris. Beta blockers and ACE inhibitors have been shown to be beneficial in myocardial infarction survivors. In patients with hypertension and heart failure, diuretics are particularly effective but ACE inhibitors and beta blockers are indicated in those with ventricular dysfunction and/or end-stage heart failure. A variety of antihypertensive drugs, including diuretics, have been demonstrated to be beneficial in patients with hypertension and diabetes. ACE inhibitors and ARBs are effective in reducing albuminuria and progression of renal disease in patients with diabetic nephropathy, but multidrug combinations involving these agents and diuretics typically are required to normalize BP. When a patient's glomerular filtration rate falls below 30 ml/min/m^2, corresponding to a serum creatinine of 2.5 to 3.0 mg/mL, loop diuretics should be used in place of thiazide-type agents.

Guidelines for Management of Hypertension

A variety of national and international organizations, including government agencies and professional societies, have published guidelines for prevention, detection, evaluation, and treatment of hypertension. The best known and most widely used are the National Heart, Lung, and Blood Institute's Reports of the Joint National Committee for Prevention, Detection, Evaluation and Treatment of High Blood Pressure (JNC reports) and the World Health Organization/International Society of Hypertension's Guidelines for Management of Hypertension (WHO/ISH reports).[46,91] The most recent 2003 JNC VII and 1999 WHO/ISH reports provide similar guidance, with the exception that diuretics are recommended as first-line drugs for patients with uncomplicated hypertension in the JNC VII report, whereas a broad array of drug classes are recommended for the same purpose in the WHO/ISH report.

SUMMARY

A substantial body of experience supports the importance of high BP as a risk factor for vascular damage to the heart, brain, kidney, and other organs. Likewise, clinical trials have repeatedly demonstrated the wisdom of antihypertensive drug therapy in patients with hypertension. Pooling of information from trials that have already published their results indicates that approximately 5 years of first-step therapy with a diuretic or a beta blocker virtually eliminates the BP-related risk of stroke and substantially reduces the corresponding BP-related risk of CHD. Pooling of clinical trial experience also suggests that treatment with ACE inhibitors or a CCB results in a substantial reduction in the risk of major CVD events. ALLHAT provides strong evidence in favor of diuretics as first-step therapy in antihypertensive drug therapy and suggests caution should be exercised in using an alpha₁-receptor blocker unless there is an additional specific indication, such as prostatic hypertrophy, for its use. More intensive BP reduction seems to lead to a greater decline in CVD risk, but this conclusion is based on analyses with limited statistical power. Primary prevention of hypertension is a logical extension of efforts aimed at detection and treatment of hypertension.[11] An increasing body of evidence from clinical trials has demonstrated the efficacy of hypertension prevention interventions aimed at modifications in diet and physical activity.[92] Although difficult to implement in practice, interventions aimed at primary prevention of hypertension have great potential for reducing the burden of illness resulting from high BP and provide an opportunity to reduce the costly cycle of managing hypertension and its complications.

REFERENCES

1. Whelton PK, He J, Klag MJ: Blood pressure in westernized populations. In Swales JD (ed). Textbook of Hypertension. Oxford, Blackwell Scientific Publications, Ltd., 1994, pp 11–21.
2. Poulter NR, Sever PS: Low blood pressure populations and the impact of rural-urban migration. In Swales JD (ed). Textbook of Hypertension. Oxford, Blackwell Scientific Publications, Ltd., 1994, pp 22–36.
3. He J, Klag MJ, Whelton PK, et al: Migration, blood pressure pattern, and hypertension. Am J Epidemiol 1991; 134:1085–1101.
4. Poulter NR, Khaw KT, Hopwood BEC, et al: The Kenyan Luo migration study: Observations on the initiation of a rise in blood pressure. Br Med J 1990; 300:967–972.
5. Burt V, Whelton PK, Roccella E, et al: Prevalence of hypertension in the US adult population: Results from the Third National Health and Nutrition Examination Survey, 1988–91. Hypertension 1995; 25:305–313.
6. Whelton PK: Epidemiology of hypertension. Lancet 1994; 344:101–106.
7. Stamler J, Stamler R, Neaton JD: Blood pressure, systolic and diastolic, and cardiovascular risks: U.S. population data. Arch Intern Med 1993; 153:598–615.
8. MacMahon S, Peto R, Cutler J, et al: Blood pressure, stroke, and coronary heart disease. I. Prolonged differences in blood pressure. prospective observational studies corrected for the regression dilution bias. Lancet 1990; 335:765–774.
9. Whelton PK, Perneger TV, He J, et al: The role of blood pressure as a risk factor for renal disease: A review of the epidemiologic evidence. J Human Hypertens 1996; 10:683–689.
10. Klag MJ, Whelton PK, Randall BL, et al: A prospective study of blood pressure and incidence of end-stage renal disease in 332,544 men. N Engl J Med 1996; 334:13–18.
11. Working Group on Primary Prevention of Hypertension: Report of the National High Blood Pressure Education Program Working Group on Primary Prevention of Hypertension. Arch Intern Med 1993; 153:186–208.
12. Harrington M, Kincaid-Smith P, McMichael J: Results of treatment of malignant hypertension. Br Med J 1959; 2:969–989.
13. Mohler ER, Freis ED: Five-year survival of patients with malignant hypertension treated with antihypertensive agents. Am Heart J 1960; 60:329–335.
14. Bjork S, Sannerstedt R, Falkheden T, et al: The effect of active drug treatment in severe antihypertensive disease. Acta Med Scand 1961; 169:673–689.
15. Hamilton M, Thompson EW, Wisniewski TKM: The role of blood pressure control in preventing complications of hypertension. Lancet 1964; 1:235–238.
16. Wolff FW, Lindeman RD: Effects of treatment in hypertension: Results of a controlled study. J Chron Dis 1966; 19:227–240.
17. Veterans Administration Cooperative Study Group on Antihypertensive Agents: Effects of treatment on morbidity in hypertension: Results in patients with diastolic blood pressure averaging 115 through 129 mm Hg. JAMA 1967; 202:1028–1034.
18. Veterans Administration Cooperative Study Group on Antihypertensive Agents: Effects of treatment on morbidity in hypertension: II. Results in patients with diastolic blood pressure averaging 90 through 114 mm Hg. JAMA 1970; 213:1143–1152.
19. Carter AB: Hypotensive therapy in stroke survivors. Lancet 1970; 1:485–489.
20. Barraclough M, Bainton D, Joy MD, et al: Control of moderately raised blood pressure: Report of a co-operative randomized controlled trial. BMJ 1973; 3:434–436.
21. Hypertension-Stroke Cooperative Study Group: Effect of antihypertensive treatment on stroke recurrence. JAMA 1974; 229:409–418.
22. US Public Health Service Hospitals Cooperative Study Group: Treatment of mild hypertension: Results of a ten-year intervention trial. Circ Res 1977; 40:I-98-I-105.
23. Veterans Administration National Heart, Lung, and Blood Institute Study Group for Cooperative Studies on Antihypertensive Therapy: Mild Hypertension (Perry HM): Treatment of mild hypertension: Preliminary results of a two-year feasibility trial. Circ Res 1977; 40(Suppl 1):180–187.
24. Veterans Administration National Heart, Lung, and Blood Institute Study Group for Evaluating Treatment in Mild Hypertension: Evaluation of drug treatment in mild hypertension: VA-NHLBI Feasibility Trial. Ann NY Acad Sci 1978; 304:267–288.
25. Hypertension Detection and Follow-up Program Cooperative Group: Five-year findings of the hypertension detection and follow-up program: I. Reduction in mortality of persons with high blood pressure, including mild hypertension. JAMA 1979; 242:2562–2571.
26. Hypertension Detection and Follow-up Program Cooperative Group: Five-year findings of the hypertension detection and follow-up program. II. Mortality by race-sex and age. JAMA 1979; 242:2572–2577.
27. Helgeland A: Treatment of mild hypertension: A five-year controlled drug trial. The Oslo Study. Am J Med 1980; 69:725–732.

28. Leren P, Helgeland A: Oslo Hypertension Study. Drugs 1986; 31(Suppl 1):41–45.
29. Australian National Blood Pressure Study Management Committee: The Australian therapeutic trial in mild hypertension. Lancet 1980; i:1261–1267.
30. Medical Research Council Working Party: MRC trial of treatment of mild hypertension: principal results. Br Med J 1985; 291:97–104.
31. Amery A, Birkenhager W, Brixko P, et al: Mortality and morbidity results from the European working party on high blood pressure in the elderly trial. Lancet 1985; i:1349–1354.
32. Cooper J, Warrender TS: Randomized trial of treatment of hypertension in elderly patients in primary care. Br Med J 1986; 293: 1145–1151.
33. SHEP Cooperative Research Group: Prevention of stroke by antihypertensive drug treatment in older persons with isolated systolic hypertension: Final results of the Systolic Hypertension in the Elderly Program (SHEP). JAMA 1991; 265:3255–3264.
34. Dahlof B, Lindholm LH, Hansson L, et al: Morbidity and mortality in the Swedish Trial in Old Patients with Hypertension (STOP-Hypertension). Lancet 1991; 338:1281–1285.
35. MRC Working Party: Medical research council trial of treatment of hypertension in older adults: principal results. BMJ 1992; 304: 405–412.
36. Cutler JA, MacMahon SW, Furberg CD: Controlled clinical trials of drug treatment for hypertension: A review. Hypertension 1989; 13(suppl I):I-36-I-44.
37. Collins R, Peto R, MacMahon SW, et al: Blood pressure, stroke, and CHD: II. Short-term reductions in blood pressure: Overview of randomized drug trials in their epidemiological context. Lancet 1990; 335:827–838.
38. Hebert PR, Moser M, Mayer J, et al: Recent evidence on drug therapy of mild to moderate hypertension and decreased risk of CHD. Arch Intern Med 1993; 153:578–581.
39. Collins R, MacMahon S: Blood pressure, antihypertensive drug treatment and the risks of stroke and of CHD. Br Med Bull 1994; 50:272–298.
40. Lipid Research Clinics Program: The Lipid Research Clinics Coronary Primary Prevention Trial results: I. Reduction in incidence of CHD. JAMA 1984; 251:351–364.
41. Frick MH, Elo O, Haapa K, et al: Helsinki Heart Study: Primary-prevention trial with gemfibrozil in middle-aged men with dyslipidemia: Safety of treatment, changes in risk factors, and incidence of CHD. N Engl J Med 1987; 317:1237–1245.
42. Multiple Risk Factor Intervention Trial Research Group: Mortality rates after 10.5 years for participants in the Multiple Risk Factor Intervention Trial: Findings related to a priori hypotheses of the trial. JAMA 1990; 263:1795–1801.
43. IPPPSH Collaborative Group: Cardiovascular risk and risk factors in a randomized trial of treatment based on the beta-blocker oxprenolol: The International Prospective Primary Prevention Study in Hypertension (IPPPSH). J Hypertens 1985; 3:379–392.
44. Wilhelmsen L, Berglund G, Elmfeldt D, et al: Beta-blockers versus diuretics in hypertensive men: Main results from the HAPPHY trial. J Hypertens 1987; 5:561–572.
45. The seventh in JAMA report of the Joint National Committee on Prevention, Detection, Evaluation, and Treatment of High Blood Pressure. Arch Intern Med 1997; 157:2413–2446.
46. Kaplan NM, Gifford RW: Choice of initial therapy for hypertension. JAMA 1996; 275:1577–1580.
47. Dzau VJ: Tissue angiotensin and pathobiology of vascular disease: A unifying hypothesis. Hypertension 2001; 37:1047–1052.
48. Manolio TA, Cutler JA, Furberg CD, et al: Trends in pharmacologic management of hypertension in the United States. Arch Intern Med 1995; 155:829–837.
49. Blood Pressure Lowering Treatment Trialists' Collaboration: Effects of ACE inhibitors, calcium antagonists, and other blood-pressure-lowering drugs: Results of prospectively designed overviews of randomised trials. Lancet 2000; 355:1955–1964.
50. Pahor M, Psaty BM, Alderman MH, et al: Health outcomes associated with calcium antagonists compared with other first-line antihypertensive therapies: A meta-analysis of randomised controlled trials. Lancet 2000; 355:1949–1954.
51. Staessen JA, Wang J-G, Thijs L: Cardiovascular protection and blood pressure reduction: A meta-analysis. Lancet 2001; 358:1305–1315.
52. HOPE (Heart Outcomes Prevention Evaluation) Study Investigators: Effects of an angiotensin-converting-enzyme-inhibitor, ramipril, on cardiovascular events in high-risk patients. N Engl J Med 2000; 342:145–153.
53. MacMahon S, Sharpe N, Gamble G, et al: Randomized, placebo-controlled trial of an angiotensin-converting enzyme inhibitor, ramipril, in patients with coronary or other occlusive arterial disease. J Am Coll Cardiol 2000; 36:438–443.
54. Cashin-Hemphill L, Holmvang G, Chan R, et al: Angiotensin converting enzyme inhibition as antiatherosclerotic therapy: No answer yet. Am J Cardiol 1999; 83:43–47.
55. Teo KK, Burton JR, Buller CE, et al: Long-term effects of cholesterol lowering and angiotensin-converting enzyme inhibition on coronary atherosclerosis: The Simvastatin/Enalapril Coronary Atherosclerosis Trial (SCAT). Circulation 2000; 102:1748–1754.
56. Pitt B, Byington RP, Furberg CD, et al: Effect of amlodipine on the progression of atherosclerosis and the occurrence of clinical events: PREVENT Investigators. Circulation 2000; 102:1503–1510.
57. Staessen JA, Fagard R, Thijs L, et al: Randomized double-blind comparison of placebo and active treatment for older patients with isolated systolic hypertension: The Systolic Hypertension in Europe (Syst-Eur) Trial Investigators. Lancet 1997; 350:757–764.
58. Hansson L, Lindholm LH, Niskanen L, et al: Effect of angiotensin-converting-enzyme inhibition compared with conventional therapy on cardiovascular morbidity and mortality in hypertension: The Captopril Prevention Project (CAPPP) randomised trial. Lancet 1999; 353:611–616.
59. Hansson L, Lindholm LH, Ekbom T, et al: Randomised trial of old and new antihypertensive drugs in elderly patients: Cardiovascular mortality and morbidity: The Swedish Trial in Old Patients with Hypertension-2 study. Lancet 1999; 354:1751–1756.
60. UK Prospective Diabetes Study Group: Efficacy of atenolol and captopril in reducing risk of macrovascular and microvascular complications in type two diabetes: UKPDS 39. BMJ 1998; 317:713–720.
61. Brown MJ, Palmer CR, Castaigne A, et al: Morbidity and mortality in patients randomised to double-blind treatment with a long-acting calcium-channel blocker or diuretic in the International Nifedipine GITS study: Intervention as a Goal in Hypertension Treatment (INSIGHT). Lancet 2000; 356:366–372.
62. National Intervention Cooperative Study in Elderly Hypertensives Study Group: Randomized double-blind comparison of a calcium antagonist and a diuretic in elderly hypertensives. Hypertension 1999; 34:1129–1133.
63. Hansson L, Hedner T, Lund-Johansen P, et al: Randomised trial of effects of calcium antagonists compared with diuretics and beta-blockers on cardiovascular morbidity and mortality in hypertension: The Nordic Diltiazem (NORDIL) study. Lancet 2000; 356:359–365.
64. Agabiti Rosei E, Dal Palu C, Leonetti G, et al: Clinical results of the Verapamil in Hypertension and Atherosclerosis Study. J Hypertens 1997; 15:1337–1344.
65. Zanchetti A, Rosei EA, Dal Palu C, et al: The Verapamil in Hypertension and Atherosclerosis Study (VHAS): results of long-term randomized treatment with either verapamil or chlorthalidone on carotid intima-media thickness. J Hypertens 1998; 16:1667–1676.
66. Estacio RO, Jeffers BW, Hiatt WR, et al: The effect of nisoldipine as compared with enalapril on cardiovascular outcomes in patients with non-insulin dependent diabetes and hypertension. N Engl J Med 1998; 338:645–652.
67. Hansson L, Zanchetti A, Carruthers SG, et al: Effects of intensive blood-pressure lowering and low-dose aspirin in patients with hypertension: Principal results of the Hypertension Optimal Treatment (HOT) randomized trial. HOT Study Group. Lancet 1988; 351:1755–1762.
68. UK Prospective Diabetes Study Group: Tight blood pressure control and risk of macrovascular and microvascular complications in type-2 diabetes. UKPDS 37. BMJ 1998; 317:703–713.
69. PROGRESS Collaborative Group: Randomised trial of a perindopril-based blood-pressure-lowering regimen among 6105 individuals with previous stroke or transient ischemic attack. Lancet 2001; 358:1033–1041.
70. Dahlof B, Devereux RB, Kjeldsen SE, et al: Cardiovascular morbidity and mortality in the Losartan Intervention For Endpoint reduction in hypertension study (LIFE): a randomised trial against atenolol. Lancet 2002; 359:995–1003.
71. Stumpe KO, Ludwig M, Heagerty AM, et al: Vascular wall thickness in hypertension: The perindopril regression of vascular thickening European Community trial (PROTECT). Am J Cardiol 1995; 76: 50E–54E.

72. Casiglia E, Spolaore P, Mazza A, et al: Effect of two different thera-peutic approaches on total and cardiovascular mortality in a car-diovascular study in the elderly (CASTEL). Jpn Heart J 1994; 35:270:713-724.

73. Tatti P, Pahor M, Byington RP, et al: Outcome results of the Fosino-pril versus Amlodipine Cardiovascular Events randomized Trial (FACET) in patients with hypertension and NIDDM. Diabetes Care 1998; 21:597-560.

74. Borhani NO, Mercuri M, Borhani PA, et al: Final outcome results of the Multicenter Isradipine Diuretic Atherosclerosis Study (MIDAS): A randomized controlled trial. JAMA 1996; 276:785-791.

75. The ALLHAT Officers and Coordinators for the ALLHAT Collabora-tive Research Group: Major cardiovascular events in hypertensive patients randomized to doxazosin vs chlorthalidone: The Antihy-pertensive and Lipid-Lowering Treatment to Prevent Heart Attack Trial (ALLHAT). JAMA 2000; 283:1967-1975.

76. He J, Whelton PK: Selection of initial antihypertensive drug ther-apy. Lancet 2000; 356:1942-1943.

77. Davis BR, Cutler JA, Gordon DJ, et al: Rationale and design for the Antihypertensive and Lipid Lowering Treatment to Prevent Heart Attack Trial (ALLHAT). Am J Hypertens 1996; 9:342-360.

78. The ALLHAT Officers and Coordinators for the ALLHAT Investiga-tive Research Group: Major outcomes in high-risk hypertensive patients randomized to angiotensin-converting enzyme inhibitor or calcium channel blocker vs diuretic: The Antihypertensive and Lipid Lowering Treatment to Prevent Heart Attack Trial (ALLHAT). JAMA 2002; 288:2981-2997.

79. Wing LMH, Reid CM, Ryan P, et al: A comparison of outcomes with angiotensin-converting-enzyme inhibitors and diuretics for hyper-tension in the elderly. N Engl J Med 2003; 348:583-592.

80. Black HR, Elliott WJ, Grandits G, et al: Principal results of the con-trolled onset verapamil investigation of cardiovascular end points (CONVINCE) trial. JAMA 2003; 289:2073-2082.

81. Blood Pressure Lowering Treatment Trialists' Collaboration: Effects of different blood-pressure-lowering regimens in cardiovascular events: Results of prospectively-designed overviews of randomised trials. Lancet 2003; 362:1527-1535.

82. Psaty BM, Lumley T, Furberg CD, et al: Health outcomes associated with various antihypertensive therapies used as first-line agents: A network meta-analysis. JAMA 2003; 2534-2544.

83. Sever PS, Dahlof B, Poulter NR, et al: Rationale, design, methods and baseline demography of participants of the Anglo-Scandinavian Cardiac Outcomes Trial. ASCOT investigators. J Hypertens 2001; 19: 1139-1147.

84. Frohlich ED: Reappearance of the J-shaped curve. Hypertension 1999; 34:1179-1180.

85. Coresh J, Whelton PK, Mead LA, et al: Increased cardiovascular disease risk in treated hypertensive men. J Hypertens 1994; 12 (Suppl 3):S73.

86. Lindholm L, Ejlertsson G, Scherstein B: High risk of cerebro-cardiovascular morbidity in well treated male hypertensives: A retrospective study of 40-59-year-old hypertensives in a Swedish primary care district. Acta Med Scand 1984; 216:251-259.

87. Samuelsson O: Hypertension in middle-aged men: management, morbidity and prognostic factors during long-term hypertensive care. Acta Med Scand 1985; 218(Suppl 702):1-79.

88. Isles CG, Walker LM, Beevers DG, et al: Mortality in patients of the Glasgow Blood Pressure Clinic. J Hypertens 1986; 4:141-156.

89. Wright JT, Bakris GL, Green T, et al: Effect of blood pressure lower-ing and antihypertensive drug class on progression of hyperten-sive kidney disease: Results from the AASK trial. JAMA 2002; 288:2421-2431.

90. Agodoa LY, Appel LJ, Bakris GL, et al: Effect of ramipril vs amlodip-ine on renal outcomes in hypertensive nephrosclerosis: A random-ized controlled trial. JAMA 2001; 285:2719-2728.

91. Chalmers J, MacMahon S, Mancia G, et al: 1999 World Health Orga-nization—International Society of Hypertension Guidelines for the management of hypertension. Guidelines sub-committee of the World Health Organization. Clinical & Experimental Hyperten-sion 1999; 21:1009-1060.

92. Whelton PK, He J, Appel LJ, et al: Primary prevention of hypertension: Clinical and public health advisory from the National High Blood Pressure Education Program. JAMA 2002; 288:1882-1888.

■ ■ ■ c h a p t e r **24**

Smoking Cessation

Paul B. Yu
Richard C. Pasternak
Nancy A. Rigotti

Tobacco smoking remains the leading preventable cause of death in the United States.[1-3] Of the more than 2 million U.S. deaths annually from 1995 to 1999, 442,398, or more than 1 in 5, were attributable to cigarette smoking, with an estimated economic impact of $157 billion in annual health-related economic losses.[3] Ischemic heart disease was the cause of 33% of these smoking-related deaths, with all cardiovascular diseases accounting for 42% of these deaths and with 8% of the total being attributed to second-hand smoke exposure. Smoking prevalence has declined dramatically since its peak in 1965, at which time 40% of adults (50% of men and 32% of women) smoked.[2,4] Nonetheless, in 2000, approximately 23% of adult Americans (26% of men and 21% of women) smoked cigarettes.[5] Nearly 90% of them began to smoke before the age of 20.[5,6] In the United States, smoking prevalence is highest among young adults (aged 18–24 years) and among individuals with less education and lower socioeconomic status.[2,5]

This chapter begins with a review of the pathophysiologic effects of tobacco use, establishing the biologic plausibility of a relationship to heart disease. It then summarizes the compelling epidemiologic evidence of a relationship between tobacco use and cardiovascular disease, particularly coronary heart disease (CHD), and reviews the evidence that smoking cessation prevents cardiovascular morbidity and mortality. The strength, abundance, and consistency of this evidence, derived almost entirely from observational studies, is such that large-scale randomized trials are not needed to demonstrate a causal relationship between tobacco smoking and cardiovascular disease.

PATHOPHYSIOLOGY

Tobacco smoking influences a vast array of physiologic and biochemical factors that act together to inflict a considerable burden on the cardiovascular system. The physiologic effects of tobacco smoke and its components on the cardiovascular system have been studied extensively, providing a number of mechanisms to account for the epidemiologic associations. Acutely, tobacco smoking alters coronary and peripheral vascular tone and cardiac output, depresses the oxygen-carrying capacity of blood, and affects the thrombotic and rheologic state of the vascular system.[7] Chronically, smoking appears to inflict oxidant injury and stress, cause endothelial cell injury and dysfunction, and generally promote atherosclerosis. Many studies have examined the role of nicotine, but it is important to note that a multitude of other cardiotoxic components of tobacco smoke exist, including carbon monoxide, oxidant and free radical gases, and polycyclic aromatic compounds, which may be as or more important in the pathogenesis of cardiac disease.[7,8]

Systemic Effects

Smoking cigarettes, both acutely and chronically, unfavorably alters the critical balance between myocardial oxygen supply and demand. The smoke of one cigarette rapidly increases blood pressure and heart rate,[9,10] with corresponding increases in sympathetic outflow and plasma levels of norepinephrine.[11] The hemodynamic response is directly related to the increase in plasma nicotine concentration,[12] suggesting that nicotine, a potent adrenergic agonist,[13] is a primary mediator of the hemodynamic response. Either as a consequence of these hemodynamic changes, or as a result of the nicotine-related increase in plasma catecholamines, or both, smoking decreases the threshold for cardiac arrhythmias and has been shown to be associated with a higher incidence of sudden cardiac arrest.[14,15] By this mechanism and by mismatches in demand and supply, the acute hemodynamic response associated with smoking may be a major component of the link between smoking and acute cardiovascular events. The effects are not limited to these transient ones, however, because long-term tobacco use increases average heart rate and blood pressure throughout the day.[16,17]

Other components of cigarette smoke may also have important systemic effects. Carbon monoxide, which composes 2% to 6% of cigarette smoke, binds to hemoglobin, reducing oxygen-carrying capacity among smokers. A direct dose-response relationship has been demonstrated between carbon monoxide concentrations and ischemic threshold,[18,19] and increased carboxyhemoglobin levels are associated with impaired ventricular function and ventricular arrhythmias.[20,21] Cigarette smoke contains a multitude of free radicals and oxidant molecules, which may impair the body's antioxidant capacity by depleting glutathione. Systemic oxidant stress likely promotes atherosclerosis by oxidation of LDL,[22] as well as by oxidative damage directly to the endothelium. Oxidative stress from smoking may exert chronic effects on microvascular endothelial function. Consistent with this idea, smoking is correlated with a decrease in the circulating levels of endogenous antioxidants vitamins C and E.[23] Large doses of intravenous vitamin C can reverse the impairment of coronary flow reserve seen in long-term smokers versus normal controls as measured by positron emission tomography scan measurement of coronary flow.[24] However, the use of typical doses of oral antioxidants for cardiovascular risk reduction in smokers has failed to demonstrate benefit in large clinical trials.[25]

Vascular Effects

The acute and chronic effects of cigarette smoking on the peripheral and coronary vasculature have been well studied. In the presence of coronary and peripheral atherosclerosis, the normal vascular dilating capacity is impaired and vasoconstrictive responses are potentiated. Acutely, a decrease in the distensibility of both carotid and brachial arteries occurs following exposure to cigarette smoke,[26] and the smoke of a single cigarette increases coronary vascular resistance and decreases coronary flow velocity.[27] In susceptible individuals, smoke from a single cigarette is capable of producing a sudden marked epicardial coronary vasoconstriction.[27] The vasoactive effects of smoking may trigger plaque rupture in patients with underlying substrate and produce acute coronary events. Further evidence of the direct vascular effect of smoking comes from the observation that smoking directly exacerbates vasospastic angina in patients without obstructive epicardial coronary artery lesions[28] and that "silent" ischemia occurs among cigarette smokers in association with demonstrable regional myocardial perfusion abnormalities.[29] A distinction is made between endothelial-dependent (e.g., nitric oxide–mediated) vasoactive effects and endothelial-independent (e.g., vascular smooth muscle) effects. Chronically, long-term smokers have evidence of impaired endothelially mediated vasodilator function but preserved responses at the smooth-muscle level, reflecting endothelial dysfunction that demonstrably impairs myocardial blood flow regulation.[30]

The direct effects of smoking on vascular endothelium is seen in several circumstances. Endothelial-dependent flow-mediated vascular forearm dilation is impaired in smokers.[31] Abnormalities in endothelium-derived relaxing factor (nitric oxide) have been detected in smokers,[32,33] and coronary vasodilation is abnormal in smokers.[34,35] Cigarette smoking appears to perturb endothelial function in many ways beyond the regulation of vasomotor tone (e.g., its role in regulating thrombosis and thrombolysis). Chronically, tobacco accelerates the progression of atherosclerotic disease, probably as a result of the manifold metabolic effects as well as toxicity to the endothelium. This relationship was demonstrated prospectively in a large cohort study (Atherosclerosis Risk in Communities [ARIC]) in which the use of tobacco was associated with increased intimal-medial thickness measured by carotid ultrasound.[36]

Metabolic Effects

Smoking induces a small to moderate change in serum lipids.[37] In general, the most marked change is in triglyceride level (approximate increase of 9%), with lesser changes in high-density lipoprotein (HDL) cholesterol (6% decrease) and total cholesterol (3% increase). Although smoking does not alter low-density lipoprotein (LDL) cholesterol levels directly, it increases the susceptibility of the LDL molecule to oxidative modification,[38] with damaging consequences in augmenting the response of scavenger cells and local inflammatory and proliferative reactions. The effect of cigarette smoking on lipid peroxidation may be one of its single most important effects in promoting atherosclerosis.[7] Smoking cessation is associated with a modest increase in HDL cholesterol and improvement in both insulin and glucose metabolism.[10,39]

Thrombosis

Acute thrombus formation at the site of a ruptured plaque is responsible for the majority of coronary disease events, whereas chronic thrombotic activity is associated with atherosclerotic progression. Smoking appears to influence both acute and chronic aspects of the thrombotic process. The influence of smoking on the clotting system includes demonstrable changes in the fibrinolytic system, the clotting cascade, and platelet function.[10,40,41] Fibrinogen and factor VII levels are higher in smokers than in nonsmokers, and both gradually normalize with smoking cessation,[10] but fibrinogenemia persists at least through 2 months after smoking cessation after an acute myocardial infarction (MI).[42] Smoking increases the production of platelet-derived growth factor (PDGF) an atherogenic mitogen.[43] Smoking has been shown to increase a number of proaggregatory prostanoids, an effect likely responsible for the observation that smoking as few as two cigarettes can increase platelet activation more than 100-fold.[44] The influence of smoking on clotting function has been shown to be both nicotine dependent and independent,[7,40] and the complexity of the clotting system itself suggests that many different components of cigarette smoke are likely to influence the pathophysiology of clotting. The toxicity of smoking on the endothelium and resulting endothelial dysfunction may also manifest as dysregulation of thrombosis and thrombolysis. Coronary plasminogen activator release is impaired in habitual smokers, particularly those with significant atherosclerotic burden.[45] Atheromatous plaques obtained from smokers after carotid endarectomy demonstrate elevated levels of tissue factor, a procoagulant substance expressed by damaged or activated vascular endothelium, versus those of nonsmokers.[46] These studies clearly support the notion that habitual smoking alters the balance of thrombosis and thrombolysis, at least in part by impairing endothelial regulatory function.

In summary, smoking tobacco influences the cardiovascular system through the interplay of a wide range of pathophysiologic and biochemical factors.[7] Some of these effects, such as increased platelet activation and vascular tone are more likely to be reversible following smoking cessation. Other effects, such as the accellerated development of atherosclerosis, may at best revert to normal only gradually after smoking cessation. Hence, there is a biologic rationale for both an initial rapid decline and a later gradual fall in cardiovascular disease risk among former smokers compared with continuing smokers.

Direct Effects of Nicotine

Nicotine appears to affect adversely several of the systems that contribute to cardiovascular risk, including lipid and glucose metabolism, and perhaps more important, the adrenergic state, vascular tone, and endothelial function.[7,47-49] It is not clear to what extent these effects are cardiotoxic absent the other components of cigarette smoking. For example, relatively little is known about the safety of long-term use of nicotine replacement in smokers who are unable or unwilling to stop nicotine use otherwise. There are isolated reports of instances in which nicotine replacement therapy is associated with adverse cardiac events.[47] While the use of nicotine replacement in individuals who continue to smoke appears to increase cardiac risk, there is presently no clear evidence that nicotine itself, as a replacement therapy, causes cardiac events.[7]

CIGARETTE SMOKING AND CARDIOVASCULAR DISEASE RISK

The epidemiologic evidence supporting a conclusion that cigarette smoking causes cardiovascular disease is overwhelming. Multiple observational epidemiologic studies conducted in many nations have demonstrated a relationship between smoking and various measures of cardiovascular disease morbidity and mortality. The evidence is consistent, the relationship is strong, the relationship is biologically plausible, and a dose-response relationship has been demonstrated between CHD and the duration and intensity of smoking. These facts meet the epidemiologic criteria for establishing causality[2,4,50,51] and have been verified consistently in many populations such that further demonstration is not needed.

The causal relationship of tobacco use to cardiovascular disease and a dose-response effect was first observed among men but has since been amply demonstrated in women.[52] Smoking is a major risk factor for cardiovascular disease in general, including MI, sudden death, stroke, peripheral vascular disease, and aortic aneurysm.[2,42,53-55] Compared with nonsmokers, current smokers have a 70% increased risk of fatal CHD and a twofold to fourfold higher risk of nonfatal CHD and sudden death.[51] There is no safe level of tobacco use. The risk of MI and cardiovascular mortality is increased in individuals who smoke as few as one to four cigarettes daily.[53] Smoking cigarettes with lower tar and nicotine content does not reduce the smoking-related risk of cardiovascular disease.[2]

Cigarette smoking synergizes with the CHD risk factors of hypertension, hyperlipidemia, and diabetes to increase markedly the risk of CHD.[36,52,53,56] Oral contraceptive use is also synergistic with smoking to increase substantially the risk of MI, subarachnoid hemorrhage, and stroke in women.[51,57]

PASSIVE SMOKING AND CARDIOVASCULAR RISK

Nonsmokers can be harmed by chronic environmental exposure to tobacco smoke, also known as *passive smoking*.[58] A substantial body of epidemiologic evidence demonstrates that regular passive smoke exposure increases the risk of lung cancer among nonsmokers. Estimates by the Environmental Protection Agency in 1992 and the Centers for Disease Control and Prevention in 2002 identify passive smoke as a carcinogen responsible for approximately 3000 lung cancer deaths per year in U.S. nonsmokers.[3,58] Evidence exists for a multitude of harmful effects of passive smoke on the developing child. For example, children whose parents smoke have more serious respiratory infections during infancy and childhood and a greater risk of asthma and chronic otitis media than the children of nonsmokers.[59] A substantial body of epidemiologic evidence indicates that passive smoke exposure increases the risk of death from ischemic heart disease among nonsmokers living with smokers by approximately 30%.[60-64] Between 1995 and 1999, it is estimated that passive smoking was responsible for approximately 35,000 cardiovascular deaths per year in the United States[3] based on increased relative risk and wide prevalence of exposure.

Mechanistically, little doubt exists that passive smoking can produce the same pathophysiologic effects as direct smoking. The biologic mechanism is plausible because the doses of exposure attained by passive exposure have similar biologic effects to direct exposure. Two recent studies demonstrated that nominal doses of environmental smoke clearly perturb coronary endothelial and other peripheral arterial endothelial function in nonsmokers.[65,66] With respect to standard endpoints of cardiovascular disease, a meta-analysis of 10 cohort and 8 case-control studies of environmental smoke exposure yielded an increase in relative risk for CHD of approximately 1.25 (95% CI 1.17-1.32), with a significant dose-response relationship to the amount of exposure, with relative risks of 1.23 and 1.31 in nonsmokers exposed to the smoke of 1 to 19 cigarettes and greater than 20 cigarettes each day (P = 0.006).[67] This analysis demonstrated similar relative risks for home and work exposure to environmental smoke, the comparison of which has been the subject of systematic review.[68] The increased cardiac risk incurred from environmental smoke exposure is sufficient to warrant similar attention.

SMOKING CESSATION AND CARDIOVASCULAR DISEASE RISK REDUCTION

Randomized controlled clinical trials provide the highest quality of evidence for demonstrating conclusively that altering a cardiac risk factor reduces cardiovascular disease morbidity or mortality. For example, the value for cardiovascular disease prevention of treating hypertension or reducing hyperlipidemia was widely accepted only after benefits had been demonstrated in randomized clinical trials. In contrast, no randomized controlled trial to assess the effect of smoking cessation as a single intervention to reduce cardiovascular morbidity or mortality or overall mortality has ever been conducted. Nonetheless, an extensive and impressive body of epidemiologic evidence supports a strong conclusion that smoking cessation reduces cardiovascular morbidity and mortality.

The strongest evidence for the benefits of smoking cessation for the primary prevention of cardiovascular disease derives from a series of large prospective observational epidemiologic studies with a decade or more of follow-up. These have compared the frequency of cardiovascular events and mortality among cohorts of current smokers, former smokers, and nonsmokers without cardiovascular disease at study entry (Table 24-1). The largest and longest of these primary prevention studies include cohorts of British physicians (40-year follow-up),[50] U.S. veterans (26-year follow-up),[69] volunteers recruited by the American

TABLE 24-1   COHORT STUDIES OF CORONARY HEART DISEASE RISK AMONG CURRENT AND FORMER SMOKERS

Reference	Population	Follow-up	RELATIVE RISKS COMPARED WITH NEVER SMOKERS*	
			Former smokers	**Current smokers**
Doll and Peto,[144] 1976	British physicians: 34,440 men	20 yr for CHD deaths	Age 30-54: 1.3-1.9 depending on years quit Age 55-64: 1.3-1.9 depending on years quit Age ≥65: 1.0-1.3 depending on years quit	3.5 1.7 1.3
Doll et al,[145] 1980	British physicians: 6194 women	22 yr for CHD deaths	0.91	1.0-2.2 depending on amount smoked
Doll et al,[50] 1994	British physicians: 34,439 men	40 yr for CHD deaths	1.2	1.6
Hammond and Horn,[146] 1958	187,783 men aged 50-60	44 mo for CHD deaths	Previously ≥1 ppd Quit <1 yr: 3.00 1-10 yr: 2.06 >10 yr: 1.60	2.20
Hammond and Garfinkel,[147] 1969	ACS CPS-I: 358,534 men free of diagnosed CHD	6 year for CHD mortality	Previously ≥1 ppd Quit <1 yr: 1.61 1-4 yr: 1.51 5-9 yr: 1.16 10-14 yr: 1.25 ≥15 yr: 1.05	2.55
Burns et al,[71] 1997	ACS CPS-I: 1,051,042 men and women aged ≥30	12 yr for CHD mortality	Years Quit Males Females 2-4 2.66 2.23 5-9 1.64 1.53 0-14 1.37 0.98 15-19 1.13 0.84 20-24 0.99 0.88 25-29 0.96 0.96	Males 1.85 Females 1.68
Thun et al,[70] 1997	ACS CPS-I and CPS-II men and women aged >30 yr CPS-I: 786,387 CPS-II: 711,363	6 yr for CHD mortality		Males CPS-I: 1.7 (1.6-1.8) CPS-II: 1.9 (1.8-2.0) Females CPS-I: 1.4 (1.3-1.5) CPS-II: 1.8 (1.7-2.0)
Kahn,[148] 1966; Rogot and Murray,[149] 1980	U.S. veterans: 248,046 men	16 yr for cardiovascular deaths	Overall: 1.15 <5 yr: 1.40 5-9 yr: 1.40 10-14 yr: 1.30 15-19 yr: 1.20 ≥20 yr: 1.00	1.58
Hrubec and McLaughlin,[69] 1997	U.S. veterans: 248,046 men	26 yr for CHD deaths	Overall: 1.2 (1.2-1.2) <5 yr: 1.7 (1.5-1.9) 5-9 yr: 1.5 (1.4-1.6) 10-19 yr: 1.4 (1.3-1.4) 20-29 yr: 1.2 (1.1-1.2) 30-39 yr: 1.1 (1.0-1.1) ≥40 yr: 1.0 (1.0-1.1)	

TABLE 24-1 COHORT STUDIES OF CORONARY HEART DISEASE RISK AMONG CURRENT AND FORMER SMOKERS—cont'd

Reference	Population	Follow-up	RELATIVE RISKS COMPARED WITH NEVER SMOKERS* Former smokers	Current smokers
Doyle et al,[150] 1962	Framingham and Albany cohorts of 4120 healthy men aged 30-62 yr	10 yr (Framingham) 8 yr (Albany) MI and CHD deaths	1.1 (0.5-2.2)	2.0-3.0 depending on amount smoked
Rosenman et al,[151] 1975	3154 healthy California men aged 39-59 yr	8-9 yr for fatal and nonfatal CHD	Aged 39-40 yr: 1.9 Aged 50-59 yr: 1.1	2.5
Cederlof et al,[74] 1975	51,911 Swedish men aged 18-69 yr	10 yr	Quit 1-9 yr: 1.5 Quit ≥10 yr: 1.0	1.7
Fuller et al,[56] 1983	Whitehall civil servants: 18,403 men aged 40-64 yr	10 yr for CHD deaths	Normoglycemic: 1.3 Glucose intolerant: 0.7 Diabetics: 3.8	2.5 1.5 2.9
Friedman et al,[152] 1981	25,917 Kaiser-Permanente subscribers in the San Francisco area aged 20-79 yr	4 yr for CHD deaths	0.9	1.6
Friedman et al,[75] 1997	60,838 Kaiser Permanente subscribers in San Francisco area, aged ≥35 yr	6.1 yr for CHD deaths	Years Quit Males Females 2-20 1.3 1.4 >20 1.0 1.1	<20 cigarettes/ day: 1.4 ≥20 cigarettes/ day: males, 2.0; females, 2.2
Keys,[73] 1980	Seven-Countries Study of 12,096 men free of CHD	10 yr for CHD deaths	2.3 (Northern Europe) 0.8 (Italy, Greece, Yugoslavia) 0.7 (United States)	2.4-4.5 depending on amount 0.7-1.8 depending on amount 1.6-3.0 depending on amount
Floderus et al,[153] 1988	10,495 Swedish twins aged 36-75 yr	21 yr for CHD deaths	Men: 1.0 (0.8-1.1) Women: 0.6 (0.4-1.0)	1.4-1.8 depending on amount smoked
Netterstrom and Juel,[154] 1988	2465 Danish bus drivers	7.75 yr for MI and CHD death	3.2 (0.4-25.6)	5.0 (0.7-6.0)
Kawachi et al,[55,60] 1993, 1997	Nurses' Health Study: 121,700 U.S. women aged 30-55 yr	12 yr for cardiovascular mortality	1.6 (1.2-21)	3.7 (2.9-4.9)
Al-Delaimy et al,[52] 2002	Nurses' Health Study: 121,700 U.S. women aged 30-55 yr	20 yr for cardiovascular mortality	1.21 (0.97-1.51) DM FS compared to DM NS: 1.01 (0.73-1.38)	1.66 (1.10-2.52) [1-14 cigarettes/day] 2.68 (2.07-3.48) [>15 cigarettes/day] DM smokers compared with DM NS: 7.67 (5.88-10.01)
Tervahauta et al,[89] 1995	647 Finnish men aged 65-84 yr; 171 with CHD at baseline, 476 without CHD	5 yr for fatal MI	1.3 (0.4-3.9) with CHD 1.1 (0.4-2.7) without CHD	>9 cigarettes/day 6.0 (1.4-25.0) with CHD 1.6 (0.4-5.7) without CHD
Qiao et al,[79] 2000	1711 Finnish men aged 40-60 yr	35 yr	1.13 (0.93-1.36) all cause 1.39 (1.00-1.94) CHD	1.62 (1.40-1.88) 1.63 (1.24-2.13)
Gupta et al,[77] 1993	524 Indian men and women; 173 with CHD, 351 without CHD; 299 NS, 173 FS, 52 smokers	6-11 yr		1.28 (1.01-1.09)†
Lam et al,[78] 2002	1268 Chinese men >60 yr	12 yr	1.11 (0.51-2.39)	2.50 (1.18-5.30) <14 cigarettes/day: 1.52 (0.58-4.02) 15-24 cigarettes/day: 2.66 (1.18-5.99) >25 cigarettes/day: 1.85 (0.68-5.06) >40 yr: 3.36 (1.46-7.76)

Modified from Cigarette smoking among adults—United States, 2000. MMWR Morb Mortal Wkly Rep 2002; 51(29):642–645.
CHD, coronary heart disease; ppd, packs/day; ACS CPS-I and II, American Cancer Society Prevention Studies I and II; HIP, health insurance plan; MI, myocardial infarction; DM, diabetes mellitus; NS, nonsmoker; FS, former smoker.
*95% confidence intervals shown in parentheses when available.
†After Cox proportional hazards model adjustment for hypertension, diabetes, age, cholesterol, congestive heart failure, and coronary disease status.

Cancer Society (12-year follow-up),[70-72] men in seven countries (10-year follow-up),[73] British civil servants (10-year follow-up),[56] Swedish twin pairs (10-year follow-up),[74] and Northern California Kaiser Permanente subscribers (6-year follow-up).[75] Early cohorts consisted of middle-aged white men, but substantial numbers of women have since been the subject of cohort studies such as the Nurses' Health Study (12 and 20 years of follow-up).[52,55,76] The results from British and American cohorts appear to be generalizable to other countries, including nonwhite populations in India and China[77-79] and tra-

ditionally lower-risk Mediterranean populations.[80] Case-control studies comparing the smoking history of patients with and without cardiovascular disease provide further support for a cardiovascular benefit of smoking cessation (Table 24-2). A third line of evidence derives from randomized controlled trials comparing the effect of a multiple risk-factor intervention including smoking cessation with usual care. These trials have the advantage of randomized allocation of treatment, but the presence of the other interventions complicates the interpretation of the independent effect of smoking cessation on cardiovascular outcomes.

TABLE 24-2   CASE-CONTROL STUDIES OF CORONARY HEART DISEASE RISK AMONG FORMER SMOKERS

Reference	Population	Number of cases	Number of controls	Number of cases among former smokers	RELATIVE RISK AS COMPARED WITH NEVER SMOKERS* Former smokers	Current smokers
Willett et al,[155] 1981	Nurses' Health Study: women aged 30-55 yr	263	5260	29	1.0 (0.7-1.6)	3.0 (2.3-4.0)
Rosenberg, et al,[82] 1985	Eastern U.S. men aged <55 yr	1873	2775	348	1.1 (0.9-1.4)	2.9 (2.4-3.4)
Rosenberg, et al,[156] 1985	Eastern U.S. women aged <50 yr	555	1864	35	1.0 (0.7-1.6)	1.4-7.0 depending on cigarettes/day
LaVecchia et al,[157] 1987	Italian women aged <55 yr	168	251	3	0.8 (0.2-3.8)	3.6-13.1 depending on cigarettes/day
Rosenberg, et al,[83] 1990	Eastern U.S. women aged <65 yr	910	2375	149	1.2 (1.0-1.7)	3.6 (3.0-4.4)
Dobson et al,[84] 1991	Australian men aged 35-69 yr	895	1039	374	1.3 (0.9-1.6)	2.7 (2.1-3.5)
	Australian women aged 35-69 yr	387	1031	86	1.5 (1.1-2.2)	4.7 (3.4-6.6)
Negri et al,[158] 1994	Italian men and women aged <75 yr	916	1106		Years quit 1: 1.6 (0.8-3.2) 2-5: 1.4 (0.9-2.1) 6-10: 1.2 (0.7-2.1) >10: 1.1 (0.8-1.8)	2.9 (2.2-3.9)
Von Eyben et al,[159] 2001	Danish men and women aged <41 yr	35	70			6.4 (1.7-24.1)
Pais et al,[160,161] 1996, 2001	Indian men and women (93% men) aged 30-60 yr	300	300		1.9 (0.93-3.90)	Overall: 3.6 (2.20-6.03) <10/day: 1.6 (0.84-3.07) >10/day: 6.7 (3.51-12.8)
McElduff et al,[81] 1998	Australian, and New Zealand men and women aged 35-69 yr	5572	6268		Quit 1-3 yr: 1.5 (1.1-1.9) Women 1-3 yr: 1.6 (1.0-2.5) Quit 4-6 yr: same as nonsmokers	Overall: 3.5 (3.0-4.0) Women: 4.8 (4.0-5.9)
Bosetti et al,[86] 1999	Italian men and women	1230	1839		Women: 2.0 (1.2-3.4) <5 yr: 2.9 (1.3-6.7) >5 yr: 1.13 (0.6-2.7) Men: 1.3 (0.9-1.9) <5 yr: 1.5 (0.9-2.5) >5 yr: 1.2 (0.8-1.7)	Women: 4.1 (2.3-5.7) <15/day: 2.4 15-24: 5.6 >24: 9.8 Men: 3.3 (2.4-4.6) <15: 2.1 15-24: 3.2 >24: 5.4

Modified from Cigarette smoking among adults—United States, 2000. MMWR Morb Mortal Wkly Rep 2002; 51(29):642-645.
95% confidence interval shown in parentheses when available.

The value of smoking cessation for the secondary prevention of cardiovascular disease (e.g., the prevention of recurrent events and death among individuals with diagnosed heart disease) has been demonstrated by longitudinal observational studies of cohorts of smokers with established CHD (Table 24-3). Outcomes are compared between smokers who stop smoking and those who continue smoking after entry into the cohort. Randomized clinical trials of therapeutic interventions (e.g., bypass surgery or angioplasty) provide additional evidence to support the benefit of smoking cessation in patients with established CHD. In these studies, the survival of smokers who quit has been compared with that of continuing smokers, adjusting for the effect of the intervention tested in the trial.

The lack of randomized controlled clinical trial data, the highest standard of epidemiologic evidence, should not preclude a firm conclusion that smoking cessation reduces cardiovascular disease risk. Rose defined a standard "Rule of Prevention," namely that the benefit of a

■ ▪ ■

TABLE 24-3 MAJOR STUDIES OF THE EFFECT OF SMOKING CESSATION ON PERSONS WITH DIAGNOSED CORONARY HEART DISEASE

Reference	Population	Follow-up	Cases among former smokers	Reduction in risk compared with persistent smokers*
Mulcahy et al,[166] 1977	190 Dublin men aged <60 yr who smoked at time of first MI or unstable angina	5 yr	13 deaths	50%
Sparrow et al,[95] 1978	195 smokers after MI	≤5 yr	10 deaths	38%
Salonen,[167] 1980	North Karelia, Finland: 523 men aged <65 yr who smoked at first MI	3 yr	22 CHD deaths	40% (0–60)
Hubert et al,[168] 1982	Framingham Heart Study: subjects with angina	≤26 yr	NR	10-yr follow-up: age <60 yr: 90% age ≥60 yr: 60%
Rodda et al,[169] 1983	918 smokers at the time of first MI	≤3 yr	37 deaths	15%
Aberg et al,[170] 1983	983 Göteborg male smokers at time of MI	≤10.5 yr	104 recurrent nonfatal MI; 80 CHD deaths	30%; difference between groups increased with time
Perkins and Dick,[171] 1985	119 smokers at the time of first MI	5 yr	9 deaths	61%
Johansson et al,[172] 1985	161 Göteborg female smokers at the time of first MI	5 yr	14 deaths	52%
Rønnevik et al,[173] 1985	1330 participants in the Norwegian timolol trial who smoked at time of MI	17 mo	44 recurrent nonfatal MI	33% reduction; 8% in quitters, 12% in persistent smokers
Hallstrom et al,[15] 1986	310 survivors of out-of-hospital arrest, smokers at that time	Mean 47.5 mo	NR	35% for fatal recurrent cardiac arrest
Vlietstra et al,[103] 1986	11,605 patients in CASS who smoked at time CHD was diagnosed with angiography	5 yr	234	40% (20–50)
Daly et al,[174] 1987	373 men aged <60 yr who smoked at time of first MI or unstable angina and survived 2 yr	Average 9.4 yr; ≤16 yr	NR	10% for sudden death; 40% for total mortality
Green,[100] 1987	2199 men who smoked at time of MI	2 yr	NR	30% for CHD
Hermanson et al,[175] 1988	3045 CASS patients with CHD aged 35–54 yr	5.3 yr for MI or death	35–54 yr: NR	40% (30–50)
	1893 CASS patients with CHD aged ≥55		55–69 yr: 239 >70 yr: 29	30% (20–50) 70% (30–80)
Cavender et al,[104] 1992	780 CASS patients	10 yr or death	NR	35%
Burr et al,[176] 1992	1186 British smokers after MI	2 yr	27 deaths	57%
Hedback et al,[177] 1993	157 Swedish smokers after MI	10 yr	31 deaths	31%
Tofler et al,[178] 1993	702 U.S. smokers after MI	4 yr	25 deaths	51%
Greenwood et al,[179] 1995	532 British smokers after MI	5 yr	64 deaths	24%
Phillips et al,[180] 1988	530 male British former smokers with non-MI CHD	Mean 7.5 yr	NR	33% for fatal or nonfatal CHD
Herlitz et al,[96,181] 1995, 2000	862 post-MI patients in Sweden	4 yr		45% reduction in risk of death
	4553 post-acute chest pain patients in Sweden	5 yr		44% reduction in risk of death

Modified from The health benefits of smoking cessation: A report of the Surgeon General. U.S. Department of Health and Human Services, Centers for Disease Control, Office on Smoking and Health, 1990; and Wilson, K, Gibson N, Willan A, et al: Effect of smoking cessation on mortality after myocardial infarction: Meta-analysis of cohort studies. Arch Intern Med, 2000;. 160(7):939–944.
MI, myocardial infarction; CHD, coronary heart disease; NR, not reported; CASS, Coronary Artery Surgery Study.
*95% confidence intervals reported in parentheses where available.

preventive therapy must exceed the risk as shown in randomized clinical trials, unless the intervention itself equals restoration of a biologic or evolutionary norm. Smoking cessation certainly meets the latter criteria. The consistency, strength, and biologic plausibility of the observational epidemiologic data collected from males and females, as well as the clear dose-response relationship between reduction in risk and years of tobacco abstinence, make a conclusive case for the benefits of smoking cessation for cardiovascular disease prevention.[4] Given the clear consensus on the benefits of smoking cessation, a randomized trial would be unethical.

PRIMARY PREVENTION OF CARDIOVASCULAR DISEASE

Observational Epidemiologic Evidence

The 1990 Surgeon General's Report on the Health Consequences of Smoking[4] reviewed the evidence and summarized the health benefits for smoking cessation for individuals of all ages. It concluded that overall mortality of former smokers declines gradually, approaching that of never-smokers, after 10 to 15 years of abstinence or perhaps sooner.[4,81] In otherwise healthy individuals, smoking cessation reduces cardiovascular disease risk more rapidly than the risk of lung cancer or overall mortality. Tables 24-1 and 24-2 summarize the major cohort and case-control studies, respectively, including those reviewed in the Surgeon General's report and several published subsequently. These tables demonstrate that despite diversity of design and geographic location, the risk of CHD is consistently lower among former smokers compared with individuals who continue to smoke.

Less clear from these data is how much time is required for total mortality and cardiovascular mortality among former smokers to decline to the level of never-smokers. The initial benefit is rapid, with a great deal of the risk reduction occurring within the first 1 to 3 years of smoking cessation. Excess risk continues to decline, albeit more gradually, over the following 10 to 15 years. Four case-control studies suggested that approximately half of the excess risk of nonfatal MI is eliminated within the first year of quitting smoking, and the risk of former smokers approaches that of never-smokers within 5 years.[81-84] Cohort studies in middle-aged men also suggest that the excess risk of heart disease is halved within 1 year, but most have observed a more gradual decline in risk, reaching the level of never-smokers after 10 to 15 years of abstinence, although in a few studies a small excess risk persists for 20 years or more.[4] More recent studies in women generally confirm this finding. An analysis of the Nurses' Health Study, the largest cohort study in women, reported that cessation reduced one third of the excess risk of CHD over 2 years and that the excess risk disappears over 10 to 14 years of abstinence.[76,85] Two more recent case-control studies by Bosetti and colleagues and McElduff and colleagues, which examined separately the relative risks of men and women in a given population, have found a significant excess of risk among women versus men smokers given comparable exposure (see Table

24-2).[81,86] These findings have been attributed variously to either a lower baseline of cardiovascular risk in women; to interactions between smoking, thrombotic risks, and gender hormonal differences; or to the known differential impact of smoking on HDL levels between the sexes.[86]

The evidence also demonstrates that the degree to which smokers benefit from cessation depends on their total exposure to tobacco, the time since quitting, and the presence or absence of comorbid conditions. In general, the observational studies cited in Tables 24-1 and 24-2 support a dose-response relationship among all aspects of smoking and outcomes.[4] The Nurses' Health Study confirms both a dose and duration effect in women. The highest mortality and cardiovascular risks were seen among women who began smoking before the age of 15.[55]

Many of the studies cited attempted to adjust for the potentially confounding effects of demographic and other risk factors that could independently influence CHD mortality and morbidity. The Surgeon General's report analysis concludes that, "in the studies of primary prevention, none of these differences could explain even a minor portion of the decreased risk among quitters."[4] Nonetheless, like all observational studies, these have the inherent limitation that an unknown confounding factor could theoretically be responsible for different outcomes among smokers and ex-smokers.

The evidence that elderly individuals benefit from smoking cessation has been less certain. A study conducted among 7178 men and women older than age 65 in three cities examined smoking behavior and resulting cardiovascular mortality.[87] Former smokers had rates of cardiovascular mortality similar to those who had never smoked, regardless of the age of cessation. Jajich and associates, who studied 2674 Chicago residents aged 64 to 75 at study entry, reached a similar conclusion. Over 4 years of follow-up, former smokers had a relative risk of 1.1 for CHD mortality, compared with 1.9 for current smokers.[88] A more recent follow-up from the Finnish Cohort of the Seven Countries Study addressed the influence of classic risk factors on coronary risk and total mortality among elderly men. For those without coronary disease at the 25-year follow-up, smoking more than nine cigarettes a day suggested higher risks of developing coronary disease events in the subsequent 5 years, but this association was not statistically significant, and the risk of relationship was less strong than that seen for elevated serum cholesterol.[89]

Randomized Controlled Clinical Trials

Only one of the many randomized, controlled trials of smoking cessation as a single-factor intervention has reported long-term health outcomes. In the early 1970s, Rose and Hamilton tested the impact of smoking cessation advice versus no advice in 1445 British male civil servants at high risk of heart disease based on a risk-factor assessment.[90] Men in the intervention group received individualized information on the health risks of smoking and strong advice to quit. Over 10 years, the self-reported daily cigarette consumption was 53% lower in the intervention group than it was in the control group, but in the next 10 years of follow-up, this difference narrowed as increasing numbers of men in the control group reduced their cigarette use. At 20-year follow-up, the intervention group, compared with controls, had a 7% lower overall mortality rate, a 13% lower CHD mortality rate, and an 11% lower lung cancer incidence rate. The differences were not statistically significant, reflecting the lower power in a trial not designed to detect differences in disease rates and a smaller-than-expected difference in exposure to tobacco because of the intervention group's imperfect compliance with smoking cessation advice and the control group's cessation over time.

Several other clinical trials have evaluated the effect of simultaneously altering several cardiovascular risk factors including smoking (Table 24-4). The Multiple Risk Factor Intervention Trial (MRFIT) is the best known of these trials.[91] Its design most clearly approaches the standard now common for randomized controlled clinical trials. More than 12,000 high-risk men, aged 35 to 57, were randomized to a special intervention or usual care and followed for 10.5 years. Participants in the special intervention group underwent intensive, consistent, and recurring instructions regarding diet and smoking and aggressive, standardized hypertension therapy. Mortality at the study's end was slightly but not significantly lower (7%) in the intervention group compared to usual care. A separate analysis of those who quit smoking during the trial suggested a powerful benefit of smoking cessation. After adjustment for the presence of other risk factors, CHD risk was 42% lower among participants who had quit at the first annual follow-up visit.[92] Persistent quitters had a 65% 3-year risk reduction compared to persistent smokers. A smaller but similar study from Oslo that enrolled normotensive men aged 40 to 49 with other cardiac risk factors demonstrated a 44% decline in coronary disease events 102 months after institution of the diet and smoking intervention.[93] It was estimated that smoking cessation was responsible for 25% of the difference between the intervention and usual-care groups.

■ ■ ■

TABLE 24-4   SINGLE AND MULTIPLE RISK-FACTOR INTERVENTION TRIALS OF SMOKING CESSATION AND CORONARY HEART DISEASE RISK

Reference	Population	Intervention	Outcome	Overall effect of intervention	Effect of smoking cessation (nonrandomized)
Single risk factor					
Rose and Colwell,[162] 1992	1445 healthy British civil servants at high CHD risk	Antismoking advice	CHD deaths	13% reduction in intervention group at 20 yr (not statistically significant)	NR
Multiple risk factors					
MRFIT Research Group,[91] 1982	MRFIT: 12,866 healthy U.S. men aged 35-57 yr at high CHD risk	Diet, weight control, hypertension, and smoking	CHD deaths	7% decline in intervention group	44% reduction compared with persistent smokers
Ockene et al,[92] 1990	MRFIT: 6943 participant smokers at entry	Diet, weight control, hypertension, and smoking	CHD deaths	—	At 3-yr follow-up, quitters had 65% reduction (37%-80%) compared with persistent smokers
Hjermann et al,[93] 1986	Oslo study: 1232 healthy men aged 40-49 yr at high CHD risk	Diet and smoking	Fatal and nonfatal MI	44% decline in intervention group at 102 mo	Smoking cessation accounted for about 25% of the difference between groups
Kornitzer et al,[163] 1983	19,409 male Belgian factory workers, aged 40-59 yr	Smoking and hypertension	Fatal and nonfatal MI	25% reduction in intervention group	No specific analysis for effect of smoking cessation
Rose et al,[164] 1983	12 pairs of factories in UK, 18,210 men aged 40-59 yr	Diet, smoking, hypertension control	Nonfatal MI and CHD deaths	4% net reduction in prevalence of current smoking, virtually no difference in outcome between the two groups	No specific analysis of ex-smokers
Wilhelmsen et al,[165] 1986	10,004 Göteborg men aged 45-55 yr	Hypertension control, dietary, and antismoking advice	Major CHD	No difference	Intervention achieved only small differences between groups for any risk factor

Modified from Department of Health and Human Services. The Health Benefits of Smoking Cessation: A Report of the Surgeon General. DHHS Publication No. (CDC) 90-8416. U.S. DHHS, Public Health Service, Centers for Disease Control, Office on Smoking and Health. Washington, DC, U.S. Government Printing Office, 1990.

CHD, coronary heart disease; MRFIT, Multiple Risk Factor Intervention Trial; MI, myocardial infarction; NR, not reported.

SECONDARY PREVENTION OF CARDIOVASCULAR DISEASE

Observational epidemiologic studies demonstrate that the favorable impact of smoking cessation extends to individuals who quit following the diagnosis of CHD. Most studies have focused on survivors of MI and out-of-hospital cardiac arrest. It has been possible to demonstrate the benefit of smoking cessation in the secondary prevention setting with smaller sample sizes because the risk of future CHD events is substantially higher than it is for those without clinical evidence of coronary artery disease. Nonetheless, the dependence on observational studies for secondary prevention poses the same limitations and methodologic considerations as discussed in the case of trials of primary prevention.

The 1990 Surgeon General's report reviewed studies of smoking cessation with diagnosed CHD.[4] Subsequently Wilson and colleagues performed a formal meta-analysis of cohort studies examining the relationship between smoking cessation and mortality after MI.[94] The combined odds ratio for death was 0.54 (95% CI 0.46-0.62; see Fig. 24-1). The benefit of smoking cessation was seen in all studies and was consistent in both men and women. These studies, summarized in Table 24-3, demonstrate that survivors of MI or cardiac arrest benefit from stopping smoking, with a mortality advantage of up to 60%.[4,15,95] As in primary prevention, the reduction in risk is most pronounced earlier (at 6-12 months), with lesser risk reduction in later follow-up periods. Studies published after 1990 have reached similar conclusions. In the study of an unselected population of MI patients in Sweden, Herlitz and colleagues found smoking cessation following the index event was associated with 17% 5-year mortality, compared with 31% mortality among patients who continued to smoke.[96] Much of this benefit was accounted for by higher baseline risk among those who failed to quit, including history of prior MI and congestive heart failure. This is in contrast to most other studies in Table 24-3, which have demonstrated higher baseline risk among quitters compared with nonquitters.[4] It has been observed by others that smokers with greater degrees of coronary artery disease are more likely to stop smoking in the long term.[97]

It has been suggested[4] that observational studies of patients with coronary disease are likely to underestimate the favorable effect of quitting for two reasons. First, as noted earlier, smokers who quit after MI often have a greater disease burden, which may provide them with a greater motivation to quit compared with less severely ill individuals but also gives them a worse prognosis at the time of cessation. Second, most observational studies of quitting after a cardiac event have not routinely used biochemical validation of smoking cessation. The individuals classified as "quitters" likely include some who continue to smoke despite a self-report of cessation,[4] because nearly 7% of self-reported quitters in a recent Swedish study had contradictory biochemical markers.[98]

Additional evidence to support the benefit of smoking cessation derives from several controlled trials of therapeutic interventions for CHD. These studies have analyzed the effect of smoking cessation on risk among former smokers, independent of the intervention being studied. In the Norwegian Timolol Post-MI Trial, smoking cessation was associated with a 33% reduction in the risk of reinfarction, at an average of 17 months follow-up.[99] At this early follow-up, no difference in total mortality was seen. Interestingly, follow-up from a similarly designed trial of practolol demonstrated a benefit of smoking cessation beginning at 18 months, and by 24 months, a 30% risk reduction in coronary disease events was demonstrated.[100]

In a prospectively planned analysis of the Cardiac Arrhythmia Suppression Trial (CAST), a study evaluating patients with ventricular ectopic activity and left-ventricular dysfunction after acute MI, smoking cessation was associated with a marked reduction in arrhythmic death as well as total mortality.[101] This major benefit

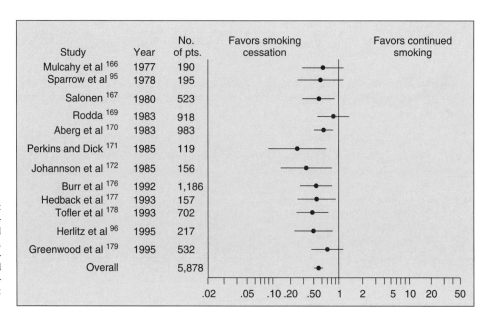

FIGURE 24-1. Meta-analysis of cohort studies on the effect of smoking cessation on mortality after myocardial infarction. (From Wilson K, Gibson N, Willan A, et al: Effect of smoking cessation on mortality after myocardial infarction: meta-analysis of cohort studies. Arch Intern Med 2000; 160[7]: 939-944.)

Study	Year	No. of pts.
Mulcahy et al [166]	1977	190
Sparrow et al [95]	1978	195
Salonen [167]	1980	523
Rodda [169]	1983	918
Aberg et al [170]	1983	983
Perkins and Dick [171]	1985	119
Johannson et al [172]	1985	156
Burr et al [176]	1992	1,186
Hedback et al [177]	1993	157
Tofler et al [178]	1993	702
Herlitz et al [96]	1995	217
Greenwood et al [179]	1995	532
Overall		5,878

occurred in patients not receiving thrombolytic therapy or undergoing coronary revascularization. These results are consistent with earlier studies of cardiac arrest survivors whose long-term prognosis is apparently improved by smoking cessation.[15] Similarly, in an analysis of the effect of smoking among participants of the Study of Left-Ventricular Dysfunction (SOLVD), all of whom had a left-ventricular ejection fraction of less than 35%, smoking cessation was associated with substantially decreased all-cause mortality, recurrent congestive heart failure, and MI within 2 years of quitting.[102] Although there were no significant differences in the deaths or hospitalizations from heart failure between ex-smokers and never-smokers, the magnitude of the benefit of smoking cessation was comparable to that achieved by several drug therapies for ventricular dysfunction.

In the Coronary Artery Surgical Study (CASS), death rates at follow-up were compared among never-smokers, persistent smokers, and persistent quitters. At baseline, quitters had a worse prognosis than did persistent smokers. However, at every level of risk, after adjustment for baseline characteristics, 5-year survival was better for quitters compared with smokers, with a risk reduction of 40% (see Table 24-3).[103] A subsequent CASS follow-up communication reported 10-year total mortality of smokers and quitters.[104] Survival was better among smokers who stopped smoking during follow-up compared with those who continued to smoke (82% vs. 77%, P = 0.025). The difference in survival was more pronounced for patients randomized to coronary artery bypass graft surgery (84% among quitters vs. 68% among nonquitters, P = 0.018) than among medically treated patients (75% for quitters vs. 71% for nonquitters, P = NS). Most other cardiac endpoints were considerably more frequent among nonquitters in both medical and surgical groups, including hospitalizations for MI, stroke, cardiac catheterization, and peripheral vascular surgery.

THE EFFECT OF PERSISTENT SMOKING ON OUTCOMES AFTER REVASCULARIZATION

Observational studies of patients undergoing bypass surgery and coronary angioplasty provide further support for a long-term benefit of smoking cessation among patients undergoing revascularization. Smoking cessation following bypass surgery appears to substantially reduce the risk of MI, repeat bypass surgery, and angina pectoris at 15 years.[105] An observational study of almost 5000 patients from the Mayo Clinic following coronary angioplasty demonstrated a much higher relative risk of mortality (RR 1.76) and of Q-wave MI (RR 2.08) in persistent smokers compared with nonsmokers. The need for repeat revascularization, either by percutaneous transluminal coronary angioplasty or surgery, was reduced by as much as one-third.[106] This effect was also observed in the Netherlands, where among 1041 patients undergoing bypass surgery with a median 20 years of follow-up, persistent smokers had an increased relative risk of mortality (RR = 1.68, 95% CI 1.33–2.13), cardiac

death (RR = 1.75, 95% CI 1.30–2.37), and requirement for subsequent angioplasty or repeat bypass (RR = 1.41, 95% CI 1.02–1.94) compared with those who quit within 1 year after surgery.[107]

The effect of smoking cessation on restenosis following coronary angioplasty has been somewhat less straightforward. In 1988, Galan and colleagues found increased frequency of restenosis following successful angioplasty in persistent smokers versus quitters, which was significant even after correction for other variables.[108] Another early study suggested a 17% higher absolute rate of restenosis among those who continued to smoke compared with quitters. An early trial of multivessel balloon angioplasty showed similar results.[109] Some subsequent studies have not regularly detected such an effect. In several randomized trials of interventions to reduce restenosis, smoking has not influenced the restenosis rate.[110-112] In a retrospective analysis of 2948 patients combined from four randomized trials of intervention, Violaris and associates found no difference between current, ex-smokers, and nonsmokers in the rate of restenosis at 6 months.[113] Some isolated studies surprisingly have suggested that persistent smoking may be associated with lower restenosis 6 months after angioplasty.[114] These negative findings have been attributed to either type I errors or differences in the composition of the populations that have not been adjusted, as the results otherwise violate conclusions considering the totality of evidence linking smoking and cardiovascular disease.[115] Cases in which the contradiction cannot be resolved by methodologic or epidemiologic explanations may in fact represent a phenomenon known as the "smoker's paradox."

THE SMOKER'S PARADOX

A surprising finding with respect to outcomes in smokers compared to nonsmokers emerged from several studies in the thrombolytic era. Smoking predicted a better prognosis following interventions done after acute MI, particularly at early follow-up.[116-118] In some studies, even smokers not actually undergoing thrombolytic therapy appeared to have better in-hospital and 6-month prognosis.[119,120] Studies of interventions after acute MI have shown better early coronary flow following thrombolytic therapy in smokers compared with nonsmokers, suggesting a greater clot burden or thrombogenicity in smokers with, perhaps, less severe underlying atherosclerosis.[121,122] It has been suggested that this "smoker's paradox" could be explained by the development of MI at younger ages with a more favorable risk-factor pattern in smokers compared with nonsmokers who develop MI.[123] This hypothesis is largely confirmed by large observational studies of MI,[118,119] including one from Israel in which the better prognosis of smokers disappeared following adjustment for age and baseline clinical variables including risk factors.[124] Cohort studies in which the short-term "benefit" conferred by smoking was not abolished by adjustment for baseline characteristics have not adjusted for atherosclerotic risk factors, which are likely to more accurately reflect underlying atherosclerotic burden than do clinical characteristics (such as history of previous MI or angina) at the time of MI presentation. Furthermore, studies showing an "advantage" for smoking were not generally consecutive series of patients but rather studies of patients eligible for thrombolytic therapy, who are generally younger with better baseline characteristics than those not eligible for thrombolytic therapy. The apparent advantage of smokers in terms of mortality and other outcomes in studies such as the Global Utilization of Streptokinase and Tissue Plasminogen Activator for Occluded Coronary Arteries trial (GUSTO) has been effectively explained by the age difference because an adjustment for the age differences between smoking and nonsmoking causes differences in outcomes in these studies to be nonsignificant.[107,116] However, analysis of the large (510,044 cases) National Registry of Myocardial Infarction (NRMI 2) database, which included rigorous adjustment for differences in age and cardiovascular risk factors between the two groups, found that a significant (RR = 0.86, 95% CI 0.83–0.89) decrease in mortality for smokers compared with nonsmokers remained that could not be explained. In this database, the smoker's advantage is not resolved by the presence of other known confounding variables.[125] Whether the residual small difference in mortality constitutes a genuine smoker's paradox or whether it is attributable to other, unmeasured confounding factors is not clear. The epidemiologic and methodologic debate is likely to continue.

The "paradox" may be more subtle at times. Although persistent smoking clearly had adverse effects on long-term outcomes after bypass surgery in the Netherlands,[107] it was noted that active smoking at the time of surgery in this study did not increase subsequent adverse events compared with never-smokers. In this study, age differences (mean of 4 years between the groups) alone could not account for the "paradox," although selection biases could have enriched the bypass candidates with healthier patients among the smoking population.

SMOKING CESSATION INTERVENTIONS

A large number of randomized controlled trials have assessed proposed smoking cessation treatments. This body of evidence was reviewed systematically by two independent U.S. and British scientific panels, each of which released an evidence-based clinical practice guideline for treating tobacco use in 2000.[126-129] Both groups found that the strongest evidence for efficacy existed for two methods: counseling and pharmacotherapy. Each of these was effective by itself, but combinations provided the highest smoking cessation rates. The success of treatment increases as the intensity of treatment increases, but even brief interventions that physicians can accomplish in office practice promote cessation.

Counseling

In primary care offices, trials demonstrate that a physician's stop-smoking advice increases patients' smoking cessation rates by approximately 30%.[126,127] Brief counseling, lasting 3 minutes or less, is more effective than advice alone and doubles cessation rates compared with no intervention. Outside the physician office, smoking cessation counseling is effective when delivered by trained counselors with repeated contacts over at least 4 weeks.[126,127] This can be done in person (in group or individual settings) or by telephone. The efficacy of treatment increases with increasing contact time. Most counseling programs use cognitive-behavioral counseling methods. The content of programs found to be effective typically combines practical problem solving, coping skills for behavior change, and social support to increase a smoker's confidence in the ability to quit.

Pharmacotherapy

Six drugs have been approved by the U.S. Food and Drug Administration (FDA) for the treatment of tobacco use: five nicotine replacement products (gum, transdermal patch, nasal spray, vapor inhaler, and lozenge) and bupropion, an antidepressant with dopaminergic and noradrenergic activity.[126,127,130] Each approximately doubles the long-term cessation rates compared with placebo in randomized double-blind trials that usually also include smoking cessation counseling. Few randomized controlled trials have directly compared these drugs with each other. One randomized controlled trial directly compared bupropion with the nicotine patch.[131] Bupropion produced a significantly higher 1-year cessation rate than either nicotine patch or placebo. Combining bupropion and the nicotine patch was safe but not significantly more effective than using bupropion alone. Another randomized trial compared four nicotine replacement products with each other and reported equivalent efficacy at short-term follow-up.[132] The U.S. clinical guideline recommended nicotine replacement products and bupropion as roughly equal in efficacy and considered them appropriate for first-line treatment.[126,127]

Two other drugs, nortriptyline and clonidine, have demonstrated some efficacy for smoking cessation but are not approved by the FDA for this indication and are regarded as second-line agents in the U.S. guidelines.[126,127] Nortriptyline was effective for smoking cessation in two small studies.[133,134] No other antidepressant has demonstrated efficacy for smoking cessation in a published trial, nor have the few trials of anxiolytics found them to be effective for smoking cessation.[127] Clonidine reduces nicotine withdrawal symptoms and demonstrates efficacy for smoking cessation in meta-analyses, but frequent adverse effects limit its use.[127]

Hypnosis and acupuncture have also been tested for smoking cessation. There is little support for hypnosis because few controlled trials have been conducted, whereas acupuncture has been ineffective in randomized trials.[127]

PUBLIC HEALTH IMPLICATIONS

The public health impact of smoking cessation on CHD events was estimated by Tosteson and colleagues, who used epidemiologic data and a complex computer simulation of the U.S. male population.[135] The analysis suggests

■ ■ ■

TABLE 24-5 PROJECTED PERCENT CHANGES (IN PARENTHESES) OVER BASELINE VALUES FOR ABSOLUTE CHD INCIDENCE AMONG MALES FREE OF CHD, 25 YEARS AFTER EACH LEVEL OF SMOKING REDUCTION IS ACHIEVED

	CHANGE IN ABSOLUTE INCIDENCE FOR EACH LEVEL OF SMOKING REDUCTION		
Age (yr)	25%	50%	75%
35-44	(−9)	(−16)	(−22)
45-54	(−4)	(−8)	(−11)
55-64	(0)	(−1)	(−1)
65-74	(+1)	(+2)	(+4)
75-84	(+1)	(+2)	(+3)

Modified from Tosteson AN, Weinstein MC, Williams LW, et al: Long-term impact of smoking cessation on the incidence of coronary heart disease. Am J Public Health 1990; 80(12):1481–1486.

that interventions that would reduce the prevalence of smoking by 25% would generate a significant decrease in the incidence of CHD among men younger than 65 years (Table 24-5). A 50% reduction in smoking in a group of 50-year-olds brings about an 8% lower incidence of CHD. This analysis suggests a large impact of smoking cessation in preventing premature cardiovascular disease in the U.S. population. In this model, there is a paradoxic slight increase in projected CHD among men age 65 or older who have quit smoking, explained by a decrease in noncoronary disease mortality that allows more former smokers to survive beyond age 65. This larger cohort of former smokers continues to manifest their underlying risks for coronary disease events over a longer period, and therefore smoking cessation prior to the age of 65 is likely to be beneficial. In fact, the benefit of smoking cessation beyond the age of 65 can be quantified. In a very large cohort of the American Cancer Society after 12 years of follow-up,[72] it appears there are still significant overall mortality benefits to be derived from quitting smoking even at the age of 65, although the proportion of lives saved as a result of the prevention of cardiac disease is unknown (Table 24-6). Similarly, in a

reanalysis of the British Doctors Study, all-cause mortality was still improved with cessation at the age of 65.[136]

The results of large-scale, well-funded public health initiatives to curtail the prevalence of smoking have been encouraging. These initiatives include raising the price of tobacco by increasing tobacco excise taxes and using a portion of the funds generated to fund mass media anti-tobacco advertising along with school-based tobacco prevention programs, and increasing the availability of smoking cessation services. The experiences in California and Oregon showed at least transient improvements in the prevalence of smoking in younger individuals during the periods of active campaigning.[137-139] However, in the case of the older initiative in California, improvement was followed by plateauing of the smoking prevalence after spending was decreased on public service announcements and other interventions.[138] Tobacco industry-funded lobbying and advertising can limit the gains made from these publicly funded initiatives.[140-142] Not surprisingly, tobacco industry-funded public health initiatives appear to promote positive attitudes toward smoking and promote smoking behavior, in contrast to independently funded campaigns.[140,143] The experience from the statewide initiatives demonstrates that independently funded campaigns can have a significant impact on the "denormalization" of tobacco use if they are empowered financially to a sufficient degree.

CONCLUSION

Despite the absence of data from randomized, controlled clinical trials, a large body of prospective observational epidemiologic data regarding the effect of smoking cessation on cardiovascular disease has been collected over more than 40 years. The evidence is diverse in design and site and includes cohort studies of both primary and secondary prevention, risk-factor intervention trials, and subgroup analyses of cardiovascular treatment trials. The overwhelming totality of this evidence demonstrates that smoking cessation promptly, dependably, and substantially lowers morbidity and mortality from coronary artery disease, compared with continuing to smoke, regardless of how long or how much one has smoked.

■ ■ ■

TABLE 24-6 LIFE EXPECTANCIES, BY SMOKING BEHAVIOR, FOR MEN AND WOMEN AGED 35 IN 1990

	MEN			WOMEN		
Smoking behavior	Expected survival (yr)	Unadjusted gain relative to continuing smoker	Adjusted* gain relative to continuing smoker	Expected survival (yr)	Unadjusted gain relative to continuing smoker	Adjusted* gain relative to continuing smoker
Never smoked	78.2	8.9	10.5	81.2	7.4	8.9
Smoked until death	69.3	...	...	73.8	...	...
Quit age 35	76.2	6.9	8.5	79.9	6.1	7.7
Quit age 45	74.9	5.6	7.1	79.4	5.6	7.2
Quit age 55	72.7	3.4	4.8	78.0	4.2	5.6
Quit age 65	70.7	1.4	2.0	76.5	2.7	3.7
No intervention†	72.9	3.6	4.6	77.7	3.9	5.1

Modified from Taylor DH Jr, Hasselblad V, Henley SJ, et al: Benefits of smoking cessation for longevity. Am J Public Health 2002; 92(6):990–996.
*Adjusted for cessation rates during course of follow-up from 1982 to 1996, as estimated by resurvey of Cancer Prevention Study II respondents in 1992.
†No intervention indicates that age- and sex-specific cessation and relapse rates were as observed in the 1990 National Health Interview Survey and the 1991 National Health and Nutrition Examination Survey I.

The effect is present in both men and women and at all ages, but little information is available about nonwhites. The data suggest that there is a rapid initial decline in excess cardiovascular risk within the first 1 to 3 years after a cardiac event. The risk among former smokers approaches that of never-smokers over approximately 10 to 15 years of abstinence. The benefit of smoking cessation persists even after the diagnosis of cardiovascular disease; a risk reduction of up to 50% has been reported. This pattern is consistent with the multiple effects of smoking on the pathogenesis of cardiovascular disease, which includes both short- and long-term effects. Given the broad consensus about the benefit of smoking cessation, the issue is not likely to be testable for ethical reasons in any future prospective randomized clinical trial. Such data are not necessary to guide medical and public health practice. The substantial prevalence of tobacco smoking and the epidemiologic evidence of the magnitude of the benefit of smoking cessation indicate that it is a leading modifiable risk factor for cardiovascular disease and that efforts to reduce smoking prevalence deserve a high priority.

REFERENCES

1. McGinnis JM, Foege WH: Actual causes of death in the United States. JAMA 1993; 270(18):2207-2212.
2. Reducing the health consequences of smoking: 25 years of progress: A report of the surgeon general. U.S. Department of Health and Human Services, Centers for Disease Control, Office on Smoking and Health, 1989.
3. Annual smoking-attributable mortality, years of potential life lost, and economic costs—United States 1995-1999. MMWR Morb Mortal Wkly Rep 2002; 51(14):300-303.
4. The health benefits of smoking cessation: A report of the surgeon general. U.S. Department of Health and Human Services, Centers for Disease Control, Office on Smoking and Health, 1990.
5. Cigarette smoking among adults—United States, 2000. MMWR Morb Mortal Wkly Rep 2002; 51(29):642-645.
6. Youth tobacco surveillance—United States, 2000. MMWR CDC Surveill Summ 2001; 50(4):1-84.
7. Benowitz NL, Gourlay SG: Cardiovascular toxicity of nicotine: implications for nicotine replacement therapy. J Am Coll Cardiol 1997; 29(7):1422-1431.
8. Benowitz NL: Drug therapy. Pharmacologic aspects of cigarette smoking and nicotine addition. N Engl J Med 1988; 319(20): 1318-1330.
9. Cellina GU, Honour AJ, Littler WA: Direct arterial pressure, heart rate, and electrocardiogram during cigarette smoking in unrestricted patients. Am Heart J 1975; 89(1):18-25.
10. McBride PE: The health consequences of smoking. Cardiovascular diseases. Med Clin North Am 1992; 76(2):333-353.
11. Narkiewicz K, van de Borne PJ, Hausberg M, et al: Cigarette smoking increases sympathetic outflow in humans. Circulation 1998; 98(6):528-534.
12. Kurihara S: Effect of age on blood pressure response to cigarette smoking. Cardiology 1995; 86(2):102-107.
13. Cryer PE, Hammond MW, Santiago JV, et al: Norepinephrine and epinephrine release and adrenergic mediation of smoking-associated hemodynamic and metabolic events. N Engl J Med 1976; 295(11):573-577.
14. Ekelund LG, Haskell WL, Johnson JL, et al: Physical fitness as a predictor of cardiovascular mortality in asymptomatic North American men: The Lipid Research Clinics Mortality Follow-up Study. N Engl J Med 1988; 319(21):1379-1384.
15. Hallstrom AP, Cobb LA, Ray R: Smoking as a risk factor for recurrence of sudden cardiac arrest. N Engl J Med 1986; 314(5): 271-275.
16. Palatini P, Pessina AC, Graniero GR, et al: [The relationship between overweight, life style and casual and 24-hour pressures in a population of male subjects with mild hypertension: The results of the HARVEST study]. G Ital Cardiol 1995; 25(8):977-989.
17. Pickering TG, Schwartz JE, James GD: Ambulatory blood pressure monitoring for evaluating the relationships between lifestyle, hypertension and cardiovascular risk. Clin Exp Pharmacol Physiol 1995; 22(3):226-231.
18. Allred EN, Bleecker ER, Chaitman BR, et al: Short-term effects of carbon monoxide exposure on the exercise performance of subjects with coronary artery disease. N Engl J Med 1989; 321(21): 1426-1432.
19. Anderson EW, Andelman RJ, Strauch JM, et al: Effect of low-level carbon monoxide exposure on onset and duration of angina pectoris: A study in ten patients with ischemic heart disease. Ann Intern Med 1973; 79(1):46-50.
20. Sheps DS, Herbst MC, Hinderliter AL, et al: Production of arrhythmias by elevated carboxyhemoglobin in patients with coronary artery disease. Ann Intern Med 1990; 113(5):343-351.
21. Adams KF, Koch G, Chatterjee B, et al: Acute elevation of blood carboxyhemoglobin to 6% impairs exercise performance and aggravates symptoms in patients with ischemic heart disease. J Am Coll Cardiol 1988; 12(4):900-909.
22. Morrow JD, Frei B, Longmire AW, et al: Increase in circulating products of lipid peroxidation (F2-isoprostanes) in smokers: Smoking as a cause of oxidative damage. N Engl J Med 1995; 332(18):1198-1203.
23. Winkelmann BR, Boehm BO, Nauck M, et al: Cigarette smoking is independently associated with markers of endothelial dysfunction and hyperinsulinaemia in nondiabetic individuals with coronary artery disease. Curr Med Res Opin 2001; 17(2):132-141.
24. Kaufmann PA, Gnecchi-Ruscone T, di Terlizzi M, et al: Coronary heart disease in smokers: Vitamin C restores coronary microcirculatory function. Circulation 2000; 102(11):1233-1238.
25. Clarke RA: Antioxidant vitamins and risk of cardiovascular disease: Review of large-scale randomised trials. Cardiovasc Drugs Ther 2002; 16(5):411-415.
26. Kool MJ, Hoeks AP, Struijker Boudier HA, et al: Short- and long-term effects of smoking on arterial wall properties in habitual smokers. J Am Coll Cardiol 1993; 22(7):1881-1886.
27. Quillen JE, Rossen JD, Oskarsson HJ, et al: Acute effect of cigarette smoking on the coronary circulation: Constriction of epicardial and resistance vessels. J Am Coll Cardiol 1993; 22(3):642-647.
28. Sugiishi M, Takatsu F: Cigarette smoking is a major risk factor for coronary spasm. Circulation 1993; 87(1):76-79.
29. Deanfield JE, Shea MJ, Wilson RA, et al: Direct effects of smoking on the heart: Silent ischemic disturbances of coronary flow. Am J Cardiol 1986; 57(13):1005-1009.
30. Campisi R, Czernin J, Schoder H, et al: Effects of long-term smoking on myocardial blood flow, coronary vasomotion, and vasodilator capacity. Circulation 1998; 98(2):119-125.
31. Celermajer DS, Sorensen KE, Georgakopoulos D, et al: Cigarette smoking is associated with dose-related and potentially reversible impairment of endothelium-dependent dilation in healthy young adults. Circulation 1993; 88(5 Pt 1):2149-2155.
32. Blann AD: The acute influence of smoking on the endothelium. Atherosclerosis 1992; 96(2-3):249-250.
33. McVeigh GE, et al: Cigarette smoking inhibits basal but not stimulated release of nitric oxide from the forearm vasculature. J Am Coll Cardiol 1995; 337A.
34. Heitzer T, Yla-Herttuala S, Luoma J, et al: Cigarette smoking potentiates endothelial dysfunction of forearm resistance vessels in patients with hypercholesterolemia: Role of oxidized LDL. Circulation 1996; 93(7):1346-1353.
35. Zeiher AM, Schachinger V, Minners J: Long-term cigarette smoking impairs endothelium-dependent coronary arterial vasodilator function. Circulation 1995; 92(5):1094-1100.
36. Howard G, Wagenknecht LE, Burke GL, et al: Cigarette smoking and progression of atherosclerosis: The Atherosclerosis Risk in Communities (ARIC) Study. JAMA 1998; 279(2):119-124.
37. Craig WY, Palomaki GE, Haddow JE: Cigarette smoking and serum lipid and lipoprotein concentrations: An analysis of published data. BMJ 1989; 298(6676):784-788.
38. Harats D, Ben-Naim M, Dabach Y, et al: Cigarette smoking renders LDL susceptible to peroxidative modification and enhanced metabolism by macrophages. Atherosclerosis 1989; 79(2-3):245-252.

39. Stamford BA, Matter S, Fell RD, et al: Effects of smoking cessation on weight gain, metabolic rate, caloric consumption, and blood lipids. Am J Clin Nutr 1986; 43(4):486-494.

40. Benowitz NL, Fitzgerald GA, Wilson M, et al: Nicotine effects on eicosanoid formation and hemostatic function: Comparison of transdermal nicotine and cigarette smoking. J Am Coll Cardiol 1993; 22(4):1159-1167.

41. Eliasson M, Asplund K, Evrin PE, et al: Relationship of cigarette smoking and snuff dipping to plasma fibrinogen, fibrinolytic variables and serum insulin. The Northern Sweden MONICA Study. Atherosclerosis 1995; 113(1):41-53.

42. Fisher SD, Zareba W, Moss AJ, et al: Effect of smoking on lipid and thrombogenic factors two months after acute myocardial infarction. Am J Cardiol 2000; 86(8):813-818.

43. Shah PK, Helfant RH: Smoking and coronary artery disease. Chest 1988; 94(3):449-452.

44. Pittilo RM, Clarke JM, Harris D, et al: Cigarette smoking and platelet adhesion. Br J Haematol 1984; 58(4):627-632.

45. Newby DE, McLeod AL, Uren NG, et al: Impaired coronary tissue plasminogen activator release is associated with coronary atherosclerosis and cigarette smoking: Direct link between endothelial dysfunction and atherothrombosis. Circulation 2001; 103(15):1936-1941.

46. Matetzky S, Tani S, Kangavari S, et al: Smoking increases tissue factor expression in atherosclerotic plaques: Implications for plaque thrombogenicity. Circulation 2000; 102(6):602-604.

47. Mathew TP, Herity NA: Acute myocardial infarction soon after nicotine replacement therapy. QJM 2001; 94(9):503-504.

48. Neunteufl T, Heher S, Kostner K, et al: Contribution of nicotine to acute endothelial dysfunction in long-term smokers. J Am Coll Cardiol 2002; 39(2):251-256.

49. Benowitz NL, Hansson A, Jacob P III: Cardiovascular effects of nasal and transdermal nicotine and cigarette smoking. Hypertension 2002; 39(6):1107-1112.

50. Doll R, Peto R, Hall E, et al: Mortality in relation to smoking: 40 years' observations on male British doctors. BMJ 1994; 309 (6959):901-911.

51. Jonas MA, Oates JA, Ockene JK, et al: Statement on smoking and cardiovascular disease for health care professionals. American Heart Association. Circulation 1992; 86(5):1664-1669.

52. Al-Delaimy WK, Manson JE, Solomon CG, et al: Smoking and risk of coronary heart disease among women with type 2 diabetes mellitus. Arch Intern Med 2002; 162(3):273-279.

53. Willett WC, Green A, Stampfer MJ, et al: Relative and absolute excess risks of coronary heart disease among women who smoke cigarettes. N Engl J Med 1987; 317(21):1303-1309.

54. Kawachi I, Colditz GA, Stampfer MJ, et al: Smoking cessation and decreased risk of stroke in women. JAMA 1993; 269(2):232-236.

55. Kawachi I, Colditz GA, Stampfer MJ, et al: Smoking cessation in relation to total mortality rates in women. A prospective cohort study. Ann Intern Med 1993; 119(10):992-1000.

56. Fuller JH, Shipley MJ, Rose G, et al: Mortality from coronary heart disease and stroke in relation to degree of glycaemia: The Whitehall study. BMJ (Clin Res Educ) 1983; 287(6396):867-870.

57. Beral V: Mortality among oral-contraceptive users. Royal College of General Practitioners' Oral Contraception Study. Lancet 1977; 2(8041):727-731.

58. Respiratory health effects of passive smoking: Lung cancer and other disorders. Washington, DC, Environmental Protection Agency: Office of Health and Environmental Assessment, 1992,

59. Charlton A: Children and passive smoking: a review. J Fam Pract 1994; 38(3):267-77.

60. Kawachi I, Colditz GA, Speizer FE, et al: A prospective study of passive smoking and coronary heart disease. Circulation 1997; 95(10):2374-2379.

61. Glantz SA, Parmley WW: Passive smoking and heart disease. Mechanisms and risk. JAMA 1995; 273(13):1047-1053.

62. Glantz SA, Parmley WW: Passive smoking and heart disease. Epidemiology, physiology, and biochemistry. Circulation 1991; 83(1):1-12.

63. Steenland K: Passive smoking and the risk of heart disease. JAMA 1992; 267(1):94-99.

64. Taylor AE, Johnson DC, Kazemi H: Environmental tobacco smoke and cardiovascular disease: A position paper from the Council on Cardiopulmonary and Critical Care, American Heart Association. Circulation 1992; 86(2):699-702.

65. Woo KS, Chook P, Leong HC, et al: The impact of heavy passive smoking on arterial endothelial function in modernized Chinese. J Am Coll Cardiol 2000; 36(4):1228-1232.

66. Otsuka R, Watanabe H, Hirata K, et al: Acute effects of passive smoking on the coronary circulation in healthy young adults. JAMA 2001; 286(4):436-441.

67. He J, Vuppuputri S, Allen K, et al: Passive smoking and the risk of coronary heart disease: A meta-analysis of epidemiologic studies. N Engl J Med 1999; 340(12):920-926.

68. Wells AJ: Heart disease from passive smoking in the workplace. J Am Coll Cardiol 1998; 31(1):1-9.

69. Hrubec Z, McLaughlin JK: Former cigarette smoking and mortality among U.S. veterans: A 26 year follow-up 1954-1980. In National Cancer Institute. Changes in cigarette-related disease risks and their implication for prevention and control, Smoking and Tobacco Control Monograph, National Cancer Institute. 1997, pp 501-530.

70. Thun MJ, Day-Lally C, Myers DG: Trends in tobacco smoking and mortality from cigarette use in Cancer Prevention Studies I (1959 through 1965) and II (1982 through 1988). In Changes in cigarette-related disease risks and their implication for prevention and control, Smoking and Tobacco Control Monograph, National Cancer Institute. 1997.305-382.

71. Burns DM, et al: The American Cancer Society Cancer Prevention Study I: 12-year follow-up of 1 million men and women. In National Cancer Institute. Changes in cigarette-related disease risks and their implication for prevention and control. Smoking and Tobacco Control Monograph, National Cancer Institute, 1997 pp 113-304.

72. Taylor DH Jr, Hasselblad V, Henley SJ, et al: Benefits of smoking cessation for longevity. Am J Public Health 2002; 92(6):990-996.

73. Keys A: Smoking habits. In A Multivariate Analysis of Death and Coronary Heart Disease. Cambridge, Harvard University Press: 1980, pp 136-160.

74. Cederlof R, Friberg L, Hrubec Z, et al: The relationship of smoking and some social covariables to mortality and cancer morbidity. A ten year follow-up in a probability sample of 55,000 Swedish subjects age 18-69, Part 1 of 2. 1975, Karolinska Institute, Dept. of Environmental Hygiene: Stockholm, Sweden.

75. Friedman GD, et al: Smoking and mortality: the Kaiser Permanente experience. In National Cancer Institute. Changes in cigarette-related disease risks and their implication for prevention and control, Smoking and Tobacco Control Monograph, National Cancer Institute, 1997; 477-497.

76. Kawachi I, Colditz GA, Stampfer MJ: Smoking cessation and decreased risks of total mortality, stroke, and coronary heart disease incidence among women: a prospective cohort study. In Changes in cigarette-related disease risks and their implication for prevention and control, Smoking and Tobacco Control Monograph, National Cancer Institute, 1997.

77. Gupta R, Gupta KD, Sharma S, et al: Influence of cessation of smoking on long term mortality in patients with coronary heart disease. Indian Heart J 1993; 45(2):125-129.

78. Lam TH, et al: Smoking, quitting, and mortality in a Chinese cohort of retired men. Ann Epidemiol 2002; 12(5):316-320.

79. Qiao Q, Tervahauta M, Nissinen A, et al: Mortality from all causes and from coronary heart disease related to smoking and changes in smoking during a 35-year follow-up of middle-aged Finnish men. Eur Heart J 2000; 21(19):1621-1626.

80. Tomas Abadal L, Varas Lorenzo C, Perez I, et al: [Risk factors and coronary morbimortality in a Mediterranean industrial cohort over 28 years of follow-up. The Manresa Study]. Rev Esp Cardiol 2001; 54(10):1146-1154.

81. McElduff P, Dobson A, Beaglehole R, et al: Rapid reduction in coronary risk for those who quit cigarette smoking. Aust N Z J Public Health 1998; 22(7):787-791.

82. Rosenberg L, Kaufman DW, Helmrich SP, et al: The risk of myocardial infarction after quitting smoking in men under 55 years of age. N Engl J Med 1985; 313(24):1511-4.

83. Rosenberg L, Palmer JR, Shapiro S: Decline in the risk of myocardial infarction among women who stop smoking. N Engl J Med 1990; 322(4):213-7.

84. Dobson AJ, Alexander HM, Heller RF, et al: How soon after quitting smoking does risk of heart attack decline? J Clin Epidemiol 1991; 44(11):1247-1253.

85. Kawachi I, Colditz GA, Stampfer MJ, et al: Smoking cessation and time course of decreased risks of coronary heart disease in middle-aged women. Arch Intern Med 1994; 154(2):169-175.

86. Bosetti C, Negri E, Tavani A, et al: Smoking and acute myocardial infarction among women and men: A case-control study in Italy. Prev Med 1999; 29(5):343-348.

87. LaCroix AZ, Lang J, Scherr P, et al: Smoking and mortality among older men and women in three communities. N Engl J Med 1991; 324(23):1619-1625.

88. Jajich CL, Ostfeld A, Freeman DH Jr: Smoking and coronary heart disease mortality in the elderly. JAMA 1984; 252(20):2831-2834.

89. Tervahauta M, Pekkanen J, Nissinen A: Risk factors of coronary heart disease and total mortality among elderly men with and without preexisting coronary heart disease. Finnish cohorts of the Seven Countries Study. J Am Coll Cardiol 1995; 26(7): 1623-1629.

90. Rose G, Hamilton PJ: A randomised controlled trial of the effect on middle-aged men of advice to stop smoking. J Epidemiol Community Health 1978; 32(4):275-281.

91. Multiple risk factor intervention trial: Risk factor changes and mortality results. Multiple Risk Factor Intervention Trial Research Group. JAMA 1982; 248(12):1465-1477.

92. Ockene JK, Kuller LH, Svendsen KH, et al: The relationship of smoking cessation to coronary heart disease and lung cancer in the Multiple Risk Factor Intervention Trial (MRFIT). Am J Public Health 1990; 80(8):954-958.

93. Hjermann I, Holme I, Leren P: Oslo Study Diet and Antismoking Trial. Results after 102 months. Am J Med 1986; 80(2A):7-11.

94. Wilson K, Gibson N, Willan A, et al: Effect of smoking cessation on mortality after myocardial infarction: Meta-analysis of cohort studies. Arch Intern Med 2000; 160(7):939-944.

95. Sparrow D, Dawber TR: The influence of cigarette smoking on prognosis after a first myocardial infarction. A report from the Framingham study. J Chronic Dis 1978; 31(6-7):425-432.

96. Herlitz J, Bengtson A, Hjalmarson A, et al: Smoking habits in consecutive patients with acute myocardial infarction: Prognosis in relation to other risk indicators and to whether or not they quit smoking. Cardiology 1995; 86(6):496-502.

97. Rosal MC, Ockene JK, Ma Y, et al: Coronary Artery Smoking Intervention Study (CASIS): 5-year follow-up. Health Psychol 1998; 17(5):476-478.

98. Attebring M, Herlitz J, Berndt AK, et al: Are patients truthful about their smoking habits? A validation of self-report about smoking cessation with biochemical markers of smoking activity amongst patients with ischaemic heart disease. J Intern Med 2001; 249(2):145-151.

99. Von Der Lippe G: Reduction of sudden deaths after myocardial infarction by treatment with beta-blocking drugs in Advances in Beta-Blocker Therapy II. Proceedings of the Second International Bayer Beta-Blocker Symposium. Venice, 1981.

100. Green KG: Falsely favourable early prognosis for continuing smokers following recovery from acute myocardial infarction. Information from the multi-centre practolol trial. Br J Clin Pract 1987; 41(6):785-788.

101. Peters RW, Brooks MM, Todd L, et al: Smoking cessation and arrhythmic death: The CAST experience. The Cardiac Arrhythmia Suppression Trial (CAST) Investigators. J Am Coll Cardiol 1995; 26(5):1287-1292.

102. Suskin N, Sheth T, Negassa A, et al: Relationship of current and past smoking to mortality and morbidity in patients with left ventricular dysfunction. J Am Coll Cardiol 2001; 37(6):1677-1682.

103. Vlietstra RE, Kronmal RA, Oberman A, et al: Effect of cigarette smoking on survival of patients with angiographically documented coronary artery disease. Report from the CASS registry. JAMA 1986; 255(8):1023-1027.

104. Cavender JB, Rogers WJ, Fisher LD, et al: Effects of smoking on survival and morbidity in patients randomized to medical or surgical therapy in the Coronary Artery Surgery Study (CASS): 10-year follow-up. CASS Investigators. J Am Coll Cardiol 1992; 20(2):287-294.

105. Voors AA, van Brussel BL, Plokker HW, et al: Smoking and cardiac events after venous coronary bypass surgery. A 15-year follow-up study. Circulation 1996; 93(1):42-47.

106. Hasdai D, Garratt KN, Grill DE, et al: Effect of smoking status on the long-term outcome after successful percutaneous coronary revascularization. N Engl J Med 1997; 336(11):755-761.

107. van Domburg RT, Meeter K, van Berkel DF, et al: Smoking cessation reduces mortality after coronary artery bypass surgery: A 20-year follow-up study. J Am Coll Cardiol 2000; 36(3): 878-883.

108. Galan KM, Deligonul U, Kern MJ, et al: Increased frequency of restenosis in patients continuing to smoke cigarettes after percutaneous transluminal coronary angioplasty. Am J Cardiol 1988; 61(4):260-263.

109. Myler RK, Topol EJ, Shaw RE, et al: Multiple vessel coronary angioplasty: Classification, results, and patterns of restenosis in 494 consecutive patients. Cathet Cardiovasc Diagn 1987; 13(1):1-15.

110. Macdonald RG, Henderson MA, Hirshfeld JW Jr, et al: Patient-related variables and restenosis after percutaneous transluminal coronary angioplasty: A report from the M-HEART Group. Am J Cardiol 1990; 66(12):926-931.

111. Gurlek A, Dagalp Z, Oral D, et al: Restenosis after transluminal coronary angioplasty: a risk factor analysis. J Cardiovasc Risk 1995; 2(1):51-55.

112. Moliterno D, Topol EJ: Clinical evaluation of restenosis. In Fuster VR, Topol EJ (eds): Atherosclerosis and Coronary Artery Diseases. Philadelphia, Lippincott-Raven Publishers, 1996, pp 1505-1526.

113. Violaris AG, Thury A, Regar E, et al: Influence of a history of smoking on short term (six month) clinical and angiographic outcome after successful coronary angioplasty. Heart 2000; 84(3): 299-306.

114. Melkert R, Violaris AG, Serruys PW: Luminal narrowing after percutaneous transluminal coronary angioplasty. A multivariate analysis of clinical, procedural and lesion related factors affecting long-term angiographic outcome in the PARK study. Post-Angioplasty Restenosis Ketanserin. J Invasive Cardiol 1994; 6(5): 160-171.

115. Pell JP: Does smoking cessation reduce the risk of restenosis following coronary angioplasty? Heart 2000; 84(3):233-234.

116. Barbash GI, White HD, Modan M, et al: Significance of smoking in patients receiving thrombolytic therapy for acute myocardial infarction. Experience gleaned from the International Tissue Plasminogen Activator/Streptokinase Mortality Trial. Circulation 1993; 87(1):53-58.

117. Lee KL, Woodlief LH, Topol EJ, et al: Predictors of 30-day mortality in the era of reperfusion for acute myocardial infarction. Results from an international trial of 41,021 patients. GUSTO-I Investigators. Circulation 1995; 91(6):1659-1668.

118. Maggioni AP, Maseri A, Fresco C, et al: Age-related increase in mortality among patients with first myocardial infarctions treated with thrombolysis. The Investigators of the Gruppo Italiano per lo Studio della Sopravvivenza nell'Infarto Miocardico (GISSI-2). N Engl J Med 1993; 329(20):1442-1448.

119. Maynard C, Weaver WD, Litwin PE, et al: Hospital mortality in acute myocardial infarction in the era of reperfusion therapy (the Myocardial Infarction Triage and Intervention Project). Am J Cardiol 1993; 72(12):877-882.

120. Molstad P: First myocardial infarction in smokers. Eur Heart J 1991; 12(7):753-9.

121. Zahger D, Cercek B, Cannon CP, et al: How do smokers differ from nonsmokers in their response to thrombolysis? (the TIMI-4 trial). Am J Cardiol 1995; 75(4):232-236.

122. Grines CL, Topol EJ, O'Neill WW, et al: Effect of cigarette smoking on outcome after thrombolytic therapy for myocardial infarction. Circulation 1995; 91(2):298-303.

123. Ockene IS, Ockene JK: Smoking after acute myocardial infarction. A good thing? Circulation 1993; 87(1):297-299.

124. Gottlieb S, Boyko V, Zahger D, et al: Smoking and prognosis after acute myocardial infarction in the thrombolytic era (Israeli Thrombolytic National Survey). J Am Coll Cardiol 1996; 28(6): 1506-1513.

125. Gourlay SG, Rundle AC, Barron HV: Smoking and mortality following acute myocardial infarction: Results from the National Registry of Myocardial Infarction 2 (NRMI 2). Nicotine Tob Res 2002; 4(1):101-107.

126. A clinical practice guideline for treating tobacco use and dependence: A US Public Health Service report. The Tobacco Use and Dependence Clinical Practice Guideline Panel, Staff, and Consortium Representatives. JAMA 2000; 283(24):3244-3254.

127. Fiore MC: Treating tobacco use and dependence: An introduction to the US Public Health Service Clinical Practice Guideline. Respir Care 2000; 45(10):1196-1199.

128. West R, McNeill A, Raw M: Smoking cessation guidelines for health professionals: an update. Health Education Authority. Thorax 2000; 55(12):987-999.

129. Lancaster T, Stead L, Silagy C, et al: Effectiveness of interventions to help people stop smoking: Findings from the Cochrane Library. BMJ 2000; 321(7257):355-358.

130. Hughes JR, Goldstein MG, Hurt RD, et al: Recent advances in the pharmacotherapy of smoking. JAMA 1999; 281(1):72-76.

131. Jorenby DE, Leischow SJ, Nides MA, et al: A controlled trial of sustained-release bupropion, a nicotine patch, or both for smoking cessation. N Engl J Med 1999; 340(9):685-691.

132. Hajek P, West R, Foulds J, et al: Randomized comparative trial of nicotine polacrilex, a transdermal patch, nasal spray, and an inhaler. Arch Intern Med 1999; 159(17):2033-2038.

133. Hall SM, Reus VI, Munoz RF, et al: Nortriptyline and cognitive-behavioral therapy in the treatment of cigarette smoking. Arch Gen Psychiatry 1998; 55(8):683-690.

134. Prochazka AV, Weaver MJ, Keller RT, et al: A randomized trial of nortriptyline for smoking cessation. Arch Intern Med 1998; 158(18):2035-2039.

135. Tosteson AN, Weinstein MC, Williams LW, et al: Long-term impact of smoking cessation on the incidence of coronary heart disease. Am J Public Health 1990; 80(12):1481-1486.

136. Peto R, Darby S, Deo H, et al: Smoking, smoking cessation, and lung cancer in the UK since 1950: combination of national statistics with two case-control studies. BMJ 2000; 321(7257): 323-329.

137. Bal DG, Lloyd JC, Roeseler A, et al: California as a model. J Clin Oncol 2001; 19(18 Suppl):69S-73S.

138. Pierce JP, Gilpin EA, Emery SL, et al: Has the California tobacco control program reduced smoking? JAMA 1998; 280(10): 893-899.

139. Effectiveness of school-based programs as a component of a statewide tobacco control initiative—Oregon 1999-2000; MMWR Morb Mortal Wkly Rep 2001; 50(31):663-666.

140. Landman A, Ling PM, Glantz SA: Tobacco industry youth smoking prevention programs: Protecting the industry and hurting tobacco control. Am J Public Health 2002; 92(6):917-930.

141. Ling PM, Glantz SA: Why and how the tobacco industry sells cigarettes to young adults: evidence from industry documents. Am J Public Health 2002; 92(6):908-916.

142. Neuman M, Bitton A, Glantz S: Tobacco industry strategies for influencing European Community tobacco advertising legislation. Lancet 2002; 359(9314):1323-1330.

143. Farrelly MC, Healton CG, Davis KC, et al: Getting to the truth: Evaluating national tobacco countermarketing campaigns. Am J Public Health 2002; 92(6):901-907.

144. Doll R, Peto R: Mortality in relation to smoking: 20 years' observations on male British doctors. BMJ 1976; 2(6051): 1525-1536.

145. Doll R, Gray R, Hafner B, et al: Mortality to relation to smoking: 22 years' observations on female British doctors. BMJ 1980; 280(6219):967-971.

146. Hammond EC, Horn D: Smoking and death reatesrates—Report on forth-four months of follow-up of 187,783 men. I. Total Mortality. JAMA 1958; 166:1159-1172 1294-1308.

147. Hammond EC, Garfinkel L. Coronary heart disease, stroke, and aortic aneurysm. Factors in the etiology. Arch Environ Health 1969; 19(2):167-182.

148. Kahn HA: The Dorn study of smoking and mortality among U.S. veterans: Report on eight and one-half years of observation., in Epidemiological approaches to the study of cancer and other chronic disease. NCI Monograph No. 19, W. Haenszel, Editor. 1966, U.S. Department of Health, Education and Welfare, U.S. Public Health Service, National Cancer Institute, 1-125.

149. Rogot E, Murray JL: Smoking and causes of death among U.S. veterans: 16 years of observation. Public Health Rep 198-; 95(3): 213-222.

150. Doyle JT, Dawber TR, Kannel WB, et al: Cigarette smoking and coronary heart disease. Combined experience of the Albany and Framingham studies. N Engl J Med 1962; 266:796-801.

151. Rosenman RH, Brand RJ, Jenkins D, et al: Coronary heart disease in Western Collaborative Group Study. Final follow-up experience of 81/2 years. JAMA 1975; 233(8):872-877.

152. Friedman GD, Petitti DB, Bawol RD, et al: Mortality in cigarette smokers and quitters. Effect of base-line differences. N Engl J Med 1981; 304(23):1407-1410.

153. Floderus B, Cederlof R, Friberg L: Smoking and mortality: a 21-year follow-up based on the Swedish Twin Registry. Int J Epidemiol 1988; 17(2):332-340.

154. Netterstrom B, Juel K: Impact of work-related and psychosocial factors on the development of ischemic heart disease among urban bus drivers in Denmark. Scand J Work Environ Health 1988; 14(4):231-238.

155. Willett WC, Hennekens CH, Bain C, et al: Cigarette smoking and non-fatal myocardial infarction in women. Am J Epidemiol 1981; 113(5):575-582.

156. Rosenberg L, Kaufman DW, Helmrich SP, et al: Myocardial infarction and cigarette smoking in women younger than 50 years of age. JAMA 1985; 253(20):2965-2969.

157. La Vecchia C, Franceschi S, Decarli A, et al: Risk factors for myocardial infarction in young women. Am J Epidemiol 1987; 125(5):832-843.

158. Negri E, La Vecchia C, D'Avanzo B, et al: Acute myocardial infarction: association with time since stopping smoking in Italy. GISSI-EFRIM Investigators. Gruppo Italiano per lo Studio della Sopravvivenza nell'Infarto. Epidemiologia dei Fattori di Rischio dell'Infarto Miocardico. J Epidemiol Community Health 1994; 48(2):129-133.

159. von Eyben FE, von Eyben R: Smoking and other major coronary risk factors and acute myocardial infarction before 41 years of age: two Danish case-control studies. Scand Cardiovasc J 2001; 35(1):25-29.

160. Pais P, Pogue J, Gerstein H, et al: Risk factors for acute myocardial infarction in Indians: a case-control study. Lancet 1996; 348(9024):358-363.

161. Pais P, Fay MP, Yusuf S: Increased risk of acute myocardial infarction associated with beedi and cigarette smoking in Indians: final report on tobacco risks from a case-control study. Indian Heart J 2001; 53(6):731-735.

162. Rose G, Colwell L: Randomised controlled trial of anti-smoking advice: final (20 year) results. J Epidemiol Community Health 1992; 46(1):75-77.

163. Kornitzer M, De Backer G, Dramaix M, et al: Belgian heart disease prevention project: incidence and mortality results. Lancet 1983; 1(8333):1066-1070.

164. Rose G, Tunstall-Pedoe HD, Heller RF: UK heart disease prevention project: incidence and mortality results. Lancet 1983; 1(8333):1062-1066.

165. Wilhelmsen L, Berglund G, Elmfeldt D, et al: The multifactor primary prevention trial in Goteborg, Sweden. Eur Heart J 7(4): 279-288.

166. Mulcahy R, Hickey N, Graham IM, et al: Factors affecting the 5 year survival rate of men following acute coronary heart disease. Am Heart J 1977; 93(5):556-559.

167. Salonen JT: Stopping smoking and long-term mortality after acute myocardial infarction. Br Heart J 1980; 43(4):463-469.

168. Hubert HB, Holford TR, Kannel WB: Clinical characteristics and cigarette smoking in relation to prognosis of angina pectoris in Framingham. Am J Epidemiol 1982; 115(2):231-242.

169. Rodda BE: The Timolol Myocardial Infarction Study: an evaluation of selected variables. Circulation 1983; 67(6 Pt 2):I101-I106.

170. Aberg A, Bergstrand R, Johansson S, et al: Cessation of smoking after myocardial infarction. Effects on mortality after 10 years. Br Heart J 1983; 49(5):416-422.

171. Perkins J, Dick TB: Smoking and myocardial infarction: secondary prevention. Postgrad Med J 1985; 61(714):295-300.

172. Johansson S, Bergstrand R, Pennert K, et al: Cessation of smoking after myocardial infarction in women. Effects on mortality and reinfarctions. Am J Epidemiol 1985; 121(6):823-831.

173. Ronnevik PK, Gundersen T, Abrahamsen AM: Effect of smoking habits and timolol treatment on mortality and reinfarction in patients surviving acute myocardial infarction. Br Heart J 1985; 54(2):134-139.

174. Daly LE, Hickey N, Graham IM, et al: Predictors of sudden death up to 18 years after a first attack of unstable angina or myocardial infarction. Br Heart J 1987; 58(6):567-571.

175. Hermanson B, Omenn GS, Kronmal RA, et al: Beneficial six-year outcome of smoking cessation in older men and women with coronary artery disease. Result from the CASS registry. N Engl J Med 1988; 319(21):1365-1369.

176. Burr ML, Holliday RM, Rehily AM, et al: Haematological prognostic indices after myocardial infarction: evidence from the diet and reinfarction trial (DART). Eur Heart J 1992; 13(2): 166-170.

177. Hedback B, Perk J, Wodlin P: Long-term reduction of cardiac mortality after myocardial infarction: 10-year results of a comprehensive rehabilitation programme. Eur Heart J 1993; 14(6):831–835.

178. Tofler GH, Muller JE, Stone PH, et al: Comparison of long-term outcome after acute myocardial infarction in patients never graduated from high school with that in more educated patients. Multicenter Investigation of the Limitation of Infarct Size (MILIS). Am J Cardiol 1993; 71(12):1031–1035.

179. Greenwood DC, Muir KR, Packham CJ, et al: Stress social support, and stopping smoking after myocardial infarction in England. J Epidemiol Community Health 1995; 49(6):583–587.

180. Phillips AN, Shaper AG, Pocock SJ, et al: The role of risk factors in heart attacks occurring in men with pre-existing ischaemic heart disease. Br Heart J 1988; 60(5):404–410.

181. Herlitz J. Karlson BW, Sjolin M, et al: Five-year mortality in patients with acute chest pain in relation to smoking habits. Clin Cardiol 2000; 23(2):84–90.

■ ■ ■ c h a p t e r **25**

Physical Activity and Weight Loss

Marcia L. Stefanick

INTRODUCTION

Reviews of the epidemiologic literature[1-4] and subsequent prospective cohort studies[5-9] have concluded that physical activity is strongly and inversely related to cardiovascular disease risk, in particular, coronary heart disease (CHD), in both men and women, leading to a strongly held belief that physical inactivity plays a major causal role in cardiovascular disease.[4] A large number of observational studies have also reported that increasing levels of body mass index (BMI), calculated as weight (kg)/height squared (m^2), are associated with an increased risk of nonfatal myocardial infarction (MI) and CHD death and that both overweight (BMI of 25-29.9 kg/m^2) and obesity (BMI of $\geq$30 kg/m^2) are associated with increased CHD morbidity and mortality relative to normal weight.[10]

Although there continues to be debate about whether there is a causal relationship of obesity to CHD, data from both observational studies and clinical trials support the direct relationship of obesity to type 2 diabetes mellitus (DM), which has been designated as a CHD risk equivalent because of the high risk of new CHD it confers within 10 years,[11] and to several other specific cardiovascular risk factors that are now regarded as obesity comorbidities (e.g., impaired glucose tolerance [IGT] and insulin resistance; hypertension; and dyslipidemias, in particular, low high-density lipoprotein-cholesterol [HDL-C] and high triglyceride levels).[10,12]

The cumulative effect of these studies has been the promotion of physical activity and weight control as part of cardiovascular health.[1,10] Specifically, the 1996 Surgeon General's Report recommended that every American adult accumulate at least 30 minutes of moderate-intensity physical activity on most, preferably all, days of the week,[1] and 1998 guidelines for treating overweight and obese, from the National Heart, Lung and Blood Institute (NHLBI) Obesity Education Initiative (OEI) Expert Panel, included a reduction in energy intake of 500 to 1000 kcal/day, to elicit a weight loss of approximately 0.5 to 0.9 kg/wk (1-2 pounds/wk) for up to 6 months, combined with a minimum of 150 minutes of moderate exercise per week.[10] Nonetheless, as of 2004, there is no randomized, controlled trial (RCT) evidence that either increased physical activity by sedentary men or women or weight loss by overweight or obese individuals prevents or reduces combined cardiovascular disease, CHD, or stroke. However, an increasing number of reasonably sized RCTs have assessed the effect of physical activity and/or weight loss on type 2 diabetes and the major CHD risk factors, which have been recognized as obesity-related comorbidities, many of which are described in this chapter. The strength of these trials provides support for the endorsement of health policies aimed at increasing the proportion of the population that is physically active and of normal weight.

PREVALENCE OF OBESITY AND PHYSICAL ACTIVITY

Determining whether physical activity and/or weight loss reduce CHD has enormous public health significance, not only because CHD is the leading cause of death in both men and women in the United States[1] but also because physical inactivity and obesity are highly prevalent in the United States,[1,10] resulting in a high risk of subsequent chronic disease. Obesity, in particular, has increased markedly over the past several decades; between the second (1976-1980) and third (1988-1994) National Health and Nutrition Examination Surveys (NHANES II and III), the percent of the U.S. population aged 20 years or older that was obese increased from 14.5% to 22.5% as a result of an increase from 12% to 19.5% in men and from 16.3% to 25.0% in women. With approximately 40% of men and 25% of women also being overweight at each survey (i.e., a total of 32.0% of all adults surveyed), an estimated 54.5% of U.S. adults were overweight or obese by 1994.[10] More recent reports, using a continuous survey approach, suggest continued increases such that an estimated 30.5% of the U.S. adult population was obese in 1999 and 2000, and the prevalence of overweight plus obese was 64.5%.[13] Furthermore, extreme obesity (BMI $\geq$40 kg/m^2) increased from 2.9% (NHANES III) to 4.7% in the 1999 and 2000 surveys.[13]

Data collected by the 1996 U.S. Behavioral Risk Factor Surveillance System (BRFSS) indicated that 29.2% of U.S. adults are inactive in their leisure time, 43.1% participate in some activity but not enough to ensure health benefits, and 27.8% are physically active at recommended levels.[14] Gender differences in participation

■ ■ ■

TABLE 25-1   RANDOMIZED TRIALS OF EXERCISE OR WEIGHT LOSS (BY DIET OR EXERCISE) FOR TYPE 2 DIABETES MELLITUS

Study title or key feature of study (reference)	Intervention(s) Treatment groups	Study population	Length	Primary outcome (secondary outcomes)	Major results
Da Qing Impaired Glucose Tolerance and Diabetes Study (Pan et al, 1997)	1: Diet, 2: Exercise, 3: Diet + exercise, 4: Control	577 men and women; Age: >25 yr, impaired glucose tolerance	6 yr	Type 2 diabetes mellitus	Cumulative incidence of type 2 diabetes mellitus: C: 67.7%, D: 43.8%, E:41.1%; D + E: 46.0%
Finnish Diabetes Prevention Trial (Tuomilehto et al, 2001)	1: Intervention: Weight loss ≥5%; <30% fat; <10% saturated fat; fiber ≥15 g/day; exercise ≥30 min/day; 2: Control	522 men and women (350 + 177); Age: 40-65 yr, obese, sedentary	Average 3.2 yr	Type 2 diabetes mellitus	Cumulative incidence of type 2 diabetes mellitus: C: 23% I: 11% (58% reduction)
Diabetes Prevention Program (DPP); DPP Research Group, 2002	1: Intense lifestyle: Weight loss ≥7% body weight (diet + exercise), 2: Metformin, 3: Placebo	3234 men and women (68% women); elevated fasting and postload glucose; Age: 51 (mean)	Average 2.8 yr	Type 2 diabetes mellitus	Cumulative incidence of type 2 diabetes mellitus: P: 11%, M: 7.8% (31% reduction); weight loss (D + E): 4.5% (58% reduction)

in physical activity are relatively minor in the United States, with levels of vigorous, moderate, and total (recommended) activity being quite similar, although more women (30.9%) than men (27.2%) report no activity.[14] The prevalence of physical inactivity was high in both normal-weight and overweight men (26.8% and 25.6%, respectively) and normal-weight and overweight women (27.8% and 31.7%, respectively); however, inactivity was even higher in obese men (32.7%) and women (40.9%).[15] Participation in recommended levels of physical activity (i.e., ≥150 minutes per week of moderate-intensity exercise)[1] was also low in both normal-weight and overweight men (29.3% and 29.2%, respectively) and women (30.7% and 26.0%, respectively) but was substantially lower among obese men (23.5%) and women (18.9%).[15]

Clinical trials are presented in this chapter that include increases in physical activity and/or weight loss in overweight or obese adults as intervention goals and specific or multiple cardiovascular outcomes or CHD risk factors as primary or key secondary outcomes. Trials are grouped by risk-factor outcomes—that is, type 2 diabetes or IGT (Table 25-1), hypertension and elevated blood pressure (BP) (Table 25-2), and dyslipidemias and lipoprotein effects (Table 25-3). The metabolic syndrome, defined by the third National Cholesterol Education Program (NCEP) Adult Treatment Panel (ATP-III),[10] is discussed briefly. Finally, evidence for a role of physical activity and/or weight loss in secondary prevention and cardiac rehabilitation is also addressed briefly (Table 25-4).

CLINICAL TRIALS OF PHYSICAL ACTIVITY AND/OR WEIGHT LOSS FOR PREVENTING CARDIOVASCULAR DISEASE OR TYPE 2 DIABETES MELLITUS

The first U.S. lifestyle-induced (diet and exercise) weight loss trial that will have cardiovascular disease (including fatal MI and stroke) and nonfatal MI and stroke as primary outcomes is the **Look AHEAD (Action for Health in Diabetes) trial,**[16] which is being conducted by the National Institutes of Diabetes and Digestive and Kidney Diseases (NIDDK).

The Look AHEAD trial has initiated recruitment of an expected 5000 overweight men and women with type 2 diabetes, aged 45 to 75 years (33% minority), for a study designed to last 9 to 11.5 years. Participants are being randomly assigned to one of the following:

1. Lifestyle intervention: diet modification and increased physical activity with a goal of sustained weight loss.
2. Control: diabetes education (emphasizing management of hypoglycemia and the importance of eating a healthy diet and being physically active for both weight loss and improving glycemic control) and support.

The lifestyle intervention is designed to achieve a minimum weight loss of 7% of initial body weight during the first year, although individual participants will be encouraged to lose 10% or more of the weight initially by restricting caloric intake to 1200 to 1500 kcal/day for individuals weighing 250 pounds (114 kg) or less

■■■

TABLE 25-2   RANDOMIZED TRIALS OF EXERCISE OR WEIGHT LOSS (BY DIET OR EXERCISE) FOR BLOOD PRESSURE

Study title or key feature of study (reference)	Intervention(s) #: treatment groups	Study population	Length	Primary outcome (secondary outcomes)	Major results
Hypertension Prevention Trial (HPT Research Group, 1990)	(If obese, 1–5; otherwise, only 2 or 5), 1: Diet (reduced calories), 2: Low sodium, 3: Diet + low sodium, 4: Low sodium, high potassium 5: Control	549 men, 292 women; Age: 25–49, DBP: 78–89 mm Hg	3 yr	DBP; SBP (weight loss)	BP decreases in all groups vs. baseline, most in 1 + 3 (Weight decreases most in 1 + 3)
Trials of Hypertension Prevention (TOHP) (Stevens et al, 1993)	1: Weight loss, diet (cal) + exercise, behavior, 2: Control	385 men, 179 women; Age: 30–54, DBP: 80–89 mm Hg, obese	18 mo	DBP; SBP (weight loss)	BP reduced more with greater weight loss (Weight decreases 1 vs. 2)
Trial of Antihypertensive Interventions and Management (TAIM) (Wassertheil-Smoller, 1992)	9 Groups: 1 of **3 drugs** (chlorthalidone atenolol, or placebo) combined with 1 of **3 diets**: Weight loss (calories), Low sodium + increased potassium, usual	878 men and women (more than 50% men); Age: 21–65, DBP: 90–100 mm Hg, obese	6 mo	DBP; SBP (weight loss)	BP decreased more with: drugs vs. diet; drugs + diet vs. drugs alone; low calorie vs. usual or low sodium/increased potassium diet
Treatment of Mild Hypertension Study (Neaton et al, 1993)	Lifestyle (low calorie, salt, and alcohol + exercise) + 1: Chlorthalidone, 2: Acebutol, 3: Doxazosin mesylate, 4: Amlodipine maleate, 5: Enalapril maleate, 6: Placebo	557 men, 345 women; Age: 45–69, Stage 1 hypertension (DBP < 100 mm Hg)	4 yr	DBP; SBP (other CHD risk factors)	BP decreased 1–5 vs. 6; DBP, SBP decreased (and lipoproteins improved) in all groups vs. baseline
Exercise for Mild Hypertension (Blumenthal et al, 1991)	1: Exercise (aerobic), 2: Strength and flexibility training, 3: Control	57 men, 42 women; Age: 29–59, SBP: 140–180 mm Hg, DBP: 90–105 mm Hg	4 mo	DBP; SBP (weight loss)	SBP, DBP, (weight), NS; SBP, DBP decrease in all from baseline
Steffen et al, 2001	1: Exercise + weight management, 2: Exercise, 3: Control	112 men and women, high normal BP or stage 1 or 2 hypertension	6 mo	Resting BP and 15-hr daytime ambulatory BP	Resting BP (NS); DBP reduced during physical activity and behavioral stress 1 vs. 3, but 2 not different from 1 or 3

DBP, diastolic blood pressure; SBP, systolic blood pressure; BP, blood pressure, CHD, coronary heart disease.

at baseline and 1500 to 1800 kcal/day for those who weigh more, with plans to restrict calories further if participants do not lose weight. The composition of the diet is structured to enhance glycemic control and improve cardiovascular risk factors and is based on guidelines of the American Diabetes Association[17] and NCEP,[11] which include a maximum of 30% of calories from total fat, a maximum of 10% from saturated fat, and a minimum of 15% of total calories from protein. The physical activity program will rely heavily on home-based exercise, with gradual progression toward a goal of 175 minutes of moderate-intensity physical activity per week for the first 6 months (with exercise bouts of 10 minutes or longer counting toward this goal and participants being directed to exercise on at least 5 days per week).

This study is built on the success of at least three completed trials of diet and exercise interventions for preventing type 2 diabetes, listed in Table 25-1. The first of these trials was the Da Qing IGT and Diabetes Study[18]

in China, which included diet only, exercise only, and combined diet and exercise interventions. This was followed by the Finnish Diabetes Prevention Trial,[19] which was followed by the U.S. Diabetes Prevention Program (DPP),[20] the latter of which was also conducted by the NIDDK. All three of these trials, described in the following paragraphs, provide strong evidence that type 2 diabetes can be prevented or delayed by weight loss and/or physical activity in persons at high risk.

The **Da Qing IGT and Diabetes Study**[18] followed 577 nondiabetic men and women who met the World Health Organization criteria for IGT at 33 Chinese clinics that were randomized to carry out one of four specified intervention protocols on each eligible subject attending that clinic:

1. Diet only: 55% to 65% carbohydrate, 10% to 15% protein, and 25% to 30% fat, and for participants with BMI of less than 25 kg/m², 25 to 30 kcal/kg body

TABLE 25-3 RANDOMIZED TRIALS OF EXERCISE OR WEIGHT LOSS (BY DIET OR EXERCISE) FOR LIPOPROTEINS

Study title or key feature of study (reference)	Intervention(s), # treatment groups	Study population	Length	Primary outcome (secondary outcomes)	Major results
(Huttenen et al, 1979)	1: Exercise (aerobic) 2: Control	90 middle-aged men, sedentary	6 mo	HDL-C (other lipoproteins)	HDL-C increases and TG decreases in 1 vs. 2
Stanford Exercise Study (Wood et al, 1983)	1: Exercise (aerobic), 2: Control	81 men; age: 30–55, sedentary	1 yr	HDL-C (other CHD risk factors)	HDL-C, NS, 1 vs. 2 (weight decreases in 1 vs. 2, no other differences)
Stanford Weight Control Project, I (Wood et al, 1988)	1: Weight loss, exercise (aerobic), 2: Weight loss, diet (calories), 3: Control	155 men; age: 35–59, obese, sedentary	1 yr	HDL-C (other CHD risk factors)	HDL-C increases and TG decreases in 1 and 2 vs. 3 (LDL-C, NS)
Overweight, Middle-aged and Older Men (Katzel et al,1995)	1: Weight loss, diet (low fat), 2: Exercise (aerobic), 3: Control	170 men; age: 46–80, obese, sedentary	9 mo	CHD risk factors: HDL-C, LDL-C, TG, BP, glucose	HDL-C increases, BP and glucose decrease in 1 vs. 3, not 2 vs. 3; glucose decreases in 1 vs. 2; LDL-C and TG decrease in 1 and 2 vs. 3; overall, 1 decreased CHD risk more than 2
Stanford Weight Control Project, II (Wood et al, 1991)	1: Weight loss, diet (low fat), 2: Weight loss, diet (low fat) + Exercise (aerobic), 3: Control	132 men, 132 women (premenopausal); age: 25–49, obese, sedentary	1 yr	HDL-C (other CHD risk factors)	Men: HDL-C increases, 2 vs. 3, not 1 vs. 2 or 3; (LDL-C, NS) Women: HDL-C increases 2 vs. 1, not 1 or 2 vs. 3; (LDL-C decreases 1 and 2 vs. 3)
Stanford-Sunnyvale Health Improvement Project (Older Adults) (King et al, 1991, 1995)	1–3: Exercise (aerobic: group vs. home-based; high vs. low-intensity), 4: Control	197 men, 160 women (postmenopausal); Age: 50–64, sedentary	1 yr; 2nd yr, w/o control	Treadmill Exercise Test Performance, VO$_{2max}$ (CHD risk factors)	VO$_{2max}$ increases 1,2,3, vs. 4 in both sexes (Lipoproteins, BP, NS); Yr 2: HDL increases from baseline in both low-intensity exercise groups
Aerobic + Anaerobic Exercise + Diet, (Svendsen et al, 1993)	1: Weight loss, diet (calories), 2: Weight loss, diet + exercise (aerobic + anaerobic), 3: Control	121 women; age: 45–54, obese	12 wk	CHD risk factors (weight loss)	HDL-C NS; LDL-C, TG decrease 1 and 2 vs. 3, not 1 vs. 2 (Weight decreases 1 and 2 vs. 3)
(Boyden et al, 1993)	1. Exercise (anaerobic) 2. Control	103 women; age 28–39	5 mo	HDL-C, LDL-C, TG (weight)	HDL-C, TG (weight) NS; LDC-C, TC reduced in 1 vs. 2
Slight to moderately elevated CHD risk (Hellenius et al, 1993)	1: Diet (low fat), 2: Exercise (aerobic), 3: Diet + exercise, 4: Control	158 men; age: 35–60, elevated total cholesterol	6 mo	CHD risk factors (weight loss)	Lipoproteins, NS; BP decreases 1 and 2 vs. 4, not 3 vs. 4 (Weight decreases 1–3 vs. 4)
Diet and Exercise for Elevated Risk (DEER) (Stefanick et al, 1996)	1: Diet (low fat), 2: Exercise (aerobic), 3: Diet + exercise, 4: Control	197 men, 180 women (postmenopausal); age: 30–64, men; 45–64, women; Low HDL + High LDL	12 mo	HDL-C (other CHD risk factors)	HDL-C (TG, BP) NS, either sex (LDL-C decreases 3 vs. 4, both sexes; not 1 vs. 4, either sex; glucose decreases, 1 and 3 vs. 4, both sexes)
Campbell's Center for Nutrition & Wellness (McCarron et al, 1997)	1: Diet (CCNW Plan), 2: Diet (AHA Step I/II)	246 men, 314 women; age: 26–70; CHD risk factors	10 wk	CHD risk factors (body weight)	SBP, DBP decrease 1 vs. 2; HDL-C, LDL-C, TG, NS (1 and 2 improved vs. baseline)
Diet and Moderate Exercise Trial, South Asian population (Singh et al, 1992)	1: Diet (AHA Step I + fruit + vegetables) + Exercise, 2: Diet (AHA Step I only)	419 men, 44 women; age: 25–65; CHD risk factors	24 wk	CHD risk factors (body weight)	LDL-C, TG, BP, glucose decrease, HDL-C increases, 1 vs. 2 (weight decreases 1 vs. 2)
STRRIDE (Kraus et al, 2002)	Exercise: 1: High amount-high intensity, 2: Low amount-high intensity, 3: Low amount-moderate intensity, 4: Wait-list control	159 men and women, age: 40–65, moderately overweight or mildly obese	8 mo	Lipoproteins	NS differences between any of the groups; Lipoprotein improvements in 1, 2, and 3 vs. baseline

HDL-C, high-density lipoprotein cholesterol; CHD, coronary heart disease; TG, triglyceride; LDL-C, low-density lipoprotein cholesterol; NS, not significant (among all groups, if not specified); BP, blood pressure; VO$_{2max}$, maximal oxygen consumption; AHA, American Heart Association.

■ ■ ■

TABLE 25-4 RANDOMIZED TRIALS WITH EXERCISE OR WEIGHT LOSS INTERVENTIONS IN INDIVIDUALS WITH CARDIOVASCULAR DISEASE

Study title or key feature of study (reference)	Intervention(s) (treatment groups)	Study population	Length	Primary outcome (secondary outcomes)	Major results
Lifestyle Heart Trial (Ornish et al, 1990)	1: Lifestyle (low-fat, vegetarian diet, stop smoking, exercise + stress reduction), 2: Usual care	36 men, 5 women; age: 35–75 yr; angiographically documented CAD	12 mo	Coronary lesions (progression, regression) (CHD risk factors)	Less progression, more regression, and reduced symptoms, 1 vs. 2 (HDL-C, TG, BP, NS; LDL-C, weight decreases, 1 vs. 2)
(Singh et al, 1992)	1: Diet (low fat), 2: Diet (low fat + fruits, vegetables, nuts)	505 people; age: unspecified; definite/possible myocardial infarction	12 mo	Cardiac events, mortality (CHD risk factors)	Incidence and mortality lower, 2 vs. 1 (LDL-C, TG, SBP, SBP, DBP, glucose decreases, HDL-C increases, 2 vs. 1)
(Schuller et al, 1992)	1: Exercise + diet (low-fat), 2: Usual care	113 people; age: unspecified; stable angina pectoris	12 mo	Coronary lesions (CHD risk factors)	Less progression, more regression, 1 vs. 2 (HDL-C, LDL-C, SBP, NS; weight decreases, 1 vs. 2)
Stanford Coronary Risk Intervention Project (Haskell et al, 1994)	1: Multifactorial risk reduction, including diet + exercise + smoking cessation, 2: Usual care	259 men, 41 women; age: 25–65 yr; angiographically documented CAD	4 yr	Coronary lesions (progression, regression) (CHD risk factors)	Lower rate of narrowing and fewer hospitalizations for cardiac events, 1 vs. 2 (LDL-C, TG, weight, glucose decreases, HDL-C increases, 1 vs. 2)

CHD, CAD, coronary heart disease, coronary artery disease; HDL-C, high-density lipoprotein cholesterol; TG, triglyceride; BP, blood pressure; NS, not significantly different; LDL-C, low-density lipoprotein cholesterol.

weight; participants with BMI ≥ 25 kg/m^2 were encouraged to reduce calorie intake so as to gradually lose weight at a rate of 0.5 to 1.0 kg/month until they achieved a BMI of 23 kg/m^2.

2. Exercise only: individuals increased leisure physical exercise by at least 1 unit (U)/day and 2 U/day for those younger than 50 years of age with no evidence of cardiovascular disease or arthritis (one U = 30 minutes mild-intensity activities such as slow walking, housecleaning; 20 minutes of moderate-intensity activities, such as faster walking, cycling; 10 minutes strenuous activity, such as slow running, table tennis; or 5 minutes of very strenuous activity, such as jumping rope, basketball, swimming).

3. Diet plus exercise.

4. Control: general information about diabetes.

The cumulative incidence of diabetes at 6 years for the 530 (92%; 283 men, 247 women) completing the trial was 67.7% in the control group, 43.8% in the diet group, 41.1% in the exercise group, and 46.0% in the diet-plus-exercise group (P < 0.05). Incidence rates of diabetes in the control group of overweight participants were higher than those in the control group of lean subjects (17.2 vs. 13.3/100 person years; P < 0.05). However, there were significantly lower incidence rates in all but one of the intervention groups. For the lean groups, diet, 8.3 (not significant); exercise, 5.1 (P < 0.01); and diet plus exercise, 6.8 (P < 0.05). For overweight group: incidence rates were 11.5, 10.8, and 11.4, respectively (P < 0.05 for all). The relative decrease in rate of development of diabetes in the active treatment groups was similar when subjects were stratified as lean (BMI < 25 kg/m^2; n = 208) or overweight (n = 322). Changes in BMI were minimal in

all four lean groups; in the overweight groups, changes in BMI were −0.9 kg/m^2 for both control and exercise only, −1.1 kg/m^2 for diet only, and −1.6 kg/m^2 for diet plus exercise. In a proportional hazards analysis adjusted for differences in baseline BMI and fasting glucose, the diet, exercise, and diet-plus-exercise interventions were associated with 31% (P < 0.03), 46% (P < 0.0005), and 42% (P < 0.0005) reductions in risk of developing diabetes, respectively. This trial is unique among the diabetes prevention trials by its inclusion of diet-only and exercise-only intervention groups, in addition to the combined group; furthermore, weight loss was not stated as an intervention goal.

The **Finnish Diabetes Prevention Trial**[19] randomly assigned 522 middle-aged (40–65 years of age) overweight men (n = 172) and women (n = 350) with IGT (plasma glucose of 140–200 mg/dl 2 hours after consuming 75 g of glucose in subjects whose plasma glucose after an overnight fast was <140 mg/dl) to:

1. Intervention: individualized counseling aimed at reducing weight by ≥5%, total fat intake to <30% of calories, and saturated fat intake to <10% of calories and increasing fiber to ≥15 g/1000 kcal and moderate physical activity to at least 30 min/day.

2. Control: no change in diet or exercise.

The mean amount of weight lost by 1 year was 0.8 kg in the control group and 4.2 kg in the intervention group (P < 0.0001); at 2 years, it was 0.8 kg in controls and 3.5 kg in the intervention group (P < 0.0001). The percentage of participants who reported more than 4 hours of exercise per week was 86% in the intervention group and 71% in the controls, which, although high, was significantly less than that in the intervention group (P < 0.001). The cumulative incidence of diabetes after 4 years (with an average of 3.2 years of follow-up) was 23% in the control group and 11% in the intervention group (i.e., a 58% reduction vs. control, P < 0.0001). Furthermore, the reduction in incidence of diabetes was directly associated with changes in lifestyle. Also noted, diabetes had not developed in any of the subjects who reached four of the five intervention goals (49 subjects in the intervention group and 15 in the control group).

The **Diabetes Prevention Program (DPP) trial**[20] randomly assigned 3234 nondiabetic persons (68% women; 45% minority; mean age of 51 years) with elevated fasting (95–125 mg/dl, 5.3–6.9 mmol/L) and postload (140–199 mg/dl, 7.8–11.0 mmol/L) plasma glucose and BMI of 24 kg/m^2 or more (≥22 kg/m^2 in Asians) to one of the following groups:

1. Intense lifestyle-modification program: with goals of at least 7% weight loss through a healthy low-calorie, low-fat diet and at least 150 min/wk of moderate-intensity physical activity, such as brisk walking (n = 1079).
2. Metformin: 850 mg twice daily plus standard lifestyle recommendations (n = 1073).
3. Placebo: standard lifestyle recommendations (n = 1082).
4. Troglitazone: The study originally included a fourth arm, troglitazone, which was discontinued because of the drug's liver toxicity.

At the close of the study 99.6% of participants were alive and 92.5% had attended scheduled visits within the previous 5 months. After an average of 2.8 years, the incidence of diabetes was 11.0% in the placebo group; 7.8% in the metformin group (31% reduction vs. placebo); and 4.8% in the lifestyle-modification group (58% reduction vs. placebo), which was significantly lower than in the metformin group. Of the lifestyle-intervention group, 50% had achieved the weight loss goal of 7% or more by week 24 and 38% had a weight loss of at least 7% at their most recent visit; the proportion who had met the physical activity goal was 74% at 24 weeks and 58% at the most recent visit. Daily energy intake at 1 year decreased by about 250 kcal in the placebo group, 300 kcal in the metformin group, and 450 kcal in the lifestyle group; average fat intake, which was 34.1% at baseline, decreased by 0.8% in the placebo and metformin groups and by 6.6% in the lifestyle-intervention group (P < 0.001). The average weight loss was 0.1, 2.1, and 5.6 kg in the placebo, metformin, and lifestyle-intervention group, respectively (P < 0.001). Metformin and lifestyle were similarly effective in restoring normal fasting glucose values, but lifestyle was more effective in restoring normal postload glucose values. Finally the effects were similar for men and women and in all racial and ethnic groups, and the lifestyle intervention was at least as effective in older versus younger participants. This study was, therefore, enormously successful both in achieving the lifestyle-intervention goals and in demonstrating their value. The independent role of weight loss and physical activity cannot be determined from this study.

A meta-analysis of controlled clinical trials of exercise on glycemic control and body mass in type 2 DM identified 12 other aerobic training studies and 2 resistance training studies, involving a total of 504 participants; this analysis concluded that exercise training reduces HbA$_{1c}$ by an amount that should decrease the risk of diabetic complications, but no significantly greater change in body mass was found when exercise groups were compared with control groups.[21] An earlier review of the effects of physical activity on insulin action and glucose tolerance in the obese concluded that the evidence is reasonably strong that insulin resistance will be reduced in the obese and among patients with type 2 DM, whereas improvements in glucose tolerance is less consistently observed and is related to exercise intensity, changes in adiposity, the interval between exercise and glucose tolerance testing, and severity of glucose intolerance before initiating an exercise training program.[22] A subsequent review by the same authors focused on possible dose-response effects of exercise on glucose homeostasis in type 2 DM and suggested that increasing levels of physical activity contribute to better diabetes prevention; however, no randomized controlled trials were identified that specifically addressed this.[23]

CLINICAL TRIALS OF PHYSICAL ACTIVITY AND/OR WEIGHT LOSS FOR REDUCING HYPERTENSTION OR MANAGING BLOOD PRESSURE

Prospective studies of factors that influence BP regulation have consistently identified weight or BMI as the strongest predictor of human BP; furthermore, it has been estimated that in up to 50% of the U.S. adults whose hypertension is being pharmacologically managed, the need for drug therapy could be alleviated with only modest reductions in body weight.[24] Although the inverse association between BP and physical activity, which generally accompanies weight loss efforts, is less clear, the NHLBI Joint National Committee on Detection, Evaluation, and Treatment of High Blood Pressure recommended that all patients with hypertension who weigh more than their ideal weight be placed on individualized, monitored weight-reduction programs involving restriction of energy intake and regular physical activity.[25]

Weight loss has been investigated in a number of trials focusing on prevention of hypertension. A decrease in BP with weight loss through calorie restriction was noted in five of the weight reduction, randomized, controlled trials involving patients with hypertension reviewed by MacMahon and colleagues in the late 1980s.[26] A more recent review of 68 study groups of both normotensive and hypertensive men and women reported an average 3.4/2.4 mm Hg (P < 0.001) weighted net reduction of BP in response to dynamic physical training that was unrelated to initial BMI.[27] It was also concluded that exercise seems to be less effective than diet in lowering BP (P < 0.02) and adding exercise to diet yields no further benefit.[27]

Several major trials, listed in Table 25-2, merit detailed review. The **Hypertension Prevention Trial (HPT)**[28] randomly assigned 841 healthy adults (549 men and 292 women), aged 25 to 49 years, who had diastolic blood pressures (DBPs) of 78 to 89 mm Hg to 3-year treatment groups, depending on BMI. Specifically, men with BMIs less than 25 kg/m² and women with BMIs less than 23 kg/m² (n = 211 total) were not assigned to calorie restriction. Otherwise, people were assigned to the following groups:

1. Reduced calories: to achieve desirable body weight (n = 125).
2. Reduced sodium: to reduce urine sodium excretion to 70 mmol or less per day (n = 196).
3. Reduced calories and reduced sodium (n = 129).
4. Reduced sodium and increased potassium: to also increase urine potassium excretion to 100 mmol or more per day and achieve a group mean 24-hour sodium-potassium excretion ratio of 1:1 (n = 195).
5. Control: no dietary counseling (n = 196).

About 90% of subjects in each group completed the 3-year visit, and 88% of all follow-up visits were completed. The treatment groups with the largest weight changes were the two calorie-restriction groups (3.4 kg vs. control for the group instructed to reduce calories only and somewhat less for those also reducing sodium). Net weight reductions attributable to calorie counseling were 3.5 kg (P < 0.001) at 3 years. BP, relative to baseline, decreased in all treatment groups, including control; however, the largest reduction was in the calorie-restricted group. The net effect of calorie counseling was to reduce mean DBP by 1.8 mm Hg and mean systolic blood pressure (SBP) by 2.4 mm Hg at 3 years (P < 0.05). At 6 months, the net effect of calorie counseling on DBP and SBP was greater than it was at 3 years (2.8 and 5.1 mm Hg, respectively), as was weight loss attributable to calorie counseling (5.8 kg; P < 0.001). The results are consistent with a beneficial effect on BP of counseling overweight people on calorie restriction; however, they also highlight the importance of maintaining weight loss.

The **Trials of Hypertension Prevention (TOHP)**[29] was a randomized, controlled clinical trial designed to determine the feasibility and efficacy of weight loss in reducing or preventing an increase in DBP. Participants, aged 30 to 54 years, who had a high-normal DBP (80 to 89 mm Hg) and were 115% to 165% of desirable body weight were randomly assigned for 18 months to:

1. Weight loss intervention, consisting of counseling on nutrition and calorie restriction; increasing physical activity by increasing daily energy expenditure, starting with walking 20 minutes at least 3 days per week and increasing to 30 to 45 minutes of activity at 40% to 55% heart rate reserve 4 or 5 times per week; and behavioral self-management techniques (n = 308).
2. Usual-care control condition (n = 256)

Compared with the usual-care group, the average weight losses in the intervention group at 6, 12, and 18 months of follow-up were 6.5 kg, 5.6 kg, and 4.7 kg, respectively, for men (P < 0.001) and 3.7 kg, 2.9 kg, and

1.8 kg, respectively, for women (P < 0.01). Mean changes in DBP and SBP for the weight loss group compared with controls at 18 months were −2.8 and −3.1 mm Hg for men and −1.1 and −2.0 mm Hg for women, respectively. BP reductions were greater for those who lost more weight. Sex-related differences in BP reduction were largely the result of a smaller amount of weight loss by women, and sex differences in weight loss could be accounted for by higher baseline body weight in men. Therefore, this trial demonstrated that weight loss, achieved by a combination of caloric restriction and physical exercise, is an effective means to reduce BP in overweight adults with high-normal BP. The independent contribution of exercise cannot be determined from these data.

Kumanyaka and colleagues examined race-specific weight loss results from these two trials and reported that mean weight change from baseline averaged 2.7 kg less in black women than in white women and 1.4 kg less in black men versus white men during the 36-month follow-up in HPT and 2.2 kg less in black women versus white women and 2.0 kg less in black versus white men during 18 months of follow-up in TOHP.[30]

The **Trial of Antihypertensive Interventions and Management (TAIM)**[31] was a multicenter, double-blind, placebo-controlled, clinical trial of drug and diet combinations for the treatment of mild hypertension among 878 participants, aged 21 to 65 years, who were 110% to 160% of ideal weight with a baseline DBP of 90 to 100 mm Hg. Individuals were randomly assigned, after stratification by center and race, to take one of three drugs for 6 months:

1. Chlorthalidone; diuretic: (25 mg/day).
2. Atenolol; beta-blocker: (50 mg/day).
3. Placebo pills.

Individuals were randomly assigned again to combine their drug with one of three diets:

A. Weight reduction.
B. Sodium restriction and potassium increase.
C. Usual (no change in diet).

Of the 878 patients randomized, 787 (89.6%) had BP readings at both baseline and 6 months; more than half were men, about one third were black, and about two-thirds had been on drug therapy at entry that was withdrawn prior to randomization. DBP fell in all nine diet/drug combination groups. Drugs outperformed diet in terms of antihypertensive effect; however, the weight loss diet was significantly better than usual diet or sodium restriction with increased potassium, and the addition of weight loss to either drug regimen resulted in a greater BP reduction, by 4 mm Hg for the diuretic and 2 mm Hg for the beta blocker. Subjects on placebo and assigned to weight reduction who lost more than 4.5 kg (and those on sodium restriction who reduced sodium to <70 mEq/day) lowered BP to a similar extent as those on either of the two drugs alone. The TAIM investigators concluded that weight loss added to either drug provided the most beneficial regimen.

The **Treatment of Mild Hypertension Study (TOMHS)**[32-34] was a 4-year randomized, double-blind, placebo-controlled clinical trial in 557 men and 345 women, aged 45 to 69 years, with stage 1 hypertension

(DBP < 100 mm Hg), assigned to one of six antihypertensive treatments, all of which were combined with sustained nutritional-hygienic advice to reduce weight, dietary sodium intake, and alcohol intake and to increase physical activity.

1. Chlorthalidone, diuretic (n = 136).
2. Acebutolol, beta blocker (n = 132).
3. Doxazosin mesylate, α_1-antagonist (n = 134).
4. Amlodipine maleate, calcium antagonist (n = 131).
5. Enalapril maleate, angiotensin-converting enzyme inhibitor (n = 135).
6. Placebo (n = 234).

On average, participants were obese at baseline, being 30% over desirable weight, with a mean BMI of 28.9 kg/m². Lifestyle intervention was identical for all groups, resulting in an average loss of 3.6 kg in participants overall, with significant decreases from baseline in reported energy intake, dietary cholesterol, and intake of fats.[33] BP reductions were sizable in all six groups but were significantly (P < 0.001) greater for participants assigned to drug treatment than placebo (SBP, −15.9 vs. −9.1 mm Hg; DBP, −12.3 vs. −8.6 mm Hg); however, the lifestyle intervention was associated with substantial reductions in SBP and DBP, so fewer than one third of participants assigned to the placebo group were taking antihypertensive drugs after 4 years of follow-up. Mean changes in all plasma lipids were also favorable in all groups, and the degree of weight loss was significantly related to favorable lipid changes, although there were significant differences (P < 0.01) among treatment groups for average lipid changes.[33,34] Reported leisure time physical activity increased by 86% at 1 year and remained 50% above baseline at 4 years.[34] Although the independent contribution of physical activity to weight loss and changes in BP or lipids is unclear in TOMHS, the fact that more than 50% of initial weight loss was maintained during the 4 years of the trial is consistent with the concept that adoption of exercise improves long-term maintenance of weight loss.

Blumenthal and colleagues[35] assessed the independent effects of exercise training in patients with mild, untreated hypertension (SBP: 140–180 mm Hg; DBP: 90–105 mm Hg) by assigning 57 men and 42 women to 4 months of one of the following:

1. Aerobic exercise training: 3 sessions per week of warm-up and 35 minutes of walking or jogging at 70% of baseline aerobic capacity (n = 39).
2. Strength and flexibility training: 20 minutes of flexibility exercises, followed by 30 minutes of circuit training, 2 or 3 times per week (n = 31).
3. Wait-list control group: no changes in exercise; (n = 22).

With 93% of subjects completing the study, aerobic exercisers increased aerobic capacity (mL/kg/min) by 15.6% (5.1), which was significant (P < 0.01) compared with small increases in strength trainers (4.4%; 1.1) and controls (0.8%; 0.2), which did not differ from each other. There were no changes in diet or weight within or between groups. All groups showed significant (P < 0.001) decreases from baseline in SBP (−7 to

−9 mm Hg) and DBP (−6 mm Hg in all); however, there were no significant differences between groups, suggesting that a program of moderate exercise without dietary changes in hypertensive patients of normal body weight and average level of fitness offers relatively little benefit to BP reduction.

Steffen and colleagues[36] investigated the BP effects of exercise training and weight loss associated with physical activity and emotional stress in daily life by randomizing 112 participants with unmedicated high normal or stage 1 to stage 2 hypertension to one of the following:

1. Combined exercise and behavioral weight management (WM): same exercise as in 2 plus a weight loss goal of 1 to 2 lb/wk by reducing caloric intake, with 15% to 20% of calories coming from fat.
2. Exercise only (EX): 35 minutes, plus 10 minute warm-up and 10 minute cool-down, supervised exercise 3 to 4 times/wk at 70% to 85% of initial heart rate (HR), with no change in diet.
3. Wait-list control: no change in exercise for 6 months.

BP was assessed in the clinic and during 15-hour daytime ambulatory BP monitoring at baseline and 6 months of treatment. Both WM and EX increased VO₂max and treadmill time versus control. WM also increased treadmill time versus EX. Subjects in WM lost significantly more weight (−7.9 kg) than EX (−1.8 kg) or control (0.7 kg). Increased physical activity and emotional distress measured during daily life were associated with increases in SBP, DBP, HR, and rate pressure product (RPP). After treatment the WM group had significantly lower DBP, HR, and RPP response during both high and low levels of physical activity and emotional distress compared with the control group. The EX group had similar BP levels as the WM group, although the EX group had significantly lower BP versus the control group during low but not high levels of physical activity and emotional distress. These findings indicate that exercise may not be as effective in reducing BP during activities of daily life as is adding weight loss with regular exercise.

CLINICAL TRIALS OF PHYSICAL ACTIVITY AND/OR WEIGHT LOSS FOR MANAGING DYSLIPIDEMIAS AND CHANGING LIPOPROTEINS

Cross-sectional and observational studies in the mid-1970s generated the hypothesis that physical activity increased HDL-C and decreased triglycerides (TG),[37] which prompted the initiation of RCTs to test this hypothesis.[38,39] Several of the larger trials over the past 25 years are presented in table 25-3. The two earliest RCTs[40,41] involved men who were neither overweight nor characterized by having low HDL-C (i.e., ≤40 mg/dl [≤1.03 mmol/L]), or elevated TG (i.e., ≥200 mg/dl [≥2.26 mmol/L]), as defined by NCEP ATP III.[11] Nonetheless, Huttenen and colleagues[40] reported a significant increase in HDL-C and a decrease in TG in 90 men randomized to aerobic exercise or control, with no weight loss.

The **Stanford Exercise Study,**[41] randomly assigned 81 middle-aged men for 1 year to:

1. Aerobic exercise: approximately 45 minutes of supervised walking or jogging three times per week (n = 48).
2. Control: no change in exercise (n = 33).

This study, which offered no instruction on diet for either group, was completed by 93% of subjects and found no significant changes in any lipoproteins, but the exercisers lost 2.5 kg (P < 0.001) and reduced percent body fat by 3.8% (P < 0.0001). Secondary analyses that separated exercisers into four "treatment-dose" groups (based on weekly mileage achieved: 0-3.9; 4-7.9; 8-12.9; and 13 + miles) revealed significant treatment effects for HDL-C (Spearman's rho = 0.48; P < 0.001) and for low-density lipoprotein cholesterol (LDL-C) (R = −0.31; P = 0.04). In exercisers who averaged at least 8 miles (12.9 km) per week (n = 25), HDL-C increased by 4.4 mg/dl (P < 0.05) compared with controls. Further exploratory analyses, which excluded exercisers who reported active dieting, showed that the weekly mileage correlated significantly with body fat changes (R = −0.49; P = 0.002), which were significantly related to HDL-C changes (R = −0.47; P = 0.004), suggesting that weight loss could be responsible for the HDL-C increases seen with increased physical activity.[42]

The first **Stanford Weight Control Project (SWCP-I)**[43] was designed to address this question by randomly assigning 155 sedentary, moderately overweight (20% to 50% above ideal body weight) men, aged 35 to 59 years, to one of three groups for 1 year:

1. Weight loss by increased aerobic exercise: consisting of approximately 45 minutes of supervised walking or jogging three times per week, with no dietary changes (n = 52).
2. Weight loss by caloric restriction: without changing diet composition or activity level (n = 51).
3. Control: no change in caloric intake, diet composition, or physical activity.

One-year measurements were made on 81% of controls, 82% of dieters, and 90% of exercisers. Caloric reduction was significant (P < 0.01) in dieters versus controls at 7 months (about 335 kcal/day) and 1 year (about 240 kcal/day), whereas caloric intake did not differ between exercisers and controls at either time point. At 1 year, VO₂max had increased in exercisers, compared with controls (6.5 mL/kg/min; P < 0.001) and dieters (4.1 mL/kg/min; P < 0.001). Compared with controls, total and fat weight losses were significantly greater (P < 0.001) in both dieters (7.8 kg and 6.2 kg, respectively) and exercisers (4.6 kg and 4.4 kg). Lean mass loss was greater only in dieters (2.1 kg), who also lost more lean weight than exercisers (1.4 kg; P < 0.01). Fat weight loss did not differ significantly between dieters and exercisers. HDL-C was elevated (P < 0.01) in both dieters (4.2 mg/dl) and exercisers (4.6 mg/dl) at 1 year, compared with controls, whereas TG was reduced (−23.9 and −14.2 mg/dl, respectively; P < 0.05). These changes did not differ significantly between the two weight loss groups.

LDL-C did not differ significantly across groups. Thus, weight loss achieved by caloric restriction alone, with no change in the proportion of calories from fat, or by exercise with no dietary changes, improved HDL-C and TG levels but did not alter LDL-C, and there was no greater benefit of weight loss by exercise versus caloric restriction.

Katzel and colleagues[44] pursued the question of the role of weight loss by exercise further by randomly assigning 170 sedentary, obese (120% to 160% of ideal body weight) men, aged 46 to 80 years, for 1 year to one of three groups:

1. Weight loss: hypocaloric NCEP Step I diet,[45] with total fat less than 30% of calories, saturated fat less than 10% of calories, and dietary cholesterol less than 300 mg/day (n = 73)
2. Aerobic exercise: consisting of 45 minutes of treadmill and cycle ergometer workouts, three times per week (n = 71).
3. Control: no weight loss or change in activity level (n = 26).

Prior to baseline testing, all three groups were instructed for 3 months on an isoenergetic reduced-fat diet, and men in both the aerobic exercise and control groups were encouraged to continue this diet, without losing weight, throughout the trial. One-year measurements were made on 69% of controls, 60% of men assigned to weight loss, and 69% of men assigned to exercise. Men assigned to weight loss lost about 9.5 kg, 75% of which was fat mass, and did not change VO₂max; whereas exercisers did not change average weight, although percent body fat was decreased 0.8% (P < 0.005), but did increase VO₂max (about 7.0 mL/kg of fat-free mass per minute, i.e., 17% above baseline) compared with the other two groups (P < 0.001). Compared with controls, HDL-C was significantly (P < 0.01) increased (about 4.6 mg/dl) in the weight loss group but not in the exercise group, whereas TG, total cholesterol (TC), and LDL-C were decreased (P < 0.05) in both the weight loss and exercise groups, with no differences between them. SBPs and DBPs were reduced in men in the weight loss group compared with controls (P < 0.01) and with exercisers (P < 0.05), whereas BP changes did not differ between the exercisers and controls. There were also significant reductions in fasting plasma glucose and insulin in the weight loss group versus controls (P < 0.01) and the exercise group (P < 0.05). In summary, weight loss by a hypocaloric, reduced-fat diet resulted in significantly greater CHD risk-factor reduction than was achieved by increasing physical activity without substantial weight loss.

The second **Stanford Weight Control Project (SWCP-II)**[46] pursued the question of weight loss by a reduced-fat diet, with and without exercise, in women as well as men, by randomly assigning moderately overweight premenopausal women (BMI = 24–30 kg/m²) and men (BMI = 28–34 kg/m²), aged 25 to 49 years, to one of three groups for 1 year:

1. Weight loss by a hypocaloric, reduced-fat diet: specifically reducing fat calories to achieve an NCEP Step I diet[45] and weight loss.
2. Weight loss by the hypocaloric, reduced-fat diet plus aerobic exercise: identical diet combined with

approximately 45 minutes of supervised walking or jogging, 3 times per week.
3. Control: no changes in diet or physical activity level.

One-year measurements were completed on about 90% of men and women in each treatment group, except diet-only women (74%; $P < 0.052$ vs. other female groups). Total calories, percentage of calories from total and saturated fat, and dietary cholesterol were reduced in both diet-only and diet-plus-exercise groups of men and women versus control ($P < 0.001$). Aerobic capacity (ml/kg/min) improved significantly ($P < 0.001$) in men in the diet-plus-exercise group compared with control (8.8) and men in the diet-only group (7.0) and in women in the diet-plus-exercise group versus control (6.4) and women in the diet-only group (5.0).

In SWCP-II women,[46] weight loss was significant ($P < 0.001$) in both dieters (5.4 kg) and dieting exercisers (6.4 kg) versus control, as was fat weight loss (4.5 kg and 6.0 kg, respectively), with no significant differences between weight loss groups. Lean mass loss did not differ between groups. Compared with controls, diet-only women had decreases in HDL-C (-3.9 mg/dl; NS), HDL_2-C (-4.3 mg/dl; $P < 0.05$), and apolipoprotein AI (-8.8 mg/dl; $P < 0.05$), whereas women in the diet-plus-exercise group increased HDL-C (2.7 mg/dl; NS) and apolipoprotein AI (1.9 mg/dl; NS) and decreased TG (-13.3 mg/dl; $P < 0.05$). HDL-C thus was increased significantly in women in the diet-plus-exercise group (6.6 mg/dl; $P < 0.01$) versus women in the diet-only group. Both dieters and dieting exercisers reduced TC (-13.9 and -9.7 mg/dl, respectively; $P < 0.05$), LDL-C (-9.7 and -10.1 mg/dl; $P < 0.05$), and apolipoprotein B (-5.8 and -6.0 mg/dl; $P < 0.01$) versus control and there were no differences between dieters and dieting exercisers. Neither the LDL-C-to-HDL-C ratio nor the apolipoprotein B-to-AI ratio were improved in dieters, whereas both ratios were reduced in dieting exercisers ($P < 0.05$) versus controls.

In SWCP-II men,[46] weight loss was significant ($P < 0.001$) in both dieters (6.8 kg) and dieting exercisers (10.4 kg) compared with controls, as was fat weight loss (5.5 kg and 9.0 kg, respectively), which was greater in dieting exercisers versus diet-only ($P < 0.001$). Lean mass loss was also significant ($P < 0.05$) in dieters (1.3 kg) and dieting exercisers (1.4 kg) versus control but did not differ between intervention groups. HDL-C was significantly increased in dieting exercisers (7.3 mg/dl; $P < 0.001$), as was apolipoprotein AI (7.2 mg/dl; $P < 0.01$), compared with controls, whereas HDL-C was not significantly increased in dieters (2.7 mg/dl), so HDL-C increased in dieting exercisers versus diet-only ($P < 0.01$). Diet-plus-exercise men also decreased TG versus control (-58.5 mg/dl; $P < 0.001$) and diet-only (-31.9 mg/dl; $P < 0.05$); however, LDL-C decreases were not significant in either dieters (-7.4 mg/dl) or dieting exercisers (-2.8 mg/dl) versus controls, who decreased LDL-C by about 5% from baseline; however, apolipoprotein B was reduced ($P < 0.01$) in both dieters (-5.8 mg/dl) and dieting exercisers (-6.0 mg/dl) versus controls. Reductions in the LDL-C-to-HDL-C ratio were significant in both diet-only and diet-plus-exercise men

versus control ($P < 0.05$), with no differences between them. There was also a significant reduction in the ratio of apolipoprotein B to apolipoprotein AI in dieters ($P < 0.01$) and dieting exercisers ($P < 0.001$) versus control, and this reduction was greater in the men who were assigned to diet plus exercise versus those who were assigned only to diet ($P < 0.05$). Resting systolic and diastolic BP were significantly reduced in both diet-only and diet-plus-exercise women and men versus controls, with no differences between groups.

Therefore, in both men and women, the addition of exercise to a reduced-fat, weight-reducing diet improved HDL-C compared with diet alone and improved the lipoprotein profile compared with controls but did not produce further reductions in BP. The facts that the diet-only women had reductions in HDL-C, despite weight loss, which did not differ significantly from the diet-plus-exercise group, and that SWCP-II[46] men lost only slightly less total (6.2 kg) and fat (5.5 kg) body weight than SWCP-I[43] men (7.8 vs. 6.8 kg, respectively), but did not have HDL-C increases, were interpreted as an HDL-lowering effect of a reduced-fat diet. These data suggested that greater weight loss, or the addition of exercise, might be necessary to raise HDL-C with a reduced-fat diet compared with caloric restriction without changing diet composition. Thus, the significant HDL-C increases in the men who lost weight with a hypocaloric NCEP Step I diet[45] in the Katzel study[44] may be explained by the fact that the men who completed that trial lost more weight (9.5 kg) than diet-only men in the SWCP-II[46] (7.1 kg).

The **Stanford-Sunnyvale Health Improvement Program (SSHIP)**[47] focused on adherence to home- versus group-based exercise programs and different training intensities in older women and men by randomly assigning 197 men and 160 women, aged 50 to 65 years, to one of four 1-year groups:

1. High-intensity, group-based aerobic exercise: involving three 40-minute endurance training sessions per week at 73% to 88% of peak treadmill heart rate.
2. High-intensity, home-based aerobic exercise: the same prescription but performed by people from their home.
3. Low-intensity home-based aerobic exercise: five 30-minute sessions per week at 60% to 73% of maximum heart rate.
4. Control: no change in activity level.

One-year assessments were completed on 85% of randomized subjects. All three exercise-training conditions resulted in significant ($P < 0.03$) improvements in VO_2max, averaging a 5% increase, compared with controls, with no significant weight or body composition changes. Neither men nor women in any of the exercise conditions showed significant changes, versus control, in HDL-C, LDL-C, TC, TG, or resting BP, providing further evidence that aerobic exercise training may not bring about significant improvements in lipid levels or BP in the absence of substantial weight loss or dietary change.

At the end of the 1-year, controlled trial, SSHIP controls were offered an exercise program, whereas men and women randomized into the three exercise groups were encouraged to continue their originally assigned exercise prescriptions for a second year.[48] At the end of this year, significant HDL-C increases (P < 0.01) were seen within each of the two home-based groups (sexes combined) compared with their baseline values. These increases were especially pronounced for the lower-intensity, home-based group, despite greater exercise adherence rates in the higher-intensity, home-based group (P < 0.003), who also most successfully maintained their treadmill exercise test performance. The investigators suggested that the frequency of exercise bouts might be particularly important for achieving such changes. For all exercise conditions, HDL-C increases were associated with decreases in waist-to-hip ratio in both men and women (P < 0.04).

Svendsen and associates[49] studied the effects of combined aerobic and anaerobic exercise added to a weight loss diet in a trial of 121 overweight (self-reported BMI ≥25 kg/m²) postmenopausal women, aged 45 to 54 years, who were randomly assigned for 12 weeks to:

1. Energy-restricted diet: a formula diet (NUPO) within which all international recommendations for proteins, essential amino acids, vitamins, minerals, and trace elements were met, with additional energy consumption of food not to exceed a total of about 1000 kcal/day (n = 51).
2. Diet plus combined aerobic and anaerobic exercise: the NUPO diet plus three sessions per week of 1 to 1.5 hours of aerobic exercise, such as bicycling, stair climbing, or treadmill running, and resistance training (n = 49).
3. Control: no change in diet or exercise (n = 21).

More than 97% of women completed the trial. Total energy intake and percentage of calories from fat decreased in the two dieting groups versus controls but did not differ between them. Aerobic capacity (mL/kg/min) increased in the dieting exercisers compared with controls (5.1) and dieters (4.6). Total weight loss was significant in both diet-only (10.0 kg) and diet-plus-exercise (10.8 kg) women compared with controls and did not differ between them; however, the dieting exercisers lost more fat weight (1.8 kg; P < 0.001) than diet only, who also lost 1.2 kg lean weight, whereas dieting exercisers did not. Despite considerable weight loss in the diet and diet-plus-exercise groups, HDL-C changes did not differ among groups; however, TG, TC, and LDL-C decreased in dieters and dieting exercisers compared with controls (P < 0.001) and did not differ between the two weight loss groups. Therefore, the addition of combined aerobic and anaerobic exercise to a hypocaloric, reduced-fat diet that effected substantial weight loss produced no greater CHD risk-factor reduction in postmenopausal women than what was seen with the diet alone.

Boyden and colleagues[50] studied anaerobic exercise in eumenorrheic, premenopausal women, aged 28 to 39 years, who were randomly assigned for 5 months to:

1. Supervised resistance exercise training: (n = 56).
2. Control: no exercise (n = 47).

With 89% of controls and 82% of exercisers completing the trial. Fat-free mass increased 1.2 kg in exercisers relative to controls (P < 0.001); however, there were no significant changes in total body weight, HDL-C, or TG. Exercisers, however, reduced TC (about 9.5 mg/dl) and LDL-C (about 11.5 mg/dl) significantly versus controls (P < 0.04). Further clinical trials designed to investigate differences between aerobic and resistance exercise seem warranted.

Hellenius and associates[51] focused on individuals with slightly adverse lipoproteins by randomly assigning 158 normoglycemic, middle-aged, nonobese men who had slightly to moderately elevated TC to 6 months of one of the following:

1. Reduced-fat diet: including advice on caloric intake to reach or maintain desirable body weight (n = 40).
2. Aerobic exercise: 30 to 45 minutes of activities such as walking and jogging at 60% to 80% of maximal heart rate, two or three times per week (n = 39).
3. Diet plus exercise: same diet as 1, same exercise as 2 (n = 39).
4. Control: no further diet intervention and no exercise (n = 40).

With 99% of the men completing 6-month assessments, total energy intake was reduced only in the dieting exercisers, whereas the percentage of calories from fat was significantly reduced in diet-only and diet-plus-exercise men versus control. Exercise and diet-plus-exercise men reported more activity than control and diet-only men; however, aerobic capacity was not measured. Reductions in BMI (kg/m²) were slight but significant (P < 0.01) versus control and in diet only (−0.6), exercise only (−0.6), and diet plus exercise (−0.9); however, there were no significant differences in lipoprotein changes between groups.

The **Diet and Exercise for Elevated Risk (DEER) trial**[52] also focused on individuals with adverse lipoproteins by randomly assigning 197 men, aged 30 to 64 years, and 180 postmenopausal women, aged 45 to 64 years, who had HDL-C levels below the sex-specific mean of the population (≤44 mg/dl for men; ≤59 mg/dl for women) combined with moderately elevated LDL-C (125–189 mg/dl for men; 125–209 mg/dl for women) and were not severely overweight (BMI ≤34 kg/m² for men; ≤32 kg/m² for women) for 1 year to one of four groups:

1. NCEP Step II diet[45] (total fat <30% of calories, saturated fat <7% of calories, dietary cholesterol <200 mg/day, and advice on caloric intake to reach or maintain desirable body weight) (n = 49 men; 47 women).
2. Aerobic exercise: 45 minutes of walking, jogging, or comparable activity at 60% to 80% of maximum heart rate at least three times per week (n = 50 men; 44 women).
3. NCEP Step II diet plus aerobic exercise (n = 51 men; 43 women)
4. Control: no change in caloric intake or activity (n = 47 men; 46 women).

More than 95% of men and women completed 1-year tests in each group. Mean dietary goals were achieved in all diet groups and aerobic capacity (mL/kg/min) was increased in all exercise groups, whereas controls made no changes. At 1 year, total and fat weight losses were significant compared with controls in dieters and dieting exercisers in both sexes but did not differ between diet only and diet plus exercise in either sex.

In DEER men, dieters lost a mean of 3.3 kg (2.1 kg fat weight) and dieting exercisers lost 4.7 kg (3.5 kg fat weight) compared with controls, whereas weight loss in exercisers (1.2 kg, 1.0 kg fat weight) was not significant. Lean mass loss did not differ between dieters or dieting exercisers and control men but was significantly greater in both dieting groups compared with exercise only (1.3 kg for both). In DEER women, dieters lost a mean of 3.5 kg and dieting exercisers lost 3.9 kg compared with controls, whereas weight loss in exercisers (1.2 kg) was not significant. Lean mass losses were minimal and did not differ between groups.

HDL-C changes did not differ between any treatment groups, in men or women; therefore, neither the modest weight loss achieved by the diet nor the increased physical activity increased HDL-C in men or women who would be encouraged to adopt these lifestyle changes to improve their lipoprotein profile. Furthermore, compared with controls, LDL-C reductions were not significant in men or women who adopted the NCEP Step II diet without increasing activity level or in men or women who increased their exercise level without altering their diet; however, significant LDL-C reductions were seen in both men and women assigned to the diet plus aerobic exercise ($P < 0.01$). (Even when analyses combined men and women, thereby increasing the number of subjects per treatment group, LDL-C decreases were not significant in the diet-only group versus control, nor did HDL-C changes differ significantly among groups.) Neither TGs nor BP changes differed significantly in men or women among DEER groups, whereas fasting glucose was reduced in both diet-only and diet-plus-exercise men and women, relative to controls ($P < 0.01$), and in men, glucose was reduced 2 hours after consumption of oral glucose in both dieters and dieting exercisers versus controls. (This was not seen in women.) Neither fasting nor 2-hour glucose reductions differed between dieters and dieting exercisers in either sex.

McCarron and colleagues[53] also focused on individuals at elevated CHD risk by randomly assigning 246 men and 314 women, aged 26 to 70 years, who had one or more CHD risk factors: dyslipidemia (TC 220 to 300 mg/dl or TG levels 200 to 1000 mg/dl), hypertension (sitting SBP of 140 to 180 mm Hg and/or DBP of 90 to 105 mm Hg), or noninsulin-dependent diabetes mellitus (fasting glucose >140 mg/dl but not taking hypoglycemic agents) to one of the following:

1. Campbell's Center for Nutrition and Wellness (CCNW) plan: composed of prepackaged breakfast, lunch, and dinner meals provided to participants.
2. Nutritionist-guided AHA Step I and Step II diet[45]: participants self-selected foods to meet their nutrition prescription for 10 weeks.

Mean weight loss with the CCNW and self-selected AHA Step I/II plans, respectively, was as follows: men, −4.5 kg and −3.5 kg; women, −4.8 and −2.8 kg, which was significant between groups when sexes were combined ($P = 0.03$). The 10-week visit was completed by 92.6% of the CCNW group and 96.8% of the self-selected diet group. Participants in both groups decreased energy intake and significantly changed intake of most nutrients compared with baseline, with greater reduction in percentage of calories from fat in the CCNW versus self-selected AHA Step I/II group ($P < 0.001$). There was no group that did not change their diet (or weight). Compared with their baseline values, both diet groups had significant ($P < 0.01$) decreases in TC, HDL-C, LDL-C, and TG, but not LDL-C/HDL-C, and fasting glucose, insulin, glycosylated hemoglobin, hemoglobin A_{Ic}, and fructosamine, but none of these changes differed between groups. It was unclear whether risk reduction was specific to those at elevated risk for a given factor; however, this study demonstrated CHD risk reduction with two different diet-induced weight loss programs.

The **Diet and Moderate Exercise Trial (DAMET)**[54] also focused on individuals with one or more CHD risk factors: BP 150/95 mm Hg or higher; DM by a positive glucose tolerance test; TC level higher than 250 mg/dl; TG level higher than 190 mg/dl; smoking fewer than 10 cigarettes per day; obesity more than 10% of normal weight for that age, sex, and height (per LIC, India); physical inactivity less than 1 km walking per day; family history of CHD; or personal history of CHD. DAMET randomly assigned 419 men and 44 women from a South Asian population, with stratification for each risk factor, to one of two groups for 24 weeks:

1. Group A: AHA Step I (reduced-fat) diet plus fruits and vegetables plus exercise: AHA Step I diet plus 400 g/day of fruits and vegetables rich in dietary fiber and antioxidants (vitamins A, C, E, carotene, copper, selenium, and magnesium), plus, after 4 weeks of diet only, moderate exercise was added, consisting of brisk walking 3 to 4 km per day or spot running 10 to 15 minutes per day (n = 231).
2. Group B: AHA Step I diet only (n = 232).

Data were analyzed at 4 weeks, when the two interventions differed only by the fruit-and-vegetable component of the diet, at which time no significant differences were seen between groups for changes in body weight or CHD risk-factor status. At 24 weeks, after 20 weeks of exercise in addition to the dietary regimen, group A had lost 6.5 kg (9.8% reduction from baseline), whereas group B had lost only 0.3 kg ($P < 0.01$ vs. A). Group A showed significantly ($P < 0.01$) greater decreases in TC, LDL-C, TG, fasting blood glucose, and BPs and a greater increase in HDL-C compared with group B. Whether these differences were due to differences in diet composition between groups, to the addition of moderate exercise in group A, or to the greater weight loss in group A is unclear.

The **Studies of Targeted Risk Reduction Interventions through Defined Exercise (STRRIDE)**[55] focused on the amount and intensity of exercise required to benefit lipoproteins by randomly assigning 159 sedentary overweight or mildly obese men and women, aged 40 to 65, with mild-to-moderate dyslipidemia (either LDL 130-190 mg/dl, i.e., 3.4-4.9 mmol/L, or HDL <40 mg/dl for men, i.e., <1.0 mmol/L, or <45 mg/dl for women, i.e., <1.2 mmol/L) to one of the following:

1. High-amount, high intensity (HH) exercise: (8 months) caloric equivalent of jogging 20 mi (32.0 km) per week at 65% to 80% VO$_2$max.
2. Low-amount, high intensity (LH) exercise: (8 months) equivalent of jogging 12 mi (19.5 km) per week at 65% to 80% VO$_2$max.
3. Low-amount, moderate-intensity (LM) exercise: (8 months) equivalent of jogging 12 mi (19.5 km) per week at 40% to 55% VO$_2$max.
4. Control: no exercise for 6 months.

Subjects were encouraged to maintain baseline body weight. Of subjects, 70% completed the trial; however, analyses excluded an additional 10.7% of subjects because of low adherence or excessive weight loss, in addition to 6.3% because of incomplete data, so analyses included only 53% of randomized subjects. Exercise training had no effect on total or LDL cholesterol, but HH reduced the concentrations of small LDL particles, measured by nuclear magnetic resonance spectroscopy, as did LH. Only HH had significant HDL-C increases, with minimal weight; however, there were improvements in TG concentrations and large very-low–density lipoprotein particles in all three exercise groups (although not significant in LH). The authors suggested that the effect on lipids of the intensity of exercise was small compared with that of the amount of exercise.

Taken together, these trials suggest that physical activity accompanied by weight loss has HDL-C-raising and TG-lowering effects, but there is little trial evidence that LDL-C is reduced by physical activity or weight loss without a reduction in dietary (saturated) fat. A reduced-fat diet, however, also has an HDL-lowering effect; furthermore, it is not very effective at lowering LDL-C in men or postmenopausal women who have low HDL-C in addition to mildly elevated LDL-C, unless they increase physical activity (and/or lose at least a modest amount of weight). In the absence of substantial weight loss, physical activity might need to be of higher intensity, greater volume, or conducted on a more regular basis (i.e., 5 days/wk rather than 3) to bring about significant HDL elevation (and/or TG reduction).

PHYSICAL ACTIVITY OR WEIGHT LOSS FOR MANAGING THE METABOLIC SYNDROME

The NCEP ATP-III[11] defined a constellation of CHD risk factors that enhance the risk of CHD at any given LDL level, the "metabolic syndrome," which is characterized by having any three of the following five risk factors: abdominal obesity (waist circumference in men >102 cm [40 in] and in women >88 cm [35 in]); elevated triglycerides (≥150 mg/dl); low HDL-C (<40 mg/dl in men; <50 mg/dl in women); raised BP (≥130/≥85 mm Hg); and fasting glucose of 110 mg/dl or more. This "syndrome" is closely linked to the generalized metabolic disorder, insulin resistance. The first-line therapies for all lipid and nonlipid the risk factors associated with the metabolic syndrome are weight reduction and increased physical activity.[11] The prevalence of metabolic syndrome is quite high in the United States,[56] and since the NCEP ATP-III was released (2001), there has been considerable interest in the effects of weight loss and/or physical activity on this constellation of risk factors and on abdominal obesity. Visceral fat and central adiposity have been shown to be substantially reduced by weight loss achieved by regular increased physical activity in men and women[57-59]; furthermore, exercise without weight loss reduced abdominal fat and prevented further weight gain in men.[58] It is unclear whether this is true for women as well.[59,60] Several trials have been initiated in adults who meet the criteria of metabolic syndrome since ATP-III's release, and these results will be published over time.

TRIALS OF PHYSICAL ACTIVITY AND WEIGHT LOSS IN INDIVIDUALS WITH PRE-ESTABLISHED CARDIOVASCULAR DISEASE

Several clinical trials have been designed to determine whether lifestyle changes, such as exercise and diets that may cause weight loss, can facilitate secondary prevention of CHD. Four are reviewed here and presented in Table 25-4.

In the **Lifestyle Heart Trial**,[61] patients with angiographically documented coronary artery disease were assigned for 1 year to one of the following:

1. Experimental group: (n = 22), involving adopting a low-fat, vegetarian diet (about 10% calories from fat, with no animal products, including fruits, vegetables, grains, legumes, and soybean products, without calorie restriction) and engaging in moderate exercise (typically walking at 50% to 80% of maximum heart rate) as well as stopping smoking and undergoing stress management training.
2. Usual-care control group: (n = 19).

The experimental group lost significant weight (10.1 kg) compared with controls (P < 0.0001), who gained 1.4 kg, and the lifestyle change group decreased LDL-C (37.4%) versus control (P < 0.01); however, HDL-C, TG, and BP changes were minimal and did not differ between groups. CHD symptoms decreased markedly in the experimental group, whereas they increased in the usual-care group. Moreover, the average percentage diameter stenosis regressed in the experimental group but progressed in the control group. Overall, 82% of experimental group patients had an average change toward regression, and adherence to the lifestyle changes was reported to be strongly related to changes in lesions in a "dose-response" manner. Although the independent contribution of weight loss or exercise on CHD risk reduction cannot be determined, these data are consistent with the concept that these lifestyle changes are beneficial, even in the absence of BP reduction that would have been expected to occur with the major weight loss seen in the trial, or HDL-C elevation, which might be related to the extreme reduction in dietary fat.

Singh and colleagues conducted another randomized trial that involved increasing fruit and vegetable intake and reducing fat intake, without other lifestyle interventions, in patients with a definite or possible acute MI.[62] Patients were randomly assigned to:

1. AHA Step I dietary recommendations: advice on how to adopt a reduced-fat diet, followed by usual care (n = 202).
2. AHA Step I/II reduced-fat diet: with the addition of increased fruits, vegetables, and nuts and regular reinforcement (n = 204).

Adherence to the diet was significantly higher in the group that received the more intensive counseling, and after 1 year this group had lost 6.3 kg, compared with 2.4 kg in the less-intensive group (P < 0.01). The intensive-diet group showed significant reductions in LDL-C, TG, fasting blood glucose, and SBP and DBP and increases in HDL-C compared with the less-intensive group; furthermore, the incidence of cardiac events was significantly lower in the intensive-diet group (50 vs. 82; P < 0.001), who also had lower total mortality (21 vs. 38; P < 0.01). The differences were attributed to the more comprehensive dietary changes and greater weight loss of the group that reduced fat intake and increased fruits, vegetables, and nuts intake.

Schuller and colleagues investigated the effects of intensive physical exercise and low-fat diet on coronary morphology and myocardial perfusion in patients who were recruited after routine coronary angiography for stable angina pectoris[63] and randomized to:

1. Intervention: group exercise training at least two times per week and daily home exercise on a bicycle ergometer, 30 minutes a day at 75% maximum heart rate, and an AHA Phase 3 low-fat (<20% of calories), low-cholesterol (<200 mg/day) diet (n = 56).
2. Usual care control (n = 57).

Patients in the intervention group decreased total calories and decreased body weight (by 5%), which was significant versus the usual-care group (P < 0.001). Fat consumption and dietary cholesterol were also significantly reduced versus control, as were TC and TG. Change in body weight was significantly correlated to change in cholesterol (P < 0.001), as was compliance with attending group exercise sessions. HDL-C, LDL-C, and resting SBP changes did not differ between groups. Progression of coronary artery disease was reduced in patients in the diet and exercise group, while regression was greater, compared with usual care (P < 0.001).

The **Stanford Coronary Risk Intervention Project (SCRIP)** randomly assigned 259 men and 41 women with angiographically defined coronary atherosclerosis[64] to 4 years of one of the following:

1. Multifactorial risk reduction: which included instruction on a low-fat (<20% of calories; <6% of calories from saturated fat), low-cholesterol (<75 mg/day) diet and caloric restriction to reduce weight to 100%

to 110% of ideal body weight; a physical activity program consisting of an increase in daily activities such as walking, climbing stairs, and household chores; and a stop-smoking and relapse-prevention program for smokers. If LDL-C goals (110 mg/dL) were not likely to be achieved in a risk-reduction participant within the first year without drug therapy, a cholesterol-lowering drug regimen was added. (n = 145).
2. Usual care: (n = 155).

Of 300 patients randomized, 274 (91.3%) had follow-up arteriograms, 28 of which could not be analyzed. The risk-reduction group significantly reduced dietary fat, including saturated fat, and cholesterol and improved exercise test performance compared with usual care. Body weight was significantly reduced in the risk-reduction group versus usual care (3.9 kg; P < 0.001). Significant differences were achieved in TC, LDL-C, HDL-C, TG, and apolipoprotein B in the risk-reduction group compared with control, as well as in fasting and 1-hour postload glucose levels. The risk-reduction group showed a rate of narrowing of diseased coronary artery segments that was 47% less than that for usual care (−0.024 vs. −0.045 mm/yr change in minimal diameter; P < 0.02), and there were fewer hospitalizations initiated by clinical cardiac events in the risk-reduction group than usual care (25 vs. 44; rate ratio, 0.61; P = 0.05). The independent contribution of weight loss and exercise could not be determined within this multiple-risk-factor intervention; however, the data are consistent with the concept that weight loss and exercise contribute to the secondary prevention of CHD.

TRIALS OF CARDIAC REHABILITATION EXERCISE TRAINING

Cardiac rehabilitation exercise training is also generally incorporated into a multifactorial approach. Randomized trials of cardiac rehabilitation following MI typically demonstrate a lower mortality in treated patients. To overcome problems of not being able to detect small but clinically important benefits in mortality in RCTs of exercise and risk-factor rehabilitation after MI with small numbers of patients, Oldridge and colleagues[65] published a meta-analysis on 10 randomized clinical trials that included 4347 patients (2145 control; 2202 rehabilitation patients). The pooled odds ratios of 0.76 (95% confidence intervals, 0.63 to 0.92) for cardiovascular death were significantly lower in the rehabilitation group than in the control group, with no significant difference for nonfatal recurrent MI. The results suggest that comprehensive cardiac rehabilitation has a beneficial effect on mortality by not on nonfatal recurrent MI.

The reader is also referred to a U.S. Department of Health and Human Services review of randomized, controlled trials of cardiac rehabilitation exercise training.[66] Of 11 trials that reported on body weight changes, most were multifactorial; it was concluded that exercise is not recommended as a sole intervention for controlling weight in cardiac patients. Eighteen trials reported changes in lipid and lipoprotein levels (TC, LDL-C,

HDL-C, TG); of 26 significant favorable changes reported, 22 resulted from multifactorial rehabilitation (i.e., dietary and behavioral strategies in addition to exercise training). Likewise, of 20 lipid comparisons that showed no significant differences, 13 came from multifactorial interventions. Thus, favorable changes in lipid levels were reported to result primarily from multifactorial rehabilitation, so exercise training was not recommended as a sole intervention for lipids. However, 8 of 12 randomized, controlled trials that addressed the effect of exercise training on symptoms reported significant improvement in cardiovascular symptoms (decreased angina pectoris in patients with disease and decreases in symptoms of heart failure in patients with left-ventricular systolic dysfunction) in intervention groups versus controls, and seven of these had exercise as the sole intervention.

Fifteen randomized trials pertained to cardiovascular morbidity, including 10 involving only exercise training and five multifactorial studies.[66] None of these reported significant differences in rates of reinfarction for rehabilitation compared with control patients; therefore, there was no evidence for reduction in cardiac morbidity, most specifically nonfatal reinfarction. The safety of moderate exercise postinfarction is well established, however, with rates of infarction and cardiovascular complications during exercise being quite low. The scientific evidence pertaining to the relationship of cardiac rehabilitation exercise training with mortality included 16 randomized, controlled trials,[65] which suggested a survival benefit among patients participating in exercise training as a component of multifactorial cardiac rehabilitation. The benefit, however, could not be attributed solely to exercise.

EFFECTS OF PHYSICAL ACTIVITY COUNSELING IN PRIMARY CARE

As the medical profession embraces the need to promote physical activity to reduce CHD risk and risk for other diseases, the value of testing counseling approaches has become evident. The NHLBI, multicenter **Activity Counseling Trial (ACT)**,[67] conducted in a primary care, practice-based setting, randomly assigned 395 inactive women and 479 men to one of three groups:

1. Advice: physician advice and written educational materials (recommended care; n = 292).
2. Assistance: all the components received by the advice group plus interactive mail and behavioral counseling at physician visits (n = 263).
3. Counseling: advice and assistance components plus regular telephone counseling and behavioral classes (n = 289).

The primary outcomes were cardiorespiratory fitness (i.e., VO$_2$max) and self-reported total physical activity. At 24 months, 91.4% had completed physical activity and 77.6% had completed cardiorespiratory fitness measurements. For women, VO$_2$max was significantly higher in both the assistance group and counseling group versus advice group, with no differences between assistance and counseling and no difference in total physical activity. In men, neither of the two counseling interventions was more effective than recommended care.

GUIDELINES

Physical activity, defined as "bodily movements produced by skeletal muscles that require energy expenditure,"[68] includes many different types of exercise (both aerobic and anaerobic) that can be performed at different intensity levels with a wide range of doses (i.e., frequency per week [or day] and duration of exercise bouts). Since the release of the Surgeon General's Report on Physical Activity and Health[1] and the NHLBI Obesity Education Initiative Expert Panel treatment guidelines,[10] there has been considerable interest in the amount of physical activity that is needed to reduce weight in most persons, with and without concomitant caloric restriction,[69,70] as well as the amount needed to bring about specific health benefits in people of different body weight status. In fact, two important roundtables have been convened by the American College of Sports Medicine (ACSM) in recent years to apply an evidence-based approach to review more carefully the literature pertaining to the role of physical activity in the prevention and treatment of obesity and its comorbidities[12,71,72] and to dose-response relationships of physical activity to health,[73,74] including cardiovascular disease[4] and total and regional obesity.[75]

The minimum physical activity goal promoted by the 1996 Surgeon General's Report[1] was based on recommendations from the Centers for Disease Control and Prevention and the ACSM[68] that were subsequently endorsed by the National Institutes of Health Consensus Development Panel on Physical Activity and Cardiovascular Health[76] (i.e., that every American adult should accumulate at least 30 minutes of moderate-intensity physical activity on most, preferably all, days of the week). The ACSM acknowledged, in a 1998 position stand that replaced its 1990 position, that lower levels of physical exercise (particularly intensity) are generally insufficient to improve cardiorespiratory fitness, as assessed by maximal oxygen consumption (VO$_2$max); therefore, it recommended a frequency of 3 to 5 days/wk at an intensity of 65% to 90% of maximum heart rate (HR$_{max}$) or 50% to 85% of VO$_2$max, with lower intensity values (i.e., 55% to 64% HR$_{max}$ or 40–49 of VO$_2$max) for individuals who are unfit, and a duration of 20–60 minutes of continuous or intermittent (minimum of 10-minute bouts accumulated throughout the day) aerobic activity, with lower-intensity activity to be conducted over a longer period of time (i.e., ≥30 minutes).[77] (The mode of activity is any activity that uses large muscle groups, can be maintained continuously, and is rhythmic and aerobic in nature). Nonetheless, the ACSM position recognized that the quantity and quality of exercise needed to attain health-related benefits may differ from what is recommended for fitness and that lower activity levels may reduce the risk for certain chronic degenerative diseases and improve "metabolic fitness," referring to variables predictive of diabetes and cardiovascular disease.[77]

A later (2001) ACSM position stand focused on intervention strategies for weight loss, in overweight and obese adults, and prevention of weight regain.[78] After acknowledging that exercise alone, without dieting (caloric restriction), is unlikely to result in more than a modest (if any) effect on total body mass and fat mass loss unless other factors that affect energy balance are well-controlled,[9,68,69] the ACSM supported the OEI Expert Panel recommendation to elicit a weight loss of approximately 0.5 to 0.9 kg/wk (1-2 pounds/wk) for up to 6 months by reducing energy intake by 500 to 1000 kcal/day and accumulating 150 minutes of moderate exercise per week.[9] It further promoted progress to more than 200 minutes per week and recommended that endurance exercise be supplemented by resistance exercise to preserve fat-free mass while maximizing fat loss.[78]

The need for more than 30 min/day of regular activity to lose weight, or even maintain body weight in adults in the recommended body mass range (18.5-25 kg/m^2), was also highlighted in a 2002 report from the Institute of Medicine, which recommended that total energy expended to maintain body weight in the ideal range be at least 1.6 to 1.7 times an individual's resting energy expenditure.[79] This would require about 60 minutes of moderately intense physical activity throughout each day (i.e., twice the daily energy expenditure promoted by current national guidelines, which the vast majority of the general population are not meeting).[14] At present, there is virtually no RCT evidence to support widespread promotion of this greater amount of physical activity to reduce the prevalence of obesity or to improve cardiovascular health or reduce CHD risk; however, few RCTs have demonstrated significant weight loss with lower levels of activity.[10,69,70] Well-designed trials that address these questions are clearly warranted. Equally important is the need to determine behavioral strategies that will improve adherence to exercise programs and maintenance of fat weight loss.

SUMMARY AND CONCLUSION

A number of trials of physical activity and weight loss have been conducted to determine the value of these lifestyle changes on risk of CHD. These studies vary considerably in design, both with respect to specific exercise interventions or weight loss strategies, and study populations, but on the whole demonstrate benefits of increasing physical activity or weight loss (for people who need to lose weight) on several specific CHD risk factors, particularly IGT and type 2 DM, BP, and lipoproteins. As the prevalence of obesity increases, obesity-related comorbidities will continue to increase, as has happened for type 2 DM; therefore, it is increasingly important that we understand whether these lifestyle approaches are effective in the most susceptible populations (i.e., those with CHD risk factors, the obese, and ethnic populations of lower socioeconomic and educational status who have been underrepresented in RCTs of physical activity and weight loss). Despite our need

for much more information, the potential benefits of exercise and weight control seem well enough supported and the risks seem small enough to justify endorsement of these lifestyle interventions by the medical community for improving the cardiovascular health of men and women across a wide age range.

REFERENCES

1. U.S. Department of Health and Human Services: Physical Activity and Health: A Report of the Surgeon General. Atlanta, GA: U.S. Department of Health and Human Services, Centers for Disease Control and Prevention, National Center for Chronic Disease Prevention and Health Promotion, 1996.
2. Powell KE, Thompson PD, Caspersen CJ, et al: Physical activity and the incidence of coronary heart disease. Annu Rev Public Health 1987; 8:253-287.
3. Fletcher GF, Blair SN, Blumenthal J, et al: Statement on exercise: Benefits and recommendations for physical activity programs for all Americans: A statement for health professionals by the Committee on Exercise and Cardiac Rehabilitation of the Council on Clinical Cardiology, American Heart Association. Circulation 1992; 86: 340-344.
4. Kohl HW: Physical activity and cardiovascular disease: Evidence for a dose response. Med Sci Sports Exerc 2001; 33:S472-483.
5. Tanasescu M, Leitzmann MF, Rimm EB, et al: Exercise type and intensity in relation to coronary heart disease in men. JAMA 2002; 288:1994-2000.
6. Manson JE, Hu FB, Rish-Edwards JW, et al: A prospective study of walking as compared with vigorous exercise in the prevention of coronary heart disease in women. N Engl J Med 1999; 341:50-58.
7. Lee IM, Rexrode KM, Cook NR, et al: Physical activity and coronary heart disease in women: Is "no pain, no gain" passé? JAMA 2001; 285:1447-1454.
8. Manson JE, Greenland P, LaCroix AZ, et al: Walking compared with vigorous exercise for the prevention of cardiovascular events in women. N Engl J Med 2002; 347:716-725.
9. Gregg EW, Cauley JA, Stone K, et al: Relationship of changes in physical activity and mortality among older women. JAMA 2003; 289: 2379-2386.
10. National Institutes of Health and National Heart, Lung, and Blood Institute: Clinical guidelines on the identification, evaluation, and treatment of overweight and obesity in adults: The Evidence Report. Obes Res 1998; 6:51S-209S.
11. Third Report of the National Cholesterol Education Program (NCEP) Expert Panel on Detection, Evaluation, and Treatment of High Blood Cholesterol in Adults (Adult Treatment Panel III). NIH Publication No. 02-5215. Bethesda, MD, National Institutes of Health, 2002.
12. Pi-Sunyer FX: Comorbidities of overweight and obesity: Current evidence and research issues. Med Sci Sports Exerc 1999; 31: S602-608.
13. Flegal KM, Carroll MD, Ogden CL, et al: Prevalence and trends in obesity among US adults, 199-2000. JAMA 2002; 288:1723-1727.
14. Stephens T, Caspersen CJ: The demography of physical activity. In Physical Activity, Fitness, and Health: International Proceedings and Consensus Statement, Ed. Bouchard C, Shephard RJ, Stephens T. Champaign, IL: Human Kinetics, 1994; 204-213.
15. DiPietro L: Physical activity in the prevention of obesity: current evidence and research issues. Med Sci Sports Exerc 1999; 31:S542-546.
16. Look AHEAD: Action for Health in Diabetes. http://www.clinicaltrials.gov/ct/show/NCT00017953?order = 1. Accessed August 18, 2003.
17. American Diabetes Association: Nutritional recommendations and principles for people with diabetes mellitus. Diabetes Care 2000; 23:S43-S49.
18. Pan XR, Li GW, Hu YH, et al: Effects of diet and exercise in preventing NIDDM in people with impaired glucose tolerance the Da Qing IGT and Diabetes Study. Diabetes Care 1997; 20: 537-544.
19. Tuomilehto J, Lindstrom J, Eriksson JG, et al: Prevention of type 2 diabetes mellitus by changes in lifestyle among subjects with impaired glucose tolerance. N Engl J Med 2001; 344:1343-1350.

20. Diabetes Prevention Program Research Group: Reduction in the incidence of type 2 diabetes with lifestyle intervention or metformin. N Engl J Med 2002; 346:393–403.

21. Boule NG, Haddad E, Kenny GP, et al: Effects of exercise on glycemic control and body mass in type 2 diabetes mellitus: A meta-analysis of controlled clinical trials. JAMA 2001; 286:1218-1227.

22. Kelley DE, Goodpaster BH: Effects of exercise on glucose homeostasis in type 2 diabetes mellitus. Med Sci Sports Exerc 2001; 33:S495–S501.

23. Kelley DE, Goodpaster BH: Effects of physical activity on insulin action and glucose tolerance in obesity. Med Sci Sports Exerc 1999; 31:S619–S623.

24. McCarron DA, Reusser ME: Body weight and blood pressure regulation. Am J Clin Nutr 1996; 63(Suppl):423S–425S.

25. Joint National Committee on Detection, Evaluation, and Treatment of High Blood Pressure: The fifth report of the Joint National Committee on Detection, Evaluation, and Treatment of High Blood Pressure (JNC-V). Arch Intern Med 1993; 153: 154–183.

26. MacMahon S, Cutler J, Brittain E, et al: Obesity and hypertension: Epidemiological and clinical issues. Eur Heart J 1987; 8(Suppl B):57–70.

27. Fagard RH: Physical activity in the prevention and treatment of hypertension in the obese. Med Sci Sports Exerc 1999; 31:S624–630.

28. Hypertension Prevention Trial Research Group: The Hypertension Prevention Trial: Three-year effects of dietary changes on blood pressure. Arch Intern Med 1990; 150:153–162.

29. Stevens VJ, Corrigan SA, Obarzanek E, et al: Weight loss intervention in phase 1 of the Trials of Hypertension Prevention: The TOHP Collaborative Research Group. Arch Intern Med 1993; 153: 849–858.

30. Kumanyaka SK, Obarzanek E, Stevens VJ, et al: Weight-loss experience of black and white participants in NHLBI-sponsored clinical trials. Am J Clin Nutr 1991; 53:1631S–1638S.

31. Wassertheil-Smoller S, Blaufox MD, Oberman AS, et al: The Trial of Antihypertensive Interventions and Management (TAIM) Study: Adequate weight loss, alone and combined with drug therapy in the treatment of mild hypertension. Arch Intern Med 1992; 152:131–136.

32. Neaton JD, Grimm RH, Prineas RJ, et al: Treatment of mild hypertension study: Final results. JAMA 1993; 270:713–724.

33. Grimm RH, Flack JM, Grandits GA, et al: Long-term effects on plasma lipids of diet and drugs to treat hypertension: Treatment of Mild Hypertension Study (TOMHS) Research Group. JAMA 1996; 275:1549–1556.

34. Elmer PJ, Grimm R, Laing B, et al: Lifestyle intervention: Results of the Treatment of Mild Hypertension Study (TOMHS). Prev Med 1995; 24:378–388.

35. Blumenthal JA, Siegel WC, Appelbaum M: Failure of exercise to reduce blood pressure in patients with mild hypertension: Results of a randomized controlled trial. JAMA 1991; 266:2098–2104.

36. Steffen PR, Sherwood A, Gullette ECD, et al: Effects of exercise and weight loss on blood pressure during daily life. Med Sci Sports Exerc 2001; 33:1635–1640.

37. Stefanick ML: Exercise, lipoproteins and cardiovascular disease. In Fletcher G (ed). Cardiovascular Response to Exercise. Mount Kisco, NY, Futura Publishing Company, Inc, 1994, pp 325–345.

38. Stefanick ML: Physical activity for preventing and treating obesity-related dyslipoproteinemias. Med Sci Sports Exerc 1999; 31:S609–618.

39. Leon AS, Sanchez OA: Response of blood lipids to exercise training alone or combined with dietary intervention. Med Sci Sports Exerc 2001; 33:S502–S515.

40. Huttenen JK, Lansimies E, Voutilainen E, et al: Effect of moderate physical exercise on serum lipoproteins: A controlled clinical trial with special reference to serum high-density lipoproteins. Circulation 1979; 60: 1220–1229.

41. Wood PD, Haskell WL, Blair SN, et al: Increased exercise level and plasma lipoprotein concentrations: A one-year, randomized, controlled study in sedentary, middle-aged men. Metabolism 1983; 32:31–39.

42. Williams PT, Wood PD, Krauss RM, et al: Does weight loss cause the exercise-induced increase in plasma high density lipoproteins? Atherosclerosis 1983; 47:173–185.

43. Wood PD, Stefanick ML, Dreon DM, et al: Changes in plasma lipids and lipoproteins in overweight men during weight loss through dieting as compared with exercise. N Engl J Med 1988; 319: 1173–1179.

44. Katzel LI, Bleecker ET, Colman EB, et al: Effects of weight loss versus aerobic exercise training on risk factors for coronary disease in healthy, obese, middle-aged and older men: A randomized controlled trial. JAMA 1995; 274:1915-1921.

45. Expert Panel on Detection, Evaluation, and Treatment of High Blood Cholesterol in Adults: Summary of the second report of the National Cholesterol Education Program (NCEP) Expert Panel on Detection, Evaluation, and Treatment of High Blood Cholesterol in Adults (Adult Treatment Panel II). JAMA 1993; 269:3015.

46. Wood PD, Stefanick ML, Williams PT, et al: The effects on plasma lipoproteins of a prudent weight-reducing diet, with or without exercise, in overweight men and women. N Engl J Med 1991; 325:461–466.

47. King AC, Haskell WL, Taylor CB, et al: Group- versus home-based exercise training in healthy older men and women: A community-based clinical trial. JAMA 1991; 266:1535–1542.

48. King AC, Haskell WL, Young DR, et al: Long-term effects of varying intensities and formats of physical activity on participation rates, fitness, and lipoproteins in men and women aged 50-65 years. Circulation 1995; 91:2596–2604.

49. Svendsen OL, Hassager C, Christiansen C: Effect of an energy-restrictive diet with or without exercise on lean tissue, resting metabolic rate, cardiovascular risk factors, and bone in overweight postmenopausal women. Am J Med 1993; 95:131–140.

50. Boyden TW, Pamenter RW, Going SB, et al: Resistance exercise training is associated with decreases in serum low-density lipoprotein cholesterol levels in premenopausal women. Arch Intern Med 1993; 153:97–100.

51. Hellenius ML, de Faire UH, Berglund BH, et al: Diet and exercise are equally effective in reducing risk for cardiovascular disease: Results of a randomized controlled study in men with slightly to moderately raised cardiovascular risk factors. Atherosclerosis 1993; 103: 81–91.

52. Stefanick ML, Mackey S, Sheehan M, et al: Effects of the NCEP Step 2 diet and exercise on lipoproteins in postmenopausal women and men with low HDL-cholesterol and high LDL-cholesterol. N Engl J Med 1998; 339:12–20.

53. McCarron DA, Oparil S, Chait A, et al: Nutritional management of cardiovascular risk factors: A randomized clinical trial. Arch Intern Med 1997; 157:169–177.

54. Singh RB, Rastogi SS, Ghosh S, et al: The Diet and Moderate Exercise Trial (DAMET): Results after 24 weeks. Acta Cardiol 1993; 48: 543–557.

55. Kraus WE, Houmard JA, Duscha, et al: Effects of the amount and intensity of exercise on plasma lipoproteins. J Engl J Med 2002; 347:1483–1492.

56. Ford ES, Giles WH, Dietz WH: Prevalence of the metabolic syndrome among US adults: Findings from the third National Health and Nutrition Examination Survey. JAMA 2002; 287:356–359.

57. Ross R, Janssen I: Is abdominal fat preferentially reduced in response to exercise-induced weight loss? Med Sci Sports Exerc 1999; 31: S568–S572.

58. Ross R, Dagnone D, Jones JH, et al: Reduction in obesity and related comorbid conditions after diet-induced weight loss or exercise-induced weight loss in men. Ann Intern Med 2000; 1333: 92–103.

59. Janssen I, Hudson R, Fortier A, et al: Effects of an energy-restrictive diet with or without exercise on abdominal fat, intermuscular fat, and metabolic risk factors in obese women. Diabetes Care 2002; 25:431–438.

60. Irwin JL, Yasui Y, Ulrich CM, et al: Effect of exercise on total and intra-abdominal body fat in postmenopausal women: A randomized controlled trial. JAMA 2003; 289:323–330.

61. Ornish D, Brown SE, Scherwitz LW, et al: Can lifestyle changes reverse coronary heart disease? Lancet 1990; 336:129–133.

62. Singh RB, Rastogi SS, Verma R, et al: Randomized controlled trial of cardioprotective diet in patients with recent acute myocardial infarction: Results of one-year follow-up. BMJ 1992; 304:1015–1019.

63. Schuller G, Hambrecht R, Schlierf G, et al: Regular physical exercise and low-fat diet: Effects on progression of coronary artery disease. Circulation 1992; 86:1–11.

64. Haskell WL, Alderman EL, Fair JM, et al: Effects of intensive multiple risk factor reduction on coronary atherosclerosis and clinical cardiac effects in men and women with coronary artery disease: The Stanford Coronary Risk Intervention Project (SCRIP). Circulation 1994; 89:975–990.

65. Oldridge NB, Guyatt GH, Fischer ME, et al: Cardiac rehabilitation after myocardial infarction: combined experience of randomized clinical trials. JAMA 1988; 260:945–950.

66. Wenger NK, Froelicher ES, Smith LK, et al: Cardiac Rehabilitation. Clinical Practice Guideline No. 17. AHCPR Publication No. 96-0672. Rockville, MD, US Department of Health and Human Services, Public Health Service, Agency for Health Care Policy and Research and the National Heart, Lung, and Blood Institute, October 1995.

67. The Writing Group for the Activity Counseling Trial Research Group: Effects of physical activity counseling in primary care: The Activity Counseling Trial: A randomized controlled trial. JAMA 2001; 286:677–687.

68. Pate RR, Pratt M, Blair SN, et al: Physical activity and public health: A recommendation from the Centers for Disease Control and Prevention and the American College of Sports Medicine. JAMA 1995; 273:402–407.

69. Ross R, Freeman JA, Janssen I: Exercise alone is an effective strategy for reducing obesity and related comorbidities. Exerc Sport Sci Rev 2000; 28:165–170.

70. Stefanick ML: Obesity: Role of physical activity. In Coulston AM, Rock CL, Monsen ER (eds). Nutrition in the Prevention and Treatment of Disease. San Diego, Academic Press, 2001, pp 481–497.

71. Bouchard C, Blair SN: Introductory comments for the consensus on physical activity and obesity. Med Sci Sports Exerc 1999; 31:S498–501.

72. Grundy SM, Blackburn G, Higgins M, et al: Physical activity in the prevention and treatment of obesity and its comorbidities: Evidence report of independent panel to assess the role of physical activity in the treatment of obesity and its comorbidities. Med Sci Sports Exerc 1999; 31:S502–508.

73. Bouchard C: Physical activity and health: introduction to the dose-response symposium. Med Sci Sports Med 2001; 33:S347–S350.

74. Kesaniemi YA, Danforth E, Jensen MD, et al: Dose-response issues concerning physical activity and health: An evidence-based symposium. Med Sci Sports Med 2001; 33:S351–S358.

75. Ross R, Janssen I: Physical activity, total and regional obesity: dose-response considerations. Med Sci Sports Med 2001; 33: S521–S527.

76. National Institutes of Health Consensus Development Panel on Physical Activity and Cardiovascular Disease: Physical activity and cardiovascular health. JAMA 1996; 276:241–246.

77. American College of Sports Medicine: The recommended quantity and quality of exercise for developing and maintaining cardiorespiratory and muscular fitness, and flexibility in healthy adults. Med Sci Sports Exerc 1998; 30:975–991.

78. American College of Sports Medicine: The appropriate intervention strategies for weight loss and prevention of weight regain for Adults. Med Sci Sports Exerc 2001; 33:2145–2156.

79. Institute of Medicine Panel on Dietary Reference Intakes for Macronutrients: Dietary reference intakes for energy, carbohydrate, fiber, fat, fatty acids, cholesterol, protein and amino acids. Washington, DC, National Academics Press, 2002.

Chapter 26

Aspirin, Other Antiplatelet Agents, and Anticoagulants

Tobias Kurth
Julie E. Buring
Paul M. Ridker
J. Michael Gaziano

Thrombosis clearly plays an important role in cardiovascular events. Over the past half century, numerous clinical trials have addressed the benefit-risk ratio of antithrombotic and anticoagulant therapies among individuals at high and low risk, focusing mainly on the endpoints of all-cause mortality, coronary mortality, myocardial infarction (MI), and stroke. This chapter reviews trials of aspirin, other antiplatelet agents, and anticoagulants in the primary and secondary prevention of cardiovascular disease (CVD), as well as their meta-analyses. Evidence on the role of aspirin and thienopyridine derivatives in the treatment of the acute phase of an evolving MI is presented in Chapter 5.

MECHANISM

The history of aspirin dates to the fifth century BC, when Hippocrates discovered that an extract of white willow bark had analgesic properties. The painkilling effect was the result of salicin, a naturally occurring chemical in willow bark, which is closely related to acetylsalicylic acid, the synthetic aspirin available today. Aspirin was synthesized in 1897, but it is only over the past few decades that attention has focused on the potential role of aspirin in reducing the risks of occlusive vascular disease.

The hypothesized mechanism for aspirin's benefit derives from its ability to decrease platelet aggregation and thereby reduce the risk of thrombotic vascular events. The disruption of platelet- and fibrin-rich atherosclerotic plaque may lead to aggressive platelet deposition and, ultimately, to the formation of a thrombus, which can precipitate an acute clinical event. Findings from basic research demonstrate that, in platelets, small amounts of aspirin (i.e., 50–80 mg/day) irreversibly acetylate the active site of the isoenzyme cyclooxygenase-1 (COX-1),[1] which is required for the production of thromboxane A_2,[2] a powerful promoter of aggregation.[3] This effect persists for the entire life of the platelet (about 10–12 days) and is so pronounced that higher dosages of aspirin appear to yield no additional benefit. Indeed, the basic research findings raise the possibility that less than daily frequency of administration (e.g., alternate-day dosing) might be as effective as a daily regimen, whereas more frequent dosing might, in theory, compromise the favorable effects of aspirin by activating reversible vessel wall enzymes.

Nonselective, nonaspirin, nonsteroidal anti-inflammatory drugs (NSAIDs), such as ibuprofen or naproxen, as well as other drugs, such as sulfinpyrazone, also inhibit the COX-1 isoenzyme.[4] Unlike aspirin, however, these agents bind reversibly at the active site of the isoenzyme, leading to impaired platelet function for only a portion of the dosing interval.[5] Although it has been suggested that the effect of the nonselective NSAID naproxen on COX-1 persists throughout the dosing interval,[6] its cardioprotective effect remains controversial. Results from a post-hoc analysis of a randomized trial[7] and from case-control studies[8-10] found a reduced risk of cardiovascular events among naproxen users, whereas other studies found no association.[11,12]

More recently, new antiplatelet drugs with a defined mechanism of action have been developed. These include the thienopyridine derivatives, such as ticlopidine and clopidogrel, which inhibit platelet aggregation by inhibiting adenosine diphosphate-dependent activation of the platelet glycoprotein IIb/IIIa complex.

The anticoagulant effect of warfarin, a coumarin derivative, results from its interference with the cyclic interconversion of vitamin K and its 2,3-epoxide.[13,14] Vitamin K is a cofactor for the carboxylation of glutamate residues of the four vitamin K–dependent proteins, which include the coagulation factors II, VII, IX, and X. These coagulation factors need vitamin K for their activity. By inhibiting the vitamin K conversion cycle, warfarin induces hepatic production of partially decarboxylated proteins with reduced coagulant activity.

According to the dose administered, an anticoagulant effect is observed within 2 to 7 days after beginning oral warfarin therapy.[14]

TRIALS OF ASPIRIN AND OTHER ANTIPLATELET AGENTS IN SECONDARY PREVENTION

Although the pathophysiologic basis for antiplatelet agents in the secondary prevention of MI is well established, the initial randomized controlled trials designed to evaluate the clinical efficacy of these agents were inconclusive. For example, the first completed trial of antiplatelet therapy among patients with prior MI randomized 1239 men in the Cardiff region of Wales to 300 mg of aspirin daily or placebo (Cardiff-I trial).[15] Patients assigned to aspirin experienced a 25% mortality reduction compared with those assigned placebo (8.3% vs. 10.9%), but this did not achieve statistical significance.

This seminal trial was followed by a number of moderate-sized trials in the late 1970s and early 1980s. These trials showed similar nonsignificant reductions in mortality for aspirin, dipyridamole, or sulfinpyrazone, alone or in combination, including Cardiff-II,[16,17] Coronary Drug Project,[18] Aspirin Myocardial Infarction Study (AMIS),[19] Persantine-Aspirin Reinfarction Study (PARIS-I),[20] PARIS-II,[21] German-Austrian Myocardial Infarction Study (GAMIS),[22] Anturane Reinfarction Trial,[23,24] and the Anturane Italian Reinfarction Trial (AIRT).[25]

These early studies tested aspirin doses between 300 and 1500 mg/day. Although none of these studies showed statistically significant reductions in mortality, the mortality rates and rates of nonfatal events were lower among those assigned to the active agents. For example, in AIRT, which randomized 727 patients 15 to 25 days after infarction to sulfinpyrazone (400 mg twice daily) or placebo, there was no difference in total mortality after a mean treatment period of 19.2 months. Sulfinpyrazone treatment, however, was associated with a significant 56% reduction in total reinfarction (P < 0.01) and a 66% reduction in all fatal and nonfatal events judged to be thromboembolic (P < 0.001).[25]

Meta-Analysis of Antithrombotic Trials

Over the last three decades, several hundred trials of antiplatelet agents in secondary prevention have been conducted. These included trials of aspirin and other antiplatelet agents (alone or in combination) versus placebo, and trials of antiplatelet agents (alone or in combination) versus other agents. The trials were conducted among a wide range of patients at high risk of occlusive vascular events.

Although many of the early individual randomized trials of antiplatelet therapy following MI (primarily with aspirin) suggested a benefit of this treatment, most trials were unable to provide definitive answers, because the sample sizes were too small to have adequate statistical power to provide reliable results. In this circum-

stance, considering the studies in aggregate can provide a more stable estimate of the most likely magnitude of the effect. To this end, the Antiplatelet Trialists' Collaboration, whose investigators have directed randomized trials of antiplatelet therapy worldwide, conducted meta-analyses in 1988, 1994, and 2002.

In 1988, the first meta-analysis was conducted on 25 completed trials of antiplatelet therapy among individuals with a prior history of CVD.[26] This overview included the results of the 10 completed trials among approximately 18,000 post-MI patients, 13 completed trials among approximately 9000 patients with prior cerebrovascular disease (stroke or transient ischemic attack [TIA]), and 2 trials among approximately 2000 patients with unstable angina.

When all 25 secondary prevention trials were considered together, antiplatelet therapy was associated with statistically significant reductions of 32% in nonfatal MI (standard deviation [SD] 5%), 27% in nonfatal stroke (SD 6%), 15% in total vascular mortality (SD 4%), and 25% (SD 3%) in the combined endpoint of important vascular events (a composite outcome that comprised nonfatal MI, nonfatal stroke, and vascular mortality). There was no apparent effect of antiplatelet treatment on nonvascular death. Therefore, the statistically significant (P = 0.0003) benefit observed on total mortality was largely explained by the significant reduction in vascular death.

When the 10 post-MI trials were considered by patient entry criteria, the overview demonstrated statistically significant reductions from antiplatelet treatment of 31% in nonfatal MI (SD 5%), 42% in nonfatal stroke (SD 11%), 13% in total vascular mortality (SD 5%), and 25% (SD 4%) in important vascular events. The 13 trials of patients with cerebrovascular disease demonstrated statistically significant reductions of 35% for nonfatal MI, 22% for subsequent nonfatal stroke, 15% for vascular death, and 22% for important vascular events. Finally, for the two trials of unstable angina patients, there were statistically significant decreases of 35% in nonfatal MI, 37% in total vascular mortality, and 36% in important vascular events. There were too few strokes in these trials to provide meaningful data on that endpoint.

In regard to the different antiplatelet agents tested, there was no clear evidence that aspirin plus dipyridamole was any more effective than aspirin alone. The indirect comparison between the risk reductions of the two agents on new vascular events was not significant, and the overview of the direct comparisons indicated no difference whatsoever. There was also no evidence that sulfinpyrazone was superior to aspirin or that daily aspirin doses of 900 to 1500 mg were any more effective in reducing vascular events than 300 mg/day, the lowest dosage tested.

The 1988 meta-analysis provided reliable evidence of the benefit of aspirin therapy in patients with prior MI, stroke, TIA, or unstable angina. On the other hand, it did not address directly whether such therapy would benefit other patient populations at increased risk for occlusive vascular disease, such as those with chronic stable angina or peripheral vascular disease, or patients undergoing revascularization procedures. The report also did not address the question of aspirin's benefit in certain subgroups of high-risk patients, such as women, elderly persons, or individuals with hypertension or diabetes.

In 1994, an updated meta-analysis was published that included subsequently completed trials among a broader range of patients with prior manifestations of vascular disease (e.g., prior coronary revascularization, peripheral vascular disease, atrial fibrillation).[27] This overview included a total of 145 trials of antiplatelet therapy among 51,144 patients with prior vascular disease and about 28,000 low-risk subjects in primary prevention trials.

The findings among patients with prior MI, stroke, TIA, and unstable angina were similar to the 1988 overview. With respect to new patient populations in the updated overview, the report included the experience of approximately 22,000 patients at high risk for occlusive vascular events due to atrial fibrillation, valve surgery, peripheral vascular disease, chronic stable angina, and coronary revascularization (either coronary artery bypass graft [CABG] or percutaneous transluminal coronary angioplasty [PTCA]). When the trials of these various high-risk patients were considered in aggregate, antiplatelet therapy was associated with a highly statistically significant reduction in vascular occlusions, with similar proportional reductions in several different types of patients.

With respect to the absolute benefits of antiplatelet treatment, the risk reductions for patients with prior MI translated to avoidance of approximately 40 vascular events per 1000 patients treated over 2 years. Among other patient categories, the risk reductions correspond to avoidance of approximately 50 vascular events per 1000 unstable angina patients treated for 6 months, 40 events per 1000 patients with prior stroke or TIAs treated for 3 years, and 20 events per 1000 patients among other high-risk patients treated for 1 year.

The 1994 meta-analysis also provided reliable data that antiplatelet treatment in high-risk patients produces vascular event reductions of similar size in various patient subgroups. Specifically, separate data for men and women were available from 29 trials conducted among approximately 40,000 men and 10,000 women. There were comparable benefits on vascular events, with reductions per 1000 patients treated of 37 events for men (SD 4; $P < 0.00001$) and 33 events for women (SD 7; $P < 0.0001$). The data from these 29 trials also demonstrate similar reductions in vascular events for middle-aged and older patients, for hypertensive and normotensive groups, and for diabetic and nondiabetic persons.

The trials that were included in this meta-analysis tested aspirin doses ranging from 75 to 1500 mg/day. As in the 1988 overview, there was no evidence that higher dosages were any more effective in reducing the risk of occlusive vascular events than were lower dosages. Although 300 mg was the lowest daily dose tested in trials in the original overview, the updated analysis included approximately 5000 patients in trials testing 75 mg of aspirin daily. When analyzed separately, the trials testing daily doses of 75 mg demonstrated a statistically significant 29% reduction in vascular events associated with aspirin ($P < 0.0001$). The updated analysis also included three trials that tested ticlopidine versus aspirin, with

no significant differences in the effectiveness of the antiplatelet agents. Finally, with respect to duration, the investigators stated that further studies are still needed to determine exactly when antiplatelet therapy should start and for how long it should be continued.

In 2002, the Antithrombotic Trialists' Collaboration published its third major meta-analysis.[28] This meta-analysis included all new trials through September 1997 among high-risk patients, which included additional trials of aspirin at various doses, other antiplatelet drugs, the combination of aspirin with other antiplatelet drugs with a different mechanism of action, and the addition of anticoagulants to antiplatelet drugs. This meta-analysis included data from 287 studies involving 135,640 patients at high risk of occlusive arterial disease of antiplatelet therapy, and 77,000 patients in comparison of different antiplatelet regimens. Overall, among these high-risk patients, there was a highly significant reduction in the proportion of the combined outcome of any serious vascular event among patients assigned to antiplatelet therapy compared with those assigned to the control group (10.7% vs. 13.2%, $P < 0.0001$). Antiplatelet therapy was protective in most types of patients at increased risk of occlusive vascular events, including those with an acute MI or ischemic stroke, unstable or stable angina, previous MI, stroke or cerebral ischemia, peripheral artery disease, or atrial fibrillation.

With respect to specific outcomes, antiplatelet therapy was associated with a 34% proportional reduction in nonfatal MI ($P < 0.0001$), a 26% reduction in nonfatal MI or fatal coronary heart disease (CHD) ($P < 0.0001$), and a 25% reduction in nonfatal stroke ($P < 0.0001$). When strokes were classified by type, antiplatelet treatment was associated with a 30% decrease in total ischemic stroke ($P < 0.0001$) and a 22% increase in total hemorrhagic stroke ($P < 0.01$). Antiplatelet therapy also reduced the risk of fatal or nonfatal pulmonary embolism by 25% ($P < 0.01$).

The magnitude of the overall treatment effect on serious vascular events varied across the five categories of high-risk patients studied (previous MI, acute MI, previous stroke/TIA, acute stroke, other high risk) and ranged from a proportional reduction of 11% (standard error [SE] 4%) for patients with acute stroke to 30% (SE 4%) in patients with acute MI. Overall, there was a 22% reduction (SE 2%). The heterogeneity was related primarily to the somewhat smaller (but still significant) reduction in risk of serious vascular events among patients treated for acute stroke. In these patients, antiplatelet treatment was associated with a benefit of 9 events (SE 3) per 1000 treated patients ($P < 0.0009$), whereas among other high-risk patients, the corresponding benefits were 22 to 38 fewer vascular events per 1000 patients allocated antiplatelet therapy. Among patients with any high-risk condition other than acute stroke, antiplatelet therapy produced a 25% (SE 2%) proportional reduction in serious vascular events that was similar in each of the four categories.

Among the 18,788 patients with prior MI, antiplatelet therapy (mean duration of 27 months) resulted in 36 (SE 5) fewer serious vascular events per 1000 patients. This benefit was due to large reductions in nonfatal MI (18 [SE 3] fewer events per 1000 patients, P < 0.0001) and vascular death (14 [SE 4] fewer events per 1000, P = 0.0006) as well as a smaller but still significant reduction in nonfatal stroke (5 [SE 1] fewer events per 1000, P < 0.002). These benefits exceeded the small increase in risk of major extracranial bleeding, estimated at 3 per 1000 patients allocated antiplatelet therapy or 1 bleed per 1000 patients per year.

Among the 19,288 patients with suspected acute MI in 15 trials, 1 month of antiplatelet therapy resulted in 38 (SE 5) fewer serious vascular events per 1000 treated patients. This reflected significant reductions in nonfatal reinfarction (13 fewer events [SE 2], P < 0.0001) and in vascular death (23 [SE 4] fewer events, P < 0.0001), as well as a small but significant reduction in nonfatal stroke (2 [SE 1] fewer events, P = 0.02). The net benefit is substantially larger then the excess risk of major extracranial bleeds, estimated to be 1 to 2 additional per 1000 patients allocated antiplatelet therapy.

Compared with the 1994 meta-analysis, the available information in the 2002 meta-analysis on the effects of prolonged antiplatelet therapy among patients with a history of stroke or TIA increased substantially. Overall, 21 trials were evaluated, including 18,270 patients with a mean duration of antiplatelet therapy of 29 months. Antiplatelet therapy resulted in 36 (SE 6) fewer serious vascular events per 1000 patients. This benefit was mainly attributable to the large and highly significant reduction in nonfatal stroke recurrence (25 [SE 5] fewer per 1000 patients, P < 0.0001) and a smaller reduction in nonfatal MI (6 [SE 2] fewer per 1000, P < 0.0009). Although the reduction in vascular mortality was only marginally significant (7 [SE 4] fewer per 1000, P = 0.04), total mortality was reduced by 15 (SE 5) events per 1000 (P < 0.002). These benefits exceeded the estimated excess risk of serious bleedings of about 1 to 2 additional major extracranial bleeds per 1000 patients per year.

Almost no information concerning the effects of antiplatelet therapy in acute ischemic stroke was available for the earlier meta-analyses. Most of the available data in the 2002 meta-analysis on antiplatelet therapy in acute stroke were derived from two large, randomized trials—the International Stroke Trial (IST),[29] which examined the efficacy of 300 mg/day of aspirin in an open-label setting, and the Chinese Acute Stroke Trial (CAST),[30] which tested 160 mg/day of aspirin in a double-blind design. Each trial enrolled approximately 20,000 patients with suspected acute ischemic stroke. Combining the results of these two large trials with five smaller trials yielded an analytic sample of 40,821 patients, in which allocation to a mean duration of 3 weeks of antiplatelet therapy led to an 11% (SE 3%) proportional reduction in vascular events. This reflected an absolute reduction of 9 (SE 3) vascular events per 1000 patients: 4 (SE 2) fewer nonfatal strokes (P = 0.003) and 5 (SE 2) fewer vascular deaths (P = 0.05) per 1000 patients. Data on nonfatal MI were not provided in either IST or CAST.

Patients in the "other high-risk" category included those with coronary artery disease (CAD), higher risk of embolism, peripheral artery disease, and other high-risk conditions. Among the 15,828 patients with coronary artery disease from 55 trials, there was a highly significant 37% (SE 5%) proportional reduction in serious vascular events (P < 0.0001). Among 5162 patients at high risk of embolism in 14 trials, there was a highly significant risk reduction of 26% (SE 7%; P = 0.0003) in serious vascular events. Among those with atrial fibrillation, the most common cardiac condition increasing risk for embolism, the risk reduction was 24% (SE 9%). Among 9214 patients with peripheral artery disease in 42 trials, the proportional risk reduction in serious vascular events was 23% (SE 8%; P = 0.004); antiplatelet therapy appeared equally beneficial to individuals with intermittent claudication, peripheral grafting, and peripheral angioplasty.

With respect to dose, daily aspirin doses of 75 to 150 mg appeared to confer the same level of cardioprotective benefit as did larger doses. Indirect comparisons using data from trials testing a particular aspirin dose versus no aspirin estimated a proportional reduction in serious vascular events of 19% (SE 3%) for dosages of 500 to 1500 mg/day, 26% (SE 3%) for dosages of 160 to 325 mg/day, and 32% (SE 6%) for dosages of 75 to 150 mg/day. Dosages below 75 mg/day had a somewhat smaller effect (13% [SE 8%]). On the other hand, a combined analysis of the three trials that directly compared doses of 75 mg/day or greater with dosages less than 75 mg/day found no significant difference in efficacy. Therefore, more data are needed to determine conclusively whether doses of less than 75 mg/day offer as comparable a protection against vascular events as dosages exceeding that amount.

Effects of Dipyridamole, Clopidogrel, and Ticlopidine

The 2002 Antithrombotic Trialists' Collaboration directly compared data from three trials of dipyridamole and aspirin and found no difference between the two agents with respect to vascular events. An indirect comparison yielded similar proportional reductions of dipyridamole and 75 mg aspirin when compared with placebo.[28] The addition of dipyridamole to aspirin has not been clearly shown to produce additional reductions in serious vascular events, but there is a suggestion of a further benefit of combined use in the secondary prevention of stroke. The second European Stroke Prevention Study (ESPS 2)[31] randomized 6602 patients to aspirin (25 mg twice daily), dipyridamole (200 mg twice daily), both, or neither. After 2 years of follow-up, the study found that compared with placebo, there was a statistically significant relative risk reduction of stroke of 16% in the dipyridamole group, 18% in the aspirin group, and 37% in the combined group. In addition, the combined administration of aspirin plus dipyridamole was significantly more effective than either agent prescribed alone. The forthcoming results of the European/Australian Stroke Prevention in Reversible Ischaemia Trial (ESPRIT)[32] will provide further information about the efficacy of aspirin versus aspirin plus dipyridamole in secondary prevention of ischemic stroke.

The thienopyridine derivatives clopidogrel and ticlopidine are antiplatelet agents that inhibit the platelet aggregation induced by adenosine diphosphate–dependent activation of the platelet glycoprotein IIb/IIIa complex. Thus, these agents have a different action on platelets than aspirin, and combining one of these agents with aspirin, which blocks the thromboxane-mediated pathway, may have an additive effect. However, initial trials examined the thienopyridines against aspirin, not in combination. Most importantly, a large-scale randomized secondary prevention trial comparing clopidogrel versus aspirin alone has been reported by the Clopidogrel Versus Aspirin in Patients at Risk of Ischemic Events (CAPRIE) investigators.[33] A total of 19,185 patients with atherosclerotic vascular disease were randomized to clopidogrel (75 mg/day) or to aspirin (325 mg/day). As compared with aspirin alone, clopidogrel alone was associated with an 8.7% reduction in the annual risk of the composite endpoint of vascular death, MI, or ischemic stroke (5.3 vs. 5.8%; P = 0.043). The reduction of events in patients with MI was 5.03% in the clopidogrel group and 4.84% in the aspirin group (P = 0.66). In CAPRIE the benefit was most prominent for patients with peripheral arterial disease.

The effect of clopidogrel plus aspirin versus placebo plus aspirin was tested in the Clopidogrel in Unstable Angina to Prevent Recurrent Events (CURE) trial.[34] In this multicenter trial, 12,562 patients with acute coronary syndrome without ST-segment elevation were randomized to receive clopidogrel (300 mg immediately, followed by 75 mg once daily) or placebo in addition to aspirin (daily recommended dose of 75–300 mg) for 3 to 12 months. Compared with the combination of aspirin and placebo, the combination of active clopidogrel and aspirin was associated with a statistically significant 20% reduction (relative risk [RR] = 0.80; 95% CI 0.72–0.90; P < 0.001) of death from cardiovascular causes, nonfatal MI, or stroke. However, major bleeding complications were significantly more common in the clopidogrel plus aspirin group as compared with the aspirin and placebo group (RR = 1.38; 95% CI 1.13–1.67; P < 0.001). Whether the combination of clopidogrel plus aspirin is superior to aspirin alone in secondary prevention of ischemic stroke is currently under investigation in the Management of Atherothrombosis with Clopidogrel in High-risk Patients with Recent Transient Ischemic Attack or Ischemic Stroke (MATCH) trial.[35]

The cost-effectiveness of aspirin, clopidogrel, or both was the focus of a recent simulation model,[36] which yielded evidence that increased prescription of aspirin for all eligible patients for secondary prevention of CHD is attractive from a cost-effectiveness perspective. Because clopidogrel is more costly, the incremental cost-effectiveness is currently unattractive, unless its use is restricted to patients with contraindications to aspirin.

With respect to ticlopidine versus aspirin, the 2002 Antithrombotic Trialists' Collaboration meta-analysis found a nonsignificant proportional reduction in serious vascular events of 12% (SE 7%).[28] This is similar to the 10% reduction of clopidogrel compared with aspirin as reported from the CAPRIE study.[28]

One trial randomized 1965 patients with coronary stenting to aspirin (325 mg) alone, aspirin plus ticlopidine (250 mg twice daily), or aspirin plus warfarin (target international normalized ratio [INR] of 2.0–2.5). Although the risk of recurrent MI was significantly lower in the combined aspirin and ticlopidine group (RR = 0.20; 95% CI 0.07–0.62, P = 0.014), the reduction of serious vascular events was nonsignificant (proportional reduction of 21% [SE 24%]).[28] In addition, there was a nonsignificant increase in risk of major extracranial bleeds in the combined group. In another study of patients who received Palmaz-Schatz coronary artery stents, the combination of ticlopidine and aspirin was more effective than the combination of heparin, phenprocoumon, and aspirin in the prevention of the combination of death, MI, CABG, or repeat PTCA.[37] Ticlopidine was, however, associated with gastrointestinal side effects such as diarrhea and has the potentially serious complication of bone marrow depression.

Duration, Side Effects, and Dosage of Aspirin in Secondary Prevention

There is no direct evidence on the question of optimal duration of treatment in secondary prevention, because no large-scale randomized trials have compared different durations of treatment. For trials of patients with prior MI, stroke, or TIA that provided individual patient data, information is available on events occurring in the first, second, and subsequent years of scheduled treatment. These trials show an apparent trend toward greater effect during the earlier years. However, there are difficulties in interpreting these data because noncompliance with treatment tends to increase with time (i.e., some treatment group members stop antiplatelet therapy and some control group members start such treatment). Therefore, the underestimation of the effect of actual treatment tends to increase over time. In addition, even with no further divergence in event rates after the first few years, continued aspirin therapy may be preventing survival and event rate curves from converging. For this reason, without direct evidence otherwise from randomized comparisons of different durations of treatment and absent the development of a contraindication to its use in individual patients, indefinite continuation of aspirin therapy in those patients who are at high risk of occlusive vascular events may be advisable. This conclusion is supported if the evidence from primary and secondary prevention trials of aspirin is considered, because participants benefit at any time from the use of aspirin.

Although aspirin's benefits in reducing occlusive vascular events may be approximately equal over the wide dose range tested in trials to date, the principal adverse side effects of aspirin appear to be strongly dose-related. The United Kingdom Transient Ischemic Attack (UK-TIA) trial, which tested two daily dosages of aspirin, provides the most informative direct comparison of the side effects of different aspirin dosages.[38] This trial among 2345 patients with a history of TIA tested 300 and 1200 mg/day of aspirin against placebo. The percentage of participants reporting upper gastrointestinal symptoms and bleeding was lowest in the placebo group (26%), somewhat higher in the group receiving 300 mg/day (31%), and highest among the group receiving 1200 mg/day (41%). The differences between the two aspirin dosages were statistically significant. For gastrointestinal bleeding, the percentages were 1% for the placebo, 3% for the 300-mg group, and 5% for the 1200-mg group. In a review of population-based observational studies, regular use of 300 mg or more of aspirin daily was associated with an approximately twelvefold increase in risk of upper gastrointestinal bleeding or perforations.[39] For hemorrhagic stroke—the most severe potential adverse effect of aspirin—the totality of randomized trial evidence in both secondary and primary prevention indicates a small but significant increase with aspirin treatment recipients versus the control group. Its overall occurrence, however, was very low (0.3% vs. 0.2%) and was substantially outweighed by the definite reduction in the far more common strokes of nonhemorrhagic etiology.[27] The evidence from the 2002 Antithrombotic Trialists' Collaboration meta-analysis supports daily doses of aspirin in the range of 75 to 150 mg for the long-term prevention of serious vascular events in high-risk patients.

Role of Nonsteroidal Antiinflammatory Drugs in Prevention of Cardiovascular Disease

As described earlier, nonselective NSAIDs also inhibit COX-1, but the COX-1 blocking activity does not persist throughout the dosing interval[5] and thus a sustained cardioprotective effect is not expected. Although it has been suggested that the effect of the nonselective NSAID naproxen on COX-1 persists throughout the dosing interval,[6] its cardioprotective effect remains controversial. Results from a post-hoc analysis of a randomised trial[7] and from case-control studies[8-10] found a reduced risk of cardiovascular events among naproxen users, whereas other studies found no association.[11,12]

There is recent evidence that aspirin and other non-aspirin NSAIDs may interact because both medications share a common docking site on COX-1.[40,41] Basic research findings,[42,43] a crossover study in healthy subjects,[44] and one observational study in secondary prevention[45] support this hypothesis. In the crossover study by Catella-Lawson and colleagues, concomitant administration of 400 mg ibuprofen every morning antagonized the irreversible platelet inhibition of COX-1 induced by 81 mg aspirin. This inhibition could be bypassed, such as when aspirin was given before a single dose of ibuprofen. Intake of enteric-coated ibuprofen three times a day inhibited the effect of aspirin on platelets, even when the aspirin was taken before the ibuprofen. No interaction was found between concomitant intake of aspirin and rofecoxib, acetaminophen, or diclofenac. The recent observational study of secondary prevention by MacDonald and Wei identified 7107 patients from Scotland who were discharged after first admission for CVD and followed for 8 years.[45] Four discharge groups were compared: low-dose (<325 mg/day) aspirin alone, aspirin plus ibuprofen, aspirin plus diclofenac, and aspirin plus another NSAID. Compared with aspirin-only users, ibuprofen users had a relative risk of 1.73 (95% CI 1.05-2.84) for cardiovascular mortality. Combined use of aspirin and diclofenac or other NSAIDs did not increase the risk. Although the authors could control for several potential confounding factors, the nature of their data did not allow them to control for lifestyle factors such as smoking and exercise.

A recent study from the randomized aspirin arm of the Physicians' Health Study[46] suggested that the clinical benefit of aspirin in the primary prevention of MI is inhibited by regular but not intermittent use of NSAIDs.[47] Among participants randomized to aspirin, use of NSAIDs 1 to 59 days per year was not associated with risk of MI (RR = 1.21; 95% CI 0.78-1.87), whereas the use of NSAIDs on 60 days or more per year was associated with an increased risk of MI (RR = 2.86; 95% CI 1.25-6.56) when compared with no use of NSAIDs. In the placebo group, the RRs for MI across the same categories of NSAID use were 1.14 (95% CI 0.81-1.60), and 0.21 (95% CI 0.03-1.48), respectively. A limitation of the study was that no information could be provided about dosing and brand of NSAIDs. However, ibuprofen was one of the most often used NSAIDs during the period of the study (1982-1988). Although the information from the secondary prevention study on NSAIDs was observational, the most plausible interpretation of the available data is that the regular use of the NSAID ibuprofen may inhibit the clinical benefit of aspirin in secondary prevention of CVD and in the primary prevention of MI.

There is an ongoing controversy about whether the COX-2 selective NSAIDs have an effect on CVD risk. Basic research findings supported the potential of a small increased risk of CVD.[48] Results of the Vioxx Gastrointestinal Outcomes Research Study (VIGOR) tested in a randomized, double-blind, stratified, parallel group trial the long-term treatment effects and the gastrointestinal toxicity of rofecoxib (50 mg/day) or naproxen (1000 mg/day) in patients with rheumatoid arthritis.[7] Patients on aspirin therapy were excluded from the trial. In a post-hoc analysis, the rates of nonfatal MI, nonfatal stroke, and death from any vascular event were higher in the rofecoxib group (0.8% vs. 0.4%, P < 0.05). The interpretation of this finding is problematic since it is unclear if the difference occurred because of a protective effect of naproxen or if rofecoxib use is associated with an increased risk of CVD. Also, the role of chance, small numbers of endpoints in exposure subgroups, and other limitations have been pointed out.[49] In contrast to the VIGOR trial, the Celecoxib Long-term Arthritis Safety Study (CLASS) showed no difference in cardiovascular events between users of celecoxib (400 mg twice daily) and ibuprofen (800 mg 3 times per day).[50] Overall, there is no consistent evidence that either nonselective or selective NSAIDs affect CVD risk, but there is a suggestion of interaction between the nonselective NSAID ibuprofen and aspirin with respect to CVD events.

Further prospective studies are needed to clarify the role of NSAIDs in cardioprotection and their combination with antiplatelet drugs.[49]

TRIALS OF ANTICOAGULANTS IN SECONDARY PREVENTION

In contrast with the clinical trials of antiplatelet therapy in the secondary prevention of MI, which have largely been conducted over the past 25 years, trials of oral anticoagulant therapy have been carried out for more than a half century. In 1946, the Board of Directors of the American Heart Association (AHA) established a Committee for the Evaluation of Anticoagulants in the Treatment of Coronary Thrombosis with Myocardial Infarction. Two years later, this panel reported results from a multicenter trial involving 800 patients hospitalized with acute MI.[51] The trial, which used a nonrandomized treatment allocation scheme, reported significant benefits of 30 days of anticoagulation on rates of subsequent mortality (24% vs. 15%; P < 0.01) and total thromboembolic events (36% vs. 14%; P < 0.01). The authors concluded that "anticoagulant therapy should be used in all cases of coronary thrombosis with MI unless a definite contraindication exists."[51]

After this early assessment, a number of trials of anticoagulant therapy following acute MI were subsequently conducted during the 1950s, 1960s, and 1970s.[52-63] Their findings, however, were not consistent, and, overall, it appeared the benefits were greatest in trials that lacked randomized treatment assignment. Benefits were also generally more pronounced for thromboembolic events than for mortality; however, many of the studies were conducted at a time when prolonged bed rest and delayed ambulation were the standard of care for MI patients, practices that would be expected to increase the overall rate of thromboembolic events. Many of the trials also predated the introduction of the coronary care unit, tested a number of orally active anticoagulants, and used a variety of assays with reagents of varying strengths and sources to determine the degree of anticoagulation. Thus, the applicability of many of these trials to current medical management was limited.

In contrast with the large number of trials performed during this early phase of the anticoagulant era, recent years have been characterized by the performance of fewer trials of overall higher quality, with greater definition of patient entry requirements and more rigorous control and reporting of the degree of anticoagulation.

Three more recent, large-scale trials have more firmly established the benefits of anticoagulant therapy in post-MI patients, demonstrating reductions in mortality, reinfarction, and stroke using moderate-intensity anticoagulation.[64-67] As with antiplatelet therapy, the optimal duration of anticoagulation is uncertain, although the results of the Sixty-Plus Reinfarction Study[64] suggest that it extends beyond 1 year post-MI.

A recent meta-analysis pooled the evidence from 31 trials published between 1960 and 1999 of patients with CAD who were treated for 3 months or more with anticoagulation therapy.[68] The rates of MI and stroke were significantly reduced with high-intensity (INR 2.8–4.8) and moderate-intensity (INR 2–3) oral anticoagulation, but the bleeding risk was increased 6.0- to 7.7-fold. When low-intensity (INR < 2.0) anticoagulation was combined with aspirin, there was no superior effect compared with aspirin alone.

In the Sixty-Plus Reinfarction Study, a multicenter trial carried out in The Netherlands, 878 patients older than 60 years who had been placed on anticoagulant therapy following a first transmural MI were randomly assigned to continue anticoagulant treatment or to receive placebo.[64,65] The average duration of prerandomization treatment with anticoagulants was 6 years. Patients allocated to active treatment received either acenocoumarol or phenprocoumon, with a target thrombotest of 5% to 10%, corresponding to an INR of 2.7 to 4.5. After 2 years of treatment, continued anticoagulant therapy was associated with an apparent, but not statistically significant, reduction in total mortality (15.7% vs. 11.6%; P = 0.071) compared with placebo. "On-treatment" analysis revealed a greater mortality reduction difference (13.4% vs. 7.6%; P = 0.017). For reinfarction, there was a highly significant benefit of continued anticoagulation (15.2% vs. 6.9%; P = 0.0005). With respect to intracranial events, all but 2 of which (1 in treatment, 1 in control) were classified as cerebrovascular in origin, there were fewer among the treatment group than placebo (13 vs. 21). This difference, however, was not statistically significant (P = 0.16). There were apparent competing effects on such events when divided by etiology, with an excess of hemorrhagic events in the anticoagulant group (7 vs. 1) and a deficit of events classified as nonhemorrhagic (2 vs. 13). Regarding major extracranial hemorrhage (i.e., events leading to protocol deviation), there were 3 events in placebo versus 27 in the anticoagulant group. Minor extracranial hemorrhage was reported for 7 patients assigned placebo compared with 57 patients assigned active treatment.

Thus, the Sixty-Plus Reinfarction Study demonstrated a possible mortality benefit of continued anticoagulation, a more definite reduction in reinfarction, and possible competing effects on cerebral thrombosis and hemorrhage, with somewhat fewer total intracranial events among treated patients than control subjects. Because all patients were exposed to an extensive period of pretrial anticoagulant treatment, however, the study actually examined the effect of maintaining versus discontinuing anticoagulation and, therefore, did not address directly the question of the benefits of initiating anticoagulation in the period just following infarction.

To address this issue directly, the Warfarin Reinfarction Study (WARIS) in Norway randomized 1214 male and female patients, 75 years of age and younger, soon after acute MI (mean interval from infarct symptoms to randomization, 27 days) to warfarin or placebo.[66] Warfarin was dosed to a target range INR of 2.8 to 4.8. The average duration of trial treatment was 37 months. With this relatively intense dosing of anticoagulant therapy, compared with placebo warfarin, treatment was associated with statistically significant reductions of 24% in total mortality (123 vs. 94 deaths; P = 0.027), 34% in reinfarction

(124 vs. 82 events; P = 0.0007), and 55% in total cerebrovascular accidents (44 vs. 20 events; P = 0.0015).

A second post-MI trial of anticoagulants in The Netherlands, the Anticoagulants in the Secondary Prevention of Events in Coronary Thrombosis (ASPECT) study, randomized 3404 hospitalized male and female survivors of acute MI, with treatment initiated as soon as possible following hospital discharge, but not more than 6 weeks later.[67] Patients were allocated at random to anticoagulation with nicoumalone or phenprocoumon or to placebo, with a target INR of 2.8 to 4.8. Following an average treatment duration of 37 months, anticoagulant-treated patients had experienced a nonsignificant 10% decrease in mortality (hazard ratio = 0.90; 95% CI 0.73-1.11). Anticoagulant treatment was associated with significant reductions in reinfarction (114 vs. 242; hazard ratio = 0.47 [95% CI 0.38-0.59]) and cerebrovascular events (37 vs. 62; hazard ratio = 0.60 [95% CI 0.40-0.90]). There was, however, an excess in cerebral hemorrhage among those allocated anticoagulant treatment (17 cases, 8 fatal) compared with those assigned placebo (2 cases, neither fatal). The numbers of fatal strokes were similar (11 in anticoagulant, 8 in placebo), so the reduction in total cerebrovascular events associated with active treatment largely reflects a decrease in nonfatal events. There were major bleeding complications in 73 patients allocated to anticoagulants and 19 assigned placebo. In on-treatment analyses, 55 major bleeds occurred in the anticoagulant group and 6 in the placebo group. This corresponds to a rate for anticoagulant therapy of 1.5 bleeds per 100 patient-years, a rate similar to that in earlier trials and one that supports the relative safety of long-term anticoagulation.

Trials of Aspirin Versus Anticoagulant Therapy in Secondary Prevention

Although a number of large-scale, randomized trials and overviews of trials have demonstrated net benefits of antiplatelet therapy with aspirin as well as anticoagulant regimens in long-term therapy of post-MI patients, these data do not address directly whether one of these forms of therapy is superior or whether a combined regimen of aspirin and anticoagulation confers any net benefit over that achieved using monotherapy with either treatment alone. Several randomized trials have evaluated these questions, and the available trial data comparing anticoagulant and aspirin regimens in post-MI patients do not provide clear evidence for the superiority of one form of antithrombotic therapy.

An early trial that compared directly antithrombotic therapy with aspirin and anticoagulant therapy was the previously described German-Austrian Reinfarction Study.[22] This trial randomized 946 patients, 45 to 70 years old, to aspirin (1500 mg/day), phenprocoumon (target thrombotest value 5%–12%), or placebo, 30 to 42 days after MI. The trial was double-blind with respect to aspirin assignment but was open-label for phenprocoumon. After 2 years of treatment, there were nonsignificant mortality reductions for aspirin versus placebo and for aspirin versus phenprocoumon, and reductions that approached borderline significance among those assigned aspirin versus phenprocoumon in coronary death (46.3% reduction; P < 0.07), and among those assigned aspirin versus placebo in coronary events (nonfatal reinfarction plus coronary death) (36.6% reduction; P < 0.06). Thus, although this early comparison of aspirin and oral anticoagulation did not yield clear results, it did suggest a possible advantage of aspirin.

The French Enquête de Prévention Secondaire de l'Infarctus du Myocarde (EPSIM) study compared aspirin (500 mg three times daily) with oral anticoagulation (acenocoumarol, luindione, ethylbiscoumacetate, phenindione, or tioclomarol) in 1303 post-MI men and women.[69] Participants were 30 to 70 years old, and the mean interval from infarction to study entry was 11 days. Following an average duration of treatment of 29 months, there were no statistically significant differences between treatment groups in mortality or reinfarction. The occurrence of at least one bleeding episode was far more common among patients assigned oral anticoagulants than aspirin (104 vs. 35 patients), whereas aspirin-allocated patients experienced excesses in reported gastritis (18 vs. 4) and confirmed peptic ulcer (22 vs. 6).

Whether differences exist in the relative efficacy of aspirin and anticoagulants in patients following thrombolysis was the focus of a recent multicenter, international trial. The Aspirin/Anticoagulants following Thrombolysis with Eminase in Recurrent Infarction (AFTER) Study randomized 1036 patients who had been treated with the thrombolytic drug Eminase (anistreplase) to aspirin (150 mg/day) or anticoagulation (intravenous heparin followed by oral anticoagulation, target INR 2.0-2.5).[70] For the primary outcome of reinfarction plus cardiac death, there were no significant differences between treatments at 30 days (11.2% for aspirin vs. 11.0% for anticoagulation) or 3 months (12.1% for aspirin vs. 13.2% for anticoagulation). Patients assigned anticoagulation were significantly more likely to have had severe bleeding or a stroke by 3 months (3.6% vs. 1.7%; P = 0.04), but most of this excess occurred in the first 3 days, a period during which anticoagulant patients were still receiving heparin.

A second trial among patients following thrombolysis, the Antithrombotics in the Prevention of Reocclusion in Coronary Thrombolysis (APRICOT) Study, enrolled 300 patients with patent infarct-related arteries following thrombolysis and initiation of intravenous heparin.[71] Participants were allocated to one of three treatment groups: continuation of heparin and initiation of warfarin (open label), a discontinuation of heparin with initiation of either aspirin (325 mg/day) or aspirin-placebo (double-blind). The initial warfarin dose was at the discretion of the attending physician, with dosage adjustments made until the INR was between 2.8 and 4.0. The primary endpoint for the trial was patency of the infarct-related artery 3 months following hospital discharge.

A total of 300 patients were randomized, with angiographic follow-up data available for 248 subjects. Reocclusion rates were not significantly different among the three groups (25% with aspirin, 30% with warfarin, and 32% with placebo). Mortality rates also did not differ. Reinfarction occurred in 3% of patients assigned aspirin,

8% of those allocated warfarin, and 11% of those receiving placebo (aspirin vs. placebo; P < 0.025; other comparisons not significant). Similarly, revascularization was lower in the aspirin group (6%) than in warfarin (13%) and placebo (16%) (aspirin vs. placebo; P < 0.05; other comparisons NS).

Trials of Combined Anticoagulant/Aspirin Therapy Versus Aspirin Monotherapy

Because the pathogenesis of thrombosis is multifactorial, it has been postulated that combined therapy with aspirin and anticoagulants might inhibit both platelet activation and thrombin generation, thereby providing greater clinical benefit than monotherapy with either regimen. Trials in unstable angina patients[72] and recipients of mechanical heart valves[73] have provided some support for use of full-dose anticoagulation plus aspirin rather than therapy with either antithrombotic regimen alone. However, the increased bleeding risks observed with this dual regimen, as well as the added clinical burden and financial costs of monitoring INR values, raised the question of whether comparable benefit might be achieved, with less bleeding and clinical monitoring, using lower, fixed doses of anticoagulants as well as lower-dose aspirin.

The Coumadin Aspirin Reinfarction Study (CARS) was designed to address this question.[74] This multicenter, North American trial randomly assigned 8803 post-MI patients to daily treatment with 160 mg aspirin alone, 3 mg warfarin plus 80 mg aspirin, or 1 mg warfarin plus 80 mg aspirin. INR values were assessed at weeks 1, 2, 3, 4, 6, and 12, and then at 3-month intervals, but the only dosage adjustments made were reductions for patients with values of 3.5 or higher. Thus, for most patients the CARS trial represents an evaluation of "fixed-dose" rather than "targeted-dose" warfarin.

The primary study endpoint was first occurrence of reinfarction, nonfatal ischemic stroke, or cardiovascular death. The trial was terminated early, at the recommendation of the Data and Safety Monitoring Committee, based on the apparent comparable efficacy of the three treatments and an estimate that there was less than 1% chance that a statistically significant 20% difference for any comparison would emerge with additional enrollment or follow-up. At the trial termination, after a median treatment of 14 months, the relative risk of the primary endpoint for the aspirin-only group compared with the group taking 3 mg warfarin plus aspirin was 0.95 (95% CI 0.81-1.12; P = 0.57). For the aspirin alone group compared with the 1 mg warfarin plus aspirin group, the relative risk was 1.03 (95% CI 0.87-1.22; P = 0.74). For the low- versus high-dose warfarin regimens, the relative risk was 0.93 (95% CI 0.78-1.11; P = 0.41). With respect to individual outcomes, there was a reduction in ischemic stroke in the aspirin-only group compared with both of the combined regimens, and the comparison with 1 mg warfarin plus 80 mg aspirin was of borderline significance (P = 0.05). The authors suggest this finding may support the possibility of greater benefit in preventing stroke with the higher

160-mg dose used in the aspirin-only arm, but this finding was based on small numbers of events (21 vs. 28 ischemic strokes). Overall, however, the CARS results demonstrated no clinical benefit of low, fixed doses of warfarin combined with 80 mg of aspirin over the results achieved with 160 mg of aspirin alone. The investigators cited evidence that mechanical heart value patients benefit from combined moderate-dose anticoagulation and aspirin, with low bleeding risk,[75] to support the possible use of higher-dose anticoagulation with aspirin in post-MI patients.

The recent Combined Hemotherapy and Mortality Prevention (CHAMP) study,[76] a Veterans Affairs Cooperative Studies Program trial, was a multicenter, open-label study comparing all-cause mortality in 5059 survivors of acute MI randomized within 14 days of their index MI to either combined warfarin (target INR 1.5-2.5) and aspirin (81 mg/day) therapy or aspirin (162 mg/day) monotherapy. Median follow-up was 2.75 years (range 1.0-6.0). Mean achieved INR in the warfarin/aspirin group was 1.8. The study showed no benefit of combined therapy relative to aspirin monotherapy, with increased major bleeding in the combined therapy group. Similar null data were observed in the multinational OASIS-II trial, which evaluated long-term, moderate intensity oral anticoagulation in addition to aspirin in the setting of unstable angina.[77] However, in this latter trial, patients randomized in countries where good compliance was achieved (majority of participants with INR >2.0) appeared to have a benefit of combined therapy of almost 30% for the endpoint of death, myocardial infarction, and stroke.

In marked contrast to CHAMP and OASIS-II, the benefit of anticoagulation alone or combined anticoagulation plus aspirin after acute coronary syndromes was observed in the second Aspirin and Coumadin After Acute Coronary Syndromes (ASPECT II) trial.[78] In this trial, 999 patients with acute MI or unstable angina in the preceding 8 weeks were treated with either high-intensity oral anticoagulation (coumadin, target INR 3.0-4.0), combined low-dose aspirin (80 mg), and moderate-intensity oral anticoagulation (coumadin, target INR 2.0-2.5), or low-dose aspirin alone. This open-label study followed participants for a maximum of 26 months. The endpoint was reached in 9% of patients on aspirin, 5% in patients taking anticoagulants (HR = 0.55 [95% CI, 0.30-1.00; P = 0.048]), and in 5% of patients receiving combination therapy (HR = 0.50 [95% CI 0.27-0.92; P = 0.03]). The authors concluded that therapy with high-intensity warfarin alone or medium-intensity warfarin plus aspirin was superior to aspirin alone in the reduction of subsequent cardiovascular events and death. There was no difference in bleeding risk between the treatment groups. For the endpoint of all-cause mortality, coumadin alone appeared to provide the greatest relative benefit (see Fig. 26-1).

The Warfarin, Aspirin Reinfarction Study II (WARIS II)[79] randomized 3630 subjects upon hospital discharge with clinically stabilized acute MI to one of three regimens: aspirin 160 mg/day, combined aspirin 75 mg/day and warfarin with a target INR of 2 to 3, or warfarin alone with a target INR of 2.8 to 4.2. The average follow-up

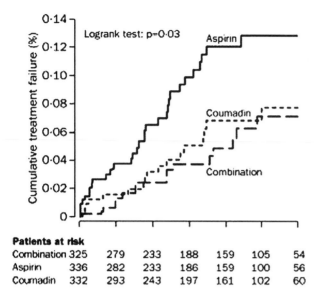

Patients at risk

Combination	325	279	233	188	159	105	54
Aspirin	336	282	233	186	159	100	56
Coumadin	332	293	243	197	161	102	60

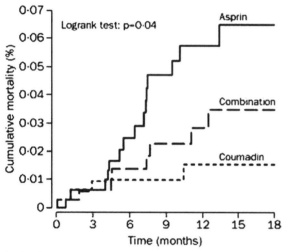

Patients at risk

Combination	332	287	299	196	165	108	61
Aspirin	336	291	242	197	165	104	55
Coumadin	325	281	237	190	166	103	58

FIGURE 26-1. Cumulative occurrence of primary events *(upper)* and mortality *(lower)* by treatment group, from the ASPECT II study. (Reprinted from van Es RF, Jonker JJ, Verheugt FW, et al: Aspirin and Coumadin after acute coronary syndromes (the ASPECT-2 study): a randomized controlled trial. Lancet 2002; 360:109–113. Copyright © 2002 Elsevier Ltd. Used with permission.)

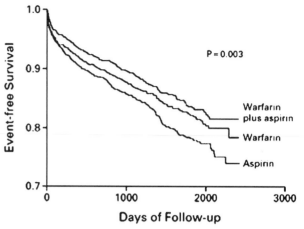

FIGURE 26-2. Event-free survival curves for the composite end point of death, nonfatal reinfarction, and thromboembolic stroke, from the WARIS II study. (Reprinted from Hurlen M, Abdelnoor M, Smith P, et al: Warfarin, aspirin, or both after myocardial infarction. N Engl J Med 2002; 347:969–974. Copyright © 2002 Massachusetts Medical Society. Used with permission.)

period was 4 years. The primary endpoint was a composite of death, nonfatal reinfarction, and nonfatal thromboembolic stroke. Warfarin, in combination with aspirin or given alone, was superior to aspirin alone in reducing the incidence of the composite endpoint. Specifically, compared with aspirin alone, warfarin alone was associated with a 19% reduction in the primary outcome (rate ratio 0.81, 95% CI 0.69 to 0.95), while the combination of warfarin plus aspirin was associated with a 29% reduction in events (rate ratio 0.71, 95% CI 0.60 to 0.83, see Fig. 26-2). There was no significant difference between the two study groups allocated warfarin. The reduction was driven primarily by a reduction in nonfatal reinfarction with little impact on mortality. Bleeding rates in the

two warfarin arms were 0.62% per treatment-year. While low, this rate was significantly higher than among those allocated aspirin alone (0.17%).

Aspirin plus coumadin versus aspirin alone has also been evaluated in the APRICOT-2 trial of patients with acute myocardial infarction treated with fibrinolysis, a setting where reocclusion of the infarct related artery is of major concern.[80] The APRICOT-2 investigators enrolled 308 patients within 48 hours of successful fibrinolysis to either short-term heparin plus aspirin, or to a 3-month course of aspirin combined with moderate intensity warfarin with a target INR between 2.0 and 3.0. Overall, reocclusion of the infarct related artery at 3 months was observed in 15% of patients receiving aspirin and coumadin as compared to 28% receiving aspirin alone. This benefit was associated with improved survival rates and reduced rates of target lesion revascularization without a significant increase in hemorrhage. The Thrombosis Prevention Trial (TPT) reported results of a 2 × 2 factorial trial of low-intensity warfarin and low-dose aspirin in men without prior events but at high risk of ischemic heart disease.[81] Although this was not a trial of secondary prevention, the findings added important new data to the totality of evidence on combination versus monotherapy with anticoagulants and aspirin to prevent occlusive vascular events. The trial randomized 5085 men in the United Kingdom, 45 to 69 years of age, who were at high risk for ischemic heart disease based on a risk score that considered family history, smoking history, body mass index, blood pressure, cholesterol, plasma fibrinogen, and plasma factor VII activity. Anticoagulation with warfarin was adjusted toward a target INR of 1.5; aspirin was given at 75 mg/day in a controlled-release preparation. The trial accrued a median treatment duration of 6.8 years. The mean warfarin INR and dosage were 1.47 and 4.1 mg/day, respectively. The primary endpoint was total ischemic heart disease, defined as nonfatal MI plus coronary death.

Warfarin-treated participants experienced a 21% reduction in ischemic heart disease (95% CI 4-35; P = 0.02),

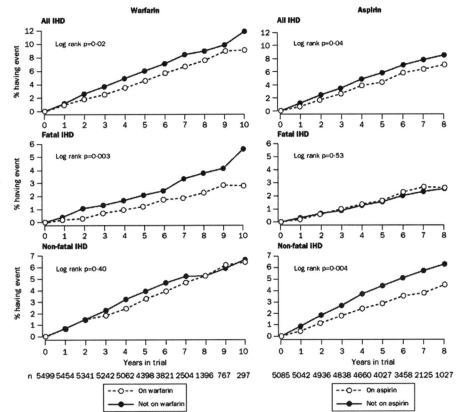

FIGURE 26-3. Cumulative proportion (%) of men with IHD, main effects (n = number) in trial for specified duration of follow-up, from the TPT study. (Reprinted from Medical Research Council's General Practice Research Framework: Thrombosis Prevention Trial: Randomized trial of low-intensity oral anticoagulation with warfarin and low-dose aspirin in the primary prevention of ischemic heart disease in men at increased risk. Lancet 1998; 351:233–241. Copyright © 2002 Elsevier Ltd. Used with permission.)

chiefly because of a statistically significant 39% reduction in fatal events. Aspirin treatment was associated with a similar 20% reduction in ischemic heart disease (95% CI 1–35; P =0.04) almost entirely because of a significant 32% reduction in nonfatal MI. Combined treatment yielded a 34% reduction in ischemic heart disease (95% CI 11–51; P =0.006). There was an excess of hemorrhagic stroke and total fatal strokes among those participants assigned combined therapy. The number of hemorrhagic stroke events was 7 in the combined treatment group, 1 in the warfarin-only group, 2 in the aspirin-only group, and 0 in the placebo group; for fatal strokes, there were 12 in combined therapy, 5 in the warfarin-only group, 2 in the aspirin-only group, and 1 in the placebo group. Taking into account the relative incidence of ischemic heart disease and stroke, the trial reported that combined therapy prevented approximately 12 times as many episodes of ischemic heart disease as it caused strokes, although the strokes tended to be hemorrhagic and fatal. Thus, the trial demonstrated that combined therapy with warfarin and aspirin may have added benefits on vascular disease events, and it further suggested that the failure to observe such an effect in the CARS investigation may have been related to that trial's use of a fixed, low dosage of warfarin (see Fig. 26-3).

Direct Thrombin Inhibition in Secondary Prevention

Despite data from WARIS-II and ASPECT-II, which have increased the use of aspirin and/or coumadin in secondary prevention, the risk of recurrent ischemia remains high following myocardial infarction. Because of continued concerns about bleeding risk and drug interactions, many investigators have sought alternative methods for anticoagulation and antithrombotic therapy in this setting. Data on the potential use of oral direct thrombin inhibition with ximelagatran have recently been provided in the ESTEEM trial.[82] In this study, 1883 patients with recent MI were randomly assigned to ximelagatran at one of 4 doses or to placebo, with all participants receiving 160 mg/day of aspirin. Compared with aspirin alone, those receiving any dose of ximelagatran had a 24% relative risk reduction (95% CI 0.59 to 0.98) in the combined endpoint of nonfatal MI, severe recurrent ischemia, or death. The benefit of ximelagatran given twice daily came at an increased risk of liver function test abnormalities, a finding consistent across ximelagatran trials. Thus, while this approach shows considerable promise, oral ximelagatran therapy may require monitoring, an issue that reduces its overall clinical attractiveness. Ongoing studies comparing oral ximelagatran therapy with warfarin will also be needed to fully evaluate this novel therapeutic approach.

Guidelines for Use of Antiplatelet and Anticoagulant Therapy in Secondary Prevention of Cardiovascular Disease

In 2001, the AHA and the American College of Cardiology (ACC) updated their Guidelines for Preventing Heart Attack and Death in Patients with Atherosclerotic Cardiovascular Disease.[83] This revision of the 1995 guidelines reflects the strong evidence from clinical trials that has emerged since that time, which further supports the benefit of aggressive risk factor management. With regard to antiplatelet agents and anticoagulants, AHA/ACC recommends that a daily dose of 75 to 325 mg aspirin be initiated and continued indefinitely if not contraindicated, and if contraindicated, that clopidogrel (75 mg/day) or warfarin be considered. Warfarin should be managed to an INR of 2.0 to 3.0 in post-MI patients when clinically indicated or for patients unable to take aspirin or clopidogrel. In the context of the fact that a larger proportion of patients in whom these therapies are indicated are not receiving them in practice, the AHA and ACC urge all medical care providers to organize specific plans to identify such patients, initiate appropriate therapy, and assess the success achieved in providing appropriate therapies.

ASPIRIN IN PRIMARY PREVENTION

The data discussed in the previous sections do not address the role of aspirin in the primary prevention of CVD among individuals at usual risk. In primary prevention, the benefit-risk ratio for aspirin must be even more carefully weighed than in secondary prevention settings. Any agent that inhibits platelet aggregation may pose a risk of increased bleeding. Although these risks may be deemed acceptable for those at high risk of a CVD event because of acute MI or other prior CVD history, they must be carefully weighed against the likely benefits for those at lower baseline risk of occlusive vascular events. The dosage of aspirin must also be carefully considered; although the benefits on CVD appear comparable over the wide dose range tested in trials to date, the major side effects of the drug are dose dependent.[38] The goal for primary prevention is to choose the lowest dosage of aspirin that has a cardioprotective effect while minimizing side effects.

Aspirin has been evaluated in five completed primary prevention trials. The British Doctors' Trial (BDT) trial was conducted among 5139 apparently healthy male physicians aged 50 to 78 years in Great Britain.[84] The treatment group was assigned to a daily dose of 500 mg of aspirin, and the control group was asked to avoid aspirin and aspirin-containing compounds. After 6 years of treatment and follow-up, there were no significant differences between the two groups with respect to nonfatal MI, nonfatal stroke, vascular death, or all important vascular events combined. It was not possible to distinguish reliably between thrombotic and hemorrhagic strokes. There was an increase of borderline statistical significance in the aspirin group of the subgroup of strokes that were self-reported as "disabling." It is difficult to determine whether this finding reflects a true increase in such events, which might be more likely to be hemorrhagic in origin, or is the result of bias in the self-reporting of residual impairment given the study's open-label design without placebo control.

The Physicians' Health Study (PHS) was a randomized, double-blind, placebo-controlled trial of 325 mg of aspirin on alternate days (as well as 50 mg of beta-carotene on alternate days) conducted among 22,071

apparently healthy U.S. male physicians, 40 to 84 years of age.[46] The trial was stopped prematurely by the Data and Safety Monitoring Board after a mean treatment period of 60.2 months, primarily because of a 44% reduction in risk of first MI among those randomized to aspirin (RR = 0.56; 95% CI 0.45-0.70, P < 0.00001). There was a 22% increased risk of total stroke among those assigned to aspirin, which was not statistically significant (RR = 1.22; 95% CI 0.93-1.60). This was primarily due to an increased risk of hemorrhagic stroke in the aspirin group (23 vs. 12 events in placebo, P = 0.06). There was no benefit observed for aspirin on cardiovascular mortality (RR = 0.96; 95% CI 0.60-1.54), although the findings for both mortality and stroke were inconclusive because of inadequate numbers of events.

The benefit of aspirin on MI emerged in the early months of the trial, and its magnitude did not change during 5 years of treatment.[85] In contrast, long-term aspirin use did not reduce the development of angina pectoris during the trial.[86]

The Thrombosis Prevention Trial (TPT) used a factorial design to randomize 5085 men aged 45 to 69 years who were at elevated risk for ischemic heart disease based on a risk score that included family history, smoking history, body mass index, blood pressure, cholesterol, plasma fibrinogen, and plasma factor VII activity, to either low-dose aspirin (75 mg/day), warfarin (target INR 1.5), both agents, or placebo.[81] After a median treatment duration of 6.8 years, aspirin was associated with a 20% reduction in the primary endpoint of ischemic heart disease, defined as coronary death and nonfatal MI (95% CI 1% to 35%). This benefit resulted primarily from a 32% reduction in nonfatal MI (95% CI 12% to 48%). There was a nonsignificant 3% aspirin-associated reduction in total stroke. There was no significant effect on fatal events, and there was an excess of hemorrhagic stroke and total fatal strokes among those assigned to both agents (hemorrhagic stroke: 7 events in combined therapy, 1 in warfarin alone, 2 in aspirin alone, and none in placebo; fatal stroke: 12, 5, 2, and 1, respectively).

In the 26-country Hypertension Optimal Treatment (HOT) trial, 18,790 persons (47% of whom were women) with elevated diastolic blood pressure (between 100 and 115 mm Hg) were randomly assigned to one of three target diastolic blood pressure ranges (≤80, ≤85, and ≤90 mm Hg) and to either controlled-release aspirin (75 mg/day) or placebo.[87] The antihypertensive agent felodipine was given as baseline therapy to all participants, with the addition of ACE inhibitors, beta blockers, or diuretics as needed to reach target blood pressure. After 3.8 years of treatment, aspirin reduced the incidence of major cardiovascular events (MI, stroke, cardiovascular death) by 15% (P = 0.03) and of MI by 36% (P = 0.002), with no effect on the incidence of total stroke or fatal bleeds. Nonfatal major bleeds, however, were more common in the aspirin group than in the placebo group (RR = 1.8, P < 0.001).

The Primary Prevention Project (PPP) trial was a randomized, open-label 2 × 2 factorial trial of enteric-coated, low-dose aspirin (100 mg/day) and vitamin E in 4495 individuals (58% women) 50 years or older who had one or more cardiovascular risk factors.[88] After a mean of 3.6 years, the trial was prematurely stopped because interim analyses were consistent with the newly available TPT and HOT results. Aspirin assignment was associated with a significantly reduced risk of the combined endpoint of cardiovascular death, nonfatal MI, and nonfatal stroke (RR = 0.77, 95% CI 0.62-0.95). Examination of specific endpoints showed an aspirin-associated risk reduction for cardiovascular death (RR = 0.56, 95% CI 0.31-0.99). No major differences were seen between the aspirin and nonaspirin groups with respect to stroke type. Severe bleeds were more frequent in the aspirin group (1.1% vs. 0.3%, P < 0.0008).

Despite design differences between the five primary prevention trials, the trials have been generally consistent in showing that aspirin therapy reduces the incidence of first CHD. A recent meta-analysis by Hayden and associates[89] of pooled data from the five trials suggests that aspirin lowers incidence of nonfatal MI or death from CHD by 28% (summary odds ratio = 0.72, 95% CI 0.60-0.87) and cumulative CHD mortality by 13% (odds ratio = 0.87, 95% CI 0.70-1.09). Limiting the meta-analysis to the three trials that used a double-blind, placebo-controlled design (PHS, TPT, and HOT) showed a slightly larger protective effect of aspirin on total CHD incidence: the summary odds ratio was 0.65 (95% CI 0.56-0.75). For total stroke, the summary odds ratio was 1.02 (95% CI 0.85-1.23). However, compared with the findings for CHD, the results for stroke were more heterogeneous across the five trials. This heterogeneity may relate to the wide range of aspirin doses tested or, alternatively, because data from secondary prevention trials suggest that aspirin prevents ischemic stroke but increases the risk of hemorrhagic stroke. Thus, the net effect of aspirin on total stroke incidence in a given population may be partly a function of its underlying risk for each stroke subtype.

A meta-analysis of the BDT, PHS, TPT, and PPP trials reported a relative risk of ischemic stroke of 1.03 (95% CI 0.87-1.21),[90] suggesting that aspirin has little effect on reducing ischemic stroke among individuals with no history of prior CVD. As to the potential adverse effects of aspirin in such populations, a meta-analysis of all five trials by Sudlow and colleagues[91] indicated a nonsignificant increased risk of hemorrhagic stroke (summary odds ratio = 1.4; 95% CI 0.9-2.0; excess risk of 0.1 event per 1000 persons per year) and a statistically significant increase in the risk of major extracranial (primarily gastrointestinal) bleeding (summary odds ratio = 1.7; 95% CI 1.4-2.1; excess risk of 0.7 per 1000 persons per year).

Using these summary estimates, Hayden and associates[89] estimated the net impact of aspirin therapy in populations at different levels of risk for CHD. The risk estimates for CHD were taken from the primary prevention trials. Treating 1000 individuals without CHD who have a 5-year risk of CHD of 5% with 5 years of aspirin therapy would prevent 14 (95% CI 6-20) events. The preventive effect for 1000 participants with a 5-year CHD risk of 3% would prevent 8 (95% CI 4-12) events, and for those with a 5-year risk of CHD of 1%, 3 (95% CI 1-4) events. On the other side, 5-year aspirin therapy would lead to 1 (95% CI 0-2) hemorrhagic stroke and 3 (95% CI 2-4) major gastrointestinal bleeds in all risk groups. Thus, aspirin therapy is likely to provide a net

benefit to persons at elevated risk of CHD but a net harm to those at low risk.

A recent update on the role of aspirin in primary prevention of CVD took all five primary prevention trials into account.[92] Among the 55,580 randomized participants, aspirin was associated with a statistically significant 32% (RR = 0.68, 95% CI 0.59-0.79) reduction in the risk of first MI and a significant 15% (RR = 0.85, 95% CI 0.79-0.93) reduction in the risk of all important vascular events. However, there were no significant effects on nonfatal stroke or vascular death. With respect to hemorrhagic stroke, although based on a small number of events, there was a 56% increase, which was of borderline statistical significance (RR = 1.56, 95% CI 0.99-2.46).

Additional data from primary prevention trials are needed for the complete assessment of aspirin's benefit-risk ratio in apparently healthy persons. None of these trials had an adequate number of women to evaluate the role of aspirin in this group. The primary concern in extrapolating findings to women from trial data in men is that the benefit-risk ratio for prophylactic aspirin use in women may differ from that in men. Women's risk of MI, the principal outcome that aspirin may prevent, is lower at almost all ages than men's risk, whereas women and men have roughly comparable rates of stroke, the hemorrhagic forms of which may be increased by aspirin.

Gender-specific subgroup analyses of data from the HOT trial among hypertensives suggested that women may not benefit from aspirin therapy to the same degree as their male counterparts.[93] In women, aspirin was associated with a nonsignificant 19% reduction in MI incidence (RR = 0.81, 95% CI 0.49-1.31; 1.7 vs. 2.1 events per 1000 person-years of observation), whereas in men, a highly significant 42% reduction was achieved (RR = 0.58, 95% CI 0.41-81; 2.9 vs. 5.0 events per 1000 person-years of observation). Gender differences in the effect of aspirin were not found for stroke or total mortality, however. Gender-stratified analyses were not provided in the PPP trial, the only other completed primary prevention trial that included women. The ongoing Women's Health Study (WHS),[94] which randomized 39,876 U.S. female health professionals 45 years and older to low-dose aspirin (100 mg every other day) or placebo, as well as 600 IU of vitamin E every other day or placebo, was begun in 1992 to evaluate directly the balance of benefits and risks of low-dose aspirin in the primary prevention of CVD among apparently healthy women. The trial is scheduled to end in 2004, at which time the average length of treatment and follow-up will be approximately 10 years.

Clinical data from primary prevention trials also support a role for antiplatelet and anticoagulant therapies as potential modifiers of novel markers of cardiovascular risk, including intrinsic fibrinolytic function and inflammation. For example, data indicate that fibrinolytic capacity as measured by baseline antigen levels of tissue plasminogen activator (t-PA) inhibitor, and D-dimer are associated with increased risks of first or recurrent MI.[95-98] However, aspirin appears to attenuate this effect, at least when fibrinolytic capacity is assessed with t-PA antigen.[96] Aspirin may also modify the risk of MI associated with elevated levels of C-reactive protein, a marker of inflammation that appears to be an independent predictor for MI, stroke, and peripheral vascular disease.[99-101] Additional support regarding aspirin, CRP, and outcomes in acute coronary syndromes has also been provided.[102]

In summary, there is conclusive evidence of a reduction associated with low-dose aspirin in the risk of a first MI in men without a prior history of CVD. However, the evidence concerning stroke and vascular mortality remains inconclusive owing to inadequate numbers of endpoints in individual primary prevention trials as well as in the meta-analytic overview of their findings. The ongoing WHS trial in women at usual risk will provide data useful for the reexamination of current policy recommendations for the role of aspirin in apparently healthy women. In any event, use of aspirin in primary prevention of MI should remain an individual clinical judgment, initiated only on the recommendation of a physician or other primary health care provider, and should be viewed as an adjunct, not an alternative, to management of other coronary risk factors.

Guidelines for Use of Aspirin for Primary Prevention of Cardiovascular Disease

In 2002, the U.S. Preventive Services Task Force (USPSTF)[103] reviewed the available data from primary prevention trials and found "good" evidence that aspirin decreases the incidence of CHD in adults at high risk for heart disease, "good" evidence that aspirin increases the incidence of gastrointestinal bleeding, and "fair" evidence that aspirin increases the incidence of hemorrhagic strokes. For primary prevention, the USPSTF concluded that aspirin may be beneficial for those whose risk of CHD is sufficiently high (i.e., 5-year risk $\geq 3\%$ and 10-year risk $\geq 6\%$) to warrant exposure to any risks of long-term administration of the drug. Thus, clinicians should discuss aspirin therapy with patients at increased risk for CHD, including men older than 40 years of age; postmenopausal women; and younger persons with CHD risk factors, such as hypertension, diabetes, or smoking. (The USPSTF noted that statistical prediction tools, such as that provided at www.med-decisions.com,[104] are likely to produce a more accurate estimate of CHD risk than is a simple count of coronary risk factors.) Discussions with patients should focus on both benefit and harm of aspirin and should consider individual preferences and risk aversions with respect to MI, stroke, and gastrointestinal bleeding. Although the benefit-risk balance is most favorable in individuals whose 5-year CHD risk exceeds 3%, some lower-risk individuals may want to consider the potential benefits to outweigh the potential harm.

Although the optimal dose of aspirin for the primary prevention of CVD is not known at this time, the USPSTF noted that dosages of 75 mg/day appear to be as effective as higher dosages. Whether dosages lower than 75 mg/day are also effective has not been determined, however.

In 2002, the AHA also updated its Guidelines for Primary Prevention of Cardiovascular Disease and Stroke.[105] The AHA recommended the use of low-dose aspirin, 75 to 160 mg/day, in men and women with a 10-year risk of CHD $\geq 10\%$ who are not at increased risk for gastrointestinal bleeding or hemorrhagic stroke. On the basis of these guidelines, a middle-aged man who is a current smoker and has a strong family history of premature CHD would be a strong candidate for prophylactic aspirin use. Similarly, aspirin may be warranted for a 60-year-old woman with a cholesterol level of 250 mg/dL and a recent diagnosis of type 2 diabetes. On the other hand, aspirin would not be indicated—and may even be contraindicated—in a 44-year-old premenopausal woman whose only cardiovascular risk factor is poorly controlled hypertension (average readings of 160/100-mm Hg), because she is at greater risk of hemorrhagic stroke than MI.

Acknowledgement

The authors thank David M. Kerins, MD for his contribution to a previous version of this chapter.

REFERENCES

1. Funk CD, Funk LB, Kennedy ME, et al: Human platelet/erythroleukemia cell prostaglandin G/H synthase: cDNA cloning, expression, and gene chromosomal assignment. FASEB J 1991; 5:2304-2312.
2. FitzGerald GA: Mechanisms of platelet activation: Thromboxane A2 as an amplifying signal for other agonists. Am J Cardiol 1991; 68:11B-15B.
3. Vane JR: Inhibition of prostaglandin synthesis as a mechanism of action for aspirin-like drugs. Nat N Biol 1971; 231:232-235.
4. Schafer AI: Effects of nonsteroidal anti-inflammatory drugs on platelet function and systemic hemostasis. J Clin Pharmacol 1995; 35:209-219.
5. Pedersen AK, FitzGerald GA: Cyclooxygenase inhibition, platelet function, and metabolite formation during chronic sulfinpyrazone dosing. Clin Pharmacol Ther 1985; 37:36-42.
6. Van Hecken A, Schwartz JI, Depre M, et al: Comparative inhibitory activity of rofecoxib, meloxicam, diclofenac, ibuprofen, and naproxen on COX-2 versus COX-1 in healthy volunteers. J Clin Pharmacol 2000; 40:1109-1120.
7. Bombardier C, Laine L, Reicin A, et al: Comparison of upper gastrointestinal toxicity of rofecoxib and naproxen in patients with rheumatoid arthritis: VIGOR Study Group. N Engl J Med 2000; 343:1520-1258.
8. Solomon DH, Glynn RJ, Levin R, et al: Nonsteroidal anti-inflammatory drug use and acute myocardial infarction. Arch Intern Med 2002; 162:1099-1104.
9. Rahme E, Pilote L, LeLorier J: Association between naproxen use and protection against acute myocardial infarction. Arch Intern Med 2002; 162:1111-1115.
10. Watson DJ, Rhodes T, Cai B, et al: Lower risk of thromboembolic cardiovascular events with naproxen among patients with rheumatoid arthritis. Arch Intern Med 2002; 162: 1105-1110.
11. Ray WA, Stein CM, Hall K, et al: Non-steroidal anti-inflammatory drugs and risk of serious coronary heart disease: An observational cohort study. Lancet 2002; 359:118-123.
12. Garcia Rodriguez LA, Varas C, Patrono C: Differential effects of aspirin and non-aspirin nonsteroidal antiinflammatory drugs in the primary prevention of myocardial infarction in postmenopausal women. Epidemiology 2000; 11:382-387.
13. Whitlon DS, Sadowski JA, Suttie JW: Mechanism of coumarin action: Significance of vitamin K epoxide reductase inhibition. Biochemistry 1978; 17:1371-1377.
14. Hirsh J, Fuster V, Ansell J, et al: American Heart Association/American College of Cardiology Foundation guide to warfarin therapy. J Am Coll Cardiol 2003; 41:1633-1652.
15. Elwood PC, Cochrane AL, Burr ML, et al: A randomized controlled trial of acetyl salicylic acid in the secondary prevention of mortality from myocardial infarction. BMJ 1974; 1:436-440.

16. Elwood PC, Sweetnam PM: Aspirin and secondary mortality after myocardial infarction. Lancet 1979; 2:1313–1315.
17. Elwood PC, Sweetnam PM: Aspirin and secondary mortality after myocardial infarction. Circulation 1980; 62:V53–V58.
18. Coronary Drug Project Research Group: Aspirin in coronary heart disease. J Chronic Dis 1976; 29:625–642.
19. Aspirin Myocardial Infarction Study Research Group: A randomized, controlled trial of aspirin in persons recovered from myocardial infarction. JAMA 1980; 243:661–669.
20. Persantine-Aspirin Reinfarction Study Research Group: Persantine and aspirin in coronary heart disease. Circulation 1980; 62:449–461.
21. Klimt CR, Knatterud GL, Stamler J, et al: Persantine-Aspirin Reinfarction Study. Part II. Secondary coronary prevention with persantine and aspirin. J Am Coll Cardiol 1986; 7:251–269.
22. Breddin K, Loew D, Lechner K, et al: Secondary prevention of myocardial infarction: A comparison of acetylsalicylic acid, placebo and phenprocoumon. Haemostasis 1980; 9:325–344.
23. Anturane Reinfarction Trial Group. Sulfinpyrazone in the prevention of cardiac death after myocardial infarction. N Engl J Med 1978; 298:289–295.
24. Anturane Reinfarction Trial Research Group. Sulfinpyrazone in the prevention of sudden death after myocardial infarction. N Engl J Med 1980; 302:250–256.
25. Anturane Reinfarction Italian Study Group. Sulfinpyrazone in post-myocardial infarction. Report from the Anturane Reinfarction Italian Study. Lancet 1982; 1:237–242.
26. Antiplatelet Trialists' Collaboration. Secondary prevention of vascular disease by prolonged antiplatelet therapy. BMJ 1988; 296:320–332.
27. Antiplatelet Trialists' Collaboration. Collaborative overview of randomised trials of antiplatelet treatment: I. Prevention of death, myocardial infarction, and stroke by prolonged antiplatelet therapy in various categories of patients. BMJ 1994; 308:81–106.
28. Antithrombotic Trialists' Collaboration. Collaborative meta-analysis of randomised trials of antiplatelet therapy for prevention of death, myocardial infarction, and stroke in high risk patients. BMJ 2002; 324:71–86.
29. International Stroke Trial Collaborative Group. The International Stroke Trial (IST): A randomised trial of aspirin, subcutaneous heparin, both, or neither among 19435 patients with acute ischaemic stroke. Lancet 1997; 349:1569–1581.
30. CAST (Chinese Acute Stroke Trial) Collaborative Group. CAST: Randomised placebo-controlled trial of early aspirin use in 20,000 patients with acute ischaemic stroke. Lancet 1997; 349: 1641–1649.
31. Diener HC, Cunha L, Forbes C, et al: European Stroke Prevention Study. 2. Dipyridamole and acetylsalicylic acid in the secondary prevention of stroke. J Neurol Sci 1996; 143:1–13.
32. De Schryver EL: Design of ESPRIT: An international randomized trial for secondary prevention after non-disabling cerebral ischaemia of arterial origin. European/Australian Stroke Prevention in Reversible Ischaemia Trial (ESPRIT) group. Cerebrovasc Dis 2000; 10:147–150.
33. CAPRIE Steering Committee. A randomised, blinded, trial of clopidogrel versus aspirin in patients at risk of ischaemic events (CAPRIE). Lancet 1996; 348:1329–1339.
34. CURE I. Effects of clopidogrel in addition to aspirin in patients with acute coronary syndromes without ST-segment elevation. N Engl J Med 2001; 345:494–502.
35. Hacke W: From CURE to MATCH: ADP receptor antagonists as the treatment of choice for high-risk atherothrombotic patients. Cerebrovasc Dis 2002; 13(Suppl 1):22–26.
36. Gaspoz JM, Coxson PG, Goldman PA, et al: Cost effectiveness of aspirin, clopidogrel, or both for secondary prevention of coronary heart disease. N Engl J Med 2002; 346:1800–1806.
37. Schomig A, Neumann FJ, Kastrati A, et al: A randomized comparison of antiplatelet and anticoagulant therapy after the placement of coronary-artery stents. N Engl J Med 1996; 334:1084–1089.
38. UK-TIA Study Group. United Kingdom Transient Ischemic Attack (UK-TIA) aspirin trial: Final results. J Neurol Neurosurg Psychiatry 1991; 54:1044–1054.
39. Garcia Rodriguez LA, Hernandez-Diaz S, de Abajo FJ: Association between aspirin and upper gastrointestinal complications: Systematic review of epidemiologic studies. Br J Clin Pharmacol 2001; 52:563–571.
40. Loll PJ, Picot D, Ekabo O, et al: Synthesis and use of iodinated nonsteroidal antiinflammatory drug analogs as crystallographic probes of the prostaglandin H2 synthase cyclooxygenase active site. Biochemistry 1996; 35:7330–7340.
41. Loll PJ, Picot D, Garavito RM: The structural basis of aspirin activity inferred from the crystal structure of inactivated prostaglandin H2 synthase. Nat Struct Biol 1995; 2:637–643.
42. Livio M, Del Maschio A, Cerletti C, et al: Indomethacin prevents the long-lasting inhibitory effect of aspirin on human platelet cyclo-oxygenase activity. Prostaglandins 1982; 23:787–796.
43. Rao GH, Johnson GG, Reddy KR, et al: Ibuprofen protects platelet cyclooxygenase from irreversible inhibition by aspirin. Arteriosclerosis 1983; 3:383–388.
44. Catella-Lawson F, Reilly MP, Kapoor SC, et al: Cyclooxygenase inhibitors and the antiplatelet effects of aspirin. N Engl J Med 2001; 345:1809–1817.
45. MacDonald TM, Wei L: Effect of ibuprofen on cardioprotective effect of aspirin. Lancet 2003; 361:573–574.
46. Steering Committee of the Physicians' Health Study Research Group: Final report on the aspirin component of the ongoing Physicians' Health Study. N Engl J Med 1989; 321:129–135.
47. Kurth T, Glynn RG, Walker AM, et al: Inhibition of clinical benefits of aspirin on first myocardial infarction by nonsteroidal antiinflammatory drugs. Circulation 2003; 108:1191–1195.
48. Murata T, Ushikubi F, Matsuoka T, et al. Altered pain perception and inflammatory response in mice lacking prostacyclin receptor. Nature. 1997; 388:678–682.
49. FitzGerald GA, Patrono C. The coxibs, selective inhibitors of cyclooxygenase-2. N Engl J Med. 2001; 345:433–442.
50. Silverstein FE, Faich G, Goldstein JL, et al: Gastrointestinal toxicity with celecoxib vs nonsteroidal anti-inflammatory drugs for osteoarthritis and rheumatoid arthritis: the CLASS study: A randomized controlled trial. Celecoxib Long-term Arthritis Safety Study. JAMA. 2000; 284:1247–1255.
51. Wright IS, Marple CD, Beck DF: Report of the Committee for the Evaluation of Anticoagulants in the Treatment of Coronary Thrombosis with Myocardial Infarction. Am Heart J 1948; 36: 801–815.
52. Tulloch JA, Gilchrist AR: Anticoagulants in treatment of coronary thrombosis. BMJ 1950; 2:965–71.
53. Wright IS: The use of anticoagulants in coronary heart disease: Progress and problems—1960. Circulation 1960; 22:608–618.
54. Wasserman AJ, Gutterman LA, Yoe KB, et al: Anticoagulants in acute myocardial infarction. The failure of anticoagulants to alter mortality in a randomized series. Am Heart J 1966; 71:43–49.
55. Loeliger EA, Hensen A, Kroes F, et al: A double-blind trial of long-term anticoagulant treatment after myocardial infarction. Acta Med Scand 1967; 182:549–566.
56. Borchgrevink CF, Bjerkelund C, Abrahamsen AM, et al: Long-term anticoagulant therapy after myocardial infarction in women. BMJ 1968; 3:571–574.
57. Drapkin A, Merskey C: Anticoagulant therapy after acute myocardial infarction: Relation of therapeutic benefit to patient's age, sex, and severity of infarction. JAMA 1972; 222:541–548.
58. Ritland S, Lygren T: Comparison of efficacy of 3 and 12 months' anticoagulant therapy after myocardial infarction: A controlled clinical trial. Lancet 1969; 1:122–124.
59. Working Party on Anticoagulant Therapy in Coronary Thrombosis to the Medical Research Council: Assessment of short-anticoagulant administration after cardiac infarction. Report of the Working Party on Anticoagulant Therapy in Coronary Thrombosis to the Medical Research Council. BMJ 1969; 1:335–342.
60. Ebert RV: Long-term anticoagulant therapy after myocardial infarction: Final report of the Veterans Administration cooperative study. JAMA 1969; 207:2263–2267.
61. Seaman AJ, Griswold HE, Reaume RB, et al: Long-term anticoagulant prophylaxis after myocardial infarction. N Engl J Med 1969; 281:115–119.
62. Meuwissen OJ, Vervoorn AC, Cohen O, et al: Double blind trial of long-term anticoagulant treatment after myocardial infarction. Acta Med Scand 1969; 186:361–368.
63. Mitchell JR. Anticoagulants in coronary heart disease: Retrospect and prospect. Lancet 1981; 1:257–262.
64. Sixty Plus Reinfarction Study Research Group: A double-blind trial to assess long-term oral anticoagulant therapy in elderly patients after myocardial infarction. Lancet 1980; 2:989–994.

65. Sixty Plus Reinfarction Study Research Group: Risks of long-term oral anticoagulant therapy in elderly patients after myocardial infarction. Second report of the Sixty Plus Reinfarction Study Research Group. Lancet 1982; 1:64-68.

66. Smith P, Arnesen H, Holme I: The effect of warfarin on mortality and reinfarction after myocardial infarction. N Engl J Med 1990; 323:147-152.

67. Anticoagulants in the Secondary Prevention of Events in Coronary Thrombosis (ASPECT) Research Group: Effect of long-term oral anticoagulant treatment on mortality and cardiovascular morbidity after myocardial infarction. Lancet 1994; 343:499-503.

68. Anand SS, Yusuf S: Oral anticoagulant therapy in patients with coronary artery disease: A meta-analysis. JAMA 1999; 282: 2058-2067.

69. EPSIM Research Group: A controlled comparison of aspirin and oral anticoagulants in prevention of death after myocardial infarction. N Engl J Med 1982; 307:701-708.

70. Julian DG, Chamberlain DA, Pocock SJ: A comparison of aspirin and anticoagulation following thrombolysis for myocardial infarction (the AFTER study): A multicentre unblinded randomised clinical trial. BMJ 1996; 313:1429-1431.

71. Meijer A, Verheugt FW, Werter CJ, et al: Aspirin versus Coumadin in the prevention of reocclusion and recurrent ischemia after successful thrombolysis: A prospective placebo-controlled angiographic study: Results of the APRICOT Study. Circulation 1993; 87:1524-1530.

72. Cohen M, Adams PC, Parry G, et al: Combination antithrombotic therapy in unstable rest angina and non-Q-wave infarction in non-prior aspirin users: Primary end points analysis from the ATACS trial. Antithrombotic Therapy in Acute Coronary Syndromes Research Group. Circulation 1994; 89:81-88.

73. Altman R, Boullon F, Rouvier J, et al: Aspirin and prophylaxis of thromboembolic complications in patients with substitute heart valves. J Thorac Cardiovasc Surg 1976; 72:127-129.

74. Coumadin Aspirin Reinfarction Study (CARS) Investigators: Randomised double-blind trial of fixed low-dose warfarin with aspirin after myocardial infarction. Lancet 1997; 350:389-396.

75. Altman R, Rouvier J, Gurfinkel E, et al: Comparison of two levels of anticoagulant therapy in patients with substitute heart valves. J Thorac Cardiovasc Surg 1991; 101:427-431.

76. Fiore LD, Ezekowitz MD, Brophy MT, et al: Department of Veterans Affairs Cooperative Studies Program clinical trial comparing combined warfarin and aspirin with aspirin alone in survivors of acute myocardial infarction: Primary results of the CHAMP Study. Circulation 2002; 105:557-563.

77. The Organization to Assess Strategies for Ischemic Syndromes (OASIS) Investigators: Effects of long-term, moderate-intensity oral anticoagulation in addition to aspirin in unstable angina. J Am Coll Cardiol. 2001; 37:475-484.

78. van Es RF, Jonker JJ, Verheugt FW, et al: Aspirin and Coumadin after acute coronary syndromes (the ASPECT-2 study): A randomised controlled trial. Lancet 2002; 360:109-113.

79. Hurlen M, Abdelnoor M, Smith P, et al: Warfarin, aspirin, or both after myocardial infarction. N Engl J Med 2002; 347:969-974.

80. Brouwer MA, van den Bergh PJPC, Aengevaeren WRM, et al: Aspirin plus coumarin versus aspirin alone in the prevention of reocclusion after fibrinolysis for acute myocardial infarction: Results of the Antithrombotics in the Prevention of Reocclusion in Coronary Thrombosis (APRICOT)-2 trial. Circulation 2002; 106:659-665.

81. Medical Research Council's General Practice Research Framework. Thrombosis Prevention Trial: Randomised trial of low-intensity oral anticoagulation with warfarin and low-dose aspirin in the primary prevention of ischaemic heart disease in men at increased risk. Lancet 1998; 351:233-241.

82. Wallentin L, Wilcox RG, Weaver WD, et al. Oral ximelagatran for secondary prophylaxis after myocardial infarction: The ESTEEM randomised controlled trial. Lancet. 2003; 362:789-797.

83. Smith SCJ, Blair SN, Bonow O, et al: AHA/ACC Guidelines for preventing heart attack and death in patients with atherosclerotic cardiovascular disease: 2001 update. Circulation 2001; 104: 1577-1579.

84. Peto R, Gray R, Collins R, et al: A randomised trial of the effects of prophylactic daily aspirin among male British doctors. BMJ 1988; 296:313-316.

85. Ridker PM, Manson JE, Buring JE, et al: The effect of chronic platelet inhibition with low-dose aspirin on atherosclerotic progression and acute thrombosis: Clinical evidence from the Physicians' Health Study. Am Heart J 1991; 122:1588-1592.

86. Manson JE, Grobbee DE, Stampfer MJ, et al: Aspirin in the primary prevention of angina pectoris in a randomized trial of US physicians. Am J Med 1990; 89:772-776.

87. Hansson L, Zanchetti A, Carruthers SG, et al: Effects of intensive blood pressure lowering and low-dose aspirin in patients with hypertension: Principal results of the Hypertension Optimal Treatment (HOT) randomized trial. Lancet. 1998; 351: 1755-1762.

88. deGaetano G, for the Collaborative Group of the Primary Prevention Project (PPP): Low-dose aspirin and vitamin E in people at cardiovascular risk: A randomised trial in general practice. Lancet 2001; 357:89-95.

89. Hayden M, Pignone M, Phillips C, et al: Aspirin for the primary prevention of cardiovascular events: A summary of the evidence for the US Preventive Services Task Force. Ann Intern Med 2002; 136:161-172.

90. Hart RG, Halperin JL, McBride R, et al: Aspirin for the primary prevention of stroke and other major vascular events: Meta-analysis and hypotheses. Arch Neurol 2000; 57:326-332.

91. Sudlow C. Antithrombotic treatment. In: American College of Physicians-American Society of Internal Medicine, ed. Clinical Evidence. London, BMJ Publishing Group: 2001.

92. Eidelman RS, Hebert PR, Weisman SM, et al: An update on aspirin in the primary prevention of cardiovascular disease. Arch Intern Med. 2003; 163:2006-2010.

93. Kjeldsen SE, Kolloch RE, Leonetti G, et al: Influence of gender and age on preventing cardiovascular disease by antihypertensive treatment and acetylsalicylic acid: The HOT Study. J Hypertens 2000; 18:629-642.

94. Rexrode KM, Lee IM, Cook NR, et al: Baseline characteristics of participants in the Women's Health Study. J Women's Health Gender-Based Med 2000; 9:19-27.

95. Hamsten A, de Faire U, Walldius G, et al: Plasminogen activator inhibitor in plasma: Risk factor for recurrent myocardial infarction. Lancet 1987; 2:3-9.

96. Ridker PM, Vaughan DE, Stampfer MJ, et al: Endogenous tissue-type plasminogen activator and risk of myocardial infarction. Lancet 1993; 341:1165-1168.

97. Thompson SG, Kienast J, Pyke SD, et al: Hemostatic factors and the risk of myocardial infarction or sudden death in patients with angina pectoris: European Concerted Action on Thrombosis and Disabilities Angina Pectoris Study Group. N Engl J Med 1995; 332:635-641.

98. Ridker PM, Hennekens CH, Cerskus A, et al: Plasma concentration of cross-linked fibrin degradation product (D-dimer) and the risk of future myocardial infarction among apparently healthy men. Circulation 1994; 90:2236-2240.

99. Ridker PM, Cushman M, Stampfer MJ, et al: Inflammation, aspirin, and the risk of cardiovascular disease in apparently healthy men. N Engl J Med 1997; 336:973-979.

100. Ridker PM, Cushman M, Stampfer MJ, et al: Plasma concentration of C-reactive protein and risk of developing peripheral vascular disease. Circulation 1998; 97:425-428.

101. Ridker PM, Rifai N, Rose L, et al: Comparison of C-reactive protein and low-density lipoprotein cholesterol levels in the prediction of first cardiovascular events. N Engl J Med 2002; 347: 1557-1565.

102. Kennon S, Price CP, Mills PG, et al: The effect of aspirin on C-reactive protein as a marker of risk in unstable angina. J Am Coll Cardiol. 2001; 37:1266-1270.

103. US Preventive Services Task Force: Aspirin for the primary prevention of cardiovascular events: Recommendation and rationale. Ann Intern Med 2002; 136:157-160.

104. Wilson PW, D'Agostino RB, Levy D: et al: Prediction of coronary heart disease using risk factor categories. Circulation 1998; 97:1837-1847.

105. Pearson TA, Blair SN, Daniels SR, et al: AHA guidelines for primary prevention of cardiovascular disease and stroke: 2002 update. Circulation 2002; 106:388-391.

Postmenopausal Hormone Replacement Therapy

Claudia U. Chae
JoAnn E. Manson

Postmenopausal hormone replacement therapy (HRT) in the primary and secondary prevention of cardiovascular disease (CVD) is a compelling example of the importance of randomized clinical trials and the evolution of understanding of a given medical therapy. Nearly 40% of women in the United States are older than 45 years of age,[1] with increasing female life expectancy resulting in more than one third of life being spent in the postmenopausal state. Because CVD is the leading cause of mortality in women in developed countries, causing 500,000 deaths annually among women in the United States,[2] and because HRT is hypothesized to reduce CVD risk in postmenopausal women, HRT has a potentially profound impact on public health.

Epidemiologic evidence supporting a cardioprotective effect of estrogen includes the low coronary heart disease (CHD) risk in premenopausal women, greater CHD risk in young women with bilateral oophorectomy who are not taking HRT, closing of the gender gap in CHD risk after menopause, and the reduced risk of CHD and mortality with HRT seen in most observational studies. Plausible biologic mechanisms supported these epidemiologic observations because estrogen may favorably influence a diverse array of mechanisms, including lipid metabolism and oxidative status, vascular tone, intimal hyperplasia, and insulin sensitivity, all of which are involved in the pathogenesis of atherosclerosis and acute coronary syndromes. Based on these factors, HRT was a widely accepted therapy in CVD prevention by women and physicians, despite the lack of randomized clinical trial data assessing clinical outcomes and limited data about the effects of combined estrogen–progestin therapy and the net benefit/risk profile of long-term HRT. Approximately 38% of postmenopausal women in the United States use HRT,[3] and in 2000, Premarin (oral conjugated estrogen) was the second most commonly prescribed medication in the United States.[4]

However, formal testing of the estrogen hypothesis awaited the initiation of several large randomized clinical trials to assess the role of HRT in primary and secondary prevention of CHD. The results thus far have been unexpected. In 1998, the Heart and Estrogen/progestin Replacement Study (HERS) trial[5] found possible early harm and an overall null effect of oral estrogen–progestin HRT on recurrent cardiac events in postmenopausal women with coronary artery disease. Other secondary prevention trials, testing different regimens of estrogen alone or combined with progestin, have subsequently also found no benefit of HRT in postmenopausal women with CHD[6] or a recent first myocardial infarction (MI)[7] or stroke[8] or on atherosclerosis progression on angiography.[9,10] Finally, in July 2002, the estrogen–progestin component of the Women's Health Initiative (WHI), a large primary prevention trial, was stopped as a result of an excess of breast cancer risk, lack of cardiovascular benefit and overall increase in global risk.[11] The estrogen-only component of this trial has reported preliminary findings of an increased risk of stroke and no overall effect on CHD. These clinical trial findings have significantly altered current thinking about the clinical role of HRT in prevention of CVD, intensifying the debate and underscoring the need for further study of HRT's biologic actions, potential benefits and risks, and net impact on clinical outcomes.

PHYSIOLOGIC EFFECTS OF ESTROGEN

There are two distinct estrogen receptors, α and β.[12,13] Found in vascular cells, reproductive tissues, liver, bone, and brain, they classically function as ligand-activated transcription factors that alter gene expression in target cells[14] and mediate many of estrogen's protean biologic effects.

Lipid Effects

High-Density Lipoprotein and Low-Density Lipoprotein

In examining the effect of HRT and biologic intermediates of cardiovascular disease, the most extensive data involve lipids. Menopause is associated with adverse changes in the lipid profile, including increased levels of low-density lipoprotein (LDL) and decreased levels of high-density lipoprotein (HDL).[15] Oral estrogen replacement therapy (ERT) favorably affects lipids, raising HDL and reducing LDL by about 10% to 15%, via a first-pass hepatic effect.[16] These lipid effects of estrogen will be influenced by the dose and duration of treatment, as well as the mode of administration, because transdermal ERT has little impact on HDL and LDL,[16,17] perhaps because of the lack of first-pass hepatic effect or lower systemic estrogen levels. Furthermore, combined therapy with progestin will attenuate some of the benefit of estrogen on lipids because progesterone decreases HDL to a degree directly related to the progestin's dose and degree of androgenicity.[18,19]

The Postmenopausal Estrogen/Progestin Interventions (PEPI) trial is an important study of HRT and biologic intermediates such as lipids.[20] In this 3-year, randomized, double-blind, placebo-controlled trial, 875 postmenopausal women aged 45 to 64 were randomized to placebo; 0.625 mg/day of conjugated equine estrogen (CEE) alone; or CEE (0.625 mg/day) combined with different progestin regimens. These regimens include the following: (1) cyclic medroxyprogesterone acetate (MPA), 10 mg/day for 12 days/month; (2) consecutive MPA, 2.5 mg/day; or (3) cyclic micronized progesterone (MP), 200 mg/day for 12 days/month. All HRT groups had similar, significant reductions in LDL (−15.9 mg/dl on average, or 11.4%). Although HDL levels were significantly higher in all HRT groups, the degree of benefit varied depending on the presence and type of progestin regimen. CEE alone or in combination with cyclic MP had the greatest effects on HDL, with increases from baseline of +5.6 mg/dl (9%) and +4.1 mg/dl (6.6%), respectively, which were not significantly different. MPA, which is more androgenic than MP, attenuated estrogen's HDL effect, whether administered cyclically (+1.6 mg/dl) or continuously (+1.2 mg/dl).

Other trials, although limited by small size[16] or lack of placebo controls,[21,22] found similar lipid effects of estrogen-only and combined HRT to the PEPI trial. The importance of the specific progestin regimen chosen for use in combined HRT, which exerted a significant influence in PEPI, was also seen in trials of combined HRT using relatively androgenic progesterones, such as norgestrel[22] or norethindrone acetate,[23,24] in which HDL was unchanged or fell below baseline levels. Further studies of combined HRT using micronized progesterone are warranted, given its minimal effect on HDL[17,20] and the desirability of retaining progestin's protective effects on the endometrium without adversely affecting estrogen's HDL benefit.

Triglycerides

In contrast to its favorable effects on HDL and LDL, estrogen therapy causes an increase in triglycerides. In PEPI,[20] triglycerides were elevated in all HRT groups to a similar degree (mean +12.8 mg/dl from baseline, or 13.1%). The clinical impact is uncertain because the role of triglycerides as an independent CHD risk factor in women remains controversial and because it may be associated with a less atherogenic form of VLDL.[25]

Lipoprotein(a)

Estrogen is one of the few therapies known to reduce levels of lipoprotein(a) [Lp(a)], which is proposed to be a novel atherothrombotic risk factor. It should be noted, however, that the role of Lp(a) as an independent CHD risk factor in women is controversial[26,27] and it is unknown if lowering Lp(a) will translate into decreased CHD risk. In a substudy of the PEPI trial involving 366 women, Lp(a) levels decreased by 17% to 23% in all HRT groups (P < 0.0001), which was not substantially affected by concomitant progestin therapy.[28] In the HERS secondary prevention trial of combined HRT,[29] the baseline Lp(a) level was independently associated with risk of recurrent CHD events. Women randomized to HRT had a significant reduction in Lp(a) at 1 year compared to those in the placebo group (−5.8 ± 15 vs. 0.34 ± 17 mg/dl, P < 0.001). Although reduction of Lp(a) was not associated with overall decreased risk of CHD, there was the suggestion of benefit from HRT in those in the highest quartile of Lp(a). Further study regarding the relationship between HRT, Lp(a), and CHD risk is needed.

Summary and Clinical Implications of Lipoprotein Effects

ERT thus is associated with potentially beneficial increases in HDL and reductions in LDL and lipoprotein(a), offset by a moderate increase in triglycerides. Combined therapy with a progestin attenuates the impact of estrogen on HDL, to a degree dependent on the progestin's androgenicity. In small trials, compared to statins, HRT reduced LDL and triglycerides to a lesser degree, more consistently increased HDL, lowered Lp(a), and had comparable effects on brachial artery flow-mediated vasodilation.[30-32] Combined HRT and statin treatment has an additive effect on LDL reduction[30,31] and negated the increase in triglycerides seen with HRT,[32] but whether combined therapy will translate into greater clinical benefit is unknown. Furthermore, the reduction in coronary[33-35] and aortic atherosclerosis[36,37] with ERT or combined HRT observed in some animal studies was not attributable to measured changes in serum lipid levels. This suggests estrogen may also be antiatherogenic by functional changes in lipids, such as an antioxidant effect, although this has not been well demonstrated in humans at physiologic dose.[38,39] In two small trials, acute intravenous or several weeks of transdermal estrogen replacement inhibited LDL oxidative lag time,[40,41] but no effect on oxidative status was seen with oral CEE or CEE plus MPA.[40] Alternatively, estrogen's effects on atherosclerosis may be mediated by other mechanisms unrelated to lipid lowering.

Hemostatic Effects

The effects of HRT on thrombosis, which plays an integral role in atherosclerosis progression and acute coronary syndromes, are in need of further study. Menopause is a potentially hypercoagulable state, associated with increases in fibrinogen, factor VII, and plasminogen activator inhibitor-1 (PAI-1),[42,43] which may be countered by increases in natural anticoagulants such as antithrombin III (AT-III).[44] In isolation, oral estrogen appears to have potential fibrinolytic effects, related to decreases in fibrinogen[20,45] and short-term reductions in PAI-1, which are unaffected by added progestin,[40,46,47] although the latter trials were small and lacked placebo controls. However, oral ERT may also have potential procoagulant effects, as suggested by increased levels of factor VII, although these trials lacked placebo controls.[21,22,46] This effect may be attenuated by an added progestin[21,22] and/or transdermal estrogen administration.[45]

Because of the complex dynamics of the clotting system in determining the net balance between thrombosis and fibrinolysis, measurement of coagulation activation peptides (e.g., fibrinopeptide A [FPA] and prothrombin fragment 1 + 2 [F1 + 2]) and enzyme-inhibitor complexes (e.g., thrombin–antithrombin-III complex [TAT]) may be more sensitive than changes in individual hemostatic factors in detecting the prothrombotic state.[48] Limited trial data suggest that oral estrogen is associated with dose-dependent increases in thrombin and fibrin generation consistent with coagulation activation. In a randomized, double-blind, placebo-controlled, crossover trial involving 29 postmenopausal women,[49] after 3 months of oral CEE (0.625 mg or 1.25 mg/day), there were significant dose-dependent increases in thrombin production (F1 + 2) and activity (FPA), and decreases in AT-III and protein S. In an open-label crossover trial,[46] 23 women with surgical menopause were given oral CEE (0.625 mg/day) or transdermal E_2 (0.05 mg/day) for 6 weeks, then crossed over. Both estrogen treatments had potentially prothrombotic effects, with significant increases in FVII and F1 + 2 levels and a decrease in AT-III in the CEE group. However, both groups had lower TAT levels, and the CEE group had significant decreases in PAI. This trial was limited by its lack of a placebo control group and omission of a washout period.

Data regarding the effect of combined HRT on markers of thrombin production and activity are also limited. In a double-blind, randomized trial, 42 postmenopausal women were given oral combined HRT with estradiol and norethisterone or placebo.[50] At 6 weeks, there were significantly increased levels of F1 + 2, soluble fibrin, and D-dimer, indicating increased thrombin generation, fibrin generation, and breakdown and decreased PAI-1 activity. The 25% reduction in PAI-1 activity was similar to that seen in other studies using estrogen only or combined HRT.[40,46,47] Previous studies with combined HRT have had conflicting results; in one study, 6 months of estradiol (2 mg/day) plus cyclic MP resulted in a 14% increase in F1 + 2,[51] whereas others found a nonsignificant increase in F1 + 2 after 3 to 6 months of treatment with CEE (0.625 mg/day) and continuous MPA (2.5 mg/day).[52]

Therefore, small numbers, weaknesses in study design, and short duration of treatment limit the existing clinical trial data examining the effects of HRT on thrombosis. Variation in findings may also be related to the different doses and types of the estrogens and progestins used, duration of treatment, and differences in study design. The available data suggest both prothrombotic and fibrinolytic effects of HRT. However, the twofold to threefold excess risk of venous thromboembolic events (VTE) with HRT[5,11] as well as the possible increased risk of MI seen early with HRT,[5,11] lend support to a clinically meaningful, potential prothrombotic risk with HRT. Identification of particularly susceptible populations, such as those with mutations such as factor V Leiden,[53,54] and its clinical implications are in need of further study.

Inflammatory Effects

Inflammation appears to play a critical role in atherogenesis,[55] and the possible effect of HRT on inflammatory markers is under current study. Both oral estrogen and combined HRT are associated with elevated levels of the proinflammatory marker C-reactive protein (CRP) in cross-sectional studies[56,57] and in the PEPI trial.[58] In a prospective, nested, case-control study of postmenopausal women in the observational component of the WHI,[59] current use of HRT was associated with elevation in levels of CRP but not interleukin-6 (IL-6). After multivariate adjustment, those in the highest quartile of CRP and IL-6 had a twofold increased risk of CHD events. When stratified by HRT, a positive relationship between the inflammatory markers and CHD risk persisted, suggesting that HRT status had less importance as a risk predictor than baseline CRP or IL-6 levels. Limited data suggest that transdermal estradiol does not elevate CRP levels after 1 year.[60] In the context of the increased risk in CHD events seen in the HERS and WHI trials, these data suggest a possible explanation for early adverse effects of oral ERT, perhaps via proinflammatory effects that increase plaque vulnerability or disease progression.[57,58]

Insulin

Hyperinsulinemia appears to be an independent risk factor for CHD[61] that may be modifiable by HRT. In the PEPI trial,[20] the HRT groups had significant decreases in fasting glucose but postchallenge insulin levels did not differ by treatment groups. However, fasting insulin levels, which may be a better marker for insulin resistance than postchallenge insulin levels, were also lower in the HRT groups, although this was not statistically significant. Further study is needed to clarify the effects of HRT on glucose metabolism.

Vascular Effects

Estrogen appears to have direct and beneficial effects on vascular tone, inhibition of remodeling injury, and endothelial and vascular smooth-muscle cell proliferation.[62,63] Estrogen's vascular effects can be separated into two types: nongenomic and genomic.[62,63] **Nongenomic** effects, such as rapid vasodilation occurring within minutes after estrogen administration, are not dependent on changes in gene expression and appear to occur by both **endothelium-dependent** and **endothelial-independent** mechanisms. Estrogen acutely improves endothelial-dependent coronary vasodilation,[64-67] which appears to be mediated by estrogen receptor alpha (ERα) functioning in a novel, nongenomic manner to directly activate endothelial nitric oxide synthase (eNOS) and increase nitric oxide (NO) release.[68-70] Furthermore, both ERα and ERβ are also expressed on cell membranes,[71] suggesting another pathway by which short-term nongenomic effects may occur such as via activation of intracellular second messenger pathways.[72] Endothelium-independent vasodilation appears to be mediated via ion channels.[73,74]

Genomic effects occur over hours to days and involve the classical estrogen receptor signaling pathway with receptor activation and gene transcription. This includes modulation of the basal release of vasodilators from vessel walls by upregulation of gene expression for biosynthesis of vasodilatory substances such as prostacyclin[75] and NO.[62,63,76-78] Long-term estrogen administration increases endothelium-dependent vasodilation in aortic rings[78-80] and in primates.[81] This may be mediated by effects of estrogen via augmentation of NOS activity or NO synthesis and release[62,63,68,76,78,82,83] or alternatively may be mediated by antioxidant effects.[84,85] However, little data exist as to estrogen's longer-term effects on endothelial-dependent vasodilation in humans; 9 weeks of oral estradiol[86] or 12 weeks of oral, but not transdermal, estrogen[87] improved endothelium-dependent, flow-mediated vasodilation. Finally, the vasoactive effects of estrogen may be mediated by enhanced production or release by the endothelium of other vasodilators, such as prostacyclin,[75] or inhibition of vasoconstrictors, such as endothelin-1.[88,89]

Progesterone may attenuate the beneficial effects of unopposed estrogen replacement on vasoreactivity, as seen in female canine coronary artery rings,[80] hypercholesterolemic primates,[90] and limited data in humans.[91,92] In postmenopausal women, 2.5 or 5 mg/day of MPA for 3 months reversed the effect of CEE on flow-mediated dilation in brachial artery in a dose-dependent fashion.[92] Whether less androgenic progestins have lesser impact on vasoreactivity is unknown; in a study of 17 postmenopausal women, micronized progesterone did not attenuate the effect of transdermal estrogen on brachial artery reactivity.[93]

Clinical data regarding the coronary vasodilatory effects of ERT are limited. Small trials reported a reduction in the frequency of angina with ERT in postmenopausal women with syndrome X,[94] a condition hypothesized to result from endothelial dysfunction in the absence of angiographic CAD. Small trials testing the effects of acute sublingual 17β-estradiol[95] and transdermal estradiol[96] on treadmill performance in postmenopausal women with CHD have had conflicting results. The effects of long-term ERT or an added progestin on functional measures of myocardial ischemia are unknown.

Genomic effects of estrogen also include inhibitory effects on vascular cell proliferation and remodeling after injury. In animal models, estrogen appears to inhibit the neointimal proliferation seen in response to vascular injury[97-102] via an ER-dependent mechanism[63,97,98,103,104]; the effect appears to be antagonized by progesterone.[101,105] Previous studies also demonstrated reduction in atherosclerotic plaque accumulation with estrogen treatment in ovariectomized, hyperlipidemic animals,[33-37] independent of lipid levels. In some[33-36] but not all[37,106] animal models, reduced atherosclerosis with estrogen was unaffected by an added progestin. Possible underlying mechanisms include direct effects of estrogen on inhibition of vascular smooth-muscle cell proliferation,[97,99] reduction of collagen and elastin synthesis,[107] promotion of angiogenesis,[108] alterations in endothelial cell growth,[108,109] inhibition of endothelial cell apoptosis,[110] and inhibition of expression of cellular adhesion molecules.[111]

EPIDEMIOLOGIC OVERVIEW

Primary Prevention

In addition to plausible biologic mechanisms involving beneficial effects on lipids and the vasculature, observational epidemiologic data consistently supported a 35% to 50% lower risk of CHD with postmenopausal HRT in primary prevention.[112,113] It should be noted that most of these studies examined estrogen-only HRT. Observational data regarding the use of combined estrogen–progestin HRT are much more limited, but the available observational data suggested similar significant reductions in CHD risk as with ERT.[112,114] In terms of other cardiovascular outcomes such as stroke, little data existed but suggested little effect of ERT on risk of stroke.[112] The relative risk of venous thromboembolic events with HRT is consistently elevated by twofold to threefold in observational data, although the absolute risk is low,[115-117] with no apparent differences in risk of venous thromboembolic events between ERT and combined HRT.[116]

Secondary Prevention

Limited epidemiologic data suggested that ERT was associated with decreased risk of recurrent CHD events, predicting improved survival in postmenopausal women with CHD on angiography,[118] and in retrospective studies, improved outcomes after coronary angioplasty[119] or coronary artery bypass surgery.[120] Current use of HRT at time of hospitalization with acute MI, after controlling for the hormone users' healthier status and more aggressive treatment, was associated with an adjusted 35% reduction in mortality.[121] After the HERS trial results were published, epidemiologic analyses from the Nurses' Health Study[122] and Group Health Cooperative[123] suggested transient increases in risk in the short term, with reduced risk seen with longer use.

Thus, the available epidemiologic data consistently supported a reduction in CHD risk among users of postmenopausal HRT. In analyses of HRT's potential benefits (CHD, osteoporosis, menopausal symptoms) versus potential risks (endometrial cancer, breast cancer, gallstones, venous thromboembolism), the net benefit/risk for an individual woman was driven predominantly by risk of CHD versus risk of breast cancer.[112,124] In white women aged 50 to 94, the cumulative absolute risk of cause-specific death is far greater from CHD (31%) compared to that from breast cancer (2.8%), hip fractures (2.8%), and endometrial cancer (0.7%) combined.[125] The risk of breast cancer increases with ERT, especially beyond 5 years in duration.[126] However, because CVD accounts for such a large proportion of morbidity and mortality in women, and because of the significant reduction in CHD risk seen with HRT in observational studies, these analyses found a net benefit with HRT.[112,124]

CLINICAL TRIALS OF HORMONE REPLACEMENT THERAPY

Large randomized clinical trials were needed to confirm or refute the potential cardioprotective effect of HRT suggested by beneficial effects on biologic intermediates such as lipids, the vasculature and atherosclerosis in animal models, and the risk reduction observed in observational studies (Tables 27-1 and 27-2).

TABLE 27-1   RANDOMIZED CLINICAL TRIALS OF POSTMENOPAUSAL HORMONE REPLACEMENT THERAPY IN PRIMARY PREVENTION OF CARDIOVASCULAR DISEASE

	Number	Population	Intervention	Follow-up	Primary outcome	Main results
WHI[11,127]	16,608	Postmenopausal women aged 50–79; mean age 63.3 years	Oral CEE 0.625 mg/day, CEE plus MPA 2.5 mg/day, or placebo	8.5 years (projected); CEE + MPA trial terminated at 5.2 years	CHD (nonfatal MI or CHD death)	Increase in risk of CHD and stroke; increase in risk of breast cancer and VTE and in global index of risk with CEE-MPA
			Oral CEE only 0.625 mg/day or placebo	CEE only terminated at 7.0 years		Estrogen-only preliminary findings: increased risk of stroke; no overall effect on CHD
WISDOM[129]	22,000 (projected) 5,700 (recruited)	Postmenopausal women aged 50–69	Oral CEE 0.625 mg/day with or without MPA	10 years (planned); terminated at approximately 3 years	CHD	Trial was terminated early after WHI results were released in 2002

CEE, conjugated equine estrogen; MPA, medroxyprogesterone acetate; CHD, coronary heart disease; MI, myocardial infarction; VTE, venous thromboembolism.

Primary Prevention of Cardiovascular Disease

The Women's Health Initiative (WHI)[11] enrolled 16,608 healthy postmenopausal women aged 50 to 79 years with an intact uterus at baseline, who were randomized to placebo or oral estrogen (CEE 0.625 mg/day) and progestin (MPA 2.5 mg/day) in one tablet. The primary outcome was CHD (nonfatal MI and CHD death). The primary adverse outcome was invasive breast cancer. A global index summarizing the net benefits and risks included CHD, invasive breast cancer, stroke, pulmonary embolism, endometrial cancer, colorectal cancer, hip fracture, and death from other causes. Planned duration of follow-up was 8.5 years. However, on May 31, 2002, after a mean of 5.2 years of follow-up, the trial's data safety and monitoring board recommended early termination of the

TABLE 27-2   RANDOMIZED CLINICAL TRIALS OF POSTMENOPAUSAL HORMONE REPLACEMENT THERAPY IN SECONDARY PREVENTION OF CARDIOVASCULAR DISEASE

	Number	Population	Intervention	Follow-up	Primary outcome	Main results
HERS[5]	2763	Postmenopausal women with CHD, mean age 66.7 years	Oral CEE 0.625 mg/day plus MPA 2.5 mg/day, or placebo	4.1 years (mean)	Nonfatal MI or CHD death	No difference in nonfatal MI or CHD death (RR 0.99, 95% CI 0.81–1.22); possible early harm
Papworth[6]	255	Postmenopausal women with angiographic CHD	Transdermal 17β-estradiol alone, with norethisterone, or control	2.6 years (mean)	Hospitalization with unstable angina, MI, or death	No difference in unstable angina, MI, or death (RR 1.29, 95% CI 0.84–1.95); possible early harm.
ESPRIT[7]	1017	Postmenopausal women who survived recent first MI, mean age 62.6 years	Oral estradiol valerate (2 mg/day) or placebo	2 years	Reinfarction or cardiac death	No difference in reinfarction or cardiac death (RR 0.99, 95% CI 0.70–1.41).
ERA[9]	309	Postmenopausal women with angiographic CHD, mean age 65.8 years	Oral CEE 0.625 mg/day, CEE plus MPA 2.5 mg/day, or placebo	3.2 years (mean)	Mean minimal coronary artery diameter	No difference in mean minimal coronary artery diameter on angiography
WAVE[10]	423	Postmenopausal women with angiographic CHD, mean age 65 years	Oral CEE 0.625 mg/day, CEE plus MPA 2.5 mg/day, or placebo	2.8 years (mean)	Annualized mean change in minimal lumen diameter	No difference in annualized mean change in minimal lumen diameter on angiography
WEST[8]	664	Postmenopausal women with stroke or TIA, mean age 71 years	Oral 17β estradiol 1.0 mg/day or placebo	2.8 years (mean)	Stroke or death	No difference in death (RR 1.2, 95% CI 0.8–1.8) or nonfatal stroke (RR 1.0, 95% CI 0.7–1.4); increase in fatal stroke (RR 2.9, 95% CI 0.9–9.0)

CHD, coronary heart disease; CEE, conjugated equine estrogen; MPA, medroxyprogesterone acetate; MI, myocardial infarction; RR, relative risk; CI, confidence interval; TIA, transient ischemic attack.

combined estrogen–progestin component of the trial because the test statistic for invasive breast cancer exceeded the stopping boundary and the global index supported an excess of risks compared to benefits. A parallel component of the trial of estrogen alone in women who have had a hysterectomy was recently terminated and reported preliminary findings of increased risk of stroke and no overall effect on CHD.

In WHI, the mean (SD) age at time of enrollment was 63.3 (±7.1) years. Only 7.7% of participants reported having had prior CVD, and the prevalence of cardiac risk factors was comparable to a generally healthy population of postmenopausal women. Dropout rates of approximately one third were comparable to adherence rates with HRT seen in the community; 42% of women in the active treatment arm and 38% of those in the placebo arm stopped taking study drugs at some time. Data were analyzed as intention-to-treat, which may have

underestimated the effect sizes if participants were fully adherent.

The major clinical outcomes of WHI are presented in Table 27-3. Overall rates of CHD were low (0.3% per year). There was a 29% increased risk of CHD events in the estrogen–progestin arm compared to placebo (95% CI 2% to 63%, 37 vs. 30 cases per 10,000 person-years), which was nominally statistically significant at the 0.05 level; most of the excess risk was in nonfatal MI. There was a 41% increased risk of stroke in the estrogen–progestin group (95% CI 7% to 85%, 29 vs. 21 cases per 10,000 person-years), again with most of the events in the nonfatal group. A significant, 2.11-fold greater risk of thromboembolic events was observed (34 vs. 16 cases per 10,000 person-years). There was a 26% increase in risk of invasive breast cancer (38 vs. 30 cases per 10,000 person-years), which was nominally statistically significant (95% CI 0 to 59%) but with a highly significant weighted test

■ ▧ ■

TABLE 27-3   CLINICAL OUTCOMES IN THE WOMEN'S HEALTH INITIATIVE TRIAL, COMPARING ESTROGEN–PROGESTIN HORMONE REPLACEMENT THERAPY TO PLACEBO IN PRIMARY PREVENTION

Outcome	Hazard ratio	95% CI	Events per 10,000 person-years
Cardiovascular disease			
CHD*	1.29	1.02–1.63	+7
CHD death	1.18	0.70–1.97	
Nonfatal MI	1.32	1.02–1.72	
CABG/PTCA	1.04	0.84–1.28	
Stroke†	1.41	1.07–1.85	+8
Fatal	1.20	0.58–2.50	
Nonfatal	1.50	1.08–2.80	
Venous thromboembolic	2.11	1.58–2.82	+18
DVT	2.07	1.49–2.87	
PE	2.13	1.39–3.25	
Total cardiovascular	1.22	1.09–1.36	
Cancer			
Invasive breast	1.26	1.00–1.59	+8
Endometrial	0.83	0.47–1.47	
Colorectal	0.63	0.43–0.92	−6
Total	1.03	0.90–1.17	
Fractures			
Hip	0.66	0.45–0.98	−5
Vertebral	0.66	0.44–0.98	
Other osteoporotic	0.77	0.69–0.86	
Total	0.76	0.69–0.85	
Death			
From other causes	0.92	0.74–1.14	
Total	0.98	0.82–1.18	
Global index‡	1.15	1.03–1.28	+19

*Updated CHD outcomes from WHI, using centrally adjudicated endpoints through July 2002, were as follows: **Total CHD**, RR 1.24 (95% CI 1.00-1.54); **nonfatal MI**, RR 1.28 (95% CI 1.00-1.63); **CHD death**, RR 1.10 (955 CI 0.70-1.75); CABG/PTCA, RR 1.01 (95% CI 0.83-1.22). Manson JE, Hsia J, Johnson KC, et al.: Estrogen plus progestin and the risk of coronary heart disease. N Engl J Med 2003; 349:523–524.

†Updated stroke outcomes from WHI, using centrally adjudicated endpoints through July 2002, were as follows: **Total stroke**, RR 1.31 (95% CI 1.02-1.68); **ischemic stroke**, RR 1.44 (95% CI 1.09-1.90); **hemorrhagic stroke**, RR 0.89 (0.43-1.56). Wassertheil-Smoller S, Hendrix SL, Limacher M, et al.: Effect of estrogen plus progestin on stroke in postmenopausal women: The Women's Health Initiative: A randomized trial. JAMA 2003; 289:2673–2684.

‡Global index represents the first event for each participant among the following types: CHD, stroke, pulmonary embolism, breast cancer, endometrial cancer, colorectal cancer, hip fracture, and death from other causes.

CI, confidence interval; CHD, coronary heart disease; MI, myocardial infarction; CABG, coronary artery bypass grafting; PTCA, percutaneous transluminal coronary angioplasty; DVT, deep venous thrombosis; PE, pulmonary embolus.

(Adapted with permission from Writing Group for the Women's Health Initiative Investigators: Risks and benefits of estrogen plus progestin in healthy postmenopausal women: principal results from the Women's Health Initiative randomized controlled trial. JAMA 2002; 288:321–333.)

statistic for monitoring. Colorectal cancer was reduced by 37% (10 vs. 16 cases per 10,000 person-years), which was nominally statistically significant. Hip fractures were reduced by 34% (10 vs. 15 cases per 10,000 person-years). The global index showed a 15% increase in risk in the estrogen–progestin group compared to the placebo group (170 vs. 151 cases per 10,000 person-years). There were no differences in mortality between the active treatment and placebo groups. As demonstrated in Fig. 27-1, the Kaplan-Meier cumulative hazard curves for cardiovascular

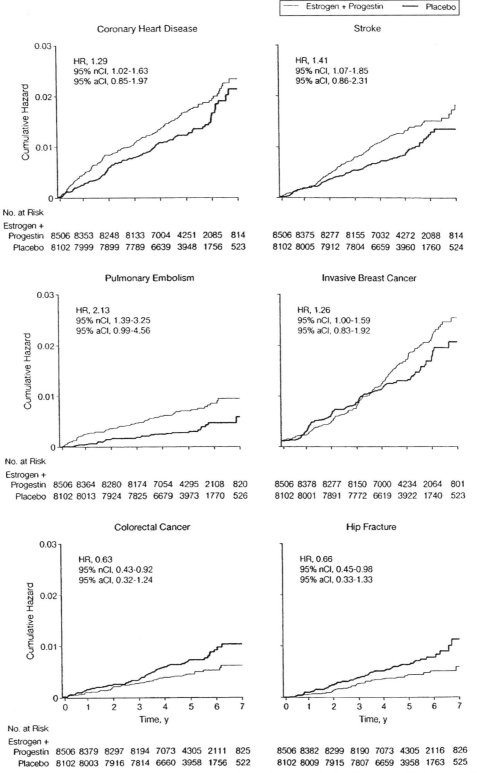

FIGURE 27-1. Kaplan-Meier estimates of cumulative hazards for selected clinical outcomes in the Women's Health Initiative trial. HR, hazard ratio; nCI, nominal confidence interval; aCI, adjusted confidence interval. (From the Writing Group for the Women's Health Initiative Investigators. Risks and benefits of estrogen plus progestin in healthy postmenopausal women: principal results from the Women's Health Initiative randomized controlled trial. JAMA 2002; 288:321–333. Copyright 2002, American Medical Association.)

outcomes diverged soon after randomization. For breast cancer, the curves began to diverge after year 4.

In an updated analysis including all centrally adjudicated CHD endpoints through July 2002,[127] combined HRT was associated with a hazards ratio for CHD of 1.24 (nominal 95% CI 1.00 to 1.54). The slight increase in risk occurred predominantly for myocardial infarction, with no increase in risk of coronary revascularization, angina or congestive heart failure. The elevation in risk was most apparent at one year (HR 1.81, 95% CI 1.09-3.01), with smaller and nonsignificant risks in years two through five, and a statistically significant trend (P = 0.02) towards a decreasing relative risk over time. Extensive subgroup analyses failed to show any important differences, except in women with higher baseline LDL levels who had augmented risk (P for interaction = 0.01); however, this must be interpreted with caution, given the large number of comparisons tested.

Thus, the WHI, which is the first large randomized clinical trial assessing the use of HRT in primary prevention, had several important conclusions. Initiated at the average age of 63 years, combined HRT with estrogen– progestin (using CEE 0.625 mg/day and MPA 2.5 mg/day) had no cardiovascular benefit in more than 5 years of follow-up. In fact, it was associated with an increase in risk of CHD and stroke, extending the results of the HERS trial in secondary prevention (see later in this chapter). The risk of stroke in WHI was greater than that seen in secondary prevention trials.[5,8] It confirmed the previously observed twofold elevation in risk of VTE seen in observational studies[115-117] and in HERS[5] and the increase in breast cancer risk suggested in observational studies.[126] The WHI trial data also definitively demonstrated significant reductions in osteoporotic fractures with HRT. Although the absolute risks and benefits of HRT in WHI were small in magnitude, over the 5.2 years of the trial, about one more in 100 women taking HRT experienced a global index event than those taking placebo. The net risk-benefit ratio was therefore unfavorable, particularly for primary prevention of chronic diseases. Furthermore, despite the low absolute risks involved, given that 38% of postmenopausal women in

the United States use HRT,[3] the potential public health impact is substantial.[128]

The Women's International Study of long-Duration Oestrogen after Menopause (WISDOM) was a large primary prevention trial aiming to recruit 22,000 postmenopausal women aged 50 to 69, with active treatment being 0.625 mg of CEE with or without MPA for 10 years. However, the WISDOM trial was terminated shortly after the WHI results were released.[129]

SECONDARY PREVENTION TRIALS

Secondary Prevention of Coronary Heart Disease

Published in 1998, the HERS trial was the first large trial to address the role of HRT in secondary prevention of CHD.[5] In HERS, 2763 postmenopausal women (mean age 66.7 years) with preexisting CHD (defined by history of MI [17%], ≥50% stenosis in at least one coronary artery on angiography, CABG [42%], or percutaneous transluminal coronary angioplasty [45%]), and who had not had a hysterectomy were randomized to placebo or 0.625 mg of oral CEE plus 2.5 mg of medroxyprogesterone daily. Over 4.1 years of mean follow-up, 361 women reached the primary combined endpoint of nonfatal MI or CHD death. There was no difference in overall risk between the two randomized comparison groups (RR 0.99, 95% CI 0.81-1.22) (Fig. 27-2). Kaplan-Meier curves of time to revascularization or hospitalization with unstable angina diverged, but the differences were not statistically significant (HR 0.89, P = 0.15). There was an excess of risk of venous thromboembolic events in the HRT group compared to placebo (43 vs. 13 events, RR 2.66, 95% CI 1.40-5.04, P = 0.003). A time-trend analysis of the data suggested a possible increase in risk of CHD events in the first year with a decrease in risk in subsequent years. In year 1, there was a 52% increase in risk of CHD events (95% CI 1.01-2.29, P = 0.03). In years 2, 3, 4, and 5, the RRs were 0.98 (95% CI 0.66-1.46), 0.85 (95% CI 0.54-1.33), and 0.75 (95% CI 0.50-1.13), respectively. The study was not

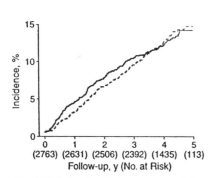
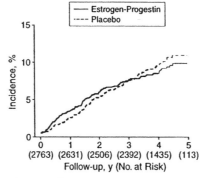
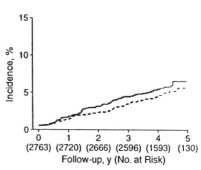

FIGURE 27-2. Kaplan-Meier estimates of the cumulative incidence of primary coronary heart disease (CHD) events *(left)*, nonfatal myocardial infarction (MI) *(center)* and CHD death *(right)* in the Heart and Estrogen/progestin Replacement Study (HERS). The number of women observed at each year of follow-up and still free of an event are provided in parentheses, and the curves become fainter when this number drops below half of the cohort. Log-rank P values are 0.91 for primary CHD events, 0.46 for nonfatal MI, and 0.23 for CHD death. (From Hulley S, Grady D, Bush T, et al: Randomized trial of estrogen plus progestin for secondary prevention of coronary heart disease in postmenopausal women. JAMA 1998; 280:605-613. Copyright 1998, American Medical Association.)

adequately powered to detect differences in other endpoints such as cancer or total mortality. Extensive post-hoc subgroup analyses failed to identify any subgroup of HERS participants in whom HRT was clearly beneficial or harmful.[130]

In HERS II, unblinded follow-up of the HERS trial participants was extended for an additional 2.7 years, with open-label treatment at the discretion of the participants' personal physicians.[131] Among women randomly assigned to HRT in HERS, 81% reported at least 80% adherence to HRT in year 1; this declined to 45% by year 6. In the placebo group, none were taking hormones in year 1, and 8% were taking hormones by year 6. There were no differences in CHD events in HERS II (HR 1.00, 95% CI 0.77-1.29) or when the results of HERS I and II were examined together (HR 0.99, 95% CI 0.84-1.17) (Fig. 27-3). When analyses were limited to those who were at least 80% adherent to the originally assigned treatment regimen, the overall HR was 0.96 (95% CI 0.77-1.19). No time trend toward lower CHD risk with longer duration of treatment with HRT was apparent in HERS II. Thus, the data from HERS II do not support the hypothesis that cardiovascular benefit would become apparent with longer duration of treatment, as originally suggested by the time-trend analysis in HERS I.

In the Papworth HRT Atherosclerosis trial, 255 postmenopausal women with angiographically proven CHD were randomized to transdermal HRT (17β-estradiol alone or in combination with cyclic norethisterone) or control.[6] After 2.6 (mean) years of follow-up, there was no benefit seen with HRT in terms of the primary combined endpoint of hospitalization with unstable angina, MI, or cardiac death. The HRT group had 15.4 events per 100 patient-years, compared to 11.9 per 100 patient-

years in the control group (RR 1.29, 95% CI 0.84-1.95). The event rates were highest in the first 2 years of follow-up, although this was not statistically significant.

In the oEStrogen in the Prevention of ReInfarction Trial (ESPRIT), 1017 postmenopausal women (mean age 62.6 years) who had survived a first MI were randomized to oestradiol valerate (2 mg/day) or placebo.[7] The majority of participants began the trial medication on hospital discharge. After 2 years, there were no significant differences in the primary combined endpoint of reinfarction or cardiac death (RR 0.99, 95% CI 0.70-1.41, P = 0.97) or in all-cause mortality (RR 0.79, 95% CI 0.50-1.27, P = 0.34). ESPRIT was the first large trial to address the role of estrogen alone in the secondary prevention of cardiac events. However, the interpretability of these results is hindered by limited statistical power, because the trial failed to reach its target recruitment goal of 1700 participants, and by poor compliance. Only 43% of those assigned to estrogen and 63% of those assigned to placebo were compliant with treatment by the end of the trial; the particularly poor compliance in the active treatment group was at least in part attributable to the high rate of vaginal bleeding. In contrast to other primary and secondary prevention trials such as WHI,[11,127] HERS,[5] and WEST,[8] however, there was no suggestion of increased short-term risk with estrogen treatment in ESPRIT.

Secondary Prevention Trials of Hormone Replacement Therapy Using Angiographic Endpoints

The Estrogen Replacement and Atherosclerosis trial (ERA)[9] was a secondary prevention trial using angiographic outcomes as the primary endpoint. Postmenopausal women (N = 309; mean age 65.8 years) with one or more coronary artery stenoses of at least 30% were randomized to oral CEE (0.625 mg daily), CEE (0.625 mg daily) plus 2.5 mg daily of MPA, or placebo and were followed for 3.2 years. Complete angiographic data were available in 80%. There was no difference in the primary outcome of mean minimal coronary artery diameter, severity of stenosis, or change in minimal diameter from baseline. There were no significant differences in CVD events between the treatment groups, although the trial was not powered to detect effects on clinical outcomes. In interpreting the ERA trial results, several issues should be considered. Using an angiographic, rather than clinical, outcome as the endpoint has potential limitations. As has been seen in lipid-lowering trials, there may be important treatment effects on plaque stability or on the vascular wall, which are independent of reduction in plaque size.[132] In addition, in this trial, HRT was started many years after the onset of menopause. Finally, any potential benefits on atherogenesis may not be detectable in 3 years of follow-up. Nevertheless, in conjunction with the HERS trial results, the ERA results cast additional doubt regarding the role of HRT in secondary prevention of CHD.

The Women's Angiographic Vitamin and Estrogen (WAVE) Trial was a randomized, double-blind trial of 423

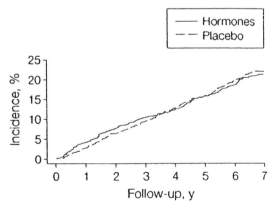

No. at Risk
Hormones 1380 1303 1247 1196 1133 1043 984 354
Placebo 1383 1334 1269 1209 1122 1039 976 336

FIGURE 27-3. Kaplan-Meier estimates of the cumulative incidence of coronary heart disease events (death and nonfatal myocardial infarction) in the Heart and Estrogen/progestin Replacement Study II. The curves are truncated at year 7 when less than half of the cohort remains in follow-up. (From Grady D, Herrington D, Bittner V, et al: Cardiovascular disease outcomes during 6.8 years of hormone therapy: Heart and Estrogen/progestin Replacement Study follow-up (HERS II). JAMA 2002; 288:49-57. Copyright 2002, American Medical Association.)

postmenopausal women (mean age 65 years) with at least one coronary stenosis (15% to 75%) at baseline.[10] Participants were randomly assigned in a 2 × 2 factorial design to receive 0.625 mg/day CEE (plus 2.5 mg/day MPA for those with an intact uterus), or matching placebo, and vitamin E (400 IU twice daily) plus vitamin C (500 mg twice daily) or placebo. Follow-up angiograms were conducted in 76% of the participants at an average of 2.8 years of follow-up. There was no significant difference in the primary outcome of annualized mean change in minimal lumen diameter from baseline. When patients with intercurrent death or MI were included, for whom the worst angiographic outcomes were imputed, there was the suggestion of increased risk in the HRT group (P = 0.045), but this was no longer statistically significant (P = 0.07) after adjustment for diabetic status. There was no interaction between the HRT and vitamin interventions.

Trials of Hormone Replacement Therapy and Subclinical Atherosclerosis

Two studies examining the effect of HRT on carotid intimal media thickness (IMT), a measure of subclinical atherosclerosis, have had conflicting results. In the Estrogen in the Prevention of Atherosclerosis Trial (EPAT),[133] 222 postmenopausal women without known cardiovascular disease and with LDL of more than 130 mg/dl were randomized to unopposed micronized 17β estradiol (1 mg/day) or placebo and followed for 2 years. The average rate of progression of IMT was slower in those taking estradiol, although it was of borderline statistical significance (P = 0.046). This effect was not apparent in women who received lipid-lowering medication and was most marked in those who did not. It should be noted that the women enrolled in EPAT were, on average, 10 years younger than those in HERS and ERA. Furthermore, they were treated with unopposed estradiol, leaving unanswered the question of whether an added progestin may counteract any beneficial effects of estrogen on subacute atherosclerosis. In contrast to the EPAT findings, in another trial of 321 postmenopausal women with increased IMT at baseline, 1 year of combined HRT treatment with 17β-estradiol (1 mg/day) with 0.025 mg gestodene 12 days/month (standard) or every third month (low-dose progestin group) failed to show any changes in IMT progression.[134]

Trials of Hormone Replacement Therapy in Unstable Angina

In one trial,[135] 293 postmenopausal women with unstable angina, who were receiving standard anti-ischemic therapy, were treated with an intravenous estradiol infusion for 30 minutes, followed by oral estrogen (1.25 mg/day), estrogen combined with MPA (2.5 mg/day), or placebo for 21 days. No differences were observed between groups in terms of the primary endpoint (the number of ambulatory electrocardiographic ischemic events over the first 48 hours), or in 6 months of follow-up.

Secondary Prevention of Stroke

Previous observational epidemiologic data regarding HRT and risk of stroke have been inconsistent. Animal models of cerebral ischemia suggest a protective effect with estrogen.[136,137] The Women's Estrogen for Stroke (WEST) trial examined the effect of estradiol in the secondary prevention of stroke.[8] This trial enrolled 664 postmenopausal women (mean age 71 years; 26% of eligible women) who had had an ischemic stroke (75%) or transient ischemic attack (TIA) in the prior 90 days. They were randomly assigned to receive 17β-estradiol, 1 mg/day, or matching placebo. The primary endpoint was death from any cause or nonfatal stroke; secondary outcomes included TIA and nonfatal MI. Mean follow-up was 2.8 years. Overall compliance was 70%. There was no significant difference in death (RR 1.2, 95% CI 0.8-1.8) or nonfatal stroke (RR 1.0, 95% CI 0.7-1.4) between treatment groups. Death from stroke (predominantly ischemic) was more common in the estradiol group (RR 2.9, 95% CI 0.9-9.0), although not statistically significant. There was an increase in risk of stroke seen in the first 6 months of treatment in post-hoc analysis (RR 2.3, 95%, CI 1.1-5.0). In a secondary analysis of the HERS trial, no reduction in stroke risk was observed (RR 1.23, 95% CI 0.89-1.70) and there was no relation between use of HRT and stroke risk over time.[138]

INTERPRETATION OF CLINICAL TRIALS OF HORMONE REPLACEMENT THERAPY

The results of WHI, HERS, and other trials in the primary and secondary prevention of CVD were unexpected and have provoked intense debate as to their implications for the estrogen hypothesis. In WHI and HERS, postmenopausal women who were about 20 years past menopause were not protected from CVD or recurrent CVD events if they were newly initiated on combination therapy with CEE and MPA.[139] Although ERA and WEST also examined the effects of unopposed estrogen, their study populations were also at least 20 years past menopause. It remains unknown if initiation of HRT immediately after menopause, and specifically prior to the development of significant atherosclerotic disease, would be beneficial. This may be particularly important if HRT is more effective at preventing development of atherosclerosis, rather than slowing the progression of preexisting subclinical or overt disease, as suggested in animal studies.[33-37,140] The effects of estrogen on atherogenesis may depend on the state of the underlying arterial endothelium,[140,141] with inhibition of cholesterol accumulation in healthy areas of a balloon-injured aorta, and paradoxical accelerated atherogenesis in de-endothelialized areas.[141] This suggests that preexisting atherosclerotic disease may influence the degree of subsequent protection from estrogen in secondary prevention. It has also been suggested that if the predominant mechanisms of benefit are through antiatherogenesis, a beneficial effect of HRT may become evident with longer duration of follow-up. However, this possibility seems less likely given the overall increase in CHD risk in WHI and the results of the HERS II follow-up data.

The WHI and HERS trials tested only combined HRT with oral CEE and continuous MPA, the latter of which may attenuate estrogen's beneficial effects on HDL,[20] atherosclerosis,[37,106] endothelial-dependent vasodilation,[80,81] and NO production.[91] The role of estrogen monotherapy remains uncertain because the estrogen-only component of WHI has reported only preliminary findings, and the ESPRIT trial was limited by methodologic issues. Whether other dosing regimens, specific formulations of estrogens and progestins, or modes of administration (such as transdermal estrogen) would have different clinical effects remains unknown.

However, despite the previously mentioned possible explanations for the disappointing trial results of HRT in primary and secondary prevention of CVD, it is possible that there is no net cardiovascular benefit with HRT and that observational data led us astray because of bias and uncontrolled confounding. Observational studies are vulnerable to several types of bias. Women who take HRT are generally healthier (selection bias), have greater access to health care and are monitored more closely (prevention bias), and are more compliant than nonusers.[142] Survivor bias may not be detected in observational studies because women who become ill may stop taking HRT and then be misclassified as nonusers.[142] Furthermore, susceptible women may die from early adverse effects of HRT but remain unaccounted as such in the cohort (prevalence-incidence bias).[142] In concordance with these possibilities, the WHI and HERS data raised the possibility of early harm with HRT, which may be the result of an early increased risk of thrombosis, plaque destabilization, or proischemia[5,57,58,143] (Subsequent epidemiologic analyses from the Nurses' Health Study[122] and Group Health Cooperative[123] also suggested transient increases in risk in the short term in secondary prevention, with reduced risk seen with longer use.) This may also explain the discordant results of clinical trials and observational studies because the latter may not detect early adverse effects of treatment that result in discontinuation of therapy or death; any subsequent risk reduction may not be real but could reflect attrition of a susceptible cohort, resulting in observation of lower risk survivors.[144]

Subgroups of women, as yet unidentified, may be more likely to benefit or be more vulnerable to the adverse effects of HRT. Extensive subgroup analyses in WHI[127] and post-hoc subgroup analyses in HERS[130] failed to identify any subgroup in whom HRT was clearly beneficial. However, in WHI, women with higher LDL cholesterol levels at baseline appeared to have an augmented risk of a CHD event with estrogen-progestin.[127] Additionally, those with the factor V Leiden mutation may be at increased risk of thrombotic complications because of its potential interaction with ERT.[53,54] Other studies suggest that postmenopausal women with CHD who have ER-αIVS1-401 C/C genotype or several closely related genotypes have an augmented response of HDL cholesterol to HRT[145] and have greater reductions in soluble adhesion molecule E-selectin without increases in CRP.[146] However, it remains unknown if these effects on intermediate phenotypes will affect clinical outcomes.

CURRENT GUIDELINES

In the wake of the release of the results of HERS, WHI, and other trials, clinical guidelines regarding the use of HRT in postmenopausal women have been revised. The U.S. Preventive Services Task Force (USPSTF) recommends against the routine use of estrogen combined with progestin for the prevention of chronic conditions in postmenopausal women; this was a grade D recommendation, with at least fair evidence that this is ineffective or that harms outweigh benefits.[147] The USPSTF found insufficient evidence to recommend for or against the use of unopposed estrogen for prevention of chronic disease in women who have had a hysterectomy (grade I recommendation).[147] With specific regard to CVD, the American Heart Association,[142,148] the North American Menopause Society (NAMS),[149] and the American College of Obstetricians and Gynecologists (ACOG)[150] recommend that HRT should not be used for primary or secondary prevention. The NAMS Advisory Panel and ACOG note that treatment of menopausal symptoms (e.g., vasomotor and urogenital) remains the primary indication for HRT, but consideration of shorter duration of treatment and lower doses of HRT were warranted. Caution was advised in using HRT solely to prevent osteoporosis, and alternative treatments should also be considered.

In January 2003, after reviewing the data from the WHI, the U.S. Food and Drug Administration approved new labels for estrogen and estrogen–progestin products.[151] The new boxed warnings, the highest level of warning information in labeling, state that estrogens with or without progestins should not be used for prevention of cardiovascular disease. The new labeling also highlights the increased risks of MI, stroke, thromboembolic events, and breast cancer observed with estrogen–progestin HRT in WHI.

SELECTIVE ESTROGEN RECEPTOR MODULATORS

Selective estrogen receptor modulators (SERMs), such as raloxifene, bind to the estrogen receptor and function as an antiestrogen in breast and uterine tissue but as an estrogen agonist in bone and lipid metabolism.[152] This selectivity of action may provide advantages over estrogen and suggests a possible role of SERMS in postmenopausal treatment. In clinical trials,[52,153,154] raloxifene reduces LDL to a similar degree as HRT but has no effect on HDL or triglycerides. Raloxifene was less effective in reducing Lp(a)[52] but, unlike estrogen, did not increase CRP levels.[154] In secondary analysis of data from the Multiple Outcomes of Raloxifene Evaluation trial,[155] in which 7705 osteoporotic postmenopausal women were randomly assigned to receive raloxifene 60 mg/day, 120 mg/day or placebo for 4 years, there were no overall differences in CVD events. Among the subset of 1035 women with increased CVD risk at baseline (202 with prior CHD, the remainder with multiple risk factors), raloxifene was associated with lower risk of CVD events (RR 0.60, 95%

CI 0.38-0.95). The ongoing RUTH trial (Raloxifene Use for the Heart), involving 10,101 postmenopausal women with CHD or multiple CHD risk factors randomized to raloxifene, 60 mg/day or placebo, will provide further data about the potential role of SERMS in prevention of CVD.

Although SERMs are potentially promising new therapies in HRT, more data are needed, particularly because the clinical benefit of estrogen in reducing CVD risk remains unproved. Compared to estrogen, raloxifene has a less pronounced effect on lipids, particularly because it does not increase HDL. Reduction in aortic atherosclerosis with raloxifene has been observed in animal studies but to a lesser degree than with estrogen.[156,157] Whether raloxifene will prove to have advantages over traditional HRT for some or all women remains to be determined.

CONCLUSION

The role of HRT in the primary and secondary prevention of cardiovascular disease has undergone a sea change in the last several years. Observational epidemiologic data had consistently demonstrated benefit, as further supported by studies of biologic intermediates suggesting beneficial effects on lipoproteins, vasomotor tone, decreased vascular response to injury, and antiatherosclerotic effects. These effects may be countered by prothrombotic or proinflammatory effects or by the impact of concomitant progestin therapy. However, testing of the HRT hypothesis in large randomized clinical trials has so far demonstrated no evidence of benefit and some evidence of harm. Additional data are needed regarding the effects of estrogen-only HRT; the optimal timing of initiation of treatment; and dose, type, and duration of hormones used. However, at the present time, HRT should not be initiated or continued for the express purpose of preventing cardiovascular disease or its complications. This dramatic evolution in our understanding of HRT has also provided the medical community with valuable lessons, reinforcing the critical need for clinical trials to test the net benefits and risks of therapeutic interventions and the importance of emphasizing and applying well-proven methods of risk reduction in cardiovascular disease prevention.

REFERENCES

1. U.S. Senate Special Committee on Aging: Aging America: Trends and Projections. Washington DC, US Department of Health and Human Services, 1988.
2. Heart and Stroke Facts. Dallas, American Heart Association, 1992
3. Keating N, Cleary P, Aossi A, et al: Use of hormone replacement therapy by postmenopausal women in the United States. Ann Intern Med 1999; 130:545-553.
4. Kreling D, Mott D, Wiederholt J, et al: Prescription drug trends: A chartbook update. Menlo Park, CA: Kaiser Family Foundation: November 2001.
5. Hulley S, Grady D, Bush T, et al: Randomized trial of estrogen plus progestin for secondary prevention of coronary heart disease in postmenopausal women. JAMA 1998; 280:605-613.
6. Clarke SC, Kelleher J, Lloyd-Jones H, et al: A study of hormone replacement therapy in postmenopausal women with ischaemic heart disease: The Papworth HRT atherosclerosis study. BJOG 2002; 109:1056-1062.

7. The ESPRIT team: Oestrogen therapy for prevention of reinfarction in postmenopausal women: A randomized placebo controlled trial. Lancet. Published online December 17, 2002. http:/image.thelancet.com/extras/02art11268web.pdf. Accessed August 19, 2003.
8. Viscoli CM, Brass LM, Kernan WN, et al: A clinical trial of estrogen replacement therapy after ischemic stroke. N Engl J Med 2001:345:1243-1249.
9. Herrington DM, Reboussin DM, Brosnihan KB, et al: Effects of estrogen replacement on the progression of coronary artery atherosclerosis. N Engl J Med 2000; 343:522-529.
10. Waters DD, Alderman EL, Hsia J, et al: Effects of hormone replacement therapy and antioxidant vitamin supplements on coronary atherosclerosis in postmenopausal women: A randomized controlled trial. JAMA 2002; 288:2432-2440.
11. Writing Group for the Women's Health Initiative Investigators: Risks and benefits of estrogen plus progestin in healthy postmenopausal women: Principal results from the Women's Health Initiative randomized controlled trial. JAMA 2002; 288:321-333.
12. Walter P, Green S, Greene G, et al: Cloning of the human estrogen receptor cDNA. Proc Natl Acad Sci USA 1985; 82:7889-7993.
13. Kuiper GGJM, Enmark E, Pelto-Huikko M, et al: Cloning of a novel receptor expressed in rat prostate and ovary. Proc Natl Acad Sci USA 1996; 93:5925-5930.
14. Tsai MJ, O'Malley BW: Molecular mechanisms of actions of steroid/thyroid receptor superfamily members, Ann Rev Biochem 1994; 63:451-486.
15. Matthews KA, Meilahn E, Kuller LH, et al: Menopause and risk factors for coronary artery disease. New Engl J Med 1989; 321: 641-646.
16. Walsh BW, Schiff I, Rosner B, et al: Effects of postmenopausal estrogen replacement on the concentrations and metabolism of plasma lipoproteins. N Engl J Med 1991; 325:1196-204.
17. Moorjani S, Dupont A, Labrie F, et al: Changes in lipoprotein and apolipoprotein composition in relation to oral versus percutaneous administration of estrogen alone or in cyclic association with utrogestan in menopausal women. J Clin Endocrinol Metab 1991; 73:373-379.
18. Sacks FM, Walsh BW: The effects of reproductive hormones on serum lipoproteins: Unresolved issues in biology and clinical practice. Ann NY Acad Sci 1990; 592: 272-285.
19. Miller VT, Muesing RA, LaRosa JC, et al: Effects of conjugated equine estrogen with and without three different progestogens on lipoproteins, high-density lipoprotein subfractions, and apoplipoprotein A-1. Obstet Gynecol 1991; 77:235-240.
20. The Writing Group for the PEPI Trial: Effects of estrogen or estrogen/progestin regimens on heart disease risk factors in postmenopausal women: The Postmenopausal Estrogen/Progestin Interventions (PEPI) Trial. JAMA 1995; 273:199-208.
21. Lobo RA, Pickar JH, Wild RA, et al: Metabolic impact of adding medroxyprogesterone acetate to conjugated estrogen therapy in postmenopausal women. Obstet Gynecol 1994; 84:987-995.
22. Medical Research Council's General Practice Research Framework: Randomized comparison of oestrogen versus oestrogen plus progestogen hormone replacement therapy in women with hysterectomy. BMJ 1996; 312:473-478.
23. Speroff L, Rowan J, Symons J, et al: The comparative effect on bone density, endometrium, and lipids of continuous hormones as replacement therapy (CHART Study). JAMA 1996; 276:1397-1403.
24. Munk-Jensen N, Ulrich LG, Obel EB, et al: Continuous combined and sequential estradiol and norethindrone acetate treatment of postmenopausal women: Effect on plasma lipoproteins in a two-year placebo-controlled trial. Am J Obstet Gynecol 1994; 171:132-138.
25. Walsh BW, Sacks FM: Effects of low dose oral contraceptives on very low density and low density lipoprotein metabolism. J Clin Invest 1993; 91:2126-2132.
26. Bostom AG, Gagnon DR, Cupples LA, et al: A prospective investigation of elevated lipoprotein(a) detected by electrophoresis and cardiovascular disease in women: The Framingham Heart Study. Circulation 1994; 90:1688-1695.
27. Orth-Gomér K, Mittleman MA, Schenck-Gustafsson K, et al: Lipoprotein(a) as a determinant of coronary heart disease in young women. Circulation 1997; 95:329-334.

28. Espeland MA, Marcovina SM, Miller V, et al: Effect of post-menopausal hormone therapy on lipoprotein(a) concentration. Circulation 1998; 97:979-986.

29. Shlipak MG, Simon JA, Vittinghoff E, et al: Estrogen and progestin, lipoprotein(a) and the risk of recurrent coronary heart disease events after menopause. JAMA 2000; 283:1845-1852.

30. Koh KK, Cardillo C, Bui MN, et al: Vascular effects of estrogen and cholesterol lowering therapies in hypercholesterolemic postmenopausal women. Circulation 1999; 99:354-360.

31. Darling GM, Johns JA, McCloud PI, et al: Estrogen and progestin compared with simvastatin for hypercholesterolemia in postmenopausal women. N Engl J Med 1997; 337:595-601.

32. Herrington DM, Werbel BL, Riley WA, et al: Individual and combined effects of estrogen/progestin therapy and lovastatin on lipids and flow-mediated vasodilation in postmenopausal women with coronary artery disease. J Am Coll Cardiol 1999; 33: 2030-2037.

33. Adams MR, Kaplan JR, Manuck SB, et al: Inhibition of coronary artery atherosclerosis by 17-beta estradiol in ovariectomized monkeys: Lack of an effect of added progesterone. Arteriosclerosis 1990; 10:1051-1057.

34. Wagner JD, Clarkson TB, St. Clair RW, et al: Estrogen and progesterone replacement therapy reduces low density lipoprotein accumulation in the coronary arteries of surgically postmenopausal cynomolgus monkeys. J Clin Invest 1991; 88: 1995-2002.

35. Clarkson TB, Shively CA, Morgan TM, et al: Oral contraceptives and coronary artery atherosclerosis of cynomolgus monkeys. Obstet Gynecol 1990; 75:217-222.

36. Haarbo J, Leth-Espensen P, Stender S, et al: Estrogen monotherapy and combined estrogen-progestogen replacement therapy attenuate aortic accumulation of cholesterol in ovariectomized cholesterol-fed rabbits. J Clin Invest 1991; 87:1274-1279.

37. Hanke H, Hanke S, Finking G, et al: Different effects of estrogen and progesterone on experimental atherosclerosis in female versus male rabbits: Quantification of cellular proliferation by bromodeoxyuridine. Circulation 1996; 94:175-181.

38. Mazière C, Auclair M, Ronveaux M-F, et al: Estrogens inhibit copper and cell-mediated modification of low density lipoprotein. Atherosclerosis 1991; 89:175-182.

39. Nègre-Salvayre A, Pieraggi M-T, Mabile L, et al: Protective effect of 17β-estradiol against the cytotoxicity of minimally oxidized LDL to cultured bovine aortic endothelial cells. Atherosclerosis 1993; 99:207-217.

40. Koh KK, Minemoyer R, Bui MN, et al: Effects of hormone-replacement therapy on fibrinolysis in postmenopausal women. N Engl J Med 1997; 336:683-690.

41. Sack MN, Rader DJ, Cannon RO: Oestrogen and inhibition of oxidation of low-density lipoproteins in postmenopausal women. Lancet 1994; 343:269-270.

42. Scarabin P-Y, Plu-Bureau G, Bara L, et al: Haemostatic variables and menopausal status: Influence of hormone replacement therapy. Thromb Haemost 1993; 70:584-587.

43. Scarabin P-Y, Vissac A-M, Kirzin J-M, et al: Population correlates of coagulation factor VII: Importance of age, sex, and menopausal status as determinants of activated factor VII. Arterioscler Thromb Vasc Biol 1996; 16:1170-1176.

44. Meade TW, Dyer S, Howarth DJ, et al: Antithrombin III and procoagulant activity: Sex differences and effects of the menopause. Br J Haematol 1990; 74:77-81.

45. The Writing Group for the Estradiol Clotting Factors Study: Effects on haemostasis of hormone replacement therapy with transdermal estradiol and oral sequential medroxyprogesterone acetate: A 1-year, double-blind, placebo-controlled study. Thromb Haemost 1996; 75:476-480.

46. Kroon U-B, Silfverstolpe G, Tengborn L: The effects of transdermal estradiol and oral conjugated estrogens on haemostasis variables. Thromb Haemost 1994; 71:420-423.

47. Sporrong T, Mattsson L-A, Samsioe G, et al: Haemostatic changes during continuous oestradiol-progestogen treatment of postmenopausal women. Br J Obstet Gynaecol 1990; 97:939-944.

48. Mannucci PM, Giangrande PLF: Detection of the prethrombotic state due to procoagulant imbalance. Eur J Haematol 1992; 48:65-69.

49. Caine YG, Bauer KA, Barzegar S, et al: Coagulation activation following estrogen administration to postmenopausal women. Thromb Haemost 1992; 68:392-395.

50. Teede HJ, McGrath BP, Smolich JJ, et al: Postmenopausal hormone replacement therapy increases coagulation activity and fibrinolysis. Arterioscler Thromb Vasc Biol 2000; 20:1404-1409.

51. Scarabin PY, Alhenc-Gelas M, Plu-Bureau, et al: Effects of oral and transdermal estrogen/progesterone regimens on blood coagulation and fibrinolysis in postmenopausal women: A randomized controlled trial. Arterioscler Thromb Vasc Biol 1997; 17:3071-3078.

52. Walsh B, Kuller L, Wild R, et al: Effects of raloxifene on serum lipids and coagulation factors in healthy postmenopausal women. JAMA 1998; 279:1445-1451.

53. Herrington DM, Vittinghoff E, Howard TD, et al: Factor V Leiden, hormone replacement therapy, and risk of venous thromboembolic events in women with coronary disease. Arterioscler Thromb Vasc Biol 2002; 22:1012-1017.

54. Rosendaal FR, Vessey M, Daly E, et al: Hormone replacement therapy, prothrombic mutations and the risk of venous thrombosis. Br J Haematol 2002; 116:851-854.

55. Ross R: Atherosclerosis: An inflammatory disease. N Engl J Med 1998; 340:115-127.

56. Cushman M, Meilahn EN, Psaty BM, et al: Hormone replacement therapy, inflammation, and hemostasis in elderly women. Arterioscler Thromb Vasc Biol 1999; 19:893-899.

57. Ridker PM, Hennekens CH, Rifai N, et al: Hormone replacement therapy and increased plasma concentration of C-reactive protein. Circulation 1999; 100:713-716.

58. Cushman M, Legault C, Barrett-Connor E, et al: Effect of postmenopausal hormones on inflammation-sensitive proteins: The Postmenopausal Estrogen/Progestin Interventions (PEPI) Study. Circulation 1999; 100:717-722.

59. Pradhan AD, Manson JE, Roussow JE, et al: Inflammatory biomarkers, hormone replacement therapy, and incident coronary heart disease: Prospective analysis from the Women's Health Initiative Observational Study. JAMA 2002; 288:980-987.

60. Decensi A, Omodei U, Robertson C, et al: Effect of transdermal estradiol and oral conjugated estrogen on C-reactive protein in retinoid-placebo trial in healthy women. Circulation 2002; 106:1224-1228.

61. Despres J-P, Lamarche B, Mauriege P, et al: Hyperinsulinemia as an independent risk factor for ischemic heart disease. N Engl J Med 1996; 334:952-957.

62. Farhat MY, Kavigne MC, Ramwell PW: The vascular protective effects of estrogen. FASEB J 1996; 10:615-624.

63. Mendelsohn ME, Karas RH: The protective effects of estrogen on the cardiovascular system. N Engl J Med 1999; 340:1801-1811.

64. Reis SE, Gloth ST, Blumenthal RS, et al: Ethinyl estradiol acutely attenuates abnormal coronary vasomotor responses to acetylcholine in postmenopausal women. Circulation 1994; 89:52-60.

65. Gilligan DM, Quyyumi AA, Cannon RO: Effects of physiological levels of estrogen on coronary vasomotor function in postmenopausal women. Circulation 1994; 89:2545-2551.

66. Collins P, Rosano GMC, Sarrel PM, et al: 17β-Estradiol attenuates acetylcholine-induced coronary arterial constriction in women but not men with coronary heart disease. Circulation 1995; 92:24-30.

67. Gilligan DM, Badar DM, Panza JA, et al: Acute vascular effects of estrogen in postmenopausal women. Circulation 1994; 90: 786-791.

68. Mendelsohn ME: Nongenomic estrogen receptor-mediated activation of endothelial nitric oxide synthase: How does it work? What does it mean? Circ Res 2000; 87:677-682.

69. Chen Z, Yuhanna IS, Galcheva-Gargova Z, et al: Estrogen receptor α mediates the nongenomic activation of endothelial nitric oxide synthase by estrogen. J Clin Invest 1999; 103:401-406.

70. Caulin-Glaser T, García-Cardeña G, Sarrel P, et al: 17β-Estradiol regulation of human endothelial cell basal nitric oxide release, independent of cytosolic Ca^{2+} mobilization. Circ Res 1997; 81:885-892.

71. Razandi M, Pedram A, Greene GL, et al: Cell membrane and nuclear estrogen receptors (ERs) originate from a single transcript: Studies of ER-alpha and ER-beta expressed in Chinese hamster ovary cells. Mol Endocrinol 1999; 13:307-319.

72. Hardy SP, Valverde MA: Novel plasma membrane action of estrogen and antiestrogens revealed by their regulation of a large conductance chloride channel. FASEB J 1994; 8:760-765.

73. White RE, Darkow DJ, Falvo Lang JL: Estrogen relaxes coronary arteries by opening BK_{Ca} channels through a cGMP-dependent mechanism. Circ Res 1995; 77:936-942.

74. Wellman GC, Bonev AD, Nelson MT, et al: Gender differences in coronary artery diameter involve estrogen, nitric oxide, and Ca^{2+} dependent K$^+$ channels. Circ Res 1996; 79:1024–1030.

75. Chang W-C, Nakao J, Orimo H, et al: Stimulation of prostaglandin cyclooxygenase and prostacyclin synthetase activities by estradiol in rat aortic smooth muscle cells. Biochim Biophys Acta 1980; 620:472–482.

76. Weiner CP, Lizasoain I, Baylis SA, et al: Induction of calcium-dependent nitric oxide synthases by sex hormones. Proc Natl Acad Sci USA 1994; 91:5212–526.

77. Hayashi T, Fukuto JM, Ignarro LJ, et al: Basal release of nitric oxide from aortic rings is greater in female rabbits than in male rabbits: Implications for atherosclerosis. Proc Natl Acad Sci USA 1992; 89: 11259–11263.

78. Binko J, Majewski H: 17β-Estradiol reduces vasoconstriction in endothelium-denuded rat aortas through inducible NOS. Am J Physiol 1998; 274:H853–H859.

79. Gisclard V, Miller VM, Vanhoutte PM: Effect of 17β-estradiol on endothelium-dependent responses in the rabbit. J Pharmacol Exp Ther 1988; 244:19–22.

80. Miller VM, Vanhoutte PM: Progesterone and modulation of endothelium-dependent responses in canine coronary arteries. Am J Physiol 1992; 261:R1022–R1027.

81. Williams JK, Adams MR, Herrington DM, et al: Short-term administration of estrogen and vascular responses of atherosclerotic coronary arteries. J Am Coll Cardiol 1992; 20:452–457.

82. Guetta V, Quyyumi AA, Prasad A, et al: The role of nitric oxide in coronary vascular effects of estrogen in postmenopausal women. Circulation 1997; 96:2795–2801.

83. Hayashi T, Yamada K, Esaki T, et al: Estrogen increases endothelial nitric oxide by a receptor-mediated system. Biochem Biophys Res Commun 1995; 214:847–855.

84. Arnal JF, Clamens S, Pechet C, et al: Ethinylestradiol does not enhance the expression of nitric oxide synthase in bovine endothelial cells but increases the release of bioactive nitric oxide by inhibiting superoxide anion production. Proc Natl Acad Sci USA 1996; 93:4108–4113.

85. Keaney JF, Shwaery GT, Xu A, et al: 17β-Estradiol preserves endothelial vasodilator function and limits low-density lipoprotein oxidation in hypercholesterolemic swine. Circulation 1994; 89:2251–2259.

86. Lieberman EH, Gerhard MD, Uehata A, et al: Estrogen improves endothelium-dependent, flow-mediated vasodilation in postmenopausal women. Ann Intern Med 1994; 121:936–941.

87. Vekhavaara S, Hakala-Ala-Pietilä T, Virkamäki A, et al: Differential effects of oral and transdermal estrogen replacement therapy on endothelial function in postmenopausal women. Circulation 2000; 102:2687–2693.

88. Sudhir K, Ko E, Zellner C, et al: Physiological concentrations of estradiol attenuate endothelin 1-induced coronary vasoconstriction in vivo. Circulation 1997; 96:3626–3632.

89. Webb CM, Ghatei MA, McNeill JG, et al: 17β-Estradiol decreases endothelin-1 levels in the coronary circulation of postmenopausal women with coronary artery disease. Circulation 2000; 102:1617–1622.

90. Williams JK, Honoré EK, Washburn SA, et al: Effects of hormone replacement therapy on reactivity of atherosclerotic coronary arteries in cynomolgus monkeys. J Am Coll Cardiol 1994; 24:1757–1761.

91. Sorenson KE, Dorup I. Hermann AP, et al: Combined hormone replacement therapy does not protect women against the age-related decline in endothelium-dependent vasomotor function. Circulation 1998; 97:1234–1238.

92. Wakatsuki A, Okatani Y, Ikenoue N, et al: Effect of medroxyprogesterone acetate on endothelial-dependent vasodilation in postmenopausal women receiving estrogen. Circulation 2001; 104:1773–1778.

93. Gerhard M, Walsh B, Tawakol A, et al: Estradiol therapy combined with progesterone and endothelial dependent vasodilation in postmenopausal women. Circulation 1998; 98:1158–1163.

94. Rosano GMC, Peters NS, Lefroy D, et al: 17-Beta estradiol therapy lessens angina in postmenopausal women with syndrome X. J Am Coll Cardiol 1996; 28:1500–1505

95. Rosano GMC, Sarrel PM, Poole-Wilson PA, et al: Beneficial effect of oestrogen on exercise-induced myocardial ischaemia in women with coronary artery disease. Lancet 1993; 342:133–1336.

96. Holdright DR, Sullivan AK, Wright CA, et al: Acute effect of oestrogen replacement on treadmill performance in postmenopausal women with coronary artery disease. Eur Heart J 1995; 16: 1566–1570.

97. Iafrati MD, Karas RH, Aronovitz M, et al: Estrogen inhibits the vascular injury response in estrogen receptor α-deficient mice. Nat Med 1997; 3:545–548.

98. Lindner V, Kim SK, Karas RH, et al: Increased expression of estrogen receptor β mRNA in male blood vessels after vascular injury. Circ Res 1998; 83:224–229.

99. Sullivan TR, Karas RH, Aronovitz M, et al: Estrogen inhibits the response-to-injury in a mouse carotid artery model. J Clin Invest 1995; 96:2482–2488.

100. Chen S-J, Li H, Durand J, et al: Estrogen reduces myointimal proliferation after balloon injury of rat carotid artery. Circulation 1996; 93:577–584.

101. Levine RL, Chen SJ, Durand J, et al: Medroxyprogesterone attenuates estrogen-mediated inhibition of neointima formation after balloon injury of the rat carotid artery. Circulation 1996; 94:2221–2227.

102. Bourassa PAK, Milos PM, Gaynor BJ, et al: Estrogen reduces atherosclerotic lesion development in apolipoprotein-E deficient mice. Proc Natl Acad Sci USA 1996; 93:10022–10027.

103. Karas RH, Hodgin JB, Kwoum M, et al: Estrogen inhibits the vascular injury response in estrogen receptor β-deficient mice. Proc Natl Acad Sci USA 1999; 96:15133–15136.

104. Bakir S, Mori T, Durand J, et al: Estrogen-induced vasoprotection is estrogen receptor dependent: Evidence from the balloon-injured rat carotid artery model. Circulation 2000; 101:2342–2344.

105. Oparil S, Levine RL, Chen S-J, et al: Sexually dimorphic response of the balloon-injured rat carotid artery to hormone treatment. Circulation 1997; 95:1301–1307.

106. Adams MR, Register TC, Golden DL, et al: Medroxyprogesterone acetate antagonizes inhibitory effects of conjugated equine estrogens on coronary atherosclerosis. Arterioscler Thromb Vasc Biol 1997; 27:217–221.

107. Fischer GM, Swain ML: Effects of estradiol and progesterone on the increased synthesis of collagen in atherosclerotic rabbit aortas. Atherosclerosis 1985; 54:1770–1785.

108. Morales DE, McGowan KA, Grant DS, et al: Estrogen promotes angiogenic activity in human umbilical vein endothelial cells in vitro and in a murine model. Circulation 1995; 91:755–763.

109. Krasinski K, Spyridopoulos I, Asahara T, et al: Estradiol accelerates functional endothelial recovery after arterial injury. Circulation 1997; 95:1768–1772.

110. Spyridopoulos I, Sullivan AB, Keraney M, et al: Estrogen-receptor-mediated inhibition of human endothelial cell apoptosis. Circulation 1997; 95:1505–1514.

111. Caulin-Glaser T, Watson CA, Pardi R, et al: Effects of 17β-Estradiol on cytokine-induced endothelial cell adhesion molecule expression. J Clin Invest 1996; 98:36–42.

112. Grady D, Rubin SM, Pettiti DB, et al: Hormone therapy to prevent disease and prolong life in postmenopausal women. Ann Int Med 1992; 117: 1016–1037.

113. Grodstein F, Stampfer M: The epidemiology of coronary heart disease and estrogen replacement in postmenopausal women. Prog Cardiovasc Dis 1995; 38:199–210.

114. Grodstein F, Stampfer MJ, Manson JE, et al: Postmenopausal estrogen and progestin use and the risk of cardiovascular disease. N Engl J Med 1996; 335:453–461.

115. Jick H, Derby LE, Myers MW, et al: Risk of hospital admission for idiopathic venous thromboembolism among users of postmenopausal oestrogens. Lancet 1996; 348:981–983.

116. Daly E, Vessey MP, Hawkins MM, et al: Risk of venous thromboembolism in users of hormone replacement therapy. Lancet 1996; 348:977–980.

117. Grodstein F, Stampfer MJ, Goldhaber SZ, et al: Prospective study of exogenous hormones and risk of pulmonary embolism in women. Lancet 1996; 348:983–987.

118. Sullivan JM, Vander Zwaag R, Hughes JP, et al: Estrogen replacement and coronary artery disease: Effect on survival in postmenopausal women. Arch Intern Med 1990; 150:2557–2562.

119. O'Keefe JH, Kim SC, Hall RR, et al: Estrogen replacement therapy after coronary angioplasty. J Am Coll Cardiol 1997; 29:1–5.

120. Sullivan JM, El-Zeky F, Zwaag Z, et al: Effect on survival of estrogen replacement therapy after coronary artery bypass grafting. Am J Cardiol 1997; 79:847–850.

121. Shlipak MG, Angeja BG, Go AS, et al: Hormone therapy and in-hospital survival after myocardial infarction in postmenopausal women. Circulation 2001; 104:2300-2304.

122. Grodstein F, Manson JE, Stampfer MJ: Postmenopausal hormone use and secondary prevention of coronary events in the Nurses' Health Study: A prospective observational study. Ann Intern Med 2001:135:1-8.

123. Heckbert SR, Kaplan RC, Weiss NS, et al: Risk of recurrent coronary events in relation to use and recent initiation of postmenopausal hormone therapy. Arch Intern Med 2001; 1709-1713.

124. Col NF, Eckman MH, Karas RH, et al: Patient-specific decisions about hormone replacement therapy in postmenopausal women. JAMA 1997; 277:1140-1147.

125. Cummings SR, Black DM, Rubin SM: Lifetime risks of hip, Colles', or vertebral fracture and coronary heart disease among white postmenopausal women. Arch Intern Med 1989; 149: 2445-2448.

126. Collaborative Group on Hormonal Factors in Breast Cancer: Breast cancer and hormone replacement therapy: Collaborative reanalysis of data from 51 epidemiological studies of 52,705 women with breast cancer and 108,411 women without breast cancer. Lancet 1997; 350:1047-1059.

127. Manson JE, Hsia J, Johnson KC, et al. Estrogen plus progestin and risk of coronary heart disease. N Engl J Med 2003; 349:523-534.

128. Fletcher SW, Colditz GA: Failure of estrogen plus progestin therapy for prevention. JAMA 2002; 288:366-367.

129. MRC stops study of long-term use of HRT. London: MRC press release, http://www.mrc.ac.uk/index/public-interest/public-press_office/public-press_releases_2002/public-23_october_2002.htm. Accessed January 6, 2003.

130. Furberg CD, Vittinghoff E, Davidson M, et al: Subgroup interactions in the Heart and Estrogen-progestin Replacement Study: Lessons learned. Circulation 2002; 105:917-922.

131. Grady D, Herrington D, Bittner V, et al: Cardiovascular disease outcomes during 6.8 years of hormone therapy: Heart and Estrogen/progestin Replacement Study follow-up (HERS II). JAMA 2002; 288:49-57.

132. Nabel EG: Coronary heart disease in women: An ounce of prevention. N Engl J Med 2000; 343:572-574.

133. Hodis HN, Mack WJ, Lobo RA, et al: Estrogen in the prevention of atherosclerosis: A randomized, double-blind, placebo-controlled trial. Ann Intern Med 2001; 135:939-953.

134. Angerer P, Störk S, Kothny W, et al: Effects of postmenopausal hormone replacement on progression of atherosclerosis: A randomized, controlled trial. Arterioscler Thromb Vasc Biol 2001; 21:262-268.

135. Schulman SP, Thiemann DR, Ouyang P, et al: Effects of acute hormone replacement therapy on recurrent ischemia on postmenopausal women with unstable angina. J Am Coll Cardiol 2002; 39:231-237.

136. Simpkins JW, Rajakumar G, Zhang Y, et al: Estrogens may reduce mortality and ischemic damage caused by middle cerebral artery occlusion in the female rat. J Neurosurg 1997; 87:724-730.

137. Yang SH, Shi J, Day AL, et al: Estradiol exerts neuroprotective effects when administered after ischemic insult. Stroke 2000; 31:745-750.

138. Simon JA, Hsia J, Cauley JA, et al: Postmenopausal hormone replacement therapy and risk of stroke: The Heart and Estrogen-progestin Replacement Study (HERS). Circulation 2001:103:638-642.

139. Mendelsohn ME, Karas RH: The time has come to stop letting the HERS tale wag the dogma. Circulation 2001; 104:2256-2259.

140. Hanke H, Kamenz J, Hanke S, et al: Effect of 17-beta estradiol on preexisting atherosclerotic lesions: Role of the endothelium. Atherosclerosis 1999; 147:123-132.

141. Holm P, Andersen HL, Andersen MR, et al: The direct antiatherogenic effect of estrogen is present, absent, or reversed, depending on the state of the arterial endothelium: A time course-study in cholesterol-clamped rabbits. Circulation 1999; 100:1727-1733.

142. Mosca L, Collins P, Herrington DM, et al: Hormone replacement therapy and cardiovascular disease: A statement for healthcare professionals from the American Heart Association. Circulation 2001; 104:499-503.

143. Herrington DM: The HERS trial results: Paradigms lost? Ann Intern Med 1999; 131:463-466.

144. Blakely JA: The Heart and Estrogen/Progestin Replacement Study revisited: Hormone replacement therapy produced net harm, consistent with the observational data. Arch Intern Med 2000; 160:2897-2900.

145. Herrington DM, Howard TD, Hawkins GA, et al: Estrogen receptor polymorphisms and effects of estrogen replacement on high-density lipoprotein cholesterol in women with coronary disease. N Engl J Med 2002; 346:967-974.

146. Herrington DM, Howard TD, Brosnihan B, et al: Common estrogen receptor polymorphism augments effects of hormone replacement therapy on E-selectin but not C-reactive protein. Circulation 2002; 105:1879-1882.

147. U.S. Preventive Services Task Force: Postmenopausal hormone replacement therapy for primary prevention of chronic conditions: Recommendations and rationale. Ann Intern Med 2002; 137:834-839.

148. American Heart Association: Q & A about hormone replacement therapy. http://216.185.112.5/presenter.jhtml?identifier = 3004068. Accessed January 6, 2003.

149. North American Menopause Society: Amended report from the NAMS advisory panel on postmenopausal hormone replacement therapy. http://www.menopause.org/news.html#advisory. Accessed December 9, 2002.

150. American College of Obstetricians and Gynecologists: Guidelines for Women's Health Care. 2nd ed. Washington, DC, ACOG 2002, pp 130-133, 171-176, 314-318.

151. FDA Approves New Labels for Estrogen and Estrogen with Progestin Therapies for Postmenopausal Women Following Review of Women's Health Initiative Data. http://www.fda.gov/cder/drug/infopage/estrogens_progestins/default.htm. Accessed January 10, 2003.

152. Fuchs-Young R, Glasebrook AL, Short LL, et al: Raloxifene is a tissue-selective agonist/antagonist that functions through the estrogen receptor. Ann NY Acad Sci 1995; 761:355-60.

153. Delmas PD, Bjarnason NH, Mitlak BH, et al: Effects of raloxifene on bone mineral density, serum cholesterol concentrations, and uterine endometrium in postmenopausal women. N Engl J Med 1997; 337:1641-1647.

154. De Valk-de Roo GW, Stehouwer CD, Meijer P, et al: Both raloxifene and estrogen reduce major cardiovascular risk factors in healthy postmenopausal women: A 2-year, placebo-controlled trial. Arterioscler Thromb Vasc Biol 1999; 19: 2993-3000.

155. Barrett-Connor E, Grady D, Sashegyi A, et al: Raloxifene and cardiovascular events in osteoporotic postmenopausal women: Four-year results from the MORE (Multiple Outcomes of Raloxifene Evaluation) randomized trial. JAMA 2002; 287: 847-857.

156. Bjarnason NH, Haarbo J, Byrjalsen I, et al: Raloxifene inhibits aortic accumulation of cholesterol in ovariectomized, cholesterol-fed rabbits. Circulation 1997; 96:1964-1969.

157. Clarkson TB, Anthony MS, Jerome CP: Lack of effect of raloxifene on coronary artery atherosclerosis of postmenopausal monkeys. J Clin Endocrinol Metab 1998; 83:721-726.

■■■chapter **28**

Antioxidant Vitamins

Shari S. Bassuk
JoAnn E. Manson
J. Michael Gaziano

Prospective observational studies have found consistent associations between higher intakes of fruit and vegetables and reduced rates of coronary heart disease (CHD)[1-4] and ischemic stroke.[4-6] The precise mechanisms for these apparent protective effects are not entirely clear. Possible explanations include the association between higher fruit and vegetable intake and higher dietary fiber intake or the replacement of fats and cholesterol. Alternative hypotheses focus on the micronutrient content of fruits and vegetables. A great deal of attention has centered on the notion that micronutrients with antioxidant properties might be responsible for the lower rates of cardiovascular disease (CVD) associated with higher fruit and vegetable consumption.

Basic research has identified a plausible mechanism—the inhibition of oxidative damage—by which antioxidants might reduce the risk of atherosclerosis. Moreover, data from a large number of cross-sectional, case-control, and cohort studies suggest that antioxidant vitamin consumption is associated with a reduced risk of CVD. These findings raise the question of a possible role of antioxidants, such as β-carotene, vitamin E, and vitamin C, in the prevention of CVD but do not provide a definitive answer. Results from several large-scale, randomized trials of antioxidant supplements are now available, but they are not entirely consistent. This chapter discusses the rationale for conducting large-scale trials of antioxidant vitamins and reviews completed and ongoing trials.

BASIC LABORATORY RESEARCH

Basic research findings suggest that oxidative damage plays a role in the pathogenesis of many chronic diseases, including atherosclerosis, cancer, arthritis, eye disease, and reperfusion injury during myocardial infarction (MI). Data from in vitro and in vivo studies suggest that oxidative damage to low-density lipoprotein (LDL) promotes several steps in atherogenesis,[7] including endothelial cell damage,[8,9] foam cell accumulation,[10-12] and growth[13,14] and synthesis of autoantibodies.[15] In addition, animal studies suggest that free radicals may directly damage arterial endothelium,[16] promote thrombosis,[17] and interfere with normal vasomotor regulation.[18] There-

fore, oxidative damage may enhance atherogenesis by a cascade of reactions.

Elaborate systems have evolved in aerobic organisms to minimize the damaging effects of uncontrolled oxidation (Table 28-1). First, there are several mechanisms to prevent the formation of unintended free radicals. Oxidative metabolism is carefully compartmentalized, and molecular oxygen and its highly reactive species are tightly bound to enzymes involved in that process. Biologic systems bind heavy metal ions such as copper and iron to storage or transport proteins to prevent the catalytic reactions with oxygen species that could lead to the formation of free radicals. Second, enzymatic (e.g., superoxide dismutase, catalase, glutathione peroxidase) and nonenzymatic (e.g., vitamins E and C, urate) antioxidants scavenge free radicals, thereby minimizing the damage they can cause once they have been formed. Finally, there are mechanisms for repairing the damage resulting from unintended oxidative reactions.

Antioxidant vitamins represent one of the many nonenzymatic antioxidant defense mechanisms. Vitamin C (ascorbic acid), vitamin E (of which α-tocopherol is the major component), and β-carotene (a provitamin A) are among the most abundant and most widely studied natural antioxidants. However, there are hundreds or thousands of other dietary compounds that may function as antioxidants. In vitro data have demonstrated the possible role of these antioxidants in preventing or retarding various steps in atherogenesis by inhibiting oxidation of LDL or other free radical reactions. These antioxidants have also been shown to prevent experimental atherogenesis in many but not all animal models of atherosclerosis.

OBSERVATIONAL EPIDEMIOLOGY

Although basic research provides a plausible mechanism for a reduction in risk of CVD by antioxidant vitamins, the efficacy of any intervention must rely on data from human studies. The hypothesis that antioxidant vitamins might reduce CVD risk has been explored in a number of observational epidemiologic studies in humans. Results from these cross-sectional, case-control, and cohort studies suggest that consumption

■ ■ ■

TABLE 28-1 NATURAL DEFENSE MECHANISMS AGAINST OXIDATIVE DAMAGE

Compartmentalization of oxidative metabolism
Binding of molecular oxygen and reactive species to proteins to prevent random oxidative reactions
Binding of transition metals (e.g., iron and copper) to transport and storage proteins to prevent involvement in free radical reactions
Enzymatic antioxidants (e.g., superoxide dismutase, catalase, and glutathione peroxidase)
Nonenzymatic antioxidants (e.g., vitamin C, vitamin E, β-carotene, urate, bilirubin, and ubiquinols)
Mechanisms to repair or dispose of damaged DNA, proteins, lipids, and carbohydrates

of antioxidant vitamins reduces the risks of developing heart disease and stroke.[19] Prospective data are more consistent for vitamin E than for either vitamin C or β-carotene.[20]

Several large cohort studies have evaluated the relationship between vitamin E intake and incidence of coronary disease. The largest of these is the Nurses' Health Study (NHS), in which the association was analyzed among more than 87,000 U.S. female nurses aged 34 to 59 years with no history of CVD at baseline.[21] Dietary antioxidant intake and use of antioxidant vitamin supplements were ascertained through a semiquantitative food-frequency questionnaire administered at baseline; information on antioxidant supplements was updated biennially. After 8 years, women in the highest quintile of vitamin E intake had a 34% lower risk of coronary disease (defined as nonfatal MI and fatal CHD) compared with those in the lowest quintile (P for trend <0.001). When vitamin E intake was examined separately by source (food or supplements), an inverse association emerged only for supplements. Women who took at least 100 IU of vitamin E supplements per day for more than 2 years experienced reductions of 40% or more in the risk of coronary disease, after adjustment for age and multiple cardiac risk factors.

Similar findings were observed in the Health Professionals' Follow-up Study (HPFS), a 4-year follow-up of nearly 40,000 U.S. male health professionals aged 40 to 75 who were free of CHD, diabetes, or hypercholesterolemia at baseline.[22] After adjustment for cardiac risk factors, the relative risk (RR) of major coronary disease for those in the highest versus lowest quintile of vitamin E intake was 0.60 (95% confidence interval [CI] 0.44–0.81; P for trend = 0.01). As in the NHS, the relation was strongest for supplement use. Men who took at least 100 IU per day for at least 2 years had a multivariate risk of coronary disease of 0.63 (95% CI, 0.47–0.84) compared with men who did not take vitamin E supplements. A weak association was found for dietary vitamin E intake alone; among men who did not take vitamin supplements, the relative risk comparing the extreme quartiles was 0.79 (95% CI, 0.54–1.15; P for trend = 0.11).

The Iowa Women's Health Study evaluated the association between antioxidant vitamin intake and CHD mortality among 34,486 postmenopausal women with no history of CVD who were followed for 7 years.[23] In contrast to the NHS and HPFS findings, vitamin E intake from food but not from supplements was strongly associ-

ated with CHD mortality; among individuals who did not use vitamin supplements, those in the highest quintile of dietary vitamin E intake had a relative risk of 0.38 as compared with those in the lowest quintile (P for trend = 0.004). The relationship persisted after controlling for other dietary factors associated with vitamin E intake, such as intake of linoleic acid, folate, fiber, and other antioxidant vitamins. The Iowa results are in agreement with a Finnish study that also found a significant inverse association between dietary intake of vitamin E and coronary mortality among 2385 women 30 to 69 years of age over a 14-year period.[1]

The relationship between vitamin E and CVD has also been examined in two elderly cohorts. The Established Populations for Epidemiologic Studies of the Elderly program, a 10-year study of 11,178 U.S. men and women aged 67 to 105 years, found a decreased risk of CHD mortality (RR, 0.53; 95% CI, 0.34–0.84) and overall mortality (RR, 0.66; 95% CI, 0.53–0.83) among those reporting vitamin E supplement use.[24] However, no association between dietary vitamin E intake (as assessed by a semiquantitative food-frequency questionnaire) and MI was observed in the Rotterdam Study, which followed 4802 Dutch men and women aged 55 to 95 years, none of whom had a history of MI at baseline, for 4 years.[25]

In contrast to studies of vitamin E intake, studies of vitamin E blood levels, conducted as nested case-control studies within large cohorts, have generally yielded null results. For example, a study of 734 U.S. men enrolled in the Multiple Risk Factor Intervention Trial found no association between serum vitamin E levels and risk of nonfatal MI or coronary death over a 20-year follow-up period.[26]

RATIONALE FOR RANDOMIZED TRIALS

Observational data raise the question of a possible role of antioxidants in the prevention of cardiovascular events but do not provide a definitive answer. Regardless of the number or sample size of such studies or the consistency of their findings, observational studies are limited in their ability to provide reliable estimates of the antioxidant–CVD relationship because the amount of uncontrolled confounding inherent in such studies may be as large as or larger than the most plausible small-to-moderate health benefits (or risks) conferred by antioxidant vitamins. Although observational studies can at least partly control for the effects of known potential confounding variables in the analysis, they cannot adjust for the effects of unknown or unmeasured confounders. A high antioxidant vitamin intake via either foods or supplements may simply be a marker for some other dietary practice or even a nondietary lifestyle variable that is truly cardioprotective. The apparent health benefits of antioxidant-rich foods may result not from their antioxidant properties but rather from some other component these foods have in common. In addition, intakes of individual dietary antioxidants tend to be highly correlated with each other, making it difficult to determine the specific benefit of any one antioxidant.

Thus, reliable data on the relationship of antioxidants and CVD can be obtained only from large-scale randomized trials of adequate dose and duration, in which investigators allocate subjects at random to either active treatment or placebo. When the sample size is sufficient, randomized trials can avoid some limitations of observational studies by distributing the known and unknown confounding variables equally among the treatment groups.

Antioxidant vitamins are among the most widely consumed nutritional supplements, and their use is rapidly increasing. Spending on dietary supplements, including antioxidants, by the American public nearly doubled during the late 1990s, to more than $13 billion annually, and will likely reach $20 billion in 2003.[27] A definitive evaluation of the benefits and risks of such supplements is essential to establish prudent recommendations for clinical decision making and public health policy. Well-designed, large-scale randomized trials can provide "informative" results on which clinical and policy decisions can be based. Informative positive results would justify at least part of the current enthusiasm for so-called "nutraceuticals," whereas informative null results would permit the rechanneling of limited resources to other, more promising areas of research.

In 1991, the U.S. National Heart, Lung, and Blood Institute's (NHLBI) conference, "Antioxidants in the Prevention of Human Atherosclerosis," concluded that data from large-scale randomized trials were required to test the hypothesis that dietary antioxidants reduce the risk of CVD and recommended the initiation of randomized trials to examine the role of vitamin C, vitamin E, and β-carotene in the primary and secondary prevention of CVD.[28] Even at that time, researchers were aware that if the trend toward increasing use of antioxidants continued, it would soon be difficult to conduct randomized trials with sufficient numbers of participants willing to be assigned to placebo. This chapter reviews the large-scale clinical trials that have been initiated and/or completed in the years since the NHLBI issued its recommendation. Except as noted, all trials used a randomized, double-blinded, placebo-controlled design.

PRIMARY PREVENTION TRIALS

Randomized trials of vitamin E and β-carotene in the primary prevention of CVD are summarized in Tables 28-2 and 28-3, respectively. Many of these trials

■ ■ ■

TABLE 28-2   COMPLETED AND ONGOING RANDOMIZED CLINICAL TRIALS OF VITAMIN E ALONE OR IN COMBINATION WITH OTHER ANTIOXIDANTS IN THE PRIMARY PREVENTION OF CARDIOVASCULAR DISEASE (CVD)

Study	Population; country	Agent(s)*	Duration of treatment (years)	Endpoint†	Effect of vitamin E supplementation RR (95% CI)
Chinese Cancer Prevention Trial	29,584 men and women; China	Cocktail of vitamin E (30 mg/day), β-carotene (15 mg/day), and selenium (50 mg/day)	5	Cerebrovascular mortality	0.90 (0.76–1.07)
Alpha-Tocopherol, Beta-Carotene Cancer Prevention Trial (ATBC)	29,133 male smokers aged 50–69; Finland	Vitamin E (50 mg/day), β-carotene (20 mg/day), or both	6.1	CVD mortality Fatal ischemic heart disease Fatal ischemic stroke Fatal hemorrhagic stroke	0.98 (0.89–1.08) 0.95 (0.85–1.05) 0.84 (0.59–1.19) 1.50 (1.03–2.20)
Primary Prevention Project (PPP)	4495 men and women aged ≥50, with ≥1 CVD risk factor; Italy	Vitamin E (300 mg/day); open-label design	3.6	CVD mortality + MI + stroke CVD mortality Nonfatal MI Nonfatal stroke	1.07 (0.74–1.56) 0.86 (0.49–1.52) 1.01 (0.56–2.03) 1.56 (0.77–3.13)
Women's Health Study (WHS)	39,876 female health professionals aged ≥45; United States	Vitamin E (600 IU alternate days), aspirin (100 mg alternate days) or both‡	12	CVD mortality + MI + stroke	Ongoing
Physicians' Health Study II (PHS II)	15,000 male physicians aged ≥55; United States	Vitamin E (400 IU alternate days), β-carotene (50 mg alternate days), vitamin C (500 mg/day), multivitamin (daily), or a combination (2 × 2 × 2 × 2 factorial design)	8	CVD mortality + MI + stroke	Ongoing
Supplémentation en Vitamines et Minéraux AntioXydants Study (SU.VI.MAX)	12,375 men and women aged 35–60; France	Cocktail of vitamin E (30 mg/day), vitamin C (120 mg/day), β-carotene (6 mg/day), selenium (100 μg/day), zinc (20 mg/day)	8	Ischemic heart disease	Ongoing

RR, relative risk; CI, confidence interval; MI, myocardial infarction.
*All trials were placebo controlled, except for the Primary Prevention Project (PPP), which used an open-label design.
†Outcome listed first is the trial's primary endpoint.
‡β-carotene (50 mg alternate days) component was discontinued after 2.1 yr.

■ ■ ■

TABLE 28-3 COMPLETED AND ONGOING RANDOMIZED CLINICAL TRIALS OF β-CAROTENE ALONE OR IN COMBINATION WITH OTHER ANTIOXIDANTS IN THE PRIMARY PREVENTION OF CARDIOVASCULAR DISEASE (CVD)

Study	Population; country	Agent(s)*	Duration of treatment† (years)	Endpoint	Effect of β-carotene supplementation RR (95% CI)
Chinese Cancer Prevention Trial	29,584 men and women; China	Cocktail of vitamin E (30 mg/day), β-carotene (15 mg/day), and selenium (50 mg/day)	5	Cerebrovascular mortality	0.90 (0.76–1.07)
Alpha-Tocopherol, Beta-Carotene Cancer Prevention Trial (ATBC)	29,133 male smokers aged 50–69; Finland	β-carotene (20 mg/day), vitamin E (50 mg/day), or both	6.1	Fatal ischemic heart disease Fatal ischemic stroke Fatal hemorrhagic stroke	1.12 (1.00–1.25) 1.23 (CI not avail.) 1.17 (CI not avail.)
Skin Cancer Prevention Study	1805 men and women with history of skin cancer; United States	β-carotene (50 mg/day)	4.3‡	CVD mortality	1.15 (0.81–1.63)
Beta-Carotene and Retinol Efficacy Trial (CARET)	18,314 men and women who were smokers or had been exposed to asbestos; United States	β-carotene (30 mg/day) and retinol (25,000 IU/day)	4	CVD mortality	1.26 (0.99–1.61)
Physicians' Health Study I (PHS I)	22,071 male physicians aged 40–84; United States	β-carotene (50 mg alternate days), aspirin (325 mg alternate days), or both	12	CVD mortality MI Stroke CVD mortality + MI + stroke *Nonsmokers:* CVD mortality MI Stroke CVD mortality + MI + stroke *Former smokers:* CVD mortality MI Stroke CVD mortality + MI + stroke *Current smokers:* CVD mortality MI Stroke CVD mortality + MI + stroke	1.09 (0.93–1.27) 0.96 (0.84–1.09) 0.96 (0.83–1.11) 1.00 (0.91–1.09) 1.00 (0.78–1.29) 0.88 (0.72–1.07) 0.92 (0.73–1.16) 1.00 (0.91–1.09) 1.16 (0.92–1.48) 1.00 (0.82–1.22) 0.90 (0.72–1.12) 1.00 (0.87–1.15) 1.13 (0.80–1.61) 1.08 (0.80–1.48) 1.18 (0.83–1.67) 1.15 (0.93–1.43)
Women's Health Study (WHS)	39,876 female health professionals aged ≥45; United States	β-carotene (50 mg alternate days), vitamin E (600 IU alternate days), aspirin (100 mg alternate days), or a combination (2 × 2 × 2 factorial design)	2.1§	CVD mortality MI Stroke CVD mortality + MI + stroke *Smokers:* CVD mortality + MI + stroke	1.17 (0.54–2.53) 0.84 (0.56–1.27) 1.42 (0.96–2.10) 1.14 (0.87–1.49) 1.01 (0.62–1.63)
Physicians' Health Study II (PHS II)	15,000 male physicians aged ≥55; United States	β-carotene (50 mg alternate days), vitamin E (400 IU alternate days), vitamin C (500 mg/day), multivitamin (daily), or a combination (2 × 2 × 2 × 2 factorial design)	8	CVD mortality MI Stroke	Ongoing
Supplémentation en Vitamines et Minéraux AntioXydants Study (SU.VI.MAX)	12,375 men and women aged 35–60; France	Cocktail of vitamin E (30 mg/day), vitamin C (120 mg/day), β-carotene (6 mg/day), selenium (100 µg/day), zinc (20 mg/day)	8	Ischemic heart disease	Ongoing

RR, relative risk; CI, confidence interval; MI, myocardial infarction.
*All trials were placebo controlled.
†Except as indicated, duration of treatment equals duration of follow-up.
‡In the Skin Cancer Prevention Study, duration of treatment was 4.3 years, but duration of follow-up was 8.2 years.
§In the Women's Health Study, duration of treatment was 2.1 years, but duration of follow-up was 4.1 years.

were originally designed to test the hypothesis that various antioxidant vitamin supplements (individually or in combination) reduce the risk of cancer and were thus conducted among persons at elevated risk for various epithelial cancers.[29-31] With the emergence of the hypothesis that antioxidants might prevent or retard atherogenesis, these cancer prevention trials also provided an excellent opportunity to assess the role of antioxidants in the primary prevention of CVD.

Vitamin E

Although vitamin E is a mixture of tocopherols and tocotrienols, clinical trials have focused on α-tocopherol, the major component of vitamin E and the predominant antioxidant in circulating lipoproteins.[32] The form of α-tocopherol that occurs in nature is RRR-α-tocopherol. The synthetic form is a mixture of eight stereoisomers known as all-rac-α-tocopherol. Vitamin E supplements generally contain all-rac-α-tocopherol, although natural supplements containing RRR-α-tocopherol are available.

The **Chinese Cancer Prevention Trial** was conducted among a poorly nourished population in Linxian, China, who were at high risk of upper gastrointestinal cancers.[29] Nearly 30,000 men and women were randomized to one of eight treatment arms comprised of various combinations of nine vitamins and minerals. There was an apparent, although insignificant, reduction in cerebrovascular mortality among participants assigned to a cocktail of synthetic vitamin E (30 mg daily), β-carotene (15 mg daily), and selenium (50 μg daily) (RR, 0.90; 95% CI, 0.76-1.07). This vitamin combination was also associated with a significant reduction in total mortality, a finding largely attributable to a reduction in stomach cancer deaths. Unfortunately, the effects of individual micronutrients could not be disentangled because of the cocktail design. Also, coronary artery disease rates in the study population were too low to assess the effect of vitamin supplementation on this endpoint.

The **Alpha-Tocopherol, Beta-Carotene (ATBC) Cancer Prevention Study** was the first large-scale randomized trial of antioxidant vitamins in a well-nourished population. This 2×2 factorial trial tested the effect of synthetic vitamin E (50 mg/day) and β-carotene (20 mg/day) in the prevention of lung cancer among 29,133 Finnish male smokers aged 50 to 69 years.[30] After a treatment period of 6.1 years, there was no reduction in lung cancer incidence, the primary endpoint under investigation, associated with vitamin E supplementation. There was also no clear reduction in risk of death from ischemic heart disease (RR, 0.95; 95% CI, 0.85-1.05) or ischemic stroke (RR, 0.84; 95% CI, 0.59-1.19),[30] although the risk of developing angina was lower among those assigned to vitamin E (RR, 0.91; 95% CI, 0.83-0.99).[33] Moreover, there was a disturbing increase in the risk of fatal hemorrhagic stroke in the vitamin E group compared to the placebo group (RR, 1.50; 95% CI, 1.03-2.20), although the association was attenuated after statistical adjustment for multiple comparisons. However, observational research suggests that supplementation at doses higher than the 50 mg used in this trial may be required to reduce risk of coronary disease. As noted earlier, the apparent benefits

associated with vitamin E supplementation in the NHS[21] and the HPFS[22] were largely confined to respondents who reported an average daily dose of 100 IU or more.

The **Primary Prevention Project (PPP)** was an open-label 2×2 factorial trial of 300 mg synthetic vitamin E and aspirin in 4495 Italian men and women with one or more of the following cardiovascular risk factors: hypertension, hypercholesterolemia, diabetes, obesity, family history of premature MI, or age 65 years or older.[34] Because of a strong treatment effect for aspirin, the PPP was stopped early, after 3.6 years of follow-up. Vitamin E showed no effect on any of the three prespecified endpoints: cardiovascular death, nonfatal MI, or nonfatal stoke. It has been suggested that the null findings may be the result of the inadequate power of this prematurely terminated trial.

Although more data are needed to draw definitive conclusions, the available trial results provide scant support for the hypothesis that vitamin E is protective against CVD in individuals with no history of CVD.

β-Carotene

β-Carotene occurs in nature as an all cis isomer, whereas synthetic β-carotene is a mixture of cis and trans isomers. Most clinical trials have tested synthetic β-carotene.

Results from large-scale randomized trials of β-carotene in the primary prevention of CVD have been disappointing. In the previously described **ATBC trial** among 29,133 male smokers, there was an insignificant increase in ischemic heart disease mortality (RR, 1.12; 95% CI, 1.00-1.25) and no reduction in the risk of angina (RR, 1.06; 95% CI, 0.97-1.16) among those assigned to 20 mg/day of β-carotene. There was also no reduction in lung cancer incidence, the primary endpoint under investigation. Rather, β-carotene assignment was associated with a statistically significant elevation in this endpoint (RR, 1.18; 95% CI 1.03-1.36).

The **Skin Cancer Prevention Study** randomized 1805 men and women with a history of skin cancer to 50 mg of β-carotene daily or placebo.[35] After a median treatment period of 4.3 years and median follow-up of 8.2 years, there was no significant reduction in cardiovascular mortality (RR, 1.15; 95% CI, 0.81-1.63), cancer mortality (RR, 0.86; 95% CI, 0.56-1.32), or total mortality (RR, 1.05; 95% CI, 0.83-1.32) associated with β-carotene supplementation.

The **β-Carotene and Retinol Efficacy Trial (CARET)** evaluated a combined treatment of β-carotene (30 mg/day) and retinol (25,000 IU/day) among 18,314 men and women at elevated risk of lung cancer resulting from cigarette smoking and/or occupational exposure to asbestos.[31] The trial was stopped prematurely because of an inability to detect a benefit over the projected funding period and an increased incidence of lung cancer in the active treatment group (RR, 1.28; 95% CI, 1.04-1.57). After 4 years, there was an excess of total deaths (RR, 1.17; 95% CI, 1.03-1.33) and a trend toward excess cardiovascular deaths (RR, 1.26; 95% CI, 0.99-1.61) among individuals assigned to β-carotene and retinol.

The **Physicians' Health Study (PHS I)** was a randomized, double-blind, placebo-controlled trial of β-carotene (50 mg on alternate days) and low-dose aspirin among

22,071 U.S. male physicians aged 40 to 84 years, of whom 11% were current smokers and 39% were former smokers.[36] After 12 years, there were no differences in cardiovascular mortality (RR, 1.09; 95% CI, 0.93–1.27), MI (RR, 0.96; 95% CI, 0.84–1.09), stroke (RR, 0.96; 95% CI, 0.83–1.11), or a composite of the three endpoints (RR, 1.00; 95% CI, 0.91–1.09) associated with β-carotene assignment. There was also no relationship between β-carotene and cancer mortality, malignant neoplasms, or lung cancer. In analyses limited to current or former smokers, no significant early or late effects of β-carotene on any endpoint of interest were detected.

A companion trial to the PHS, the **Women's Health Study (WHS)**, was designed to evaluate the effect of β-carotene (50 mg on alternate days), vitamin E, and low-dose aspirin on the development of CVD and cancer in 39,876 healthy U.S. women health professionals.[37] Although the other two components of the trial will last a mean of 10 years, the β-carotene arm was terminated after only 2.1 years, primarily because of the null findings on β-carotene and cancer incidence in the PHS. After an additional 2 years of follow-up, β-carotene supplementation had no effect on cardiovascular mortality (RR, 1.17; 95% CI, 0.54–2.53), MI (RR, 0.84; 95% CI, 0.56–1.27), stroke (RR, 1.42; 95% CI, 0.96–2.10), or a composite of these endpoints (RR, 1.14; 95% CI, 0.87–1.49). β-carotene was also not associated with cancer incidence (RR, 1.03; 95% CI 0.89–1.18). Among smokers at baseline, there were no differences between the β-carotene and placebo groups with respect to incidence of CVD (RR, 1.01; 95% CI, 0.62–1.63) or cancer (RR, 1.11; 95% CI, 0.78–1.58).

These randomized trials, taken as a whole, provide convincing evidence of no benefit of β-carotene in the primary prevention of CVD or cancer. Indeed, the ATBC and CARET trials raise the possibility of harm among smokers, a finding that highlights the need for randomized trials even for putatively harmless agents.

Vitamin C

In the **Chinese Cancer Prevention Trial**, no reduction in cerebrovascular mortality was found among participants assigned a combination of vitamin C (125 mg) and molybdenum (30 μg). Data from large-scale randomized trials on the role of vitamin C in primary prevention of CVD in well-nourished Western populations are not yet available.

Ongoing Trials

The findings to date suggest that the cardiovascular benefits of antioxidants reported in observational studies may have been overestimates and raise the possibility that supplementation may even have some deleterious effects not previously considered. Three ongoing large randomized trials are testing the role of antioxidant vitamins in the primary prevention of CVD and should provide more conclusive answers as to the balance of benefits and risks of antioxidant supplementation. The **WHS** is testing vitamin E (600 IU of natural vitamin E on alternate days) and low-dose aspirin in the primary prevention of CVD and cancer in approximately 40,000 healthy U.S. women

health professionals.[38] Results are expected in 2004. **PHS II** has randomized nearly 15,000 healthy U.S. male physicians in a factorial design to β-carotene (50 mg on alternate days), vitamin E (400 IU on alternate days), vitamin C (500 mg daily), and a daily multivitamin.[39] The β-carotene component ended in 2003 (results were unavailable at press time); the remaining three interventions will continue until 2007. The 8-year **SUpplémentation en VItamines et Minéraux AntioXydants (SU.VI.MAX) Study**, begun in 1994, is testing the efficacy of daily supplementation at nutritional doses of antioxidant vitamins (120 mg vitamin C, 30 mg vitamin E, and 6 mg β-carotene) and minerals (100 μg selenium and 20 mg zinc) in reducing the risks of CVD and cancer among 12,375 French men and women aged 35 to 60 years.[40] The antioxidant doses being tested in the SU.VI.MAX trial are lower than the doses associated with benefit in the major observational studies, which may limit the trial's ability to provide informative answers to the questions raised by the observational studies.

SECONDARY PREVENTION TRIALS

Primary prevention trials do not address whether antioxidants may benefit patients with established CVD or those at high risk for developing CVD. As with cholesterol-lowering interventions (see Chapter 22), antioxidant vitamin supplementation may provide greater benefits in secondary prevention than in primary prevention settings. Secondary prevention trials of vitamin E and β-carotene that utilize clinical CVD endpoints are shown in Tables 28-4 and 28-5, respectively.

Vitamin E

Small-scale trials using surrogate CVD endpoints have tested the effects of supplemental vitamin E among people with various forms of atherosclerotic disease, including claudication and angina. One such trial tested the effect of vitamin E supplementation (400 IU/day) on restenosis rates following percutaneous transluminal coronary angioplasty.[41] There was a nonsignificant 30% reduction in the risk of restenosis as measured by subsequent catheterization or exercise test. Benefits of supplemental vitamin E were also found in early trials among claudication patients,[42,43] although the inferences that can be drawn from these trials are limited by small sample sizes, high dropout rates, and lack of blinding. Indeed, more recent trials have yielded conflicting data. A study of 120 men and women with intermittent claudication randomized to antioxidants or placebo found little improvement in lower limb function and similar rates of cardiovascular events and death in both groups,[44] and a substudy of the ATBC trial found that low-dose vitamin E did not affect the development of claudication.[45]

Trials have also tested whether vitamin E supplementation is an effective treatment for angina pectoris. Two early trials reported equivocal results, with one reporting a nonsignificant trend toward improved angina pain score in a 9-week placebo-controlled trial among stable angina patients consuming 3200 IU/day of vitamin E as

TABLE 28-4   COMPLETED AND ONGOING RANDOMIZED CLINICAL TRIALS OF VITAMIN E SUPPLEMENTATION ALONE OR IN COMBINATION WITH OTHER ANTIOXIDANTS IN THE SECONDARY PREVENTION OF CARDIOVASCULAR DISEASE (CVD)

Study	Population; country	Agent(s)*	Duration (years)	Endpoint†	Effect of vitamin E supplementation RR (95% CI)
Cambridge Heart Antioxidant Study (CHAOS)	2002 men and women with atherosclerosis, mean age = 62; United Kingdom	Vitamin E (400 or 800 IU/day)	1.4	Nonfatal MI + CVD mortality Nonfatal MI CVD mortality	0.53 (0.34–0.83) 0.23 (0.11–0.47) 1.18 (0.62–2.27)
Alpha-Tocopherol, Beta-Carotene Cancer Prevention Trial (ATBC) substudy	1862 male smokers aged 50–69 with prior MI; Finland	Vitamin E (50 mg/day), β-carotene (20 mg/day), or both	6	Major coronary event Nonfatal MI CHD mortality	0.90 (0.67–1.22) 0.62 (0.41–0.96) 1.33 (0.86–2.05)
Gruppo Italiano per lo Studio della Sopravvivenza nell' Infarto miocardico Prevenzione trial (GISSI)	11,324 men and women with prior MI; Italy	Vitamin E (300 mg/day), n-3 polyunsaturated fatty acids (1 g/day), or both (open-label design)	3.5	CVD mortality + MI + stroke CVD mortality	0.98 (0.87–1.10) 0.80 (0.65–0.99)‡
Heart Outcomes Prevention Evaluation trial (HOPE)	9541 men and women age ≥55, at high risk of CVD; N. America, S. America, Europe	Vitamin E (400 IU/day)	4.5	CVD mortality + MI + stroke CVD mortality MI Stroke	1.05 (0.95–1.16) 1.05 (0.90–1.22) 1.02 (0.90–1.15) 1.17 (0.95–1.42)
Secondary Prevention with Antioxidants of Cardiovascular disease in Endstage renal disease (SPACE)	196 hemodialysis patients with CVD, mean age = 65; Israel	Vitamin E (800 IU/day), ramipril, or both	1.4	MI + ischemic stroke + peripheral vascular disease + unstable angina MI	0.46 (0.27–0.78) 0.30 (0.10–0.80)
HDL-Atherosclerosis Treatment Study (HATS)	142 men and 18 women with CHD, low HDL, and normal LDL levels, mean age = 53; United States	Simvastatin and niacin;§ AO cocktail of vitamin E (800 IU/day), vitamin C (1000 mg/day), β-carotene (25 mg/day), selenium (100 μg/day); or both	3	MI + stroke + revascularization + death	Simvastatin/niacin alone: 3%‖ AO alone: 21% Simvastatin/niacin + AO: 14% Placebo: 24%
Heart Protection Study (HPS)	20,536 men and women aged 40–80 with previous CVD or diabetes; United Kingdom	Simvastatin (40 mg/day); cocktail of vitamin E (600 mg/day), β-carotene (20 mg/day), and vitamin C (250 mg/day); or both	>5	Nonfatal MI + CHD mortality Nonfatal MI + CHD mortality + stroke + revascularization	1.02 (0.94–1.11) 1.00 (0.94–1.06)
Women's Antioxidant Cardiovascular Study (WACS)	8171 female health professionals aged ≥40, with CVD or diabetes or ≥3 coronary risk factors; United States	Vitamin E (600 IU every other day), other antioxidant,¶ or a combination (2 × 2 × 2 factorial design)	8	MI + stroke + revascularization + CVD mortality	Ongoing

RR, relative risk; CI, confidence interval; MI, myocardial infarction; AO, antioxidant; LDL, low-density lipoprotein cholesterol; HDL, high-density lipoprotein cholesterol; CHD, coronary heart disease.

*All trials were placebo controlled, except for the Gruppo Italiano per lo Studio dell Sopravvienza nell'Infarto miocardico Prevenzione (GISSI) trial, which used an open-label design.

†Outcome listed first is the trial's primary endpoint.

‡Secondary four-way analysis.

§Initial simvastatin dose was 10 mg if baseline LDL ≤110 mg/dL and 20 mg if LDL >110 mg/dL, with subsequent dose adjustment dependent on LDL level. Initial niacin dose was 250 mg twice per day, increasing to 1000 mg twice per day over a 4-week period.

‖The comparison between simvastatin/niacin alone with placebo was statistically significant (P < 0.05); other comparisons were not.

¶β-carotene (50 mg on alternate days); vitamin C (500 mg daily); or a combination of folic acid (2.5 mg daily), vitamin B_6 (50 mg daily), and vitamin B_{12} (1 mg daily).

compared with placebo[46] and the other finding no benefit of 1600 IU/d of vitamin E on angina symptoms, left-ventricular function, or exercise tolerance.[47] The small sample size and the short duration of treatment may have limited the ability of these studies to detect small-to-moderate benefits. Nevertheless, the larger subgroup analyses of the ATBC trial found only a very small decrease in the incidence of angina associated with low-dose vitamin E supplementation[33] and no evidence that such supplementation affected the symptoms or

■ ■ ■

TABLE 28-5 COMPLETED AND ONGOING RANDOMIZED CLINICAL TRIALS OF β-CAROTENE ALONE OR IN COMBINATION WITH OTHER ANTIOXIDANTS IN THE SECONDARY PREVENTION OF CARDIOVASCULAR DISEASE (CVD)

Study	Population; country	Agent(s)*	Duration of tx† (years)	Endpoint	Effect of β-carotene supplementation RR (95% CI)
Alpha-Tocopherol, Beta-Carotene Cancer Prevention Trial (ATBC) substudy	1862 male smokers aged 50-69 with prior MI; Finland	β-carotene (20 mg/day), vitamin E (50 mg/day), or both	5.3	Major coronary event Nonfatal MI CHD mortality	1.11 (0.84-1.49) 0.67 (0.44-1.02) 1.75 (1.16-2.64)
Physicians' Health Study I (PHS I) substudy	333 male physicians aged 40-84 with angina or coronary revascularization; United States	β-carotene (50 mg/day), aspirin (325 mg alternate days), or both	12	CVD mortality + MI + stroke	0.71 (0.24-1.07)
HDL-Atherosclerosis Treatment Study (HATS)	142 men and 18 women with CHD, low HDL, and normal LDL levels, mean age = 53; United States	Simvastatin and niacin;‡ AO cocktail of vitamin E (800 IU/day), vitamin C (1000 mg/day), β-carotene (25 mg/day), selenium (100 μg/day); or both	3	MI + stroke + revascularization + death	Simvastatin/niacin alone: 3% § AO alone: 21% Simvastatin/niacin + AO: 14% Placebo: 24%
Heart Protection Study (HPS)	20,536 men and women aged 40-80, with previous CVD; United Kingdom	Simvastatin (40 mg/day); cocktail of vitamin E (600 mg/day), β-carotene (20 mg/day), and vitamin C (250 mg/day); or both	>5	CHD mortality + nonfatal MI CHD mortality + nonfatal MI + stroke + revascularization	1.02 (0.94-1.11) 1.00 (0.94-1.06)
Women's Antioxidant Cardiovascular Study (WACS)	8171 female health professionals aged ≥40, with CVD or diabetes, or ≥3 coronary risk factors; United States	β-carotene (50 mg alternate days), other antioxidant,‖ or a combination (2 × 2 × 2 × 2 factorial design)	8	CVD mortality + MI + stroke + revascularization	Ongoing

RR, relative risk; CI, confidence interval; MI, myocardial infarction; CHD, coronary heart disease; CVD, cardiovascular disease, HDL, high-density lipoprotein cholesterol; LDL, low-density lipoprotein cholesterol; AO, antioxidant.
*All trials were placebo controlled.
†Duration of treatment equals duration of follow-up.
‡Initial simvastatin dose was 10 mg if baseline LDL ≤110 mg/dL and 20 mg if LDL >110 mg/dL, with subsequent dose adjustment dependent on LDL level. Initial niacin dose was 250 mg twice per day, increasing to 1000 mg twice per day over a 4-week period.
§The comparison between simvastatin/niacin alone with placebo was statistically significant (P < 0.05); other comparisons were not.
‖Vitamin E (600 IU alternate days); vitamin C (500 mg daily); or a combination of folic acid (2.5 mg daily), vitamin B_6 (50 mg daily), and vitamin B_{12} (1 mg daily).

progression of angina in male smokers with a history of angina at baseline.[48]

In the **Cambridge Heart Antioxidant Study (CHAOS)**, 2002 patients with angiographically proven coronary artery disease were randomly assigned to receive supplemental natural vitamin E (400 or 800 IU/day) or placebo for a median treatment duration of 1.4 years.[49] Compared with those assigned to placebo, patients in the vitamin E group had a significantly lower risk of subsequent nonfatal MI (RR, 0.23; 95% CI, 0.11-0.47) and a combined endpoint of nonfatal MI and cardiovascular death (RR, 0.53; 95% CI, 0.34-0.83). However, there was a nonsignificant increase in cardiovascular deaths (RR, 1.18; 95% CI, 0.62-2.27) and total mortality (3.5 vs. 2.7%; P = 0.31) among those assigned to vitamin E. Because of the relatively small sample size, there were imbalances in various baseline characteristics between the treatment groups, including trends toward fewer women, lower cholesterol levels, and lower systolic blood pressure levels in the placebo group. However, the explanation for the disparity between nonfatal and fatal cardiovascular outcomes is unclear. It is interesting that similar disparities were observed in subgroup analyses of the **ATBC trial**. Among the 1862 men who entered the

trial with a history of MI, vitamin E was associated with a reduction in subsequent risk of nonfatal MI (RR, 0.62; 95% CI, 0.41-0.96) but a nonsignificant increased risk of fatal CHD (RR, 1.33; 95% CI, 0.86-2.05).[50] Similar findings were observed for β-carotene (see later in this chapter) and for the combination of vitamin E and β-carotene. Compared with those assigned to neither agent, men assigned to both agents were less likely to experience nonfatal MI (RR, 0.86; 95% CI, 0.58-1.26) but more likely to have fatal CHD (RR, 1.75; 95% CI, 1.16-2.64). Data on stroke outcomes were not provided.

In the **Gruppo Italiano per lo Studio della Sopravvivenza nell'Infarto miocardico (GISSI) Prevention Trial**, 11,324 men and women who survived an acute MI were randomized to synthetic vitamin E (300 mg/day), n-3 polyunsaturated fatty acids (1 g/day), both, or neither in an open-label design.[51] After 3.5 years of treatment, vitamin E had no impact on risk of the combined primary endpoint of cardiovascular death, nonfatal MI, and nonfatal stroke (RR, 0.98; 95% CI 0.87-1.10). However, secondary analyses of the individual components of cardiovascular death outcomes revealed significant declines—ranging from 20% for all cardiovascular deaths to 35% for sudden death—associated with vitamin E assignment.

In the **Heart Outcomes Prevention Evaluation (HOPE) trial**, 9541 men and women at high risk of cardiovascular events as a result of existing CVD or diabetes plus at least one additional risk factor (hypertension, hypercholesterolemia, smoking, low high-density lipoprotein (HDL), or microalbuminuria) were randomized in a 2×2 factorial design to natural vitamin E (400 IU daily), the angiotensin-converting enzyme inhibitor ramipril, both agents, or neither agent.[52] The ramipril arm was terminated early as a result of unequivocal reductions in cardiovascular death, MI, and stroke. In the vitamin E arm, however, no significant differences between the active agent and placebo groups with respect to cardiovascular death, nonfatal MI, nonfatal stroke, or a variety of secondary endpoints (including claudication, angina, and revascularization) emerged after 4 to 6 years of treatment.

The **Secondary Prevention with Antioxidants of Cardiovascular disease in Endstage renal disease (SPACE)** trial randomized 196 hemodialysis patients with CVD to natural vitamin E (800 IU/day) or placebo.[53] After 1.4 years of treatment, vitamin E was associated with significant reductions in the composite endpoint of MI (fatal and nonfatal), ischemic stroke, peripheral vascular disease, and/or unstable angina (RR, 0.46; 95% CI, 0.27-0.78). Those in the vitamin E group also were less likely to experience the specific endpoint of MI (RR, 0.30; 95% CI, 0.10-0.80). The results of this small Israeli trial are consistent with those of CHAOS, which also used a higher dose of vitamin E than GISSI or HOPE and which was also of 1.4 years duration.

The **HDL-Atherosclerosis Treatment Study (HATS)**, a trial that enrolled 160 CHD patients with normal levels of LDL cholesterol but low levels of HDL cholesterol, suggested that antioxidants may blunt the benefits of statins and/or niacin, which are used to lower LDL and raise HDL, respectively.[54] Patients were randomly assigned in a 2×2 factorial design to simvastatin plus niacin or to an antioxidant combination (800 IU of vitamin E, 1000 mg of vitamin C, 25 mg of natural β-carotene, and 100 µg selenium). (The initial statin dose was 10 mg if baseline LDL $\leq$110 mg/dL, and 20 mg if LDL $>$110 mg/dL, with doses adjusted depending on LDL level. The initial niacin dose was 250 mg twice per day, gradually increasing to 1000 mg twice per day over a 4-week period.) After 3 years, 3% of the simvastatin/niacin group had died or experienced MI, stroke, or revascularization. In contrast, 14% of those who also took an antioxidant had these outcomes (P = 0.13 for the interaction between the two treatments). Arterial plaques shrank slightly in those assigned to simvastatin plus niacin, whereas they increased slightly in those who were also assigned to antioxidant therapy (P = 0.02 for the interaction). The worse outcomes in the antioxidant group were attributed to a smaller increase in HDL-2, an HDL subfraction thought to be especially cardioprotective.

Several issues must be considered when interpreting these findings. Because the sample size was small and because there are no known biologic mechanisms that can convincingly account for the observed interaction between antioxidants and lipid-modifying agents, these unexpected results could well be to the result of chance and thus require replication in larger studies. In addition, the study was limited to a specific population—that is, CHD patients with normal LDL but low HDL levels. Because this cholesterol pattern is more common among men than among women, few women were included in the sample. Thus, the applicability of these results to women is questionable. Finally, because simvastatin was administered in combination with niacin, it is not clear whether the blunting as a result of antioxidants, if it exists, is related to the statin or the niacin. Because statins are not known to increase HDL levels appreciably, the antioxidant blunting may be specific to niacin and may not occur in patients taking statins without niacin.

Indeed, no interaction between antioxidant and simvastatin therapy was found in the **Heart Protection Study (HPS)**, which used a 2×2 factorial design to test a daily antioxidant cocktail (600 mg of synthetic vitamin E, 250 mg of vitamin C, and 20 mg of β-carotene) and simvastatin (40 mg) among 20,536 men and women with CVD, diabetes, or, if male and age 65 or older, treated hypertension. Simvastatin appeared to be equally beneficial in reducing the risk of major cardiovascular events—a combined endpoint of nonfatal MI, CHD death, stroke, and revascularization—among individuals randomized to the antioxidant group and those who were not.[55] Main-effects analyses showed neither a beneficial nor a deleterious effect of the antioxidant cocktail on cardiovascular outcomes over 5 years of follow-up.[56]

β-Carotene

β-carotene supplementation has been less well studied in secondary prevention than in primary prevention settings. Although no data are yet available from randomized trials specifically designed to answer whether β-carotene supplementation alone (as opposed to in combination with other antioxidants) is effective in secondary prevention of CVD, subgroup analyses from the ATBC trial and PHS I allow an empiric examination of this issue. Table 28-5 lists completed and ongoing trials testing the efficacy of β-carotene alone or in combination with other antioxidants in the secondary prevention of CVD.

Among the 1862 men who entered the **ATBC trial** with a history of MI, β-carotene was associated with a reduction in subsequent risk of nonfatal MI (RR, 0.67; 95% CI, 0.44-1.02) but an increased risk of fatal CHD (RR, 1.75; 95% CI, 1.16-2.64) after 5.3 years of treatment.[50] A similar pattern of findings was observed for the combination of vitamin E and β-carotene, as noted earlier.

In **PHS I**, data from the 333 men with a history of chronic stable angina or a coronary revascularization procedure prior to randomization were analyzed.[57] Among those in the β-carotene group, a dramatic reduction (RR = 0.46; 95% CI, 0.24-0.85) in the risk of major cardiovascular events was observed after 5 years, and a persistent although attenuated reduction was also found after 12 years (RR = 0.71; 95% CI, 0.47-1.07). Of note, at 12 years, there was a similar divergence of findings between nonfatal and fatal cardiovascular events as in the ATBC trial—that is, β-carotene supplementation was associated with a reduced risk of nonfatal events (specifically, nonfatal MI [RR, 0.76; 95% CI, 0.36-1.60], nonfatal stroke [RR, 0.66; 95% CI, 0.28-1.58], and revascularization [RR, 0.66; 95% CI, 0.34–1.30]), but it was also associated with an increased risk of cardiovascular mortality (RR, 1.42; 95% CI, 0.72–2.80).

As discussed earlier, the **HATS** and **HPS** trials found no benefit of a daily antioxidant cocktail containing β-carotene at doses of 25 and 20 mg, respectively, in the secondary prevention of CVD.

Vitamin C

Vitamin C supplementation has not been adequately tested in secondary prevention trials. Vitamin C was included in the antioxidant cocktail administered in the **HATS** and **HPS** trials, both of which found that antioxidant supplementation did not reduce recurrent cardiovascular events.

Ongoing Trials

One large-scale secondary prevention trial is in progress. The **Women's Antioxidant Cardiovascular Study (WACS)** is a trial of natural vitamin E (600 IU on alternate days), β-carotene (50 mg on alternate days), and vitamin C (500 mg daily) in a factorial design that has randomized 8171 female health professionals with preexisting CVD or with several coronary risk factors.[58] The trial is scheduled to end in 2005. The factorial design of WACS—and of the PHS II in primary prevention—will allow for an exploration of possible interactions between various antioxidants. In recent years, a growing appreciation of the complex interrelationships between naturally occurring antioxidant networks, with their highly specialized arrangement of recycling and sparing capabilities within specific cell components,[59] has led some researchers to suggest that supplementing high-risk individuals with high doses of one antioxidant without concurrent administration of complementary antioxidants could in fact be deleterious. It has been proposed that such supplementation could promote rather than reduce lipid peroxidation.[60] For example, when functioning as an antioxidant, vitamin E is itself oxidized to harmful α-tocopheroxyl radicals; vitamin C reduces these radicals back to α-tocopherol.[61] In the recent **Antioxidant Supplementation in Atherosclerosis Prevention (ASAP) trial**, 3 years of supplementation with both vitamin E (136 IU twice per day) and vitamin C (250 mg twice per day), but not with either vitamin alone, significantly slowed the progression of common carotid atherosclerosis among 256 middle-aged Finnish men, a finding that may imply benefits with regard to subsequent cardiovascular events.[60] Supplementation with a combination of vitamin E (400 IU twice per day) and vitamin C (500 mg twice per day) has also been shown to reduce the early progression of transplant-associated coronary arteriosclerosis in a small trial of 40 cardiac-transplant recipients, most of whom were men.[62]

However, studies of postmenopausal women to date have not found cardiovascular benefits for antioxidant combinations. Among the 264 postmenopausal women participating in the ASAP trial, no protective effect of the vitamin E–vitamin C combination was observed.[60] In the **Women's Angiographic Vitamin and Estrogen (WAVE) trial**, a combination of vitamin E (400 IU twice per day) and vitamin C (500 mg twice per day) did not retard the progression of coronary atherosclerosis over a 2.8-year follow-up among 423 postmenopausal women.[63]

CONCLUSIONS

Basic research findings strongly suggest that oxidative stress may play an important role in the development of atherosclerotic disease and that antioxidant vitamins may delay or prevent various steps in atherogenesis. Human observational data are compatible with the possibility that antioxidant intake either from foods or supplements may reduce the risk of CVD. However, neither basic laboratory nor human observational research has yielded conclusive evidence. Results from such studies, however, together with the increasingly widespread use of antioxidant supplements despite lack of documented benefit, have provided the impetus to conduct large-scale trials of antioxidant supplements.

Clinical trials in primary prevention settings raise the possibility that some of the cardiovascular benefits of antioxidant vitamins reported by observational epidemiologic studies may have been overestimates. Methodologic limitations in available primary prevention studies preclude a definite conclusion regarding the cardioprotective potential of vitamin E. The doses of vitamin E used in the ATBC and the Chinese Cancer Prevention Trials may have been too low for cardioprotection, and the PPP, which used a higher dose of vitamin E, was terminated prematurely. There appears to be no overall benefit for β-carotene in the primary prevention of CVD among well-nourished Western populations. Whether there is a risk reduction among individuals with very low baseline blood levels of β-carotene or when β-carotene is administered in combination with other micronutrients remains unclear, however. To date, the Chinese Cancer Prevention Trial is the only completed large trial of vitamin C in primary prevention; it found no effect on cerebrovascular mortality but did not have adequate power to analyze coronary artery disease outcomes. Several large primary prevention trials are ongoing and may yet show benefit for one or more of these antioxidant vitamins.

Secondary prevention trials have tended to show minimal benefit from vitamin E supplementation. The promising findings of the seminal CHAOS trial have generally not been confirmed in subsequent large trials. However, it is possible that vitamin E supplementation may benefit certain groups at high risk for future cardiovascular events, such as patients undergoing hemodialysis. The CHAOS and SPACE results suggested that vitamin E supplementation reduces risks of nonfatal MI and other selected cardiovascular endpoints, although an elevated cardiovascular mortality rate was also observed in the CHAOS trial. Both trials had follow-up periods averaging less than 2 years, however, and it is surprising that a risk reduction was observed in such a short time. Conversely, if there is risk from vitamin E supplementation, then this may more clearly emerge in trials of longer duration. Yet the longer-term (and larger) GISSI, HOPE, and HPS trials found neither cardiovascular benefit nor harm associated with vitamin E

■■■

TABLE 28-6　DIETARY REFERENCE INTAKES FOR ADULTS AGED 19 YEARS AND OLDER*

	VITAMIN A[†]		VITAMIN C		VITAMIN E, AS α-TOCOPHEROL	
	RDA	UL	RDA	UL	RDA	UL
Men	900 μg/day	3000 μg/day	90 mg/day	2000 mg/day	15 mg/day	1000 mg/day
Women	700 μg/day	3000 μg/day	75 mg/day	2000 mg/day	15 mg/day	1000 mg/day
During pregnancy	770 μg/day	3000 μg/day	85 mg/day	2000 mg/day	15 mg/day	1000 mg/day
During lactation	1300 μg/day	3000 μg/day	120 mg/day	2000 mg/day	19 mg/day	1000 mg/day

*Recommended Dietary Allowances (RDAs) are set to meet the needs of almost all (97% to 98%) individuals in the stated group. Tolerable Upper Intake Level (UL) is the maximum level of daily intake that is likely to pose no risk of adverse effects.
[†]Includes provitamin A carotenoids such as β-carotene that are dietary precursors of retinol.
(Adapted from Institute of Medicine. Dietary Reference Intakes for Vitamin C, Vitamin E, Selenium, and Carotenoids. Washington DC: National Academy Press, 2000.)

supplementation. Additional data from randomized trials of sufficient sample size, dose, and duration of treatment and follow-up are needed to resolve the question of whether the long-term effects of antioxidant supplementation in secondary prevention are favorable, unfavorable, or neither.

No randomized trial has addressed whether antioxidant vitamins from natural food sources are cardioprotective. Dietary vitamin E is a mixture of tocopherols and tocotrienols, whereas vitamin E supplements generally contain only α-tocopherol. It has been suggested that the absence of other tocopherols, particularly γ-tocopherol, may explain some of the disappointing trial results.[64-66] Thus, a cardioprotective role for dietary vitamin E or for alternative formulations of vitamin E supplements cannot be eliminated. Similar issues have been raised regarding β-carotene. β-carotene is only one of some 600 carotenoids, and it may be that a collection of carotenoids is required for cardiovascular health. Moreover, there may be differences between *cis* and *trans* isomers with respect to bioavailability or bioconversion; however, the impact this might have on efficacy is unclear.[67]

RECOMMENDATIONS

According to the American Heart Association (AHA), there are insufficient efficacy and safety data from completed randomized trials to justify the establishment of populationwide recommendations regarding the use of vitamin E supplements for disease prevention.[68] Similarly, the AHA discourages the use of β-carotene supplements.[69] Instead, the AHA's dietary guidelines recommend a balanced diet with an emphasis on antioxidant-rich fruits and vegetables and whole grains.[69] Such foods are likely to provide a wide range of nutritional benefits beyond any potential antioxidant effects. In 2002, the influential Institute of Medicine (IOM) concurred with this recommendation and concluded that available empiric evidence indicates that the relationship between vitamin E supplement use and CHD prevention is "uncertain."[70]

The IOM has issued a comprehensive set of dietary standards known as Dietary Reference Intakes.[70,71] The new standards provide recommended dietary allowances (RDA) and designate tolerable upper intake levels (UL) for various nutrients. Table 28-6 lists the RDA and UL for the antioxidant vitamins reviewed in this chapter.

Even if future clinical trials demonstrate that antioxidant vitamin supplements reduce the risks of CVD, the use of such supplements should be considered an adjunct, not an alternative, to other established cardioprotective measures, such as smoking abstention, avoidance of obesity, adequate physical activity, and control of high blood pressure and dyslipidemia.

REFERENCES

1. Knekt P, Reunanen A, Jarvinen R, et al: Antioxidant vitamin intake and coronary mortality in a longitudinal population study. Am J Epidemiol 1994; 139:1180-1189.
2. Liu S, Manson JE, Lee IM, et al: Fruit and vegetable intake and risk of cardiovascular disease: The Women's Health Study. Am J Clin Nutr 2000; 72:922-928.
3. Joshipura KJ, Hu FB, Manson JE, et al: The effect of fruit and vegetable intake on risk for coronary heart disease. Ann Intern Med 2001; 134:1106-1114.
4. Bazzano LA, He J, Ogden LG, et al: Fruit and vegetable intake and risk of cardiovascular disease in US adults: The first National Health and Nutrition Examination Survey Epidemiologic Follow-up Study. Am J Clin Nutr 2002; 76:93-99.
5. Gillman MW, Cupples LA, Gagnon D, et al: Protective effect of fruits and vegetables on development of stroke in men. JAMA 1995; 273:1113-1117.
6. Joshipura KJ, Ascherio A, Manson JE, et al: Fruit and vegetable intake in relation to risk of ischemic stroke. JAMA 1999; 282:1233-1239.
7. Steinberg D, Parthasarathy S, Carew TE, et al: Beyond cholesterol. Modifications of low-density lipoprotein that increase its atherogenicity. N Engl J Med 1989; 320:915-924.
8. Hessler JR, Morel DW, Lewis LJ, et al: Lipoprotein oxidation and lipoprotein-induced cytotoxicity. Arteriosclerosis 1983; 3:215-222.
9. Yagi K: Increased serum lipid peroxides initiate atherogenesis. Bioessays 1984; 1:58-60.
10. Quinn MT, Parthasarathy S, Steinberg D: Endothelial cell-derived chemotactic activity for mouse peritoneal macrophages and the effects of modified forms of low density lipoprotein. Proc Natl Acad Sci USA 1985; 82:5949-5953.
11. Schaffner T, Taylor K, Bartucci EJ, et al: Arterial foam cells with distinctive immunomorphologic and histochemical features of macrophages. Am J Pathol 1980; 100:57-80.
12. Gerrity RG: The role of the monocyte in atherogenesis: I. Transition of blood-borne monocytes into foam cells in fatty lesions. Am J Pathol 1981; 103:181-190.
13. Fogelman AM, Shechter I, Seager J, et al: Malondialdehyde alteration of low density lipoproteins leads to cholesteryl ester accumulation in human monocyte-macrophages. Proc Natl Acad Sci USA 1980; 77:2214-2218.
14. Goldstein JL, Ho YK, Basu SK, et al: Binding site on macrophages that mediates uptake and degradation of acetylated low density lipoprotein, producing massive cholesterol deposition. Proc Natl Acad Sci USA 1979; 76:333-337.
15. Salonen JT, Yla-Herttuala S, Yamamoto R, et al: Autoantibody against oxidised LDL and progression of carotid atherosclerosis. Lancet 1992; 339:883-887.
16. Beckman JS, Beckman TW, Chen J, et al: Apparent hydroxyl radical production by peroxynitrite: Implications for endothelial injury from nitric oxide and superoxide. Proc Natl Acad Sci USA 1990; 87:1620-1624.

17. Marcus AJ, Silk ST, Safier LB, et al: Superoxide production and reducing activity in human platelets. J Clin Invest 1977; 59:149-158.

18. Saran M, Michel C, Bors W: Reaction of NO with O₂: Implications for the action of endothelium-derived relaxing factor (EDRF). Free Radic Res Commun 1990; 10:221-226.

19. Gaziano JM, Steinberg D: Natural antioxidants. *In* Manson JE, Ridker PM, Gaziano JM, et al (eds). Prevention of myocardial infarction. New York, Oxford University Press, 1996:321-350.

20. Albert CM, Manson JE: Aspirin, antioxidants, and alcohol. In Charney P, ed. Coronary artery disease in women. Philadelphia, American College of Physicians, 1999:236-263.

21. Stampfer MJ, Hennekens CH, Manson JE, et al: Vitamin E consumption and the risk of coronary disease in women. N Engl J Med 1993; 328:1444-1449.

22. Rimm EB, Stampfer MJ, Ascherio A, et al: Vitamin E consumption and the risk of coronary heart disease in men. N Engl J Med 1993; 328:1450-1456.

23. Kushi LH, Fee RM, Sellers TA, et al: Intake of vitamins A, C, and E and postmenopausal breast cancer: The Iowa Women's Health Study. Am J Epidemiol 1996; 144:165-174.

24. Losonczy KG, Harris TB, Havlik RJ: Vitamin E and vitamin C supplement use and risk of all-cause and coronary heart disease mortality in older persons: The Established Populations for Epidemiologic Studies of the Elderly. Am J Clin Nutr 1996; 64: 190-196.

25. Klipstein-Grobusch K, Geleijnse JM, den Breeijen JH, et al: Dietary antioxidants and risk of myocardial infarction in the elderly: The Rotterdam Study. Am J Clin Nutr 1999; 69:261-266.

26. Evans RW, Shaten BJ, Day BW, et al: Prospective association between lipid soluble antioxidants and coronary heart disease in men: The Multiple Risk Factor Intervention Trial. Am J Epidemiol 1998; 147:180-186.

27. Industry works to size up growing nutraceutical market. The Food and Drug Letter 2002; 649.

28. Steinberg D: Antioxidants in the prevention of human atherosclerosis: Summary of the proceedings of a National Heart, Lung, and Blood Institute Workshop: September 5-6, 1991, Bethesda, Maryland. Circulation 1992; 85:2337-2344.

29. Blot WJ, Li JY, Taylor PR, et al: Nutrition intervention trials in Linxian, China: Supplementation with specific vitamin/mineral combinations, cancer incidence, and disease-specific mortality in the general population. J Natl Cancer Inst 1993; 85: 1483-1492.

30. Alpha-Tocopherol Beta Carotene Cancer Prevention Study Group: The effect of vitamin E and beta carotene on the incidence of lung cancer and other cancers in male smokers. The Alpha-Tocopherol, Beta Carotene Cancer Prevention Study Group. N Engl J Med 1994; 330:1029-1035.

31. Omenn GS, Goodman GE, Thornquist MD, et al: Effects of a combination of beta carotene and vitamin A on lung cancer and cardiovascular disease. N Engl J Med 1996; 334:1150-1155.

32. Esterbauer H, Gebicki J, Puhl H, et al: The role of lipid peroxidation and antioxidants in oxidative modification of LDL. Free Radic Biol Med 1992; 13:341-390.

33. Rapola JM, Virtamo J, Haukka JK, et al: Effect of vitamin E and beta carotene on the incidence of angina pectoris: A randomized, double-blind, controlled trial. JAMA 1996; 275:693-698.

34. de Gaetano G: Low-dose aspirin and vitamin E in people at cardiovascular risk: A randomised trial in general practice: Collaborative Group of the Primary Prevention Project. Lancet 2001; 357: 89-95.

35. Greenberg ER, Baron JA, Karagas MR, et al: Mortality associated with low plasma concentration of beta carotene and the effect of oral supplementation. JAMA 1996; 275:699-703.

36. Hennekens CH, Buring JE, Manson JE, et al: Lack of effect of long-term supplementation with beta carotene on the incidence of malignant neoplasms and cardiovascular disease. N Engl J Med 1996; 334:1145-1149.

37. Lee IM, Cook NR, Manson JE, et al: Beta-carotene supplementation and incidence of cancer and cardiovascular disease: The Women's Health Study. J Natl Cancer Inst 1999; 91:2102-2106.

38. Buring JE, Hennekens CH: The Women's Health Study: summary of the study design. J Myocardial Ischemia 1992; 4:27-29.

39. Christen WG, Gaziano JM, Hennekens CH: Design of Physicians' Health Study II: A randomized trial of beta-carotene, vitamins E and C, and multivitamins, in prevention of cancer, cardiovascular disease, and eye disease, and review of results of completed trials. Ann Epidemiol 2000; 10:125-134.

40. Hercberg S, Preziosi P, Briancon S, et al: A primary prevention trial using nutritional doses of antioxidant vitamins and minerals in cardiovascular diseases and cancers in a general population: The SU.VI.MAX study—Design, methods, and participant characteristics. SUpplémentation en VItamines et Minéraux AntioXydants. Control Clin Trials 1998; 19:336-351.

41. DeMaio SJ, King SB, 3rd, Lembo NJ, et al: Vitamin E supplementation, plasma lipids and incidence of restenosis after percutaneous transluminal coronary angioplasty (PTCA). J Am Coll Nutr 1992; 11:68-73.

42. Williams HT, Fenna D, Macbeth RA: Alpha tocopherol in the treatment of intermittent claudication. Surg Gynecol Obstet 1971; 132:662-666.

43. Haeger K: Long-time treatment of intermittent claudication with vitamin E. Am J Clin Nutr 1974; 27:1179-1181.

44. Leng GC, Lee AJ, Fowkes FG, et al: Randomized controlled trial of antioxidants in intermittent claudication. Vasc Med 1997; 2: 279-285.

45. Tornwall M, Virtamo J, Haukka JK, et al: Effect of alpha-tocopherol (vitamin E) and beta-carotene supplementation on the incidence of intermittent claudication in male smokers. Arterioscler Thromb Vasc Biol 1997; 17:3475-3480.

46. Anderson TW, Reid DB: A double-blind trial of vitamin E in angina pectoris. Am J Clin Nutr 1974; 27:1174-1178.

47. Gillilan RE, Mondell B, Warbasse JR: Quantitative evaluation of vitamin E in the treatment of angina pectoris. Am Heart J 1977; 93:444-449.

48. Rapola JM, Virtamo J, Ripatti S, et al: Effects of alpha tocopherol and beta carotene supplements on symptoms, progression, and prognosis of angina pectoris. Heart 1998; 79:454-8.

49. Stephens NG, Parsons A, Schofield PM, et al: Randomised controlled trial of vitamin E in patients with coronary disease: Cambridge Heart Antioxidant Study (CHAOS). Lancet 1996; 347:781-786.

50. Rapola JM, Virtamo J, Ripatti JK, et al: Randomized trial of α-tocopherol and β-carotene supplements on incidence of major coronary events in men with previous myocardial infarction. Lancet 1997; 349:1715-1720.

51. GISSI-Prevenzione Investigators: Dietary supplementation with n-3 polyunsaturated fatty acids and vitamin E after myocardial infarction: Results of the GISSI-Prevenzione trial. Gruppo Italiano per lo Studio della Sopravvivenza nell'Infarto miocardico. Lancet 1999; 354:447-55.

52. Yusuf S, Dagenais G, Pogue J, et al: Vitamin E supplementation and cardiovascular events in high-risk patients: The Heart Outcomes Prevention Evaluation Study Investigators. N Engl J Med 2000; 342:154-160.

53. Boaz M, Smetana S, Weinstein T, et al: Secondary prevention with antioxidants of cardiovascular disease in endstage renal disease (SPACE): Randomised placebo-controlled trial. Lancet 2000; 356:1213-1218.

54. Brown BG, Zhao XQ, Chait A, et al: Simvastatin and niacin, antioxidant vitamins, or the combination for the prevention of coronary disease. N Engl J Med 2001; 345:1583-1592.

55. Heart Protection Study Collaborative Group: MRC/BHF Heart Protection Study of cholesterol lowering with simvastatin in 20,536 high-risk individuals: A randomised placebo-controlled trial. Lancet 2002; 360:7-22.

56. Heart Protection Study Collaborative Group: MRC/BHF Heart Protection Study of antioxidant vitamin supplementation in 20,536 high-risk individuals: A randomised placebo-controlled trial. Lancet 2002; 360:23-33.

57. Gaziano JM, Manson JE, Ridker PM, Buring JE, Hennekens CH. Beta carotene therapy for chronic stable angina [abstract]. Circulation 1990; 82:III-202.

58. Manson JE, Gaziano JM, Spelsberg A, et al: A secondary prevention trial of antioxidant vitamins and cardiovascular disease in women: Rationale, design, and methods: The WACS Research Group. Ann Epidemiol 1995; 5:261-269.

59. Upston JM, Terentis AC, Stocker R: Tocopherol-mediated peroxidation of lipoproteins: Implications for vitamin E as a potential antiatherogenic supplement. 1999; 13:977-994.

60. Salonen JT, Nyyssonen K, Salonen R, et al: Antioxidant Supplementation in Atherosclerosis Prevention (ASAP) study: A randomized trial of the effect of vitamins E and C on 3-year progression of carotid atherosclerosis. J Intern Med 2000; 248:377-386.

61. Packer JE, Slater TF, Willson RL: Direct observation of a free radical interaction between vitamin E and vitamin C. Nature 1979; 278: 737-738.

62. Fang JC, Kinlay S, Beltrame J, et al: Effect of vitamins C and E on progression of transplant-associated arteriosclerosis: A randomised trial. Lancet 2002; 359:1108-1113.

63. Waters DD, Alderman EL, Hsia J, et al: Effects of hormone replacement therapy and antioxidant vitamin supplements on coronary atherosclerosis in postmenopausal women: A randomized controlled trial. JAMA 2002; 288:2432-2440.

64. Jiang Q, Christen S, Shigenaga MK, et al: gamma-tocopherol, the major form of vitamin E in the US diet, deserves more attention. Am J Clin Nutr 2001; 74:714-722.

65. Liu M, Wallmon A, Olsson-Mortlock C, et al: Mixed tocopherols inhibit platelet aggregation in humans: Potential mechanisms. Am J Clin Nutr 2003; 77:700-706.

66. Devaraj S, Traber MG: Gamma-tocopherol, the new vitamin E? Am J Clin Nutr 2003; 77:530-531.

67. Patrick L: Beta-carotene: The controversy continues. Altern Med Rev 2000; 5:530-545.

68. Tribble DL: AHA Science Advisory. Antioxidant consumption and risk of coronary heart disease: emphasis on vitamin C, vitamin E, and beta-carotene: A statement for healthcare professionals from the American Heart Association. Circulation 1999; 99:591-595.

69. Krauss RM, Eckel RH, Howard B, et al: AHA Dietary Guidelines: Revision 2000: A statement for healthcare professionals from the Nutrition Committee of the American Heart Association. Circulation 2000; 102:2284-2299.

70. Institute of Medicine: Evolution of evidence for selected nutrient and disease relationships. Washington, DC: National Academy Press, 2002.

71. Institute of Medicine: Dietary reference intakes for vitamin C, vitamin E, selenium, and carotenoids. Washington DC: National Academy Press, 2000.

■ ■ ■ c h a p t e r **29**

Dietary Factors

Frank M. Sacks

Definitive trials using 3-hydroxy-3-methylglutaryl coenzyme A reductase inhibitors to lower blood low-density lipoprotein (LDL) cholesterol have now proved the LDL theory of coronary heart disease (CHD).[1-4] The causal relationship between LDL levels and CHD had been supported strongly by a consistent body of evidence from observational epidemiologic studies,[5-8] trials that used coronary angiography to assess change in atherosclerosis,[9] and early clinical trials that used treatments that had less effect on LDL cholesterol than the reductase inhibitors.[10] Lowering LDL cholesterol reduces coronary events in populations with or without clinical CHD and in populations with hypercholesterolemia or high-risk patients with average or below-average cholesterol levels.[1-4] For every 40 mg/dL drop in LDL cholesterol, coronary incidence decreases by 25%.[1-4] Clearly, average blood cholesterol level in Western societies is too high[11,12] and is likely to cause coronary events. Because most adults could conceivably benefit from a lower cholesterol level, the importance of nonpharmacologic approaches is great. This chapter reviews the considerable body of evidence that dietary modification can prevent CHD.

National health organizations advocate dietary changes that decrease intake of saturated fat and cholesterol to prevent CHD.[13] A point of controversy concerns the nutrient that should replace the energy provided by saturated fat—that is, either carbohydrate or unsaturated oils.[14] Moreover, the *trans*-unsaturated fatty acids, produced during the industrial hydrogenation of vegetable oil to make shortenings and margarine, have been shown to have adverse effects on serum lipid levels and to be associated with CHD. The relationship between dietary fat and serum lipoprotein levels is central to understanding the link between diet and CHD and to evaluate different dietary approaches.

In addition to the dietary fats, evidence from epidemiologic studies and clinical trials suggests that dietary factors other than fats may protect against CHD. These include antioxidant vitamins (discussed in Chapter 28), folic acid, and vitamin B_6. The possible role of these nutrients in dietary therapy is discussed.

DIETARY FAT AND SERUM LIPOPROTEIN CONCENTRATIONS

Thirty years ago, experiments conducted on metabolic wards established that intake of saturated fatty acids having 12, 14, or 16 carbon atoms (lauric, myristic, and palmitic acids, respectively) raised serum total cholesterol levels.[15,16] Myristic and palmitic acids are the most common saturated fatty acids in Western diets; lauric acid is the major fatty acid in coconut and palm kernel oils. More recent studies confirmed that these saturated fatty acids raised LDL cholesterol levels; descending order of potency is myristic, lauric, and palmitic.[17] Meta-analysis of controlled dietary trials demonstrated that the average effect of replacing 10% of energy from saturated fat by either carbohydrate or monounsaturated or polyunsaturated fat in groups of persons is a decrease in LDL of 13 mg/dL, 15 mg/dL, or 18 mg/dL, respectively.[17] Therefore, exchanging any of these nutrients for saturated fat lowers LDL cholesterol levels. Monounsaturated and particularly polyunsaturated fatty acids accentuate this effect compared with carbohydrate.

In contrast to their differential effects on LDL, all three major classes of fatty acids raise high-density lipoprotein (HDL) levels compared with carbohydrate, with saturated fat having the most and polyunsaturated fat having the least effect.[17] HDL is well established as an independent protective factor for coronary disease worthy for consideration as a therapeutic target.[18] In clinical trials of drug therapy, increases in HDL have been correlated with reductions in coronary events[19,20] or with decreases in coronary stenosis.[21] The ratio of total cholesterol to HDL cholesterol concentrations is often used as a summary measure of blood lipid changes to estimate change in risk of CHD.[22,23] The ratio shows little change when saturated fat is replaced with carbohydrate because the percentage decreases in total cholesterol and HDL are about the same; however, the ratio is improved with monounsaturated or polyunsaturated fat, which lowers LDL and very-low-density lipoprotein (VLDL) more than HDL.[17]

Plasma triglycerides are an independent risk factor for coronary disease when measured in the fasting[24-27] or nonfasting states.[28] Carbohydrate increases fasting triglyceride levels when it replaces any type of fat.[17] A meal with mainly carbohydrate, compared with monounsaturated fat, increases postprandial triglyceride levels.[29-30] However, carbohydrate foods such as whole grains and vegetables that are slowly digested and absorbed have little or no hypertriglyceridemic effect.[31]

Examples of changes in dietary intake with a high-carbohydrate/low-fat diet compared with a high-unsaturated-fat diet are shown in Table 29-1. In the first instance, a relatively high total fat intake, 38%, is reduced to 25% solely by decreasing saturated fat and increasing carbohydrate. In the other instance, saturated fat is decreased by replacing it with primarily monounsaturated but also polyunsaturated fats, resulting in a diet similar to that eaten traditionally in Greece.[32] The dietary cholesterol intake is reduced similarly in both diets. Changes in intake of types of foods are shown in Table 29-2. The predicted percentage changes in blood lipids are calculated in a patient with mild combined hyperlipidemia who is at high risk for coronary events (Fig. 29-1). Both diets reduce LDL by similar amounts, 17% to 21%. However, the low-fat diet would reduce HDL by 18% compared with 6% with the high-unsaturated-fat diet. The total cholesterol-to-HDL ratio would increase by 5% on the low-fat diet compared with a decrease of 9% with the high-unsaturated-fat diet. Moreover, the low-fat diet would increase fasting triglycerides by 17%

TABLE 29-1 EXAMPLES OF TWO DIETARY APPROACHES TO LOWER BLOOD CHOLESTEROL LEVELS

	Low-fat/high-carbohydrate diet (NCEP step 2*)	High-unsaturated-fat diet (Mediterranean)
Total fat	38% → 25%	38% → 38%
Saturated fat	20% → 6%	20% → 6%
Monounsaturated	11% → 12%	11% → 22%
Polyunsaturated	7% → 7%	7% →10%
Carbohydrate	42% → 55%	42% → 42%
Cholesterol	400 mg → 100 mg	400 mg → 100 mg

*NCEP Step 2 recommends total fat ≤30%, saturated fat <7%, carbohydrate ≥55%, and cholesterol intake <200 mg/day.
NCEP, National Cholesterol Education Program

TABLE 29-2 CHANGES IN FOODS TO ACHIEVE NUTRITIONAL GOALS TO PREVENT CARDIOVASCULAR DISEASE

Increase	Decrease
Vegetables	Animal fats
Fruits	Hydrogenated vegetable oils (*trans*-fatty acids)
Whole grains	Sugar
Fish	Refined (low-fiber) cereal grains
Nuts	Red meat
Low-fat dairy foods	

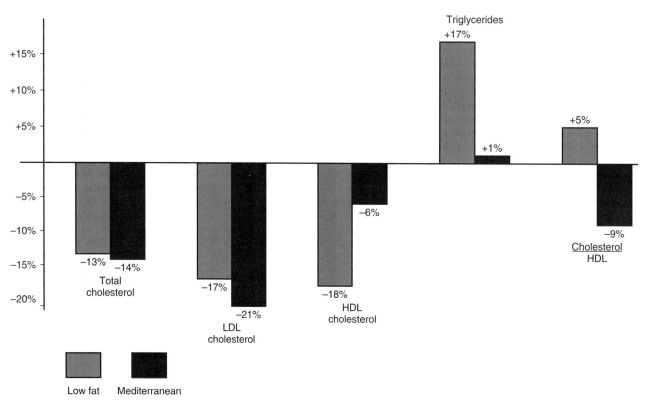

FIGURE 29-1. Changes in blood lipids with low-fat or Mediterranean diets. Dietary composition shown in Table 29-1.

compared with 1% on the high-unsaturated-fat diet, unless the carbohydrate was not from sugar or refined grains but from vegetables and whole grains. Such decreases in HDL and increases in triglycerides with the low-fat diet raise questions about the eventual effects on risk of CHD.[14]

The effects of *trans*-unsaturated fatty acids (*trans*-fatty acids) on lipoproteins and CHD need to be considered separately from the natural *cis*-unsaturated oils. Oils from plants have double bonds between carbon atoms that are exclusively in the *cis* orientation, and their effects have been discussed earlier. *Trans*-fatty acids are produced during industrial hydrogenation of vegetable oil in the manufacturing of vegetable shortening and margarine. The hydrogenation process uses high temperature, metallic catalysts, and hydrogen gas to reduce the double bonds between carbon atoms to single bonds; a by-product of this process is the isomerization of *cis* to *trans* double bonds. *Trans*-fatty acids have a higher melting point than *cis*-isomers and contribute to solidity of these products. Hydrogenation does not occur during cooking with vegetable oil. *Trans*-fatty acids are also produced by bacteria in the gut of ruminant animals and are found in red meat and dairy fat. Many careful dietary studies have shown that intake of *trans*-fatty acids has several harmful effects on plasma lipoprotein concentrations: LDL increases; HDL decreases; and lipoprotein(a), a potentially atherogenic lipoprotein, also increases.[33,34] These adverse effects on plasma lipoproteins may explain why epidemiologic studies found an association between intake of *trans*-fatty acids and incidence of CHD.[35-37] Although a clinical endpoint trial has not, and probably never will be, conducted that alters *trans*-fatty acids as a single nutrient, the evidence for harmful effects is strong and should lead to avoidance of foods that contain hydrogenated oils. Food labeling now separately lists the *trans*-fatty acids, also the term *partially hydrogenated* in the list of ingredients indicates that *trans*-fatty acids are present. In the United States, they are ubiquitous in baked goods.

CONTROLLED TRIALS OF DIETARY THERAPY AND CORONARY EVENTS

Controlled dietary trials show a clear pattern of benefit in relation to CHD events. For this analysis, I have considered randomized dietary trials with at least 2 years of average follow-up[38-43] because, in cholesterol-lowering therapy, 2 years appears to be the average duration before the treatment group begins to show a reduction in coronary events.[44] The Indian Heart Study,[45,46] a controlled dietary trial with several unique aspects, is discussed separately. Multifactorial intervention programs are also considered separately because it is impossible to distinguish the effect of the diet from that of the other treatments. Two dietary approaches have been tested: one to lower total and saturated fat[38,39] and the other to replace saturated with unsaturated fats, leaving total fat unchanged.[40-43] The high-unsaturated-fat diets were more successful than the low-fat diets in lowering serum

■ ■ ■

TABLE 29-3 CLINICAL TRIALS OF DIET THERAPY TO LOWER BLOOD CHOLESTEROL LEVELS AND REDUCE CORONARY EVENTS

Trials[†]	N	Dietary fat (% energy)	Duration (yr)	ΔCholesterol (%)	ΔCHD (%)
Reduction in Total Fat					
MRC[38]	123	22	3	−5	+4
DART[39]	1015	"low fat"	2	−3.5	−9
Substitution of Unsaturated Fat for Saturated Fat					
Turpeinen[42]	676	34	6	−15*	−43*
Leren[43]	206	39	5	−14*	−25*
MRC soy oil[41]	194	46	4	−15*	−14
Dayton[40]	424	40	8	−13*	−23*

*$P < 0.05$.
†Trials with at least 2 years of average follow-up were included.
ΔCholesterol refers to the percentage change in serum cholesterol in the treatment group compared with the change in the control group. ΔCHD refers to the percentage difference in coronary event rates in the treatment group compared with the control group.

cholesterol (mean 14% vs. 4%) and in lowering CHD (Table 29-3). Reduction in CHD in the high-unsaturated-fat diets averaged 21% and ranged from 14% to 43%, as opposed to −9% to +4% in the low-fat diet trials. Because, theoretically, the two types of diets should lower serum total cholesterol levels to a similar extent,[17] one must conclude that adherence to the low-fat diet was poorer than for the high-unsaturated-fat diets. To summarize, coronary events decreased significantly in all trials in which the diet lowered plasma total cholesterol by at least 10% (see Table 29-3). Overall, in these trials of patients with hypercholesterolemia, the mean reductions in coronary events in the trials of unsaturated fat diets[40-43] averaged 21% and compare favorably with that achieved with nicotinic acid[47] or cholestyramine,[19] but the magnitude of effect was less than that observed for pravastatin[1,4] or simvastatin.[2,3]

In the St. Thomas Atherosclerosis Regression Study (STARS), coronary arteriography was used to measure the luminal diameter or luminal obstruction of diseased coronary arteries, as the primary study endpoints, in a trial that compared dietary therapy with or without cholestyramine[48] (Table 29-4). The diet was designed to lower total and saturated fat and increase unsaturated oils and vegetables and fruits. LDL significantly decreased by 16%, but contrary to expectation,[17] HDL did not decrease, and triglycerides actually decreased rather than increased. Because the patients did not lose weight, it seems likely that saturated fat was replaced more by unsaturated oils than by carbohydrate; the specific dietary changes made by the patients were not reported. Relative to the control group, the dietary groups with or without cholestyramine both showed significant improvement in coronary stenosis, and there was little difference between the two treatments. One could speculate that the beneficial effects on coronary stenosis of the decrease in LDL caused by cholestyramine were counterbalanced by the increase in triglyceride levels relative to the diet-only group. In this trial, the improvement in coronary stenosis with diet alone was greater than in other angiographic studies of

■■ ■

TABLE 29-4   EFFECTIVENESS OF DIET THERAPY ON CORONARY STENOSIS IN MEN WITH COMBINED HYPERLIPIDEMIA: THE ST. THOMAS ATHEROSCLEROSIS REGRESSION STUDY (STARS)[48]

	Control (%)	Diet (%)	Diet + cholestyramine (%)
Change in Blood Lipids			
Total cholesterol	−2	−14*	−25*
LDL cholesterol	−3	−16*	−36*
HDL cholesterol	−1	0	−4
Triglycerides	+1	−20*	0
Coronary Atherosclerosis			
Change in stenosis†	+6	−1*	−2*

*P < 0.05 compared with control.
†For change in stenosis, a positive sign indicates worsening and a negative sign indicates improvement.
LDL, low-density lipoprotein; HDL, high-density lipoprotein.

diet or drug therapy.[49] Again, the evidence supports the conclusion that effective diet therapy produces considerable benefit to coronary disease.

The Lyon Diet Heart Study,[50] a secondary prevention trial, tested the effects of a "Mediterranean" diet compared with a standard low-fat diet (Table 29-5). The specific dietary changes were substitution of animal fat with polyunsaturated vegetable oil rich in α-linolenic acid (ALA) and replacement of meat, butter, and cream with fish, legumes, bread, fruits, and vegetables. Total fat intake

did not change. Surprisingly, there were no changes in plasma lipid levels. Nonetheless, coronary events were reduced in the treatment group by 73%. Adherence to the diet was confirmed by increases in blood levels of oleic acid, the omega-3 fatty acids, ALA and eicosapentaenoic acid (EPA), and antioxidant vitamins. This trial suggests that aspects of the diet besides those that affect blood lipids can prevent coronary events. Which of these nutritional changes were responsible for the benefit cannot be determined.

FISH AND FISH OIL

A British trial tested the effects of three dietary therapies for 2 years in men with myocardial infarction (MI): reducing fat, eating high-fiber cereal, or increasing fatty fish consumption.[39] In these men who usually did not eat much fatty fish, only two fish meals per week significantly reduced total mortality by 29% (Fig. 29-2) and coronary mortality by 33%. In contrast, neither the reduced-fat nor the increased-fiber diets showed any tendency to produce benefit. These results have been much reinforced by GISSI (Gruppo Italiano per lo Studio della Sopravvivenza nell'Infarcto Miocardico) Prevenzione trial, a randomized controlled trial in 11,324 Italian patients surviving a recent MI.[51] Treatment with 1 gram per day of omega-3 polyunsaturated fatty acids from fish lowered the overall risk of death and of cardiovascular events. In both trials, the death rate began to lessen in the fish oil group as early as 3 months after treatment was started. As with the Lyon Heart Study[50]

■■ ■

TABLE 29-5   MEDITERRANEAN DIETARY APPROACH TO PREVENT DEATH AFTER MYOCARDIAL INFARCTION: THE LYON HEART STUDY[50]

Dietary Changes

Increased: fruits, vegetables, beans, bread, vegetable oil
Decreased: meats, butter, cream
Unchanged: total fat (31%)

Body Weight:

Decreased

Fatty Acid Changes

Increased: oleic, α-linolenic, ω-3 (EPA, DHA)
Decreased: linoleic, saturated
Unchanged: trans

Blood Levels

Increased: ascorbic acid, α-tocopherol, oleic acid, α-linolenic, EPA, DHA
Decreased: none
Unchanged: cholesterol, LDL, HDL, blood pressure, platelet aggregation

Coronary Events (*n*)

Control: 33/303
Experimental: 8/302
Change: −73% (P = 0.001)

EPA, eicosapentaenoic acid; DHA, docosahexaenoic acid; LDL, low-density lipoprotein; HDL, high-density lipoprotein.

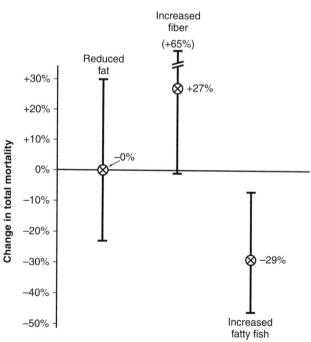

FIGURE 29-2. Effects of reduced fat, increased fiber, or increased fatty fish in the diet on mortality in British men.[39]

(see Table 29-5), these trials suggests that omega-3 fatty acids could be beneficial against CHD.

The omega-3 fatty acids that are found in fish, EPA and docosahexaenoic acid (DHA), have several effects that could contribute to reducing clinical coronary events. In relatively high amounts, 3 to 12 g daily, as in 200 to 800 g of fatty fish, they lower the plasma triglyceride concentration,[52] raise HDL_2 cholesterol concentration,[53] and lower blood pressure in patients with mild to moderate hypertension but not in patients with normal or high normal blood pressure.[53,54] Recent evidence is consistent with an antiarrhythmic action of omega-3 fatty acids. In dogs who had sustained experimental MI, intravenous infusion of omega-3 fatty acids raised the threshold for ischemia-induced ventricular fibrillation.[55] In a double-blind trial in patients who had ventricular premature complexes, fish oil supplementation using 16 mL of cod liver oil daily for 16 weeks reduced the daily incidence of such events.[56] In agreement with this hypothesis, a case-control study found that dietary intake of omega-3 fatty acids was very low in persons who experienced sudden death.[57] Perhaps this antiarrhythmic action could have contributed to the reduction in coronary death in the Lyon Heart Study,[50] in the Diet and Reinfarction Trial (DART),[39] and the GISSI trial,[51] all of which increased intake of omega-3 fatty acids in patients who had acute MI.

DIET AND EXERCISE

Diet and vigorous exercise therapy for 1 year improved coronary stenosis in angiographic trials (Table 29-6). In one trial, adherence was enhanced by providing the patients with all of their food, and yoga and stress management training were integral components.[58] Adherence to the entire program was correlated with improvement in stenosis. In the other trial, improvement in exercise capacity was the most significant variable that predicted improved stenosis.[59] Comparing the various diet and drug trials, the diet trials with or without

TABLE 29-6 DIETARY AND EXERCISE PROGRAMS TO IMPROVE CORONARY ATHEROSCLEROSIS

Trial	Lifestyle heart study (Ornish[58])	Schuler[59]
Location	San Francisco, USA	Heidelberg, Germany
Intervention	Low-fat, strict vegetarian diet Exercise Stress management, yoga	Low-fat diet Exercise
Duration	1 yr	1 yr
Blood Cholesterol*	−19	−10
Coronary Stenosis*,†	−5.6	−4

*Change in blood cholesterol level and coronary stenosis in treatment group compared with control group.
†For coronary stenosis, the change is expressed in percentage points of luminal narrowing. A negative sign indicates improvement.

exercise had a greater benefit on coronary stenosis than could be expected from the reductions in LDL cholesterol.[49] Thus it seems likely that nonpharmacologic therapy has benefits that are independent of effects on LDL concentration. However, long-term adherence and clinical outcomes in these rigorous programs need to be studied.

EARLY BENEFITS FROM PROMPT INITIATION OF DIET THERAPY AFTER MYOCARDIAL INFARCTION

Several studies enrolled patients soon after MI: 2 days,[45,46] 2 weeks,[50,60] and 6 weeks[39] (Table 29-7). Diet therapy was used in three of the trials,[39,45,50] whereas diet, exercise, and smoking cessation were used in one.[60] All demonstrated reduction in coronary death at the end of the trials, which ranged from 1 to 3 years in average duration. However, the striking finding in these trials was the early benefit. The curves of the event rates of the treated groups began

TABLE 29-7 EFFECT ON RECURRENT CORONARY EVENTS OF DIET AND OTHER NONPHARMACOLOGICAL THERAPY INITIATED EARLY AFTER MYOCARDIAL INFARCTION

Trial	N	Therapy	When started (post-MI)	Duration	CORONARY EVENTS Death (N)	CORONARY EVENTS Nonfatal MI (N)	Time to earliest discernible benefit*
WHO Finland[60]	375	Diet, exercise, no smoking	2 wk	3 yr	35 vs. 55‖	34 vs. 21	≤3 mo
DART[39]	1015	Fatty fish	6 wk	2 yr	78 vs. 116‖	49 vs. 33	<2 mo
Indian Heart Study[45,46]	406	Diet†	2 days	1 yr	21 vs. 38‖	29 vs. 44‖	12 wk§
Lyon Heart Study[50]	606	Mediterranean diet‡	2 wk	27 mo	3 vs. 6‖	5 vs. 17	<6 mo

*Earliest discernible benefit is defined as the point at which the event rate of the treatment group began to diverge from that of the control group, as estimated from Kaplan-Meier or survival curves.
†Increased fruits and vegetables, decreased saturated fat, cholesterol, and refined carbohydrate.
‡See Table 29.5 for description of diet.
§Significant reduction in coronary events by 12 weeks.
‖P <0.05.
MI, myocardial infarction.

diverging from the control groups within 2 to 3 months of randomization[39,45,60] or before 6 months.[50]

The Indian Heart Study[45,46] was unique in its population and intervention and in the demonstration of a significant reduction in coronary events after only 12 weeks of treatment. In this 1-year dietary trial in India,[45,46] patients during hospitalization with acute MI were taught to increase intake of vegetables, fruits, and whole grains and to decrease saturated fat and cholesterol. Unique to this trial, the patients were eating a low-fat, mainly vegetarian diet before treatment, and the total fat in both treatment groups was maintained at the customarily low level of 24% to 26%. Several coronary risk factors were significantly improved in the treatment group compared with the control group. Serum cholesterol decreased by 8%, body weight decreased by 4 kg, blood pressure decreased by 8 mm Hg systolic and 6 mm Hg diastolic, and fasting glucose level was reduced. Coronary death was reduced by 41% and nonfatal MI was reduced by 38% at the end of the trial. After 12 weeks, coronary events were reduced by 36% (P < 0.01).

The early benefit in these trials that started dietary therapy soon after MI contrasts with a generally longer duration of latency, 2 years on average, in secondary prevention trials in which therapy is started later after MI or in most primary prevention trials.[44] This analysis suggests that timing of diet therapy after MI is important to produce early benefit.

DIETARY FACTORS THAT COULD BE PROTECTIVE AGAINST CORONARY HEART DISEASE

The diets that were used in CHD prevention trials usually made changes in many nutrients that could have been responsible for the reduction in CHD. Reduction in saturated fat and cholesterol lowers LDL-cholesterol concentrations, and this has the most well-established relationship to coronary events. Increases in omega-3 fatty acids either from vegetable oils or fish oils favorably affect lipoproteins, blood pressure, and the threshold for ventricular arrhythmia. Intake of fruits and vegetables is often increased in diets to prevent CHD, which increases antioxidant vitamins, folic acid, vitamin B_6, and fiber that are associated with a lower CHD event rate in epidemiologic studies. Dietary antioxidants are discussed in Chapter 28.

Plasma homocysteine concentration is a risk factor for CHD.[61,62] Folic acid, vitamin B_6, and vitamin B_{12} are cofactors for enzymes that convert homocysteine to methionine, thereby lowering plasma concentrations. Elevated plasma homocysteine levels occur mainly in persons whose daily intake of folic acid is below 400 μg.[63] Primary sources of folic acid are vegetables and fruits. A standard multivitamin contains enough folic acid to normalize folic acid levels, as well as supply the other cofactors, vitamins B_6 and B_{12}. The homocysteine hypothesis of atherosclerosis has not been examined in a controlled clinical trial by supplementing folic acid or the other cofactors. However, in view of the strength of the available evidence, it would appear reasonable to recommend daily use of a standard multivitamin in a program to prevent CHD.

Epidemiologic studies have found an inverse association between fiber intake and CHD.[64] Fruits, vegetables, and whole cereal grains are good sources of dietary fiber. Fiber is divided into two general categories: soluble and insoluble. Soluble fibers are like gels and gums and absorb water in the intestine. This may affect intestinal cholesterol and bile-acid metabolism and result in lowered plasma LDL cholesterol.[65] However, the effect on LDL is small within practical ranges of intake[65-67] and cannot explain the inverse association between fiber and CHD in populations. Moreover, the protective association with CHD was found mainly with cereal fiber,[64] which is mostly insoluble and does not lower LDL concentrations. High intake of soluble fiber may reduce the glycemic index of foods to improve postprandial glucose and insulin levels,[68] although this effect is not fully established.[69] Only one clinical trial exists that increased dietary fiber, and it showed no effect on recurrent coronary events in patients with recent MI.[39] Therefore, the causal role for fiber is not supported by clinical outcome trials, and its inverse association with CHD in epidemiologic studies may be partly because high fiber intake occurs in persons with an entire constellation of healthy behaviors, dietary and other.[64,70] Fiber should increase as a by-product of adhering to diets that are recommended to prevent CHD. Eating foods that are high in fiber supplies other important nutrients such as antioxidants and folic acid that could be protective, as well as displaces foods that contain saturated fat and cholesterol.

MULTIFACTORIAL TRIALS

Multifactorial approaches to prevent cardiovascular disease have been difficult to interpret in view of conflicting results. Certain trials combined nonpharmacologic and pharmacologic therapy to treat hyperlipidemia,[71] others combined various nonpharmacologic interventions,[72] whereas still other trials combined diet and drug therapy to treat simultaneously both hyperlipidemia and hypertension.[73-75] Variable compliance to the nonpharmacologic intervention, and possible toxicity from drug therapies such as clofibrate[71] or high-dose diuretics,[75] confound conclusions as to the benefits, if any, that can be expected. The Oslo Study Group[72] and the World Health Organization (WHO) Collaborative Program for primary prevention of cardiovascular disease[73,74] both provide insight into such programs. The Oslo study intervened with diet to reduce serum cholesterol and body weight and with smoking cessation. Each risk factor was significantly improved, and coronary events were reduced by 47%. The investigators estimated that lowered serum cholesterol was responsible for at least 75% of the benefit and smoking cessation was responsible for no more than 25%.[72] The WHO Collaborative Program was carried out with closely comparable methods for 5 to 6 years in 18,210 persons in Belgium[73] and

19,409 persons in the United Kingdom.[74] The intervention consisted of diet therapy and exercise to reduce blood cholesterol and body weight, smoking cessation, and hypertension control by diuretics with potassium supplementation. The Belgian program was successful in reducing significantly the coronary event rate by 25% and total mortality by 18% in the intervention compared with the control group, whereas in the United Kingdom, the coronary event rate was 6% higher (not significant) in the intervention group. The favorable result in Belgium compared to United Kingdom was attributed to better adherence as shown by greater improvements in risk factors. Finally, the perplexing Helsinki Businessmen Study of primary prevention[71] deserves comment. In this trial, 1222 men were randomized to a control group or to a multifactorial program of diet with or without clofibrate and/or probucol for hyperlipidemia, or diuretics and/or beta blockers for hypertension. The treated men were "frequently" given four or five agents.[76] The results were inconclusive after the 5-year planned duration of the randomized trial, but 10 years after the trial ended, coronary deaths were higher in the previously treated group. However, the patients who received only diet treatment did not have a higher death rate, and it may be considered that an adverse effect of the particular combination of drugs used could have been responsible. In conclusion, as regards multifactorial programs, good adherence to effective therapy for elevated blood cholesterol and/or blood pressure that does not have major side effects, as well as smoking cessation, produces the desired benefits for CHD.

GUIDELINES AND SUMMARY

A consensus conference was held on the role of diet in preventing chronic disease, including cardiovascular disease and cancer, in London in January 2000. The international group of nutrition experts attending the conference devised the following consensus statement on dietary fat, the Mediterranean diet, and health:

> There is increasing scientific evidence of positive health effects from diets which are high in fruits, vegetables, legumes, and whole grains, and which include fish, nuts and low-fat dairy products. Such diets need not be restricted in total fat as long as there is not an excess of calories, and emphasize predominantly vegetable oils that are low in saturated fats and free of partially hydrogenated oils. The traditional Mediterranean Diet, whose principal source of fat is olive oil, encompasses these dietary characteristics.[77]

See also the dietary guidelines discussed in Chapter 31.

Evidence-based medicine requires that guidelines for treatment be based on randomized clinical trials that show improvement in clinical event rates or in risk factors that are known to be in the causal pathway. Clinical trials demonstrate that diets that increase unsaturated fat and decrease saturated fat reduce coronary events without increasing other causes of morbidity or mortality. In contrast, the standard low-fat approach for diet therapy has not shown efficacy either for improving the lipid profile or reducing coronary events either because of low adherence or adverse metabolic effects. Clinicians can recommend to patients or to dietitians who work with them cookbooks on Mediterranean-type diets to assist them in making diet changes. The use of unsaturated oils expands the range of cooking styles that are compatible with the dietary goals. Other dietary approaches that have reduced coronary events in single trials are increased intake of fatty fish,[39] increased fruits and vegetables,[45] and a Mediterranean diet.[50] Initiation of dietary therapy soon after MI may produce early benefits. Multifactorial programs for hyperlipidemia and hypertension are more complicated to evaluate, but programs that demonstrably improve risk factors with diet therapy and use simple drug regimens that are known individually to reduce cardiovascular events and are not a cause of toxicity are likely to be effective.

REFERENCES

1. Shepherd J, Cobbe SM, Ford I, et al: Prevention of coronary heart disease with pravastatin in men with hypercholesterolemia. N Engl J Med 1995; 333:1301-1307.
2. Scandinavian Simvastatin Survival Study Group (4S): Randomized trial of cholesterol lowering in 4444 patients with coronary heart disease: The Scandinavian Simvastatin Survival Study (4S). Lancet 1994; 344:1383-1389.
3. Sacks FM, Pfeffer MA, Moye LA, et al: The effect of pravastatin on coronary events after myocardial infarction in patients with average cholesterol levels. N Engl J Med 1996; 335:1001-1009.
4. Heart Protection Study Collaborative Group: MRC/BHF Heart Protection Study of cholesterol lowering with simvastatin in 20,356 high-risk individuals: A randomised placebo-controlled trial. Lancet 2002; 360:7-22.
5. Martin MJ, Hulley SB, Browner WS, et al: Serum cholesterol, blood pressure, and mortality: Implications from a cohort of 361,662 men. Lancet 1986; 2:933-936.
6. Pekkanen J, Linn S, Heiss G, et al: Ten-year mortality from cardiovascular disease in relation to cholesterol level among men with and without preexisting cardiovascular disease. N Engl J Med 1990; 322:1700-1707.
7. Rose G, Reid DD, Hamilton PJ, et al: Myocardial ischemia, risk factors and death from coronary heart disease. Lancet 1977; 1:105-109.
8. Kannel WB: Range of serum cholesterol values in the population developing coronary artery disease. Am J Cardiol 1995; 76:69C-77C.
9. Rossouw JE: Lipid-lowering interventions in angiographic trials. Am J Cardiol 1995;76:86C-92C.
10. Holme I: Cholesterol reduction and its impact on coronary artery disease and total mortality. Am J Cardiol 1995;76:10C-17C.
11. Rubins HB, Robins SJ, Collins C, et al: Distribution of lipids in 8,500 men with coronary artery disease. Am J Cardiol 1995; 75:1196-1201.
12. Johnson CL, Rifkind BM, Sempos CT, et al: Declining serum total cholesterol levels among US adults: The National Health and Nutrition Examination Surveys. JAMA 1993; 269:3002-3008.
13. Expert Panel on Detection, Evaluation, and Treatment of High Blood Cholesterol: Executive Summary of the Third Report of the National Cholesterol Education Program (NCEP) Expert Panel on Detection, Evaluation, and Treatment of High Blood Cholesterol in Adults (Adult Treatment Panel III). JAMA 2001; 285:2486-2497.
14. Sacks FM, Willett WC: More on chewing the fat: The good fat and the good cholesterol [Editorial]. N Engl J Med 1991; 325:1740-1742.
15. Keys A, Anderson JT, Grande F: Serum cholesterol response to changes in the diet. Metabolism 1965;14:747-787.
16. Hegsted DM, McGandy RB, Myers ML, et al: Quantitative effects of dietary fat on serum cholesterol in man. Am J Clin Nutr 1965; 17:281-295.
17. Mensink RP, Katan MB: Effect of dietary fatty acids on serum lipids and lipoproteins: A meta-analysis of 27 trials. Arterioscl Thromb 1992;12:911-919.

18. Sacks FM: The role of high-density lipoprotein (HDL) cholesterol in the prevention and treatment of coronary heart disease: Expert group recommendations. Am J Cardiol 2002; 90:139-143.

19. Lipid Research Clinics Program: The Lipid Research Clinics Coronary Primary Prevention Trial Results: II. The relationship of reduction of incidence of coronary heart disease to cholesterol lowering. JAMA 1984; 251:365-374.

20. Manninen V, Elo O, Frick H, et al: Lipid alterations and decline in the incidence of coronary heart disease in the Helsinki Heart Study. JAMA 1988; 260:641-651.

21. Brown G, Albers JJ, Fisher LD, et al: Regression of coronary artery disease as a result of intensive lipid-lowering therapy in men with high levels of apolipoprotein B. N Engl J Med 1990; 323: 1289-1298.

22. Kinosian B, Glick H, Garland G: Cholesterol and coronary heart disease: Predicting risks by levels and ratios. Ann Intern Med 1994; 121:641-647.

23. Stampfer MJ, Sacks FM, Salvini S, et al: A prospective study of lipids, apolipoproteins, and risks of myocardial infarction. N Engl J Med 1991; 325:373-381.

24. Manninen V, Tenkanen L, Koskinen P, et al: Joint effects of serum triglyceride and LDL cholesterol and HDL cholesterol concentrations on coronary heart disease risk in the Helsinki Heart Study. Circulation 1992; 85:37-45.

25. Austin M: Plasma triglyceride and coronary heart disease. Arterioscler Thromb 1991; 11:2-13.

26. Criqui MH, Heiss G, Cohn R, et al: Plasma triglyceride level and mortality from coronary heart disease. N Engl J Med 1993; 328: 120-125.

27. Assmann G, Schulte H: Relation of HDL cholesterol and triglycerides to incidence of atherosclerotic coronary artery disease: The PROCAM experience. Am J Cardiol 1992; 70:733-737.

28. Stampfer MJ, Krauss RM, Ma J, et al: A prospective study of triglycerides, LDL particle diameter, and risk of myocardial infarction. JAMA 1996; 276:882-888.

29. Chen YD, Skowronski R, Coulston AM, et al: Effect of acute variations in dietary fat and carbohydrate intake on retinyl ester content of intestinally derived lipoproteins. J Clin Endocrinol Metab 1992; 74:28-32.

30. Lichtenstein AH, Ausman LM, Carrasco W, et al: Effects of canola, corn, and olive oils on fasting and postprandial plasma lipoproteins in humans as part of a National Cholesterol Education Program Step 2 diet. Arterioscler Thromb 1993; 13:1533-1542.

31. Obarzanek E, Sacks FM, Vollmer WM, et al: Effects on blood lipids of a blood pressure lowering diet: The Dietary Approaches to Stop Hypertension (DASH) Trial. Am J Clin Nutr 2001; 74:80-89.

32. Tzonou A, Kalandidi A, Trichopoulou A, et al: Diet and coronary heart disease: A case-control study in Athens, Greece. Epidemiology 1993; 4:511-516.

33. Mensink RP, Zock PL, Katan MB, et al: Effect of dietary cis and trans fatty acids on serum lipoprotein(a) in humans. J Lipid Res 1992; 33:1493-1501.

34. Nestel P, Noakes M, Belling B, et al: Plasma lipoprotein and Lp(a) changes with substitution of elaidic acid for oleic acid in the diet. J Lipid Res 1992; 33:1029-1036.

35. Willett WC, Stampfer MJ, Colditz GA, et al: Intake of trans fatty acids and risk of coronary heart disease among women. Lancet 1993; 341:581-585.

36. Ascherio A, Hennekens CH, Buring JE, et al: Trans fatty acids and risk of myocardial infarction. Circulation 1994; 89:969-974.

37. Siguel EN, Lerman RH: Trans fatty acid patterns in patients with angiographically documented coronary artery disease. Am J Cardiol 1993; 71:916-920.

38. Research Committee: Low-fat diet in myocardial infarction. Lancet 1965; 2:501-504.

39. Burr ML, Fehily AM, Gilbert JF, et al: Effects of changes in fat, fish, and fibre intakes on death and myocardial infarction: Diet and Reinfarction Trial (DART). Lancet 1989; 2:757-761.

40. Dayton S, Pearce ML, Hashimoto S, et al: A controlled clinical trial of a diet high in unsaturated fat in preventing complications of atherosclerosis. Circulation 1969; 40(Suppl II):II1-II63.

41. Research Committee: Controlled trial of soya-bean oil in myocardial infarction. Lancet 1968; 2:693-700.

42. Turpeinen O, Karvonen MJ, Pekkarinen M, et al: Dietary prevention of coronary heart disease: The Finnish Mental Hospital Study. Int J Epidemiol 1979; 8:99-118.

43. Leren P: The Oslo Diet-Heart Study: Eleven-year report. Circulation 1970; 42:935-942.

44. Law M, Wald NJ, Thompson NJ: By how much and how quickly does reduction in serum cholesterol concentration lower risk of ischaemic heart disease? BMJ 1994; 308:367-372.

45. Singh RB, Rostogi SS, Verma R, et al: Randomised, controlled trial of cardioprotective diet in patients with recent acute myocardial infarction: Results of one-year follow-up. BMJ 1992; 304:1015-1019.

46. Singh RB, Niaz MA, Ghosh S, et al: Effect on mortality and reinfarction of adding fruits and vegetables to a prudent diet in the Indian Experiment of Infarct Survival. J Am Coll Nutr 1993; 12:255-261.

47. The Coronary Drug Project Research Group: Clofibrate and niacin in coronary heart disease. JAMA 1975; 231:360-381.

48. Watts GF, Lewis B, Brunt JN, et al: Effects on coronary artery disease of lipid-lowering diet, or diet plus cholestyramine, in the St Thomas' Atherosclerosis Regression Study (STARS). Lancet 1992; 339:563-569.

49. Sacks FM, Gibson CM, Rosner B, et al: The influence of pretreatment low-density lipoprotein cholesterol concentrations on the effect of hypocholesterolemic therapy on coronary atherosclerosis in angiographic trials. Am J Cardiol 1995; 76:78C-85C.

50. De Lorgeril M, Renaud S, Mamelle N, et al: Mediterranean alpha-linolenic acid-rich diet in secondary prevention of coronary heart disease. Lancet 1994; 343:1454-1459.

51. GISSI-Prevenzione Investigators: Dietary supplementation with n-3 polyunsaturated fatty acids and vitamin E after myocardial infarction: results of the GISSI-Prevenzione trial. Lancet 1999; 354:447-455.

52. Harris WS: Fish oils and plasma lipid and lipoprotein metabolism in humans: A critical review. J Lipid Res 1989; 30:785-807.

53. Sacks FM, Hebert P, Appel LJ, et al: The effect of fish oil on blood pressure and high-density lipoprotein cholesterol levels in phase 1 of the Trials of Hypertension Prevention. J Hypertension 1994; 12(Suppl 7):S23-S31.

54. Morris MC, Sacks F, Rosner B: Does fish oil lower blood pressure? A meta-analysis of controlled trials. Circulation 1993; 88:523-533.

55. Billman GE, Hallaq H, Leaf A: Prevention of ischemia-induced ventricular fibrillation by omega-3 fatty acids. Proc Natl Acad Sci USA 1994; 91:4427-4430.

56. Sellmayer A, Witzgall H, Lorenz RL, et al: Effects of dietary fish oil on ventricular premature complexes. Am J Cardiol 1995; 76: 974-976.

57. Siscovic DS, Raghunathan TE, King I, et al: Dietary intake and cell membrane levels of long-chain n-3 polyunsaturated fatty acids and the risk of primary cardiac arrest. JAMA 1995; 274:1363-1367.

58. Ornish D, Brown SE, Scherwitz LW, et al: Can lifestyle changes reverse coronary heart disease? The Lifestyle Heart Trial. Lancet 1990; 336:129-133.

59. Schuler G, Hambrecht R, Schlierf G, et al: Regular physical exercise and low-fat diet: Effects on progression of coronary artery disease. Circulation 1992; 86:1-11.

60. Kallio V, Hamalainen H, Hakkila J, et al: Reduction in sudden deaths by a multifactorial intervention programme after acute myocardial infarction. Lancet 1979; 2:1091-1094.

61. Clarke R, Daly L, Robinson D, et al: Hyperhomocysteinemia: An independent risk factor for vascular disease. N Engl J Med 1991; 324:1149-1155.

62. Stampfer MJ, Malinow MR, Willett WC, et al: A prospective study of plasma homocysteine and risk of myocardial infarction. JAMA 1992; 268:877-881.

63. Selhub J, Jacques PF, Wilson PW, et al: Vitamin status and intake as primary determinants of homocystenemia in elderly populations. JAMA 1993; 270:2693-2698.

64. Rimm EB, Ascherio A, Giovannucci E, et al: Vegetable, fruit, and cereal fiber intake and risk of coronary heart disease among men. JAMA 1996; 275:447-451.

65. Jenkins DJ, Wolever TM, Rao AV, et al: Effect on blood lipids of very high intakes of fiber in diets low in saturated fat and cholesterol. N Engl J Med 1993; 329:21-26.

66. Ripsin CM, Keenan JM, Jacobs DR, et al: Oat products and lipid lowering: A meta-analysis. JAMA 1992; 267:3317-3325.

67. Brown L, Rosner B, Willett WC, et al: Cholesterol lowering effects of dietary fiber: a meta-analysis. Am J Clin Nutr 1999; 69:30-42.

68. Jenkins DJ, Leeds AR, Gassull MA, et al: Unabsorbable carbohydrate and diabetes: Decreased postprandial hyperglycemia. Lancet 1976; 2:172-174.

69. Hollenbeck CB, Coulston AM, Reaven GM: To what extent does increased dietary fiber improve glucose and lipid metabolism in patients with noninsulin-dependent diabetes mellitus (NIDDM)? Am J Clin Nutr 1986; 43:16–24.

70. Wynder EL, Stellman SD, Zang EA: High-fiber intake: Indicator of a healthy lifestyle [Editorial]. JAMA 1996; 275:486–487.

71. Strandberg TE, Salomaa VV, Naukkarinen VA, et al: Long-term mortality after 5-year multifactorial primary prevention of cardiovascular diseases in middle-aged men. JAMA 1991; 266:1225–1229.

72. Hjermann I, Velve Byre K, Holme I, et al: Effect on diet and smoking intervention on the incidence of coronary heart disease. Lancet 1981; 2:1303–1309.

73. Kornitzer M, DeBacker G, Dramaix M, et al: Belgian Heart Disease Prevention Project: Incidence and mortality results. Lancet 1983; 1:1066–1070.

74. Rose G, Tunstall-Pedoe HD, Heller RF: UK Heart Disease Prevention Project: Incidence and mortality results. Lancet 1983; 1:1062–1066.

75. The Multiple Risk Factor Intervention Trial Research Group: Mortality after 16 years for participants randomized to the Multiple Risk Factor Intervention Trial. Circulation 1996; 94:946–951.

76. Strandberg TE, Miettinen TA: Multifactorial primary prevention: Exploring the failures. J Myocard Ischemia 1994; 6:15–23.

77. Dietary fat consensus statements. Am J Med 2002; 113:5S–8S.

Cardiac Psychology: Psychosocial Factors

Robert Allan
Stephen Scheidt

There has been much recent research on psychosocial factors for heart disease, sufficient to merit a name for this emerging field. In fact, two names have evolved: **cardiac psychology**[1] and **behavioral cardiology**. Each of these terms is imperfect, however. Psychologists cannot call themselves "behavioral cardiologists," nor will physicians refer to themselves as "cardiac psychologists." Moreover, the term "behavioral" emphasizes that which is observable and does not necessarily include emotions or presumed underlying motivations for behavior. However, **cardiac psychology** and **behavioral cardiology** are two new, closely related subspecialties in mental health and cardiology, respectively, summarized in this chapter.

Cardiac psychology has evolved with a unifying hypothesis that psychologic and social factors, together termed "psychosocial factors," can affect the development of and outcome from coronary heart disease (CHD), the leading cause of death and disability for men and women in the United States. In the late 1950s, some of the earliest research linked stress, such as the loss of a loved one or job, with increased risk of CHD. Subsequently, a number of psychosocial factors, including the type A behavior pattern (TABP), depression, social isolation, anger, anxiety, and job strain, among others, have attained some degree of empiric validity as CHD risk factors. Although improvement in psychosocial CHD risk factors has been considered a goal in and of itself, because of their generally negative impact on quality of life, the as-yet-unrealized "holy grail" of behavioral cardiology is a reduction in cardiac morbidity or mortality with intervention directed at presumed adverse psychosocial or behavioral characteristics.

Behavioral cardiology is evolving rapidly. A number of important studies have led to a changing emphasis in the relative importance ascribed to putative psychosocial CHD risk factors. **Depression** and **social isolation** have emerged from the literature as consistent and powerful risk factors. Type A behavior pattern seems of less importance than previously believed. Recent research on type A behavior has been quite limited, with the focus having shifted from the total behavior pattern to **hostility**, one of its major components, which in 1987 Redford Williams suggested might be its "toxic core."[2] A constellation of "negative emotions" (depression and chronic anger) and one possible consequence of such negativity (social isolation) have emerged with striking predictive power from a number of studies. A provocative twin study reported in 2002 a possible genetic basis for the relationship between depression, anger, and social isolation.[3]

Over the past few years, behavioral cardiology/cardiac psychology has attained considerable credibility in medicine, as evidenced by many recent studies published in cardiology and other medical journals where they may be expected to have greater impact on patient care than in the past. Review articles on psychosocial risk factors abound, and the interested reader is referred to these sources for comprehensive summaries. In 1999, Rozanski, Blumenthal, and Kaplan[4] published a "new frontiers" article in **Circulation**, which was an exhaustive review of psychosocial factors associated with CHD. Since then, two additional general reviews of the literature have appeared[5,6] as well as numerous reviews on specific psychosocial risk factors, including: depression,[7,8] anxiety and depression[9]; psychologic factors for sudden cardiac death (SCD)[10] and in heart failure[11]; and psychosocial risk factors in women.[12] Two additional reviews of the depression literature provide detailed psychotherapy case presentations.[13,14] Social isolation is another important psychosocial factor associated with excess cardiac events as well as increased all-cause mortality. See Eng and colleagues[15] for the most recent database in the introduction to their large-scale study of social ties and CHD.

An area of emerging importance is psychosocial adjustment in implantable cardioverter defibrillator (ICD) patients, a population that has greatly expanded in the past few years. Many ICD patients are sudden death survivors, and significant numbers suffer from depression, anxiety, and posttraumatic stress disorder. See Sears and colleagues[16] for a review of the ICD psychosocial literature.

Autonomic imbalance may be a major physiologic mechanism responsible for the harmful effects from psychosocial factors. Among many others, Curtis and O'Keefe[17] have discussed the hypothesis that heightened sympathetic and reduced parasympathetic nervous system activity are the major underlying links between mind and behavior and CHD. Chronic overactivation of the "fight or flight" response is believed to be the principal behavioral mechanism for heightened sympathetic nervous system activity. The "fight or flight" metaphor, coined more than 60 years ago by Cannon, is easily understood by patients and can form the nucleus of psychologic treatment strategies aimed at reducing stress: many individuals tend to perceive objectively innocuous situations, such as differences of opinion and automobile traffic, as personally threatening and respond with exaggerated cardiovascular reactivity. In addition to direct effects of increased sympathetic or decreased parasympathetic activity, which include increased blood pressure, heart rate, and myocardial contractility—all of which increase cardiac oxygen needs—there are indirect effects of autonomic imbalance, including platelet and clotting system reactivity, predisposition to thrombosis, and increased propensity to arrhythmia. The renin-angiotensin axis can be stimulated, and cortisol production can be increased. Unfortunately, far too little work has been done on explaining mechanisms by which psychologic factors might affect the cardiovascular system—and it seems likely that this serious gap in our knowledge is at least partly responsible for the hesitant acceptance by many health care professionals of a possible causal relationship between psychosocial factors and various manifestations of cardiac disease.

HIGHLIGHTS FROM THE RECENT CARDIAC PSYCHOLOGY LITERATURE: DEPRESSION, SOCIAL ISOLATION, AND ANGER

Depression

Data on depression can be subdivided into research on initially healthy subjects and studies of patients who already have CHD. A number of prospective studies have noted an increased relative risk (approximately 1.5 to 2.0) of acute myocardial infarction (MI) and cardiovascular mortality in depressed but otherwise healthy individuals.[18-25] This area was reviewed in 2003.[26] The data linking depression with adverse events among patients with established cardiac disease are particularly striking, with a 1998 review noting that 11 of 11 studies reported a positive relationship between depression and worsened outcome.[7] The relative risk of future adverse cardiac events and cardiovascular mortality in depressed patients is increased approximately threefold to fourfold.[7,8] Between 35% and 45% of post-MI and post-coronary artery bypass graft surgery (CABG) patients suffer from some level of depression, ranging from a few symptoms to major depressive disorder. A suggestion from two intervention trials is that much cardiac depression (approximately 50%) may remit spontaneously within a few months of the cardiac event.[27,28]

The practicing physician would do well to pay more attention to depression, an often debilitating condition, which has been shown to respond well to psychotherapy, psychotropic medication, or a combination of both. Autonomic dysfunction, reflected by reduced heart rate variability, is the physiologic mechanism most often cited as linking depression to increased cardiac mortality.[29] **An important cautionary note: nortriptyline (and likely other tricyclic antidepressants), compared with paroxetine (and likely other selective serotonin reuptake inhibitors [SSRIs]), has been shown to reduce heart rate variability and increase both heart rate and adverse cardiac events in depressed cardiac patients[30]; tricyclics cannot be recommended for cardiac patients with depression.** Whether SSRIs are helpful in reducing future cardiac events remains to be proved.

Social Isolation

Early anecdotal evidence in the area of social isolation noted increased mortality among widows and widowers. In 1984, Ruberman and colleagues[31] were among the first to provide evidence of increased mortality in socially isolated cardiac patients among 2320 male survivors of acute MI in the Beta Blocker Heart Attack Trial (BHAT). Since then, there have been many studies supporting a connection between social isolation with both the initial development of and the subsequent outcome from CHD. Lack of social support has also been associated with increased all-cause mortality. Several large studies have supplied convincing evidence that social isolation or lack of social support is an important predictor of adverse outcome after MI. In 1992, Case and colleagues[32] reported on 1234 patients 6 months after acute MI; the recurrent event rate for nonfatal MI or cardiac death was nearly double for those living alone compared to those living with a companion. Similarly, Williams and colleagues[33] followed a consecutive sample of 1368 patients undergoing cardiac catheterization over 5 years. Unmarried individuals without a confidant had more than three times the increased risk of death compared to those who were married or had a close friend. Most studies of socially isolated individuals have reported a twofold to threefold increased risk of adverse cardiac events or mortality.

In a study of 430 patients with CHD, Brummett and colleagues[34] reported that the **most isolated** individuals, those with 3 or fewer people in their social support network, had the worst outcome, with a relative risk of 2.43 (P = 0.001) for cardiac and 2.11 (P = 0.001) for all-cause mortality. Once past a threshold of minimal support, additional social ties did not appear to provide extra benefit.

Although poor health habits and lower socioeconomic status have been linked with social isolation, little is known about possible underlying physiologic pathways linking social isolation to increased CHD or all-cause mortality.

Hostility and Anger

Hostility and anger have long been suspected of playing a role in CHD. Free-floating, or easily aroused, hostility is one of the two major symptoms of the TABP (the other being time pressure), which is one of the first psychosocial conditions suggested as a risk factor for CHD. Likely because of strong social undesirability, assessment of hostility and anger has been more difficult than assessment of other psychosocial factors. Many individuals are not eager to acknowledge that they have "anger problems." Hence, structured interviews of "potential for hostility" have generally found stronger associations with CHD than self-report questionnaires. Hostility is a complex phenomenon and has been noted to have emotional, cognitive, trait, and behavioral components. Anger, the emotional component, varies from mild annoyance to rage. The cognitive aspect, a cynical and pessimistic world view, has generally been assessed by the Cook-Medley Scale of the Minnesota Multiphasic Personality Inventory (MMPI). "Trait" anger is a predisposition to become easily and intensely angered and hold grudges. Behavioral components include tendencies to inhibit or express anger outwardly as well as engage in violence. Each of the questionnaires used for assessment of hostility emphasizes one or another of these components, which has led to confusion and controversy in the literature.

A 1996 meta-analysis of 45 studies by Miller and colleagues[35] suggests that chronic hostility is indeed an independent risk factor for CHD as well as all-cause mortality, with the relationship strongest among younger patients.

In 2000, JE Williams and colleagues[36] reported on 12,986 Americans without known CHD at baseline, aged 45 to 64 years at entry, who were followed for a median of 53 months. Anger was assessed by the Spielberger Trait Anger Scale (Table 30-1). There was a strong graded relationship between increasing "trait anger" and subsequent MI and CHD mortality. The increased multivariate-adjusted hazard ratio (HR) of "hard events," (nonfatal and fatal MI) was 2.69 (95% confidence interval [CI] 1.48-4.90) for high versus low anger and 1.35 (95% CI 0.87-2.10) for moderate versus low anger. It is puzzling, however, that results were significant for only normotensive individuals, approximately two thirds of the population under investi-

gation. A similar relationship between scores on the Spielberger Trait Anger Scale and increased risk of hemorrhagic and ischemic stroke was found in a sample of 13,851 men and women followed for a median of 77.3 months.[37] Although Cox proportional hazards regression analyses showed a modest increased risk of stroke for the entire cohort, after multivariate adjustment results were statistically significant for only those younger than 60 years of age (high trait anger vs. low trait anger [relative risk, or RR = 2.82; 95% CI 1.65-4.80]).

The largest study of anger to date failed to confirm these results. Eng and colleagues[38] administered a slightly different measure of anger, the Spielberger Anger-Out Expression Scale, to 23,552 health professionals (primarily dentists, veterinarians, pharmacists, and other nonphysicians), who were then followed for 2 years. Moderate, compared to low, expressed anger conferred a **protective effect** on both MI (RR = 0.56; 95% CI 0.32-0.97) and stroke (RR = 0.42; 95% CI 0.20-0.88) in this large sample. It is remarkable that these three large studies have come to inconsistent conclusions about the expression of anger using very similar anger measurement instruments. Hence, research on anger, its expression, and cardiovascular disease is still fraught with conflicting findings.

Other Psychosocial Risk Factors

In addition to depression, social isolation, and hostility, there is some evidence that several other psychosocial factors increase risk of CHD. These include job strain (a combination of high job demands and low decision latitude),[39] anxiety (a relationship between "phobic anxiety" and SCD, but not MI or overall CHD, has been noted in a study of about 40,000 initially healthy men),[40] "type D" (distressed) personality,[41] and "vital exhaustion" (a debilitating condition of chronic fatigue and depression).[42]

TRIGGERING OF ACUTE CARDIAC EVENTS

Beginning in biblical times, anecdotes have suggested a causal relationship between stressful life events and sudden death. Within the past several decades, observational studies of both natural and manmade disasters, such as earthquakes[43] and the Iraqi SCUD missile attacks on Israel,[44] have reported higher rates of both MI and SCD than during normal times. We have also learned a great deal from the recently completed Determinants of Time of Myocardial Infarction Onset Study (MI Onset Study), resolving a long-standing, contentious debate about whether MI and SCD are precipitated by identifiable specific physical, behavioral, or psychologic events. The MI Onset Study used a "case-crossover" design, in which patients serve as their own controls by completing diaries for their activities prior to symptoms and comparing activities just prior to their MI to similar days and times during weeks when they did not have an MI. In addition, diaries and interviews of age- and sex-matched neighborhood controls who wore beepers that were activated at the same time of day and day of the week that the MI occurred in the patient were used to support the data analysis.

■ ■ ■

TABLE 30-1

Spielberger Trait Anger Scale

1. I am quick tempered.
2. I have a fiery temper.
3. I am a hotheaded person.
4. I get angry when I am slowed down by others' mistakes.
5. I feel annoyed when I am not given recognition for doing good work.
6. I fly off the handle.
7. When I get angry, I say nasty things.
8. It makes me furious when I am criticized in front of others.
9. When I get frustrated, I feel like hitting someone.
10. I feel infuriated when I do a good job and get a poor evaluation.

Answers

(1) Almost never, (2) Sometimes, (3) Often, (4) Almost always.

Spielberger Anger-Out Expression Scale

1. I express my anger.
2. I make sarcastic remarks to others.
3. I do things like slam doors.
4. I argue with others.
5. I strike out at whatever infuriates me.
6. I say nasty things.
7. I lose my temper.
8. If someone annoys me, I'm apt to tell him how I feel.

Answers

(1) Almost never, (2) Sometimes, (3) Often, (4) Almost always.

In the MI Onset study, most myocardial infarcts and SCDs could not be attributed to a specific cause. It should be noted that the **absolute risk** of MI in any given hour for a healthy 50-year-old man is quite low—only 1 in 1 million.[45] A number of behavioral "triggers," some potentially avoidable, were identified, including strenuous exertion,[46] intense anger,[47] sexual activity,[48] assuming the upright posture on awakening,[45] and use of marijuana[49] and cocaine.[50] A small but statistically significant Monday morning peak in MI, presumably related to beginning the work week, has also been noted by other investigators.[51]

All told, triggers are suggested in approximately 17% of cases of MI.[45,52] Strenuous exertion is the most potent trigger, particularly for sedentary individuals; however, most Americans do not spend very many hours per week in strenuous exercise. In the MI Onset Study, only 4.4% of patients engaged in strenuous activity in the hour prior to their infarction.[45,46] For healthy individuals who exercise regularly there was a 5.6 × relative risk of MI during exercise and for the hour afterward, compared with hours when such individuals were not exercising. Strenuous exercise does increase the risk of acute MI from about 1 in 1 million to 1 in 200,000 during exercise and for 1 hour afterward in a healthy 50-year-old (i.e., strenuous exercise is a statistically significant "trigger" of acute MI, yet its clinical and epidemiologic importance is negligible). Moreover, the increased risk during and immediately following exercise is more than offset by a reduction in cardiac events during the rest of the week in active versus sedentary people. For sedentary individuals without a history of CHD, the relative risk of MI with strenuous exertion is increased from 1 in 1 million to approximately 1 in 14,000,[45,52] but again, sedentary individuals spend even less overall time per week doing strenuous exercise. Nevertheless, this is important information for public health: **sedentary mid-life individuals should be discouraged from engaging in occasional strenuous activities such as snow shoveling, moving heavy furniture, and the like.**

Intense anger has also been found to be a trigger for MI. In the MI Onset Study, 8% of patients reported an episode in which they were at least "very angry" in the 24 hours prior to MI and 2.4% reported such anger in the 2 hours preceding their infarction.[47] Each time an individual becomes angry there is a 2.3 × increased risk of triggering a cardiac event during the angry episode and for a 2-hour hazard period afterward. For those who become angry only occasionally, this added risk is modest. For those who become angry repeatedly throughout the day, however, a 2.3 × increased risk per episode of intense anger can be multiplied many fold. Modifying chronic anger is an attractive psychologic treatment goal because it can often enhance an individual's well-being. It should be noted that regular aspirin use, a far simpler, although arguably less life-enhancing treatment than anger management, eliminated the added triggering risk from anger in the MI Onset Study cohort.

Sexual activity, it turns out, is indeed a modest trigger, accounting for fewer cases of MI than assuming the upright posture on awakening.[48] This is reassuring information for cardiac patients with an active love life. The slightly increased risk is lessened with regular physical exercise.[48]

Among the 3882 patients interviewed in the MI Onset Study, 124 (3.2%) reported using marijuana in the previous year, 37 within 24 hours and 9 within 1 hour of MI symptoms.[49] The MI Onset Study identified a 1-hour hazard period after marijuana use with a 4.8-fold increased relative risk (95% CI 2.4-9.5). Similarly, 38 (approximately 1%) of 3946 patients interviewed reported using cocaine within the prior year, and 9 reported use within 60 minutes prior to symptoms of MI, elevating risk of MI 23.7 times over baseline (95% CI 8.5-66.3). Other potentially important information from the MI Onset Study is that beta blockers diminish the morning peak in cardiac events and aspirin reduces the morning peak in nonfatal MI.[52]

Two small studies have reported that physical and psychologic stress, as well as anger, can serve as "triggers" for discharge from ICDs.[53,54] Both studies used a "case-crossover" design, similar to the MI Onset Study. Fries and colleagues[53] reported prior physical and mental stress in 26% and 24%, respectively, of 95 ICD-documented tachyarrhythmic events. Relative risks in this sample of 43 consecutive patients with ICD discharge were 7.5 for physical activity (95% CI 5.2-11.1), 9.5 (6.3-14.5) for psychologic stress, and 7.5 (2.3-24.8) for sexual activity. In a similar series of 107 confirmed ventricular shocks among 42 patients, Lampert and colleagues[54] reported increased anger in the 15 minutes preceding shocks 15% of the time, compared with 3% during control periods (P < 0.04; odds ratio 1.83; 95% CI 1.04-3.16). As in the previous citation, patients were more physically active prior to shock than during control periods. ICD discharge is an important surrogate marker for ventricular tachycardia and/or ventricular fibrillation, the physiologic mechanisms for most SCD. Whether ICD discharge might be reduced with psychosocial intervention has not, to our knowledge, been reported.

CARDIAC DENIAL AND PREHOSPITAL DELAY IN SEEKING TREATMENT FOR ACUTE MYOCARDIAL INFARCTION

Prompt medical attention for MI has never been more important. With widespread availability of thrombolytic therapy and emergent ("primary") percutaneous transluminal angioplasty (PTCA), myocardial necrosis can often be limited and sometimes eliminated—if individuals obtain prompt medical attention. Significant percentages of patients, however, fail to do so. Ironically, in one study of 100 consecutive patients with suspected MI in Wales, the United Kingdom, and British Columbia, Canada, those with a history of CHD actually arrived at the hospital **later** than those without prior CHD.[55]

A number of community interventions have attempted to educate the public about the importance of early intervention. One of the largest, the Rapid Early Action for Coronary Treatment (REACT), was conducted in 20 pair-matched communities in the United States.[56,57] One community from each pair received extensive education for the general public, health professionals, and those with a history of CHD or CHD risk factors. After 18 months of intervention, there was a 34% increase in the use of Emergency Medical Services to provide transportation to the hospital. However, the community intervention **did not improve** the time from symptom onset to hospital arrival.

Similarly disappointing results also occurred after an intensive 3-week multimedia campaign undertaken in Göteborg, Sweden.[58] The "HJARTA-SMARTA" program provided newspaper articles, ads on radio and public transportation, and leaflets distributed twice to all 200,000 households. Median delay time **was** reduced, albeit modestly, from 3 hours to 2 hours and 20 minutes. However, neither in-hospital nor 1-year mortality were improved by this ambitious effort. The lack of success of both REACT and "HJARTA-SMARTA" suggests that some factor(s) other than lack of knowledge may play a crucial role in preventing individuals from seeking prompt medical attention for symptoms of MI.

In our clinical experience, **cardiac denial** is a powerful **emotional factor** that we have frequently observed in individuals who were intelligent and educated enough so that they would be expected to obtain prompt attention for their cardiac symptoms. One aspect of cardiac denial is a tendency to minimize or ignore the significance of chest pains. This process is generally **not** volitional. Denial, as with most psychologic defense mechanisms, does diminish anxiety, which can be profound with the sense that one's life is in danger. In addition, acknowledging a serious threat to one's health may result in concerns about personal weakness, embarrassment, and expense, all factors that can have strong emotional overtones. A 1992 review reported on 21 studies and concluded that cardiac denial has a long-term negative effect on health outcome.[59] A scale has also been developed for assessment.[60] This is an area worthy of future research, in light of both the enormous potential health benefits as well as the failure of public education trials as large and expensive as REACT and "HJARTA-SMARTA."

PSYCHOSOCIAL INTERVENTIONS

Despite the increasing strength of the database linking psychosocial factors with CHD, there have been only a limited number of clinical trials, many with small numbers of subjects. Three meta-analyses of the psychosocial intervention literature have been published. In 1987, Nunes, Frank, and Kornfeld[61] reviewed 18 controlled studies for treatment of the TABP. Of these, only two provided sufficient data for analysis of "hard" cardiac endpoints: a 1979 study by Rahe and colleagues[62] and the 1986 Friedman and associates' Recurrent Coronary Prevention Project (RCPP)[63] together reduced recurrent MI and cardiac mortality by approximately 50% over 3 years. A 1996 meta-analysis by Linden, Stossel, and Maurice[64] examined 23 randomized clinical trials, with a total of 2024 patients and 1156 control subjects, and reported that when added to standard cardiac rehabilitation, psychosocial intervention reduced some biologic risk factors and psychologic distress, as well as cardiac morbidity and mortality, with benefits evident within the first 2 years, although less marked afterward. The most recent meta-analysis, a review of 37 studies published by Dusseldorp and colleagues[65] in 1999, concluded that psychosocial interventions provided a significant positive effect on cardiac risk factors, a 29% reduction in recurrent MI, and a 34% reduction in cardiac mortality.

It should be noted that the three meta-analyses included studies going back as far as 1974, when the understanding and treatment of CHD were far different from today. Furthermore, there has been little in the way of a standardized intervention. Indeed, most researchers developed their own treatment strategies loosely based on health education and "stress management" models. Such heterogeneity undoubtedly contributes to the continuing controversy in this area. Since publication of the three meta-analyses, the most recent and largest interventions to date have produced modest results. Following is a brief description of the trials that we consider the most noteworthy (Table 30-2).

The Recurrent Coronary Prevention Project

Meyer Friedman, a cardiologist, was one of the originators of the TABP and a founding father of cardiac psychology. The Friedman and associates' RCPP[63] was the "grand daddy" of psychosocial intervention studies, the first large post-MI type A behavior modification program. The RCPP randomized 862 post-MI patients (n = 592 treatment; 270 controls) to group counseling for modification of the TABP, along with standard risk factors, or to control groups that received counseling for only standard factors. After 4.5 years of counseling, initially weekly and then monthly, there was a 44% reduction in second MI, which was associated with reductions in type A behavior. The control group was subsequently offered type A counseling and showed a similar reduction in MI recurrence rates over an additional year.[66] The RCPP also determined that type A counseling was most protective against cardiac death for patients with less severe MI,[67] suggesting that psychosocial intervention is most effective when individuals are still relatively healthy but less beneficial when disease is advanced and physiologic processes predominate. Further, there was a significant reduction in sudden, but not nonsudden, cardiac death,[68] providing support for the hypothesis that behavioral factors may precipitate lethal arrhythmias. Criticisms of the RCPP include more counseling sessions for TABP groups than controls (likely providing added social support), a lack of information about possible confounding improvements in lifestyle between groups, and difficulty in replicating both diagnosis and treatment of TABP at other institutions.

Enhancing Recovery in Coronary Heart Disease Patients

Over the past decade, as the data linking depression and social isolation with adverse cardiac outcome became more compelling, it seemed promising to treat these conditions in a clinical trial. Accordingly, the Enhancing

■ ▪ ■

TABLE 30-2   NOTEWORTHY CLINICAL TRIALS

Study	Year published	N	Intervention	Follow-up duration	Psychologic outcome	Cardiac outcome
Psychologic interventions						
Recurrent Coronary Prevention Project	1986	862 270C 592E	Group therapy for type A behavior	4.5 yr	Reductions in type A behavior	44% reduction in 2nd MI; reductions in SCD
ENRICHD	2003	2481 1238C 1243E	Cognitive-behavioral group + individual psychology + sertraline (as needed)	41 mo	Improvement in depression and social isolation at 6 mo	No differences in morbidity or mortality
Jones and West	1996	2328 1155C 1159E	Seven 2-hr group sessions	1 yr	No improvement	No improvement
Blumenthal et al.	1997 and 2002	107 40C 34 Exercise 33 Stress Management	4 mo group + 2 sessions biofeedback	38 mo and 5 yr, respectively	Reductions in depression + hostility	0.26 (P = 0.04) risk of adverse cardiac events in stress management group compared to controls
Denollet and Brutsaert	2001	150 72C 78E	6 weekly group sessions + selected patient individual therapy	9 yr	43% improvement, 15% worsening of mood	17% vs. 4% mortality (P = 0.009) in treated vs. control group
Hamalainen	1995	375 187C 188E	Multiple risk factor rehabilitation, including discussion of psychologic problems, for 3 mo + close contact for 3 yr	15 yr	Not reported	Lower incidence SCD (16.5% vs. 28.9%; P = 0.006); cardiac mortality (47.9% vs 58.5%; P = 0.04) in treated group
Project New Life	1996	268 133C 128E	17 3-hr group sessions + 5-6 booster	4.5 yr	Not reported	Significant difference in total (7 vs. 16; P = 0.02) deaths; fewer cardiac events (P = 0.04)
Pharmacologic intervention						
SADHART	2002	369 183C 186E	Sertraline—safety		Modest improvement, more effective if 1 prior episode or major depression	No significant difference in morbidity; not powered for mortality
Lifestyle trials with a psychologic or behavioral component						
LIFESTYLE	1990, 1993, and 1998	48 20C 28E	Major life change: Diet + yoga + exercise + group therapy	1, 4, 5 yr	Not reported	Regression of atherosclerotic plaque on quantitative angio; improved myocardial perfusion on PET scans
MULTI-CENTER LIFESTYLE	1998	333 139C 194E	As above	3 yr	Not reported	No difference in MI, stroke, or mortality; cost savings $29,528 per patient

MI, myocardial infarction; SCD, sudden cardiac death; PET, positron emission tomography; C, control group; E, experimental group.

Recovery in Coronary Heart Disease Patients (ENRICHD) study[28] was undertaken by the National Heart, Lung and Blood Institute. The largest psychosocial intervention to date, ENRICHD was a randomized clinical trial of individual and group cognitive-behavioral psychotherapy versus usual care for 2481 post-MI patients (1084 women) who met modified *Diagnostic and Statistical Manual of Mental Disorders,* Fourth Edition (DSM IV) criteria for major or minor depression or low perceived social support (LPSS), as measured by a scale specially constructed

for the study. Patients were enrolled within 28 days of MI from eight centers across the United States. At entry into the study, 39% of the cohort were depressed, 26% had LPSS, and 34% met both criteria. Intervention patients were treated with a median of 11 individual psychotherapy sessions, as well as group therapy when feasible, for 6 months and followed for a minimum of 18 months, with an average of 29 months.

Cognitive-behavioral therapy is widely regarded as well-researched and highly effective psychologic treatment for depression.[69] The psychotherapy employed in ENRICHD was developed and supervised by the Aaron Beck Institute in Philadelphia, one of the world's leading authorities in cognitive-behavioral therapy. Sertraline was provided for patients with high scores on the Hamilton Rating Scale for Depression and those who had less than a 50% reduction in Beck Depression Inventory Scores after 5 weeks.

At 6 months, the cognitive-behavioral intervention reduced the number of patients with depression, depression severity, and social isolation in the treated group, compared to usual care controls. However, group differences diminished over time and became nonsignificant for depression at 30 months and nonsignificant for LPPS by 42 months. There were no improvements in recurrent MI or cardiac death with the intervention compared to the control group.

A number of hypotheses have been suggested for the disappointing results of the ENRICHD trial. Because the psychosocial intervention was not sufficiently robust to reduce depression and social isolation by the end of the trial, improvements in cardiac morbidity or mortality from reductions in these psychosocial risk factors would not be expected. Patients were not self-referred, as in traditional psychotherapy practice, and therefore may have been less motivated to engage in therapy and make behavioral changes. It is also possible that patients were recruited too soon after their qualifying MIs (mean = 8 days, median = 6 days), as some patients may have had spontaneous, rapid remission and no need for psychosocial treatment. The intervention lasted for approximately 6 months (with some patients extending their participation in group therapy for an additional 12 weeks), and it has been suggested that 6 months may not be long enough to effect changes powerful enough to improve psychologic or cardiac outcome over the long term.

Perhaps most importantly, both depression and social isolation improved to an unexpected degree in the usual care group, confounding the design of the study. Cumulative use of antidepressants increased steadily in both treatment and control groups over time, from 9.1% at baseline in the treatment group to 28%, and from 4.8% at baseline in the usual care group to 20.6% by the end of the trial. Hence, both treated and control patients may have benefited from antidepressant medication, making the treatment and control groups more homogeneous.

Although the results of ENRICHD are disappointing, the data linking both depression and social isolation with adverse cardiac outcome remain strong.

The Sertraline Antidepressant Heart Attack Randomized Trial

The Sertraline Antidepressant Heart Attack Randomized Trial (SADHART)[27] was a drug trial, with **no psychotherapy**, for depression in post-MI (74%) and unstable angina (26%) patients, conducted to establish the safety and efficacy of sertraline in the cardiac population. SADHART randomized 369 patients to sertraline (n = 186) in flexible doses ranging from 50 to 200 mg or placebo (n = 183) for 24 weeks at 40 outpatient clinics in the United States, Canada, Europe, and Australia. The primary safety outcome measure was change in left-ventricular ejection fraction (EF). Secondary outcomes included adverse cardiac events and changes in depression, as measured by scores on the Hamilton Depression Inventory and the Clinical Global Impression Improvement scale.

Sertraline was found to be safe in this population, with no reductions in EF, even among high-risk patients with a baseline EF of less than 30%. There were also no significant changes in secondary physiologic parameters, including electrocardiograms and Holter incidence of nonsustained ventricular tachycardia. The incidence of major cardiovascular events was 14.5% in the sertraline-treated group compared with 22.4% in the placebo group, a nonsignificant difference. The study was not powered to detect differences in mortality.

As with ENRICHD, SADHART found a high rate of improvement in depression (about 50%) in the control group. Nonetheless, sertraline-treated patients showed significantly greater improvement than control subjects on the Clinical Global Impression Improvement Scale (P = 0.049), supporting a potential benefit of psychotropic intervention for depressed post-MI patients. Treatment with sertraline appeared more effective at improving depression in patients with at least one prior episode of depression (72% vs. 51%; P = 0.003) and in those with the more severe condition of major depressive disorder (78% vs. 45%; P = 0.001).

INTENSIVE LIFESTYLE CHANGES

Likely, the most controversial intervention for secondary prevention comes from the work of Dean Ornish. His first study, the Lifestyle Heart Trial,[70,71] achieved great national attention by demonstrating angiographic evidence for **reversing** coronary atherosclerosis with intensive lifestyle modification—without drugs or surgery. Additionally, positron emission tomography (PET) scans have shown improved myocardial perfusion with lifestyle change.[72]

In the Lifestyle Heart Trial, 48 patients with CHD were randomized to either intensive lifestyle intervention or routine medical care. The program began with a week-long retreat and became a major focus in participants' lives: twice-weekly sessions included exercise, stress management, yoga and meditation, a communal meal, and "group support" psychotherapy. A spouse or significant other was encouraged to attend these 4-hour evening meetings. Patients ate a vegetarian diet with only 6.8% of calories derived from fat. The program required daily yoga practice, which included stretching, relaxation, and meditation for 1 hour, as well as moderate exercise on days when there were no sessions. A minimum of 14 hours per week was required for full participation.

Patients underwent coronary arteriograms before entering the study and again at the end of 1 and 4 years with coronary artery lesions analyzed by quantitative angiography. After 1 year, 82% of experimental subjects showed regression in atherosclerotic lesions compared to 42% of controls.[70] After 4 years, average stenosis diameter decreased from 43.6% to 39.7% in experimental patients but progressed from 41.6% to 51.4% in the control group.[71] Patients in the experimental group also reported dramatic reductions in angina compared to controls. Regression of lesions was associated with overall adherence to the program in a dose-response relationship. Favorable changes in myocardial perfusion, assessed by PET scans, were reported after 5 years of intervention.[72]

Criticisms of the Lifestyle Heart Trial include the small number of subjects, possible flaws in randomization, and substantial numbers of dropouts. This study has generated enormous media attention, although it is based on a total of 48 patients—28 experimental and 20 controls.

Ornish's most recent work, the Multicenter Lifestyle Demonstration Project,[73] was a nonrandomized study of 333 patients provided by an insurance company (194 experimental, 139 controls matched for age, gender, left-ventricular EF, and severity of stenosis score) at 8 sites across the United States, designed to assess whether patients could avoid revascularization by making comprehensive lifestyle changes. Patients had angiographically documented coronary artery disease severe enough to warrant revascularization. Experimental patients underwent intensive treatment similar to the Lifestyle Heart Trial. After 3 years, there were no significant differences in MI, stroke, or deaths (cardiac or other) for treated versus control subjects. The major finding of this demonstration project was an average cost savings of $29,529 per patient because of decreased frequency of PTCA and CABG in the lifestyle group compared with the control group.

In addition to the absence of any prospective, randomized, double-blind trial showing improved outcomes in a reasonable number of patients over an adequate follow-up period, a most important unanswered question about Ornish's intensive lifestyle program is whether a significant percentage of the population can be persuaded to live in ways so far from current cultural norms—and whether favorable results could be attained with less than 14 hours per week devoted to lifestyle modification.

HOME VISITS BY NURSES

The Montreal Heart Attack Readjustment Trial (M-HART) was a novel approach to post-MI care, reported by Frasure-Smith and colleagues in 1997.[74] Post-MI patients (n = 1376, 473 women) were randomized to 1 year of usual care or special intervention with monthly telephone calls to assess patients' stress levels with the General Health Questionnaire (GHQ). Whenever symptoms exceeded a threshold score, nurses made home visits and attempted to resolve whatever problems were causing the patient's distress. Over the year, three fourths of patients had elevated stress scores on at least 1 occasion. An average of six 1-hour home visits were provided by nurses with cardiac experience who were under the supervision of psychiatrists. Individually tailored treatment consisted of education, emotional support, and

referral to other health resources. In contrast to an encouraging pilot study,[75] there was no treatment impact on psychosocial variables or mortality in men. An unexpected finding was that women who received the special treatment were marginally **more likely to die** than those in usual care (hazard ratio = 1.94; CI 0.89–3.80, P = 0.055). In many cases, death was arrhythmogenic and occurred in women with low EFs.

In a retrospective, secondary analysis of M-HART, Cosette and colleagues[76] studied 433 patients (36% women) who received 2 home visits after obtaining high psychologic distress scores on the GHQ. Patients whose distress was improved as a result of the intervention were less likely to die of cardiac causes, less likely to be readmitted to the hospital for any reason, and less likely to be depressed or anxious at 1 year than patients who did not have successful interventions. In other words, when the intervention succeeded at reducing distress there was an improvement in outcome.

The results from M-HART suggest caution in the design of future trials for certain subgroups of cardiac patients. Therefore, hypotheses should be two-sided, allowing for the possibility that outcomes from psychosocial interventions could be beneficial as well as harmful.

PSYCHOLOGIC INTERVENTIONS

A large study conducted in Wales, United Kingdom, assessed the effectiveness of psychologic intervention for cardiac patients, independent of efforts to modify the "standard" risk factors of cigarette smoking, diet, and exercise. Jones and West[77] randomized 2328 post-MI patients to either routine medical care or seven 2-hour psychologic interventions, which included education about stress and CHD, relaxation training, stress management, and individual and group counseling. Although there were encouraging reductions in angina and cardiac mortality at 6 months among intervention patients, after 1 year there were no significant differences in psychologic factors, such as depression and anxiety, or cardiac endpoints, including utilization of medical services, angina, and mortality. One question posed by these results is that because the intervention was not successful at reducing psychosocial factors, why would it be expected to improve cardiac outcome? In our clinical experience, 14 hours of patient contact over a year would not be expected to have much of an impact. In addition, patients were not preselected for any psychologic condition, such as depression or distress—all patients were included in the study.[78]

Blumenthal and colleagues[78,79] randomly assigned 107 CHD patients with evidence of ambulatory or mental stressed–induced myocardial ischemia to a 4-month program of exercise or stress management. Patients living at a great distance from the study site at Duke University Medical Center served as a usual care comparison group. Psychosocial intervention consisted of 16 1.5-hour group sessions based a "cognitive–social" model. Initial sessions provided education about heart disease and were followed by instruction in specific skills on how to avoid stress. Patients were also taught progressive relaxation techniques and had a minimum of two biofeedback sessions. Much of the treatment was modeled after the RCPP. After an average of 38 months, stress management was associated with a 0.26 (P = 0.04) relative risk of an adverse cardiac event compared with usual-care control subjects who did not live near the medical center.[78] Follow-up after 5 years showed a similar reduction in adverse cardiac events as well as considerably reduced medical costs.[79] A larger, fully randomized replication is under way.

In the Netherlands, Denollet and Brutsaert[80] studied 150 men with CHD (n = 78 experimental; n = 72 controls, not randomized) who received either usual care or special intervention that added psychotherapy to standard exercise cardiac rehabilitation. At entry, there were no significant differences between experimental or control patients in severity of cardiac disease, MI, thrombolytic therapy, or medical/surgical treatment. Intervention patients received 36 exercise sessions, as well as 6 weekly 2-hour group therapy sessions along with a significant other, designed to promote a healthy lifestyle. All patients were screened psychologically at entry into the study and, in an effort to tailor treatment to patients' particular issues, 49% (38 of 78) patients were provided weekly, individual psychotherapy by the study's lead author, a cognitive-behavioral psychologist. The intervention lasted 3 months, with 43% of patients (64) reporting improvement and 15% of patients (22) reporting worsening of distress on the Global Mood Scale. At 9-year follow-up, rate of death was 17% (12 of 72) for control patients compared to 4% (3/78) for intervention patients (P = 0.009).

Hamalainen and associates[81] studied a group of 375 acute MI patients (74 women) younger than 65 years of age at entry in Finland. Patients were provided with a comprehensive rehabilitation program that included exercise, smoking cessation, dietary advice, and discussion of psychologic problems. Intervention was most intensive during the first 3 months post-MI, but there was close contact with the health care team for 3 years. Patients were followed for 15 years, with a significantly lower incidence of sudden death (16.5% vs. 28.9%; P = 0.006) and cardiac mortality (47.9% vs. 58.5%; P = 0.04) in the intervention compared to the control group. The protective effects of the comprehensive cardiac rehabilitation program were significant 12 years after all intervention had ceased. Total mortality, however, was similar between groups as a result of excess deaths from cancer in the intervention group.

In a modified replication of the RCPP in Sweden, Burell[82] randomized 268 nonsmoking post-CABG patients to a group program for modification of the TABP and cardiac risk factor education or a control group that received routine care from their own physicians. During the first year, intervention patients met for 17 three-hour group sessions with 5 to 6 "booster sessions" in years 2 and 3. The behavioral treatment was modeled after the RCPP with patients encouraged to reduce anger, impatience, annoyance, and irritation in daily life. "Homework assignments," "drills," and relaxation techniques were provided to facilitate self-observation and reduce type A behavior. At follow-up 4.5 years after surgery, there was a significant difference in total (7 vs. 16, P = 0.02) but not in cardiovascular (5 vs. 8, NS) deaths between treatment and control patients, respectively. There were 14 fatal and nonfatal cardiovascular events (reinfarction, reoperation, or PTCA) in the intervention group versus 19 in the control group (P = 0.04). A limitation of this study is that it was published in a textbook rather than in a peer-reviewed scientific journal.

THE CURRENT STATE OF BEHAVIORAL CARDIOLOGY/CARDIAC PSYCHOLOGY

Over the past decade, the database linking psychosocial factors with the development and outcome from CHD has been greatly expanded. In particular, the evidence linking depression and social isolation with CHD appears robust. There have been numerous studies linking anger and other psychosocial factors with CHD as well, although findings have been less consistent. The current literature on clinical trials, however, is guardedly optimistic. The earliest intervention studies were characterized by few patients and nonstandardized treatments. Despite early encouraging results with type A behavior modification from the RCPP and Project New Life, several large studies were unable to implicate type A behavior as a risk factor,[83,84] and research on the TABP has been largely abandoned in favor of a more specific focus on hostility, one of its core components. Highly researched for several decades, type A behavior has always been controversial; several studies have reported that **untreated** patients with type A behavior **survived their MIs better** than untreated patients assessed with type B behavior, adding to the controversy.[85-87]

Regarding the psychosocial risk factors that have what we consider the best supporting data, assessment has been a critical methodologic issue. Most recent studies have relied on self-report questionnaires, which bias responses by limitations in subjects' self-awareness, as well as their willingness to acknowledge socially undesirable personality characteristics. Many individuals are reluctant to admit that they are depressed, hostile, or socially isolated. Some of the most robust associations in the field have come from studies in which psychosocial factors were assessed by more costly and time-consuming structured interviews. At present, there are no agreed-on standards for assessment of any of the psychosocial risk factors, although some questionnaires, such as the Beck Depression Inventory, the Cook-Medley Hostility Scale, and the Spielberger anger scales, have been used extensively.

Home visits by specially trained nurses to distressed patients used in M-HART, an initially promising and novel approach to post-MI care, not only failed to replicate the improved outcome of its precursor study with men but resulted in an increased risk of arrhythmogenic death among women.

A hopeful finding is the safety and efficacy of treating cardiac patients for depression using sertraline. Unexplained, however, is the robustness of the literature linking depression and social isolation to increased cardiac morbidity and mortality along with the failure of ENRICHD to improve cardiac outcome with intervention for these variables using cognitive-behavioral therapy, one of the most well-respected psychologic treatments for depression.

As clinical trials have become larger and interventions have become more formalized, results appear less favorable. Results from several recent small studies such as those by Denollet and Brutsaert and Hamalainen, although encouraging, lack standardized, reproducible interventions. Indeed, the techniques used in these trials have not been published. To the consternation of many physicians, it is not possible to equate psychosocial intervention with medication or invasive procedures. By its nature, psychosocial intervention is highly variable and depends in great part on the skill sets of both therapist and patient. To complicate matters further, a therapist can be very effective with some individuals and scarcely effective, and even destructive, with others. The capacity to make use of psychotherapy is a variable with tremendous individual differences. Although efforts may be made to formalize an intervention, how much of any program an individual is able to integrate into his or her life is enormously variable. Such complexity undoubtedly contributes to the confusing state of the intervention literature.

Another critical issue is the breadth and intensity of an intervention. Ornish's program requires a great deal of effort by participants—a minimum of 14 hours a week. At the other extreme, the unsuccessful study by Jones and West provided only seven 2-hour sessions over a year and showed no improvement in either quality of life or cardiac outcome. The RCPP required a full year of weekly then monthly sessions before achieving a reduction in recurrent MI; Project New Life provided 15 to 16 3-hour sessions in the first year followed by "booster sessions" in years 2 and 3 to demonstrate reduced morbidity and mortality. We find that it has been quite difficult for most cardiac patients to change lifelong health habits, and intervention, when successful, requires a sustained effort. It is interesting that Jones and West note that their patients rated their program highly but wished that it were more extensive. A dose-response to psychosocial intervention is likely. A critical issue is whether the public can be convinced to take sufficient doses of behavioral medicine to significantly impact their coronary heart disease.

It may also be noteworthy that Jones and West provided treatment for **all** patients—not just those who met eligibility requirements for a stressful condition, such as depression, social isolation, or anger. In their successful intervention, Blumenthal and colleagues chose only patients who demonstrated ambulatory or stress-induced myocardial ischemia. Similarly, Denollet and Brutsaert[80] selected patients who scored high on a distress scale. Future studies may prove to be more effective with more stringent selection criteria.

Peter Kaufmann, Health Scientist Administrator in the Behavioral Medicine Branch of the National Heart, Lung and Blood Institute, has compared the current state of cardiac psychology to the early research on the treatment of cholesterol: although cholesterol was known for quite some time to be a powerful risk factor for CHD, it was only with the advent of the statin drugs that changes in serum cholesterol and subsequent improvements in mortality were sufficiently robust to be evident in clinical trials. By analogy, although there are now considerable data in support of the importance of psychosocial factors for cardiac outcome, there is not yet a standardized treatment that has consistently improved morbidity and mortality (personal communication, 2002). It should be emphasized that most psychosocial intervention programs have reported improvements in quality of life, a worthy goal in its own right: it is not just how long one lives, but how well.

Since Freud's pioneering work at the beginning of the twentieth century, the power of the psyche has been elevated to a major position in both psychology and the popular mind. The increasing influence of Eastern philosophy has reinforced the belief in the power of the mind over the body as we have seen fakirs walk barefoot over hot coals and Buddhist monks raise their body temperature while sitting outdoors in the freezing cold. With a philosophy of "mind over matter" comes a widespread belief that a "proper" mental attitude should contribute to health and well-being and may even reduce morbidity and mortality. However, a "great debate" between longtime supporters and critics of behavioral medicine has challenged whether the power of the mind has been greatly overestimated when treating medical illness.[88]

CONCLUSIONS

1. There is no longer any question that psychosocial factors have a major influence on the onset and course of CHD—although the specific factors that seem most powerful are quite different from what was believed important for the first several decades of research in this field.
2. Depression and social isolation are the most powerful psychosocial risk factors for CHD so far confirmed—for both initial development and progression to recurrent events. Intense anger and hostility seem somewhat less powerful, but likely have some influence.
3. There are many other psychosocial factors proposed as CHD risk factors, including anxiety (particularly "phobic anxiety,"), "vital exhaustion," "job strain," "distress," type A behavior, and others. However, the weight of evidence is insufficient to validate these other psychosocial factors as important because of insufficient number or size of clinical trials, methodologic arguments, lack of standardized or validated measurement or diagnostic tools, nonstandard treatment modalities, and insufficient validation by researchers not part of the group that initially championed a particular factor's importance. This is not to deny that some of these other psychosocial factors might be important, but the current evidence is not yet sufficient to recommend diagnosis or treatment directed at any of these "other" psychosocial factors.
4. A few psychosocial factors are also clear triggers of acute coronary events including acute MI and SCD. Temporary, indeed remarkably short-lived, increases in acute coronary events have been repeatedly observed

just after natural disasters such as earthquakes. Factors that are associated with transient increased risk of acute MI in well designed clinical trials include strenuous physical exercise (especially in sedentary individuals), intense anger, marijuana and cocaine use, sexual relations, circadian rhythms (notably assuming the upright position when getting up in the morning but also a secondary circadian peak of acute events in late afternoon whose external cause is unclear), and possibly day of the week (Monday mornings, perhaps related to returning to work after a weekend off). The prevalence of these "triggers" in the population susceptible to acute CHD events is low, the persistence of risk is relatively short lived (usually 1–2 hours at most), and the total number of acute coronary events that can be related to currently known triggers is quite small. Thus, with the exception of strenuous physical activity in sedentary individuals; chronic, intense anger; and marijuana and cocaine use, elimination of currently identified triggers would not appear to yield major reductions in acute CHD.

5. The greatest current importance of cardiac psychology/behavioral cardiology is likely the improvement of CHD risk-factor modification. Lifestyle change is difficult but vitally important for the vast majority of CHD sufferers. Having cardiac psychologists, or behavioral cardiologists, or whatever the appropriate health professionals are named, as part of the cardiac "team" is, in our opinion, likely to improve currently disappointing rates of successful lifestyle modification. For this reason alone, all those who deal with patients with CHD need to develop behavioral or psychologic skills.

6. There is considerable value in training mental health providers who specialize in cardiac psychology/behavioral cardiology. Regardless of whether routine improvements in cardiac morbidity and mortality with psychosocial intervention will ultimately be demonstrated, a significant percentage of cardiac patients are distressed from this life-threatening condition. Many can benefit from the palliative care provided by mental health specialists and cardiac support groups. A good understanding of cardiology as well as cardiac psychology/behavioral cardiology will assist such psychotherapists in helping patients and their families by promoting heart-healthy living and emotional well-being. Table 30-3 describes patients who, in our opinion, are most likely to benefit from psychosocial intervention.

■ ▪ ■

TABLE 30-3   PATIENTS MOST LIKELY TO BENEFIT FROM PSYCHOSOCIAL INTERVENTION

Young
Multiple modifiable risk factors—cigarette smoker, sedentary, moderately overweight
Depressed
Socially isolated
Highly stressed
Unresolved anger issues

REFERENCES

1. Allan R, Scheidt S: Heart and mind: The practice of cardiac psychology. Washington, DC, American Psychological Association, 1996.
2. Williams RBL Refining the type-A hypothesis: Emergence of the hostility complex. Am J Cardiol 1987; 60:27J-32J.
3. Raynor DA, Pogue-Geile MF, Kamarck TW, et al: Covariation of psychosocial characteristics associated with cardiovascular disease: Genetic and environmental influences. Psychosom Med 2002; 64:191-203.
4. Rozanski A, Blumenthal JA, Kaplan J: Impact of psychological factors on the pathogenesis of cardiovascular disease and implications for therapy. Circulation 1999; 99:2192-2217.
5. Krantz DS, McCeney MK: Effects of psychological and social factors on organic disease: A critical assessment of research on coronary heart disease. Ann Rev Psychol 2002; 53:341-369.
6. Hemingway H, Marmot M: Psychosocial factors in the aetiology and prognosis of coronary heart disease: Systematic review of prospective cohort studies. BMJ 1999; 318:1460-1467.
7. Glassman AH, Shapiro PA: Depression and the course of coronary artery disease. Am J Psychiatry 1998; 155:4-11.
8. Musselman DL, Evans DL, Nemeroff CB: The relationship of depression to cardiovascular disease: Epidemiology, biology, and treatment. Arch Gen Psychiatry 1998; 55:580-592.
9. Januzzi JL, Stern TA, Pasternak RC, et al: The influence of anxiety and depression on outcomes of patients with coronary artery disease. Arch Intern Med 2000; 160:1913-1921.
10. Hemingway H, Malik M, Marmot M: Social and psychological influences on sudden cardiac death, ventricular arrhythmia and cardiac autonomic function. Eur Heart J 2001; 22:1082-1101.
11. MacMahon KMA, Lipp GY: Psychological factors in heart failure. Arch Intern Med 2002; 162:509-516.
12. Bankier B, Littman AB: Psychiatric disorders and coronary heart disease in women: A still neglected topic: Review of the literature from 1971-2000. Psychother Psychosom 2002; 71:133-140.
13. Burg M, Abrams D: Depression in chronic medical illness: The case of coronary heart disease. JCLP/In Session: Psychotherapy in Practice 2001; 57:1323-1337.
14. Ziegelstein RC: Depression in patients recovering from a myocardial infarction. JAMA 2001; 286:1621-1627.
15. Eng PM, Rimm EB, Fitzmaurice G, et al: Social ties and change in social ties in relation to subsequent total cause-specific mortality and coronary heart disease incidence in men. Am J Epidem 2002; 155:700-709.
16. Sears SF, Todaro JF, Lewis TS, et al: Examining the psychosocial impact of implantable cardioverter defibrillators: A literature review. Clin Cardiol 1999; 22:481-489.
17. Curtis BM, O'Keefe JH: Autonomic tone as a cardiovascular risk factor: The dangers of chronic fight or flight. Mayo Clin Proc 2002; 77:45-54.
18. Anda R, Williamson D, Jones D, et al: Depressed affect, hopelessness, and the risk of ischemic heart disease in a cohort of U.S. adults. Epidemiology 1993; 4:285-294.
19. Ferketich AK, Schwartzbaum JA, Frid DJ, et al: Depression as an antecedent to heart disease among women and men in the NHANES I study. Arch Intern Med 2000; 160:1261-1268.
20. Ariyo AA, Haan M, Tangen CM, et al: Depressive symptoms and risks of coronary heart disease and mortality in elderly Americans. Circulation 2000; 102:1773-1779.
21. Schultz R, Beach SR, Ives DG, et al: Association between depression and mortality in older adults: The Cardiovascular Health Study. Arch Intern Med 2000; 160:1761-1768.
22. Barefoot JC, Schroll M: Symptoms of depression, myocardial infarction, and total mortality in a community sample. Circulation 1996; 93:1976-1980.
23. Pratt LA, Ford DE, Crum RM, et al: Depression, psychotropic medication, and risk of myocardial infarction: Prospective data from the Baltimore ECA follow-up. Circulation 1996; 94:3123-3129.
24. Aromaa A, Raitasolo R, Reunanen A, et al: Depression and cardiovascular disease. Acta Psychiatr Scand Suppl 1994; 377: 77-82.
25. Ford DE, Mead LA, Chang PP, et al: Depression is a risk factor for coronary artery disease in men: The precursors study. Arch Intern Med 1998; 158:1422-1426.

26. Wulsin LR, Singal BM: Do depressive symptoms increase the risk for the onset of coronary disease? A systematic quantitative review. Psychosom Med 2003; 65:201-210.

27. Glassman AH, O'Connor CM, Califf RM, et al: Sertraline treatment of major depression in patients with acute MI or unstable angina. JAMA 2002; 288:701-709.

28. Writing Committee for the ENRICHD Investigators: Effects of treating depression and low perceived social support on clinical events after myocardial infarction: The enhancing recovery in coronary heart disease patients (ENRICHD) randomized trial. JAMA 2003; 289:3106-3116.

29. Carney RM, Blumenthal JA, Stein PK, et al: Depression, heart rate variability, and acute myocardial infarction. Circulation 2001; 104:2024-2028.

30. Roose SP, Laghrissi-Thode F, Kennedy JS, et al: Comparison of paroxetine and nortriptyline in depressed patients with ischemic heart disease. JAMA 1998; 279:287-291,

31. Ruberman W, Weinblatt E, Goldberg JD, et al: Psychosocial influences on mortality after myocardial infarction. N Engl J Med 1984; 311:552-559.

32. Case RB, Moss AJ, Case N, et al: Living alone after myocardial infarction: Impact on prognosis. JAMA 1992; 267:515-519.

33. Williams RB, Barefoot JC, Califf RM: Prognostic importance of social and economic resources among medically treated patients with angiographically documented coronary artery disease. JAMA 1992; 267:520-524.

34. Brummett BH, Barefoot JC, Siegler IC, et al: Characteristics of socially isolated patients with coronary artery disease who are at elevated risk for mortality. Psychosom Med 2001; 63:267-272.

35. Miller TQ, Smith TW, Turner CW, et al: A meta-analytic review of research on hostility and health. Psychol Bul 1996; 119:322-348.

36. Williams JE, Paton CC, Siegler IC, et al: Anger proneness predicts coronary heart disease risk: Prospective analysis from the Atherosclerosis Risk in Communities (ARIC) Study. Circulation 2000; 101:2034-2039.

37. Williams JE, Nieto FJ, Sanford CO, et al: The association between trait anger and incident stroke risk: The Atherosclerosis Risk in Communities (ARIC) Study. Stroke 2002; 33:13-20.

38. Eng PM, Fitzmaurice G, Kubzansky LD, et al: Anger expression and risk of stroke and coronary heart disease among male health professionals. Psychosom Med 2003; 65:100-110.

39. Kivimaki M, Leino-Arjas P, Luukkonen R, et al: Work stress and risk of cardiovascular mortality: Prospective cohort study of industrial employees. BMJ 2002; 325:857-860.

40. Kawachi I, Colditz GA, Ascherio A, et al: Prospective study of phobic anxiety and risk of coronary heart disease in men. Circulation 1994; 89:1992-1997.

41. Denollet J, Van Heck GL: Psychological risk factors in heart disease: What type D personality is (not) about. J Psychosom Res 2001; 51:465-468.

42. Kop WJ, Appels AP, Mendes de Leon CF, et al: Vital exhaustion predicts new cardiac events after successful coronary angioplasty. Psychosom Med 1994; 56:281-287.

43. Leor J, Poole WK, Kloner RA: Sudden cardiac death triggered by an earthquake. New Engl J Med 1996; 334:413-419.

44. Meisel SR, Kutz I, Davan KI, et al: Effect of the Iraqi missile war on incidence of acute myocardial infarction and sudden death in Israeli citizens. Lancet 1991; 338:660-661.

45. Muller JE, Kaufmann PG, Luepker RV, et al: Mechanisms precipitating acute cardiac events: Review and recommendations of an NHLBI workshop. Circulation 1997; 96:3233-3239.

46. Mittleman MA, Maclure M, Tofler GH, et al: Triggering of acute myocardial infarction by heavy physical exertion. N Engl J Med 1993; 329:1677-1683.

47. Mittleman MA, Maclure M, Sherwood JB, et al: Triggering of acute myocardial infarction onset by episodes of anger. Circulation 1995; 92:1720-1725.

48. Muller JE, Mittleman MA, Maclure M, et al: Triggering of myocardial infarction by sexual activity. Low absolute risk and prevention by regular exercise. JAMA 1996; 275:1405-1409.

49. Mittleman MA, Lewis RA, Maclure M, et al: Triggering myocardial infarction by marijuana. Circulation 2001; 103:2805-2809.

50. Mittleman MA, Mintzer D, Maclure M, et al: Triggering of myocardial infarction by cocaine. Circulation 1999; 99:2737-2741.

51. Willich SN, Lowel J, Lewis M, et al: Increased Monday risk of acute myocardial infarction in the working population. Circulation 1992; 86(Suppl 1):61.

52. Muller JE: Circadian variation and triggering of acute coronary events. Am Heart J 1999; 137 (Part 2): S1-S8.

53. Fries R, Konig J, Schafers HJ, et al: Triggering effect of physical and mental stress on spontaneous ventricular tachyarrhythmias in patients with implantable cardioverter-defibrillators. Clin. Cardiol 2002; 25:474-478.

54. Lampert R, Joska T, Burg MM, et al: Emotional and physical precipitants of ventricular arrhythmia. Circulation 2002; 106:1800-1805.

55. Mumford AD, Warr KV, Owen SJ, et al: Delays by patients in seeking treatment for acute chest pain: Implications for achieving earlier thrombolysis. Postgrad Med J 1999; 75(880):90-95.

56. Luepker RV, Raczynski JM, Osganian S, et al: Effect of a community intervention on patient delay and medical service use in acute coronary heart disease: The Rapid Early Action for Coronary Treatment (REACT) Trial. JAMA 2000; 284:60-67.

57. Osganian SK, Zapka JG, Feldman HA, et al: Use of emergency medical services for suspected acute cardiac ischemia among demographic and clinical patient subgroups: The REACT trial. Prehosp Emerg Care 2002; 6:175-185.

58. Blohm M, Herlitz J, Hartford, M, et al: Consequences of a media campaign focusing on delay in acute myocardial infarction. Am J Cardiol 1992; 69:411-413.

59. Sirous F Le: Deni dans la maladie coronarienne [Denial in coronary disease]. Canadian Med J 1992; 147:315-321.

60. Fowers BJ: The cardiac denial of impact scale: A brief, self-report research measure. J Psychosom Res 1992; 36:469-475.

61. Nunes EV, Frank KA, Kornfeld DS: Psychologic treatment for the type A behavior pattern and for coronary heart disease: A meta-analysis of the literature. Psychosomatic Med 1987; 48:159-173.

62. Rahe RH, Ward HW, Hayes V: Brief group therapy in myocardial infarction rehabilitation: Three- to four-year follow-up of a controlled trial. Psychosom Med 1979; 41:229-242.

63. Friedman M, Thoresen CE, Gill JJ, et al: Alteration of type-A behavior and its effect on cardiac recurrences in post myocardial infarction patients: Summary results of the Recurrent Coronary Prevention Project. Am Heart J 1986; ll2:653-665.

64. Linden W, Stossel C, Maurice J: Psychosocial interventions for patients with coronary artery disease. Arch Intern Med 1996; 156:745-752.

65. Dusseldorp E, van Elderen T, Maes S, et al: A meta-analysis of psychoeducational programs for coronary heart disease patients. Health Psychology 1999; 18:506-519.

66. Friedman M, Powell LH, Thoresen CE, et al: Effect of discontinuance of type-A behavioral counseling on type-A behavior and cardiac recurrence rate of post myocardial infarction patients. Am Heart J 1987; ll4:483-490.

67. Powell LH, Thoresen CE: Effects of type-A behavioral counseling and severity of prior acute myocardial infarction on survival. Am J Cardiol 1988; 62:1159-1163.

68. Brackett CD, Powell LH: Psychosocial and physiological predictors of sudden cardiac death after healing of acute myocardial infarction. Am J Cardiol 1988; 61:979-983.

69. Deckersbach T, Gershuny BS, Otto MW: Cognitive-behavioral therapy for depression: Applications and outcomes. Psychiatr Clin North Am 2000; 23:795-809.

70. Ornish D, Brown SE, Scherwitz LW, et al: Can lifestyle changes reverse coronary heart disease? Lancet 1990; 336:129-133.

71. Ornish D, Brown SE, Billings JH, et al: Can lifestyle changes reverse coronary atherosclerosis? Four-year results of the Lifestyle Heart Trial [Abstract]. Circulation 1993; 88:I-385.

72. Ornish D, Scherwitz LW, Billings JH, et al: Intensive lifestyle changes for reversal of coronary heart disease. JAMA 1998; 280:2001-2007.

73. Ornish D: Avoiding revascularization with lifestyle changes: the multicenter lifestyle demonstration project. Am J Cardiol 1998; 82:72T-76T.

74. Frasure-Smith N, Lesperance F, Prince R, et al: Randomized trial of home-based psychosocial nursing intervention for patients recovering from myocardial infarction. Lancet 1997; 350: 473-479.

75. Frasure-Smith N, Prince R: Long-term follow-up of the Ischemic Heart Disease Life Stress Monitoring Program. Psychosom Med 1989; 51:485-513.

76. Cosette S, Frasure-Smith N, Lesperance F: Clinical implications of a reduction in psychological distress on cardiac prognosis in a psychosocial intervention program. Psychosom Med 2001; 63:257-266.

77. Jones DA, West RR: Psychological rehabilitation after myocardial infarction: Multicentre randomized controlled trial. BMJ 1996; 313:1517-1521.

78. Blumenthal JA, Jiang W, Babyak M, et al: Stress management and exercise training in patients with myocardial ischemia. Arch Intern Med 1997; 157:2213-2223.

79. Blumenthal JA, Babyak M, Wei J, et al: Usefulness of psychosocial treatment of mental stress-induced myocardial ischemia in men. Am J Cardiol 2002:89:164-168.

80. Denollet J, Brutsaert DL: Reducing emotional distress improves prognosis in coronary heart disease. Circulation 2001; 104:2018-2023.

81. Hamalainen H, Luurila OJ, Kallio V, et al: Reduction in sudden deaths and coronary mortality in myocardial infarction patients after rehabilitation: 15-year follow-up study. European Heart J 1995; 16:1839-1844.

82. Burell G: Group psychotherapy in Project New Life: Treatment of coronary-prone behavior for post coronary artery bypass patients. *In* Allan R, Scheidt S (eds). Heart and mind: The practice of cardiac psychology. Washington DC, American Psychological Association, 1996.

83. Shekelle RB, Hulley SB, Neaton JD, et al: The MRFIT Behavior Pattern Study II: Type A behavior and incidence of coronary heart disease. Am J Epidemiol 1985; 122:559-570.

84. Case RB, Heller SS, Case NB, et al: Type A behavior and survival after acute myocardial infarction. New Eng J Med 1985; 312:737-741.

85. Barefoot JC, Peterson BL, Harrell FE, et al: Type A behavior and survival: A follow-up study of 1,467 patients with coronary artery disease. Am J Cardiol 1989; 64:427-432.

86. Ragland DR, Brand RJ: Type A behavior and mortality from coronary heart disease. New Engl J Med 1988; 318:65-69.

87. Ahern DK, Gorkin L, Anderson JL, et al: Biobehavioral variables and morality in the Cardiac Arrhythmia Pilot Study (CAPS). Am J Cardiol 1990; 66:59-62.

88. Markovitz JH, Williams RB, Schneiderman N, et al: The great debate. Psychosom Med 2002; 64:549-570.

chapter 31

Multiple Risk-Factor Intervention Trials

Bret Scher
Erminia M. Guarneri
Jacqueline A. Hart
Dean Ornish

INTRODUCTION

Coronary artery disease (CAD) is the leading cause of morbidity and mortality in the Western industrialized world. Approximately 12.6 million people in the United States carry the diagnosis of CAD. In 1999, there were 1.1 million heart attacks, 355,000 coronary bypass operations, and 600,000 percutaneous transluminal coronary angioplasties (PTCA) in Americans, with a total estimated cost of $329.2 billion.[1]

Increasing evidence supports the idea that much of this cost—both financial and in human suffering—may be greatly reduced by implementing comprehensive risk-factor intervention strategies. These strategies may include behavioral interventions for motivating patients to make and maintain comprehensive changes in lifestyle (e.g., optimal diets, exercise, smoking cessation, stress management techniques, and psychosocial support) and drug therapy (e.g., lipid-lowering drugs and antihypertensive medications).

Although more research is needed, we believe that, taken as a whole, the available body of evidence is sufficient to make clear recommendations. This is especially true given that the risks of changing diet and lifestyle are quite low, whereas the potential benefits are often substantial. In short, the limiting factor at this time is not a lack of scientific and clinical data; rather, it is a lack of education, infrastructure, and third-party reimbursement necessary to provide this information to the patients and health professionals who may benefit from it.

This chapter selectively reviews the literature. Rather than providing an encyclopedic listing of all of the multiple risk-factor intervention trials that have been conducted, we focus on a few of the most important and representative studies and synthesize their key lessons and applications to patient care. Such studies include individual-level clinical trials that use discrete clinical endpoints and/or intermediate outcomes as well as community-level intervention trials. We focus on nonpharmacologic approaches to risk-factor modification, particularly studies that affect more than one risk factor simultaneously; there is evidence that synergy often exists between various cardiac risk factors. We describe studies of pharmacologic interventions (e.g., lipid-lowering drugs, antihypertensive medications) only if they also included one or more behavioral interventions.

ISSUES IN MULTIPLE RISK-FACTOR TRIALS

Multiple risk-factor intervention trials are inherently messy. The scientific method and the randomized controlled trial are easiest to implement in animal studies, where one has complete control over the environment, or in drug studies where one can conduct double-blinded, placebo-controlled clinical trials. In a classic randomized controlled trial, the investigators study one independent variable (e.g., a drug) and one dependent variable (e.g., a disease) while balancing all other variables.

When asking patients to make multiple changes in diet and lifestyle, however, the issues are much more complex. In regards to the study design, we need to know the following:

How does one control for the competing effects of multiple interventions?

Which social factors influence and may confound the interpretation of medical outcomes?

Can one conduct a true randomized controlled trial with behavioral interventions? (By definition, double-blinded studies are usually impossible when one group of patients is asked to make diet and lifestyle changes because it is obvious to both patients and investigators which group is receiving the intervention.)

How can one assess the relative and potentially confounding contribution of each component of an intervention?

From a clinical perspective, we need to know:

How can patients be motivated to make and maintain intensive lifestyle changes?

How much change in behavior is required to achieve a significant change in a risk factor? How much change in a risk factor, in turn, is required to achieve a clinically significant effect? Which is more important—the relative reduction or absolute reduction in a risk factor?

EPIDEMIOLOGIC STUDIES AND THE DISCOVERY OF RISK FACTORS

Although the concept of "risk factors" is now widely understood, this idea has been established for only a short period. Epidemiologic studies will not be the focus of this chapter, but it is worth reviewing the early developments of epidemiology as the discipline evolved into an important tool to advance knowledge of cardiovascular disease (CVD). Starting in the late 1940s, epidemiologic prospective studies have uncovered associations between certain factors and the development and progression of CAD.

Cardiovascular risk factors can be classified as either modifiable or nonmodifiable (Table 31-1). These risk factors often confer not only an additive but also a multiplicative effect.[2] This synergy is particularly true of cigarette smoking and its relation to other risk factors.[3]

According to William Kannel, one of the principal investigators of the Framingham Heart Study, "Epidemiology has become the basic science of preventive cardiology . . . Clinicians now look to epidemiological research to provide definitive information about possible predisposing factors for cardiovascular disease and preventive measures that are justified. As a result, clinicians are less inclined to regard usual or average values as acceptable and are more inclined to regard optimal values as 'normal.' Cardiovascular events are coming to be regarded as a medical failure rather than the first indication of treatment."[4]

Cardiovascular disease epidemiology began in 1948 with the advent of the Seven Countries Study[5] and the Framingham Heart Study.[6] At that time, many researchers believed that CVD must have a single origin. Exercise was considered dangerous for most people with CVD, and the idea that dietary fat, blood pressure, elevated blood cholesterol levels, and smoking were important causes of CVD was controversial.

As the importance of these risk factors became better documented, interest grew in studying what happens when these risk factors were modified. Although advances in conventional treatments were occurring rapidly (e.g., the advent of coronary artery bypass surgery, PTCA, new categories of medications, etc.), half of coronary heart disease (CHD) deaths occur suddenly in people without prior diagnosis of heart disease, and most strokes occur without prior transient ischemic attacks.[7] Therefore, the need for prevention became increasingly understood.

INTERVENTION TRIALS

Epidemiologic studies observed associations between various risk factors and CVD. Based on these observations, a number of interventional studies were conducted to determine if some of these risk factors could be modified and, if so, what the effects on CVD incidence, mortality, or progression of atherosclerotic disease would be. Individual-level trials with hard clinical endpoints or intermediate outcomes are listed in Table 31-2.

Individual-Level Trials with Hard Clinical Endpoints

The **Multiple Risk Factor Intervention Trial (MRFIT)** was a randomized controlled clinical trial to test the effect of a multifactorial intervention program on CHD mortality in 12,866 high-risk men aged 35 to 57 years.[8] In this seminal trial, men were randomly assigned either to a special intervention (SI) program consisting of stepped-care treatment for hypertension, counseling for cigarette smoking, and dietary advice for lowering blood cholesterol levels or to their usual sources of health care in the community (UC).

The primary outcome measure was death from CAD. Additional outcome measures included death from other cerebrovascular diseases, all-cause mortality, nonfatal myocardial infarction (MI), change in lipid profiles with comparison between the SI and UC groups, change in resting electrocardiograms (ECGs), change in resting diastolic blood pressure, self-reported smoking histories with verification by serum thiocyanate levels, and change in exercise treadmill tests.

The modalities used in the SI group were as follows:

1. Weight reduction, sodium restriction, and a stepwise approach to blood pressure treatment using medications (beginning with thiazide diuretics, then adding beta blockers, and then other medications as needed).
2. Smoking cessation programs, including behavioral modification, aversive techniques, hypnosis in selected

■ ▦ ■

TABLE 31-1   RISK FACTORS FOR CARDIOVASCULAR DISEASE

Modifiable risk factors proven to reduce cardiovascular risk

1. Cigarette smoking
2. Elevated LDL cholesterol
3. Hypertension
4. Low HDL

Modifiable risk factors that may reduce cardiovascular risk

1. Physical activity
2. Obesity
3. Psychologic factors
4. Lack of social support
5. Lipoprotein (a)
6. Elevated levels of homocysteine
7. Small dense LDL
8. Low HDL 2B
9. Alcohol consumption
10. Plasma fibrinogen
11. Insulin resistance/diabetes mellitus
12. Elevated triglyceride level
13. Low educational level
14. Low socioeconomic status

Nonmodifiable risk factors

Age
Gender
Family history

LDL, low-density lipoprotein; HDL, high-density lipoprotein.

■ ■ ■

TABLE 31-2   TRIAL SUMMARIES

INDIVIDUAL-LEVEL TRIALS WITH HARD CLINICAL ENDPOINTS

Trial	Patients	Intervention	Findings
MRFIT	12,866 high-risk patients	Counseling for tobacco use and diet, medication for HTN vs. control	Both groups reduced risk factors No significant mortality difference at 7 years
Oslo	1232 patients aged 40–49 yr in upper quartile of cardiac risk	AHA step 1 diet and smoking cessation vs. control	Reduced total and LDL cholesterol Decreased composite cardiac events but increased mortality from HTN therapy

INDIVIDUAL-LEVEL TRIALS WITH INTERMEDIATE OUTCOMES

Trial	Patients	Intervention	Findings
Heidelberg	113 patients with stable CAD	AHA Step 1 diet and moderate exercise vs. more strict low-fat diet plus an organized exercise program	Fewer percentage of patients had progression of angiographic CAD with improved exercise thallium tests
SCRIP	300 patients with stable CAD	Usual care or a multifactorial risk-reduction program of diet, exercise, smoking cessation, and close follow-up	Significant reduction in LDL, TG, and increase in HDL. 47% less progression of CAD at 4 years
Lifestyle Heart	48 patients with stable CAD	Low-fat vegetarian diet, aerobic exercise, stress management, smoking cessation, and group support vs. usual care	Reduction in LDL, angina, and angiographic coronary stenosis
Stefanick et al	367 patients with dyslipidemia	NCEP step 2 diet plus aerobic exercise vs. aerobic exercise alone, diet alone, or control	Diet plus exercise significantly reduced LDL 14.5% without a change in HDL compared to control Diet alone and exercise alone did not have a significant effect
Multicenter Lifestyle Demonstration Project (not a randomized trial)	194 patients with CAD qualifying for revascularization compared to case-control	12 months of exercise; stress management; group support; and low-fat, low-calorie diet compared to matched controls	Decreased revascularization by 77% with no difference in adverse cardiac events Cost savings of $29,529

COMMUNITY-LEVEL TRIALS

Trial	Patients	Intervention	Findings
WHO	All men aged 40–59 yr in the study factories	Educational materials on smoking cessation, low-fat diet, daily exercise, hypertension treatment	Nonsignificant reduction in cardiac outcomes Only the Belgian cohort had a significant improvement, which correlated with more health provider contact
Minnesota Heart Health Program	50,000 people from 6 communities	Multiple educational interventions directed toward the community	No statistically significant difference between the groups, but both groups reduced risk factors
Stanford Five City	320,300 subjects in 2 treatment and 3 control cities	Multiple educational interventions directed toward the community	There were significant baseline differences between the groups, but the intervention group had improved knowledge and reduction in total cholesterol and fewer active smokers

HTN, hypertension; AHA, American Heart Association; CAD, coronary artery disease; LDL, low-density lipoprotein; TG, triglycerides; HDL, high-density lipoprotein.

instances, and a 10-week group support session. Group support was the most effective of these techniques for getting people to quit permanently. The investigators from MRFIT did not intervene with pipe or cigar smokers, only cigarette smokers.

3. Dietary counseling for hypercholesterolemia initially aimed to reduce saturated fat to no more than 10% of total calories and restrict cholesterol ingestion to 300 mg/day; in 1976, the study protocol was changed to no more than 8% of total calories from saturated fat and 250 mg or less of cholesterol per day. These differences reflect the American Heart Association (AHA) Step I and Step II dietary guidelines (200 mg cholesterol/day), respectively.

The SI group was seen at least every 4 months by a variety of health care professionals on a multidisciplinary team. The UC group received treatment from their usual physician(s) and yearly check-ups by health care providers of the MRFIT study. Outcome measures were examined annually for the duration of the study.[9]

Over an average follow-up period of 7 years, risk-factor levels declined in both groups but to a greater degree for the SI men. Mortality from CHD was 17.9 deaths per 1000 in the SI group and 19.3 per 1000 in the UC group, a statistically nonsignificant difference (90% confidence interval, −15%—25%). The difference in total mortality was also not statistically significant, with 41.2 per 1000 in the SI group and 40.4 per 1000 in the UC group.

The lack of a statistically significant difference was disappointing. However, a more detailed analysis of the data suggests that patients in the SI group did not change risk factors as much as intended, whereas patients in the UC group changed risk factors more than expected compared with the general population.

Despite the problems in the MRFIT study, it was a landmark trial. It was the first intensive, comprehensive, long-term intervention looking at multiple risk factors simultaneously and using a multidisciplinary approach. Given the size of the trial, the investigators did a remarkable job with recruitment and follow-up; there was less than a 10% total dropout rate over the 7-year treatment period. This study was an ambitious undertaking; only studies of this scope could begin to address questions about mortality. Finally, MRFIT illustrates that implementation of a comprehensive approach to lifestyle change can significantly affect risk-factor modification, which has been a prelude to subsequent research; the investigators of MRFIT had particular success in the area of smoking cessation.

The **Oslo Study**, started in the early 1970s, was also designed to look at the causal relationship between coronary risk-factor modification and coronary events in subjects without identified CAD. The trial enrolled 1232 male residents of Oslo, Norway between the ages of 40 and 49 years with hypercholesterolemia (serum cholesterol levels between 290 and 380 mg/dL), systolic blood pressure less than 150 mm Hg, a coronary risk score in the upper quartile of risk (based on cholesterol levels, smoking, and blood pressure), and a ECG. Participants were randomly assigned to either an intervention or control group and were followed for 5 years. The principal outcome measure was coronary events defined as nonfatal MI, fatal MI, or sudden death. The incidence of strokes was also assessed.

The intervention group received initial evaluation and educational training in a diet similar to an AHA Step 1 diet as well as in smoking cessation, with follow-up every 6 months by a multidisciplinary team. The control group received follow-up examinations once per year by a physician.

At baseline, the two groups were similar with regards to cholesterol level, tobacco consumption, and blood pressure. Following 5 years of intervention, total and low-density lipoprotein (LDL) cholesterol were both 13% lower in the intervention group compared with the control group, and triglyceride levels were 20% lower. High-density lipoprotein (HDL) levels remained unchanged in both groups. Tobacco consumption was decreased by 45% in the intervention group compared with the control group at the 5-year point. Mean body weight was also significantly reduced in the intervention group compared with control. Degree of physical activity and level of blood pressure remained unchanged in both groups compared with baseline.

Unlike MRFIT, there was a significant reduction of fatal MI, nonfatal MI, sudden death, and cerebrovascular accidents in the intervention group compared with controls. Although overall cardiac mortality was 55% lower and total mortality was 33% lower in the intervention group, these differences did not reach statistical significance.[10]

The Oslo Trial also looked at hypertension treatment in 785 men with moderately elevated blood pressure (systolic between 150 and 179 mm Hg and diastolic between 90 and 110 mm Hg). They were randomly assigned to drug treatment or usual care without a placebo intervention. As in MRFIT, there was no difference in the treatment group compared to control in terms of cardiovascular events despite a statistically significant change in both diastolic and systolic blood pressure from baseline compared with the control group.[11] Antihypertensive drugs included hydrochlorothiazide, α-methyldopa, and propranolol.

The Oslo Trial supports the impact of reducing two risk factors—cigarette smoking and hypercholesterolemia—on lowering the incidence of MIs, strokes, and cardiovascular deaths. Hypertension as a risk factor was separated in the Oslo Trial but was not in MRFIT. Although the Oslo Trial investigators achieved significant reduction in blood pressure levels, there was no significant difference between groups with regard to major cardiovascular morbidity or mortality. In fact, there was a nonsignificant trend toward higher CHD, including sudden cardiac death, in the treated group. As in the MRFIT study, antihypertensive drugs may have had unanticipated side effects that negated any potential benefit from the lower blood pressure.

A number of trials have examined various aspects of diet, an important component of lifestyle targeted by some multiple intervention trials. Dietary trials are reviewed in Chapters 29 and are not comprehensively discussed here. A few trials are highlighted here. The **Indian Heart Study**[12] found that a semivegetarian diet emphasizing fruits, vegetables, whole grains, and nuts was associated with a 41% reduction in coronary death and a 38% reduction in nonfatal MIs. The **Lyon Diet Heart Study**, a randomized, single-blind study enrolled approximately 600 patients with a recent MI and randomized them to a "Mediterranean" diet or a "prudent Western" diet.[13] The Mediterranean diet consisted of "bread, root vegetables and green vegetables, more fish, less meat, no day without fruit" in addition to olive and rapeseed oil and margarine high in alpha linolenic acid. The goal of the diet was less than 35% of calories from fat with less than 10% saturated fat, less than 4% linoleic acid, and more than 0.6% α-linolenic acid (a precursor to n-3 long-chain fatty acids).

The 27-month data showed a significant reduction in total deaths (20 vs. 8, P = 0.02), cardiovascular deaths (16 vs. 3), and combined death and nonfatal MI (33 vs. 8, P < 0.001).[14] The 46-month analysis, which had 204 control and 219 experimental subjects,[15] showed a reduction in all-cause and cardiovascular mortality as well as the combined endpoint of recurrent MI and cardiac death for the Mediterranean diet (1.24 per 100 patients per year vs. 4.07 in the control). This accounts to a 50% to 70% reduction depending on the outcome measured. When all endpoints were combined, the reduction was less impressive but still statistically significant at 37% (104 vs. 68). The biggest difference was seen in the reduction of nonfatal MIs.

A number of lessons can be derived from this study. First, the Mediterranean diet and addition of α-linolenic acid (a source of protective omega-3 fatty acids) had a significant cardioprotective effect when compared with a diet equivalent to the AHA Step 1 diet. This suggests that many physicians may not go far enough when prescribing traditional AHA diets to patients and that specific components of the diet may have as much importance as do the fat and cholesterol content. Second, the majority of subjects still complied with the diet 4 years after randomization. The authors concluded that the prevalent opinion that the Mediterranean diet is too hard to follow is not accurate as long the education and follow-up are done properly.

Other clinical trials have focused on particular nutrients rather than the overall diet. An active area of investigation is omega-3 fatty acids. Data from retrospective and case-control studies suggest that fish oil and omega-3 polyunsaturated fatty acids (n-3 PUFA) may be beneficial in preventing CVD.[16] Fish oil and n-3 PUFA have been used interchangeably in the literature, and the best study looking at this is the **GISSI Prevenzione Study**.[17] Although this was a trial of dietary supplements, it has been extrapolated to relate to n-3 PUFA from food intake as well. GISSI was a large multicenter, open-label study with more than 11,000 patients who had had a MI within the past 3 months. Patients were randomized to one of four groups: (1) 1 g/day of n-3 PUFA (ratio of EPA/DHA = 1:2), (2) 300 mg of vitamin E, (3) n-3 PUFA plus vitamin E, or (4) control group. After only 3 months there was a significant reduction in all-cause mortality in the n-3 PUFA group compared to controls (1.1 vs. 1.6, $P = 0.037$), which remained significant at the final 3.5-year follow-up (8.4% vs. 9.8%, $P = 0.006$).[18] In addition, sudden cardiac death was significantly reduced at the 4-month point (0.5% vs. 7%, $P = 0.046$) and remained significant at the 42-month point (2.0% vs. 0.7% $P = 0.0006$). Because the same beneficial effect should be seen with fatty fish consumption, those who cannot tolerate the capsules will have a good alternate source of n-3 PUFAs. Of note, vitamin E had no significant beneficial effect.

The reduction in sudden cardiac death without a change in nonfatal MIs suggests that n-3 PUFAs have an antiarrhythmic and antifibrillatory effect but not an effect on progression of atherosclerosis or plaque stabilization. This study also suggests that the effects of n-3 PUFAs are evident within 3 to 4 months of initiating them. For patients with known CAD, n-3 PUFA either in pill or food form should be routinely recommended. Studies in primary prevention are lacking, but the risk-benefit ratio suggests that n-3 PUFAs may be useful in primary prevention as well.

Individual-Level Intervention Trials with Intermediate Outcomes

Several trials have used angiography to measure changes in coronary atherosclerosis as the primary outcome variable under investigation.[19-24] A few trials were also able to look at cardiovascular morbidity and mortality, but, for the most part, these trials were not powered to examine clinical endpoints. The major risk factor examined in these trials was cholesterol, except for the Stanford Coronary Risk Intervention Project (SCRIP; see later in this chapter), which considered multiple risk factors simultaneously.

The Heidelberg Trial[25] for 1 year followed 113 subjects who were randomized to one of the following: (1) a control group that received advice about the AHA Step 1 diet and moderate aerobic exercise or (2) an intervention group that was asked to follow a lower-fat diet (20% fat, <200 mg/day dietary cholesterol, P/S ratio >1) and a specific physical activity program involving 30 minutes of exercise at home on a daily basis at 75% of the maximal heart rate plus two 60-minute group training sessions per week where they received ongoing advice and motivation for compliance. Patients assigned to the intervention group stayed on a metabolic unit during the initial 3 weeks of the program where they were specifically instructed on how to meet their new dietary requirements.

During strict supervision on the metabolic unit, total cholesterol decreased 23% in the intervention group. In the months after leaving the unit, there was a considerable erosion of dietary discipline, and average reduction of lipoproteins was only 10%. Cholesterol levels in the control group remained unchanged.

Results of quantitative coronary arteriography were analyzed on both a per-patient and a per-lesion basis using both minimum diameter and percent diameter stenosis. According to minimal diameter reduction analyzed on a per patient basis in the intervention group, 23% of patients had disease progression, 45% had no change, and 32% had a regression of disease. In the control group, the incidence of progression was noted in 48% of patients, no change in 35%, and regression in 17%. According to relative diameter reduction, progression was noted in 20% of patients, no change in 50%, and regression in 30% of the intervention group. In the control group, coronary morphology deteriorated in 42%, no change was noted in 54%, and regression was noted in 4%. Both groups differed significantly from each other ($P < 0.001$). On a per lesion basis, no significant change was noted either in relative diameter reduction ($65 \pm 24\%$ vs. $64 \pm 23\%$) or minimal diameter reduction (0.92 ± 0.72 mm vs. 0.91 ± 0.67 mm).

Exercise thallium scintigraphy performed in these patients showed statistically significant improvements in myocardial perfusion when compared with the control group. Of great interest is that this improvement occurred although, as noted earlier, there was no significant improvement in coronary atherosclerosis on a per lesion basis. Indeed, the investigators found that a decrease in myocardial ischemia was not limited to patients with regression but also occurred in individual patients with no change or significant progression. Possible mechanisms of improvement in myocardial perfusion in the absence of regression of atherosclerosis might include improved exercise-induced stimulation of growth in collateral circulation and improvements in blood rheology or endothelial dysfunction. In hindsight, this trial may have been one of the early trials to show the effect of CAD as a systemic disease and thus its response to the "systemic" therapy of lifestyle modification.

The **Stanford Coronary Risk Intervention Project (SCRIP)** applied a stepwise approach combining intensive lifestyle change and medication.[26] Quantitative coronary arteriography was the primary endpoint measure. Of the 4771 patients (recruited from four institutions) who were initially screened, 538 (11.3%) were eligible, and 300 (56%) of those eligible agreed to be randomized to either usual care with their personal physician or to an individualized, multifactorial, risk-reduction program managed by the SCRIP staff in cooperation with the subject's personal physician. Recruitment took place between 1984 and 1987, and participants were followed for 4 years. Eligibility criteria included age younger than 75 years; residence within a 5-hour drive of Stanford University; and lack of severe congestive heart failure, pulmonary disease, intermittent claudication, and noncardiac life-threatening illness.

The risk-reduction intervention included an initial risk stratification and goal-setting session with a SCRIP nurse. Follow-up for the intervention group was approximately every 2 to 3 months, whereas follow-up for the control group was determined by subjects' usual physician. As part of the intake, the SCRIP staff tried to determine how likely it would be that a particular subject would meet the maximal clinical goal of an LDL cholesterol of less than 110 mg/dL within the first year without the use of medication. If the staff determined that a person was unlikely to meet the goal by lifestyle intervention (it is not clear how that determination was made), then a lipid-lowering medication was prescribed. Such medication was also added during the trial if needed. By the end of the first year, 70.6% of the subjects in the SCRIP treatment arm were on medication; this figure reached 89.9% by the end of the fourth year. In contrast, only 11% and 22.6% of the usual-care subjects were on lipid-lowering medication by the end of the first and fourth years, respectively.

The lifestyle intervention included a moderately low-fat diet, physical activity, and counseling for smoking cessation. The recommended diet was less than 20% of calories from fat, less than 6% of calories from saturated fat, and less than 75 mg of cholesterol per day. This represented a diet more restrictive than the AHA Step 2 diet. The goal of the physical activity program for the risk-reduction group was to increase the subject's level from his or her baseline. Staff psychologists gave current and recent ex-smokers advice to stop smoking and prevent relapse. The risk-reduction subjects returned every 2 to 3 months at which time lipids, body weight, and blood pressure were measured and adherence to the individually prescribed lifestyle program was evaluated.

Data from 274 (91.3%) of the original 300 subjects randomized were available at the end of four years. At baseline, there were significant differences between the two groups, with a higher percentage of women, higher HDL, lower average weight, significantly less daily cholesterol ingestion, and a more favorable polyunsaturated to saturated fat ratio in the risk reduction group as compared with usual care. At the conclusion of the trial, there were clinically significant improvements in percent body fat, weight, blood pressure (particularly systolic), LDL cholesterol, apolipoprotein B levels, triglycerides, HDL cholesterol, and exercise capacity in the treatment group compared to controls. Overall,

these changes reduced cardiac risk based on the calculated Framingham score in the treatment arm by 22%. Although not statistically significant, risk-factor profiles in the control group worsened in the areas of smoking, blood pressure, and weight, which may be of some clinical relevance despite the lack of statistical significance. There were no significant differences between the groups in the change in percentage of smokers during the trial nor in lipoprotein(a) levels; and among the smokers in the treatment group, the number of cigarettes smoked per day decreased.

The primary endpoint for the SCRIP trial was minimum diameter as assessed by quantitative coronary arteriography. Both groups had progression of disease based on minimal diameter change, which was the factor by which the trial was powered. The risk-reduction group, however, had a 47% lower rate of progression per individual and a 58% lower rate of worsening in diseased vessel segments than the usual-care group. This difference was statistically significant. Women had the same rate of progression as men in the control group; however, women who received the treatment intervention had less progression than men did in the same arm. A multivariate analysis showed that the three variables that best predicted rate of change in minimum diameter included exercise performance by treadmill (specifically METS), Framingham risk score (based on systolic blood pressure, total cholesterol, HDL, and smoking status), and dietary fat intake.

Although not designed for this purpose, SCRIP investigators reported clinical events, which were as follows: five cardiac-related deaths (three in usual-care and two in risk-reduction); one noncardiac-related death from cancer in the risk-reduction group; and 17 nonfatal MIs (11 in usual-care, six in risk-reduction, P = 0.23). The majority of events for the risk-reduction group occurred in the first year (68%) compared with the usual-care group, which had only 20% of their coronary events occur during this period.

This trial demonstrated that a diet more restrictive than the Step 2 diet, accompanied by an increase in physical activity, smoking reduction, and close physician follow-up, produced a significant decrease in the progression of CAD. It is important to note that dietary fat and overall Framingham risk score correlated with the beneficial effects seen.

Two other studies deserve mention as multiple risk-factor interventions that have had a profound effect on establishing an effective structure for benefiting patient's cardiovascular risk and clinical condition. In 1986, the **Lifestyle Heart Trial** enrolled 48 patients with angiographically documented coronary atherosclerosis who were randomized to intensive lifestyle modification or to a usual-care group. The lifestyle modification consisted of a low-fat vegetarian diet high in complex carbohydrates and low in simple carbohydrates, moderate aerobic exercise, stress management training, smoking cessation, and group support.[27] Control group patients were not asked to make lifestyle changes, although they were free to do so. The diet contained approximately 10% of calories as fat (P/S ratio > 1), 15% to 20% protein, and 70% to 75% predominantly complex carbohydrates. Cholesterol intake was limited to no more than 10 mg/day. The stress management techniques included stretching exercises, breathing techniques, meditation, progressive relaxation, and imagery. The purpose of each technique was to increase patients' sense of relaxation, concentration, awareness, and well-being. Patients were asked to practice these stress management techniques for at least 1 hour per day. Patients were asked to exercise a minimum of 3 hours per week and to spend a minimum of 30 minutes per session exercising within their prescribed target heart rates and/or perceived exertion levels. Group support sessions were designed to increase social support and a sense of community by creating a safe environment for the expression of feelings and also to help patients adhere to the lifestyle-change program.

Entry criteria included age between 35 and 75 years; single-, double-, or triple-vessel coronary disease in non-revascularized vessel(s); no coexisting life-threatening illness; no MI within 6 weeks of the start of the trial; not currently taking lipid-lowering medication; left-ventricular ejection fraction greater than 25%; and lack of treatment with thrombolytics when treated for MI or unstable angina. The original Lifestyle Heart Trial was a 1-year study, but based on the results after 1 year, the National Heart, Lung and Blood Institute (NHLBI) provided funding to extend the trial for 4 additional years.

Endpoint measurements included the following: (1) quantitative coronary arteriography at baseline, 1 year, and 5 years to assess the extent of coronary atherosclerosis; (2) cardiac positron emission tomography (PET) scans to measure myocardial perfusion; (3) lipoprotein and apolipoprotein profiles; (4) 3-day diet diaries and other questionnaires designed to measure adherence; and (5) psychosocial questionnaires to evaluate change in quality of life.

After 5 years, experimental subjects were exercising an average of 3.6 hours per week, practicing stress management 4 hours per week, and consuming an average of 18.6 mg/day of cholesterol with 8.5% of total calories from fat.[28] Control subjects were exercising 2.9 hr/week, practicing stress management techniques 0.98 hr/week, and consuming an average of 138.7 mg/day of cholesterol with 25% of total calories from fat.

From baseline to 1 year, the experimental group decreased their LDL cholesterol by 40%, and at 5 years this reduction was 20%. The control group's LDL cholesterol decreased only 1.2% after the first year, but by the fifth year, the reduction was 19.3%. The difference between the experimental and control subjects was statistically significant at year 1, but not at year 5. The interpretation of the results is confounded by the fact that 60% of control subjects had started lipid-lowering medicines between year 1 and 5, whereas none of the experimental subjects had done so. In addition, it is important to note that the control diet was equivalent to the AHA Step 2 diet, and it was only able to decrease LDL by 1.2% in the first year. However, the more restrictive diet in the intervention group had a much more profound effect.

From baseline to 1 year, experimental group patients had a 91% reduction in reported angina frequency, and at 5 years angina frequency had decreased by 72% from baseline levels. In contrast, from baseline to 1 year, the control group had a 186% increase in reported angina frequency, and at 5 years they had a 36% decrease in frequency from baseline levels. The decrease in the control group angina was in large part because three of the five patients who reported an increase in angina episodes from baseline to 1 year underwent coronary angioplasty between years 1 and 5.

At baseline, there were no significant angiographic differences between the experimental and control groups. The intervention group had an average diameter stenosis decrease of 1.75 absolute percentage points after 1 year and 3.1% reduction at 5 years (relative reduction of 7.9%). In contrast, the average percent diameter stenosis in the control group increased by 2.3% after 1 year and increased by 11.8% after 5 years (27.7% relative worsening). The difference between the groups was statistically significant at both 1 and 5 years (P = 0.02 and 0.001, respectively).

The investigators had hypothesized they would achieve the greatest reduction of atherosclerosis in younger patients and in those with the least disease at baseline. To their surprise, they found that neither variable correlated with disease regression. Instead, they found a clear dose-response relationship between program adherence and disease regression after 1 year and also after 5 years, with the most adherent patients having the greatest degree of improvement. Additionally, at 5 years, the control group had 2.25 cardiac events per patient year (defined as MI, PTCA, coronary artery bypass grafting (CABG), cardiac death and cardiac-related hospitalization), significantly worse than the experimental group, which had 0.89 events per patient year. These data are made even more impressive when considering that 60% of the control group was on lipid-lowering therapy compared to 0% in the experimental group. Also, cardiac PET scans revealed that almost 100% of experimental group patients were able to stop or reverse the progression of CHD as measured by myocardial perfusion.[29] Therefore, lifestyle interventions were even more effective than pharmacologic therapy at reducing clinical cardiovascular events. A more recent study suggests that the benefits of lifestyle interventions and lipid-lowering drug therapy may be additive.[30]

The Lifestyle Heart Trial was the first study to show that intensive lifestyle changes and multiple risk-factor interventions decreased angiographic coronary disease, reduced cardiac events, improved myocardial perfusion, and reduced angina frequency. Based on this conclusion, every patient with CAD should be considered for such a program. However, the feasibility and cost effectiveness of this remained to be established. This led the authors to investigate if such a program was economically and medically beneficial at safely reducing the need for patients to undergo revascularization.

Although not a randomized clinical trial, the Multicenter Lifestyle Demonstration Project is of interest because it was based on the concept that intensive lifestyle intervention may decrease the need for patients to undergo costly interventional procedures such as PTCA and CABG. This was not a randomized study, but they enrolled 194 patients with angiographically proven CAD severe enough to warrant revascularization.[31] Instead of undergoing revascularization, patients agreed to participate in a year-long comprehensive lifestyle modification program, which consisted of meeting as a group with health care professionals 3 days per week for 12 weeks and then once weekly for 9 months. Each meeting lasted 4 hours and consisted of 1 hour each of exercise, stress management techniques, group support, and a meal with cooking instructions. The cost of this year-long program was $7,000. As controls, the investigators used 139 patients selected from the Mutual of Omaha database and matched them for gender, age, left-ventricular function, and angiographically determined "cardiac score." All of these patients received "usual care" without regard of being in the trial.

Although the intervention lasted only 1 year, the investigators followed the patients for 3 years. The primary endpoint was the need for revascularization. All control group patients selected from the database underwent revascularization. However, at the end of 3 years, only 44 (23%) experimental patients required revascularization. Despite the drastic difference in percentage of patients revascularized (23% vs. 100%), there was no difference in the rate of MI, cerebrovascular accident (CVA), cardiac death, or noncardiac death between the two groups. In addition, among the controls, 23 required a repeat PTCA and 11 required CABG. A conservative estimate from Mutual of Omaha calculated that the lifestyle intervention group saved an average of $29,529 per patient.

Therefore, this study concluded that intensive lifestyle modification and risk-factor reduction is medically safe and effective, as well as cost effective over a 3-year period. Many of the shortcomings of prior multiple risk-factor trials were corrected in this study. For example, the diet went beyond the Step 2 diet, there was close follow-up and good adherence, and there was no cross contamination between the groups. In addition, it went beyond diet and exercise and intervened with stress reduction and group support. We can conclude that such a program is very effective, both medically and economically. In addition, although the intervention lasted only 1 year, the results persisted for at least 3 years. It remains to be seen if these results can be duplicated in less structured settings such as private physicians' offices, or if it requires a comprehensive program structure. This could be an interesting area for future research.

More recent trials have provided further evidence that prior studies did not go far enough in their interventions to achieve maximal effect.[32,33] They also have emphasized the need for a multifaceted approach to achieve meaningful risk-factor reduction, and they suggest new monitoring parameters that may help predict the amount of intervention required to reduce cardiovascular risk.

Stefanick and colleagues conducted a **Diet and Exercise for Elevated Risk (DEER) trial** that enrolled 367 men (30–64 years old) and women (45–64 years old).[34] Participants had mildly reduced HDL, had increased LDL, did not meet criteria for drug therapy, and had no history of CAD or other significant CAD risk factor. They were randomized to one of four groups: (1) National Choles-

terol Education Program (NCEP) Step 2 diet; (2) aerobic exercise equivalent to 10 miles of brisk walking per week; (3) Step 2 diet plus aerobic exercise; (4) control group instructed to maintain their current diet and physical activity. In the experimental groups, there was an intensive educational phase of 12 weeks for dietary education and 6 weeks for exercise education, followed by a maintenance phase with monthly contact and counseling for dietary compliance and monitored exercise sessions three times weekly. Those in the diet-alone group and diet-plus-exercise group reduced the amount of cholesterol in their diet (−67% and −63%, respectively) as well as the percentage of calories from total, saturated, and monounsaturated fat. The investigators did not emphasize weight loss, because they did not want that as an uncontrolled variable. The data showed that the Step 2 diet alone did not have a beneficial or detrimental effect on lipoprotein profiles. However, when the Step 2 diet was combined with exercise, the subjects had a significant decrease in LDL (−14.5%) without a significant change in their HDL compared to controls. When compared to the patients randomized to exercise alone, only the male patients in the diet and exercise group had a significant decrease in their LDL. This is likely because of the higher cholesterol and fat content in the baseline diet of the males compared to the females.

Overall, this study suggests that the AHA Step 2 diet alone is not sufficient to improve the cardiovascular risk profiles of "average"-risk individuals. However, addressing two risk factors by adding moderate aerobic exercise to this diet did produce a beneficial effect. This could explain why many dietary intervention trials in the past have failed to show significant improvement in cholesterol profiles. This study supports the concept that physicians provide substandard care if they only address dietary changes with their patients. Fortunately, current NCEP and AHA guidelines stress the need for physicians to counsel their patients about weight loss and physical activity in addition to dietary changes. The problem arises in the practicality of teaching patients to make drastic lifestyle changes in a regular office visit. Another strength of Stefanick's study is that the patients benefited from an intensive education process as well as close follow-up throughout the study to ensure compliance and help address any problems that may have arisen. This structure is similar to what we see in our cardiac rehabilitation and prevention programs and provides much more opportunity to educate patients and ensure they incorporate their lifestyle changes long term.

Community-Level Intervention Trials

Many clinical trials have shown the greatest degree of benefit—both in risk factor and coronary event reduction—in the highest-risk population. In addition, potential unexpected adverse effects from drug treatments are more justifiable in patients who are at high risk or who have overt disease than in population-based settings in which a large number of people need to be treated to save relatively few lives. Nevertheless, from a population standpoint, most coronary events occur in the larger percentage of people with moderately increased risk rather than the smaller percentage with very high risk. The implication is that prevention efforts, therefore, should be concentrated on that larger population because there would be a greater theoretic public health and cost-effective benefit.

The first symposium defining and discussing the community trials approach was published in the *American Journal of Epidemiology* in 1978.[35] Several major community-based trials looking at prevention of CAD started around the time of that publication. Because of similarities among these studies, only selected trials are discussed here: the World Health Organization (WHO) European Collaborative Trials, the North Karelia Project, and the Minnesota Heart Health Program.

Several of the original community-based trials on multiple risk-factor modification for CAD took place in Europe and are known collectively as the **World Health Organization (WHO) European Collaborative Trial of Multifactorial Prevention of Coronary Heart Disease.** The WHO Multifactorial Trial was started in the United Kingdom in 1971; other countries, including Belgium, Italy, Poland, and Spain, joined the effort soon thereafter.[36] The locations functioned independently; however, the study design and methods of intervention at each site were virtually identical to facilitate data pooling. In addition to the collaborative analysis, each country in the WHO Collaborative was evaluated individually.

One variation between sites was how much time health care professionals spent with treatment subjects, which turned out to be a statistically significant factor. As one would expect, the more time spent with an individual or individuals by health care providers, the more clinical improvement they achieved in terms of risk-factor modification as well as morbidity and mortality reduction. This is discussed more completely with review of the results of the trial.

The two main research questions were as follows:

1. Can coronary risk factors be reduced using a population-based intervention?
2. If so, do changes in risk factors translate into decreased incidence of coronary and all-cause mortality?

Two factories in each country were paired—one received the intervention and the other acted as a control. Within study factories, all men ages 40 to 59 years were offered an initial screening examination followed by educational materials and/or individual counseling on risk-factor modification in the areas of smoking cessation, low-fat/low-cholesterol diet, daily exercise, weight reduction, and treatment of hypertension. Of those eligible, 86% agreed to participate. WHO trial authors did not discuss any particular characteristics, demographic or otherwise, regarding those who agreed to participate and how they may have differed from those who did not. There is also no comment as to whether those with already defined CAD were or were not excluded from the trial.[37]

In all centers taken together, the combined risk estimate decreased 11.1% for the entire population and decreased 19.4% for the high-risk subjects. There was a 7.4% net overall reduction for CHD, a 3.9% reduction for

death, and a 3.9% reduction for fatal CHD plus nonfatal MI. However, none of these differences was statistically significant for the whole group.[38] Only the Belgian center showed statistically significant differences, although the subjects at the Belgian intervention factory did not experience a much larger change in coronary risk factors compared with the Belgian control factory.[39] The one variable that distinguished the Belgian intervention site from the others was that the subjects received more attention from health care professionals. This suggests that the amount of time spent with subjects, and not necessarily the amount of risk reduction, was associated with a decreased incidence of CVD and death. These benefits of close personal attention may simply be reflected in better adherence. However, the effects of social support on morbidity and mortality from both cardiac and noncardiac events, independent of changes in risk factors, has been well documented.[40] These powerful social factors are often ignored as potentially confounding influences when assessing the effects of multiple risk-factor modification interventions.

The power of social support was seen in the **North Karelia Project**, which was the first population-based cardiovascular disease prevention program.[41] This educational program was designed to reduce tobacco use and improve cholesterol and blood pressure through diet and exercise modifications. Although the intervention achieved a sizeable reduction in smoking and a modest beneficial effect in both blood pressure and serum cholesterol levels as compared with the reference population, its effect on coronary disease and cardiovascular mortality remained equivocal. As seen in other community trials and in the MRFIT study, the failure to show significant differences between the groups resulted from an insufficiently rigorous intervention and from secular trends in the comparison group.

However, observational analyses of the North Karelia data demonstrated a significant association between the extent of social support and mortality from ischemic heart disease. Those who were socially isolated had a 200% to 300% increased risk of death over 5 to 9 years when compared with those who had the greatest sense of social connection and community. These results were found even when there was extensive adjustment for traditional cardiovascular risk factors. Analyses using a variety of techniques provide no evidence that this association was a result of the impact of prevalent disease on the extent of social contacts. Furthermore, changes in social connections during one 9-year period were prospectively associated with increased risk of death from ischemic heart disease in a subsequent 9-year period. Finally, the level of social connections modified the association between diastolic blood pressure and risk of death from ischemic heart disease.

The **Minnesota Heart Health Program (MHHP)** remains the largest community-based trial funded by the NHLBI to look at a community approach to primary prevention of CAD.[43] The study included 500,000 people from a total of six communities (three paired communities) in the upper Midwest. This was a community-wide intervention invoking multiple approaches to encourage changes in the population at large instead of in selected individuals. It was hoped that this type of population-based intervention would decrease the development of CAD, coronary events, and death. The intent was to decrease the **population's** risk as opposed to an **individual's** risk and to measure the resulting impact on public health.

After a few years of baseline data collection, the MHHP intervention was implemented between 1981 and 1984 and remained ongoing in the last treatment community until 1990. Each treatment community received 5 to 6 years of active intervention in the areas of hypertension prevention and control, dietary education and counseling, smoking cessation, and encouragement of physical activity. All communities were assessed for lifestyle behaviors and risk factors for up to 7 years of follow-up and for morbidity and mortality for up to 13 years. The paired communities were matched on size, character, and distance from Minneapolis-St. Paul.

The sites within each matched pair were not randomly assigned to either intervention or comparison; however, the assignments were completed prior to collection of any data. Baseline and follow-up data were collected by both **cross-sectional** and **cohort** survey methods. The **cross-sectional** surveys were conducted every 2 years on 300 to 500 randomly selected adults between the ages of 25 and 74 years in each of the six study communities. The **cohort** surveys were conducted on a group of randomly selected participants from the preintervention cross-sectional surveys who were recontacted for follow-up throughout the 6- to 7 year time course—that is, the same group was followed longitudinally over time, as opposed to the cross-sectional surveys, which were composed of different individuals at any given survey point. Each approach provides somewhat different information. The cohort surveys allow for following behavioral trends and risk-factor patterns in people over time, but they are complicated by potential bias from contact with the health care professionals conducting the surveys. Observing corresponding data from independent samples by the cross-sectional surveys controls for this contact bias. In other words, the cross-sectional surveys theoretically examine the impact of the community-based learning programs on individuals without the influence of individualized attention.

Interventions were implemented on different levels including the following: (1) individual exposure with structured programs geared toward risk-factor reduction through education and behavioral modification; (2) community organization with involvement of respected community leaders, including physicians; and (3) mass media communication. Examples of approaches used include but are not limited to those in Table 31-3.

The results of this large, comprehensive, population-based study were not as positive or promising as anticipated. For most cardiac risk factors examined (i.e., hypertension, smoking, weight, cholesterol, and physical activity), the changes in the intervention groups were in a favorable direction relative to the comparison groups; however, with a few rare exceptions, none of the changes was statistically significant. There was no significant difference in CAD mortality between

■ ▫ ■

TABLE 31-3   RISK-FACTOR REDUCTION APPROACHES

1. Adult education classes for weight control, exercise, and lowering cholesterol
2. Weight control programs at work
3. Home correspondence course for weight loss and/or smoking cessation made available to those in the intervention communities by mass mailings
4. Incentive programs for weight loss and smoking cessation (including reimbursement of the cost of the program if smoking cessation was achieved or if the weight goal was obtained; "Quit & Win" contests)
5. School interventions for primary prevention in adolescents
6. Self-help materials and pamphlets available in the intervention communities and sent by direct mailings to peoples' homes
7. Telephone support (for those participating in programs)
8. Presence of screening education centers in town for screening blood pressure, weight, and cholesterol level
9. Grocery store food labeling with education about "shopping smart for your heart"
10. Use of mass media including newspaper, radio, and television

the two groups, which is the only cardiac event data available.

As in MRFIT, (1) the experimental group was not asked to make changes large enough to cause substantial changes in risk factors, and (2) the control group began to make changes on their own, in part because of background secular trends—that is, a greater awareness in the general population of the importance of changing risk factors—and because the act of observing people in a study with surveys and questionnaires often influences their behavior. In addition, several influential events occurred during the time course of the trial, including social smoking restrictions, improved labeling of food products, and general increased availability of health information. More broadly, the existence of a trial such as MHHP influences and affects secular trends, presumably through advertising, media exposure, communication between participants and nonparticipants, communication between participating and nonparticipating health care providers, and migration of people from treatment community to nontreatment communities. It is difficult to control for these components, and their influence should not be underestimated.

There are other interesting lessons to learn from the MHHP study design and findings. The design is unusual and complicated in that communities are the units of analysis, whereas individuals within the communities are the units of observation and data collection. The investigators learned that it would have been better to have a greater number of smaller communities, maximizing both the similarities within each community and the likelihood of identifying differences between communities.

Another problem in the study design was that the communities were not randomly selected for participation in the trial; therefore, there were baseline differences between the groups that may have influenced subsequent information gathered and comparisons made. Additionally, the investigators looked at all interventional programs together despite the variety of treatment methods used. Separate analysis of distinct approaches may have yielded more valuable information about which particular methods were most effective. The more intense types of behavioral change were the most effective in eliciting clinical improvement in risk-factor modification, but recruitment to those particular interventional programs was more difficult than expected. Therefore, as the trial went on, investigators focused their promotional efforts on the programs with more "mass appeal," which were not always effective in altering cardiac risk factors or cardiac status.[44]

Understanding what is **effective** as opposed to what is **feasible** for lifestyle modification of risk factors is an extremely important concept. If a method is relatively easy to do but ineffective, it is misleading to tell people that it will help modify their risk for coronary disease. In addition, acknowledging and discussing what is effective makes that method more accessible over time by enhancing familiarity and, ultimately, changing belief patterns about what is feasible and desirable. By analogy, most physicians acknowledge to their patients the difficulty of quitting smoking, yet advise their patients to quit, not simply to cut back from three to two packs a day. It may be easier to cut back than to quit, but it may not be very effective. The same concept applies to study design. It is easier to design a study that does not control for all imaginable variables, but this makes the results less interpretable. Regardless of the design flaws, the MHHP was a remarkable undertaking at the time, and it established a potential model for implementing and evaluating cardiovascular risk-factor modification.

GUIDELINES

Based on the concepts demonstrated by the trials discussed earlier, the AHA and NCEP have modified their prior guidelines for lifestyle interventions to prevent CHD. The Adult Treatment Panel III (ATP III) guidelines propose a diet composed of less than 35% of total calories from fat, less than 7% saturated fat, and less than 200 mg/day of cholesterol and including 2g/day of plant stenols and sterols.[45] They also recognize that patients with the metabolic syndrome or diabetes should increase the proportion of polyunsaturated fats in an effort to decrease the amount of carbohydrates consumed. In addition, they recommend daily energy expenditure of "at least moderate physical activity."

The AHA has revised its prior "Step 1" and "Step 2" diets in favor of general guidelines for the whole population, which are then modified according to different patient subgroups.[46] They still differentiate between primary (those without known CVD) and secondary (those with known CVD) (primary prevention: <10% saturated fat, <300 mg/day cholesterol; secondary prevention: <7% saturated fat, <200 mg/day cholesterol), but they recommend that all patients maintain a healthy body weight and consume two servings of fish per week as well as increase their consumption of fruits, vegetables, low-fat dairy products, and whole grains. They mention potential benefits of n3-PUFA and α-linolenic acid but are unclear as to the amount recommended. Regarding exercise, they suggest "30 minutes of physical activity on most, if not all days of the week."

SUMMARY OF LESSONS LEARNED FROM MULTIPLE RISK-FACTOR INTERVENTION TRIALS

1. Multiple risk-factor intervention studies are inherently difficult to execute. One can control access to new drugs but not to behavioral changes. Therefore, it is difficult to have a true nonintervention control group because many control group patients also may begin to make lifestyle changes. In the MRFIT study, for example, subjects randomized to the control group were as aware of its goals as were the patients in the interventional group; indeed, control group patients often believed that they were in the intervention group.

2. Intensive changes in risk factors via diet and lifestyle and/or drug therapy cause improvements in morbidity and mortality that are both clinically and statistically significant. However, moderate changes in risk factors may not go far enough to cause statistically or clinically significant reductions in morbidity and mortality. This was seen in a number of studies, including the MRFIT, Lifestyle Heart Trial, and the Multicenter Lifestyle Demonstration Project. Increasing evidence indicates that the AHA/NCEP Steps 1 and 2 diets such as those used in the MRFIT study do not go far enough to stop the progression of coronary atherosclerosis in most patients, whereas more intensive changes in diet may stop or reverse the progression of atherosclerosis.[47,48]

3. Treatment of a single risk factor, such as hypertension, may not induce the expected reduction in occurrence of coronary events if other risk factors are not also adequately treated.[49] Likewise, intervention in only one aspect of life (i.e., just diet or just exercise) is frequently not adequate to see optimal effects of cardiovascular risk reduction. However, treatment of several risk factors simultaneously affords greater improvement in each compared with treatment of a single risk factor at a time, and addressing more than one aspect of life produces better adherence to the lifestyle change and much better results.

4. Intensive risk-factor modification by lifestyle changes or lipid-lowering medicines may reduce cardiac events rapidly by stabilizing the endothelium even before there is time for meaningful regression in coronary atherosclerosis.

5. Defining the exact threshold of lifestyle modification necessary for a clinical benefit is often difficult to define in trials that target multiple interventions. Therefore, it sometimes may be useful to extract data from studies that use one intervention and apply them to multiple intervention programs.

6. Social factors may play an important role in adherence to comprehensive lifestyle changes and may have powerful effects on morbidity and mortality independent of other influences.[50-52]

In summary, risk-factor intervention trials have made a major contribution to the understanding of the pathophysiology of coronary artery disease and the best ways to intervene to reduce cardiovascular risk. They have also provided a greater understanding of study design and clinical approaches that are not as effective. Further studies are necessary to understand the most cost-effective and medically effective strategies for making intensive risk-factor modification programs available to the large number of people who can benefit from them. Although initial studies suggest that this can be done cost effectively, future studies should continue to include cost-effective analysis from insurance companies, managed care organizations, and Medicare. However, it is clear that comprehensive, intensive risk-factor reduction programs provide the ideal setting for reducing cardiac morbidity and mortality through risk-factor reduction. They provide a structured environment that incorporates the necessary dietary, exercise, psychologic, and other changes that patients need to motivate lifestyle changes. The evidence strongly supports referring patients to these programs with the goals of improving cardiac outcomes and decreasing costs.

REFERENCES

1. American Heart Association: 2002 Heart and Stroke Statistical Update. Dallas, American Heart Association, 2001.
2. Kannel WB: Contributions of the Framingham Study to the conquest of artery disease. Am J Cardiol 1988; 62:1109-1112.
3. Gordon T, Kannel WB, Castelli WP, et al: Lipoproteins, cardiovascular disease, and death: The Framingham study. Arch Intern Med 1981; 141:1128-1132.
4. Kannel WB: Clinical misconceptions dispelled by epidemiological research. Circulation 1995; 92(11):3350-3360.
5. Verschuren WM, Jacobs DR, Bloemberg BP, et al: Serum total cholesterol and long-term coronary heart disease mortality in different cultures: Twenty-five-year follow-up of the Seven Countries Study. JAMA 1995; 274:131-136.
6. Kannel WB: Clinical misconceptions dispelled by epidemiological research. Circulation 1995; 92:3350-3360.
7. Kannel WB, Barry P, Dawber TR: Immediate mortality in coronary heart disease: The Framingham study. In: Proceedings of the IV World Congress of Cardiology, Mexican Intl Soc Cardiol 1963; IV-B:176-188.
8. Multiple Risk Factor Intervention Trial Research Group: Multiple Risk Factor Intervention Trial: Risk factor changes and mortality results (MRFIT). JAMA 1982; 248:1465-1477.
9. Grimm R: The Multiple Risk Factor Intervention Trial in the U.S.A.: Summary of results at four years in special intervention and usual care men. Prev Med 1983; 12:185-190.
10. Hjrmann I: A randomized primary preventive trial in coronary heart disease: The Oslo study. Prev Med 1983; 12:181-184.
11. Wihelmsen L: Risk factors for coronary heart disease in perspective: European Intervention Trials. Am J Med 1984; 76(2A):37-40.
12. Sigh RB, Rastogi SS, Verman R, et al: Randomized controlled trial of cardioprotective diet in patients with recent acute myocardial infarction: Results of one year follow-up. BMJ 1992; 304:1015-1019.
13. deLorgeril M, Renaud S, Mamelle N, et al: Mediterranean alpha-linolenic acid-rich diet in secondary prevention of coronary heart disease. Lancet 1994; 343:1454-1459.
14. deLorgeril M, Salen P, Martin J, et al: Effects of a Mediterranean type diet on the rate of cardiovascular complications in patients with coronary artery disease. JACC 1996; 28:1103-1108.
15. deLorgeril M, Salen P, Martin J, et al: Mediterranean diet, traditional risk factors, and the rate of cardiovascular complications after myocardial infarction. Circulation 1999; 99:779-785.
16. Hu FB, Willett WC: Optimal diets for prevention of coronary heart disease. JAMA 2002; 288:2569-2578.
17. GISSI-Prevenzione Investigators: Dietary supplementation with n-3 polyunsaturated fatty acids and vitamin E after myocardial infarction: Results of the GISSI-Prevenzione trial. Lancet 1999; 354:447-455.
18. Marchioli R, Barzi F, Bomba E, et al: Early protection against sudden death by n-3 polyunsaturated fatty acids after myocardial infarction. Circulation 2002; 105:1897-1903.
19. Blankenhorn DH, Nessim SA, Johnson RL, et al: Beneficial effects of combined colestipol-niacin therapy on coronary atherosclerosis and coronary venous bypass grafts. JAMA 1987; 257:3233-3240.
20. Brown GB, Albers JJ, Fisher LD, et al: Niacin or lovastatin combined with colestipol regresses coronary atherosclerosis and prevents clinical events in men with elevated apolipoprotein B. N Engl J Med 1990; 323:1289-1298.
21. Kane JP, Malloy MJ, Ports TA, et al: Regression of coronary atherosclerosis during treatment of familial hypercholesterolemia with combined drug regimens. JAMA 1990; 264:3007-3012.
22. Buchwald H, Vargo RL, et al: Effect of partial ileal bypass surgery on mortality and morbidity from coronary heart disease in patients with hypercholesterolemia. N Engl J Med 1990; 323:946-955.
23. Cashin-Hemphill L, Mack WJ, Pogoda JM, et al: Beneficial effects of colestipol-niacin on coronary atherosclerosis. JAMA 1990; 264:3013-3017.
24. Schuler G, Hambrecht R, Schlierf G, et al: Myocardial perfusion and regression of coronary artery disease in patients on a regimen of intensive physical exercise and low fat diet. J Am Coll Cardiol 1992; 19:34-42.
25. Schuler G, Hambrecht R, Schlierf G, et al: Regular physical exercise and low-fat diet effects on progression of coronary artery disease. Circulation 1992; 86:1-11.
26. Haskell WL, Alderman EL, Fair JM, et al: Effects of intensive multiple risk factor reduction on coronary atherosclerosis and clinical cardiac events in men and women with coronary artery disease: The Stanford Coronary Risk Intervention Project (SCRIP). Circulation 1994; 89:975-990.
27. Ornish D: Dr. Dean Ornish's Program for Reversing Heart Disease. New York: Random House, 1990; Ballantine Books, 1992.
28. Ornish D, Scherwitz LW, Billings JH, et al: Intensive lifestyle changes for reversal of coronary heart disease. JAMA 1998; 280:2001-2007.
29. Gould KL, Ornish D, Scherwitz L, et al: Changes in myocardial perfusion abnormalities by positron emission tomography after long-term, intense risk factor modification. JAMA 1995; 274:894-901.
30. Sdringola S, Nakagawa K, Nakagawa Y, et al: Combined intense lifestyle and pharmacologic lipid treatment further reduce coronary events and myocardial perfusion abnormalities compared with usual-care cholesterol-lowering drugs in coronary artery disease. J Am Coll Cardiol 2003; 41:263-272.
31. Ornish D: Avoiding revascularization with lifestyle changes: The Multicenter lifestyle demonstration project. Am J Cardiol 1998; 82:72T-76T.
32. Stefanick ML, Mackey S, Sheehan M, et al: Effects of diet and exercise in men and postmenopausal women with low levels of HDL cholesterol and high levels of LDL cholesterol. N Engl J Med 1998; 339:12-20.
33. Krauss WE, Houmard JA, Duscha BD, et al: Effects of the amount and intensity of exercise on plasma lipoproteins. N Engl J Med 2002; 347:1483-1492.
34. Stefanick ML, Mackey S, Sheehan M, et al: Effects of diet and exercise in men and postmenopausal women with low levels of HDL cholesterol and high levels of LDL cholesterol. N Engl J Med 1998; 339:12-20.
35. Murray D: Design and Analysis of Community Trials: Lessons From the Minnesota Heart Health Program. Am J Epidemiol 1995; 142:569-575.
36. World Health Organization European Collaborative Group: European collaborative trial of multifactorial prevention of coronary heart disease: Final report on the 6-year results. Lancet 1986; 869-872.
37. World Health Organization European Collaborative Group Multifactorial trial in the prevention of coronary heart disease: III. Incidence and mortality results. Eur Heart J 1983; 4:141-147.
38. Wilhelmsen L: Risk factors for coronary heart disease in perspective: European Intervention Trials. Am J Med 1984; 76(2A):37-40.
39. Menotti A: The European Multifactorial Preventive Trial of Coronary Heart Disease: Four-year Experience. Prev Med 1983; 12:175-180.
40. House JS, Landis KR, Umberson D: Social relationships and health. Science 1988; 241(4865):540-545.
41. Salonen JT: Prevention of coronary heart disease in Finland: Application of the population strategy. Annals of Medicine 1991; 23(6):607-612.
42. Kaplan GA: Social contacts and ischaemic heart disease. Ann Clin Res 1988; 20(1-2):131-136.

43. Murray DM, Kurth C, Mullis R, et al: Cholesterol reduction through low-intensity interventions: Results from the Minnesota Heart Health Program. Prev Med 1990; 19:181-189.

44. Murray D: Design and analysis of community trials: Lessons from the Minnesota Heart Health Program. Am J Epidemiol 1995; 142:569-575.

45. Third report of the national cholesterol education program (NCEP) expert panel on detection, evaluation, and treatment of high blood cholesterol in adults (ATP III) final report. Circulation 2002; 106:3145-3421.

46. Krauss RM, Eckel RH, Howard B, et al: AHA Dietary guidelines Revision 2000: A statement for healthcare professional from the nutrition committee of the AHA. Circulation 2000; 102:2284-2299.

47. Ornish D: Dietary treatment of hyperlipidemia. J Cardiovasc Risk 1994; 1:283-286.

48. Ornish D: Statins and the soul of medicine. Am J Cardiol 2002; 89(11):1286-1290.

49. Borghi C, Ambrosioni E: Primary and secondary prevention of myocardial infarction. Clin Exp Hypertens 1996; 18:547-558.

50. House JS, Landis KR, Umberson D: Social relationships and health. Science 1988; 241(4865):540-545.

51. Berkman LF: The role of social relations in health promotion. Psychosom Med 1995; 57(3):24-254.

52. Ruberman W, Weinblatt E, Goldberg JD, et al: Psychosocial influences on mortality after myocardial infarction. N Engl J Med 1984; 311(9):552-559.

■■■c h a p t e r **32**

Prevention Strategies: From the Office
to the Community and Beyond

David Chiriboga
Ira S. Ockene

The clinical trials described in this book represent the best that medical science can offer: teams of well-trained people led by experienced investigators and focused on the project at hand. The results of these trials inform us as to those methodologies and interventions that have the potential to be truly useful. They leave us, however, with several important problems.

How will these interventions work in the real world, as opposed to the world of the clinical trial? In the real world, health care providers may not be as well informed or trained as we would like them to be; therefore, they may not apply an intervention effectively or may fail to use it at all.

What is a population-based intervention? Is there tension between interventions carried out at the level of the individual, in traditional physician–patient interactions, and interventions carried out at the population level? Or are these activities synergistic?

In the realm of prevention, much of what needs to be done falls outside the purview of the traditional medical environment. What can be done to bring preventive interventions to the community, worksite, and school? Are there effective methodologies that will work at these levels?

Many of the public health advances in the conquest of infectious diseases in the past came from environmental and policy interventions as opposed to behavioral interventions. Are there environmental and policy interventions that might aid in confronting the ongoing epidemic of chronic disease, particularly of coronary heart disease (CHD)?

In this chapter, the issue of clinical trials in prevention is placed into the largest possible perspective, beginning with a discussion of the concept of the "population-based" approach, then considering what can be done to improve the delivery of preventive interventions in the physician's office and practice, and, finally, evaluating the available evidence for intervention at the community level and beyond.

POPULATION APPROACH VERSUS
THE HIGH-RISK APPROACH

"Population" and "high-risk," the two primary approaches to the prevention of CHD, are at times described as though they were mutually exclusive. This is not the case. Both are appropriate, although requiring differing

levels of intensity. The high-risk approach is the usual modus operandi of physicians. Patients at high risk are looked for in physicians' offices or by screening programs and, when found, are treated to reduce their risk. In contrast, the population approach aims to lower the mean level of a risk factor in the entire population and thus shift the entire risk curve to the left (Fig. 32-1). Population interventions include antismoking campaigns, efforts to reduce the use of saturated fat in fast-food restaurants, and national nutrition education programs.

These two approaches relate to two different etiologic questions. The individual-centered approach seeks the causes of cases and asks questions such as "Why does this person have an elevated cholesterol level?" The population-centered approach seeks the causes of incidence and asks the question "Why does this population of people have a higher mean cholesterol level and many individuals with elevated levels, when in other populations elevated cholesterol levels are rare?" The relative advantages and disadvantages of these approaches are summarized in Tables 32-1 and 32-2.

The high-risk strategy (i.e., centered on the individual) uses an approach that is inherently appealing to physicians. Paying special attention to those at the high end of a risk distribution is a typical medical approach. The physician is treating a person who understands the need to be treated ("I have high cholesterol, and so I need to change my diet"), and this approach also applies resources to those people who will have the highest pay-off in terms of diminished risk. Likewise, any unfavorable consequences of the treatment will be seen as being part of a favorable risk-benefit ratio.

Nonetheless, this approach has a number of drawbacks. It is difficult to screen a population. Patients at highest risk are often least likely to be reached, and the level of compliance with recommended follow-up is often poor. The younger, hyperlipidemic, smoking, physician-avoiding person is far less likely to appear at a screening site. The same logic applies to many other risk-altering situations: the population at highest risk is often least likely to voluntarily participate in risk-modifying behaviors.

There is an even more important disadvantage to the high-risk approach: treating only those most liable to be affected by a population-based condition such as a high-saturated fat diet does not affect the root cause of the problem, and the next generation will have the same burden of disease as the last. In addition, the prediction of risk for a given individual always will be poor for all

412

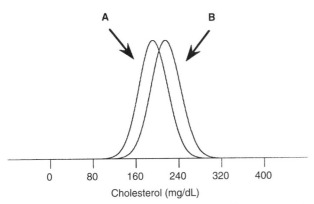

FIGURE 32-1. An example of the population-based approach to the prevention of coronary heart disease. The goal is to move the curve from B to A.

but those at highest risk. Most clinical events always will come from the middle of the risk distribution because the great bulk of the population resides here.

A study looking at the decline in CHD mortality between 1980 and 1990 in the United States reported that 25% of the decline was explained by primary prevention, whereas 29% was explained by secondary reduction in risk factors in patients with coronary disease and 43% by other improvements in treatment in patients with coronary disease. The study concluded that primary and secondary risk-factor reductions explain about 50% of the decline in coronary mortality in the United States in that period, but it stressed that more than 70% of the overall decline in mortality occurred among patients with coronary disease,[1] reinforcing the concept that the high-risk approach most benefits people at the highest end of the risk distribution, (i.e., those who already have developed disease).

The high-risk strategy also may require a person to change behavior in a fashion that is socially difficult. Eating in a different way than the rest of the family, exercising when your friends want to watch a football game—these are difficult changes to make.

The population-based strategy is quite different. Shifting the risk curve of a population can progressively lower the incidence of disease. Changes occurring in an entire population make it easier for an individual to change—it is easier to quit smoking when your workplace is smoke-free, and it is easier to follow a low-saturated–fat diet

TABLE 32-1   THE "HIGH-RISK" STRATEGY

Advantages	Disadvantages
Intervention appropriate to the individual	Difficulties and cost of screening
Subject motivation	Does not deal with the root causes of disease
Physician motivation	Limited potential for the population as a whole
Cost-effective use of resources	Imposes behavioral difficulties
Favorable risk-benefit ratio	Labels asymptomatic individuals as "sick"

TABLE 32-2   THE "POPULATION APPROACH"

Advantages	Disadvantages
Radical—can alter the root causes of the disease	Small benefit to the individual (the "prevention paradox")
Larger potential for reducing disease incidence	Poor motivation of subject
Behaviorally appropriate	Poor motivation of physician
	Problematic risk-benefit ratio if intervention may not be entirely benign
	"Blaming the victim"

when such choices are widely available in the company or school cafeteria and in fast-food restaurants.

The population-based strategy does have an inherent downside, which Rose has called the *prevention paradox:* preventive measures that greatly benefit society as a whole may bring little benefit to each person who is individually at relatively low risk.[2] Because the gain for a given person is small, motivating that person to make lifestyle changes may be difficult. All that this means, however, is that the intensity of the intervention needs to be matched to the person's level of risk: individual, high-intensity, and relatively expensive approaches for those at high levels of risk and population approaches such as those described in this chapter for the great bulk of the population at low or moderate risk. These approaches should be combined into an overall national strategy.

Another limitation of the population approach, which to some extent is shared by the high-risk approach, is that it may "blame the victim" (i.e., each individual in the society). Individuals respond to the manner in which the environment has been constructed; therefore, the results of this interaction (health or disease) are also the responsibility of the system that created the determining conditions in the first place. The behavioral approach, shared by both the high-risk and the population approaches, tends to place a disproportionate portion of the blame on the individual's will power (e.g., stop smoking, don't eat saturated fat, and start exercising).

The importance of the population approach is made clear by simulations carried out by several investigators. Kottke and colleagues tested the effects of several intervention strategies on CHD mortality rates.[3] Lowering serum cholesterol by 4%, smoking by 15%, and diastolic blood pressure by 3% in the entire population—goals that are easily achievable and, in the case of cholesterol and smoking, already surpassed in the United States— would be expected to reduce the incidence of nonfatal myocardial infarction by at least 13% and CHD deaths by at least 18%. However, lowering serum cholesterol by 34%, smoking by 20%, and diastolic blood pressure to 90 mm Hg in the subset of the population with all three risk factors in the highest quartile would result only in a 6% to 8% reduction in nonfatal myocardial infarction and a 2% to 9% reduction in deaths from CHD. Similarly, Goldman and colleagues[4] used Framingham Heart Study coefficients in a computer simulation (the Coronary Heart Disease Policy Model) to analyze the effect of a targeted program to treat all cholesterol levels of 250 mg/dL or higher, as opposed to a population-wide program to reduce everyone's cholesterol level. Their model suggests that such a targeted program would reduce CHD incidence by 8% to 10% in men 35 to 54 years of age and by 1% to 4% in men 55 to 74 years of age. A similar reduction in CHD incidence also could be achieved by a 10 mg/dL population-wide reduction in serum cholesterol. Such a decline in cholesterol already has been seen in the United States and has been associated with an unprecedented decline in CHD mortality. More recently several other methods for risk prediction have been developed and compared.[5]

Thus, it is clear that efforts targeting only high-risk segments of the overall population are inadequate to reduce significantly the population burden of disease. If we are to improve the cardiovascular health of the nation, we must develop population approaches that build on the high-risk approach offered by the individual practitioner, while fostering changes in policy to create a favorable environment for the changes to occur.

THE HEALTH-CARE PROVIDER AND THE HEALTH-CARE SYSTEM

The medical profession has an important role to play in the reduction of cardiovascular risk. Some 76% of Americans visit a physician in any given year, with many of them (59% to 85%) reporting repeat visits within that year. Appropriate counseling of these patients regarding alteration of health risk behaviors could have a substantial public health impact, yet our increasing knowledge of effective interventions for the prevention of CHD is often poorly translated into effective delivery of preventive care by the provider. Some of the existing barriers to the delivery of effective preventive care include the following:

- Traditionally, most physicians have been more interested in the delivery of therapeutic, rather than preventive, care. They often express the belief that they are ineffective in health behavior interventions and often also state that patients do not want their physicians to intervene on risk factors (such as smoking) when they are seeing them for other problems.
- Physicians (and other health care providers) often believe that they have poor intervention skills. In reality, few have had training in behavioral counseling; yet the modification of behavior is the essence of patient-oriented preventive activities.
- Physicians traditionally have prided themselves on their autonomy. Following best-practice guidelines is foreign to them and often is derided as "cookbook" medicine.
- Physicians and other providers increasingly are pressured for time in today's cost-conscious environment. Thus they often have little time to fit preventive interventions into their practices, keeping in mind that lifestyle intervention is only one of their many responsibilities.
- There are few economic incentives for prevention-oriented activities. Taking the time to counsel patients

effectively is rarely adequately reimbursed and does not yield the same financial rewards as technologic interventions do.
- Physicians' practices generally also are not set up to cue them to intervene and to facilitate integration of prevention activities with other more traditional medical needs.

Two general strategies have been shown to be effective in improving the delivery of preventive services to individual patients. These are (1) the training of individual providers in counseling methodologies in combination with office systems that facilitate the delivery of such counseling and (2) the development of case-management systems that add onto the physician's activities a systematic risk-factor modification approach that is entirely separate from the usual office activities. Examples of both follow.

Worcester-Area Trial for Counseling in Hyperlipidemia

The Worcester-Area Trial for Counseling in Hyperlipidemia (WATCH) randomized 45 primary care health maintenance organization internists by site into three conditions: (I) usual care; (II) physician nutrition counseling training; and (III) physician nutrition counseling training plus a structured office support program for nutrition management.[6] The two physician intervention groups were provided with a 3-hour training program incorporating behavioral principles for brief, patient-centered, interactive counseling. Group III also was provided with an office support program that included prompts, algorithms, and simple dietary assessment tools. Patient recruitment occurred over a 2-year period, and physician-counseling skills were maintained over this period, despite the lack of any further training. At 1 year of follow-up, significant improvement was seen in diet, weight, and blood lipid levels but was limited to patients in condition III. As compared with the control group, condition III patients had average reductions of 2.53 percentage points (an 8% decline) for energy intake from fat (P = 0.03); 1.1 percentage points for saturated fat (10.3% decline; P = 0.01); an average weight loss of 2.3 kilograms (P < 0.001); and a 3.8 mg/dL decrease in low-density lipoprotein (LDL) cholesterol (P = 0.10). When patients prescribed cholesterol-lowering medication were excluded, the LDL-cholesterol reduction increased to 9.3 mg/dL (P = 0.009) because more patients in the control condition were placed on lipid-lowering medication. Average time for the initial counseling intervention in condition III was 9.2 minutes. Patients of condition II physicians (trained but not supported) showed results no different from controls. The study demonstrated that brief physician nutrition counseling can produce beneficial changes in diet, weight, and blood lipids but only if accompanied by an office support system that facilitates the intervention.

The lipid outcomes in a diet intervention study such as this may seem modest when compared with the results of recent studies involving pharmacologic intervention. The findings, however, must be placed in context. WATCH was a primary care study involving a low-cost, minimal-effort counseling intervention. To achieve a 10% reduction in calories from saturated fat and a meaningful reduction in LDL-cholesterol levels at 1 year of follow-up in patients *not* placed on pharmacologic therapy is clearly worthwhile. Such an LDL-cholesterol change, if maintained, should lead to a significant reduction in coronary event rates.

In any analysis of the prevention literature, it is important to differentiate between primary and secondary intervention studies. In primary care the intervention needs to be of low intensity (and low cost), and the patient's motivation to change is much less than it is when a myocardial infarction or other clinical event already has occurred.

Stanford Case Management System for Coronary Risk Factor Modification After Acute Myocardial Infarction

The Stanford Case Management System for Coronary Risk Factor Modification After Acute Myocardial Infarction[7] was a secondary prevention study designed to evaluate the efficacy of a physician-directed but nurse-managed case management system for coronary risk factor modification. Patients (N = 585) with a recent myocardial infarction, all members of the Kaiser-Permanente medical system, were randomized to usual care or special intervention. Following an initial in-hospital nurse intervention for smoking cessation, diet/drug intervention for hyperlipidemia, and exercise training, follow-up intervention (approximately 9 hours of nurse contact during the 1-year follow-up) was implemented primarily by telephone and mail.

The study had a number of interesting outcomes. The intervention group made significant dietary changes, achieving a better than Step II American Heart Association (AHA) diet. Surprisingly, however, the usual-care group achieved almost the same level of dietary change. The special-care group had significantly lower 1-year plasma LDL-cholesterol levels (107 vs. 132 mg/dL special care vs. usual care, respectively), but this was primarily the result of a much greater percentage of special-care patients being placed on pharmacologic lipid-lowering therapy (66% vs. 21% at 12 months, respectively). Smoking cessation rates were 70% for the special-care group and 53% for the usual-care group. Functional capacity at 1 year was also significantly higher in the special-care group.

There was no difference in the number of coronary events seen in the 2 groups over the 1 year of follow-up. However, it is known that lipid changes generally have a 1- to 2-year lag before clinical benefit is seen, and only 43.1% of the patients were smokers. The study demonstrated that a relatively intensive case-management approach could result in significant and important changes in patients' risk-factor profiles.

For risk-factor change on the level of the health care provider and the individual patient, then, we have learned that there is value to training practitioners in behavioral counseling methodology and in setting up supportive office systems, as well as developing case-management systems that deliver a more intensive intervention that coordinates with the primary providers' efforts. It is also likely that dietitians can make an important contribution to patient behavior change, although this is not as well studied.

PREVENTION OF CARDIOVASCULAR DISEASE OUTSIDE THE TRADITIONAL HEALTH CARE ENVIRONMENT

Community Interventions

The community approach is based on the premise that interventions at the level of the community organization can change the setting in which people live so as to support healthier lifestyles and decrease in chronic disease morbidity and mortality.

In the past few decades increasing attention has been paid to community organization as a means of accomplishing large-scale change for the prevention of chronic health problems.[8] In general, community interventions for CHD attempt to reduce the prevalence of risk factors associated with the disease, such as high blood pressure, elevated serum cholesterol level, smoking, overweight, and sedentary lifestyle. Program components include community organization, needs assessment, prioritization and evaluation, and program maintenance. Activities include social marketing, direct behavior-change efforts (including skills training, health education, and contingency management), screening (including counseling and referral), and environmental and policy interventions.

As an example of such a process, King and colleagues discuss the use of policy (both legislative and regulatory) and environmental interventions in the promotion of physical activity to prevent CHD and other chronic diseases. These interventions may include federal, state, and local legislation and regulation; policy development and implementation; and environmental support.[9]

Community interventions can be applied through a variety of channels: contacting community leaders and existing formal and informal community groups (such as social, religious, ethnic, and school programs; adult education programs; and self-help programs); using the existing mass media network; and supporting community organization efforts. The core of a successful program is the community organization process. This involves identification and activation of key community leaders, stimulation of citizens and organizations to volunteer time and offer resources for CVD prevention, and the promotion of prevention as a community theme. Community health professionals play a vital role in providing program endorsement and stimulating the participation of community leaders.

Community Intervention Studies

One of the earliest community trials for the reduction of cardiovascular risk was the **Stanford Three-Community Study**[10] (Table 32-3). One community was monitored as a control site, one was assigned to media intervention only, and the third was assigned to a combination of media and face-to-face intervention. In both treatment communities

■ ■ ■

TABLE 32-3 SAMPLE COMMUNITY INTERVENTION STUDIES

Study	Strategies	Main findings
Stanford Three Community Study[10]	Mass media education campaigns and face-to-face education	Substantial and sustained decrease in cardiovascular risk factors
The North Karelia Project[11,12]	Education and building of a strong social support system to point-of-purchase advertising and television campaigns	Substantial decrease in cardiovascular risk factors and CHD mortality
Stanford Five City Project[13]	Comprehensive program using social learning theory, a communication–behavior change model, community organization principles, and social marketing methods. Exposure to multichannel and multifactor education	Significant reductions in CHD risk factors
The Minnesota Heart Health Program[8]	Risk-factor screening, mass media education, adult education classes, worksite interventions, home correspondence programs, school-based programs, restaurant programs, and point-of-purchase education in supermarkets	No overall effect on mean body mass index. However, a positive intervention effect early in the intervention among those with elevated cholesterol levels or a history of obesity-related disease
The Washington Heights-Inwood Healthy Heart Program (part of the New York State Healthy Heart Program)[15]	Community intervention in a largely Hispanic population	Description of barriers to the implementation of the intervention
The Heartbeat Wales Coronary Heart Disease Prevention Program[16]	To examine the difficulties of developing and maintaining outcome evaluation designs in long-term, community-based health promotion programs	Discussion of study contamination related to the dissemination of information across communities as a limitation of community intervention evaluation

CHD, coronary heart disease.

there was substantial and similar improvement in cardiovascular risk profiles by the end of the second year, although initially the level of improvement was greater in the community with face-to-face counseling. The study suggested that mass media campaigns could be effective in modifying risk factors at the community level.

The North Karelia project carried out in Finland yielded comparable results.[11] After 10 years of follow-up, men in the intervention group demonstrated statistically significant differences in risk factors: a 1% decrease in mean diastolic blood pressure, a 3% decrease in mean systolic blood pressure, a 28% decrease in smoking prevalence, and a 3% decrease in serum cholesterol levels. This was associated with a 22% reduction in age-standardized CHD mortality in men and 43% in women. This study used community channels for cardiovascular risk-factor modification, ranging from education and building of a strong social support system to point-of-purchase advertising and television campaigns.

The North Karelia Project has not only had an effect on reducing the mortality from CHD in all of Finland, but over a 20-year follow-up period (1972 to 1991), cancer mortality declined in North Karelia by 45.4% and in all of Finland by 32.7% (P = 0.006 for difference). The greater decline in North Karelia occurred particularly in the second decade of the follow-up period and was related particularly to a decrease in lung cancer mortality. The results support the hypothesis that reduction in the population levels of cardiovascular risk factors leads to beneficial changes in cancer mortality rates, presumably via effects on smoking and diet, but such changes take a longer time to manifest than for CHD.[12]

After these initial efforts, a second generation of studies was funded by the National Heart, Lung and Blood Institute to examine the effects of a community approach to changing cardiovascular risk factors, including the Pawtucket Heart Health Program, the Minnesota Heart Health Program, and the Stanford Five-City Project. All three studies used various community organization techniques to ensure participation by the community members.

The Stanford Five-City Project is typical of this group of studies.[13] Treatment cities received a 5-year, low-cost, comprehensive program using social learning theory, a communication–behavior change model, community organization principles, and social marketing methods that resulted in about 26 hours of exposure to multichannel and multifactor education. Surveys carried out at intervals varying from 30 to 64 months following the start of the study demonstrated significant reductions favoring the treatment communities: plasma cholesterol level (2%), blood pressure (4%), resting pulse rate (3%), and smoking rate (13%); a composite total mortality risk score fell 15%, and a CHD risk score decreased 16%. Thus, such low-cost programs can have an impact on risk factors in broad population groups.

Some studies, however, have not been able to clearly demonstrate benefit. **The Minnesota Heart Health Program** found no overall effect on mean body mass index after 7 years of community intervention activities that included risk-factor screening, mass-media education, adult education classes, worksite interventions, home correspondence programs, school-based programs, restaurant programs, and point-of-purchase education in supermarkets. However, a positive intervention effect was noted early in the intervention among those with elevated cholesterol levels or a history of obesity-related disease.[8] There was a marked secular trend for weight to increase in all study communities. The investigators note that explanations for a less-than-expected intervention effect include secular forces' overwhelming intervention effects, an inadequately focused intervention effort, a population already highly aware of the issue at baseline, and inherent limitations in educational approaches for a difficult public health problem.

In the United States, state public health departments nationwide are implementing community-based CHD prevention programs, with the development of a statewide CVD prevention plan being an important element of such efforts. These programs must attend to factors such as affordability, acceptability, and adequacy of the intervention, given that efforts sponsored at the state level rarely will have the resources of federally funded demonstration projects. A significant source of funding, particularly for smoking prevention, has been the funds paid to the states as a result of the master tobacco settlement between 46 states and the 4 largest tobacco companies in the United States.[14]

Limitations of Community Interventions

The overall results of these interventions suggest that there is great potential for community interventions. Where differences between intervention and control groups have been less than expected, the factors explained in the following paragraphs may be playing a role.

In many community interventions, an initial favorable effect in groups that already have a given risk factor for CHD seems to abate with time, despite the increased level of awareness of the community as a whole. With few exceptions,[15] most of these studies have not looked at differences in subgroups within the community. It may be that for people at risk, community interventions are useful to initiate change but that this "high risk" subgroup ultimately may need a more intensive intervention to maintain the desired behavior and to prevent a "rebound effect." However, the rest of the population (the majority) slowly may assimilate the information and work toward behavior modification. The diffusion of innovations learning theory also could explain some of the differences in adoption of new behaviors between "early" and "late" adopters.

Another problem inherent to community-based intervention projects in this age of rapid communication is that information can disseminate quickly and interfere with classic intervention/evaluation control designs through contamination. Therefore, alternative experimental designs for assessing the effectiveness of long-term intervention programs need to be considered. These should not rely solely on the use of reference populations but should balance the measurement of outcome with an assessment of the process of change in communities.[16]

Populations of low socioeconomic status or of differing cultural backgrounds may require specific approaches that differ from those applicable to the general population.[1] The Washington Heights-Inwood Healthy Heart Program, part of the New York State Healthy Heart Program, studied a population of approximately 200,000 people, predominantly Hispanic and of low socioeconomic status, living in northern Manhattan in New York City.[15] Potential barriers to diffusion of the community-based disease prevention model in disadvantaged inner-city communities were identified, including issues of scale and complexity, adaptation of the model to a "community"

without geopolitical boundaries or infrastructure, linguistic and cultural diversity, competing problems, and sustainability of the program in a poor community. Strategies used to address obstacles to model adoption included legitimizing the program, building program infrastructure, setting realistic expectations, focusing on one risk factor at a time, defining target population segments, and emphasizing a small number of communication channels. The initial experience implementing this model in a disadvantaged urban setting supports the feasibility of this approach.

Worksite Intervention

The worksite provides a vehicle for helping people reduce risk through changes in the work organization and environment. CHD risks may be reduced by eliminating or reducing exposures to hazardous substances such as cigarette smoke or by altering work conditions that are associated with increased disease incidence, such as the stressful work combination of high demand and low control.

More than three fourths (76%) of the U.S. civilian, non-institutionalized men age 20 and older currently are employed; the corresponding figure for women is 60.8%.[18] Even a small intervention effect in this large segment of the population has the potential to change health behaviors so as to result in substantial changes in CHD event rates.[2] At the same time interventions in this group can be an important window into the usefulness of worksite policy/regulation and for implementation of environmental changes, which in turn would foster changes in individual behavior.

This target population includes many people with low income and educational levels who may not be reached through other intervention channels. Interventions addressing multiple risk-related behaviors, such as smoking, diet, and exercise, can be offered in worksites repeatedly over time, thus increasing the likelihood of motivating change in persons who are at various points of readiness for such change. Increasingly, businesses themselves are taking an active role in this process because they perceive prevention as a way of holding down health care costs related to absenteeism, insurance claims, and disability.[19,20] However, the efficacy of such efforts is limited not only by their availability but also by the degree of interest that employees show in participating in these programs.

The number of health promotion programs in the worksite has increased in recent years, with most of the programs aimed at individual behavior change.[21] Results of the first National Survey of Worksite Health Promotion Activities found that 65.5% of responding worksites had one or more types of health promotion activities.[22] Worksite preventive health programs typically include, in decreasing order of frequency, smoking cessation, health risk assessment, back care regimens, stress management, exercise and fitness programs, accident prevention, nutrition education, high blood pressure treatment, and weight control. The frequency of these activities is directly related to the size of the worksite and varies by industry type.[23]

A recent study of the prevalence of workplace health promotion activities at small worksites with 15 to 99 employees used a random sample of U.S. worksites stratified by size and industry. The overall response rate for eligible worksites was 78% for a total sample of 2680 worksites. Approximately one fourth of worksites with 15 to 99 employees offered health promotion programs to their employees, compared with 44% of worksites with 100 or more employees. The study concludes that small worksites are providing programs to their employees, with a primary focus on job-related hazards. Small worksites also have formal policies regarding alcohol, drug use, smoking, and seatbelt use and offer health insurance to their employees at a rate only slightly lower than that of large worksites.[24]

Worksite Intervention Studies

A study representative of the type of research carried out in the workplace is IBM's "A Plan for Life" program (Table 32-4), which evaluated changes in blood pressure; serum total, high-density lipoprotein, and non-high-density lipoprotein cholesterol; body mass index; and cigarette smoking over a 1- to 5-year period among nonrandomized program participants and nonparticipants initially found to be at risk. After adjustment for age, sex, time to follow-up, and baseline values, the proportion of participants no longer at high risk was significantly greater than the corresponding proportion of nonparticipants, with meaningful changes occurring in blood pressure, total and non-high–density lipoprotein cholesterol, and smoking cessation.[25]

Few systematic studies have provided evidence that health promotion is a cost-effective means of decreasing health care costs, although the evidence for tangible benefits is beginning to accumulate.[26,27] A landmark study conducted at the DuPont Company compared 41 intervention sites and 19 control sites with a total of more than 40,000 hourly employees.[26] Over a 2-year period, blue-collar employees at intervention sites experienced a significant decline in disability days (14%), as compared with a smaller decline in the control sites (5.8%). Savings resulting from lower disability costs at intervention sites provided a return of $2.05 for every dollar invested in the program by the end of the second year. There is also evidence suggesting that a comprehensive health promotion program may have other benefits for employers, including improved attitudes of employees toward the company, reductions in corporate health benefits costs, and decreased utilization of inpatient services.[28] For some employers, the major motivation for sponsoring health promotion efforts may be the potential savings resulting from healthier employee lifestyles; in such cases, accurate estimates of cost savings can improve the program's chances of adoption. Other employers may be interested primarily in programs as a means to improve employee morale or the company's public image and may be especially responsive to employee requests when offering programs.

In a randomized controlled worksite nutrition intervention program that focused on promoting eating patterns low in fat and high in fiber **(The Treatwell Study)**, 16 worksites from Massachusetts and Rhode Island were randomly assigned to either an intervention or a control condition.[29] The intervention included direct education and environmental programming tailored to each worksite; control worksites received no intervention. A cohort of workers randomly sampled from each site was surveyed both prior to and following the intervention. Dietary patterns were assessed using a semiquantitative food frequency questionnaire. Adjusting for worksite, the decrease in mean dietary fat intake was 1.1% of total calories more in intervention sites than in control sites (P < 0.005). There was no difference in dietary fiber intake between intervention and control sites. Thus a worksite nutrition intervention program can effectively influence the dietary habits of workers.

■ ■ ■

TABLE 32-4   SAMPLE WORKSITE INTERVENTION STUDIES

Study	Strategies	Main findings
IBM's "A Plan for Life" program[25]	Comprehensive cardiovascular risk factor education	Significant decrease in coronary heart disease risk factors (blood pressure, hypercholesterolemia, and smoking)
DuPont Company[26]	Impact of comprehensive workplace promotion program on absenteeism	Significant reduction in absenteeism and good return on investment.
The Treatwell Study[29]	Direct education regarding eating habits, coupled with environmental programming tailored to each site	Significant decrease in dietary fat intake
The Shape Up Challenge (Part of the Minnesota Heart Health Program)[19]	A worksite exercise competition designed to increase levels of physical activity as part of community-wide annual exercise campaigns	Participating companies were more likely to offer other health promotion programs and perceived greater benefits from participation. Women and smaller companies had significantly greater participation rates than men and larger companies
Worksite nutrition intervention trial—Belgium[20]	Individualized health risk appraisal, group sessions, mass media activities, and environmental changes regarding low-fat diet	Nutrition knowledge improved significantly, reduction in total caloric intake and in the percentage of energy from total fat, significant reduction in blood cholesterol only among participants with hypercholesterolemia

School Intervention

Most adult CHD is attributable to risk factor–related behaviors that often are established in early childhood. Even a couple of decades ago, by age 12 at least one modifiable risk factor for CHD was present in 36% to 60% of children in the United States.[30] There is a general assumption that the psychosocial environment of childhood contributes to behaviors in adult life, including those related to CHD morbidity and mortality. These behavioral risks—cigarette smoking, inappropriate dietary habits, and insufficient exercise—are all difficult to modify once established. The large numbers of children who attend private and public schools 5 days a week for an average of 36 weeks a year turn schools into a major window of opportunity for promoting health-related behaviors among children.

For the most part, the model for school health services that has guided the development of school health programs in the United States includes three components: health instruction, a healthful school environment, and the provision of school health services (Table 32-5). Health instruction includes teaching health-related knowledge, attitudes, and practices. The school environment relates to the actual physical setting as well as to an awareness of its influence on the attitude and behavior of students. School health services include medical examinations, screening programs, communicable disease control, and correction of remediable problems. This model has been used to tailor CHD interventions as well as interventions for other acute and chronic diseases in the school setting.[31]

Before 1980, the goal of most school health education programs was to transmit information with the hope that increased knowledge would lead students to adopt positive health behaviors.[31] However, there is substantial evidence that such an approach is ineffective. It is clear, for example, that most adults who smoke begin smoking while in their teens, and rates of adolescent smoking have not declined as have those for other age groups. This has been particularly true for teenage girls, who now smoke more than their male counterparts. Thus a modified approach has evolved that places less emphasis on knowledge acquisition and more on skills development, social influences, and behavioral competencies, with the goal of intervening before risk behaviors become established.

Smoking Interventions

School-based smoking prevention programs incorporating these approaches have had generally positive results, the most successful being programs that are targeted to delay the onset of smoking, which is important in terms of reducing the likelihood of a person becoming a heavy smoker as an adult.[32] It is generally agreed that, at a minimum, a smoking prevention program in the school setting should offer information about the short-term physiologic effects of tobacco and the social influences that lead to smoking, training in refusal skills, and facts on the social consequences of smoking.[33]

The school environment also must support smoking prevention and a nonsmoking policy for both staff and students. In schools with the most restrictive smoking

---

◼ ◼ ◼

TABLE 32-5   SAMPLE SCHOOL INTERVENTION STUDIES

Study	Strategies	Main findings
Youth tobacco use in the United States—problem, progress, goals, and potential solutions[33]	Review of health and economic burden of tobacco use, current knowledge about youth tobacco use, and youth-related national tobacco reduction goals.	Most effective strategies include those that involve the family or health care providers and programs carried out in schools and/or through the media. Approaches such as limiting access, advertising restrictions, and increased taxes are also effective.
Ethnic and gender differences in drinking and smoking among London adolescents[32]	Confidential, self-completed questionnaire assessing onset and frequency of drinking and smoking.	White children were more likely to have ever smoked tobacco and consumed alcohol, and to progress from initiation to regular use than were black or Asian children.
Use of fat-modified food products to change dietary fat intake of young people[38]	Environmental nutrition program aimed at changing the food buying and preparation practices of school food service workers.	The diet of the students in the intervention group contained 15% to 20% less sodium and 20% less saturated fat than that of a control group.
The Heart Smart Cardiovascular School Health Promotion[39]	Environmental intervention including a school lunch program providing cardiovascular healthful food choices; a physical education program; and cardiovascular risk-factor screening.	Improvements in health knowledge, cardiovascular healthful lunch choices, lipid profile, and run/walk performance.
Child-reported family and peer influences on fruit, juice, and vegetable consumption[40]	Questionnaires to measure family and peer influences on children's fruit, juice, and vegetable consumption.	Parental modeling, peer normative beliefs, and fruit and vegetable availability were significantly correlated with fruit, juice, and vegetable consumption.
Child and Adolescent Trial for Cardiovascular Health (CATCH)[48]	School and family intervention from grades 3 through 5. Follow-up (after 3 years, without further intervention) of a randomized, controlled field trial with 56 intervention and 40 control elementary schools.	Decreased total fat intake, higher self-reported daily activity, and no impact on smoking behavior were reported. There were no significant differences in body mass index, blood pressure, or serum lipid levels. Results suggest that the behavioral changes initiated during the elementary school years persisted to early adolescence.

policies and a strong emphasis on prevention, fewer students used tobacco. Recognizing the importance of school smoking policies, the National Cancer Institute recommended establishment of restrictive smoking policies by schools as one of the essential elements of school-based tobacco use prevention programs. However, there have been reports of practical difficulties in enforcing such policies at the school level.[34]

The social-influences approach frequently is described as the most effective model for prevention of adolescent smoking, and it is the only program with demonstrated results. With up to 5 years of follow-up, these programs consistently have demonstrated the ability to delay the onset of smoking. However, there is also evidence suggesting that the benefits in early adolescence may disappear entirely by the time a student graduates from high school.

Suggestions for further research on tobacco use prevention focus on transitions from one level of tobacco use to another; use of high-quality measures and of multiple methodologies, including nonpanel longitudinal studies, intensive interview, ethnography, experimental intervention, and small exploratory studies as well as further prospective studies; inclusion of variables from multiple streams of influence to investigate interrelationships among cultural, social, and intrapersonal factors; and collection of data from multiple nested units (e.g., children within families, within schools, within neighborhoods).[35]

Dietary Interventions

Dietary recommendations are a major component of national chronic disease prevention strategies, particularly for CHD and cancer. National recommendations include reducing total, saturated fat, and trans-fatty-acid consumption; increasing the consumption of fruits, vegetables, and whole-grain products; and reducing alcohol, sugar, and salt intake. Although these recommendations are for adults, they seem to be appropriate as well for children older than 2 years of age. Parents have a powerful influence on their children's eating behavior—an influence that is probably even greater than it is for cigarette smoking. Although parents usually select most of their children's food, these selections take into account the needs and expressed demands of children. The advertising of foods on television often shapes these demands.

An analysis of school lunches carried out as part of a CHD prevention program demonstrated that total fat accounted for 38.8% of the total calories children consumed at lunch, nearly one-third more than the recommendations of the National School Lunch Program.[36] These results were consistent with the findings of other school-based heart disease prevention programs and showed little change even after the U.S. Department of Agriculture (USDA) published guidelines in 1983 for reducing the fat, sugar, and sodium content of school lunches. Because 60% of public school students participate in school lunch programs and consume 25% to 33% of their total daily calories at school, cafeteria and school lunch interventions are a common component of comprehensive school-based nutrition programs.[37]

The value of nutritional interventions in the schools has been shown in a number of studies. Ellison and colleagues[38] tested the influence of an environmental nutrition program aimed at changing the food buying and preparation practices of school food service workers. Although there was no student education component, the diet of the students in the intervention group contained 15% to 20% less sodium and 20% less saturated fat than that of a control group. A multifactorial approach as used in the Heart Smart cardiovascular school health project (a school lunch program providing cardiovascular healthful food choices, a physical education program promoting personal fitness and aerobic conditioning, and cardiovascular risk-factor screening) also has been shown to be of value.[39] Participants showed greater improvement in health knowledge than did nonparticipants. School lunch choices were altered successfully, and children whose lunch choices were more healthful demonstrated the greatest cholesterol reduction. Improvements in run/walk performance were related in predicted directions to the overall cardiovascular risk profile.

Social and Family Environment

A supportive and reinforcing school environment increases the likelihood that the students will develop health-promoting skills and attitudes. The student activities should be based on sound behavioral and learning theory and, whenever possible, should be those that already have been shown to be effective in achieving positive outcomes. However, although schools can be instrumental in promoting the health of school-aged children, they cannot be expected to do the job alone. A supportive and reinforcing family and home setting is particularly important in encouraging children to establish healthy behaviors.[40,41] Reviewing the literature on the role of families in influencing health-related behaviors, studies suggest that children also can influence their parents' health behavior, that parents are often difficult to recruit to traditional health education classes, and that more flexible learning methods are needed that can be used at home. Schools also can provide an effective channel for rural health promotion efforts, where community intervention programs face the challenge of disseminating health information to widely scattered populations.

One problem of particular concern is the relative lack of attention directed at high-risk, hard-to-reach youth. In the past, with a few exceptions,[42] most CHD prevention programs have been targeted at nonminority, middle-class populations. However, currently there is more interest in such studies.[43] Health professionals and schools continually must be alert to provide appropriate programming for high-risk, difficult-to-reach groups, particularly while they can still be reached in the formal school system.

Among adults there is substantial evidence that lack of physical activity is related to obesity, hypertension, high blood lipid levels, and early death from CHD. National physical fitness surveys indicate that only a minority of adults engage in regular physical activity at a level likely to maintain cardiac and respiratory fitness.[44]

Physical inactivity in adulthood often has its roots in childhood. Most observers have concluded that the current generation of children is not as fit as the previous one; today's youth have more body fat than children did in the 1960s. The goal of school-based physical education programs should be, at least partially, to create favorable attitudes, experiences, and skills to increase the likelihood that those children will continue being physically active as adults. At least 80% of 10- to 18-year-olds are enrolled in physical education programs at school, but these programs often do not focus on health-related fitness that is likely to lead to greater activity by adults.[45] Data from the Class of 1989 Study (part of the Minnesota Heart Health Program), however, suggest that multiple intervention components such as behavioral education in schools and complementary community-wide strategies can produce lasting improvement in adolescent physical activity.[46]

Some programs have targeted multiple cardiovascular risk factors among elementary school students, high school students, and minority populations. Most notable among these was a National Heart, Lung, and Blood Institute-funded cooperative project: the Child and Adolescent Trial for Cardiovascular Health (CATCH).[47] This study's overall goal was to determine the effect of school-based intervention on promoting healthy behavior and reducing CHD risk factors among elementary school students. It used programs promoting exercise, a healthful diet, and fitness. Interventions focus on school curricula and environment and on fostering parental involvement. Follow-up of the CATCH cohort suggests that the behavioral changes initiated during the elementary school years persisted to early adolescence for self-reported dietary and physical activity behaviors.[48] However, despite favorable reported changes in dietary fat intake and physical activity, no changes were seen in blood pressure, serum cholesterol levels, or body mass index between the intervention and control groups.

The relationship of home- and school-based programs has been examined in several studies. In the San Diego Family Health Project, Mexican-American and Anglo-American families with children in the fifth or sixth grade were randomized to either a control condition or to a year-long education program designed to change dietary and exercise habits using classes held in local schools.[42] After 1 year, positive changes had occurred in the intervention families' dietary practices, but their cardiovascular fitness levels had not changed significantly. The authors concluded that involving families in health education programs using school-based resources is effective and that this is a promising area for future research.[40]

In another study, the benefits of school-based programs were compared with those aimed directly at the home environment.[49] Conducted in Minnesota and North Dakota, the study compared the results of a 5-week school-based program for third graders with that of a 5-week program of written information sent to the homes of third graders; both programs required parental involvement. Of eligible parents, 86% participated in the home-based program and 71% completed the 5-week course. Students in the home-based program had greater reductions in dietary fat and saturated fat than did those in the school-based program. The study showed that a large number of parents are willing to participate in home-based programs and that this type of parental participation can initiate changes in the eating patterns of young children as well as the parents. There are also reports in the literature of successful dietary interventions among preschool children.[41]

One of the limitations of school-based programs is that they do not influence the high-risk adolescents who drop out of school. These adolescents are untouched by school-based interventions and their risk behaviors often exceed those of their peers who are still in school.[34] This is true for smoking and also may be the case for other cardiovascular risks. Other identified barriers to CHD prevention programs in the schools include overcrowded curricula, overburdened teachers, the desire for broad and locally controlled programs, inadequate funding, and lack of teacher training.

LIFESTYLE, ENVIRONMENT, AND POLICY ISSUES

From the preventive health perspective, the current way of life in the "developed" world is characterized by physical inactivity, overeating, and engaging in self-destructive behaviors such as smoking. Development has been responsible for many achievements benefiting the population—it has saved the modern world from most of the infectious diseases that affected our ancestors for millennia, primarily through the widespread availability of safe drinking water, sewage systems, and improved housing. However, development is also in many ways responsible for most of the chronic diseases that we face today.

From automobiles to washing machines to remote controls, technology has "developed" us into a morbidly sedentary way of life. Industry's growth, based on the population's consumption patterns, has fashioned many unessential needs. We now have widespread access to cigarettes and other tobacco products and to an unprecedented array of food items, many of which have been modified by processing techniques and by the inclusion of ingredients such as sugar, salt, and fat, making these foods more attractive, usually higher in calories, and requiring a minimum amount of time and effort for preparation and utilization. The end result is an unfortunate combination of habits: a sedentary lifestyle, excess food intake, and engagement in harmful behaviors such as smoking.

Given our current way of life, the challenge confronting us is how we, as a society, can "develop" healthier lifestyle habits. The answer probably requires an approach combining behavioral change with environmental and policy regulations. Most of the initiatives to date have centered on behavioral change geared to modifying individual undesirable habitual patterns (smoking, diet, and physical activity). However, a number of reports have appeared in the literature highlighting the importance of environmental changes supported by policy regulations as a means of enhancing and facilitating behavioral change.[50]

Behavioral change has been studied extensively, and many models have been developed around different learning theories. Behavioral change interventions for CHD are based on our understanding of the underlying science. However, as science evolves the need for consensus gains particular importance. The knowledge base underlying dietary guidelines is a special example. The relationship of dietary patterns to disease is not always clear. Thus, at present, the national dietary guidelines continue to recommend diets low in total fat, but there is substantial evidence that such diets are not effective either in lowering cholesterol or in curbing the progressive weight gain seen in our population. The balance of opinion is shifting toward diets restricted in saturated fat and trans-fatty acids, but not in total fat, where monounsaturated fats are seen as a source of calories preferable to carbohydrates, especially simple sugars, and ω-3 fatty acids are seen as clearly beneficial.[51]

Policy Interventions—Smoking, Diet, and Physical Activity

Smoking, diet, and physical activity increasingly have become a source of concern at the national level, with regulatory agencies and Congress progressively more involved in suggesting or enacting rules and regulations that respond to public concern. For smoking such approaches have included increased taxation on cigarettes, the banning of smoking in public places, the use of tobacco settlement monies for prevention efforts, and the support of media campaigns against smoking by public agencies such as the National Cancer Institute. The U.S. Department of Health and Human Services (DHHS) also has funded programs to develop interventions to improve diet and physical activity. Table 32-6 summarizes sample policy studies.

Preventing tobacco use, especially among America's youth, is one of the nation's most important health

■ ▦ ■

TABLE 32-6   SAMPLE POLICY STUDIES

Study	Strategies	Main findings
The new food label, type of fat, and consumer choice. A pilot study[54]	Cross-sectional survey in the general community and university setting regarding food labels	Current consumer choice exceedingly may be influenced by industry-directed claims placed on the front of a product package.
Counting calories—caveat emptor—NY[55]	To determine the accuracy of caloric labeling of "diet" and "health" foods and whether the accuracy differs for certain categories of food suppliers: regionally distributed, nationally advertised, or locally prepared.	All locally prepared foods had more actual than labeled calories. Regionally distributed foods had significantly more calories than were reported. Nationally advertised foods were more accurate regarding labeled caloric content.
The contribution of expanding portion sizes to the U.S. obesity epidemic[61]	Information about current and past marketplace food portion size obtained from manufacturers, from direct weighing, and from contemporary publications.	Marketplace food portions have increased in size and now exceed federal standards. Portion size increase parallels increasing body weight in the population.
Small taxes on soft drinks and snack foods to promote health[60]	Review of tax revenue information.	18 states and one major city charge special taxes on soft drinks, candy, chewing gum, or snack foods. The tax rates may be too small to affect sales, but the revenues generated may be significant. Nationally, about $1 billion is raised annually from these taxes.
Changes in physical activity patterns in the United States, by sex and cross-sectional age[58]	Review of cross-sectional data from the National Health Interview Survey, using the Youth Risk Behavior Survey supplement for adolescents and the Health Promotion/Disease Prevention supplement for adults.	Among adolescents, physical activity patterns decreased from ages 15 through 18. Young adulthood often marked continuing erosion of activity patterns, whereas middle adulthood of ten revealed relatively stable patterns. At retirement age, there was a stabilizing, tendency in activity patterns, usually followed by further decrease through the final period of life.
Physical activity interventions using mass media, print media, and information technology[64]	Literature review of 28 studies of media-based interventions of which 7 were mass media campaigns at the state or national level and the remaining 21 were delivered through health care, through the workplace, or in the community.	Recall of mass media messages generally was high, but mass media campaigns had very little impact on physical activity behavior. Interventions using print and/or telephone were effective in changing behavior in the short term. A key issue is reaching socially disadvantaged groups.
Developing principles for health impact assessment[65]	Health impact assessment using case studies comparing possible future scenarios for developing transport in Edinburgh based on funding levels and health impacts of housing investment in a disadvantaged part of Edinburgh.	Disadvantaged communities bore more detrimental effects from the low transport investment scenario in terms of accidents; pollution; access to amenities, jobs and social contacts; physical activity; and impacts on community networks. The housing investment had the greatest impact on residents' mental health by reducing overcrowding, noise pollution, stigma, and fear of crime.

challenges. According to the Department of Health and Human Services' Substance Abuse and Mental Health Administration, more than 57 million individuals currently smoke. In addition, data from HHS's Centers for Disease Control and Prevention (CDC) indicate that more than 430,000 deaths in the United States are attributable to tobacco use, making tobacco the leading preventable cause of death and disease in the country. Every day, 3000 young people become regular tobacco users, and one third of them will die from smoking-related diseases.[52] The Surgeon General's office has taken the lead in marshalling the evidence against smoking, much of which has been used in the legislative process, which has contributed to the progressive reduction in smoking rates in this country. Several states have implemented excise taxes on tobacco products and observed significant decreases in cigarette consumption.

Diet: Policy Issues Surrounding Food Labeling

The U.S. food supply is regulated by a series of laws administered by the DHHS and the USDA. The Food and Drug Administration's (FDA) requirements concerning the provision of basic, standard-format nutrition information ("nutrition labeling") on food products have changed dramatically over the past 50 years. The FDA regulations that became effective in 1994 require standardized nutrition labeling on most food products carried in interstate commerce. Under the new FDA regulations, it is illegal to use any health claim or nutrient content claim in food labeling unless the FDA has approved the claim in advance.

In 1993 the FDA promulgated regulations that described general requirements for health claims on foods and specific requirements for seven authorized health claim topics. Three authorized claims were related to heart disease: dietary saturated fat and cholesterol and CHD; fruits, vegetables, and grain products that contain fiber, particularly soluble fiber, and risk of CHD; and the relationship of sodium intake to hypertension. Approval for health claims is based on the totality of publicly available scientific evidence and significant agreement among experts qualified by scientific training and experience to evaluate the relationship.

Food labeling is an especially important and interesting interface between policy and preventive medicine. Diet is complex, and in contrast to cigarette smoking, the consumer needs a great deal of information to make intelligent choices. The awareness of the nutritional content of foods influences people's choices. A study performed at the University of Utah to estimate the effects of changing nutrition information format assessed consumer preferences for 12 label alternatives used to provide nutrition information on Campbell's Soup cans. Consumers clearly preferred the nutrition label that displayed all nutrient values using a bar graph format, offered the most information, and expressed nutrient values using both absolute numbers and percentages. Consumers also preferred nutrition information arranged in an order that grouped nutrients that should be consumed in adequate amounts on the top, calories in the middle, and nutrients that

should be consumed in lesser amounts on the bottom of the label.[53] Another study concluded that consumer choices might be overly influenced by industry-directed claims placed on the front of a product package.[54]

The use of labels seems to be an effective way to spread knowledge. At the same time, studies show that the general public currently is overloaded with nutritional information and that many basic concepts regarding healthful dietary choices are not clear. There are also problems in the implementation of labeling guidelines. A New York City study carried out to determine the accuracy of caloric labeling demonstrated that locally prepared foods had more actual than labeled kilocalories (the mean percentage of kilocalories over label, per item, was 85.42% (SD = 77.88%; P = .01).[55] Regionally distributed foods also had significantly more kilocalories than reported on the label, but the average discrepancy was considerably smaller (25.22%). However, the labeling of nationally advertised foods was quite accurate, with only a 2.2% underestimate of caloric content. These findings suggest that labels on foods produced by small enterprises without extensive resources to carry out or commission appropriate testing may be inadequate sources for nutritional information.

Changes in regulations regarding nutrition labeling are a very complex issue. As an example, the debate over labeling of hydrogenated fat, brought up because of its deleterious effects on the lipid profile and its widespread use in the food industry, will be summarized.

In 1999, a proposal for change in nutrition labeling regarding trans-fatty acids was filed by the FDA, partly in response to a citizen's petition by the Center for Science in the Public Interest (CSPI). CSPI is a Washington D.C.-based, nonprofit education and advocacy organization that focuses on improving the safety and nutritional quality of the food supply. The proposal[56] describes the relevant literature and offers a cost-benefit analysis. The cost of implementing the rule is divided into several categories, including product nutrient analysis, research costs, printing of new labels, disposal of inventory, and marketing of the new product. It also takes into account the potential health benefits by calculating the impact of the proposed rule on CHD morbidity and mortality prevention.

In the case of trans-fat, the economic and health benefits are clear, but implementation of the rule would place a burden on small businesses, with an estimated nationwide implementation cost of more than $100 million. The FDA found that this proposed rule was economically significant as defined by Executive Order 12866, thus breaking a cap on the economic cost of implementation of the rule and requiring further analysis of the feasibility of implementation of the rule.

A small business is defined here as one having 500 or fewer employees. Exempt small businesses are considered those that sell less than 100,000 units of the product per year or that have less than 100 full-time employees. For small businesses the implementation of the rule was estimated to result in an average cost of $22,600. After all the analyses are presented, the FDA opens a public forum to receive questions and concerns about the proposed rule.[56]

As a final rule, on July 11, 2003, the FDA amended its regulations on nutrition labeling to require that trans fatty acids be declared in the nutrition label of conventional foods and dietary supplements on a separate line, immediately below the line for the declaration of saturated fatty acids, which will be effective on January 1, 2006 (7 years after the proposal was presented).

Several observations are of particular interest. The interactions between the public interest and the economic interests of the industry are complex. Second, locally produced food products are minimally regulated by the FDA. Furthermore, the FDA does not regulate the food service industry. Partially hydrogenated fats and oils are used extensively in the food service industry for baking and frying. USDA data indicate that a single serving of french-fried potatoes from a fast food restaurant may contain more than 3.5 g of trans-fat per 70-g serving.[57] If the FDA were to require that content information about trans-fat be provided in food service establishments, consumers could more easily make informed menu choices. However, the FDA is not permitted to pursue this alternative. The 1990 amendments to the Nutrition Labeling Act specifically preclude the FDA from requiring nutrition labeling in food service establishments unless the food bears a nutrition claim or other nutrition information on its menu or other forms of labeling.[56]

Body Weight: A Function of Caloric Intake and Energy Expenditure

Despite the significant reduction in fat consumption in the United States in the past decades, the obesity epidemic continues to increase,[58] not only among adults but also among children. One of the proposed explanations for this phenomenon is a decrease in physical activity levels.[59] The recent Internal Revenue Service ruling considering obesity to be a disease highlights the importance of the problem and, as a policy decision, may have an impact on the entire population.

Our emphasis should be directed toward reaching and maintaining a healthy body weight. Body weight is a function of caloric intake and energy expenditure. Among factors significantly increasing caloric intake on a population basis are consumption of soft drinks and sugar [59,60] and an increase in portion size.[61] The food service industry could support efforts geared to controlling obesity by offering "petit" portions (as opposed to "king") as a menu option and by focusing on improving flavor and nutritional composition instead of increasing size.

On the energy expenditure side of the equation, exercise in all its forms should be promoted. The current decrease in physical activity primarily is related to our modern way of life, with its dependence on labor-saving technology. A small proportion of Americans (approximately 25% of all adults) participate in regular physical activity,[62] and a study evaluating cross-sectional data from the National Health Interview Survey concluded that there is a significant decline of physical activity with age.[58] Physical inactivity appears to be lower among women, minority populations, the elderly, and the less educated.[63]

Behavioral interventions in general advocate increases in all forms of exercise; however, environmental and policy interventions might significantly strengthen the effect of such behavioral endeavors by facilitating engagement in physical activity. There are comprehensive descriptions in the literature of environmental and policy approaches to CHD prevention through physical activity.[9] Some of the suggestions from the literature include the following:

- Restricting downtown centers to foot or bicycle traffic.
- Making stairways more attractive and convenient.
- Encouraging local and state health departments to collaborate with parks and education and transportation departments to facilitate physical activity.
- Developing and improving greenways.
- Creating exercise-friendly zoning regulations.
- Using vacant lots, landfill sites, and/or old railroad beds to develop exercise facilities such as parks, swimming pools, and bike paths.
- Improving access to exercise facilities (closer to home or worksite) and availability of on-site showering.
- Designing tax rebate programs for businesses that offer physical activity programs.
- Decreasing health insurance premiums for people engaged in regular physical activities.
- Implementing health center fee rebates.
- Using excise and gasoline taxes on cars, as well as highway tolls, which amount to many billions of dollars annually and now are used primarily to support road construction and repair, at the local or state levels to develop and maintain community exercise facilities, greenways, and bike paths.

Media-Based Interventions

Media-based interventions in CHD prevention are an important tool because of their potential for reaching large segments of the population.[8,64] Such interventions include a variety of printed, graphic, audiovisual, electronic, and broadcast programs intended to influence behavior change. A review of 28 studies of media-based interventions suggests that recall of mass media messages generally is high; however, mass media campaigns have had very little impact on physical activity behavior. The authors point out that a key issue is reaching socially disadvantaged groups for whom access, particularly to new forms of communication technology, may be limited.[64] Thus the provision of information alone is of limited value as a tool for behavioral change. Public mass media institutions should commit to health promotion, coordinating with local and state health officials for support of issues ranging from informational programming to a ban on advertising of nutritionally empty calories.

Call for Cost Analysis

The primary modifiable behavioral risk factors for CHD are smoking, diet, and physical activity. A number of reports have attempted to predict the change in morbidity and mortality associated with relatively small changes in these factors on a population level.[5] However, these improvements in health may result in a long-term increase in the nation's net health care costs related to the shift of health-related costs to a number of other diseases that affect people living to an older age. Therefore, it is prudent to explore the alternatives using health prediction models and, as a society, make conscious decisions as to the appropriate approach.[65] Regardless of the methodology used, the changes required at the population level to address the current CHD epidemic are complex in nature and will be accomplished only if the necessary policy and environmental steps are taken to support behavior change by the individual.[66]

CONCLUSIONS

To be truly effective, a strategy for the prevention of CHD must incorporate intervention at many levels. The physician and other health care workers remain central to this strategy, but their care needs to incorporate newer methodologies that enhance the delivery of preventive services. Beyond this, to reduce the national burden of CHD, it is necessary to intervene at the level of the school, worksite, and community and also to influence the political process so as to facilitate policy changes and changes in the environment that will foster the prevention of disease. Only by expanding our horizons in this manner will we shift the entire population risk profile in a favorable direction, so that the next generation will see a much-lessened incidence of CHD.

REFERENCES

1. Hunink MG, Goldman L, Tosteson AN, et al: The recent decline in mortality from coronary heart disease 1980-1990: The effect of secular trends in risk factors and treatment. JAMA 1997; 277(7):535-542.
2. Rose G: Strategy of prevention: Lessons from cardiovascular disease. BMJ (Clin Res Educ) 1981; 282(6279):1847-1851.
3. Kottke TE, Gatewood LC, Wu SC, et al: Preventing heart disease: Is treating the high risk sufficient? J Clin Epidemiol 1988; 41(11):1083-1093.
4. Goldman L, Weinstein MC, Williams LW: Relative impact of targeted versus populationwide cholesterol interventions on the incidence of coronary heart disease: Projections of the Coronary Heart Disease Policy Model. Circulation 1989; 80(2):254-60.
5. Durrington PN, Prais H: Methods for the prediction of coronary heart disease risk. Heart 2001; 85(5):489-490.
6. Ockene IS, Hebert JR, Ockene JK, et al: Effect of physician-delivered nutrition counseling training and an office-support program on saturated fat intake, weight, and serum lipid measurements in a hyperlipidemic population: Worcester Area Trial for Counseling in Hyperlipidemia (WATCH). Arch Intern Med 1999; 159(7):725-731.
7. DeBusk RF, Miller NH, Superko HR, et al: A case-management system for coronary risk factor modification after acute myocardial infarction. Ann Intern Med 1994; 120(9):721-729.
8. Jeffery RW, Gray CW, French SA, et al: Evaluation of weight reduction in a community intervention for cardiovascular disease risk: Changes in body mass index in the Minnesota Heart Health Program. Int J Obes Relat Metab Disord 1995; 19(1):30-39.
9. King AC, Jeffery RW, Fridinger F, et al: Environmental and policy approaches to cardiovascular disease prevention through physical activity: Issues and opportunities. Health Educ Q 1995; 22(4):499-511.
10. Farquhar JW, Maccoby N, Wood PD, et al: Community education for cardiovascular health. Lancet 1977; 1(8023):1192-1195.
11. Puska P, Nissinen A, Tuomilehto J, et al: The community-based strategy to prevent coronary heart disease: Conclusions from the ten years of the North Karelia project. Annu Rev Public Health 1985; 6:147-193.
12. Puska P, Korhonen HJ, Torppa J, et al: Does community-wide prevention of cardiovascular diseases influence cancer mortality? Eur J Cancer Prev 1993; 2(6):457-460.
13. Farquhar JW, Fortmann SP, Maccoby N, et al: The Stanford Five-City Project: Design and methods. Am J Epidemiol 1985; 122(2):323-334.
14. Kessler DA, Myers ML: Beyond the tobacco settlement. N Engl J Med 2001; 345(7):535-537.
15. Shea S, Basch CE, Lantigua R, et al: The Washington Heights-Inwood Healthy Heart Program: A third generation community-based cardiovascular disease prevention program in a disadvantaged urban setting. Prev Med 1992; 21(2):203-217.
16. Nutbeam D, Smith C, Murphy S, et al: Maintaining evaluation designs in long term community based health promotion programmes: Heartbeat Wales case study. J Epidemiol Community Health 1993; 47(2):127-133.
17. Fardy PS, Azzollini A, Magel JR, et al: Gender and ethnic differences in health behaviors and risk factors for coronary disease among urban teenagers: The PATH program. J Gend Specif Med 2000; 3(2):59-68.
18. Bureau of Labor Statistics: Report on Employment Situation. U.S. Department of Labor, 2002.
19. Blake SM, Caspersen CJ, Finnegan J, et al: The shape up challenge: A community-based worksite exercise competition. Am J Health Promot 1996; 11(1):23-34.
20. Braeckman L, De Bacquer D, Maes L, et al: Effects of a low-intensity worksite-based nutrition intervention. Occup Med (Lond) 1999; 49(8):549-555.
21. Sorensen G, Himmelstein J: Worksite intervention. In Ockene IS (ed). Prevention of Coronary Heart Disease. Boston, Little, Brown, 1992.
22. Fielding JE, Piserchia PV: Frequency of worksite health promotion activities. Am J Public Health 1989; 79(1):16-20.
23. Fisher B, Golaszewski T, Barr D: Measuring worksite resources for employee heart health. Am J Health Promot 1999; 13(6): 325-332.
24. Wilson MG, DeJoy DM, Jorgensen CM, et al: Health promotion programs in small worksites: Results of a national survey. Am J Health Promot 1999; 13(6):358-365.
25. Goetzel R, Sepulveda M, Knight K, et al: Association of IBM's "A Plan for Life" health promotion program with changes in employees' health risk status. J Occup Med 1994; 36(9):1005-1009.
26. Bertera RL: The effects of workplace health promotion on absenteeism and employment costs in a large industrial population. Am J Public Health 1990; 80(9):1101-1105.
27. Max W: The financial impact of smoking on health-related costs: A review of the literature. Am J Health Promot 2001; 15(5): 321-331.
28. Shephard RJ: Worksite fitness and exercise programs: A review of methodology and health impact. Am J Health Promot 1996; 10(6):436-452.
29. Sorensen G, Morris DM, Hunt MK, et al: Work-site nutrition intervention and employees' dietary habits: The Treatwell program. Am J Public Health 1992; 82(6):877-880.
30. Williams CL, Carter BJ, Wynder EL: Prevalence of selected cardiovascular and cancer risk factors in a pediatric population: The "Know Your Body" project, New York. Prev Med 1981; 10(2):235-250.
31. Eriksen M: School intervention. In Ockene IS (ed). Prevention of Coronary Heart Disease. Boston, Little, Brown, 1992.
32. Best D, Rawaf S, Rowley J, et al: Ethnic and gender differences in drinking and smoking among London adolescents. Ethn Health 2001; 6(1):51-57.
33. Glynn TJ, Greenwald P, Mills SM, et al: Youth tobacco use in the United States: Problem, progress, goals, and potential solutions Prev Med 1993; 22(4):568-575.
34. Pentz MA, Sussman S, Newman T: The conflict between least harm and no-use tobacco policy for youth: Ethical and policy implications. Addiction 1997; 92(9):1165-1173.
35. Flay BR, Petraitis J, Hu FB: Psychosocial risk and protective factors for adolescent tobacco use. Nicotine Tob Res 1999 (1 Suppl 1):S59-65.
36. Parcel GS, Simons-Morton BG, O'Hara NM, et al: School promotion of healthful diet and exercise behavior: An integration of organizational change and social learning theory interventions. J Sch Health 1987; 57(4):150-156.
37. Frank G: Primary prevention in the school arena: A dietary approach. Health Values 1983(7):14-21.
38. Ellison R, Goldberg RJ, Witschi JC, et al: Use of fat-modified food products to change dietary fat intake of young people. Am J Public Health 1990(80):1374-1376.

39. Arbeit ML, Johnson CC, Mott DS, et al: The Heart Smart cardiovascular school health promotion: Behavior correlates of risk factor change. Prev Med 1992; 21(1):18-32.
40. Cullen KW, Baranowski T, Rittenberry L, et al: Child-reported family and peer influences on fruit, juice and vegetable consumption: Reliability and validity of measures. Health Educ Res 2001; 16(2):187-200.
41. Nicklas TA, Baranowski T, Baranowski JC, et al: Family and childcare provider influences on preschool children's fruit, juice, and vegetable consumption. Nutr Rev 2001; 59(7):224-235.
42. Nader PR, Sallis JF, Patterson TL, et al: A family approach to cardiovascular risk reduction: Results from the San Diego Family Health Project. Health Educ Q 1989; 16(2):229-244.
43. Cullen KW, Baranowski T, Rittenberry L, et al: Social-environmental influences on children's diets: Results from focus groups with African-, Euro- and Mexican-American children and their parents. Health Educ Res 2000; 15(5):581-590.
44. Crespo C, Keteyian SJ, Heath GW, et al: Leisure-time physical activity among US adults: Results from the Third National Health and Nutrition Examination Survey. Arch Intern Med 1996(156):93-98.
45. Ross J, Pate RR: The National Children and Youth Fitness Study: II. A summary of findings. Phys Educ Recreat Dance J 1987(58):51-56.
46. Kelder SH, Perry CL, Klepp KI: Community-wide youth exercise promotion: Long-term outcomes of the Minnesota Heart Health Program and the Class of 1989 Study. J Sch Health 1993; 63(5):218-23.
47. Perry CL, Stone EJ, Parcel GS, et al: School-based cardiovascular health promotion: The child and adolescent trial for cardiovascular health (CATCH). J Sch Health 1990; 60(8):406-413.
48. Nader PR, Stone EJ, Lytle LA, et al: Three-year maintenance of improved diet and physical activity: The CATCH cohort. Child and Adolescent Trial for Cardiovascular Health. Arch Pediatr Adolesc Med 1999; 153(7):695-704.
49. Perry CL, Luepker RV, Murray DM, et al: Parent involvement with children's health promotion: A one-year follow-up of the Minnesota home team. Health Educ Q 1989; 16(2):171-180.
50. Glasgow RE, McKay HG, Piette JD, et al: The RE-AIM framework for evaluating interventions: What can it tell us about approaches to chronic illness management? Patient Educ Couns 2001; 44(2):119-127.
51. Willett WC. Eat, Drink, and Be Healthy. New York, Simon & Schuster Source, 2001.
52. U.S. Department of Health and Human Services: HSS Fact Sheet: Preventing Disease and Death from Tobacco Use. Washington, DC, U.S. Department of Health and Human Services, 2001.
53. Geiger CJ, Wyse BW, Parent CR, et al: Nutrition labels in bar graph format deemed most useful for consumer purchase decisions using adaptive conjoint analysis. J Am Diet Assoc 1991; 91(7):800-807.
54. Hrovat KB, Harris KZ, Leach AD, et al: The new food label, type of fat, and consumer choice. A pilot study. Arch Fam Med 1994; 3(8):690-695.
55. Allison DB, Heshka S, Sepulveda D, et al: Counting calories: Caveat emptor. JAMA 1993; 270(12):1454-1456.
56. Food and Drug Administration: Food Labeling: Trans Fatty Acids in Nutrition Labeling, Nutrient Content Claims, and Health Claims; Proposed Rule. Federal Register 1999; 64(221).
57. U.S. Department of Agriculture ARS: USDA Food Composition Data, Selected Foods Containing trans Fatty Acids. Washington, DC, USDA, Agricultural Research Service, 1995.
58. Caspersen CJ, Pereira MA, Curran KM: Changes in physical activity patterns in the United States, by sex and cross-sectional age. Med Sci Sports Exerc 2000; 32(9):1601-1609.
59. Nestle M, Jacobson MF: Halting the obesity epidemic: A public health policy approach. Public Health Rep 2000; 115(1):12-24.
60. Jacobson MF, Brownell KD: Small taxes on soft drinks and snack foods to promote health. Am J Public Health 2000; 90(6):854-857.
61. Young LR, Nestle M: The contribution of expanding portion sizes to the US obesity epidemic. Am J Public Health 2002; 92(2):246-249.
62. U.S. Centers for Disease Control and Prevention: Increasing Physical Activity: A Report on Recommendations of the Task Force on Community Preventive Services. MMWR 2001; 50(RR18).
63. U.S. Centers for Disease Control and Prevention: Prevalence of Sedentary Lifestyle: Behavioral Risk Factor Surveillance System, United States 1991; 1993; 42(29):576.
64. Marcus BH, Owen N, Forsyth LH, et al: Physical activity interventions using mass media, print media, and information technology. Am J Prev Med 1998; 15(4):362-378.
65. Douglas MJ, Conway L, Gorman D, et al: Developing principles for health impact assessment. J Public Health Med 2001; 23(2):148-154.
66. Schmid TL, Pratt M, Howze E: Policy as intervention: Environmental and policy approaches to the prevention of cardiovascular disease. Am J Public Health 1995; 85(9):1207-1211.

INDEX

Page numbers followed by f refer to figures; page numbers followed by t refer to tables.